Keep Your Entire Drug Reference Library Completely Up-To-Date With These

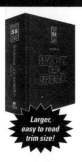
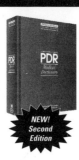
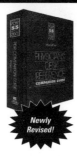
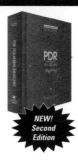
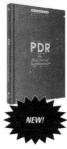
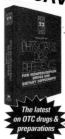
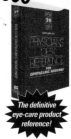

Larger, easy to read trim size!

NEW! Second Edition

Newly Revised!

NEW! Second Edition

NEW!

The latest on OTC drugs & preparations

The definitive eye-care product reference!

2001 Physicians' Desk Reference®

Physicians have turned to PDR for the latest word on prescription drugs for over 55 years! Today, PDR is still considered the standard prescription drug reference and can be found in virtually every physician's office, hospital, and pharmacy in the United States. The 55th edition is a larger, easier to read book with more information per page. PDR provides the most complete data on over 4,000 drugs by product and generic name (both in the same convenient index), manufacturer, and category. Also, product overviews that summarize listings with more than 2,100 full-size, full-color photos cross-referenced to complete drug information.

PDR® Medical Dictionary,™ 2nd Edition

Newly revised with over 2000 pages including a complete medical etymology section to help the reader understand medical/scientific word formation. Includes a comprehensive cross-reference table of generic and brand-name pharmaceuticals and manufacturers, plus an appendix containing useful charts on scales, temperatures, temperature equivalents, metric and SI units, laboratory and reference values, blood groups and more.

2001 PDR® Companion Guide

This unique, all-in-one clinical reference assures safe, appropriate drug selection with ten critical checkpoints: *Drug Imprint Identification Guide, Interactions Index, Side Effects Index, Food Interactions Cross-Reference, Indications Index, Contraindications Index, Off-label Treatment Guide, Cost of Therapy Guide, International Drug Guide, and a Generic Availability Table* showing forms and strengths of brand-name drugs dispensed generically. This time-saving complement to your 2001 *PDR, PDR for Nonprescription Drugs and Dietary Supplements* and *PDR for Ophthalmic Medicines*, will soon prove to be indispensable.

PDR® for Herbal Medicines,™ 2nd Edition

PDR for Herbal Medicines is the most comprehensive reference of its kind. Based upon the work conducted by Germany's Commission E and Jöerg Grüenwald, Ph.D. a botanist and renowned expert on herbal medicines, this detailed guide provides information on over 600 botanical remedies. Entries include: a thorough description of the plant and derived compounds... pharmacological effects of each plant... precautions, warnings and contraindications... adverse reactions and overdose data... scientific and common English names... typical dosage... and exhaustive literature citations.

PDR® for Nutritional Supplements,™ 1st Edition

The definitive information source on hundreds of nutritional supplements. Now healthcare professionals can have the facts at their fingertips with the *PDR for Nutritional Supplements*, the first comprehensive source of solid, evidence-based information covering a full range of nutritional supplements. Detailed analyses are presented in an easy-to-read format. And, in addition, a clinical research summary synthesizes all the published findings on each supplement. **The *PDR for Nutritional Supplements* provides practitioners with the most current and reliable information to help them assist their patients in making more educated choices.**

2001 PDR for Nonprescription Drugs and Dietary Supplements™

The acknowledged authority offers full FDA-approved descriptions of the most commonly used OTC medicines, four separate indices and in-depth data on ingredients, indications, and drug interactions. Includes a valuable Companion Drug Index. **Now expanded to include a section on supplements, vitamins, and herbal remedies.**

2001 PDR for Ophthalmic Medicines™

The definitive reference filled with accurate, up-to-date information specifically for the eye-care professional. It provides detailed reference data on drugs and equipment used in the fields of ophthalmology and optometry. Its comprehensive coverage includes lens types and their uses... specialized instrumentation... color product photographs... a detailed encyclopedia of pharmaceuticals in ophthalmology... five full indices... an extensive bibliography... and much more.

Complete Your 2001 PDR® Library NOW! Enclose payment and save shipping costs.

Code		Item	Price	
101006	_____ copies	**2001 Physicians' Desk Reference®**	$86.95 ea.	$_____
101022	_____ copies	**2001 PDR for Ophthalmic Medicines™**	$58.95 ea.	$_____
101139	_____ copies	**PDR® for Nutritional Supplements,™ 1st EDITION!**	$59.95 ea.	$_____
101063	_____ copies	**PDR® for Herbal Medicines,™ 2nd EDITION!**	$59.95 ea.	$_____
101048	_____ copies	**PDR® Medical Dictionary,™ 2nd EDITION!**	$49.95 ea.	$_____
101014	_____ copies	**2001 PDR® Companion Guide**	$62.95 ea.	$_____
101089	_____ copies	**2001 PDR for Nonprescription Drugs and Dietary Supplements™**	$53.95 ea.	$_____

PLEASE INDICATE METHOD OF PAYMENT: Payment Enclosed (shipping & handling FREE)

☐ **Check payable to PDR** ☐ **VISA** ☐ **MasterCard** ☐ **Discover** ☐ **American Express**

Shipping & Handling $_____

Sales Tax (FL, GA, IA, & NJ) $_____

Total Amount of Order $_____

Account No. _____

Exp. Date _____ Telephone No. _____

Signature _____

Name _____

Address _____

City/State/Zip _____

☐ **BILL ME LATER** (Add $7.95 per book for shipping and handling)

For Faster Service—FAX YOUR ORDER (515) 284-6714

Do not mail a confirmation order in addition to this fax.

Mail this order form to: **PDR**, P.O. Box 10689, Des Moines, IA 50336

e-mail: customer.service@medec.com

Valid for 2001 editions only, prices and shipping & handling higher outside U.S.

☐ **SAVE TIME AND MONEY EVERY YEAR AS A STANDING ORDER SUBSCRIBER.** Check here to enter your standing order for future editions of publications ordered. They will be shipped to you automatically, after advance notice. As a standing order subscriber, you are **guaranteed** our lowest price offer, earliest delivery and **FREE** shipping and handling.

663344

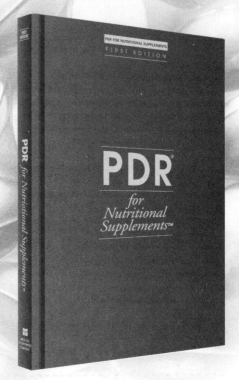

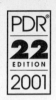

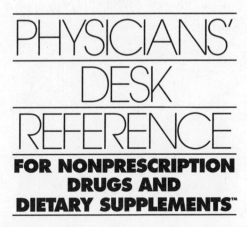

PHYSICIANS' DESK REFERENCE
FOR NONPRESCRIPTION DRUGS AND DIETARY SUPPLEMENTS™

Executive Vice President, Directory Services: Paul Walsh

Vice President, Sales and Marketing: Dikran N. Barsamian

National Sales Manager, Custom Sales: Anthony Sorce

Senior Account Managers: Marion Gray, RPh, Frank Karkowsky

Account Managers: Lawrence C. Keary, Eileen Sullivan, Suzanne E. Yarrow, RN

Director of Trade Sales: Bill Gaffney

Associate Product Manager: Jason Springer

Senior Business Manager: Mark S. Ritchin

Director, PDR Electronic Product Management: Laurie G. Murphy

Director of Direct Marketing: Michael Bennett

Direct Mail Manager: Lorraine M. Loening

Senior Marketing Analyst: Dina A. Maeder

Vice President, Clinical Communications and New Business Development: Mukesh Mehta, RPh

New Business Development Manager: Jeffrey D. Dubin

Manager, Drug Information Services: Thomas Fleming, RPh

Drug Information Specialists: Maria Deutsch, MS, PharmD, CDE; Christine Wyble, PharmD

Editor, Directory Services: David W. Sifton

Project Manager: Edward P. Connor

Senior Associate Editor: Lori Murray

Assistant Editor: Gwynned L. Kelly

Director of Production: Brian Holland

Data Manager: Jeffrey D. Schaefer

Production Manager: Amy Brooks

Production Coordinators: Gianna Caradonna, Dee Ann DeRuvo, Melissa Katz, Christina Klinger

Index Supervisor: Johanna M. Mazur

Index Editors: Noel Deloughery, Shannon Reilly

Format Editor: Stu W. Lehrer

Art Associate: Joan K. Akerlind

Digital Imaging Supervisor: Shawn W. Cahill

Digital Imaging Coordinator: Frank J. McElroy, III

Electronic Publishing Designer: Livio Udina

Fulfillment Managers: Louis J. Bolcik, Stephanie DeNardi

ISBN: 1-56363-381-7

FOREWORD

Today more than ever, we face a burgeoning array of options on our local drugstore shelves. Traditional over-the-counter drugs have been joined by a flood of new herbal remedies, nutritional supplements, and combination products. Just keeping abreast of this torrent demands increased reference resources, and Physicians' Desk Reference has moved decisively to meet this need.

Two years ago we expanded *PDR for Nonprescription Drugs* with a new section devoted to the full spectrum of dietary supplements. Last year we issued the enhanced and expanded second edition of the popular *PDR® for Herbal Medicines™*. And this year we are pleased to introduce *PDR® for Nutritional Supplements™,* a compendium of the latest data on hundreds of popular supplement products, including an array of amino acids, co-factors, fatty acids, probiotics, phytoestrogens, phytosterols, over-the-counter hormones, hormonal precursors, and more.

Focused on the scientific evidence (or lack of evidence) for each supplement's claims, this unique new reference offers you today's most detailed, informed, and objective overview of the fastest-growing area in the field of self-treatment. To protect your patients from bogus remedies and steer them towards truly beneficial products, this book is a must.

Other Prescribing Aids from *PDR*

This year for the first time, *PDR* has issued a condensed drug guide designed specifically for quick dosage checks. Entitled the *PDR Pharmacopoeia™ Pocket Edition,* this little handbook can accompany you wherever you need to go, around the office or on rounds. Only slightly larger than an index card, and a quarter of an inch thick, it fits easily into any pocket, while providing you with FDA-approved dosing recommendations for over 1,500 drugs.

For complicated cases, patients on multi-drug regimens, those with hepatic or renal conditions, and members of special populations, there's still no substitute for the detailed guidelines found in *Physicians' Desk Reference* itself. But if all you need is quick confirmation of a form, strength, or dose, the new *PDR Pharmacopoeia* may be the ideal answer for your needs.

Unlike other condensed drug references, this new handbook is drawn almost exclusively from the FDA-approved drug labeling published in *Physicians' Desk Reference,* so you can rely on it for authoritative, official dosage guidelines. Its tabular presentation makes lookups a breeze. And to expedite comparisons, it lists drugs by major category and specific indication. At $9.95 a copy, it's a tool you really can't afford to be without.

If portability is your goal, we have two other intriguing new options for you. Now you can get the full text of six key topics for every fully-described prescription drug in *PDR* and *PDR for Ophthalmic Medicines* and load it into your Palm®, Visor™, Pocket PC® or other handheld personal digital assistant (PDA). Or if you prefer, you can get a brand new Franklin eBookman® unit loaded with the same information.

Whichever handheld device you use, you'll get the complete, FDA-approved text of these six crucial topics: Indications and Usage, Contraindications, Warnings, Adverse Reactions, How Supplied, and Dosage and Administration. (These topics are also available on a traditional *Pocket PDR®* DataCard.) No matter how you choose to view it, you'll have a complete databank of prescribing information at your fingertips wherever you go!

If you haven't already encountered a copy, you should also take a look at the *PDR Companion Guide*, a 1,900-page reference that augments *PDR* with a total of 10 unique decision-making tools. In this indispensable volume, you'll find the following:

- **Interactions Index** identifies all pharmaceuticals and foods capable of interacting with a chosen medication.

- **Food Interactions Cross-Reference** lists the drugs that may interact with a given dietary item.

- **Side Effects Index** pinpoints the pharmaceuticals associated with each of 3,600 distinct adverse reactions.

- **Indications Index** presents the full range of therapeutic options for any given diagnosis.

- **Off-Label Treatment Guide** lists medications routinely used—but never officially approved—for treatment of nearly 1,000 specific disorders.

- **Contraindications Index** lists all drugs to avoid in the presence of any given medical condition.

- **International Drug Index** names the U.S. equivalents of some 15,000 foreign medications.

- **Generic Availability Guide** shows which forms and strengths of a brand-name drug are also available generically.

- **Cost of Therapy Guide** provides a quick overview of the relative expense of the leading therapeutic options for a variety of common indications.

- **Imprint Identification Guide** enables you to establish the nature of any unknown tablet or capsule by matching its imprint against an exhaustive catalog of identifying codes.

The *PDR Companion Guide* includes all drugs described in *PDR, PDR for Nonprescription Drugs and Dietary Supplements,* and *PDR for Ophthalmic Medicines.* We're certain that you'll find it makes safe, appropriate selection of drugs faster and easier than ever before.

PDR and its major companion volumes are also found in the *PDR® Electronic Library™* on CD-ROM, now used in over 100,000 practices. This Windows-compatible disc provides users with a complete database of *PDR* prescribing information, electronically searchable for instant retrieval. A standard subscription includes *PDR's* sophisticated search software and an extensive file of chemical structures, illustrations, and full-color product photographs. For anyone who wants to run a fast double check on a proposed prescription, there's also the *PDR® Drug Interactions and Side Effects System™* — sophisticated software capable of automatically screening a 20-drug regimen for conflicts, then proposing alternatives for any problematic medication. This unique decision-making tool now comes free with the *PDR Electronic Library*.

Remember, too, that the contents of *PDR* and its main companion volumes can always be found on the Internet at **www.pdr.net**. For more information on these or any other members of the growing family of *PDR* products, please call, toll-free, 1-800-232-7379 or fax 201-722-2680.

How to Use This Book
Physicians' Desk Reference for Nonprescription Drugs and Dietary Supplements is divided into two major sections. The first, entitled *Nonprescription Drug Information*, presents descriptions of conventional remedies marketed in compliance with the Code of Federal Regulations labeling requirements for over-the-counter drugs. The second section, entitled *Dietary Supplement Information*, contains information on herbal remedies and nutritional supplements marketed under the Dietary Supplement Health and Education Act of 1994. For your convenience, products in both sections are listed in the consolidated indices at the front of the book.

Physicians' Desk Reference for Nonprescription Drugs and Dietary Supplements is published annually by Medical Economics Company in cooperation with participating manufacturers. The function of the publisher is the compilation, organization, and distribution of product information obtained from manufacturers. Each product description has been prepared by the manufacturer, and edited and approved by the manufacturer's medical department, medical director, and/or medical consultant. During compilation of this information, the publisher has emphasized the necessity of describing products comprehensively, in order to provide all the facts necessary for sound and intelligent decision making. Descriptions seen here include all information made available by the manufacturer. Please note that descriptions of over-the-counter products marketed under the Dietary Supplement Health and Education Act of 1994 have not been evaluated by the Food and Drug Administration, and that such products are not intended to diagnose, treat, cure, or prevent any disease.

In organizing and presenting the material in *Physicians' Desk Reference For Nonprescription Drugs and Dietary Supplements*, the publisher does not warrant or guarantee any of the products described, or perform any independent analysis in connection with any of the product information contained herein. *Physicians' Desk Reference* does not assume, and expressly disclaims, any obligation to obtain and include any information other than that provided to it by the manufacturer. It should be understood that by making this material available the publisher is not advocating the use of any product described herein, nor is the publisher responsible for misuse of a product due to typographical error. Additional information on any product may be obtained from the manufacturer.

CONTENTS

Manufacturers' Index (White Pages)   **1**

Section 1

Lists all participating pharmaceutical manufacturers. Includes addresses, phone numbers, and emergency contacts. Shows each manufacturer's products and the page number of those described.

Product Name Index (Pink Pages)   **101**

Section 2

Gives the page number of each product description in the Nonprescription Drug and Dietary Supplement sections. Products are listed alphabetically by brand name.

Product Category Index (Blue Pages)   **201**

Section 3

Lists by prescribing category all fully-described products.

Active Ingredients Index (Yellow Pages)   **301**

Section 4

A cross-reference by generic ingredient of all product descriptions.

Companion Drug Index (Green Pages)   **401**

Section 5

Lists symptoms occurring during prescription drug therapy, and presents over-the-counter products that may be recommended for relief.

Product Identification Guide (Gray Pages)   **501**

Section 6

Shows full-color, actual-size photos of tablets and capsules, plus pictures of a variety of other dosage forms and packages. Arranged alphabetically by manufacturer.

Nonprescription Drug Information (White Pages)   **601**

Section 7

Provides information on hundreds of traditional over-the-counter medications and home testing products. Entries are arranged alphabetically by manufacturer.

Dietary Supplement Information (White Pages)   **793**

Section 8

Includes manufacturers' descriptions of a variety of natural remedies and nutritional supplements marketed under the Dietary Supplement Health and Education Act of 1994. Entries are organized alphabetically by manufacturer.

Drug Information Centers   **423**

Poison Control Centers   **428**

U.S. Food and Drug Administration Telephone Directory   **527**

SECTION 1

MANUFACTURERS' INDEX

Listed in this index are all manufacturers that have supplied information in this edition. Each company's entry includes the address, phone, and fax number of its headquarters and regional offices, as well as contacts for inquiries, orders, and emergency information.

Products with entries in the Nonprescription Drug Information section are listed with their page numbers under the heading OTC Products Described. Products with entries in the Dietary Supplement Information section are listed with their page numbers under the

heading Dietary Supplements Described. Other OTC products and dietary supplements available from the manufacturer follow these two sections.

If an entry in the index lists multiple page numbers, the first one shown refers to the photograph of the product, the last one to its prescribing information.

- The ◆ symbol marks drugs shown in the Product Identification Guide.

- *Italic page numbers* signify partial information.

A & Z PHARMACEUTICAL INC.   503, 794
180 Oser Avenue, Suite 300
Hauppauge, NY 11788
Direct Inquiries to:
Customer Service
(631) 952-3800
FAX: (631) 952-3900

Dietary Supplements Described:
◆ D-Cal Chewable Caplets **503, 794**

ADVOCARE INTERNATIONAL, L.L.C.   794
2727 Realty Road, Suite 134
Carrollton, TX 75006
Direct Inquiries to:
Medical/Scientific Advisory Board
(972) 478-4500
FAX: (972) 478-4751

Dietary Supplements Described:
ActoTherm Caplets **794**
Advantin Capsules **794**
Antioxidant Booster Caplets **794**
BodyLean Powder **795**
Brite-Life Caplets **795**
CardiOptima Drink Mix Packets **795**
Catalyst Capsules **795**
C-Grams Caplets **795**
Coffeccino Beverage Mix **796**
Cold Season Nutrition Booster
   Capsules **796**
CorePlex Capsules **796**
FemEssence Capsules **796**
Fiber 10 Packets **797**
IntelleQ Capsules **797**
LipoTrol Caplets **797**
Macro-Mineral Complex Caplets **797**
Metabolic Nutrition System **798**

MetaBoost Caplets **798**
Perfect Meal **798**
Performance Gold Caplets **798**
Performance Optimizer System **798**
ProForm Bars **799**
ProMotion Capsules **800**
ProBiotic Restore Capsules **799**
Second Look Capsules **800**
Spark! Beverage Mix **800**
System 3-4-3 Capsules **800**
Thermo-E Caplets **801**
Thermo-G Caplets **801**
ZZZ Spray Liquid **801**

AK PHARMA INC.   503, 801
P.O. Box 111
Pleasantville, NJ 08232-0111
Direct Inquiries to:
Elizabeth Klein
(609) 645-5100
FAX: (609) 645-0767
For Medical Emergencies Contact:
Alan E. Kligerman
(609) 645-5100
FAX: (609) 485-0423

Dietary Supplements Described:
◆ Prelief Tablets and Granulate **503, 801**

ALPHARMA   602
U.S. Pharmaceuticals Division
7205 Windsor Boulevard
Baltimore, MD 21244
Direct Inquiries to:
Customer Service
(800) 638-9096

OTC Products Described:
Permethrin Lotion **602**

BAYER CORPORATION CONSUMER CARE DIVISION   503, 602
P.O. Box 1910
36 Columbia Road
Morristown, NJ 07962-1910
Direct Inquiries to:
Consumer Relations
(800) 331-4536
Internet: www.bayercare.com
For Medical Emergencies Contact:
Bayer Corporation
Consumer Care Division
(800) 331-4536

OTC Products Described:
◆ Aleve Tablets, Caplets and
   Gelcaps **503, 602**
◆ Aleve Cold & Sinus Caplets **503, 603**
◆ Alka-Seltzer Original Antacid
   and Pain Reliever
   Effervescent Tablets **503, 603**
◆ Alka-Seltzer Cherry Antacid
   and Pain Reliever
   Effervescent Tablets **503, 603**
◆ Alka-Seltzer Lemon Lime
   Antacid and Pain Reliever
   Effervescent Tablets **503, 603**
◆ Alka-Seltzer Extra Strength
   Antacid and Pain Reliever
   Effervescent Tablets **503, 603**
◆ Alka-Seltzer Plus Cold
   Medicine Liqui-Gels **503, 604**
◆ Alka-Seltzer Plus Night-Time
   Cold Medicine Liqui-Gels **503, 604**
◆ Alka-Seltzer Plus Cold &
   Cough Medicine Liqui-Gels ... **503, 604**
◆ Alka-Seltzer Plus Cold & Flu
   Medicine Liqui-Gels **503, 604**
◆ Alka-Seltzer Plus Cold & Sinus
   Medicine Liqui-Gels **503, 604**

BAYER CORPORATION CONSUMER CARE DIVISION—*cont.*

◆ Alka-Seltzer Heartburn Relief Tablets **503, 604**
◆ Alka-Seltzer PM Effervescent Tablets **503, 605**
◆ Bactine First Aid Liquid **503, 611**
◆ Genuine Bayer Tablets, Caplets and Gelcaps.....**503, 606**
◆ Extra Strength Bayer Caplets and Gelcaps **504, 610**
◆ Aspirin Regimen Bayer Children's Chewable Tablets (Orange or Cherry Flavored) **504, 607**
◆ Aspirin Regimen Bayer Adult Low Strength 81 mg Tablets **503, 606**
Aspirin Regimen Bayer 81 mg Caplets with Calcium **607**
◆ Aspirin Regimen Bayer Regular Strength 325 mg Caplets....**503, 606**
Genuine Bayer Professional Labeling (Aspirin Regimen Bayer) **608**
◆ Extra Strength Bayer Arthritis Caplets **504, 610**
◆ Extra Strength Bayer Plus Caplets **504, 610**
◆ Extra Strength Bayer PM Caplets **504, 611**
◆ Domeboro Powder Packets **504, 611**
◆ Domeboro Effervescent Tablets **504, 611**
◆ Maximum Strength Midol Menstrual Caplets and Gelcaps **504, 612**
◆ Maximum Strength Midol PMS Caplets and Gelcaps.....**504, 613**
◆ Maximum Strength Midol Teen Caplets **504, 612**
Mycelex-3 Vaginal Cream with 3 Disposable Applicators **613**
Mycelex-3 Vaginal Cream in 3 Pre-filled Applicators **613**
Mycelex-7 Combination-Pack Vaginal Inserts & External Vulvar Cream **614**
Mycelex-7 Vaginal Cream **614**
Mycelex-7 Vaginal Cream with 7 Disposable Applicators **614**
◆ Neo-Synephrine Nasal Drops, Regular and Extra Strength ..**504, 614**
◆ Neo-Synephrine Nasal Sprays, Mild, Regular and Extra Strength.....................**504, 614**
◆ Neo-Synephrine 12 Hour Nasal Spray.....................**504, 615**
Neo-Synephrine 12 Hour Extra Moisturizing Nasal Spray **615**
Phillips' Chewable Tablets.............**615**
◆ Phillips' FiberCaps Caplets **505, 615**
Phillips' Liqui-Gels **616**
◆ Phillips' Milk of Magnesia Liquid (Original, Cherry, & Mint) **505, 616**
◆ Maximum Strength Rid Mousse **505, 617**
◆ Maximum Strength Rid Shampoo **505, 616**
◆ Vanquish Caplets **505, 617**

Dietary Supplements Described:
◆ Bugs Bunny Children's Multivitamin Plus Iron Chewable Tablets **504, 802**
◆ Bugs Bunny Children's Multivitamin Plus Extra C Chewable Tablets (Sugar Free) **504, 804**

◆ Bugs Bunny Complete Children's Multivitamin/ Multimineral Chewable Tablets (Sugar Free) **504, 803**
◆ Fergon Iron Tablets **504, 802**
◆ Flintstones Original Children's Multivitamin Chewable Tablets **504, 802**
◆ Flintstones Children's Multivitamin Plus Calcium Chewable Tablets **504, 804**
◆ Flintstones Children's Multivitamin Plus Extra C Chewable Tablets **504, 804**
◆ Flintstones Children's Multivitamin Plus Iron Chewable Tablets **504, 802**
◆ Flintstones Complete Children's Mutivitamin/ Multimineral Chewable Tablets **504, 803**
◆ One-A-Day Antioxidant Softgels ..**504, 805**
◆ One-A-Day Bedtime & Rest Tablets **505, 805**
◆ One-A-Day Calcium Plus Chewable Tablets **505, 805**
◆ One-A-Day Cholesterol Health Tablets **505, 805**
◆ One-A-Day Energy Formula Tablets **505, 806**
◆ One-A-Day Essential Tablets **504, 806**
◆ One-A-Day 50 Plus Tablets.......**504, 804**
◆ One-A-Day Garlic Softgels........**505, 806**
◆ One-A-Day Joint Health Tablets ..**505, 806**
◆ One-A-Day Kids Complete Tablets **505, 806**
◆ One-A-Day Maximum Tablets....**504, 807**
◆ One-A-Day Memory & Concentration Tablets **505, 807**
◆ One-A-Day Men's Tablets **504, 808**
◆ One-A-Day Menopause Health Tablets **505, 808**
◆ One-A-Day Prostate Health Softgels....................**505, 808**
◆ One-A-Day Tension & Mood Softgels....................**505, 808**
◆ One-A-Day Women's Tablets **504, 809**

Other Products Available:
Bronkaid Caplets
Campho-Phenique Antiseptic Gel
Campho-Phenique Cold Sore Gel
Campho-Phenique Maximum Strength First Aid Antibiotic Plus Pain Reliever Ointment
Campho-Phenique Liquid
Haley's M-O (Regular & Flavored)
Night Time Formula Midol PM
Miles Nervine Nighttime Sleep-Aid
Concentrated Phillips' Milk of Magnesia (Strawberry)

BEACH PHARMACEUTICALS 809

Division of Beach Products, Inc.
EXECUTIVE OFFICE:
5220 South Manhattan Avenue
Tampa, FL 33611
(813) 839-6565
Direct Inquiries to:
Richard Stephen Jenkins, Exec. V.P.:
(813) 839-6565
Clete Harmon, Dir. of Q.A.:
(864) 277-7282
Manufacturing and Distribution:
201 Delaware Street
Greenville, SC 29605
(800) 845-8210

Dietary Supplements Described:
Beelith Tablets........................**809**

BEUTLICH LP 618
PHARMACEUTICALS

1541 Shields Drive
Waukegan, IL 60085-8304
Direct Inquiries to:
(847) 473-1100
(800) 238-8542 in the U.S. and Canada
FAX: (847) 473-1122
Internet: www.beutlich.com
E-mail: fjb1541@worldnet.att.net

OTC Products Described:
Ceo-Two Evacuant Suppository........**618**
Hurricaine Topical Anesthetic Gel, 1 oz. Fresh Mint, Wild Cherry, Pina Colada, Watermelon, 1/6 oz. Wild Cherry, Watermelon........................**618**
Hurricaine Topical Anesthetic Liquid, 1 oz. Wild Cherry, Pina Colada, .25 ml Dry Handle Swab Wild Cherry, 1/6 oz. Wild Cherry **618**
Hurricaine Topical Anesthetic Spray Extension Tubes (200)......**618**
Hurricaine Topical Anesthetic Spray Kit, 2 oz. Wild Cherry **618**
Hurricaine Topical Anesthetic Spray, 2 oz. Wild Cherry..........**618**
Peridin-C Tablets.......................**618**

BLOCK DRUG COMPANY, 505, 619
INC.

257 Cornelison Avenue
Jersey City, NJ 07302
Direct Inquiries to:
Consumer Affairs/Block
(201) 434-3000, Ext. 1308
For Medical Emergencies Contact:
Consumer Affairs/Block
(201) 434-3000, Ext. 1308

OTC Products Described:
◆ Balmex Diaper Rash Ointment...**505, 619**
◆ Balmex Medicated Plus Baby Powder.....................**505, 619**
BC Powder **619**
BC Allergy Sinus Cold Powder **619**
Arthritis Strength BC Powder **619**
BC Sinus Cold Powder................**619**
Goody's Body Pain Formula Powder..........................**620**
Goody's Extra Strength Headache Powder..........................**620**
Goody's Extra Strength Pain Relief Tablets **620**
Goody's PM Powder **621**
◆ Nature's Remedy Tablets **506, 621**
◆ Nytol Natural Tablets.............**506, 622**
◆ Nytol QuickCaps Caplets **506, 622**
◆ Maximum Strength Nytol QuickGels Softgels **506, 621**
◆ Phazyme-125 mg Quick Dissolve Chewable Tablets ..**506, 622**
◆ Phazyme-180 mg Ultra Strength Softgels **506, 622**
Sensodyne Original Flavor **623**
Sensodyne Cool Gel **623**
Sensodyne Extra Whitening............**623**
Sensodyne Fresh Mint................**623**
Sensodyne Tartar Control **623**
Sensodyne Tartar Control Plus Whitening **623**
Sensodyne with Baking Soda........**623**
Tegrin Dandruff Shampoo - Extra Conditioning **623**
◆ Tegrin Dandruff Shampoo - Fresh Herbal **506, 624**
◆ Tegrin Skin Cream **506, 624**

Dietary Supplements Described:
Beano Liquid...........................809
Beano Tablets 809

BODY WISE INTERNATIONAL   810
INC.
2802 Dow Avenue
Tustin, CA 92780
Direct Inquiries to:
Wellness Research Center
(714) 505-6121
FAX: (714) 832-7247
E-mail: wellness@bodywise.com

Dietary Supplements Described:
Ag-Immune Tablets 810
Beta-C Tablets 811
Biolax.....................................*810*
Carbo Energy Bar *810*
Chito-Maxx................................*810*
CoEnzyme Q10+..........................*810*
Electro Aloe *810*
Future Perfect *810*
Mem X^2.................................*810*
Oxy-G^2.................................*810*
Relief Nasal & Throat Spray 811
Right Choice A.M. Multi Formula
    Caplets 811
Right Choice P.M. Multi Formula
    Caplets 812
St. John's Complex.....................*810*
Super Reshape Formula...............*810*
Tiger Vites *810*
Workout Formula *810*
Xtreme...................................*810*

BOEHRINGER INGELHEIM   506, 624
CONSUMER
HEALTHCARE
PRODUCTS
Division of Boehringer Ingelheim
Pharmaceuticals, Inc.
900 Ridgebury Road
P.O. Box 368
Ridgefield, CT 06877
Direct Inquiries to:
(888) 285-9159

OTC Products Described:
◆ Natru-Vent Nasal Spray, Adult
    Strength.........................**506, 624**
◆ Natru-Vent Nasal Spray,
    Pediatric Strength............**506, 625**
◆ Natru-Vent Saline Nasal Spray...**506, 625**

BOIRON, THE WORLD LEADER   625
IN HOMEOPATHY
6 Campus Blvd.
Newtown Square, PA 19073
Direct Inquiries to:
Boiron Information Center
(800) 264-7661
FAX: (888) 264-7661
E-mail: info@boiron.com
For Medical Emergencies Contact:
Boiron Information Center
(800) 264-7661
E-mail: info@boiron.com

OTC Products Described:
Oscillococcinum Pellets 625

Other Products Available:
Acidil, for Heartburn
Arnica & Calendula Gel & Ointment
Camilia, for Baby Teething
Chestal Cough Syrup
Chestal For Children Cough Syrup
Cocyntal, for Baby Colic
Coldcalm, for Cold Symptoms

Cyclease, for Menstrual Cramps
Gasalia, for Gas
Ginsenique, for Fatigue
Homeodent Toothpaste
Natural Phases, for PMS
Optique 1 Eye Drops, for Eye Irritation
Quiétude, for Sleeplessness
Roxalia, for Sore Throat
Sabadil, for Allergies
Sedalia, for Nervousness Associated with
    Stress
Sinusalia, for Sinus Pain
Sportenine, for Cramps and Muscle
    Fatigue
Yeastaway, for Vaginal Yeast Infections

BRISTOL-MYERS   506, 626
PRODUCTS
A Bristol-Myers Squibb Company
345 Park Avenue
New York, NY 10154
Direct Inquiries to:
Bristol-Myers Products Division
Consumer Affairs Department
1350 Liberty Avenue
Hillside, NJ 07207
Questions or Comments:
(800) 468-7746

OTC Products Described:
◆ Comtrex Acute Head Cold &
    Sinus Pressure Relief
    Tablets **506, 627**
◆ Comtrex Deep Chest Cold &
    Congestion Relief Softgels ..**506, 627**
◆ Comtrex Flu Therapy & Fever
    Relief Daytime Caplets **506, 628**
◆ Comtrex Flu Therapy & Fever
    Relief Nighttime Tablets **506, 628**
◆ Comtrex Maximum Strength
    Multi-Symptom Cold &
    Cough Relief Tablets and
    Caplets **506, 626**
◆ Aspirin Free Excedrin Caplets
    and Geltabs..................**507, 628**
◆ Excedrin Extra-Strength
    Tablets, Caplets, and
    Geltabs **507, 629**
◆ Excedrin Migraine Tablets,
    Caplets, and Geltabs **507, 630**
◆ Excedrin PM Tablets, Caplets,
    and Geltabs..................**506, 631**

Other Products Available:
Alpha Keri Moisture Rich Cleansing Bar
Bufferin, Arthritis Strength Caplets
Bufferin, Extra Strength Tablets
Comtrex Maximum Strength
    Multi-Symptom Allergy-Sinus Day/
    Night Caplets/Tablets
Comtrex Maximum Strength
    Multi-Symptom Allergy-Sinus
    Treatment Tablets
Comtrex Maximum Strength
    Multi-Symptom Day/Night Caplets/
    Tablets
Comtrex Maximum Strength
    Multi-Symptom Non-Drowsy Liquigels
Fostex 10% Benzoyl Peroxide Bar
Fostex 10% Benzoyl Peroxide (Vanish) Gel
Fostex 10% Benzoyl Peroxide Wash
Fostex Medicated Cleansing Bar
Fostex Medicated Cleansing Cream
4-Way Long Lasting Nasal Spray
4-Way Nasal Moisturizing Saline Mist
KeriCort-10 Cream
Pazo Hemorrhoidal Ointment
Therapeutic Mineral Ice Exercise Formula

CARE-TECH LABORATORIES,   632
INC.
Over-The-Counter Pharmaceuticals
3224 South Kingshighway Boulevard
St. Louis, MO 63139
Direct Inquiries to:
Sherry L. Brereton
(314) 772-4610
FAX: (314) 772-4613
For Medical Emergencies Contact:
Customer Service
(800) 325-9681
FAX: (314) 772-4613

OTC Products Described:
Clinical Care Antimicrobial Wound
    Cleanser **632**
Humatrix Microclysmic Burn/
    Wound Healing Gel **632**
Techni-Care Surgical Scrub, Prep
    and Wound Decontaminant........**632**

Other Products Available:
CC-500 Antibacterial Skin Cleanser for
    Dialysis Patient Care
Just Lotion - Highly Absorbent Aloe Vera
    Glycerine Based Skin Lotion
Loving Lather Collagen Enriched Geriatric
    Cleanser
Loving Lather II Antibacterial Skin
    Cleanser
Loving Lotion Antibacterial Skin & Body
    Lotion
Nex-Gen Antimicrobial Rinse/Mucosal
    Solution
Orchid Fresh Perineal/Ostomy Deodorizer
Skin Magic - Antimicrobial Body Rub &
    Emollient
Soft Skin Non-greasy Bath Oil with Rich
    Emollients for Severely Damaged
    Dermal Tissue
Surgi-Soft Alcohol Degerming Foam
Swirlsoft Whirlpool Emollient for Dry Skin
    Conditions
Tech 2000 Antimicrobial Oral Rinse (No
    Alcohol, No Sodium)
Velvet Fresh Non-irritating Cornstarch
    Baby Powder

COOKE PHARMA   812
1404 Old Country Road
Belmont, CA 94002
Direct Inquiries to:
Customer Service Dept.
(888) 808-6838

Dietary Supplements Described:
HeartBar................................812

COVEX   507, 813
Sector Oficios 33, 1-3
28760 Tres Cantos
Madrid, Spain
Direct Inquiries to:
+34-91-804-4545
FAX: +34-91-804-3030
E-mail: vinpocetin@covex.es

Dietary Supplements Described:
◆ Intelectol Tablets **507, 813**

EFFCON LABORATORIES,   507, 632
INC.
P.O. Box 7499
Marietta, GA 30065-1499
Direct Inquiries to:
J. Bradley Rivet
(800) 722-2428
FAX: (770) 428-6811

EFFCON LABORATORIES, INC.—cont.
For Medical Emergencies Contact:
J. Bradley Rivet
(800) 722-2428
FAX: (770) 428-6811

OTC Products Described:
◆ Pin-X Pinworm Treatment **507, 632**

**FISONS CORPORATION
PRESCRIPTION PRODUCTS**
(See MEDEVA PHARMACEUTICALS, INC.)

FLEMING & COMPANY   **633**
1600 Fenpark Dr.
Fenton, MO 63026
Direct Inquiries to:
Tom Fleming
(636) 343-8200
FAX: (636) 343-9865
Internet: www.flemingcompany.com
For product orders, call (800) 343-0164

OTC Products Described:
Chlor-3 Shaker..........................633
Marblen Suspension.....................633
Nicotinex Elixir.........................633
Ocean Nasal Mist.......................633
Purge Liquid 633

Dietary Supplements Described:
Magonate Liquid.......................**814**
Magonate Natal Liquid **814**
Magonate Tablets......................**814**

4LIFE RESEARCH, LC   **526, 814**
9850 South 300 West
Sandy, UT 84070
Direct Inquiries to:
(801) 562-3600
FAX: (801) 562-3670
Internet: www.4-life.com

Dietary Supplements Described:
◆ Transfer Factor Capsules **526, 814**
◆ Transfer Factor Plus Capsules.........*526*

HYLAND'S, INC.
(See STANDARD HOMEOPATHIC
COMPANY)

JOHNSON & JOHNSON •   **507, 634**
**MERCK CONSUMER
PHARMACEUTICALS
CO.**
7050 Camp Hill Road
Fort Washington, PA 19034
Direct Inquiries to:
Consumer Affairs Department
(800) 469-5268
For Medical Emergencies Contact:
(800) 462-5268

OTC Products Described:
◆ Children's Mylanta Upset
    Stomach Relief Liquid **508, 634**
◆ Children's Mylanta Upset
    Stomach Relief Tablets **508, 634**
◆ Mylanta Gelcaps **507, 637**
   Mylanta Liquid **634**
◆ Mylanta Extra Strength Liquid ...**507, 634**
◆ Mylanta Supreme Liquid.........**507, 636**
◆ Mylanta Ultra Tabs Tablets.......**507, 637**
◆ Extra Strength Mylanta Calci
    Tabs Tablets **507, 636**
◆ Ultra Mylanta Calci Tabs
    Tablets **507, 636**
◆ Mylanta Gas Softgels...........**507, 637**
   Mylanta Gas Tablets...................**637**

◆ Maximum Strength Mylanta
    Gas Tablets **507, 637**
◆ Infants' Mylicon Drops.........**508, 634**
◆ Pepcid AC Tablets, Chewable
    Tablets, and Gelcaps **508, 638**
◆ Pepcid Complete Chewable
    Tablets **508, 638**

LEDERLE CONSUMER HEALTH   **639**
A Division of Whitehall-Robins Healthcare
Five Giralda Farms
Madison, NJ 07940
Direct Inquiries to:
Lederle Consumer Product Information
(800) 282-8805

OTC Products Described:
FiberCon Caplets **639**

Dietary Supplements Described:
Caltrate 600 Tablets...................**814**
Caltrate 600 PLUS Chewables **815**
Caltrate 600 PLUS Tablets **815**
Caltrate 600 + D Tablets **814**
Caltrate 600 + Soy Tablets............**814**
Centrum Focused Formulas
    Bone Health Tablets **815**
Centrum Focused Formulas
    Energy Tablets **816**
Centrum Focused Formulas
    Heart Tablets **816**
Centrum Focused Formulas
    Mental Clarity Tablets..............**816**
Centrum Focused Formulas
    Prostate Softgels **816**
Centrum Kids Complete
    Children's Chewables **817**
Centrum Performance
    Multivitamin-Multimineral
    Tablets **817**
Centrum Tablets **815**
Centrum Silver Tablets **818**

Other Products Available:
Centrum Focused Formulas Stress Tablets
Centrum Kids Extra C Children's
    Chewables
Centrum Kids Extra Calcium Children's
    Chewables
Centrum Liquid

LEGACY FOR LIFE   **508, 818**
P.O. Box 2522
Melbourne, FL 32902-2522
Direct Inquiries to:
(800) 557-8477
Internet:
www.legacyforlife.net
   (for general information)
www.biochoice.net
   (for direct product information)

Dietary Supplements Described:
◆ BioChoice Immune[26] Powder
    and Capsules **508, 818**
   BioChoice Immune Support
    Powder...........................**818**

Other Products Available:
BioChoice FLEX
BioChoice SLIM

3M HEALTH CARE   **508, 640**
Bldg. 304-1-01
St. Paul, MN 55144-1000
Direct Inquiries to:
Customer Service
(800) 537-2191

For Medical Emergencies Contact:
(651) 733-2882 (answered 24 hrs.)

OTC Products Described:
◆ 3M Titralac Antacid Tablets......**508, 640**
◆ 3M Titralac Extra Strength
    Antacid Tablets **508, 640**
◆ 3M Titralac Plus Antacid
    Tablets **508, 640**

MANNATECH, INC.   **508, 819**
600 S. Royal Lane
Suite 200
Coppell, TX 75019
Direct Inquiries to:
Customer Service
(972) 471-8111
For Medical Information Contact:
Kia Gary, RN LNCC
(972) 471-8189
E-mail: Kgary@mannatech.com
Internet:
www.mannatech.com
(for product information)
www.glycoscience.com
(for ingredient information)

Dietary Supplements Described:
◆ Ambrotose Capsules **508, 819**
◆ Ambrotose Powder................**508, 819**
   Ambrotose with Lecithin Capsules **819**
◆ PhytAloe Capsules **508, 819**
◆ PhytAloe Powder **508, 819**
◆ Plus Caplets **508, 820**

Other Products Available:
AmbroDerm Lotion
AmbroStart Beverage Mix
EM-PACT Sports Drink
Emprizone Hydrogel
FIRM with Ambrotose Lotion
Glyco-Bears Tablets
GlycoLEAN Accelerator Capsules
GlycoLEAN Catalyst Caplets
GlycoLEAN Fiber Full Capsules
GlycoLEAN Manager Capsules
GlycoSLIM Meal Replacement Shake
ImmunoSTART Chewables
Man-Aloe (Classic Formula) Capsules
Manna-C Capsules
Manna-Cleanse Caplets
Mannatonin Tablets
MVP Caplets
Phyto-Bear Supplements
Profile Vitamin and Mineral Supplements
Protein MannaBAR Supplement Bar
Sport Capsules
Vanilla Yogurt-Coated Apple Crunch
    MannaBar Supplement Bar

MATOL BOTANICAL   **508, 640**
INTERNATIONAL, LTD.
1111, 46th Avenue
Lachine, Quebec
Canada H8T 3C5
Direct Inquiries to:
(800) 363-3890
Internet: www.matol.com

OTC Products Described:
◆ Biomune OSF Express Spray **508, 640**

Dietary Supplements Described:
◆ Biomune OSF Plus Capsules **508, 820**

MAYOR PHARMACEUTICAL   **821**
LABORATORIES
2401 South 24th Street
Phoenix, AZ 85034

Direct Inquiries to:
Medical Director
(602) 244-8899
Internet: www.vitamist.com

Dietary Supplements Described:
Vitamist Intra-Oral Spray..............**821**
　1-Before, 2-During, 3-After..........*821*
　Anti-Oxidant..........................*821*
　ArthriFlex *821*
　B12 ....*821*
　Blue-Green Sea Spray *821*
　CardioCare...........................*821*
　Colloidal Minerals *821*
　C+Zinc *821*
　DHEA *821*
　Echinacea + G *821*
　E+Selenium...........................*821*
　Ex. O *821*
　Folacin *821*
　GinkgoMist...........................*821*
　Melatonin *821*
　Multiple.............................*821*
　Osteo-CalMag.........................*821*
　Pine Bark and Grape Seed *821*
　PMS and LadyMate.....................*821*
　Re-Leaf *821*
　Revitalizer..........................*821*
　Slender-Mist.........................*821*
　Smoke-Less *821*
　St. John's Wort *821*
　Stress *821*
　VitaMotion-S.........................*821*
　VitaSight *821*

McNEIL CONSUMER HEALTHCARE　508, 640
Division of McNeil-PPC, Inc.
Camp Hill Road
Fort Washington, PA 19034
Direct Inquiries to:
Consumer Relationship Center
Fort Washington, PA 19034
(215) 273-7000
Manufacturing Divisions:
Fort Washington, PA 19034

Southwest Manufacturing Plant
4001 N. I-35
Round Rock, TX 78664

Road 183 KM 19.8
Barrios Montones
Las Piedras, Puerto Rico 00771

OTC Products Described:
◆ Maximum Strength Gas Aid
　Softgels.......................**509, 640**
◆ Imodium A-D Liquid and
　Caplets **509, 641**
◆ Imodium Advanced Chewable
　Tablets........................**509, 641**
◆ Children's Motrin Oral
　Suspension and Chewable
　Tablets........................**509, 643**
◆ Children's Motrin Cold Oral
　Suspension **509, 646**
　Children's Motrin Dosing Chart........**645**
◆ Infants' Motrin Concentrated
　Drops.........................**509, 643**
◆ Junior Strength Motrin Caplets
　and Chewable Tablets **509, 643**
◆ Motrin IB Tablets, Caplets,
　and Gelcaps...................**510, 642**
◆ Motrin Migraine Pain Caplets....**510, 646**
◆ Motrin Sinus/Headache
　Caplets **510, 643**
◆ Nizoral A-D Shampoo **510, 647**
◆ Simply Sleep Caplets **510, 647**

◆ Children's Tylenol
　Suspension Liquid
　and Soft Chews
　Chewable Tablets **510, 511, 657**
◆ Children's Tylenol Allergy-D
　Liquid **510, 658**
◆ Children's Tylenol Cold
　Suspension Liquid and
　Chewable Tablets **510, 659**
◆ Children's Tylenol Cold Plus
　Cough Suspension Liquid
　and Chewable Tablets **510, 659**
◆ Children's Tylenol Flu
　Suspension Liquid **511, 663**
◆ Children's Tylenol Sinus
　Suspension Liquid **511, 663**
　Children's Tylenol Dosing Chart.......**660**
◆ Infants' Tylenol Cold
　Decongestant & Fever
　Reducer Concentrated
　Drops **511, 659**
◆ Infants' Tylenol Cold
　Decongestant & Fever
　Reducer Concentrated
　Drops Plus Cough...........**511, 659**
◆ Infants' Tylenol Concentrated
　Drops **511, 657**
◆ Junior Strength Tylenol
　Soft Chews
　Chewable Tablets **511, 512, 657**
◆ Extra Strength Tylenol Adult Liquid
　Pain Reliever.......................**647**
◆ Extra Strength Tylenol
　Gelcaps, Geltabs, Caplets,
　and Tablets **511, 647**
◆ Regular Strength Tylenol
　Tablets....................**511, 647**
◆ Maximum Strength Tylenol
　Allergy Sinus Caplets,
　Gelcaps, and Geltabs........**511, 649**
◆ Maximum Strength Tylenol
　Allergy Sinus NightTime
　Caplets **511, 649**
◆ Tylenol Severe Allergy Caplets...**511, 649**
◆ Tylenol Arthritis Pain Extended
　Relief Caplets...............**511, 647**
◆ Multi-Symptom Tylenol Cold
　Complete Formula Caplets ..**512, 651**
◆ Multi-Symptom Tylenol Cold
　Non-Drowsy Caplets and
　Gelcaps **512, 651**
◆ Multi-Symptom Tylenol Cold
　Severe Congestion
　Non-Drowsy Caplets **512, 652**
◆ Maximum Strength Tylenol Flu
　NightTime Gelcaps...........**512, 653**
◆ Maximum Strength Tylenol Flu
　NightTime Liquid **512, 653**
◆ Maximum Strength Tylenol Flu
　Non-Drowsy Gelcaps.........**512, 653**
◆ Extra Strength Tylenol PM
　Caplets, Geltabs, and
　Gelcaps **512, 654**
◆ Maximum Strength Tylenol
　Sinus NightTime Caplets **512, 655**
◆ Maximum Strength Tylenol
　Sinus Non-Drowsy Geltabs,
　Gelcaps, Caplets, and
　Tablets....................**512, 655**
◆ Maximum Strength Tylenol
　Sore Throat Adult Liquid **512, 656**
◆ Women's Tylenol Menstrual
　Relief Caplets...............**512, 656**

Dietary Supplements Described:
◆ Aflexa Tablets **508, 821**
◆ Lactaid Original Strength
　Caplets **509, 822**
◆ Lactaid Extra Strength Caplets ..**509, 822**
◆ Lactaid Ultra Caplets and
　Chewable Tablets **509, 822**
◆ Lactaid Drops..................**509, 822**
◆ Probiotica Tablets...............**510, 822**

MEDEVA PHARMACEUTICALS, INC.　664
P.O. Box 31710
Rochester, NY 14603
Direct Inquiries to:
Customer Service Department
P.O. Box 31766
Rochester, NY 14603
(716) 274-5300
(888) 9-MEDEVA
For Emergency Medical Information Contact:
(800) 932-1950 (24 hours)
(888) 9-MEDEVA (24 hours)

OTC Products Described:
Delsym Extended-Release
　Suspension **664**

MEDTECH　664
488 Main Avenue
Norwalk, CT 06851
Direct Inquiries to:
(800) 443-4908

OTC Products Described:
APF Arthritis Pain Formula............*664*
Compound W One Step Pads for
　Kids..............................**664**
Compound W One Step Plantar
　Pads **664**
Compound W One Step Wart
　Remover Pads **664**
Compound W Wart Remover Gel **665**
Compound W Wart Remover
　Liquid **665**
Dermoplast Antibacterial Spray,
　Hospital Strength **666**
Dermoplast Hospital Strength
　Spray **666**
Freezone Corn & Callus Liquid *664*
Heet Liniment.......................*664*
Momentum Backache Relief Extra
　Strength Caplets...................**666**
New Skin Liquid Bandage **667**
Oxipor Psoriasis Lotion *664*
Percogesic Aspirin-Free Coated
　Tablets **667**
Extra Strength Percogesic
　Aspirin-Free Coated Caplets **665**
Zincon Medicated Dandruff
　Shampoo *664*

MEYENBERG GOAT MILK PRODUCTS　823
P.O. Box 934
Turlock, CA 95381
Direct Inquiries to:
(800) 343-1185
(209) 667-2019
Internet: www.meyenberg.com
Medical Professionals Contact:
Carol Jones
(209) 667-2019

Dietary Supplements Described:
Meyenberg Goat Milk **823**

MILES INC. CONSUMER HEALTHCARE PRODUCTS
(See BAYER CORPORATION CONSUMER CARE DIVISION)

MISSION PHARMACAL COMPANY　667
10999 IH 10 West, Suite 1000
San Antonio, TX 78230-1355

MISSION PHARMACAL COMPANY—
cont.
Direct Inquiries to:
P.O. Box 786099
San Antonio, TX 78278-6099
(800) 292-7364
(210) 696-8400
FAX: (210) 696-6010
For Medical Emergencies Contact:
George Alexandrides
(830) 249-9822
FAX: (830) 816-2545

OTC Products Described:
Thera-Gesic Creme 667

Dietary Supplements Described:
Citracal Liquitab Tablets 823
Citracal Tablets 823
Citracal Caplets + D 823
Citracal 250 MG + D Tablets 823
Citracal Plus Tablets 824

Other Products Available:
Calcet Triple Calcium Supplement Tablets
Calcet Plus Multivitamin/Mineral Tablets
Citracal Prenatal Rx
Compete Multivitamin/Mineral Tablets
Fosfree Multivitamin/Mineral Tablets
Iromin-G Multivitamin/Mineral Tablets
Maxilube Personal Lubricant

NOVARTIS CONSUMER   **512, 668**
HEALTH, INC.
560 Morris Ave.
Summit, NJ 07901-1312
Direct Inquiries to:
Consumer and Professional Affairs
(800) 452-0051
FAX: (800) 635-2801
Or write to the above address

OTC Products Described:
◆ Desenex Max Cream *512*
    Desenex Liquid Spray 668
◆ Desenex Shake Powder **512, 668**
◆ Desenex Spray Powder **512, 668**
    Desenex Jock Itch Spray Powder 668
◆ Dulcolax Suppositories **513, 668**
◆ Dulcolax Tablets **513, 668**
◆ Ex•Lax Gentle Strength
    Caplets **513, 670**
◆ Ex•Lax Regular Strength Pills ... **513, 670**
◆ Ex•Lax Regular Strength
    Chocolated Pieces **513, 669**
◆ Ex•Lax Maximum Strength
    Pills **513, 670**
◆ Ex•Lax Milk of Magnesia
    Liquid **513, 670**
◆ Ex•Lax Stool Softener Caplets .. **513, 671**
◆ Gas-X Chewable Tablets **513, 671**
◆ Extra Strength Gas-X Liquid...... **513, 671**
◆ Extra Strength Gas-X Softgels ... **513, 671**
◆ Extra Strength Gas-X
    Chewable Tablets **513, 671**
◆ Maximum Strength Gas-X
    Softgels **513, 671**
◆ Lamisil^AT Cream **513, 672**
◆ Lamisil^AT Solution.............. **513, 672**
◆ Maalox Antacid/Anti-Gas Oral
    Suspension **514, 673**
◆ Maalox Max Maximum
    Strength Antacid/Anti-Gas
    Liquid **514, 673**
◆ Quick Dissolve Maalox Antacid
    Chewable Tablets **514, 674**
◆ Quick Dissolve Maalox Max
    Maximum Strength
    Antacid/Antigas Chewable
    Tablets **514, 674**
◆ Perdiem Fiber Therapy
    Granules **514, 675**

◆ Perdiem Overnight Relief
    Granules **514, 674**
◆ Tavist 12 Hour Allergy Tablets ... **514, 676**
◆ Tavist Sinus Non-Drowsy
    Coated Caplets **514, 676**
◆ TheraFlu Regular Strength
    Cold & Cough Night Time
    Hot Liquid **515, 676**
◆ TheraFlu Regular Strength
    Cold & Sore Throat Night
    Time Hot Liquid **515, 676**
◆ TheraFlu Maximum Strength
    Flu & Congestion
    Non-Drowsy Hot Liquid....... **515, 677**
◆ TheraFlu Maximum Strength
    Flu & Cough Night Time
    Hot Liquid **515, 678**
◆ TheraFlu Maximum Strength
    Flu & Sore Throat Night
    Time Hot Liquid **515, 677**
◆ TheraFlu Maximum Strength
    Severe Cold & Congestion
    Night Time Caplets **515, 678**
◆ TheraFlu Maximum Strength
    Severe Cold & Congestion
    Night Time Hot Liquid....... **515, 678**
◆ TheraFlu Maximum Strength
    Severe Cold & Congestion
    Non-Drowsy Caplets **515, 679**
◆ TheraFlu Maximum Strength
    Severe Cold & Congestion
    Non-Drowsy Hot Liquid....... **515, 679**
◆ Triaminic Allergy Congestion
    Liquid **515, 680**
◆ Triaminic Chest Congestion
    Liquid **515, 680**
◆ Triaminic Cold & Allergy Liquid... **515, 681**
◆ Triaminic Cold & Allergy
    Softchews................... **515, 683**
◆ Triaminic Cold & Cough Liquid ... **515, 681**
◆ Triaminic Cold & Cough
    Softchews................... **515, 683**
◆ Triaminic Cold & Night Time
    Cough Liquid **515, 681**
◆ Triaminic Cold, Cough & Fever
    Liquid **515, 681**
◆ Triaminic Cough Liquid........... **515, 682**
◆ Triaminic Cough Softchews **515, 684**
◆ Triaminic Cough & Congestion
    Liquid **515, 682**
◆ Triaminic Cough & Sore Throat
    Liquid **515, 682**
◆ Triaminic Cough & Sore Throat
    Softchews................... **515, 684**
◆ Triaminic Vapor Patch-Cherry
    Scent **515, 684**
◆ Triaminic Vapor Patch-Menthol
    Scent **515, 684**
    Triaminicin Tablets..................... *515*

Dietary Supplements Described:
◆ ReSource Wellness AllerPro
    Capsules................... **514, 824**
◆ ReSource Wellness CalciWise
    Soft Chews **514, 824**
◆ ReSource Wellness EnVigor
    Caplets **514, 824**
◆ ReSource Wellness FlexTend
    Caplets **514, 825**
◆ ReSource Wellness ForSight
    Caplets **514, 825**
◆ ReSource Wellness
    MemorAble Softgels **514, 825**
◆ ReSource Wellness ResistEx
    Capsules................... **514, 826**
◆ ReSource Wellness 2nd Wind
    Capsules................... **514, 826**
◆ ReSource Wellness StayCalm
    Caplets **514, 826**
◆ ReSource Wellness VeinTain
    Caplets **514, 827**
◆ Slow Fe Tablets **514, 827**
◆ Slow Fe with Folic Acid Tablets .. **514, 828**

NUMARK LABORATORIES,   **828**
INC.
164 Northfield Avenue
Edison, NJ 08837
Direct Inquiries to:
Consumer Services
Phone: (800) 331-0221
FAX: (732) 225-0066

Dietary Supplements Described:
Lipoflavonoid Caplets.................. **828**

PARKE-DAVIS
(See PFIZER INC., WARNER-LAMBERT
CONSUMER HEALTHCARE)

THE PARTHENON COMPANY,   **685**
INC.
3311 West 2400 South
Salt Lake City, UT 84119
Direct Inquiries to:
(801) 972-5184
FAX: (801) 972-4734
For Medical Emergencies Contact:
Nick G. Mihalopoulos
(801) 972-5184

OTC Products Described:
Devrom Chewable Tablets **685**

PFIZER INC.,   **515, 685**
WARNER-LAMBERT
CONSUMER GROUP
Consumer Health Products Group
201 Tabor Road
Morris Plains, NJ 07950 (See also Pfizer
Inc., Warner-Lambert Consumer
Healthcare)
Direct Inquiries to:
(800) 223-0182
For Consumer Product Information Call:
(800) 524-2854 (Celestial Seasonings
Soothers only)
(800) 223-0182

OTC Products Described:
◆ Celestial Seasonings Soothers
    Throat Drops................. **515, 685**
◆ Certs Cool Mint Drops......... **515, 685**
◆ Certs Powerful Mints **516, 686**
◆ Halls Defense Drops............. **516, 687**
◆ Halls Mentho-Lyptus Drops...... **516, 686**
◆ Halls Sugar Free
    Mentho-Lyptus Drops........ **516, 686**
◆ Halls Sugar Free Squares **516, 686**
◆ Halls Plus Cough Drops **516, 686**
◆ Trident Advantage Mints **516, 687**
◆ Trident Advantage Sugarless
    Gum....................... **516, 687**
◆ Trident for Kids Sugarless
    Gum....................... **516, 687**

PFIZER INC.,   **516, 688**
WARNER-LAMBERT
CONSUMER
HEALTHCARE
201 Tabor Road
Morris Plains, NJ 07950
Address Questions & Comments to:
Consumer Affairs, Pfizer CHC
182 Tabor Road
Morris Plains, NJ 07950
**For Medical Emergencies or Information
Contact:**
(800) 223-0182
(800) 732-7529 (BenGay, Bonine,
Cortizone, Desitin, Unisom, Visine and

Wart-Off products)
(800) 378-1783 (e.p.t.)
(800) 337-7266 (e.p.t.-Spanish)

OTC Products Described:
◆ Actifed Cold & Allergy Tablets ...**516, 688**
◆ Actifed Cold & Sinus Caplets
   and Tablets **516, 688**
◆ Anusol HC-1 Hydrocortisone
   Anti-Itch Cream **516, 689**
◆ Anusol Ointment **516, 688**
◆ Anusol Suppositories **516, 689**
◆ Benadryl Allergy Chewables **517, 689**
◆ Benadryl Allergy Kapseal
   Capsules **516, 691**
◆ Benadryl Allergy Liquid **517, 690**
◆ Benadryl Allergy Ultratab
   Tablets **516, 691**
◆ Benadryl Allergy/Cold Tablets ...**517, 691**
◆ Benadryl Allergy/Congestion
   Tablets **517, 692**
  Benadryl Allergy & Sinus Liquid **693**
◆ Benadryl Allergy & Sinus
   Fastmelt Tablets **517, 693**
◆ Benadryl Allergy Sinus
   Headache Caplets &
   Gelcaps **517, 693**
◆ Benadryl Severe Allergy &
   Sinus Headache Caplets **517, 694**
◆ Benadryl Children's Allergy and
   Sinus Liquid *517*
◆ Benadryl Children's Allergy/
   Cold Fastmelt Tablets **517, 692**
◆ Benadryl Dye-Free Allergy
   Liquid **517, 690**
◆ Benadryl Dye-Free Allergy
   Liqui-Gels Softgels...........**517, 690**
· Benadryl Itch Relief Stick
   Extra Strength **517, 695**
◆ Benadryl Itch Stopping Cream
   Original Strength.............**517, 695**
◆ Benadryl Itch Stopping Cream
   Extra Strength **517, 695**
◆ Benadryl Itch Stopping Gel
   Original Strength.............**517, 695**
◆ Benadryl Itch Stopping Gel
   Extra Strength **517, 695**
◆ Benadryl Itch Stopping Spray
   Original Strength.............**517, 696**
◆ Benadryl Itch Stopping Spray
   Extra Strength **517, 696**
◆ BenGay External Analgesic
   Products **518, 696**
◆ Benylin Adult Formula Cough
   Suppressant Liquid **518, 696**
◆ Benylin Cough Suppressant/
   Expectorant Liquid **518, 697**
◆ Benylin Multi-Symptom Liquid ...**518, 697**
◆ Benylin Pediatric Cough
   Suppressant Liquid **518, 698**
◆ Bonine Chewable Tablets **518, 698**
◆ Caladryl Clear Lotion **518, 698**
◆ Caladryl Lotion.................**518, 698**
◆ Cortizone•5 Creme **518, 699**
  Cortizone•5 Ointment **699**
◆ Cortizone•10 Creme **518, 699**
  Cortizone•10 Ointment **699**
◆ Cortizone•10 Plus Creme **518, 700**
◆ Cortizone•10 Quick Shot
   Spray.........................**518, 699**
◆ Cortizone for Kids Creme........**518, 699**
◆ Desitin Baby Powder............**518, 700**
◆ Desitin Creamy Ointment **518, 700**
◆ Desitin Ointment...............**518, 700**
◆ e.p.t. Pregnancy Test **518, 701**
◆ Listerine Mouthrinse............**518, 702**
◆ Cool Mint Listerine Mouthrinse..**518, 702**
◆ FreshBurst Listerine
   Mouthrinse...................**519, 702**
◆ Tartar Control Listerine
   Mouthrinse...................**519, 702**
◆ Listermint Alcohol-Free
   Mouthrinse...................**519, 703**

◆ Lubriderm Advanced Therapy
   Creamy Lotion **519, 703**
◆ Lubriderm Daily UV Lotion **519, 703**
◆ Lubriderm Seriously Sensitive
   Lotion **519, 703**
◆ Lubriderm Skin Therapy
   Moisturizing Lotion...........**519, 703**
◆ Neosporin "Neo to Go!" Ointment.....*519*
◆ Neosporin Ointment **519, 704**
◆ Neosporin + Pain Relief
   Maximum Strength Cream ...**519, 704**
◆ Neosporin + Pain Relief
   Maximum Strength
   Ointment.....................**519, 704**
◆ Nix Creme Rinse **519, 704**
◆ Nix Spray.....................**519, 705**
  OcuHist Eye Allergy Relief Eye Drops
   (see Visine-A Eye Drops)
◆ Polysporin Ointment **519, 706**
◆ Polysporin Powder **519, 706**
◆ Rolaids Tablets **519, 706**
◆ Extra Strength Rolaids Tablets...**519, 706**
◆ Sinutab Non-Drying Liquid
   Caps **520, 706**
◆ Sinutab Sinus Allergy
   Medication, Maximum
   Strength Formula, Tablets
   & Caplets **520, 707**
◆ Sinutab Sinus Medication,
   Maximum Strength
   Without Drowsiness
   Formula, Tablets & Caplets ..**520, 707**
◆ Sudafed 12 Hour Tablets **520, 708**
◆ Sudafed 24 Hour Tablets **520, 708**
◆ Children's Sudafed Cold &
   Cough Liquid **520, 709**
◆ Children's Sudafed Nasal
   Decongestant Chewables....**520, 711**
◆ Children's Sudafed Nasal
   Decongestant Liquid
   Medication **521, 711**
◆ Sudafed Cold & Allergy Tablets ..**520, 708**
◆ Sudafed Cold & Cough Liquid
   Caps **520, 709**
◆ Sudafed Cold & Sinus Liquid
   Caps **520, 710**
◆ Sudafed Nasal Decongestant
   Tablets **520, 710**
◆ Sudafed Non-Drying Sinus
   Liquid Caps **520, 712**
◆ Sudafed Severe Cold Formula
   Caplets **520, 711**
◆ Sudafed Severe Cold Formula
   Tablets **520, 711**
◆ Sudafed Sinus Headache
   Caplets **520, 712**
◆ Sudafed Sinus Headache
   Tablets **520, 712**
◆ Tucks Pre-moistened Pads.......**521, 713**
◆ Unisom SleepTabs **521, 713**
  Unisom Maximum Strength
   SleepGels....................**521, 713**
◆ Visine Original Eye Drops **521, 715**
◆ Visine A.C. Eye Drops **521, 715**
◆ Visine L.R. Eye Drops **521, 715**
◆ Advanced Relief Visine Eye
   Drops **521, 714**
◆ Visine Tears Eye Drops **521, 716**
◆ Visine Tears Preservative Free
   Eye Drops **521, 716**
◆ Visine-A Eye Drops..............**521, 714**
◆ Wart-Off Liquid.......................**716**
◆ Zantac 75 Tablets **528, 717**

Other Products Available:
Barbasol Shaving Products
Borofax Skin Protectant Ointment
Hemorid Creme
Hemorid Ointment
Advanced Formula Plax Pre-Brushing
   Dental Rinse

**PHARMACIA CONSUMER   717
HEALTHCARE**
100 Route 206 North
Peapack, NJ 07977
**For Medical and Pharmaceutical
Information, Including Emergencies,
Contact:**
(800) 253-8600 ext. 3-8244
(616) 833-8244

OTC Products Described:
Cortaid Intensive Therapy Cream......**717**
Cortaid Maximum Strength Cream **717**
Cortaid Maximum Strength
   Ointment.........................**717**
Cortaid Sensitive Skin Cream **717**
Dramamine Original Formula
   Tablets **718**
Dramamine Chewable Formula
   Tablets **718**
Dramamine Less Drowsy Tablets......**718**
Emetrol Oral Solution
   (Lemon-Mint & Cherry Flavors) **718**
NasalCrom Nasal Spray **719**
PediaCare Cough-Cold Liquid..........**719**
PediaCare Infants' Drops
   Decongestant **719**
PediaCare Infants' Drops
   Decongestant Plus Cough **719**
PediaCare NightRest Cough-Cold
   Liquid **719**
Rogaine Extra Strength for Men
   Topical Solution..................**721**
Rogaine for Women Topical
   Solution.........................**721**
Surfak Liqui-Gels **721**

Other Products Available:
Cortaid FastStick
Doxidan Liqui-Gels
Kaopectate Anti-Diarrheal, Peppermint
   Flavor Liquid
Kaopectate Anti-Diarrheal, Regular Flavor
   Liquid
Kaopectate Maximum Strength Caplets
Children's Kaopectate Cherry Flavor Liquid
Micatin Cream
Micatin Jock Itch Cream
Micatin Jock Itch Spray Powder
Micatin Odor Control Spray Powder
Micatin Powder
Micatin Spray Liquid
Micatin Spray Powder
Progaine Conditioner
Progaine Shampoo (Extra Body)
Progaine Shampoo (Permed & Color
   Treated)
Progaine Shampoo (2 in 1)
Rogaine Regular Strength For Men Hair
   Regrowth Treatment
Unicap Capsules
Unicap M Tablets
Unicap T Tablets
Unicap Sr. Tablets

**PHARMATON NATURAL   521, 828
HEALTH PRODUCTS**
A Division of Boehringer Ingelheim
Pharmaceuticals, Inc.
900 Ridgebury Road
Ridgefield, CT 06877
Direct Inquiries to:
Consumer Affairs
(800) 451-6688
FAX: (203) 798-5771
For Medical Emergencies Contact:
David Morrison
(203) 775-7826
FAX: (203) 798-5771

PHARMATON NATURAL HEALTH PRODUCTS—*cont.*
Dietary Supplements Described:
◆ Ginkoba M/E Suppli-Cap
  Capsules........................**521, 829**
  Ginkoba Tablets **828**
  Ginsana Capsules **830**
◆ Ginsana Chewy Squares.........**521, 830**
◆ Ginsana Sport Capsules.........**521, 831**
◆ Movana Tablets...................**521, 832**
◆ Prostatonin Softgel Capsules....**521, 832**
◆ Venastat Suppli-Cap Capsules...**521, 833**
◆ Vitasana Gelcaps **521, 834**

PLOUGH, INC.
(See SCHERING-PLOUGH HEALTHCARE PRODUCTS)

PROCTER & GAMBLE   **521, 722**
P.O. Box 5516
Cincinnati, OH 45201
Direct Inquiries to:
Charles Lambert
(800) 358-8707
For Medical Emergencies Contact:
Call Collect: (513) 636-5107

OTC Products Described:
Metamucil Powder, Original
  Texture Orange Flavor..............**722**
Metamucil Powder, Original
  Texture Regular Flavor **722**
◆ Metamucil Smooth Texture
  Powder, Orange Flavor **521, 722**
Metamucil Smooth Texture
  Powder, Sugar-Free, Orange
  Flavor **722**
Metamucil Smooth Texture
  Powder, Sugar-Free, Regular
  Flavor **722**
◆ Metamucil Wafers, Apple Crisp
  & Cinnamon Spice Flavors...**521, 722**
◆ Pepto-Bismol Original Liquid,
  Original and Cherry
  Chewable Tablets &
  Caplets **521, 723**
Pepto-Bismol Maximum Strength
  Liquid **724**
Vicks 44 Cough Relief Liquid..........**724**
Vicks 44D Cough & Head
  Congestion Relief Liquid...........**724**
Vicks 44E Cough & Chest
  Congestion Relief Liquid...........**725**
Pediatric Vicks 44e Cough &
  Chest Congestion Relief
  Liquid **728**
Vicks 44M Cough, Cold & Flu
  Relief Liquid **725**
Pediatric Vicks 44m Cough &
  Cold Relief **728**
Vicks Cough Drops, Menthol and
  Cherry Flavors **726**
Vicks DayQuil LiquiCaps/Liquid
  Multi-Symptom Cold/Flu Relief **727**
Children's Vicks NyQuil Cold/
  Cough Relief **726**
Vicks NyQuil LiquiCaps/Liquid
  Multi-Symptom Cold/Flu
  Relief, Original and Cherry
  Flavors **727**
Vicks Sinex Nasal Spray and Ultra
  Fine Mist...........................**729**
Vicks Sinex 12-Hour Nasal Spray
  and Ultra Fine Mist **729**
Vicks Vapor Inhaler **730**
Vicks VapoRub Cream **730**
Vicks VapoRub Ointment **730**
Vicks VapoSteam **730**

Dietary Supplements Described:
Metamucil Dietary Fiber
  Supplement........................**834**

PRODUCTS ON DEMAND   **522, 731**
1621 East Flamingo Road
Suite 15A
Las Vegas, NV 89119
Direct Inquiries to:
Shaina M. Toppo
(702) 765-5001
FAX: (702) 765-5002
Internet: www.vitara.com
For Medical Emergencies Contact:
(702) 765-5001
FAX: (702) 765-5002

OTC Products Described:
◆ Vitara Cream......................**522, 731**

THE PURDUE FREDERICK   **522, 731**
COMPANY
One Stamford Forum
Stamford, CT 06901-3431
For Medical Information Contact:
Medical Department
(888) 726-7535

OTC Products Described:
◆ Betadine Brand First Aid
  Antibiotics + Moisturizer
  Ointment......................**522, 731**
◆ Betadine Brand Plus First Aid
  Antibiotics + Pain Reliever
  Ointment......................**522, 731**
◆ Betadine Ointment...............**522, 732**
◆ Betadine PrepStick Applicator ...**522, 732**
  Betadine Skin Cleanser **732**
◆ Betadine Solution...............**522, 732**
◆ Senokot Children's Syrup........**522, 732**
◆ Senokot Granules................**522, 732**
◆ Senokot Syrup **522, 732**
◆ Senokot Tablets **522, 732**
◆ Senokot-S Tablets **522, 732**
  SenokotXTRA Tablets **732**

RICHARDSON-VICKS, INC.
(See PROCTER & GAMBLE)

ROBERTS PHARMACEUTICAL
CORPORATION
(See SHIRE PHARMACEUTICALS)

SCHERING CORPORATION
(See SCHERING-PLOUGH HEALTHCARE PRODUCTS)

SCHERING-PLOUGH   **522, 733**
HEALTHCARE
PRODUCTS
3 Oak Way
Berkeley Heights, NJ 07922
Direct Product Requests to:
Schering-Plough HealthCare Products
Attn: Managed Care Department
3 Oak Way
Berkeley Heights, NJ 07922
(908) 679-1983
FAX: (908) 679-1776
For Medical Emergencies Contact:
Consumer Relations Department
(901) 320-2988 (Business Hours)
(901) 320-2364 (After Hours)

OTC Products Described:
◆ A + D Original Ointment.........**522, 733**
◆ A + D Ointment with Zinc
  Oxide.........................**522, 733**
Afrin Nasal Decongestant
  Children's Pump Mist..............**734**
◆ Afrin Original Nasal Spray......**522, 733**

Afrin Extra Moisturizing Nasal
  Spray **733**
Afrin Severe Congestion Nasal
  Spray **733**
Afrin Sinus Nasal Spray **733**
◆ Afrin No Drip Original Nasal
  Spray.........................**522, 735**
Afrin No Drip Extra Moisturizing
  Nasal Spray........................**735**
Afrin No Drip Severe Congestion
  Nasal Spray........................**735**
Afrin No Drip Sinus Nasal Spray......**735**
Afrin Original Pump Mist..............**733**
Afrin Saline Aromatic Mist...........**734**
◆ Afrin Extra Moisturizing Saline
  Mist..........................**522, 734**
◆ Chlor-Trimeton Allergy Tablets ...**522, 735**
◆ Chlor-Trimeton Allergy/
  Decongestant Tablets........**522, 736**
Clear Away Gel with Aloe Wart
  Remover System **736**
Clear Away Liquid Wart Remover
  System.............................**736**
◆ Clear Away One Step Wart
  Remover **522, 737**
◆ Clear Away One Step Wart
  Remover for Kids **522, 737**
Clear Away One Step Plantar Wart
  Remover **737**
◆ Coricidin 'D' Cold, Flu & Sinus
  Tablets.......................**522, 737**
◆ Coricidin HBP Cold & Flu
  Tablets.......................**523, 738**
◆ Coricidin HBP Cough & Cold
  Tablets.......................**523, 738**
◆ Coricidin HBP Maximum
  Strength Flu Tablets **523, 738**
◆ Coricidin HBP Night-Time Cold
  & Flu Tablets.................**523, 738**
◆ Correctol Laxative Tablets and
  Caplets.......................**523, 739**
◆ Drixoral Allergy/Sinus
  Extended-Release Tablets ...**523, 741**
◆ Drixoral Cold & Allergy
  Sustained-Action Tablets.....**523, 740**
◆ Drixoral Cold & Flu
  Extended-Release Tablets ...**523, 740**
◆ Drixoral Nasal Decongestant
  Long-Acting Non-Drowsy
  Tablets.......................**523, 740**
DuoFilm (see Clear Away products)
◆ Gyne-Lotrimin 3, 3-Day Cream ...**523, 741**
◆ Lotrimin AF Cream, Lotion,
  Solution, and Jock Itch
  Cream.........................**523, 742**
◆ Lotrimin AF Spray Powder,
  Spray Liquid, Spray
  Deodorant Powder, Shaker
  Powder and Jock Itch
  Spray Powder **523, 742**

SHIRE PHARMACEUTICALS   **743**
U.S. Consumer Products Division
7900 Tanners Gate Drive
Florence, KY 41042
Direct Inquiries to:
Customer Service Department
(800) 828-2088
FAX: (859) 372-7684
For Medical Emergencies Contact:
Medical Information Department
(800) 536-7878
(800) 992-9306

OTC Products Described:
Colace Capsules, Syrup and
  Drops **743**
Peri-Colace Capsules and Syrup.......**743**

Dietary Supplements Described:
Slow-Mag Tablets **835**

Other Products Available:
Cheracol Cough Syrup CV
Cheracol Cough/Sore Throat Lozenges
Squibb Cod Liver Oil
Squibb Glycerin Suppositories
Squibb Mineral Oil

SIGMA-TAU　　　　　**523, 835**
HEALTHSCIENCE, INC.
800 South Frederick Avenue
Suite 102
Gaithersburg, MD 20877
Direct Medical Inquiries to:
(877) PROXEED (776-9333)
(301) 948-1041
FAX: (301) 948-5452
E-Mail: proxeedinfo@sigmatau.com
Direct Product Orders to:
(877) PROXEED (776-9333)
Internet: www.proxeed.com

Dietary Supplements Described:
◆ Proxeed Powder..................523, 835

SMITHKLINE BEECHAM　　**523, 744**
CONSUMER
HEALTHCARE, L.P.
Unit of SmithKline Beecham Corporation
P.O. Box 1467
Pittsburgh, PA 15230
For Medical Information Contact:
(800) 245-1040 (Consumer Inquiries)
(800) 378-4055 (Healthcare Professional
Inquiries)
Direct Healthcare Professional Sample
Requests to:
(800) BEECHAM

OTC Products Described:
Abreva Cream...........................744
Citrucel Caplets 745
◆ Citrucel Orange Flavor Powder...**523, 744**
◆ Citrucel Sugar Free Orange
　Flavor Powder..................**523, 745**
◆ Contac Non-Drowsy 12 Hour
　Cold Caplets **523, 745**
◆ Contac Non-Drowsy Timed
　Release 12 Hour Cold
　Caplets **523, 746**
◆ Contac Severe Cold and Flu
　Caplets Maximum
　Strength......................**523, 746**
　Contac Severe Cold and Flu
　Caplets Non-Drowsy **746**
◆ Debrox Drops..................**523, 747**
◆ Ecotrin Enteric Coated Aspirin
　Low Strength Tablets **524, 747**
◆ Ecotrin Enteric Coated Aspirin
　Maximum Strength Tablets ...**524, 747**
◆ Ecotrin Enteric Coated Aspirin
　Regular Strength Tablets....**524, 747**
◆ Gaviscon Extra Strength Liquid ..**524, 751**
◆ Gaviscon Extra Strength
　Tablets **524, 751**
◆ Gaviscon Regular Strength
　Liquid.......................**524, 751**
◆ Gaviscon Regular Strength
　Tablets **524, 750**
◆ Gly-Oxide Liquid.................**524, 751**
　Massengill Feminine Cleansing
　Wash.............................**753**
　Massengill Disposable Douches **752**
　Massengill Baby Powder Scent
　Soft Cloth Towelette **753**
◆ Massengill Medicated
　Disposable Douche..........**524, 753**
　Massengill Medicated Soft Cloth
　Towelette **753**
◆ NicoDerm CQ Patch............**524, 754**
◆ Nicorette Gum **524, 758**

Singlet Caplets **761**
　Sominex Original Formula Tablets **761**
◆ Tagamet HB 200 Suspension ..**525, 762**
◆ Tagamet HB 200 Tablets **525, 761**
◆ Tums E-X Antacid/Calcium
　Tablets......................**525, 763**
◆ Tums E-X Sugar Free Antacid/
　Calcium Tablets..............**525, 763**
◆ Tums Regular Antacid/Calcium
　Tablets......................**525, 763**
◆ Tums ULTRA Antacid/Calcium
　Tablets......................**525, 763**
◆ Vivarin Caplets **525, 763**
◆ Vivarin Tablets **525, 763**

Dietary Supplements Described:
　Alluna Sleep Tablets..................**837**
◆ Feosol Caplets **524, 837**
◆ Feosol Tablets **524, 838**
◆ Os-Cal Chewable Tablets **525, 838**
◆ Os-Cal 250 + D Tablets.........**525, 838**
◆ Os-Cal 500 Tablets **525, 839**
◆ Os-Cal 500 + D Tablets.........**525, 839**
　Remifemin Menopause Tablets........**839**

Other Products Available:
Sominex Maximum Strength Caplets
　Nighttime Sleep Aid
Sominex Pain Relief Formula Tablets

STANDARD HOMEOPATHIC　　**764**
COMPANY
210 West 131st Street
Box 61067
Los Angeles, CA 90061
Direct Inquiries to:
Jay Borneman
(800) 624-9659, Ext. 20

OTC Products Described:
Hyland's Arnisport Tablets **764**
Hyland's Back Ache with Arnica
　Caplets..........................**764**
Hyland's Bumps 'n Bruises
　Tablets..........................**764**
Hyland's Calms Forté Tablets and
　Caplets..........................**764**
Hyland's Cold Tablets with Zinc **765**
Hyland's Colic Tablets **765**
Hyland's Earache Tablets **765**
Hyland's Leg Cramps with Quinine
　Tablets..........................**765**
Hyland's MenoCalm Tablets **765**
Hyland's Nerve Tonic Tablets and
　Caplets..........................**766**
Hyland's Teething Gel **766**
Hyland's Teething Tablets **766**
Smile's Prid Salve **766**

STRATEGIC SCIENCE &　　**525, 840**
TECHNOLOGIES, INC.
P.O. Box 395
Newton Center, MA 02459
Direct Inquiries to:
Consumer Product Information Center
(888) 408-6262

Dietary Supplements Described:
◆ Doctor Ginsberg's Psoria Rid
　Cream......................**525, 840**
◆ Natural Arousal Cream **525, 840**
　Natural Sensation Cream.............**841**
　Nature's Own Pain Expeller
　Cream...........................**841**
◆ Warm Cream...................**525, 841**

SUNPOWER　　　　**525, 841**
NUTRACEUTICAL INC.
18003 Sky Park Circle
Suite G
Irvine, CA 92614

Direct Inquiries to:
(949) 833-8899

Dietary Supplements Described:
Power Circulation Tablets..............*841*
Power Lasting Tablets *841*
Sun Beauty 1 Tablets..................*841*
Sun Beauty 2 Tablets..................*841*
Sun Beauty 3 Tablets..................*841*
Sun Cardio Tablets *841*
Sun Joint Tablets *841*
◆ Sun Liver Tablets *525, 841*

UAS LABORATORIES　　　**767**
5610 Rowland Road # 110
Minnetonka, MN 55343
Direct Inquiries to:
Dr. S.K. Dash
(612) 935-1707
FAX: (612) 935-1650
For Medical Emergencies Contact:
Dr. S.K. Dash
(612) 935-1707
FAX: (612) 935-1650

OTC Products Described:
DDS-Acidophilus Capsules,
　Tablets, and Powder..............**767**

THE UPJOHN COMPANY
(See PHARMACIA CONSUMER
HEALTHCARE)

UPSHER-SMITH　　　　**767**
LABORATORIES, INC.
14905 23rd Avenue N.
Plymouth, MN 55447
Direct Inquiries to:
Professional Services
(763) 475-3023
FAX: (763) 475-3410
For Medical Emergencies Contact:
Professional Services
(763) 475-3023
(800) 654-2299
FAX: (763) 475-3410
Branch Offices:
13700 1st Avenue N.
Plymouth, MN 55441
(763) 475-3023
FAX: (763) 475-3410

OTC Products Described:
Amlactin 12% Moisturizing Lotion
　and Cream........................*767*

WALLACE LABORATORIES　**525, 767**
P.O. Box 1001
Half Acre Road
Cranbury, NJ 08512
Direct Inquiries to:
Wallace Laboratories
Div. of Carter-Wallace, Inc.
P.O. Box 1001
Cranbury, NJ 08512
609-655-6000
For Medical Information, Contact:
Generally:
Professional Services
800-526-3840
After Hours and Weekend Emergencies:
609-655-6474

OTC Products Described:
◆ Maltsupex Powder, Liquid,
　Tablets **525, 767**
◆ Ryna Liquid **768**
◆ Ryna-C Liquid **525, 768**

WARNER-LAMBERT COMPANY
(See PFIZER INC., WARNER-LAMBERT CONSUMER GROUP)

WARNER-LAMBERT CONSUMER HEALTHCARE
(See PFIZER INC., WARNER-LAMBERT CONSUMER HEALTHCARE)

WELLNESS INTERNATIONAL NETWORK, LTD.   769
5800 Democracy Drive
Plano, TX 75024
Direct Inquiries to:
Product Coordinator
(972) 312-1100
FAX: (972) 943-5250

OTC Products Described:
Bio-Complex 5000 Gentle
  Foaming Cleanser **769**
Bio-Complex 5000 Revitalizing
  Conditioner **769**
Bio-Complex 5000 Revitalizing
  Shampoo **770**
StePHan Bio-Nutritional Daytime
  Hydrating Creme **770**
StePHan Bio-Nutritional
  Eye-Firming Concentrate........... **770**
StePHan Bio-Nutritional Nightime
  Moisture Creme **770**
StePHan Bio-Nutritional
  Refreshing Moisture Gel........... **770**
StePHan Bio-Nutritional Ultra
  Hydrating Fluid.................... **770**

Dietary Supplements Described:
BioLean Capsules and Tablets **842**
BioLean Accelerator Tablets **842**
BioLean Free Tablets **843**
BioLean LipoTrim Capsules........... **843**
DHEA Plus Capsules................. **844**
Food for Thought Drink Mix.......... **844**
Mass Appeal Tablets **845**
Phyto-Vite Tablets................... **849**
Pro-Xtreme Drink Mix **845**
Satiete Tablets...................... **846**
Sleep-Tite Caplets **850**
StePHan Clarity Capsules **844**
StePHan Elasticity Capsules **847**
StePHan Elixir Capsules.............. **848**
StePHan Essential Capsules **848**
StePHan Feminine Capsules **848**
StePHan Flexibility Capsules **848**
StePHan Lovpil Capsules **849**
StePHan Masculine Capsules **849**
StePHan Protector Capsules **850**
StePHan Relief Capsules............. **850**
StePHan Tranquility Capsules **851**
Sure2Endure Tablets **851**
Winrgy Drink Mix.................... **852**

WHITEHALL LABORATORIES INC.
(See WHITEHALL-ROBINS HEALTHCARE)

WHITEHALL-ROBINS HEALTHCARE   771
American Home Products Corporation
Five Giralda Farms
Madison, NJ 07940-0871
Direct Inquiries to:
Whitehall Consumer Product Information:
(800) 322-3129 (9-5 E.S.T.)
Robins Consumer Product Information:
(800) 762-4672 (9-5 E.S.T.)

OTC Products Described:
Advil Caplets............................ **771**
Advil Gel Caplets **771**
Advil Liqui-Gels **771**
Advil Tablets **771**
Children's Advil Oral Suspension **773**
Children's Advil Chewable Tablets..... **773**
Advil Cold and Sinus Caplets.......... **771**
Advil Cold and Sinus Tablets **771**
Advil Flu & Body Ache Caplets........ **772**
Infants' Advil Drops.................... **773**
Junior Strength Advil Tablets **773**
Junior Strength Advil Chewable
  Tablets............................. **773**
Advil Migraine Liquigels............... **772**
Baby Anbesol Gel **774**
Junior Anbesol Gel..................... **774**
Maximum Strength Anbesol Gel **774**
Maximum Strength Anbesol Liquid **774**
Dimetapp Elixir **777**
Dimetapp Cold and Fever
  Suspension **775**
Dimetapp DM Cold & Cough Elixir..... **775**
Dimetapp Nighttime Flu Liquid **776**
Dimetapp Non-Drowsy Flu Syrup...... **777**
Dimetapp Infant Drops
  Decongestant...................... **775**
Dimetapp Infant Drops
  Decongestant Plus Cough **776**
Orudis KT Tablets..................... **778**
Preparation H Cream **778**
Preparation H Cooling Gel **778**
Preparation H Ointment **778**
Preparation H Suppositories **778**
Preparation H Medicated Wipes....... **779**
Primatene Mist **779**
Primatene Tablets **780**
Robitussin Liquid **782**
Robitussin Cold Caplets Cold &
  Congestion **780**
Robitussin Cold Softgels Cold &
  Congestion **780**
Robitussin Cold Caplets
  Multi-Symptom Cold & Flu **781**
Robitussin Cold Softgels
  Multi-Symptom Cold & Flu **781**
Robitussin Cold Softgels Severe
  Congestion **782**
Robitussin Cough Drops.............. **781**
Robitussin Honey Cough Drops **784**
Robitussin Honey Cough Liquid **784**
Robitussin Cough & Cold Infant
  Drops **782**
Robitussin Maximum Strength
  Cough & Cold Liquid............... **785**
Robitussin Pediatric Cough &
  Cold Formula Liquid **785**
Robitussin Maximum Strength
  Cough Suppressant Liquid **784**
Robitussin Pediatric Cough
  Suppressant Liquid................. **784**
Robitussin Multi Symptom Honey
  Flu Liquid **785**
Robitussin Nighttime Honey Flu
  Liquid **786**
Robitussin Honey Calmers Throat
  Drops **783**
Robitussin Sugar Free Throat
  Drops **786**
Robitussin-CF Liquid.................. **783**
Robitussin DM Infant Drops **783**
Robitussin-DM Liquid **783**
Robitussin-PE Liquid.................. **782**

Dietary Supplements Described:
Centrum Echinacea Softgels **852**
Centrum Ginkgo Biloba Softgels....... **852**
Centrum Ginseng Softgels............. **853**
Centrum Saw Palmetto Softgels....... **853**
Centrum St. John's Wort Softgels..... **853**

Other Products Available:
Anacin Caplets and Tablets
Aspirin Free Anacin Tablets
Maximum Strength Anacin Tablets
Anbesol Cold Sore Therapy Ointment
Axid AR
Chapstick Flava-Craze
Chapstick Lip Balm
Chapstick Lip Moisturizer
Chapstick LipSations
Chapstick Medicated
Chapstick OverNight Lip Treatment
Chapstick Plus
Chapstick Sunblock 15 Lip Balm
Chapstick Ultra SPF 30
Denorex Advanced Formula
Denorex Extra Strength
Denorex Extra Strength with Conditioner
Denorex Mountain Fresh
Denorex Regular with Conditioner
Dimetapp Get Better Bear Sore Throat
  Pop
Dristan Cold Multi-Symptom Tablets
Dristan Maximum Strength Cold
  Non-Drowsiness Gel Caplets
Dristan Nasal Spray
Dristan Long-Lasting Nasal Spray
Dristan Sinus Caplets
Flexagen Caplets
Preparation H Hydrocortisone 1% Cream
Riopan Plus Suspension
Riopan Plus Double Strength Suspension
Robitussin Cough & Congestion
Robitussin Liquid Center Cough Drops
Robitussin Maximum Strength
Robitussin Night Relief
Robitussin Pediatric Night Relief
Robitussin Sugar-Free Cough Drops
Semicid Contraceptive Suppositories

J.B. WILLIAMS COMPANY, INC.   526, 786
65 Harristown Road
Glen Rock, NJ 07452
Direct Inquiries to:
Consumer Affairs
(800) 254-8656
(201) 251-8100
FAX: (201) 251-8097
For Medical Emergencies Contact:
(800) 254-8656

OTC Products Described:
◆ Cēpacol Antiseptic
    Mouthwash/Gargle,
    Original....................... **526, 786**
◆ Cēpacol Antiseptic
    Mouthwash/Gargle, Mint **526, 786**
Children's Cēpacol Sore Throat
    Formula, Cherry Flavor Liquid **788**
Children's Cēpacol Sore Throat
    Formula, Grape Flavor Liquid **788**
Cēpacol Maximum Strength Sugar
    Free Sore Throat Lozenges,
    Cherry Flavor **787**
Cēpacol Maximum Strength Sugar
    Free Sore Throat Lozenges,
    Cool Mint Flavor **787**
◆ Cēpacol Maximum Strength
    Sore Throat Lozenges,
    Cherry Flavor................. **526, 787**
◆ Cēpacol Maximum Strength
    Sore Throat Lozenges,
    Mint Flavor.................. **526, 787**
Cēpacol Regular Strength Sore
    Throat Lozenges, Cherry
    Flavor **787**
Cēpacol Regular Strength Sore
    Throat Lozenges, Original
    Mint Flavor........................ **787**
Cēpacol Maximum Strength Sore
    Throat Spray, Cherry Flavor........ **787**

Cēpacol Maximum Strength Sore
Throat Spray, Cool Menthol
Flavor **787**
Cēpacol Maximum Strength Sore
Throat Spray, Honey Lemon
Flavor **787**
◆ Cēpacol Viractin Cold Sore
and Fever Blister
Treatment, Cream **526, 788**
◆ Cēpacol Viractin Cold Sore
and Fever Blister
Treatment, Gel **526, 788**

WYETH-AYERST PHARMACEUTICALS   526, 788

Division of American Home Products
Corporation
P.O. Box 8299
Philadelphia, PA 19101
Direct General Inquiries to:
(610) 688-4400
For Professional Services:
(For example: Sales representative
information, product pamphlets,
educational materials):
(800) 395-9938
For Medical Information Contact:
Medical Affairs
Day: (800) 934-5556 (8:30 AM to 4:30
PM, Eastern Standard Time, Weekdays
Only)
Night: (610) 688-4400 (Emergencies
Only; non-emergencies should wait until
the next day)
WYETH-AYERST DISTRIBUTION CENTERS
(Do not use freight addresses
for mailing orders.)
Atlanta, GA – P.O. Box 1773
Paoli, PA 19301-1773
(800) 666-7248
Freight Address:
100 Union Court
Kennesaw, GA 30144

Mail DEA order forms to:
P.O. Box 4365
Atlanta, GA 30302-4365
Chicago, IL – P.O. Box 1773
Paoli, PA 19301-1773
(800) 666-7248
Freight Address:
284 Lies Road
Carol Stream, IL 60188
Mail DEA order forms to:
P.O. Box 140
Wheaton, IL 60189-0140
Dallas, TX – P.O. Box 1773
Paoli, PA 19301-1773
(800) 666-7248
Freight Address:
11240 Petal Street
Dallas, TX 75238
Mail DEA order forms to:
P.O. Box 650231
Dallas, TX 75265-0231
Sparks, NV – P.O. Box 1773
Paoli, PA 19301-1773
(800) 666-7248
Freight Address:
1802 Brierley Way
Sparks, NV 89434
Mail DEA order forms to:
1802 Brierley Way
Sparks, NV 89434
Philadelphia, PA – P.O. Box 1773
Paoli, PA 19301-1773
(800) 666-7248
Freight Address:
31 Morehall Road
Frazer, PA 19355
Mail DEA order forms to:
P.O. Box 61
Paoli, PA 19301

OTC Products Described:
◆ Amphojel Suspension (Mint
Flavor) **526, 789**
◆ Donnagel Liquid **526, 789**
◆ Mitrolan Chewable Tablets **526, 789**

YOUNGEVITY, THE ANTI-AGING COMPANY   853

3227 Skylane Drive
Dallas, TX 75006
Direct Inquiries to:
(972) 239-6864, Ext. 108
FAX: (972) 404-3067
E-mail: asd@youngevity.com
Internet: www.youngevity.com

Dietary Supplements Described:
Chitosan Fat Snatcher Capsules *853*
Fat Metabolizer + Capsules **854**
HGH-Turn Back the Hands of Time
Capsules.......................... **854**
Super Anti-Oxidant Cell Protector
Capsules.......................... **854**
Super Food Soy Shake **854**
Vitality Immunity Anti-Oxidant
Complex Capsules................. *854*

ZANFEL LABORATORIES, INC.   526, 790

P.O. Box 349
Morton, IL 61550
Direct Inquiries to:
(800) 401-4002
Internet: www.zanfel.com

OTC Products Described:
◆ Zanfel Urushiol Wash **526, 790**

ZILA CONSUMER PHARMACEUTICALS, INC.   790

5227 North 7th Street
Phoenix, AZ 85014-2800
Direct Inquiries to:
Carol Suich
Marketing Manager
(602) 266-6700
Internet: www.zila.com

OTC Products Described:
Zilactin Gel............................ **790**
Zilactin Baby Gel...................... **791**
Zilactin-B Gel **790**
Zilactin-L Liquid **790**

SECTION 2

PRODUCT NAME INDEX

This index includes all entries in the Product Information sections. Products are listed alphabetically by brand name.

If an entry in the index lists multiple page numbers, the first one shown refers to the photograph of the product, the last one to its prescribing information.

- **Bold page numbers** indicate full product information.

- *Italic page numbers* signify partial information.

A

A + D Original Ointment (Schering-Plough) **522, 733**
A + D Ointment with Zinc Oxide (Schering-Plough) **522, 733**
Abreva Cream (SmithKline Beecham Consumer) **744**
Actifed Cold & Allergy Tablets (Pfizer Inc., Warner-Lambert Healthcare) **516, 688**
Actifed Cold & Sinus Caplets and Tablets (Pfizer Inc., Warner-Lambert Healthcare) ... **516, 688**
ActoTherm Caplets (AdvoCare) **794**
Adult Strength products *(see base product name)*
Advantin Capsules (AdvoCare) **794**
Advil Caplets (Whitehall-Robins) **771**
Advil Gel Caplets (Whitehall-Robins) **771**
Advil Liqui-Gels (Whitehall-Robins) **771**
Advil Tablets (Whitehall-Robins) **771**
Children's Advil Oral Suspension (Whitehall-Robins) **773**
Children's Advil Chewable Tablets (Whitehall-Robins) **773**
Advil Cold and Sinus Caplets (Whitehall-Robins) **771**
Advil Cold and Sinus Tablets (Whitehall-Robins) **771**
Advil Flu & Body Ache Caplets (Whitehall-Robins) **772**
Infants' Advil Drops (Whitehall-Robins) **773**
Junior Strength Advil Tablets (Whitehall-Robins) **773**
Junior Strength Advil Chewable Tablets (Whitehall-Robins) **773**
Advil Migraine Liquigels (Whitehall-Robins) **772**
Aflexa Tablets (McNeil Consumer) **508, 821**

Afrin Nasal Decongestant Children's Pump Mist (Schering-Plough) **734**
Afrin Original Nasal Spray (Schering-Plough) **522, 733**
Afrin Extra Moisturizing Nasal Spray (Schering-Plough) **733**
Afrin Severe Congestion Nasal Spray (Schering-Plough) **733**
Afrin Sinus Nasal Spray (Schering-Plough) **733**
Afrin No Drip Original Nasal Spray (Schering-Plough) **522, 735**
Afrin No Drip Extra Moisturizing Nasal Spray (Schering-Plough) **735**
Afrin No Drip Severe Congestion Nasal Spray (Schering-Plough) **735**
Afrin No Drip Sinus Nasal Spray (Schering-Plough) **735**
Afrin Original Pump Mist (Schering-Plough) **733**
Afrin Saline Aromatic Mist (Schering-Plough) **734**
Afrin Extra Moisturizing Saline Mist (Schering-Plough) **522, 734**
Ag-Immune Tablets (Body Wise) **810**
Aleve Tablets, Caplets and Gelcaps (Bayer Consumer) **503, 602**
Aleve Cold & Sinus Caplets (Bayer Consumer) **503, 603**
Alka-Seltzer Original Antacid and Pain Reliever Effervescent Tablets (Bayer Consumer) **503, 603**
Alka-Seltzer Cherry Antacid and Pain Reliever Effervescent Tablets (Bayer Consumer) **503, 603**
Alka-Seltzer Lemon Lime Antacid and Pain Reliever Effervescent Tablets (Bayer Consumer) **503, 603**

Alka-Seltzer Extra Strength Antacid and Pain Reliever Effervescent Tablets (Bayer Consumer) **503, 603**
Alka-Seltzer Plus Cold Medicine Liqui-Gels (Bayer Consumer) **503, 604**
Alka-Seltzer Plus Night-Time Cold Medicine Liqui-Gels (Bayer Consumer) **503, 604**
Alka-Seltzer Plus Cold & Cough Medicine Liqui-Gels (Bayer Consumer) **503, 604**
Alka-Seltzer Plus Cold & Flu Medicine Liqui-Gels (Bayer Consumer) **503, 604**
Alka-Seltzer Plus Cold & Sinus Medicine Liqui-Gels (Bayer Consumer) **503, 604**
Alka-Seltzer Heartburn Relief Tablets (Bayer Consumer) **503, 604**
Alka-Seltzer PM Effervescent Tablets (Bayer Consumer) **503, 605**
Alluna Sleep Tablets (SmithKline Beecham Consumer) **837**
Ambrotose Capsules (Mannatech) **508, 819**
Ambrotose Powder (Mannatech) **508, 819**
Ambrotose with Lecithin Capsules (Mannatech) **819**
Amlactin 12% Moisturizing Lotion and Cream (Upsher-Smith) *767*
Amphojel Suspension (Mint Flavor) (Wyeth-Ayerst) **526, 789**
Baby Anbesol Gel (Whitehall-Robins).... **774**
Junior Anbesol Gel (Whitehall-Robins)... **774**
Maximum Strength Anbesol Gel (Whitehall-Robins) **774**
Maximum Strength Anbesol Liquid (Whitehall-Robins) **774**
Antioxidant Booster Caplets (AdvoCare) **794**

Anusol HC-1 Hydrocortisone Anti-Itch Cream (Pfizer Inc., Warner-Lambert Healthcare)...**516, 689**

Anusol Ointment (Pfizer Inc., Warner-Lambert Healthcare)...**516, 688**

Anusol Suppositories (Pfizer Inc., Warner-Lambert Healthcare) **516, 689**

APF Arthritis Pain Formula (Medtech) *664*

Arthritis Strength products *(see base product name)*

B

Bactine First Aid Liquid (Bayer Consumer) **503, 611**

Balmex Diaper Rash Ointment (Block) **505, 619**

Balmex Medicated Plus Baby Powder (Block) **505, 619**

Genuine Bayer Tablets, Caplets and Gelcaps (Bayer Consumer) **503, 606**

Extra Strength Bayer Caplets and Gelcaps (Bayer Consumer) **504, 610**

Aspirin Regimen Bayer Children's Chewable Tablets (Orange or Cherry Flavored) (Bayer Consumer)...**504, 607**

Aspirin Regimen Bayer Adult Low Strength 81 mg Tablets (Bayer Consumer) **503, 606**

Aspirin Regimen Bayer 81 mg Caplets with Calcium (Bayer Consumer)..........................**607**

Aspirin Regimen Bayer Regular Strength 325 mg Caplets (Bayer Consumer) **503, 606**

Genuine Bayer Professional Labeling (Aspirin Regimen Bayer) (Bayer Consumer).........................**608**

Extra Strength Bayer Arthritis Caplets (Bayer Consumer).....**504, 610**

Extra Strength Bayer Plus Caplets (Bayer Consumer).....**504, 610**

Extra Strength Bayer PM Caplets (Bayer Consumer).....**504, 611**

BC Powder (Block) **619**

BC Allergy Sinus Cold Powder (Block) **619**

Arthritis Strength BC Powder (Block) ..**619**

BC Sinus Cold Powder (Block) **619**

Beano Liquid (Block) **809**

Beano Tablets (Block) **809**

Beelith Tablets (Beach) **809**

Benadryl Allergy Chewables (Pfizer Inc., Warner-Lambert Healthcare) **517, 689**

Benadryl Allergy Kapseal Capsules (Pfizer Inc., Warner-Lambert Healthcare)...**516, 691**

Benadryl Allergy Liquid (Pfizer Inc., Warner-Lambert Healthcare) **517, 690**

Benadryl Allergy Ultratab Tablets (Pfizer Inc., Warner-Lambert Healthcare)...**516, 691**

Benadryl Allergy/Cold Tablets (Pfizer Inc., Warner-Lambert Healthcare) **517, 691**

Benadryl Allergy/Congestion Tablets (Pfizer Inc., Warner-Lambert Healthcare)...**517, 692**

Benadryl Allergy & Sinus Liquid (Pfizer Inc., Warner-Lambert Healthcare) **693**

Benadryl Allergy & Sinus Fastmelt Tablets (Pfizer Inc., Warner-Lambert Healthcare).....................**517, 693**

Benadryl Allergy Sinus Headache Caplets & Gelcaps (Pfizer Inc., Warner-Lambert Healthcare)...**517, 693**

Benadryl Severe Allergy & Sinus Headache Caplets (Pfizer Inc., Warner-Lambert Healthcare) **517, 694**

Benadryl Children's Allergy and Sinus Liquid (Pfizer Inc., Warner-Lambert Healthcare).........*517*

Benadryl Children's Allergy/ Cold Fastmelt Tablets (Pfizer Inc., Warner-Lambert Healthcare) **517, 692**

Benadryl Dye-Free Allergy Liquid (Pfizer Inc., Warner-Lambert Healthcare)...**517, 690**

Benadryl Dye-Free Allergy Liqui-Gels Softgels (Pfizer Inc., Warner-Lambert Healthcare) **517, 690**

Benadryl Itch Relief Stick Extra Strength (Pfizer Inc., Warner-Lambert Healthcare)...**517, 695**

Benadryl Itch Stopping Cream Original Strength (Pfizer Inc., Warner-Lambert Healthcare) **517, 695**

Benadryl Itch Stopping Cream Extra Strength (Pfizer Inc., Warner-Lambert Healthcare)...**517, 695**

Benadryl Itch Stopping Gel Original Strength (Pfizer Inc., Warner-Lambert Healthcare) **517, 695**

Benadryl Itch Stopping Gel Extra Strength (Pfizer Inc., Warner-Lambert Healthcare)...**517, 695**

Benadryl Itch Stopping Spray Original Strength (Pfizer Inc., Warner-Lambert Healthcare) **517, 696**

Benadryl Itch Stopping Spray Extra Strength (Pfizer Inc., Warner-Lambert Healthcare)...**517, 696**

BenGay External Analgesic Products (Pfizer Inc., Warner-Lambert Healthcare)...**518, 696**

Benylin Adult Formula Cough Suppressant Liquid (Pfizer Inc., Warner-Lambert Healthcare) **518, 696**

Benylin Cough Suppressant/ Expectorant Liquid (Pfizer Inc., Warner-Lambert Healthcare) **518, 697**

Benylin Multi-Symptom Liquid (Pfizer Inc., Warner-Lambert Healthcare) **518, 697**

Benylin Pediatric Cough Suppressant Liquid (Pfizer Inc., Warner-Lambert Healthcare) **518, 698**

Beta-C Tablets (Body Wise) **811**

Betadine Brand First Aid Antibiotics + Moisturizer Ointment (Purdue Frederick)...**522, 731**

Betadine Brand Plus First Aid Antibiotics + Pain Reliever Ointment (Purdue Frederick)...**522, 731**

Betadine Ointment (Purdue Frederick)...................**522, 732**

Betadine PrepStick Applicator (Purdue Frederick) **522, 732**

Betadine Skin Cleanser (Purdue Frederick).............................**732**

Betadine Solution (Purdue Frederick) **522, 732**

BioChoice Immune[26] Powder and Capsules (Legacy for Life)............................**508, 818**

BioChoice Immune Support Powder (Legacy for Life)......................**818**

Bio-Complex 5000 Gentle Foaming Cleanser (Wellness International) ...**769**

Bio-Complex 5000 Revitalizing Conditioner (Wellness International) **769**

Bio-Complex 5000 Revitalizing Shampoo (Wellness International) ..**770**

Biolax (Body Wise) *810*

BioLean Capsules and Tablets (Wellness International) **842**

BioLean Accelerator Tablets (Wellness International) **842**

BioLean Free Tablets (Wellness International) **843**

BioLean LipoTrim Capsules (Wellness International) **843**

Biomune OSF Express Spray (Matol) **508, 640**

Biomune OSF Plus Capsules (Matol) **508, 820**

BodyLean Powder (AdvoCare) **795**

Bonine Chewable Tablets (Pfizer Inc., Warner-Lambert Healthcare) **518, 698**

Brite-Life Caplets (AdvoCare) **795**

Bugs Bunny Children's Multivitamin Plus Iron Chewable Tablets (Bayer Consumer) **504, 802**

Bugs Bunny Children's Multivitamin Plus Extra C Chewable Tablets (Sugar Free) (Bayer Consumer) **504, 804**

Bugs Bunny Complete Children's Multivitamin/ Multimineral Chewable Tablets (Sugar Free) (Bayer Consumer) **504, 803**

C

Caladryl Clear Lotion (Pfizer Inc., Warner-Lambert Healthcare)........................**518, 698**

Caladryl Lotion (Pfizer Inc., Warner-Lambert Healthcare)...**518, 698**

Caltrate 600 Tablets (Lederle Consumer)..........................**814**

Caltrate 600 PLUS Chewables (Lederle Consumer)..................**815**

Caltrate 600 PLUS Tablets (Lederle Consumer)..........................**815**

Caltrate 600 + D Tablets (Lederle Consumer)..........................**814**

Caltrate 600 + Soy Tablets (Lederle Consumer)..........................**814**

Carbo Energy Bar (Body Wise) *810*

CardiOptima Drink Mix Packets (AdvoCare).............................**795**

Catalyst Capsules (AdvoCare) **796**

Celestial Seasonings Soothers Throat Drops (Pfizer Inc., Warner-Lambert Group)........**515, 685**

Centrum Echinacea Softgels (Whitehall-Robins)....................**852**

Centrum Focused Formulas Bone Health Tablets (Lederle Consumer)..........................**815**

Centrum Focused Formulas Energy Tablets (Lederle Consumer)........**816**

Centrum Focused Formulas Heart Tablets (Lederle Consumer).........**816**

Centrum Focused Formulas Mental Clarity Tablets (Lederle Consumer)...........................**816**

Centrum Focused Formulas Prostate Softgels (Lederle Consumer)........**816**

Centrum Ginkgo Biloba Softgels (Whitehall-Robins) **852**

Centrum Ginseng Softgels (Whitehall-Robins) **853**

Centrum Kids Complete Children's Chewables (Lederle Consumer) **817**

Centrum Performance Multivitamin-Multimineral Tablets (Lederle Consumer) **817**

Centrum Saw Palmetto Softgels (Whitehall-Robins) **853**

Centrum St. John's Wort Softgels (Whitehall-Robins) **853**

Centrum Tablets (Lederle Consumer) ...**815**

Centrum Silver Tablets (Lederle Consumer) **818**

Ceo-Two Evacuant Suppository (Beutlich) **618**

Cēpacol Antiseptic Mouthwash/Gargle, Original (Williams) **526, 786**

Cēpacol Antiseptic Mouthwash/Gargle, Mint (Williams) **526, 786**

Children's Cēpacol Sore Throat Formula, Cherry Flavor Liquid (Williams) **788**

Children's Cēpacol Sore Throat Formula, Grape Flavor Liquid (Williams) **788**

Cēpacol Maximum Strength Sugar Free Sore Throat Lozenges, Cherry Flavor (Williams) **787**

Cēpacol Maximum Strength Sugar Free Sore Throat Lozenges, Cool Mint Flavor (Williams) **787**

Cēpacol Maximum Strength Sore Throat Lozenges, Cherry Flavor (Williams) **526, 787**

Cēpacol Maximum Strength Sore Throat Lozenges, Mint Flavor (Williams) **526, 787**

Cēpacol Regular Strength Sore Throat Lozenges, Cherry Flavor (Williams) **787**

Cēpacol Regular Strength Sore Throat Lozenges, Original Mint Flavor (Williams) **787**

Cēpacol Maximum Strength Sore Throat Spray, Cherry Flavor (Williams) **787**

Cēpacol Maximum Strength Sore Throat Spray, Cool Menthol Flavor (Williams) **787**

Cēpacol Maximum Strength Sore Throat Spray, Honey Lemon Flavor (Williams) **787**

Cēpacol Viractin Cold Sore and Fever Blister Treatment, Cream (Williams) **526, 788**

Cēpacol Viractin Cold Sore and Fever Blister Treatment, Gel (Williams) **526, 788**

Certs Cool Mint Drops (Pfizer Inc., Warner-Lambert Group)...**515, 685**

Certs Powerful Mints (Pfizer Inc., Warner-Lambert Group)...**516, 686**

C-Grams Caplets (AdvoCare) **795**

Children's Strength products *(see base product name)*

Chito-Maxx (Body Wise).................*810*

Chitosan Fat Snatcher Capsules (Youngevity).................*853*

Chlor-3 Shaker (Fleming) **633**

Chlor-Trimeton Allergy Tablets (Schering-Plough) **522, 735**

Chlor-Trimeton Allergy/ Decongestant Tablets (Schering-Plough) **522, 736**

Citracal Liquitab Tablets (Mission) **823**

Citracal Tablets (Mission)...............**823**

Citracal Caplets + D (Mission).........**823**

Citracal 250 MG + D Tablets (Mission)...................**823**

Citracal Plus Tablets (Mission) **824**

Citrucel Caplets (SmithKline Beecham Consumer) **745**

Citrucel Orange Flavor Powder (SmithKline Beecham Consumer) **523, 744**

Citrucel Sugar Free Orange Flavor Powder (SmithKline Beecham Consumer) **523, 745**

Clear Away Gel with Aloe Wart Remover System (Schering-Plough) **736**

Clear Away Liquid Wart Remover System (Schering-Plough) **736**

Clear Away One Step Wart Remover (Schering-Plough) **522, 737**

Clear Away One Step Wart Remover for Kids (Schering-Plough) **522, 737**

Clear Away One Step Plantar Wart Remover (Schering-Plough)..........**737**

Clinical Care Antimicrobial Wound Cleanser (Care-Tech) **632**

CoEnzyme Q10+ (Body Wise) *810*

Coffeccino Beverage Mix (AdvoCare)...**796**

Colace Capsules, Syrup and Drops (Shire) **743**

Cold Season Nutrition Booster Capsules (AdvoCare) **796**

Compound W One Step Pads for Kids (Medtech)..................**664**

Compound W One Step Plantar Pads (Medtech)..................**664**

Compound W One Step Wart Remover Pads (Medtech) **664**

Compound W Wart Remover Gel (Medtech)..................**665**

Compound W Wart Remover Liquid (Medtech)..................**665**

Comtrex Acute Head Cold & Sinus Pressure Relief Tablets (Bristol-Myers).........**506, 627**

Comtrex Deep Chest Cold & Congestion Relief Softgels (Bristol-Myers) **506, 627**

Comtrex Flu Therapy & Fever Relief Daytime Caplets (Bristol-Myers) **506, 628**

Comtrex Flu Therapy & Fever Relief Nighttime Tablets (Bristol-Myers) **506, 628**

Comtrex Maximum Strength Multi-Symptom Cold & Cough Relief Tablets and Caplets (Bristol-Myers) **506, 626**

Contac Non-Drowsy 12 Hour Cold Caplets (SmithKline Beecham Consumer) **523, 745**

Contac Non-Drowsy Timed Release 12 Hour Cold Caplets (SmithKline Beecham Consumer) **523, 746**

Contac Severe Cold and Flu Caplets Maximum Strength (SmithKline Beecham Consumer) **523, 746**

Contac Severe Cold and Flu Caplets Non-Drowsy (SmithKline Beecham Consumer) **746**

CorePlex Capsules (AdvoCare)..........**796**

Coricidin 'D' Cold, Flu & Sinus Tablets (Schering-Plough)......**522, 737**

Coricidin HBP Cold & Flu Tablets (Schering-Plough).....**523, 738**

Coricidin HBP Cough & Cold Tablets (Schering-Plough).....**523, 738**

Coricidin HBP Maximum Strength Flu Tablets (Schering-Plough)............**523, 738**

Coricidin HBP Night-Time Cold & Flu Tablets (Schering-Plough)............**523, 738**

Correctol Laxative Tablets and Caplets (Schering-Plough) **523, 739**

Cortaid Intensive Therapy Cream (Pharmacia Consumer) **717**

Cortaid Maximum Strength Cream (Pharmacia Consumer) **717**

Cortaid Maximum Strength Ointment (Pharmacia Consumer) ...**717**

Cortaid Sensitive Skin Cream (Pharmacia Consumer) **717**

Cortizone•5 Creme (Pfizer Inc., Warner-Lambert Healthcare)...**518, 699**

Cortizone•5 Ointment (Pfizer Inc., Warner-Lambert Healthcare).........**699**

Cortizone•10 Creme (Pfizer Inc., Warner-Lambert Healthcare).................**518, 699**

Cortizone•10 Ointment (Pfizer Inc., Warner-Lambert Healthcare).........**699**

Cortizone•10 Plus Creme (Pfizer Inc., Warner-Lambert Healthcare) **518, 700**

Cortizone•10 Quick Shot Spray (Pfizer Inc., Warner-Lambert Healthcare) **518, 699**

Cortizone for Kids Creme (Pfizer Inc., Warner-Lambert Healthcare) **518, 699**

D

D-Cal Chewable Caplets (A & Z Pharm)...................**503, 794**

DDS-Acidophilus Capsules, Tablets, and Powder (UAS Labs) **767**

Debrox Drops (SmithKline Beecham Consumer) **523, 747**

Delsym Extended-Release Suspension (Medeva) **664**

Dermoplast Antibacterial Spray, Hospital Strength (Medtech)........**666**

Dermoplast Hospital Strength Spray (Medtech)..................**666**

Desenex Max Cream (Novartis Consumer)..................*512*

Desenex Liquid Spray (Novartis Consumer)..................**668**

Desenex Shake Powder (Novartis Consumer)...........**512, 668**

Desenex Spray Powder (Novartis Consumer)...........**512, 668**

Desenex Jock Itch Spray Powder (Novartis Consumer) **668**

Desitin Baby Powder (Pfizer Inc., Warner-Lambert Healthcare) **518, 700**

Desitin Creamy Ointment (Pfizer Inc., Warner-Lambert Healthcare) **518, 700**

Desitin Ointment (Pfizer Inc., Warner-Lambert Healthcare)...**518, 700**

Devrom Chewable Tablets (Parthenon)...........................**685**

DHEA Plus Capsules (Wellness International) **844**

Dimetapp Elixir (Whitehall-Robins) **777**

Dimetapp Cold and Fever Suspension (Whitehall-Robins) **775**

Dimetapp DM Cold & Cough Elixir (Whitehall-Robins) **775**

Dimetapp Nighttime Flu Liquid (Whitehall-Robins) **776**

Dimetapp Non-Drowsy Flu Syrup (Whitehall-Robins) **777**

Dimetapp Infant Drops Decongestant (Whitehall-Robins) ...**775**

Dimetapp Infant Drops Decongestant Plus Cough (Whitehall-Robins) **776**

Doctor Ginsberg's Psoria Rid Cream (Strategic Science)......**525, 840**

Domeboro Powder Packets (Bayer Consumer).............**504, 611**

Domeboro Effervescent Tablets (Bayer Consumer).............**504, 611**

Donnagel Liquid (Wyeth-Ayerst) ...**526, 789**

Dramamine Original Formula Tablets (Pharmacia Consumer) **718**

Dramamine Chewable Formula
Tablets (Pharmacia Consumer)...... **718**
Dramamine Less Drowsy Tablets
(Pharmacia Consumer) **718**
Drixoral Allergy/Sinus
Extended-Release Tablets
(Schering-Plough) **523, 741**
Drixoral Cold & Allergy
Sustained-Action Tablets
(Schering-Plough) **523, 740**
Drixoral Cold & Flu
Extended-Release Tablets
(Schering-Plough) **523, 740**
Drixoral Nasal Decongestant
Long-Acting Non-Drowsy
Tablets (Schering-Plough)...... **523, 740**
Dulcolax Suppositories
(Novartis Consumer).......... **513, 668**
Dulcolax Tablets (Novartis
Consumer) **513, 668**

E

Ecotrin Enteric Coated Aspirin
Low Strength Tablets
(SmithKline Beecham
Consumer) **524, 747**
Ecotrin Enteric Coated Aspirin
Maximum Strength Tablets
(SmithKline Beecham
Consumer) **524, 747**
Ecotrin Enteric Coated Aspirin
Regular Strength Tablets
(SmithKline Beecham
Consumer) **524, 747**
Electro Aloe (Body Wise)............... *810*
Emetrol Oral Solution (Lemon-Mint &
Cherry Flavors) (Pharmacia
Consumer) **718**
e.p.t. Pregnancy Test (Pfizer
Inc., Warner-Lambert
Healthcare) **518, 701**
Ex•Lax Gentle Strength
Caplets (Novartis
Consumer) **513, 670**
Ex•Lax Regular Strength Pills
(Novartis Consumer).......... **513, 670**
Ex•Lax Regular Strength
Chocolated Pieces
(Novartis Consumer).......... **513, 669**
Ex•Lax Maximum Strength
Pills (Novartis Consumer).... **513, 670**
Ex•Lax Milk of Magnesia
Liquid (Novartis Consumer) ... **513, 670**
Ex•Lax Stool Softener Caplets
(Novartis Consumer).......... **513, 671**
Aspirin Free Excedrin Caplets
and Geltabs (Bristol-Myers).... **507, 628**
Excedrin Extra-Strength
Tablets, Caplets, and
Geltabs (Bristol-Myers) **507, 629**
Excedrin Migraine Tablets,
Caplets, and Geltabs
(Bristol-Myers) **507, 630**
Excedrin PM Tablets, Caplets,
and Geltabs (Bristol-Myers).... **506, 631**
Extra Strength products
(see base product name)

F

Fat Metabolizer + Capsules
(Youngevity)........................... **854**
FemEssence Capsules (AdvoCare)...... **796**
Feosol Caplets (SmithKline
Beecham Consumer) **524, 837**
Feosol Tablets (SmithKline
Beecham Consumer) **524, 838**
Fergon Iron Tablets (Bayer
Consumer) **504, 802**
Fiber 10 Packets (AdvoCare) **797**
FiberCon Caplets (Lederle Consumer) .. **639**
Flintstones Original Children's
Multivitamin Chewable
Tablets (Bayer Consumer)..... **504, 802**

Flintstones Children's
Multivitamin Plus Calcium
Chewable Tablets (Bayer
Consumer) **504, 804**
Flintstones Children's
Multivitamin Plus Extra C
Chewable Tablets (Bayer
Consumer) **504, 804**
Flintstones Children's
Multivitamin Plus Iron
Chewable Tablets (Bayer
Consumer) **504, 802**
Flintstones Complete
Children's Mutivitamin/
Multimineral Chewable
Tablets (Bayer Consumer) **504, 803**
Food for Thought Drink Mix
(Wellness International) **844**
Freezone Corn & Callus Liquid
(Medtech)...................... *664*
Future Perfect (Body Wise) *810*

G

Maximum Strength Gas Aid
Softgels (McNeil Consumer)... **509, 640**
Gas-X Chewable Tablets
(Novartis Consumer).......... **513, 671**
Extra Strength Gas-X Liquid
(Novartis Consumer).......... **513, 671**
Extra Strength Gas-X Softgels
(Novartis Consumer).......... **513, 671**
Extra Strength Gas-X Chewable
Tablets (Novartis
Consumer) **513, 671**
Maximum Strength Gas-X
Softgels (Novartis
Consumer) **513, 671**
Gaviscon Extra Strength Liquid
(SmithKline Beecham
Consumer) **524, 751**
Gaviscon Extra Strength
Tablets (SmithKline
Beecham Consumer) **524, 751**
Gaviscon Regular Strength
Liquid (SmithKline Beecham
Consumer) **524, 751**
Gaviscon Regular Strength
Tablets (SmithKline
Beecham Consumer) **524, 750**
Ginkoba M/E Suppli-Cap
Capsules (Pharmaton)....... **521, 829**
Ginkoba Tablets (Pharmaton) **828**
Ginsana Capsules (Pharmaton) **830**
Ginsana Chewy Squares
(Pharmaton).................. **521, 830**
Ginsana Sport Capsules
(Pharmaton).................. **521, 831**
Gly-Oxide Liquid (SmithKline
Beecham Consumer) **524, 751**
Goody's Body Pain Formula Powder
(Block)............................... **620**
Goody's Extra Strength Headache
Powder (Block) **620**
Goody's Extra Strength Pain Relief
Tablets (Block)...................... **620**
Goody's PM Powder (Block)............. **621**
Gyne-Lotrimin 3, 3-Day Cream
(Schering-Plough) **523, 741**

H

Halls Defense Drops (Pfizer Inc.,
Warner-Lambert Group)........ **516, 687**
Halls Mentho-Lyptus Drops
(Pfizer Inc., Warner-Lambert
Group) **516, 686**
Halls Sugar Free
Mentho-Lyptus Drops (Pfizer
Inc., Warner-Lambert Group)... **516, 686**
Halls Sugar Free Squares
(Pfizer Inc., Warner-Lambert
Group) **516, 686**
Halls Plus Cough Drops (Pfizer
Inc., Warner-Lambert Group)... **516, 686**

HeartBar (Cooke)........................ **812**
Heet Liniment (Medtech)............... *664*
HGH-Turn Back the Hands of Time
Capsules (Youngevity) **854**
Humatrix Microclysmic Burn/Wound
Healing Gel (Care-Tech) **632**
Hurricaine Topical Anesthetic Gel, 1
oz. Fresh Mint, Wild Cherry, Pina
Colada, Watermelon, 1/6 oz.
Wild Cherry, Watermelon
(Beutlich) **618**
Hurricaine Topical Anesthetic Liquid,
1 oz. Wild Cherry, Pina Colada,
.25 ml Dry Handle Swab Wild
Cherry, 1/6 oz. Wild Cherry
(Beutlich) **618**
Hurricaine Topical Anesthetic Spray
Extension Tubes (200) (Beutlich)... **618**
Hurricaine Topical Anesthetic Spray
Kit, 2 oz. Wild Cherry (Beutlich) ... **618**
Hurricaine Topical Anesthetic Spray,
2 oz. Wild Cherry (Beutlich)......... **618**
Hyland's Arnisport Tablets (Standard
Homeopathic)........................ **764**
Hyland's Back Ache with Arnica
Caplets (Standard Homeopathic) ... **764**
Hyland's Bumps 'n Bruises Tablets
(Standard Homeopathic)............. **764**
Hyland's Calms Forté Tablets and
Caplets (Standard Homeopathic) ... **764**
Hyland's Cold Tablets with Zinc
(Standard Homeopathic)............. **765**
Hyland's Colic Tablets (Standard
Homeopathic)........................ **765**
Hyland's Earache Tablets (Standard
Homeopathic)........................ **765**
Hyland's Leg Cramps with Quinine
Tablets (Standard Homeopathic) ... **765**
Hyland's MenoCalm Tablets
(Standard Homeopathic)............. **765**
Hyland's Nerve Tonic Tablets and
Caplets (Standard Homeopathic) ... **766**
Hyland's Teething Gel (Standard
Homeopathic)........................ **766**
Hyland's Teething Tablets (Standard
Homeopathic)........................ **766**

I

Imodium A-D Liquid and
Caplets (McNeil Consumer) ... **509, 641**
Imodium Advanced Chewable
Tablets (McNeil Consumer).... **509, 641**
Infants' Strength products
(see base product name)
Intelectol Tablets (Covex) **507, 813**
IntelleQ Capsules (AdvoCare) **797**

J

Junior Strength products
(see base product name)

L

Lactaid Original Strength
Caplets (McNeil Consumer) ... **509, 822**
Lactaid Extra Strength Caplets
(McNeil Consumer)............ **509, 822**
Lactaid Ultra Caplets and
Chewable Tablets (McNeil
Consumer) **509, 822**
Lactaid Drops (McNeil
Consumer) **509, 822**
Lamisil^AT Cream (Novartis
Consumer) **513, 672**
Lamisil^AT Solution (Novartis
Consumer) **513, 672**
Lipoflavonoid Caplets (Numark)......... **828**
LipoTrol Caplets (AdvoCare)............. **797**
Listerine Mouthrinse (Pfizer
Inc., Warner-Lambert
Healthcare) **518, 702**
Cool Mint Listerine Mouthrinse
(Pfizer Inc., Warner-Lambert
Healthcare) **518, 702**

Italic Page Number **Indicates Brief Listing**

FreshBurst Listerine Mouthrinse (Pfizer Inc., Warner-Lambert Healthcare)...**519, 702**

Tartar Control Listerine Mouthrinse (Pfizer Inc., Warner-Lambert Healthcare)...**519, 702**

Listermint Alcohol-Free Mouthrinse (Pfizer Inc., Warner-Lambert Healthcare)...**519, 703**

Lotrimin AF Cream, Lotion, Solution, and Jock Itch Cream (Schering-Plough) **523, 742**

Lotrimin AF Spray Powder, Spray Liquid, Spray Deodorant Powder, Shaker Powder and Jock Itch Spray Powder (Schering-Plough) **523, 742**

Lubriderm Advanced Therapy Creamy Lotion (Pfizer Inc., Warner-Lambert Healthcare)...**519, 703**

Lubriderm Daily UV Lotion (Pfizer Inc., Warner-Lambert Healthcare) **519, 703**

Lubriderm Seriously Sensitive Lotion (Pfizer Inc., Warner-Lambert Healthcare)...**519, 703**

Lubriderm Skin Therapy Moisturizing Lotion (Pfizer Inc., Warner-Lambert Healthcare) **519, 703**

M

Maalox Antacid/Anti-Gas Oral Suspension (Novartis Consumer) **514, 673**

Maalox Max Maximum Strength Antacid/Anti-Gas Liquid (Novartis Consumer) ...**514, 673**

Quick Dissolve Maalox Antacid Chewable Tablets (Novartis Consumer) **514, 674**

Quick Dissolve Maalox Max Maximum Strength Antacid/Antigas Chewable Tablets (Novartis Consumer) **514, 674**

Macro-Mineral Complex Caplets (AdvoCare) **797**

Magonate Liquid (Fleming) **814**

Magonate Natal Liquid (Fleming) **814**

Magonate Tablets (Fleming) **814**

Maltsupex Powder, Liquid, Tablets (Wallace) **525, 767**

Marblen Suspension (Fleming) **633**

Mass Appeal Tablets (Wellness International) **845**

Massengill Feminine Cleansing Wash (SmithKline Beecham Consumer) **753**

Massengill Disposable Douches (SmithKline Beecham Consumer) ...**752**

Massengill Baby Powder Scent Soft Cloth Towelette (SmithKline Beecham Consumer) **753**

Massengill Medicated Disposable Douche (SmithKline Beecham Consumer) **524, 753**

Massengill Medicated Soft Cloth Towelette (SmithKline Beecham Consumer) **753**

Maximum Strength products *(see base product name)*

Mem X² (Body Wise) *810*

Metabolic Nutrition System (AdvoCare) **798**

MetaBoost Caplets (AdvoCare) **798**

Metamucil Dietary Fiber Supplement (Procter & Gamble) **834**

Metamucil Powder, Original Texture Orange Flavor (Procter & Gamble) ..**722**

Metamucil Powder, Original Texture Regular Flavor (Procter & Gamble)...........................**722**

Metamucil Smooth Texture Powder, Orange Flavor (Procter & Gamble) **521, 722**

Metamucil Smooth Texture Powder, Sugar-Free, Orange Flavor (Procter & Gamble) **722**

Metamucil Smooth Texture Powder, Sugar-Free, Regular Flavor (Procter & Gamble) **722**

Metamucil Wafers, Apple Crisp & Cinnamon Spice Flavors (Procter & Gamble) **521, 722**

Meyenberg Goat Milk (Meyenberg) **823**

Maximum Strength Midol Menstrual Caplets and Gelcaps (Bayer Consumer) **504, 612**

Maximum Strength Midol PMS Caplets and Gelcaps (Bayer Consumer) **504, 613**

Maximum Strength Midol Teen Caplets (Bayer Consumer)....**504, 612**

Mitrolan Chewable Tablets (Wyeth-Ayerst)..................**526, 789**

Momentum Backache Relief Extra Strength Caplets (Medtech) **666**

Children's Motrin Oral Suspension and Chewable Tablets (McNeil Consumer)....**509, 643**

Children's Motrin Cold Oral Suspension (McNeil Consumer)...........................**509, 646**

Infants' Motrin Concentrated Drops (McNeil Consumer) **509, 643**

Junior Strength Motrin Caplets and Chewable Tablets (McNeil Consumer) **509, 643**

Motrin IB Tablets, Caplets, and Gelcaps (McNeil Consumer) **510, 642**

Motrin Migraine Pain Caplets (McNeil Consumer) **510, 646**

Motrin Sinus/Headache Caplets (McNeil Consumer) **510, 643**

Movana Tablets (Pharmaton)......**521, 832**

Mycelex-3 Vaginal Cream with 3 Disposable Applicators (Bayer Consumer)...........................**613**

Mycelex-3 Vaginal Cream in 3 Pre-filled Applicators (Bayer Consumer)...........................**613**

Mycelex-7 Combination-Pack Vaginal Inserts & External Vulvar Cream (Bayer Consumer).........**614**

Mycelex-7 Vaginal Cream (Bayer Consumer)...........................**614**

Mycelex-7 Vaginal Cream with 7 Disposable Applicators (Bayer Consumer)...........................**614**

Children's Mylanta Upset Stomach Relief Liquid (J&J • Merck) **508, 634**

Children's Mylanta Upset Stomach Relief Tablets (J&J • Merck) **508, 634**

Mylanta Gelcaps (J&J • Merck) ...**507, 637**

Mylanta Liquid (J&J • Merck) **634**

Mylanta Extra Strength Liquid (J&J • Merck) **507, 634**

Mylanta Supreme Liquid (J&J • Merck) **507, 636**

Mylanta Ultra Tabs Tablets (J&J • Merck) **507, 637**

Extra Strength Mylanta Calci Tabs Tablets (J&J • Merck)....**507, 636**

Ultra Mylanta Calci Tabs Tablets (J&J • Merck) **507, 636**

Mylanta Gas Softgels (J&J • Merck)...........................**507, 637**

Mylanta Gas Tablets (J&J • Merck).....**637**

Maximum Strength Mylanta Gas Tablets (J&J • Merck)....**507, 637**

Infants' Mylicon Drops (J&J • Merck) **508, 634**

N

NasalCrom Nasal Spray (Pharmacia Consumer).............................**719**

Natru-Vent Nasal Spray, Adult Strength (Boehringer Ingelheim)....................**506, 624**

Natru-Vent Nasal Spray, Pediatric Strength (Boehringer Ingelheim).........**506, 625**

Natru-Vent Saline Nasal Spray (Boehringer Ingelheim).........**506, 625**

Natural Arousal Cream (Strategic Science)............**525, 840**

Natural Sensation Cream (Strategic Science) **841**

Nature's Own Pain Expeller Cream (Strategic Science) **841**

Nature's Remedy Tablets (Block)........................**506, 621**

Neosporin "Neo to Go!" Ointment (Pfizer Inc., Warner-Lambert Healthcare) *519*

Neosporin Ointment (Pfizer Inc., Warner-Lambert Healthcare)...**519, 704**

Neosporin + Pain Relief Maximum Strength Cream (Pfizer Inc., Warner-Lambert Healthcare) **519, 704**

Neosporin + Pain Relief Maximum Strength Ointment (Pfizer Inc., Warner-Lambert Healthcare)...**519, 704**

Neo-Synephrine Nasal Drops, Regular and Extra Strength (Bayer Consumer).............**504, 614**

Neo-Synephrine Nasal Sprays, Mild, Regular and Extra Strength (Bayer Consumer) ...**504, 614**

Neo-Synephrine 12 Hour Nasal Spray (Bayer Consumer)......**504, 615**

Neo-Synephrine 12 Hour Extra Moisturizing Nasal Spray (Bayer Consumer)...........................**615**

New Skin Liquid Bandage (Medtech) ...**667**

NicoDerm CQ Patch (SmithKline Beecham Consumer)....................**524, 754**

Nicorette Gum (SmithKline Beecham Consumer) **524, 758**

Nicotinex Elixir (Fleming) **633**

Nix Creme Rinse (Pfizer Inc., Warner-Lambert Healthcare)...**519, 704**

Nix Spray (Pfizer Inc., Warner-Lambert Healthcare)...**519, 705**

Nizoral A-D Shampoo (McNeil Consumer)...........................**510, 647**

Nytol Natural Tablets (Block)......**506, 622**

Nytol QuickCaps Caplets (Block)........................**506, 622**

Maximum Strength Nytol QuickGels Softgels (Block)....**506, 621**

O

Ocean Nasal Mist (Fleming)............**633**

One-A-Day Antioxidant Softgels (Bayer Consumer).............**504, 805**

One-A-Day Bedtime & Rest Tablets (Bayer Consumer) **505, 805**

One-A-Day Calcium Plus Chewable Tablets (Bayer Consumer) **505, 805**

One-A-Day Cholesterol Health Tablets (Bayer Consumer) **505, 805**

One-A-Day Energy Formula Tablets (Bayer Consumer) **505, 806**

One-A-Day Essential Tablets (Bayer Consumer)..............**504, 806**

One-A-Day 50 Plus Tablets
(Bayer Consumer).............504, 804
One-A-Day Garlic Softgels
(Bayer Consumer).............505, 806
One-A-Day Joint Health Tablets
(Bayer Consumer).............505, 806
One-A-Day Kids Complete
Tablets (Bayer Consumer).....505, 806
One-A-Day Maximum Tablets
(Bayer Consumer).............504, 807
One-A-Day Memory &
Concentration Tablets
(Bayer Consumer).............505, 807
One-A-Day Men's Tablets
(Bayer Consumer).............504, 808
One-A-Day Menopause Health
Tablets (Bayer Consumer).....505, 808
One-A-Day Prostate Health
Softgels (Bayer Consumer)....505, 808
One-A-Day Tension & Mood
Softgels (Bayer Consumer)....505, 808
One-A-Day Women's Tablets
(Bayer Consumer).............504, 809
Orudis KT Tablets (Whitehall-Robins) ...778
Os-Cal Chewable Tablets
(SmithKline Beecham
Consumer).....................525, 838
Os-Cal 250 + D Tablets
(SmithKline Beecham
Consumer).....................525, 838
Os-Cal 500 Tablets (SmithKline
Beecham Consumer) 525, 839
Os-Cal 500 + D Tablets
(SmithKline Beecham
Consumer).....................525, 839
Oscillococcinum Pellets (Boiron) 625
Oxipor Psoriasis Lotion (Medtech) *664*
Oxy-G² (Body Wise).....................*810*

P

PediaCare Cough-Cold Liquid
(Pharmacia Consumer) 719
PediaCare Infants' Drops
Decongestant (Pharmacia
Consumer)..........................719
PediaCare Infants' Drops
Decongestant Plus Cough
(Pharmacia Consumer).............719
PediaCare NightRest Cough-Cold
Liquid (Pharmacia Consumer) 719
Pepcid AC Tablets, Chewable
Tablets, and Gelcaps (J&J •
Merck) 508, 638
Pepcid Complete Chewable
Tablets (J&J • Merck) 508, 638
Pepto-Bismol Original Liquid,
Original and Cherry
Chewable Tablets &
Caplets (Procter & Gamble) ...521, 723
Pepto-Bismol Maximum Strength
Liquid (Procter & Gamble)...........724
Percogesic Aspirin-Free Coated
Tablets (Medtech) 667
Extra Strength Percogesic
Aspirin-Free Coated Caplets
(Medtech)............................665
Perdiem Fiber Therapy
Granules (Novartis
Consumer).....................514, 675
Perdiem Overnight Relief
Granules (Novartis
Consumer).....................514, 674
Perfect Meal (AdvoCare) 798
Performance Gold Caplets
(AdvoCare)...........................798
Performance Optimizer System
(AdvoCare)...........................798
Peri-Colace Capsules and Syrup
(Shire) 743

Peridin-C Tablets (Beutlich) 618
Permethrin Lotion (Alpharma)..........602
Phazyme-125 mg Quick
Dissolve Chewable Tablets
(Block) 506, 622
Phazyme-180 mg Ultra
Strength Softgels (Block) 506, 622
Phillips' Chewable Tablets (Bayer
Consumer)...........................615
Phillips' FiberCaps Caplets
(Bayer Consumer).............505, 615
Phillips' Liqui-Gels (Bayer Consumer) ..616
Phillips' Milk of Magnesia
Liquid (Original, Cherry, &
Mint) (Bayer Consumer).......505, 616
PhytAloe Capsules (Mannatech) ..508, 819
PhytAloe Powder (Mannatech) 508, 819
Phyto-Vite Tablets (Wellness
International) 849
Pin-X Pinworm Treatment
(Effcon) 507, 632
Plus Caplets (Mannatech).......508, 820
Polysporin Ointment (Pfizer Inc.,
Warner-Lambert Healthcare)...519, 706
Polysporin Powder (Pfizer Inc.,
Warner-Lambert Healthcare)...519, 706
Power Circulation Tablets
(Sunpower) *841*
Power Lasting Tablets (Sunpower)......*841*
Prelief Tablets and Granulate
(AK Pharma) 503, 801
Preparation H Cream
(Whitehall-Robins) 778
Preparation H Cooling Gel
(Whitehall-Robins) 778
Preparation H Hydrocortisone 1%
Cream (Whitehall-Robins)
Preparation H Ointment
(Whitehall-Robins) 778
Preparation H Suppositories
(Whitehall-Robins) 778
Preparation H Medicated Wipes
(Whitehall-Robins) 779
Prescription Strength products
(see base product name)
Primatene Mist (Whitehall-Robins)......779
Primatene Tablets (Whitehall-Robins)...780
Probiotica Tablets (McNeil
Consumer) 510, 822
ProForm Bars (AdvoCare) 799
ProMotion Capsules (AdvoCare) 800
Prostatonin Softgel Capsules
(Pharmaton)....................521, 832
Proxeed Powder (Sigma-Tau) 523, 835
Pro-Xtreme Drink Mix (Wellness
International) 845
Purge Liquid (Fleming) 633

R

Regular Strength products
(see base product name)
Relief Nasal & Throat Spray (Body
Wise) 811
Remifemin Menopause Tablets
(SmithKline Beecham Consumer) ...839
ReSource Wellness AllerPro
Capsules (Novartis
Consumer).....................514, 824
ReSource Wellness CalciWise
Soft Chews (Novartis
Consumer) 514, 824
ReSource Wellness EnVigor
Caplets (Novartis
Consumer).....................514, 824
ReSource Wellness FlexTend
Caplets (Novartis
Consumer).....................514, 825

ReSource Wellness ForSight
Caplets (Novartis
Consumer).....................514, 825
ReSource Wellness MemorAble
Softgels (Novartis
Consumer).....................514, 825
ReSource Wellness ResistEx
Capsules (Novartis
Consumer) 514, 826
ReSource Wellness 2ndWind
Capsules (Novartis
Consumer) 514, 826
ReSource Wellness StayCalm
Caplets (Novartis
Consumer) 514, 826
ReSource Wellness VeinTain
Caplets (Novartis
Consumer) 514, 827
ProBiotic Restore Capsules
(AdvoCare)...........................799
Maximum Strength Rid Mousse
(Bayer Consumer)..............505, 617
Maximum Strength Rid
Shampoo (Bayer Consumer)...505, 616
Right Choice A.M. Multi Formula
Caplets (Body Wise)................811
Right Choice P.M. Multi Formula
Caplets (Body Wise)................812
Robitussin Liquid (Whitehall-Robins) ...782
Robitussin Cold Caplets Cold &
Congestion (Whitehall-Robins)......780
Robitussin Cold Softgels Cold &
Congestion (Whitehall-Robins) 780
Robitussin Cold Caplets
Multi-Symptom Cold & Flu
(Whitehall-Robins) 781
Robitussin Cold Softgels
Multi-Symptom Cold & Flu
(Whitehall-Robins) 781
Robitussin Cold Softgels Severe
Congestion (Whitehall-Robins) 782
Robitussin Cough Drops
(Whitehall-Robins) 781
Robitussin Honey Cough Drops
(Whitehall-Robins) 784
Robitussin Honey Cough Liquid
(Whitehall-Robins) 784
Robitussin Cough & Cold Infant
Drops (Whitehall-Robins) 782
Robitussin Maximum Strength
Cough & Cold Liquid
(Whitehall-Robins) 785
Robitussin Pediatric Cough & Cold
Formula Liquid (Whitehall-Robins)...785
Robitussin Maximum Strength
Cough Suppressant Liquid
(Whitehall-Robins) 784
Robitussin Pediatric Cough
Suppressant Liquid
(Whitehall-Robins) 784
Robitussin Multi Symptom Honey Flu
Liquid (Whitehall-Robins) 785
Robitussin Nighttime Honey Flu
Liquid (Whitehall-Robins) 786
Robitussin Honey Calmers Throat
Drops (Whitehall-Robins) 783
Robitussin Sugar Free Throat Drops
(Whitehall-Robins) 786
Robitussin-CF Liquid
(Whitehall-Robins) 783
Robitussin DM Infant Drops
(Whitehall-Robins) 783
Robitussin-DM Liquid
(Whitehall-Robins) 783
Robitussin-PE Liquid
(Whitehall-Robins) 782
Rogaine Extra Strength for Men
Topical Solution (Pharmacia
Consumer)...........................721

Italic Page Number **Indicates Brief Listing**

Rogaine for Women Topical Solution
(Pharmacia Consumer) 721
Rolaids Tablets (Pfizer Inc.,
Warner-Lambert Healthcare)... 519, 706
Extra Strength Rolaids Tablets
(Pfizer Inc., Warner-Lambert
Healthcare) 519, 706
Ryna Liquid (Wallace) 768
Ryna-C Liquid (Wallace) 525, 768

S
Satiete Tablets (Wellness
International) 846
Second Look Capsules (AdvoCare)...... 800
Senokot Children's Syrup
(Purdue Frederick) 522, 732
Senokot Granules (Purdue
Frederick) 522, 732
Senokot Syrup (Purdue
Frederick) 522, 732
Senokot Tablets (Purdue
Frederick) 522, 732
Senokot-S Tablets (Purdue
Frederick) 522, 732
SenokotXTRA Tablets (Purdue
Frederick) 732
Sensodyne Original Flavor (Block) 623
Sensodyne Cool Gel (Block)............. 623
Sensodyne Extra Whitening (Block) 623
Sensodyne Fresh Mint (Block) 623
Sensodyne Tartar Control (Block)....... 623
Sensodyne Tartar Control Plus
Whitening (Block) 623
Sensodyne with Baking Soda (Block)... 623
Simply Sleep Caplets (McNeil
Consumer) 510, 647
Singlet Caplets (SmithKline Beecham
Consumer) 761
Sinutab Non-Drying Liquid Caps
(Pfizer Inc., Warner-Lambert
Healthcare) 520, 706
Sinutab Sinus Allergy
Medication, Maximum
Strength Formula, Tablets
& Caplets (Pfizer Inc.,
Warner-Lambert Healthcare)... 520, 707
Sinutab Sinus Medication,
Maximum Strength Without
Drowsiness Formula,
Tablets & Caplets (Pfizer
Inc., Warner-Lambert
Healthcare) 520, 707
Sleep-Tite Caplets (Wellness
International) 850
Slow Fe Tablets (Novartis
Consumer) 514, 827
Slow Fe with Folic Acid Tablets
(Novartis Consumer)........... 514, 828
Slow-Mag Tablets (Shire) 835
Smile's Prid Salve (Standard
Homeopathic) 766
Sominex Original Formula Tablets
(SmithKline Beecham Consumer) ... 761
Spark! Beverage Mix (AdvoCare) 800
St. John's Complex (Body Wise) *810*
StePHan Bio-Nutritional Daytime
Hydrating Creme (Wellness
International) 770
StePHan Bio-Nutritional Eye-Firming
Concentrate (Wellness
International) 770
StePHan Bio-Nutritional Nightime
Moisture Creme (Wellness
International) 770
StePHan Bio-Nutritional Refreshing
Moisture Gel (Wellness
International) 770
StePHan Bio-Nutritional Ultra
Hydrating Fluid (Wellness
International) 770

StePHan Clarity Capsules (Wellness
International) 844
StePHan Elasticity Capsules
(Wellness International) 847
StePHan Elixir Capsules (Wellness
International) 848
StePHan Essential Capsules
(Wellness International) 848
StePHan Feminine Capsules
(Wellness International) 848
StePHan Flexibility Capsules
(Wellness International) 848
StePHan Lovpil Capsules (Wellness
International) 849
StePHan Masculine Capsules
(Wellness International) 849
StePHan Protector Capsules
(Wellness International) 850
StePHan Relief Capsules (Wellness
International) 850
StePHan Tranquility Capsules
(Wellness International) 851
Sudafed 12 Hour Tablets (Pfizer
Inc., Warner-Lambert
Healthcare) 520, 708
Sudafed 24 Hour Tablets (Pfizer
Inc., Warner-Lambert
Healthcare) 520, 708
Children's Sudafed Cold &
Cough Liquid (Pfizer Inc.,
Warner-Lambert Healthcare)... 520, 709
Children's Sudafed Nasal
Decongestant Chewables
(Pfizer Inc., Warner-Lambert
Healthcare) 520, 711
Children's Sudafed Nasal
Decongestant Liquid
Medication (Pfizer Inc.,
Warner-Lambert Healthcare)... 521, 711
Sudafed Cold & Allergy Tablets
(Pfizer Inc., Warner-Lambert
Healthcare) 520, 708
Sudafed Cold & Cough Liquid
Caps (Pfizer Inc.,
Warner-Lambert Healthcare)... 520, 709
Sudafed Cold & Sinus Liquid
Caps (Pfizer Inc.,
Warner-Lambert Healthcare)... 520, 710
Sudafed Nasal Decongestant
Tablets (Pfizer Inc.,
Warner-Lambert Healthcare)... 520, 710
Sudafed Non-Drying Sinus
Liquid Caps (Pfizer Inc.,
Warner-Lambert Healthcare)... 520, 712
Sudafed Severe Cold Formula
Caplets (Pfizer Inc.,
Warner-Lambert Healthcare)... 520, 711
Sudafed Severe Cold Formula
Tablets (Pfizer Inc.,
Warner-Lambert Healthcare)... 520, 711
Sudafed Sinus Headache
Caplets (Pfizer Inc.,
Warner-Lambert Healthcare)... 520, 712
Sudafed Sinus Headache
Tablets (Pfizer Inc.,
Warner-Lambert Healthcare)... 520, 712
Sun Beauty 1 Tablets (Sunpower)....... *841*
Sun Beauty 3 Tablets (Sunpower)....... *841*
Sun Cardio Tablets (Sunpower) *841*
Sun Joint Tablets (Sunpower) *841*
Sun Liver Tablets (Sunpower) 525, *841*
Super Anti-Oxidant Cell Protector
Capsules (Youngevity) 854
Super Food Soy Shake (Youngevity).... 854
Super Reshape Formula (Body Wise) ... *810*
Sure2Endure Tablets (Wellness
International) 851
Surfak Liqui-Gels (Pharmacia
Consumer) 721
System 3-4-3 Capsules (AdvoCare) 800

T
Tagamet HB 200 Suspension
(SmithKline Beecham
Consumer) 525, 762
Tagamet HB 200 Tablets
(SmithKline Beecham
Consumer) 525, 761
Tavist 12 Hour Allergy Tablets
(Novartis Consumer)........... 514, 676
Tavist Sinus Non-Drowsy
Coated Caplets (Novartis
Consumer) 514, 676
Techni-Care Surgical Scrub, Prep
and Wound Decontaminant
(Care-Tech)......................... 632
Tegrin Dandruff Shampoo - Extra
Conditioning (Block)................ 623
Tegrin Dandruff Shampoo -
Fresh Herbal (Block)........... 506, 624
Tegrin Skin Cream (Block)......... 506, 624
TheraFlu Regular Strength Cold
& Cough Night Time Hot
Liquid (Novartis Consumer) ... 515, 676
TheraFlu Regular Strength Cold
& Sore Throat Night Time
Hot Liquid (Novartis
Consumer) 515, 676
TheraFlu Maximum Strength
Flu & Congestion
Non-Drowsy Hot Liquid
(Novartis Consumer)........... 515, 677
TheraFlu Maximum Strength
Flu & Cough Night Time
Hot Liquid (Novartis
Consumer) 515, 678
TheraFlu Maximum Strength
Flu & Sore Throat Night
Time Hot Liquid (Novartis
Consumer) 515, 677
TheraFlu Maximum Strength
Severe Cold & Congestion
Night Time Caplets
(Novartis Consumer)........... 515, 678
TheraFlu Maximum Strength
Severe Cold & Congestion
Night Time Hot Liquid
(Novartis Consumer)........... 515, 678
TheraFlu Maximum Strength
Severe Cold & Congestion
Non-Drowsy Caplets
(Novartis Consumer)........... 515, 679
TheraFlu Maximum Strength
Severe Cold & Congestion
Non-Drowsy Hot Liquid
(Novartis Consumer)........... 515, 679
Thera-Gesic Creme (Mission) 667
Thermo-E Caplets (AdvoCare) 801
Thermo-G Caplets (AdvoCare)........... 801
Tiger Vites (Body Wise) *810*
3M Titralac Antacid Tablets
(3M)........................... 508, 640
3M Titralac Extra Strength
Antacid Tablets (3M) 508, 640
3M Titralac Plus Antacid
Tablets (3M) 508, 640
Transfer Factor Capsules
(4Life)........................ 526, 814
Transfer Factor Plus Capsules
(4Life)............................ *526*
Triaminic Allergy Congestion
Liquid (Novartis Consumer)... 515, 680
Triaminic Chest Congestion
Liquid (Novartis Consumer) ... 515, 680
Triaminic Cold & Allergy Liquid
(Novartis Consumer)........... 515, 681
Triaminic Cold & Allergy
Softchews (Novartis
Consumer) 515, 683
Triaminic Cold & Cough Liquid
(Novartis Consumer)........... 515, 681

Italic Page Number **Indicates Brief Listing**

Triaminic Cold & Cough Softchews (Novartis Consumer) 515, 683

Triaminic Cold & Night Time Cough Liquid (Novartis Consumer) 515, 681

Triaminic Cold, Cough & Fever Liquid (Novartis Consumer) ... 515, 681

Triaminic Cough Liquid (Novartis Consumer).......... 515, 682

Triaminic Cough Softchews (Novartis Consumer) 515, 684

Triaminic Cough & Congestion Liquid (Novartis Consumer) ... 515, 682

Triaminic Cough & Sore Throat Liquid (Novartis Consumer) ... 515, 682

Triaminic Cough & Sore Throat Softchews (Novartis Consumer) 515, 684

Triaminic Vapor Patch-Cherry Scent (Novartis Consumer).... 515, 684

Triaminic Vapor Patch-Menthol Scent (Novartis Consumer).... 515, 684

Triaminicin Tablets (Novartis Consumer)............................ *515*

Trident Advantage Mints (Pfizer Inc., Warner-Lambert Group)... 516, 687

Trident Advantage Sugarless Gum (Pfizer Inc., Warner-Lambert Group)........ 516, 687

Trident for Kids Sugarless Gum (Pfizer Inc., Warner-Lambert Group) 516, 687

Tucks Pre-moistened Pads (Pfizer Inc., Warner-Lambert Healthcare) 521, 713

Tums E-X Antacid/Calcium Tablets (SmithKline Beecham Consumer) 525, 763

Tums E-X Sugar Free Antacid/ Calcium Tablets (SmithKline Beecham Consumer) 525, 763

Tums Regular Antacid/Calcium Tablets (SmithKline Beecham Consumer) 525, 763

Tums ULTRA Antacid/Calcium Tablets (SmithKline Beecham Consumer) 525, 763

Children's Tylenol Suspension Liquid and Soft Chews Chewable Tablets (McNeil Consumer) 510, 511, 657

Children's Tylenol Allergy-D Liquid (McNeil Consumer) 510, 658

Children's Tylenol Cold Suspension Liquid and Chewable Tablets (McNeil Consumer) 510, 659

Children's Tylenol Cold Plus Cough Suspension Liquid and Chewable Tablets (McNeil Consumer) 510, 659

Children's Tylenol Flu Suspension Liquid (McNeil Consumer) 511, 663

Children's Tylenol Sinus Suspension Liquid (McNeil Consumer) 511, 663

Infants' Tylenol Cold Decongestant & Fever Reducer Concentrated Drops (McNeil Consumer) 511, 659

Infants' Tylenol Cold Decongestant & Fever Reducer Concentrated Drops Plus Cough (McNeil Consumer) 511, 659

Infants' Tylenol Concentrated Drops (McNeil Consumer) 511, 657

Junior Strength Tylenol Soft Chews Chewable Tablets (McNeil Consumer) 511, 512, 657

Extra Strength Tylenol Adult Liquid Pain Reliever (McNeil Consumer) ... 647

Extra Strength Tylenol Gelcaps, Geltabs, Caplets, and Tablets (McNeil Consumer) 511, 647

Regular Strength Tylenol Tablets (McNeil Consumer).... 511, 647

Maximum Strength Tylenol Allergy Sinus Caplets, Gelcaps, and Geltabs (McNeil Consumer) 511, 649

Maximum Strength Tylenol Allergy Sinus NightTime Caplets (McNeil Consumer) ... 511, 649

Tylenol Severe Allergy Caplets (McNeil Consumer) 511, 649

Tylenol Arthritis Pain Extended Relief Caplets (McNeil Consumer) 511, 647

Multi-Symptom Tylenol Cold Complete Formula Caplets (McNeil Consumer) 512, 651

Multi-Symptom Tylenol Cold Non-Drowsy Caplets and Gelcaps (McNeil Consumer)... 512, 651

Multi-Symptom Tylenol Cold Severe Congestion Non-Drowsy Caplets (McNeil Consumer) 512, 652

Maximum Strength Tylenol Flu NightTime Gelcaps (McNeil Consumer) 512, 653

Maximum Strength Tylenol Flu NightTime Liquid (McNeil Consumer) 512, 653

Maximum Strength Tylenol Flu Non-Drowsy Gelcaps (McNeil Consumer) 512, 653

Extra Strength Tylenol PM Caplets, Geltabs, and Gelcaps (McNeil Consumer)... 512, 654

Maximum Strength Tylenol Sinus NightTime Caplets (McNeil Consumer) 512, 655

Maximum Strength Tylenol Sinus Non-Drowsy Geltabs, Gelcaps, Caplets, and Tablets (McNeil Consumer).... 512, 655

Maximum Strength Tylenol Sore Throat Adult Liquid (McNeil Consumer) 512, 656

Women's Tylenol Menstrual Relief Caplets (McNeil Consumer) 512, 656

U

Unisom SleepTabs (Pfizer Inc., Warner-Lambert Healthcare)... 521, 713

Unisom Maximum Strength SleepGels (Pfizer Inc., Warner-Lambert Healthcare)... 521, 713

V

Vanquish Caplets (Bayer Consumer) 505, 617

Venastat Suppli-Cap Capsules (Pharmaton).................... 521, 833

Vicks 44 Cough Relief Liquid (Procter & Gamble) 724

Vicks 44D Cough & Head Congestion Relief Liquid (Procter & Gamble) 724

Vicks 44E Cough & Chest Congestion Relief Liquid (Procter & Gamble) 725

Pediatric Vicks 44e Cough & Chest Congestion Relief Liquid (Procter & Gamble) 728

Vicks 44M Cough, Cold & Flu Relief Liquid (Procter & Gamble) 725

Pediatric Vicks 44m Cough & Cold Relief (Procter & Gamble) 728

Vicks Cough Drops, Menthol and Cherry Flavors (Procter & Gamble)........................... 726

Vicks DayQuil LiquiCaps/Liquid Multi-Symptom Cold/Flu Relief (Procter & Gamble) 727

Children's Vicks NyQuil Cold/Cough Relief (Procter & Gamble) 726

Vicks NyQuil LiquiCaps/Liquid Multi-Symptom Cold/Flu Relief, Original and Cherry Flavors (Procter & Gamble) 727

Vicks Sinex Nasal Spray and Ultra Fine Mist (Procter & Gamble) 729

Vicks Sinex 12-Hour Nasal Spray and Ultra Fine Mist (Procter & Gamble)........................... 729

Vicks Vapor Inhaler (Procter & Gamble).......................... 730

Vicks VapoRub Cream (Procter & Gamble).......................... 730

Vicks VapoRub Ointment (Procter & Gamble)........................... 730

Vicks VapoSteam (Procter & Gamble) .. 730

Visine Original Eye Drops (Pfizer Inc., Warner-Lambert Healthcare) 521, 715

Visine A.C. Eye Drops (Pfizer Inc., Warner-Lambert Healthcare) 521, 715

Visine L.R. Eye Drops (Pfizer Inc., Warner-Lambert Healthcare) 521, 715

Advanced Relief Visine Eye Drops (Pfizer Inc., Warner-Lambert Healthcare)... 521, 714

Visine Tears Eye Drops (Pfizer Inc., Warner-Lambert Healthcare) 521, 716

Visine Tears Preservative Free Eye Drops (Pfizer Inc., Warner-Lambert Healthcare)... 521, 716

Visine-A Eye Drops (Pfizer Inc., Warner-Lambert Healthcare)... 521, 714

Vitality Immunity Anti-Oxidant Complex Capsules (Youngevity) *854*

Vitamist Intra-Oral Spray (Mayor) *821*

1-Before, 2-During, 3-After (Mayor) *821*

Anti-Oxidant (Mayor) *821*

ArthriFlex (Mayor) *821*

B12 (Mayor) *821*

Blue-Green Sea Spray (Mayor) *821*

CardioCare (Mayor)................... *821*

Colloidal Minerals (Mayor) *821*

C+Zinc (Mayor)....................... *821*

DHEA (Mayor)........................ *821*

Echinacea + G (Mayor) *821*

E+Selenium (Mayor) *821*

Ex. O (Mayor) *821*

Folacin (Mayor) *821*

GinkgoMist (Mayor) *821*

Melatonin (Mayor) *821*

Multiple (Mayor) *821*

Osteo-CalMag (Mayor) *821*

Pine Bark and Grape Seed
(Mayor) *821*
PMS and LadyMate (Mayor).......... *821*
Re-Leaf (Mayor)........................ *821*
Revitalizer (Mayor) *821*
Slender-Mist (Mayor) *821*
Smoke-Less (Mayor).................... *821*
St. John's Wort (Mayor) *821*
Stress (Mayor)......................... *821*
VitaMotion-S (Mayor).................. *821*
VitaSight (Mayor)...................... *821*
Vitara Cream (Products on
Demand) **522, 731**
Vitasana Gelcaps (Pharmaton).... **521, 834**

W
Vivarin Caplets (SmithKline
Beecham Consumer) **525, 763**
Vivarin Tablets (SmithKline
Beecham Consumer) **525, 763**

W
Warm Cream (Strategic
Science) **525, 841**
Wart-Off Liquid (Pfizer Inc.,
Warner-Lambert Healthcare)........ **716**
Winrgy Drink Mix (Wellness
International) **852**
Women's Strength products
(see base product name)
Workout Formula (Body Wise)........... *810*

X
Xtreme (Body Wise) *810*

Z
Zanfel Urushiol Wash (Zanfel)..... **526, 790**
Zantac 75 Tablets (Pfizer Inc.,
Warner-Lambert Healthcare)... **528, 717**
Zilactin Gel (Zila Consumer) **790**
Zilactin Baby Gel (Zila Consumer) **791**
Zilactin-B Gel (Zila Consumer) **790**
Zilactin-L Liquid (Zila Consumer)........ **790**
Zincon Medicated Dandruff
Shampoo (Medtech) *664*
ZZZ Spray Liquid (AdvoCare) **801**

SECTION 3

PRODUCT CATEGORY INDEX

This index cross-references each brand by pharmaceutical category. All fully-described products in the Product Information sections are included.

If an entry in the index lists multiple page numbers, the first one shown refers to the photograph of the product, the last one to its prescribing information.

The classification of each product is determined by the publisher in cooperation with the product's manufacturer or, when necessary, by the publisher alone.

A

ACNE PREPARATIONS
(see under:
  SKIN & MUCOUS MEMBRANE AGENTS
    ACNE PREPARATIONS)
ALPHA ADRENERGIC AGONISTS
(see under:
  OPHTHALMIC PREPARATIONS
    SYMPATHOMIMETICS & COMBINATIONS)
ALTERNATIVE MEDICINE
(see under:
  HOMEOPATHIC REMEDIES)
AMINO ACIDS
(see under:
  DIETARY SUPPLEMENTS
    AMINO ACIDS & COMBINATIONS)
ANALEPTIC AGENTS
(see under:
  CENTRAL NERVOUS SYSTEM STIMULANTS)
ANALGESICS
(see also under:
  MIGRAINE PREPARATIONS
  RESPIRATORY AGENTS
    MISCELLANEOUS COLD & COUGH PRODUCTS WITH ANALGESICS
  SKIN & MUCOUS MEMBRANE AGENTS
    ANALGESICS & COMBINATIONS
    ANESTHETICS & COMBINATIONS
  ACETAMINOPHEN & COMBINATIONS
  (see also under:
    ANTIHISTAMINES & COMBINATIONS
    RESPIRATORY AGENTS
      DECONGESTANTS & COMBINATIONS)
Actifed Cold & Sinus Caplets and
  Tablets (Pfizer Inc.,
  Warner-Lambert Healthcare)... **516, 688**
Alka-Seltzer Plus Cold Medicine
  Liqui-Gels (Bayer Consumer)... **503, 604**
Alka-Seltzer Plus Night-Time
  Cold Medicine Liqui-Gels
  (Bayer Consumer)............... **503, 604**

Alka-Seltzer Plus Cold & Cough
  Medicine Liqui-Gels (Bayer
  Consumer)..................... **503, 604**
Alka-Seltzer Plus Cold & Flu
  Medicine Liqui-Gels (Bayer
  Consumer)..................... **503, 604**
Alka-Seltzer Plus Cold & Sinus
  Medicine Liqui-Gels (Bayer
  Consumer)..................... **503, 604**
Benadryl Allergy/Cold Tablets
  (Pfizer Inc., Warner-Lambert
  Healthcare)................... **517, 691**
Benadryl Severe Allergy & Sinus
  Headache Caplets (Pfizer
  Inc., Warner-Lambert
  Healthcare) **517, 694**
Children's Cēpacol Sore Throat
  Formula, Cherry Flavor Liquid
  (Williams)........................ **788**
Children's Cēpacol Sore Throat
  Formula, Grape Flavor Liquid
  (Williams)........................ **788**
Comtrex Acute Head Cold &
  Sinus Pressure Relief
  Tablets (Bristol-Myers)......... **506, 627**
Comtrex Deep Chest Cold &
  Congestion Relief Softgels
  (Bristol-Myers) **506, 627**
Comtrex Flu Therapy & Fever
  Relief Daytime Caplets
  (Bristol-Myers) **506, 628**
Comtrex Flu Therapy & Fever
  Relief Nighttime Tablets
  (Bristol-Myers) **506, 628**
Comtrex Maximum Strength
  Multi-Symptom Cold &
  Cough Relief Tablets and
  Caplets (Bristol-Myers)......... **506, 626**
Contac Severe Cold and Flu
  Caplets Maximum Strength
  (SmithKline Beecham
  Consumer) **523, 746**

Contac Severe Cold and Flu Caplets
  Non-Drowsy (SmithKline Beecham
  Consumer)......................... **746**
Coricidin 'D' Cold, Flu & Sinus
  Tablets (Schering-Plough)...... **522, 737**
Coricidin HBP Cold & Flu Tablets
  (Schering-Plough) **523, 738**
Coricidin HBP Maximum
  Strength Flu Tablets
  (Schering-Plough) **523, 738**
Coricidin HBP Night-Time Cold &
  Flu Tablets (Schering-Plough) .. **523, 738**
Aspirin Free Excedrin Caplets
  and Geltabs (Bristol-Myers).... **507, 628**
Excedrin Extra-Strength Tablets,
  Caplets, and Geltabs
  (Bristol-Myers) **507, 629**
Excedrin Migraine Tablets,
  Caplets, and Geltabs
  (Bristol-Myers) **507, 630**
Excedrin PM Tablets, Caplets,
  and Geltabs (Bristol-Myers).... **506, 631**
Goody's Body Pain Formula Powder
  (Block) **620**
Goody's Extra Strength Headache
  Powder (Block)................... **620**
Goody's Extra Strength Pain Relief
  Tablets (Block).................. **620**
Goody's PM Powder (Block) **621**
Maximum Strength Midol
  Menstrual Caplets and
  Gelcaps (Bayer Consumer) **504, 612**
Maximum Strength Midol PMS
  Caplets and Gelcaps (Bayer
  Consumer) **504, 613**
Maximum Strength Midol Teen
  Caplets (Bayer Consumer)..... **504, 612**
Percogesic Aspirin-Free Coated
  Tablets (Medtech) **667**

ANALGESICS—cont.

ACETAMINOPHEN & COMBINATIONS—cont.

Extra Strength Percogesic
Aspirin-Free Coated Caplets
(Medtech)..............................665
Robitussin Multi Symptom Honey Flu
Liquid (Whitehall-Robins).............785
Robitussin Nighttime Honey Flu Liquid
(Whitehall-Robins)....................786
Tavist Sinus Non-Drowsy Coated
Caplets (Novartis
Consumer)......................514, 676
TheraFlu Regular Strength Cold
& Cough Night Time Hot
Liquid (Novartis Consumer)....515, 676
TheraFlu Regular Strength Cold
& Sore Throat Night Time
Hot Liquid (Novartis
Consumer)......................515, 676
TheraFlu Maximum Strength Flu
& Congestion Non-Drowsy
Hot Liquid (Novartis
Consumer)......................515, 677
TheraFlu Maximum Strength Flu
& Cough Night Time Hot
Liquid (Novartis Consumer)....515, 678
TheraFlu Maximum Strength Flu
& Sore Throat Night Time
Hot Liquid (Novartis
Consumer)......................515, 677
TheraFlu Maximum Strength
Severe Cold & Congestion
Night Time Caplets
(Novartis Consumer)............515, 678
TheraFlu Maximum Strength
Severe Cold & Congestion
Night Time Hot Liquid
(Novartis Consumer)............515, 678
TheraFlu Maximum Strength
Severe Cold & Congestion
Non-Drowsy Caplets
(Novartis Consumer)............515, 679
TheraFlu Maximum Strength
Severe Cold & Congestion
Non-Drowsy Hot Liquid
(Novartis Consumer)............515, 679
Triaminic Cold, Cough & Fever
Liquid (Novartis Consumer)....515, 681
Triaminic Cough & Sore Throat
Liquid (Novartis Consumer)....515, 682
Triaminic Cough & Sore Throat
Softchews (Novartis
Consumer)......................515, 684
Children's Tylenol
Suspension Liquid and
Soft Chews Chewable
Tablets (McNeil
Consumer)..............510, 511, 657
Children's Tylenol Allergy-D
Liquid (McNeil Consumer).....510, 658
Children's Tylenol Cold
Suspension Liquid and
Chewable Tablets (McNeil
Consumer)......................510, 659
Children's Tylenol Cold Plus
Cough Suspension Liquid
and Chewable Tablets
(McNeil Consumer)............510, 659
Children's Tylenol Flu
Suspension Liquid (McNeil
Consumer)......................511, 663
Children's Tylenol Sinus
Suspension Liquid (McNeil
Consumer)......................511, 663
Infants' Tylenol Cold
Decongestant & Fever
Reducer Concentrated
Drops (McNeil Consumer).....511, 659

Infants' Tylenol Cold
Decongestant & Fever
Reducer Concentrated
Drops Plus Cough (McNeil
Consumer)......................511, 659
Infants' Tylenol Concentrated
Drops (McNeil Consumer).....511, 657
Junior Strength Tylenol
Soft Chews Chewable
Tablets (McNeil
Consumer)..............511, 512, 657
Extra Strength Tylenol Adult Liquid
Pain Reliever (McNeil Consumer)....647
Extra Strength Tylenol Gelcaps,
Geltabs, Caplets, and
Tablets (McNeil Consumer)....511, 647
Regular Strength Tylenol Tablets
(McNeil Consumer)............511, 647
Maximum Strength Tylenol
Allergy Sinus Caplets,
Gelcaps, and Geltabs
(McNeil Consumer)............511, 649
Maximum Strength Tylenol
Allergy Sinus NightTime
Caplets (McNeil Consumer)....511, 649
Tylenol Severe Allergy Caplets
(McNeil Consumer)............511, 649
Tylenol Arthritis Pain Extended
Relief Caplets (McNeil
Consumer)......................511, 647
Multi-Symptom Tylenol Cold
Complete Formula Caplets
(McNeil Consumer)............512, 651
Multi-Symptom Tylenol Cold
Non-Drowsy Caplets and
Gelcaps (McNeil Consumer)...512, 651
Multi-Symptom Tylenol Cold
Severe Congestion
Non-Drowsy Caplets (McNeil
Consumer)......................512, 652
Maximum Strength Tylenol Flu
NightTime Gelcaps (McNeil
Consumer)......................512, 653
Maximum Strength Tylenol Flu
NightTime Liquid (McNeil
Consumer)......................512, 653
Maximum Strength Tylenol Flu
Non-Drowsy Gelcaps (McNeil
Consumer)......................512, 653
Extra Strength Tylenol PM
Caplets, Geltabs, and
Gelcaps (McNeil Consumer)...512, 654
Maximum Strength Tylenol
Sinus NightTime Caplets
(McNeil Consumer)............512, 655
Maximum Strength Tylenol
Sinus Non-Drowsy Geltabs,
Gelcaps, Caplets, and
Tablets (McNeil Consumer)....512, 655
Maximum Strength Tylenol Sore
Throat Adult Liquid (McNeil
Consumer)......................512, 656
Women's Tylenol Menstrual
Relief Caplets (McNeil
Consumer)......................512, 656
Vanquish Caplets (Bayer
Consumer)......................505, 617

NONSTEROIDAL ANTI-INFLAMMATORY DRUGS (NSAIDS)

Advil Caplets (Whitehall-Robins).........771
Advil Gel Caplets (Whitehall-Robins).....771
Advil Liqui-Gels (Whitehall-Robins).......771
Advil Tablets (Whitehall-Robins).........771
Children's Advil Oral Suspension
(Whitehall-Robins)....................773
Children's Advil Chewable Tablets
(Whitehall-Robins)....................773

Advil Cold and Sinus Caplets
(Whitehall-Robins)....................771
Advil Cold and Sinus Tablets
(Whitehall-Robins)....................771
Advil Flu & Body Ache Caplets
(Whitehall-Robins)....................772
Infants' Advil Drops
(Whitehall-Robins)....................773
Junior Strength Advil Tablets
(Whitehall-Robins)....................773
Junior Strength Advil Chewable
Tablets (Whitehall-Robins)...........773
Advil Migraine Liquigels
(Whitehall-Robins)....................772
Aleve Tablets, Caplets and
Gelcaps (Bayer Consumer)....503, 602
Aleve Cold & Sinus Caplets
(Bayer Consumer).............503, 603
Children's Motrin Oral
Suspension and Chewable
Tablets (McNeil Consumer)....509, 643
Children's Motrin Cold Oral
Suspension (McNeil
Consumer)......................509, 646
Infants' Motrin Concentrated
Drops (McNeil Consumer).....509, 643
Junior Strength Motrin Caplets
and Chewable Tablets
(McNeil Consumer)............509, 643
Motrin IB Tablets, Caplets, and
Gelcaps (McNeil Consumer)...510, 642
Motrin Migraine Pain Caplets
(McNeil Consumer)............510, 646
Motrin Sinus/Headache Caplets
(McNeil Consumer)............510, 643
Orudis KT Tablets (Whitehall-Robins)....778

SALICYLATES

ASPIRIN & COMBINATIONS

Alka-Seltzer Original Antacid
and Pain Reliever
Effervescent Tablets
(Bayer Consumer)............503, 603
Alka-Seltzer Cherry Antacid
and Pain Reliever
Effervescent Tablets
(Bayer Consumer)............503, 603
Alka-Seltzer Lemon Lime
Antacid and Pain
Reliever Effervescent
Tablets (Bayer
Consumer)......................503, 603
Alka-Seltzer Extra Strength
Antacid and Pain
Reliever Effervescent
Tablets (Bayer
Consumer)......................503, 603
Alka-Seltzer PM
Effervescent Tablets
(Bayer Consumer)............503, 605
Genuine Bayer Tablets,
Caplets and Gelcaps
(Bayer Consumer)............503, 606
Extra Strength Bayer
Caplets and Gelcaps
(Bayer Consumer)............504, 610
Aspirin Regimen Bayer
Children's Chewable
Tablets (Orange or
Cherry Flavored) (Bayer
Consumer)......................504, 607
Aspirin Regimen Bayer Adult
Low Strength 81 mg
Tablets (Bayer
Consumer)......................503, 606
Aspirin Regimen Bayer 81 mg
Caplets with Calcium (Bayer
Consumer)............................607

Aspirin Regimen Bayer
 Regular Strength 325
 mg Caplets (Bayer
 Consumer) **503, 606**
Genuine Bayer Professional
 Labeling (Aspirin Regimen
 Bayer) (Bayer Consumer) **608**
Extra Strength Bayer
 Arthritis Caplets (Bayer
 Consumer) **504, 610**
Extra Strength Bayer Plus
 Caplets (Bayer
 Consumer) **504, 610**
Extra Strength Bayer PM
 Caplets (Bayer
 Consumer) **504, 611**
BC Powder (Block) **619**
BC Allergy Sinus Cold Powder
 (Block) **619**
Arthritis Strength BC Powder
 (Block) **619**
BC Sinus Cold Powder (Block) **619**
Ecotrin Enteric Coated
 Aspirin Low Strength
 Tablets (SmithKline
 Beecham Consumer) **524, 747**
Ecotrin Enteric Coated
 Aspirin Maximum
 Strength Tablets
 (SmithKline Beecham
 Consumer) **524, 747**
Ecotrin Enteric Coated
 Aspirin Regular Strength
 Tablets (SmithKline
 Beecham Consumer) **524, 747**
Excedrin Extra-Strength
 Tablets, Caplets, and
 Geltabs (Bristol-Myers) **507, 629**
Excedrin Migraine Tablets,
 Caplets, and Geltabs
 (Bristol-Myers) **507, 630**
Goody's Body Pain Formula
 Powder (Block)..................... **620**
Goody's Extra Strength Headache
 Powder (Block)..................... **620**
Goody's Extra Strength Pain
 Relief Tablets (Block) **620**
Vanquish Caplets (Bayer
 Consumer) **505, 617**

OTHER SALICYLATES & COMBINATIONS

Momentum Backache Relief Extra
 Strength Caplets (Medtech) **666**

ANESTHETICS
(*see under:*
 SKIN & MUCOUS MEMBRANE AGENTS
 ANESTHETICS & COMBINATIONS)

ANORECTAL PRODUCTS
(*see under:*
 SKIN & MUCOUS MEMBRANE AGENTS
 ANORECTAL PREPARATIONS)

ANTACIDS
(*see under:*
 GASTROINTESTINAL AGENTS
 ANTACID & ANTIFLATULENT COMBINATIONS
 ANTACIDS)

ANTHELMINTICS
(*see under:*
 ANTI-INFECTIVE AGENTS, SYSTEMIC
 ANTHELMINTICS)

ANTIARTHRITICS
(*see under:*
 ANALGESICS
 NONSTEROIDAL ANTI-INFLAMMATORY DRUGS (NSAIDS)
 SALICYLATES
 SKIN & MUCOUS MEMBRANE AGENTS
 ANALGESICS & COMBINATIONS)

ANTIBIOTICS
(*see under:*
 SKIN & MUCOUS MEMBRANE AGENTS
 ANTI-INFECTIVES
 ANTIBIOTICS & COMBINATIONS)

ANTIEMETICS
(*see under:*
 GASTROINTESTINAL AGENTS
 ANTIEMETICS)

ANTIFLATULENTS
(*see under:*
 GASTROINTESTINAL AGENTS
 ANTACID & ANTIFLATULENT COMBINATIONS
 ANTIFLATULENTS)

ANTIFUNGALS
(*see under:*
 SKIN & MUCOUS MEMBRANE AGENTS
 ANTI-INFECTIVES
 ANTIFUNGALS & COMBINATIONS
 VAGINAL PREPARATIONS
 ANTI-INFECTIVES
 ANTIFUNGALS & COMBINATIONS)

ANTIGLAUCOMATOUS AGENTS
(*see under:*
 OPHTHALMIC PREPARATIONS
 SYMPATHOMIMETICS & COMBINATIONS)

ANTIHISTAMINES & COMBINATIONS
(*see also under:*
 OPHTHALMIC PREPARATIONS
 ANTIHISTAMINES & COMBINATIONS
 SKIN & MUCOUS MEMBRANE AGENTS
 ANTIHISTAMINES & COMBINATIONS)

Actifed Cold & Allergy Tablets
 (Pfizer Inc., Warner-Lambert
 Healthcare) **516, 688**
Actifed Cold & Sinus Caplets
 and Tablets (Pfizer Inc.,
 Warner-Lambert Healthcare)... **516, 688**
Alka-Seltzer Plus Cold Medicine
 Liqui-Gels (Bayer Consumer)... **503, 604**
Alka-Seltzer Plus Night-Time
 Cold Medicine Liqui-Gels
 (Bayer Consumer)............... **503, 604**
Alka-Seltzer Plus Cold & Cough
 Medicine Liqui-Gels (Bayer
 Consumer) **503, 604**
BC Allergy Sinus Cold Powder (Block) ... **619**
Benadryl Allergy Chewables
 (Pfizer Inc., Warner-Lambert
 Healthcare) **517, 689**
Benadryl Allergy Kapseal
 Capsules (Pfizer Inc.,
 Warner-Lambert Healthcare)... **516, 691**
Benadryl Allergy Liquid (Pfizer
 Inc., Warner-Lambert
 Healthcare) **517, 690**
Benadryl Allergy Ultratab
 Tablets (Pfizer Inc.,
 Warner-Lambert Healthcare)... **516, 691**
Benadryl Allergy/Cold Tablets
 (Pfizer Inc., Warner-Lambert
 Healthcare) **517, 691**
Benadryl Allergy/Congestion
 Tablets (Pfizer Inc.,
 Warner-Lambert Healthcare)... **517, 692**
Benadryl Allergy & Sinus Liquid
 (Pfizer Inc., Warner-Lambert
 Healthcare) **693**
Benadryl Allergy & Sinus
 Fastmelt Tablets (Pfizer Inc.,
 Warner-Lambert Healthcare)... **517, 693**
Benadryl Allergy Sinus
 Headache Caplets &
 Gelcaps (Pfizer Inc.,
 Warner-Lambert Healthcare)... **517, 693**
Benadryl Severe Allergy & Sinus
 Headache Caplets (Pfizer
 Inc., Warner-Lambert
 Healthcare) **517, 694**

Benadryl Children's Allergy/
 Cold Fastmelt Tablets (Pfizer
 Inc., Warner-Lambert
 Healthcare) **517, 692**
Benadryl Dye-Free Allergy Liquid
 (Pfizer Inc., Warner-Lambert
 Healthcare) **517, 690**
Benadryl Dye-Free Allergy
 Liqui-Gels Softgels (Pfizer
 Inc., Warner-Lambert
 Healthcare) **517, 690**
Chlor-Trimeton Allergy Tablets
 (Schering-Plough) **522, 735**
Chlor-Trimeton Allergy/
 Decongestant Tablets
 (Schering-Plough) **522, 736**
Comtrex Acute Head Cold &
 Sinus Pressure Relief
 Tablets (Bristol-Myers) **506, 627**
Comtrex Flu Therapy & Fever
 Relief Nighttime Tablets
 (Bristol-Myers) **506, 628**
Comtrex Maximum Strength
 Multi-Symptom Cold &
 Cough Relief Tablets and
 Caplets (Bristol-Myers)......... **506, 626**
Contac Severe Cold and Flu
 Caplets Maximum Strength
 (SmithKline Beecham
 Consumer) **523, 746**
Coricidin 'D' Cold, Flu & Sinus
 Tablets (Schering-Plough) **522, 737**
Coricidin HBP Cold & Flu Tablets
 (Schering-Plough) **523, 738**
Coricidin HBP Cough & Cold
 Tablets (Schering-Plough) **523, 738**
Coricidin HBP Maximum
 Strength Flu Tablets
 (Schering-Plough)............... **523, 738**
Coricidin HBP Night-Time Cold &
 Flu Tablets (Schering-Plough) .. **523, 738**
Dimetapp Elixir (Whitehall-Robins)....... **777**
Dimetapp Cold and Fever Suspension
 (Whitehall-Robins) **775**
Dimetapp DM Cold & Cough Elixir
 (Whitehall-Robins) **775**
Dimetapp Nighttime Flu Liquid
 (Whitehall-Robins) **776**
Drixoral Cold & Allergy
 Sustained-Action Tablets
 (Schering-Plough) **523, 740**
Drixoral Cold & Flu
 Extended-Release Tablets
 (Schering-Plough) **523, 740**
PediaCare Cough-Cold Liquid
 (Pharmacia Consumer) **719**
PediaCare NightRest Cough-Cold
 Liquid (Pharmacia Consumer) **719**
Percogesic Aspirin-Free Coated
 Tablets (Medtech) **667**
Extra Strength Percogesic
 Aspirin-Free Coated Caplets
 (Medtech)........................... **665**
Robitussin Nighttime Honey Flu Liquid
 (Whitehall-Robins) **786**
Ryna Liquid (Wallace)................... **768**
Ryna-C Liquid (Wallace)......... **525, 768**
Singlet Caplets (SmithKline Beecham
 Consumer)........................... **761**
Sinutab Sinus Allergy
 Medication, Maximum
 Strength Formula, Tablets &
 Caplets (Pfizer Inc.,
 Warner-Lambert Healthcare)... **520, 707**
Sudafed Cold & Allergy Tablets
 (Pfizer Inc., Warner-Lambert
 Healthcare) **520, 708**

ANTIHISTAMINES & COMBINATIONS—cont.

Tavist 12 Hour Allergy Tablets
(Novartis Consumer)...........**514, 676**

TheraFlu Regular Strength Cold
& Cough Night Time Hot
Liquid (Novartis Consumer)....**515, 676**

TheraFlu Regular Strength Cold
& Sore Throat Night Time
Hot Liquid (Novartis
Consumer).......................**515, 676**

TheraFlu Maximum Strength Flu
& Cough Night Time Hot
Liquid (Novartis Consumer)....**515, 678**

TheraFlu Maximum Strength Flu
& Sore Throat Night Time
Hot Liquid (Novartis
Consumer).......................**515, 677**

TheraFlu Maximum Strength
Severe Cold & Congestion
Night Time Caplets
(Novartis Consumer)............**515, 678**

TheraFlu Maximum Strength
Severe Cold & Congestion
Night Time Hot Liquid
(Novartis Consumer)............**515, 678**

Triaminic Cold & Allergy Liquid
(Novartis Consumer)...........**515, 681**

Triaminic Cold & Allergy
Softchews (Novartis
Consumer).......................**515, 683**

Triaminic Cold & Cough Liquid
(Novartis Consumer)...........**515, 681**

Triaminic Cold & Cough
Softchews (Novartis
Consumer).......................**515, 683**

Triaminic Cold & Night Time
Cough Liquid (Novartis
Consumer).......................**515, 681**

Triaminic Cold, Cough & Fever
Liquid (Novartis Consumer)....**515, 681**

Children's Tylenol Allergy-D
Liquid (McNeil Consumer).....**510, 658**

Children's Tylenol Cold
Suspension Liquid and
Chewable Tablets (McNeil
Consumer).......................**510, 659**

Children's Tylenol Cold Plus
Cough Suspension Liquid
and Chewable Tablets
(McNeil Consumer) **510, 659**

Children's Tylenol Flu
Suspension Liquid (McNeil
Consumer).......................**511, 663**

Maximum Strength Tylenol
Allergy Sinus Caplets,
Gelcaps, and Geltabs
(McNeil Consumer) **511, 649**

Maximum Strength Tylenol
Allergy Sinus NightTime
Caplets (McNeil Consumer)....**511, 649**

Tylenol Severe Allergy Caplets
(McNeil Consumer) **511, 649**

Multi-Symptom Tylenol Cold
Complete Formula Caplets
(McNeil Consumer) **512, 651**

Maximum Strength Tylenol Flu
NightTime Gelcaps (McNeil
Consumer).......................**512, 653**

Maximum Strength Tylenol Flu
NightTime Liquid (McNeil
Consumer).......................**512, 653**

Extra Strength Tylenol PM
Caplets, Geltabs, and
Gelcaps (McNeil Consumer)...**512, 654**

Maximum Strength Tylenol
Sinus NightTime Caplets
(McNeil Consumer) **512, 655**

Vicks 44M Cough, Cold & Flu Relief
Liquid (Procter & Gamble) **725**

Pediatric Vicks 44m Cough & Cold
Relief (Procter & Gamble) **728**

Children's Vicks NyQuil Cold/Cough
Relief (Procter & Gamble) **726**

Vicks NyQuil LiquiCaps/Liquid
Multi-Symptom Cold/Flu Relief,
Original and Cherry Flavors
(Procter & Gamble) **727**

ANTI-INFECTIVE AGENTS
(see under:

ANTI-INFECTIVE AGENTS, SYSTEMIC

SKIN & MUCOUS MEMBRANE AGENTS
ANTI-INFECTIVES

VAGINAL PREPARATIONS
ANTI-INFECTIVES)

ANTI-INFECTIVE AGENTS, SYSTEMIC

ANTHELMINTICS
Pin-X Pinworm Treatment (Effcon) .**507, 632**

ANTI-INFECTIVES, NON-SYSTEMIC

SCABICIDES & PEDICULICIDES
(see also under:

SKIN & MUCOUS MEMBRANE AGENTS
ANTI-INFECTIVES
SCABICIDES & PEDICULICIDES)
Nix Spray (Pfizer Inc.,
Warner-Lambert Healthcare)...**519, 705**

ANTI-INFLAMMATORY AGENTS
(see under:

ANALGESICS
NONSTEROIDAL ANTI-INFLAMMATORY DRUGS (NSAIDS)
SALICYLATES

SKIN & MUCOUS MEMBRANE AGENTS
STEROIDS & COMBINATIONS)

ANTIMYCOTICS
(see under:

SKIN & MUCOUS MEMBRANE AGENTS
ANTI-INFECTIVES
ANTIFUNGALS & COMBINATIONS

VAGINAL PREPARATIONS
ANTI-INFECTIVES
ANTIFUNGALS & COMBINATIONS)

ANTIPRURITICS
(see under:

ANTIHISTAMINES & COMBINATIONS

SKIN & MUCOUS MEMBRANE AGENTS
ANTIPRURITICS)

ANTIPYRETICS
(see under:

ANALGESICS
ACETAMINOPHEN & COMBINATIONS
NONSTEROIDAL ANTI-INFLAMMATORY DRUGS (NSAIDS)
SALICYLATES)

ANTISEPTICS
(see under:

SKIN & MUCOUS MEMBRANE AGENTS
ANTI-INFECTIVES
MISCELLANEOUS ANTI-INFECTIVES &
COMBINATIONS)

ANTITUSSIVES
(see under:

RESPIRATORY AGENTS
ANTITUSSIVES)

ARTHRITIS MEDICATIONS
(see under:

ANALGESICS
NONSTEROIDAL ANTI-INFLAMMATORY DRUGS (NSAIDS)
SALICYLATES

SKIN & MUCOUS MEMBRANE AGENTS
ANALGESICS & COMBINATIONS)

ARTIFICIAL TEARS
(see under:

OPHTHALMIC PREPARATIONS
ARTIFICIAL TEARS/LUBRICANTS & COMBINATIONS)

ASTHMA PREPARATIONS
(see under:

RESPIRATORY AGENTS
BRONCHODILATORS)

ASTRINGENTS
(see under:

SKIN & MUCOUS MEMBRANE AGENTS
ASTRINGENTS)

B

BABY PRODUCTS
Desitin Creamy Ointment (Pfizer
Inc., Warner-Lambert
Healthcare) **518, 700**

Desitin Ointment (Pfizer Inc.,
Warner-Lambert Healthcare)...**518, 700**

Tucks Pre-moistened Pads
(Pfizer Inc., Warner-Lambert
Healthcare) **521, 713**

BLOOD MODIFIERS

ANTIPLATELET AGENTS
Genuine Bayer Tablets, Caplets
and Gelcaps (Bayer
Consumer).......................**503, 606**

Aspirin Regimen Bayer Adult
Low Strength 81 mg Tablets
(Bayer Consumer).............**503, 606**

Aspirin Regimen Bayer Regular
Strength 325 mg Caplets
(Bayer Consumer).............**503, 606**

Genuine Bayer Professional Labeling
(Aspirin Regimen Bayer) (Bayer
Consumer).......................**608**

Ecotrin Enteric Coated Aspirin
Low Strength Tablets
(SmithKline Beecham
Consumer).......................**524, 747**

Ecotrin Enteric Coated Aspirin
Maximum Strength Tablets
(SmithKline Beecham
Consumer).......................**524, 747**

Ecotrin Enteric Coated Aspirin
Regular Strength Tablets
(SmithKline Beecham
Consumer).......................**524, 747**

BRONCHIAL DILATORS
(see under:

RESPIRATORY AGENTS
BRONCHODILATORS)

BURN PREPARATIONS
(see under:

SKIN & MUCOUS MEMBRANE AGENTS
BURN PREPARATIONS)

C

CALCIUM SUPPLEMENTS
(see under:

DIETARY SUPPLEMENTS
MINERALS & ELECTROLYTES
CALCIUM & COMBINATIONS)

CANKER SORE PREPARATIONS
(see under:

SKIN & MUCOUS MEMBRANE AGENTS
MOUTH & THROAT PRODUCTS
CANKER SORE PREPARATIONS)

CARDIOVASCULAR AGENTS
(see under:

BLOOD MODIFIERS
ANTIPLATELET AGENTS)

CENTRAL NERVOUS SYSTEM AGENTS
(see under:

ANALGESICS

CENTRAL NERVOUS SYSTEM STIMULANTS

GASTROINTESTINAL AGENTS
ANTIEMETICS

SEDATIVES & HYPNOTICS)

CENTRAL NERVOUS SYSTEM STIMULANTS

**MISCELLANEOUS CENTRAL NERVOUS SYSTEM
STIMULANTS**
Vivarin Caplets (SmithKline
Beecham Consumer) **525, 763**

Vivarin Tablets (SmithKline
   Beecham Consumer) **525, 763**

CERUMENOLYTICS
(*see under:*
  OTIC PREPARATIONS
    CERUMENOLYTICS)

COLD & COUGH PREPARATIONS
(*see under:*
  ANTIHISTAMINES & COMBINATIONS
  NASAL PREPARATIONS
    SYMPATHOMIMETICS & COMBINATIONS
  RESPIRATORY AGENTS
    ANTITUSSIVES
    DECONGESTANTS & COMBINATIONS
    DECONGESTANTS, EXPECTORANTS & COMBINATIONS
    EXPECTORANTS & COMBINATIONS
    MISCELLANEOUS COLD & COUGH PRODUCTS WITH ANALGESICS
    MISCELLANEOUS RESPIRATORY AGENTS
  SKIN & MUCOUS MEMBRANE AGENTS
    MOUTH & THROAT PRODUCTS
      LOZENGES & SPRAYS)

COLD SORE PREPARATIONS
(*see under:*
  SKIN & MUCOUS MEMBRANE AGENTS
    MOUTH & THROAT PRODUCTS
      COLD SORE PREPARATIONS)

COLOSTOMY DEODORIZERS
(*see under:*
  DEODORANTS
    INTERNAL DEODORANTS)

CONSTIPATION AIDS
(*see under:*
  GASTROINTESTINAL AGENTS
    LAXATIVES)

COUGH PREPARATIONS
(*see under:*
  RESPIRATORY AGENTS
    ANTITUSSIVES
    DECONGESTANTS, EXPECTORANTS & COMBINATIONS
    EXPECTORANTS & COMBINATIONS
    MISCELLANEOUS COLD & COUGH PRODUCTS WITH ANALGESICS)

D

DANDRUFF PRODUCTS
(*see under:*
  SKIN & MUCOUS MEMBRANE AGENTS
    ANTISEBORRHEIC AGENTS)

DECONGESTANTS
(*see under:*
  NASAL PREPARATIONS
    SYMPATHOMIMETICS & COMBINATIONS
  OPHTHALMIC PREPARATIONS
    SYMPATHOMIMETICS & COMBINATIONS
  RESPIRATORY AGENTS
    DECONGESTANTS & COMBINATIONS
    DECONGESTANTS, EXPECTORANTS & COMBINATIONS)

DENTAL PREPARATIONS
(*see under:*
  SKIN & MUCOUS MEMBRANE AGENTS
    MOUTH & THROAT PRODUCTS
      DENTAL PREPARATIONS)

DEODORANTS
  INTERNAL DEODORANTS
  Devrom Chewable Tablets (Parthenon).. **685**

DERMATOLOGICALS
(*see under:*
  SKIN & MUCOUS MEMBRANE AGENTS)

DIAGNOSTICS
  PREGNANCY TESTS
  e.p.t. Pregnancy Test (Pfizer Inc.,
    Warner-Lambert Healthcare)... **518, 701**

DIAPER RASH RELIEF
(*see under:*
  SKIN & MUCOUS MEMBRANE AGENTS
    DIAPER RASH PRODUCTS)

DIARRHEA MEDICATIONS
(*see under:*
  GASTROINTESTINAL AGENTS
    ANTIDIARRHEALS)

DIET AIDS
(*see under:*
  DIETARY SUPPLEMENTS)

DIETARY SUPPLEMENTS
  AMINO ACIDS & COMBINATIONS
  BodyLean Powder (AdvoCare) **795**
  Catalyst Capsules (AdvoCare) **796**
  HeartBar (Cooke) **812**
  LipoTrol Caplets (AdvoCare) **797**
  Mass Appeal Tablets (Wellness
    International) **845**
  Perfect Meal (AdvoCare).................. **798**
  Proxeed Powder (Sigma-Tau)....... **523, 835**
  Pro-Xtreme Drink Mix (Wellness
    International) **845**
  Spark! Beverage Mix (AdvoCare) **800**
  StePHan Feminine Capsules
    (Wellness International) **848**
  StePHan Flexibility Capsules
    (Wellness International) **848**
  Vitamist Intra-Oral Spray (Mayor) **821**
  Winrgy Drink Mix (Wellness
    International) **852**
  AMINO ACIDS & HERBAL COMBINATIONS
  BioLean Capsules and Tablets
    (Wellness International) **842**
  BioLean Accelerator Tablets
    (Wellness International) **842**
  BioLean Free Tablets (Wellness
    International) **843**
  CardiOptima Drink Mix Packets
    (AdvoCare) **795**
  Coffeccino Beverage Mix (AdvoCare) **796**
  HGH-Turn Back the Hands of Time
    Capsules (Youngevity) **854**
  IntelleQ Capsules (AdvoCare) **797**
  Metabolic Nutrition System
    (AdvoCare)......................... **798**
  Performance Gold Caplets (AdvoCare) .. **798**
  Performance Optimizer System
    (AdvoCare)......................... **798**
  Plus Caplets (Mannatech) **508, 820**
  ProForm Bars (AdvoCare)................ **799**
  Satiete Tablets (Wellness
    International) **846**
  StePHan Clarity Capsules (Wellness
    International) **844**
  StePHan Elasticity Capsules
    (Wellness International) **847**
  StePHan Elixir Capsules (Wellness
    International) **848**
  StePHan Essential Capsules
    (Wellness International) **848**
  StePHan Lovpil Capsules (Wellness
    International) **849**
  StePHan Masculine Capsules
    (Wellness International) **849**
  StePHan Protector Capsules
    (Wellness International) **850**
  StePHan Relief Capsules (Wellness
    International) **850**
  StePHan Tranquility Capsules
    (Wellness International) **851**
  Super Food Soy Shake (Youngevity) **854**
  System 3-4-3 Capsules (AdvoCare)...... **800**
  BLOOD MODIFIERS
    IRON & COMBINATIONS
  Feosol Caplets (SmithKline
    Beecham Consumer) **524, 837**
  Feosol Tablets (SmithKline
    Beecham Consumer) **524, 838**

Fergon Iron Tablets (Bayer
    Consumer) **504, 802**
Slow Fe Tablets (Novartis
    Consumer) **514, 827**
Slow Fe with Folic Acid
    Tablets (Novartis
    Consumer) **514, 828**
  DIGESTIVE AIDS
DDS-Acidophilus Capsules, Tablets,
    and Powder (UAS Labs).............. **767**
Perfect Meal (AdvoCare).................. **798**
Probiotica Tablets (McNeil
    Consumer)..................... **510, 822**
ProBiotic Restore Capsules
    (AdvoCare)......................... **799**
  DIGESTIVE ENZYMES
Beano Liquid (Block)..................... **809**
Beano Tablets (Block).................... **809**
Fiber 10 Packets (AdvoCare) **797**
Lactaid Original Strength
    Caplets (McNeil Consumer).... **509, 822**
Lactaid Extra Strength Caplets
    (McNeil Consumer)............. **509, 822**
Lactaid Ultra Caplets and
    Chewable Tablets (McNeil
    Consumer)..................... **509, 822**
Lactaid Drops (McNeil
    Consumer)..................... **509, 822**
System 3-4-3 Capsules (AdvoCare)...... **800**
  FIBER SUPPLEMENTS
Fiber 10 Packets (AdvoCare) **797**
Metamucil Dietary Fiber Supplement
    (Procter & Gamble) **834**
System 3-4-3 Capsules (AdvoCare)...... **800**
  GARLIC & COMBINATIONS
Beta-C Tablets (Body Wise).............. **811**
  HERBAL COMBINATIONS
    DHEA & COMBINATIONS
  DHEA Plus Capsules (Wellness
    International) **844**
    ECHINACEA & COMBINATIONS
  Centrum Echinacea Softgels
    (Whitehall-Robins) **852**
  Cold Season Nutrition Booster
    Capsules (AdvoCare) **796**
  ReSource Wellness ResistEx
    Capsules (Novartis
    Consumer) **514, 826**
  System 3-4-3 Capsules
    (AdvoCare) **800**
    GARLIC & COMBINATIONS
  CorePlex Capsules (AdvoCare) **796**
  One-A-Day Garlic Softgels
    (Bayer Consumer)............ **505, 806**
  System 3-4-3 Capsules
    (AdvoCare) **800**
    GINKGO BILOBA & COMBINATIONS
  Centrum Focused Formulas
    Mental Clarity Tablets (Lederle
    Consumer)......................... **816**
  Centrum Ginkgo Biloba Softgels
    (Whitehall-Robins) **852**
  CorePlex Capsules (AdvoCare) **796**
  FemEssence Capsules (AdvoCare) **796**
  Ginkoba M/E Suppli-Cap
    Capsules (Pharmaton)....... **521, 829**
  Ginkoba Tablets (Pharmaton)......... **828**
  IntelleQ Capsules (AdvoCare) **797**
  ProForm Bars (AdvoCare).............. **799**
  ReSource Wellness EnVigor
    Caplets (Novartis
    Consumer) **514, 824**
  ReSource Wellness
    MemorAble Softgels
    (Novartis Consumer)......... **514, 825**

DIETARY SUPPLEMENTS—*cont.*

HERBAL COMBINATIONS—*cont.*

GINKGO BILOBA & COMBINATIONS—*cont.*

Right Choice A.M. Multi Formula
Caplets (Body Wise) **811**
Vitamist Intra-Oral Spray (Mayor) **821**

GINSENG & COMBINATIONS

Centrum Focused Formulas
Energy Tablets (Lederle
Consumer) **816**
Centrum Ginseng Softgels
(Whitehall-Robins) **853**
Ginkoba M/E Suppli-Cap
Capsules (Pharmaton) **521, 829**
Ginsana Capsules (Pharmaton) **830**
Ginsana Chewy Squares
(Pharmaton)...................**521, 830**
Ginsana Sport Capsules
(Pharmaton)...................**521, 831**
Metabolic Nutrition System
(AdvoCare) **798**
MetaBoost Caplets (AdvoCare).........**798**
Performance Gold Caplets
(AdvoCare) **798**
Performance Optimizer System
(AdvoCare) **798**
ReSource Wellness EnVigor
Caplets (Novartis
Consumer) **514, 824**
ReSource Wellness ResistEx
Capsules (Novartis
Consumer) **514, 826**
ReSource Wellness 2ndWind
Capsules (Novartis
Consumer) **514, 826**

HYPERICUM & COMBINATIONS

Brite-Life Caplets (AdvoCare) **795**
Centrum St. John's Wort Softgels
(Whitehall-Robins) **853**
Movana Tablets (Pharmaton) **521, 832**
ReSource Wellness
StayCalm Caplets
(Novartis Consumer).........**514, 826**
Vitamist Intra-Oral Spray (Mayor) **821**

MISCELLANEOUS HERBAL COMBINATIONS

Advantin Capsules (AdvoCare).........**794**
Alluna Sleep Tablets (SmithKline
Beecham Consumer) **837**
Ambrotose Capsules
(Mannatech) **508, 819**
Ambrotose Powder
(Mannatech) **508, 819**
Ambrotose with Lecithin Capsules
(Mannatech) **819**
Centrum Saw Palmetto Softgels
(Whitehall-Robins) **853**
Cold Season Nutrition Booster
Capsules (AdvoCare) **796**
PhytAloe Capsules
(Mannatech) **508, 819**
PhytAloe Powder
(Mannatech) **508, 819**
Prostatonin Softgel
Capsules (Pharmaton) **521, 832**
Remifemin Menopause Tablets
(SmithKline Beecham
Consumer).......................**839**
ReSource Wellness VeinTain
Caplets (Novartis
Consumer) **514, 827**
Sleep-Tite Caplets (Wellness
International) **850**
Venastat Suppli-Cap
Capsules (Pharmaton).......**521, 833**

HERBAL & MINERAL COMBINATIONS

BioLean LipoTrim Capsules (Wellness
International) **843**
Fat Metabolizer + Capsules
(Youngevity)......................**854**
LipoTrol Caplets (AdvoCare) **797**
MetaBoost Caplets (AdvoCare)..........**798**
One-A-Day Bedtime & Rest
Tablets (Bayer Consumer) **505, 805**
One-A-Day Prostate Health
Softgels (Bayer Consumer) **505, 808**
ProMotion Capsules (AdvoCare).........**800**
Second Look Capsules (AdvoCare)......**800**
StePHan Masculine Capsules
(Wellness International) **849**
Super Anti-Oxidant Cell Protector
Capsules (Youngevity) **854**

HERBAL & VITAMIN COMBINATIONS

Beta-C Tablets (Body Wise)..............**811**
Centrum Focused Formulas Energy
Tablets (Lederle Consumer) **816**
Centrum Focused Formulas Prostate
Softgels (Lederle Consumer) **816**
FemEssence Capsules (AdvoCare) **796**
IntelleQ Capsules (AdvoCare) **797**
One-A-Day Cholesterol Health
Tablets (Bayer Consumer) **505, 805**
One-A-Day Energy Formula
Tablets (Bayer Consumer) **505, 806**
One-A-Day Joint Health Tablets
(Bayer Consumer).............**505, 806**
One-A-Day Memory &
Concentration Tablets
(Bayer Consumer).............**505, 807**
One-A-Day Menopause Health
Tablets (Bayer Consumer) **505, 808**
One-A-Day Tension & Mood
Softgels (Bayer Consumer) **505, 808**
ProForm Bars (AdvoCare)...............**799**
Right Choice A.M. Multi Formula
Caplets (Body Wise) **811**
StePHan Clarity Capsules (Wellness
International) **844**

HERBAL, MINERAL & VITAMIN COMBINATIONS

ActoTherm Caplets (AdvoCare) **794**
Antioxidant Booster Caplets
(AdvoCare) **794**
BioLean Free Tablets (Wellness
International) **843**
CardiOptima Drink Mix Packets
(AdvoCare)......................**795**
Centrum Focused Formulas Heart
Tablets (Lederle Consumer) **816**
Centrum Focused Formulas Mental
Clarity Tablets (Lederle
Consumer) **816**
Centrum Performance
Multivitamin-Multimineral Tablets
(Lederle Consumer)...............**817**
Coffeccino Beverage Mix (AdvoCare)....**796**
CorePlex Capsules (AdvoCare) **796**
HGH-Turn Back the Hands of Time
Capsules (Youngevity) **854**
Macro-Mineral Complex Caplets
(AdvoCare)......................**797**
Metabolic Nutrition System
(AdvoCare)......................**798**
Performance Optimizer System
(AdvoCare)......................**798**
Phyto-Vite Tablets (Wellness
International) **849**
ReSource Wellness EnVigor
Caplets (Novartis
Consumer) **514, 824**

ReSource Wellness StayCalm
Caplets (Novartis
Consumer) **514, 826**
Satiete Tablets (Wellness
International) **846**
StePHan Elasticity Capsules
(Wellness International) **847**
StePHan Elixir Capsules (Wellness
International) **848**
StePHan Lovpil Capsules (Wellness
International) **849**
StePHan Tranquility Capsules
(Wellness International) **851**
Super Food Soy Shake (Youngevity) **854**
Sure2Endure Tablets (Wellness
International) **851**
System 3-4-3 Capsules (AdvoCare)......**800**
Thermo-E Caplets (AdvoCare) **801**
Thermo-G Caplets (AdvoCare) **801**
Vitamist Intra-Oral Spray (Mayor) **821**
Vitasana Gelcaps (Pharmaton) **521, 834**
ZZZ Spray Liquid (AdvoCare)............**801**

IMMUNE SYSTEM SUPPORT

Ag-Immune Tablets (Body Wise) **810**
Ambrotose Capsules
(Mannatech) **508, 819**
Ambrotose Powder (Mannatech)...**508, 819**
Ambrotose with Lecithin Capsules
(Mannatech) **819**
BioChoice Immune26 Powder
and Capsules (Legacy for
Life)........................**508, 818**
BioChoice Immune Support Powder
(Legacy for Life)..................**818**
Biomune OSF Plus Capsules
(Matol) **508, 820**
PhytAloe Capsules (Mannatech)...**508, 819**
PhytAloe Powder (Mannatech) **508, 819**
Plus Caplets (Mannatech) **508, 820**
ReSource Wellness ResistEx
Capsules (Novartis
Consumer) **514, 826**
Transfer Factor Capsules (4Life)...**526, 814**

MINERALS & ELECTROLYTES

CALCIUM & COMBINATIONS

Caltrate 600 Tablets (Lederle
Consumer)..................... **814**
Caltrate 600 PLUS Chewables
(Lederle Consumer)................**815**
Caltrate 600 PLUS Tablets
(Lederle Consumer)................**815**
Caltrate 600 + D Tablets (Lederle
Consumer).......................**814**
Caltrate 600 + Soy Tablets
(Lederle Consumer)................**814**
Citracal Liquitab Tablets (Mission) **823**
Citracal Tablets (Mission)...............**823**
Citracal Caplets + D (Mission).........**823**
Citracal 250 MG + D Tablets
(Mission).........................**823**
Citracal Plus Tablets (Mission) **824**
D-Cal Chewable Caplets
(A & Z Pharm)................**503, 794**
Extra Strength Mylanta Calci
Tabs Tablets (J&J •
Merck) **507, 636**
Ultra Mylanta Calci Tabs
Tablets (J&J • Merck)........**507, 636**
One-A-Day Bedtime & Rest
Tablets (Bayer
Consumer) **505, 805**
One-A-Day Calcium Plus
Chewable Tablets (Bayer
Consumer) **505, 805**
Os-Cal Chewable Tablets
(SmithKline Beecham
Consumer) **525, 838**

Os-Cal 250 + D Tablets
(SmithKline Beecham
Consumer) **525, 838**
Os-Cal 500 Tablets
(SmithKline Beecham
Consumer) **525, 839**
Os-Cal 500 + D Tablets
(SmithKline Beecham
Consumer) **525, 839**
Prelief Tablets and
Granulate (AK Pharma) **503, 801**
ReSource Wellness
CalciWise Soft Chews
(Novartis Consumer).........**514, 824**
MAGNESIUM & COMBINATIONS
Beelith Tablets (Beach) **809**
Magonate Liquid (Fleming) **814**
Magonate Natal Liquid (Fleming) **814**
Magonate Tablets (Fleming) **814**
Slow-Mag Tablets (Shire) **835**
MULTIMINERALS & COMBINATIONS
Centrum Focused Formulas Bone
Health Tablets (Lederle
Consumer).........................**815**

MISCELLANEOUS DIETARY SUPPLEMENTS
Aflexa Tablets (McNeil Consumer) . **508, 821**
Doctor Ginsberg's Psoria Rid
Cream (Strategic Science).....**525, 840**
Intelectol Tablets (Covex) **507, 813**
Meyenberg Goat Milk (Meyenberg) **823**
Natural Arousal Cream
(Strategic Science).............**525, 840**
Natural Sensation Cream (Strategic
Science) **841**
Nature's Own Pain Expeller Cream
(Strategic Science) **841**
ReSource Wellness AllerPro
Capsules (Novartis
Consumer).....................**514, 824**
ReSource Wellness FlexTend
Caplets (Novartis
Consumer) **514, 825**
Second Look Capsules (AdvoCare)......**800**
Thermo-E Caplets (AdvoCare) **801**
Warm Cream (Strategic
Science) **525, 841**

VITAMINS & COMBINATIONS
 GERIATRIC FORMULATIONS
 Centrum Silver Tablets (Lederle
 Consumer)...........................**818**
 MULTIMINERALS & COMBINATIONS
 Right Choice P.M. Multi Formula
 Caplets (Body Wise) **812**
 MULTIVITAMINS & COMBINATIONS
 Bugs Bunny Children's
 Multivitamin Plus Extra C
 Chewable Tablets (Sugar
 Free) (Bayer Consumer)......**504, 804**
 Centrum Focused Formulas
 Energy Tablets (Lederle
 Consumer).........................**816**
 Flintstones Original
 Children's Multivitamin
 Chewable Tablets (Bayer
 Consumer) **504, 802**
 Flintstones Children's
 Multivitamin Plus Extra C
 Chewable Tablets (Bayer
 Consumer) **504, 804**
 HeartBar (Cooke) **812**
 One-A-Day Essential Tablets
 (Bayer Consumer)............**504, 806**
 Right Choice A.M. Multi Formula
 Caplets (Body Wise) **811**
 MULTIVITAMINS WITH MINERALS
 BodyLean Powder (AdvoCare) **795**

Bugs Bunny Children's
Multivitamin Plus Iron
Chewable Tablets (Bayer
Consumer) **504, 802**
Bugs Bunny Complete
Children's Multivitamin/
Multimineral Chewable
Tablets (Sugar Free)
(Bayer Consumer)...........**504, 803**
Centrum Focused Formulas
Mental Clarity Tablets (Lederle
Consumer)...........................**816**
Centrum Kids Complete
Children's Chewables (Lederle
Consumer).......................**817**
Centrum Performance
Multivitamin-Multimineral
Tablets (Lederle Consumer) **817**
Centrum Tablets (Lederle
Consumer).........................**815**
Centrum Silver Tablets (Lederle
Consumer).........................**818**
Flintstones Children's
Multivitamin Plus
Calcium Chewable
Tablets (Bayer
Consumer) **504, 804**
Flintstones Children's
Multivitamin Plus Iron
Chewable Tablets (Bayer
Consumer) **504, 802**
Flintstones Complete
Children's Mutivitamin/
Multimineral Chewable
Tablets (Bayer
Consumer) **504, 803**
Food for Thought Drink Mix
(Wellness International) **844**
One-A-Day Antioxidant
Softgels (Bayer
Consumer) **504, 805**
One-A-Day 50 Plus Tablets
(Bayer Consumer)............**504, 804**
One-A-Day Kids Complete
Tablets (Bayer
Consumer) **505, 806**
One-A-Day Maximum Tablets
(Bayer Consumer)............**504, 807**
One-A-Day Men's Tablets
(Bayer Consumer)............**504, 808**
One-A-Day Women's Tablets
(Bayer Consumer)............**504, 809**
Perfect Meal (AdvoCare)...............**798**
ReSource Wellness
CalciWise Soft Chews
(Novartis Consumer).........**514, 824**
ReSource Wellness ForSight
Caplets (Novartis
Consumer) **514, 825**
Spark! Beverage Mix (AdvoCare) **800**
StePHan Flexibility Capsules
(Wellness International) **848**
Vitamist Intra-Oral Spray (Mayor) **821**
Vitasana Gelcaps
(Pharmaton)..................**521, 834**
Winrgy Drink Mix (Wellness
International) **852**
PEDIATRIC FORMULATIONS
Bugs Bunny Children's
Multivitamin Plus Iron
Chewable Tablets (Bayer
Consumer) **504, 802**
Bugs Bunny Children's
Multivitamin Plus Extra C
Chewable Tablets (Sugar
Free) (Bayer Consumer)......**504, 804**

Bugs Bunny Complete
Children's Multivitamin/
Multimineral Chewable
Tablets (Sugar Free)
(Bayer Consumer)...........**504, 803**
Centrum Kids Complete
Children's Chewables (Lederle
Consumer).......................**817**
Flintstones Original
Children's Multivitamin
Chewable Tablets (Bayer
Consumer) **504, 802**
Flintstones Children's
Multivitamin Plus Extra C
Chewable Tablets (Bayer
Consumer) **504, 804**
Flintstones Children's
Multivitamin Plus Iron
Chewable Tablets (Bayer
Consumer) **504, 802**
Flintstones Complete
Children's Mutivitamin/
Multimineral Chewable
Tablets (Bayer
Consumer) **504, 803**
One-A-Day Kids Complete
Tablets (Bayer
Consumer) **505, 806**
PRENATAL FORMULATIONS
Metamucil Dietary Fiber
Supplement (Procter &
Gamble).............................**834**
VITAMIN A & COMBINATIONS
Centrum Focused Formulas
Prostate Softgels (Lederle
Consumer).........................**816**
B VITAMINS & COMBINATIONS
Brite-Life Caplets (AdvoCare) **795**
Lipoflavonoid Caplets (Numark) **828**
Nicotinex Elixir (Fleming)...............**633**
VITAMIN C & COMBINATIONS
C-Grams Caplets (AdvoCare) **795**
Halls Defense Drops (Pfizer
Inc., Warner-Lambert
Group) **516, 687**
Peridin-C Tablets (Beutlich) **618**

E
EAR WAX REMOVAL
(*see under:*
OTIC PREPARATIONS
 CERUMENOLYTICS)
ELECTROLYTES
(*see under:*
DIETARY SUPPLEMENTS
 MINERALS & ELECTROLYTES)
EXPECTORANTS
(*see under:*
RESPIRATORY AGENTS
 DECONGESTANTS, EXPECTORANTS & COMBINATIONS
 EXPECTORANTS & COMBINATIONS)

F
FEVER PREPARATIONS
(*see under:*
ANALGESICS
 ACETAMINOPHEN & COMBINATIONS
 NONSTEROIDAL ANTI-INFLAMMATORY DRUGS (NSAIDS)
 SALICYLATES)
FOOT CARE PRODUCTS
(*see under:*
SKIN & MUCOUS MEMBRANE AGENTS
 FOOT CARE PRODUCTS)
FUNGAL MEDICATIONS
(*see under:*
SKIN & MUCOUS MEMBRANE AGENTS
 ANTI-INFECTIVES
 ANTIFUNGALS & COMBINATIONS
VAGINAL PREPARATIONS
 ANTI-INFECTIVES
 ANTIFUNGALS & COMBINATIONS)

G

GASTROINTESTINAL AGENTS

ANTACIDS

ALUMINUM ANTACIDS & COMBINATIONS
Amphojel Suspension (Mint Flavor) (Wyeth-Ayerst).......**526, 789**

CALCIUM ANTACIDS & COMBINATIONS
Quick Dissolve Maalox Antacid Chewable Tablets (Novartis Consumer)........**514, 674**
Quick Dissolve Maalox Max Maximum Strength Antacid/Antigas Chewable Tablets (Novartis Consumer)........**514, 674**
Children's Mylanta Upset Stomach Relief Liquid (J&J • Merck)..............**508, 634**
Children's Mylanta Upset Stomach Relief Tablets (J&J • Merck)..............**508, 634**
Extra Strength Mylanta Calci Tabs Tablets (J&J • Merck)........**507, 636**
Ultra Mylanta Calci Tabs Tablets (J&J • Merck)........**507, 636**
3M Titralac Antacid Tablets (3M)..............**508, 640**
3M Titralac Extra Strength Antacid Tablets (3M)........**508, 640**
3M Titralac Plus Antacid Tablets (3M)..............**508, 640**
Tums E-X Antacid/Calcium Tablets (SmithKline Beecham Consumer)........**525, 763**
Tums E-X Sugar Free Antacid/Calcium Tablets (SmithKline Beecham Consumer)..............**525, 763**
Tums Regular Antacid/Calcium Tablets (SmithKline Beecham Consumer)..............**525, 763**
Tums ULTRA Antacid/Calcium Tablets (SmithKline Beecham Consumer)..............**525, 763**

COMBINATION ANTACIDS
Alka-Seltzer Original Antacid and Pain Reliever Effervescent Tablets (Bayer Consumer)..........**503, 603**
Alka-Seltzer Cherry Antacid and Pain Reliever Effervescent Tablets (Bayer Consumer)..........**503, 603**
Alka-Seltzer Lemon Lime Antacid and Pain Reliever Effervescent Tablets (Bayer Consumer)..............**503, 603**
Alka-Seltzer Extra Strength Antacid and Pain Reliever Effervescent Tablets (Bayer Consumer)..............**503, 603**
Alka-Seltzer Heartburn Relief Tablets (Bayer Consumer)..............**503, 604**
Gaviscon Extra Strength Liquid (SmithKline Beecham Consumer) **524, 751**
Gaviscon Extra Strength Tablets (SmithKline Beecham Consumer) **524, 751**

Gaviscon Regular Strength Liquid (SmithKline Beecham Consumer) **524, 751**
Gaviscon Regular Strength Tablets (SmithKline Beecham Consumer) **524, 750**
Marblen Suspension (Fleming) **633**
Mylanta Gelcaps (J&J • Merck)..............**507, 637**
Mylanta Supreme Liquid (J&J • Merck)..............**507, 636**
Mylanta Ultra Tabs Tablets (J&J • Merck)..............**507, 637**
Pepcid Complete Chewable Tablets (J&J • Merck)........**508, 638**
Rolaids Tablets (Pfizer Inc., Warner-Lambert Healthcare)..............**519, 706**
Extra Strength Rolaids Tablets (Pfizer Inc., Warner-Lambert Healthcare)..............**519, 706**

MAGNESIUM ANTACIDS & COMBINATIONS
Ex•Lax Milk of Magnesia Liquid (Novartis Consumer)..............**513, 670**
Phillips' Chewable Tablets (Bayer Consumer)..............**615**
Phillips' Milk of Magnesia Liquid (Original, Cherry, & Mint) (Bayer Consumer)..............**505, 616**

MISCELLANEOUS ANTACID PREPARATIONS
Alka-Seltzer Heartburn Relief Tablets (Bayer Consumer) ...**503, 604**

ANTACID & ANTIFLATULENT COMBINATIONS
Maalox Antacid/Anti-Gas Oral Suspension (Novartis Consumer)..............**514, 673**
Maalox Max Maximum Strength Antacid/Anti-Gas Liquid (Novartis Consumer)..........**514, 673**
Mylanta Liquid (J&J • Merck)............**634**
Mylanta Extra Strength Liquid (J&J • Merck)..............**507, 634**
3M Titralac Plus Antacid Tablets (3M)..............**508, 640**

ANTIDIARRHEALS
Donnagel Liquid (Wyeth-Ayerst)....**526, 789**
Imodium A-D Liquid and Caplets (McNeil Consumer) **509, 641**
Imodium Advanced Chewable Tablets (McNeil Consumer) **509, 641**
Mitrolan Chewable Tablets (Wyeth-Ayerst)..................**526, 789**
Pepto-Bismol Original Liquid, Original and Cherry Chewable Tablets & Caplets (Procter & Gamble) **521, 723**
Pepto-Bismol Maximum Strength Liquid (Procter & Gamble) **724**

ANTIEMETICS
Bonine Chewable Tablets (Pfizer Inc., Warner-Lambert Healthcare) **518, 698**
Dramamine Original Formula Tablets (Pharmacia Consumer) **718**
Dramamine Chewable Formula Tablets (Pharmacia Consumer)......**718**
Dramamine Less Drowsy Tablets (Pharmacia Consumer) **718**
Emetrol Oral Solution (Lemon-Mint & Cherry Flavors) (Pharmacia Consumer)..........................**718**

Pepto-Bismol Original Liquid, Original and Cherry Chewable Tablets & Caplets (Procter & Gamble) **521, 723**
Pepto-Bismol Maximum Strength Liquid (Procter & Gamble) **724**

ANTIFLATULENTS
Maximum Strength Gas Aid Softgels (McNeil Consumer)...**509, 640**
Gas-X Chewable Tablets (Novartis Consumer)..........**513, 671**
Extra Strength Gas-X Liquid (Novartis Consumer)..........**513, 671**
Extra Strength Gas-X Softgels (Novartis Consumer)..........**513, 671**
Extra Strength Gas-X Chewable Tablets (Novartis Consumer) ..**513, 671**
Maximum Strength Gas-X Softgels (Novartis Consumer)....................**513, 671**
Imodium Advanced Chewable Tablets (McNeil Consumer) **509, 641**
Quick Dissolve Maalox Max Maximum Strength Antacid/Antigas Chewable Tablets (Novartis Consumer)..........**514, 674**
Mylanta Gas Softgels (J&J • Merck)..............**507, 637**
Mylanta Gas Tablets (J&J • Merck)......**637**
Maximum Strength Mylanta Gas Tablets (J&J • Merck)..........**507, 637**
Infants' Mylicon Drops (J&J • Merck)..............**508, 634**
Phazyme-125 mg Quick Dissolve Chewable Tablets (Block)..............**506, 622**
Phazyme-180 mg Ultra Strength Softgels (Block)................**506, 622**

HISTAMINE (H₂) RECEPTOR ANTAGONISTS
Pepcid AC Tablets, Chewable Tablets, and Gelcaps (J&J • Merck)..............**508, 638**
Tagamet HB 200 Suspension (SmithKline Beecham Consumer)....................**525, 762**
Tagamet HB 200 Tablets (SmithKline Beecham Consumer)....................**525, 761**
Zantac 75 Tablets (Pfizer Inc., Warner-Lambert Healthcare)...**528, 717**

HISTAMINE (H₂) RECEPTOR ANTAGONISTS & COMBINATIONS
Pepcid Complete Chewable Tablets (J&J • Merck)..........**508, 638**

LAXATIVES

BULK-PRODUCING LAXATIVES
Citrucel Caplets (SmithKline Beecham Consumer) **745**
Citrucel Orange Flavor Powder (SmithKline Beecham Consumer) **523, 744**
Citrucel Sugar Free Orange Flavor Powder (SmithKline Beecham Consumer) **523, 745**
FiberCon Caplets (Lederle Consumer)..........................**639**
Maltsupex Powder, Liquid, Tablets (Wallace)............**525, 767**
Metamucil Powder, Original Texture Orange Flavor (Procter & Gamble) **722**
Metamucil Powder, Original Texture Regular Flavor (Procter & Gamble) **722**

Metamucil Smooth Texture
Powder, Orange Flavor
(Procter & Gamble) **521, 722**
Metamucil Smooth Texture
Powder, Sugar-Free, Orange
Flavor (Procter & Gamble) **722**
Metamucil Smooth Texture
Powder, Sugar-Free, Regular
Flavor (Procter & Gamble) **722**
Metamucil Wafers, Apple
Crisp & Cinnamon Spice
Flavors (Procter &
Gamble)...................... **521, 722**
Mitrolan Chewable Tablets
(Wyeth-Ayerst)............... **526, 789**
Perdiem Fiber Therapy
Granules (Novartis
Consumer) **514, 675**
Perdiem Overnight Relief
Granules (Novartis
Consumer) **514, 674**
Phillips' FiberCaps Caplets
(Bayer Consumer)........... **505, 615**

FECAL SOFTENERS & COMBINATIONS
Colace Capsules, Syrup and
Drops (Shire) **743**
Ex•Lax Gentle Strength
Caplets (Novartis
Consumer) **513, 670**
Ex•Lax Stool Softener
Caplets (Novartis
Consumer) **513, 671**
Phillips' Liqui-Gels (Bayer
Consumer)........................ **616**
Senokot-S Tablets (Purdue
Frederick) **522, 732**
Surfak Liqui-Gels (Pharmacia
Consumer)........................ **721**

LAXATIVE COMBINATIONS
Perdiem Overnight Relief
Granules (Novartis
Consumer) **514, 674**
Peri-Colace Capsules and Syrup
(Shire) **743**
Senokot-S Tablets (Purdue
Frederick) **522, 732**

SALINE LAXATIVES
Ex•Lax Milk of Magnesia
Liquid (Novartis
Consumer) **513, 670**
Phillips' Chewable Tablets (Bayer
Consumer)........................ **615**
Phillips' Milk of Magnesia
Liquid (Original, Cherry,
& Mint) (Bayer
Consumer) **505, 616**

STIMULANT LAXATIVES & COMBINATIONS
Ceo-Two Evacuant Suppository
(Beutlich) **618**
Correctol Laxative Tablets
and Caplets
(Schering-Plough) **523, 739**
Dulcolax Suppositories
(Novartis Consumer)........ **513, 668**
Dulcolax Tablets (Novartis
Consumer) **513, 668**
Ex•Lax Gentle Strength
Caplets (Novartis
Consumer) **513, 670**
Ex•Lax Regular Strength
Pills (Novartis
Consumer) **513, 670**
Ex•Lax Regular Strength
Chocolated Pieces
(Novartis Consumer)........ **513, 669**

Ex•Lax Maximum Strength
Pills (Novartis
Consumer) **513, 670**
Nature's Remedy Tablets
(Block) **506, 621**
Perdiem Overnight Relief
Granules (Novartis
Consumer) **514, 674**
Purge Liquid (Fleming) **633**
Senokot Children's Syrup
(Purdue Frederick) **522, 732**
Senokot Granules (Purdue
Frederick) **522, 732**
Senokot Syrup (Purdue
Frederick) **522, 732**
Senokot Tablets (Purdue
Frederick) **522, 732**
Senokot-S Tablets (Purdue
Frederick) **522, 732**
SenokotXTRA Tablets (Purdue
Frederick) **732**

GENITAL WART PREPARATIONS
(see under:
SKIN & MUCOUS MEMBRANE AGENTS
WART PREPARATIONS)
GLAUCOMA PREPARATIONS
(see under:
OPHTHALMIC PREPARATIONS
SYMPATHOMIMETICS & COMBINATIONS)

H

HAIR GROWTH STIMULANTS
(see under:
SKIN & MUCOUS MEMBRANE AGENTS
HAIR GROWTH STIMULANTS)
HEAD LICE RELIEF
(see under:
SKIN & MUCOUS MEMBRANE AGENTS
ANTI-INFECTIVES
SCABICIDES & PEDICULICIDES)
HEMATINICS
(see under:
DIETARY SUPPLEMENTS
BLOOD MODIFIERS
IRON & COMBINATIONS)
HEMORRHOIDAL PREPARATIONS
(see under:
SKIN & MUCOUS MEMBRANE AGENTS
ANORECTAL PREPARATIONS)
HERPES TREATMENT
(see under:
SKIN & MUCOUS MEMBRANE AGENTS
MOUTH & THROAT PRODUCTS
COLD SORE PREPARATIONS)
HISTAMINE (H₂) RECEPTOR ANTAGONISTS
(see under:
GASTROINTESTINAL AGENTS
HISTAMINE (H₂) RECEPTOR ANTAGONISTS)
HOMEOPATHIC REMEDIES

COLD & FLU PRODUCTS
Biomune OSF Express Spray
(Matol) **508, 640**
Hyland's Cold Tablets with Zinc
(Standard Homeopathic)............. **765**
Oscillococcinum Pellets (Boiron) **625**

GASTROINTESTINAL AGENTS
Hyland's Colic Tablets (Standard
Homeopathic)........................ **765**

IMMUNE SYSTEM SUPPORT
Relief Nasal & Throat Spray (Body
Wise) **811**

MISCELLANEOUS HOMEOPATHIC REMEDIES
Hyland's Bumps 'n Bruises Tablets
(Standard Homeopathic)............. **764**
Hyland's Calms Forté Tablets and
Caplets (Standard Homeopathic).... **764**

Hyland's MenoCalm Tablets
(Standard Homeopathic)............. **765**
Hyland's Nerve Tonic Tablets and
Caplets (Standard Homeopathic).... **766**
PAIN RELIEVERS
Hyland's Arnisport Tablets (Standard
Homeopathic)........................ **764**
Hyland's Back Ache with Arnica
Caplets (Standard Homeopathic).... **764**
Hyland's Earache Tablets (Standard
Homeopathic)........................ **765**
Hyland's Leg Cramps with Quinine
Tablets (Standard Homeopathic) **765**
Smile's Prid Salve (Standard
Homeopathic)........................ **766**
SEDATIVES & HYPNOTICS
Nytol Natural Tablets (Block)....... **506, 622**
TEETHING REMEDIES
Hyland's Teething Gel (Standard
Homeopathic)........................ **766**
Hyland's Teething Tablets (Standard
Homeopathic)........................ **766**
HYPNOTICS
(see under:
SEDATIVES & HYPNOTICS)

I

IMMUNE SYSTEM SUPPORT
(see under:
DIETARY SUPPLEMENTS
IMMUNE SYSTEM SUPPORT
HOMEOPATHIC REMEDIES
IMMUNE SYSTEM SUPPORT)
IRON DEFICIENCY
(see under:
DIETARY SUPPLEMENTS
BLOOD MODIFIERS
IRON & COMBINATIONS)

K

KERATOLYTICS
(see under:
SKIN & MUCOUS MEMBRANE AGENTS
KERATOLYTICS)

L

LAXATIVES
(see under:
GASTROINTESTINAL AGENTS
LAXATIVES)
LICE TREATMENTS
(see under:
SKIN & MUCOUS MEMBRANE AGENTS
ANTI-INFECTIVES
SCABICIDES & PEDICULICIDES)
LUBRICANTS
(see under:
NASAL PREPARATIONS
SALINE
OPHTHALMIC PREPARATIONS
ARTIFICIAL TEARS/LUBRICANTS & COMBINATIONS
SKIN & MUCOUS MEMBRANE AGENTS
EMOLLIENTS & MOISTURIZERS)

M

MAGNESIUM PREPARATIONS
(see under:
DIETARY SUPPLEMENTS
MINERALS & ELECTROLYTES
MAGNESIUM & COMBINATIONS)
MALE PATTERN HAIR LOSS TREATMENTS
(see under:
SKIN & MUCOUS MEMBRANE AGENTS
HAIR GROWTH STIMULANTS)
MAST CELL STABILIZERS
NasalCrom Nasal Spray (Pharmacia
Consumer)........................... **719**

MIGRAINE PREPARATIONS
MISCELLANEOUS MIGRAINE PREPARATIONS
Excedrin Migraine Tablets, Caplets, and Geltabs (Bristol-Myers) **507, 630**
Motrin Migraine Pain Caplets (McNeil Consumer) **510, 646**
MINERALS
(*see under:*
DIETARY SUPPLEMENTS
MINERALS & ELECTROLYTES)
MOISTURIZERS
(*see under:*
OPHTHALMIC PREPARATIONS
ARTIFICIAL TEARS/LUBRICANTS & COMBINATIONS
SKIN & MUCOUS MEMBRANE AGENTS
EMOLLIENTS & MOISTURIZERS)
MOTION SICKNESS PRODUCTS
Bonine Chewable Tablets (Pfizer Inc., Warner-Lambert Healthcare) **518, 698**
Dramamine Original Formula Tablets (Pharmacia Consumer) **718**
Dramamine Chewable Formula Tablets (Pharmacia Consumer)......**718**
Dramamine Less Drowsy Tablets (Pharmacia Consumer) **718**
MOUTH & THROAT PRODUCTS
(*see under:*
SKIN & MUCOUS MEMBRANE AGENTS
MOUTH & THROAT PRODUCTS)
MOUTHWASHES
(*see under:*
SKIN & MUCOUS MEMBRANE AGENTS
MOUTH & THROAT PRODUCTS
ORAL RINSES)
MUCOLYTICS
(*see under:*
RESPIRATORY AGENTS
DECONGESTANTS, EXPECTORANTS & COMBINATIONS
EXPECTORANTS & COMBINATIONS)

N
NAIL PREPARATIONS
(*see under:*
SKIN & MUCOUS MEMBRANE AGENTS)
NARCOTICS
(*see under:*
RESPIRATORY AGENTS
ANTITUSSIVES
NARCOTIC ANTITUSSIVES & COMBINATIONS)
NASAL PREPARATIONS
MAST CELL STABILIZERS
NasalCrom Nasal Spray (Pharmacia Consumer)............................**719**
SALINE
Afrin Saline Aromatic Mist (Schering-Plough) **734**
Afrin Extra Moisturizing Saline Mist (Schering-Plough) **522, 734**
Natru-Vent Saline Nasal Spray (Boehringer Ingelheim).........**506, 625**
Ocean Nasal Mist (Fleming) **633**
SYMPATHOMIMETICS & COMBINATIONS
Afrin Nasal Decongestant Children's Pump Mist (Schering-Plough) **734**
Afrin Original Nasal Spray (Schering-Plough) **522, 733**
Afrin Extra Moisturizing Nasal Spray (Schering-Plough) **733**
Afrin Severe Congestion Nasal Spray (Schering-Plough) **733**
Afrin Sinus Nasal Spray (Schering-Plough) **733**
Afrin No Drip Original Nasal Spray (Schering-Plough)........**522, 735**

Afrin No Drip Extra Moisturizing Nasal Spray (Schering-Plough) **735**
Afrin No Drip Severe Congestion Nasal Spray (Schering-Plough).......**735**
Afrin No Drip Sinus Nasal Spray (Schering-Plough) **735**
Afrin Original Pump Mist (Schering-Plough) **733**
Natru-Vent Nasal Spray, Adult Strength (Boehringer Ingelheim).......................**506, 624**
Natru-Vent Nasal Spray, Pediatric Strength (Boehringer Ingelheim).........**506, 625**
Neo-Synephrine Nasal Drops, Regular and Extra Strength (Bayer Consumer)..............**504, 614**
Neo-Synephrine Nasal Sprays, Mild, Regular and Extra Strength (Bayer Consumer)....**504, 614**
Neo-Synephrine 12 Hour Nasal Spray (Bayer Consumer).......**504, 615**
Neo-Synephrine 12 Hour Extra Moisturizing Nasal Spray (Bayer Consumer).....................**615**
Vicks Sinex Nasal Spray and Ultra Fine Mist (Procter & Gamble)........**729**
Vicks Sinex 12-Hour Nasal Spray and Ultra Fine Mist (Procter & Gamble)...........................**729**
Vicks Vapor Inhaler (Procter & Gamble).............................**730**
NAUSEA MEDICATIONS
(*see under:*
GASTROINTESTINAL AGENTS
ANTIEMETICS
MOTION SICKNESS PRODUCTS)
NONSTEROIDAL ANTI-INFLAMMATORY AGENTS (NSAIDS)
(*see under:*
ANALGESICS
NONSTEROIDAL ANTI-INFLAMMATORY DRUGS (NSAIDS))
NSAIDS
(*see under:*
ANALGESICS
NONSTEROIDAL ANTI-INFLAMMATORY DRUGS (NSAIDS))
NUTRITIONALS
(*see under:*
DIETARY SUPPLEMENTS)

O
OPHTHALMIC PREPARATIONS
ADRENERGIC AGONISTS
(*see under:*
OPHTHALMIC PREPARATIONS
SYMPATHOMIMETICS & COMBINATIONS)
ANTIGLAUCOMA AGENTS
(*see under:*
OPHTHALMIC PREPARATIONS
SYMPATHOMIMETICS & COMBINATIONS)
ANTIHISTAMINES & COMBINATIONS
Visine-A Eye Drops (Pfizer Inc., Warner-Lambert Healthcare)...**521, 714**
ARTIFICIAL TEARS/LUBRICANTS & COMBINATIONS
Advanced Relief Visine Eye Drops (Pfizer Inc., Warner-Lambert Healthcare) **521, 714**
Visine Tears Eye Drops (Pfizer Inc., Warner-Lambert Healthcare) **521, 716**
Visine Tears Preservative Free Eye Drops (Pfizer Inc., Warner-Lambert Healthcare)...**521, 716**

DECONGESTANTS
(*see under:*
OPHTHALMIC PREPARATIONS
SYMPATHOMIMETICS & COMBINATIONS)
GLAUCOMA, AGENTS FOR
(*see under:*
OPHTHALMIC PREPARATIONS
SYMPATHOMIMETICS & COMBINATIONS)
LUBRICANTS
(*see under:*
OPHTHALMIC PREPARATIONS
ARTIFICIAL TEARS/LUBRICANTS & COMBINATIONS)
SYMPATHOMIMETICS & COMBINATIONS
Visine Original Eye Drops (Pfizer Inc., Warner-Lambert Healthcare) **521, 715**
Visine A.C. Eye Drops (Pfizer Inc., Warner-Lambert Healthcare) **521, 715**
Visine L.R. Eye Drops (Pfizer Inc., Warner-Lambert Healthcare) **521, 715**
Advanced Relief Visine Eye Drops (Pfizer Inc., Warner-Lambert Healthcare)...**521, 714**
Visine-A Eye Drops (Pfizer Inc., Warner-Lambert Healthcare)...**521, 714**
VASOCONSTRICTORS
(*see under:*
OPHTHALMIC PREPARATIONS
SYMPATHOMIMETICS & COMBINATIONS)
ORAL HYGIENE PRODUCTS
(*see under:*
SKIN & MUCOUS MEMBRANE AGENTS
MOUTH & THROAT PRODUCTS)
OTIC PREPARATIONS
CERUMENOLYTICS
Debrox Drops (SmithKline Beecham Consumer) **523, 747**

P
PAIN RELIEVERS
(*see under:*
ANALGESICS)
PEDICULICIDES
(*see under:*
SKIN & MUCOUS MEMBRANE AGENTS
ANTI-INFECTIVES
SCABICIDES & PEDICULICIDES)
PLATELET INHIBITORS
(*see under:*
BLOOD MODIFIERS
ANTIPLATELET AGENTS)
POISON IVY, OAK OR SUMAC PRODUCTS
(*see under:*
SKIN & MUCOUS MEMBRANE AGENTS
POISON IVY, OAK OR SUMAC PRODUCTS)
PREGNANCY TESTS
(*see under:*
DIAGNOSTICS
PREGNANCY TESTS)
PRURITUS MEDICATIONS
(*see under:*
ANTIHISTAMINES & COMBINATIONS
SKIN & MUCOUS MEMBRANE AGENTS
ANTIPRURITICS)
PSORIASIS AGENTS
(*see under:*
SKIN & MUCOUS MEMBRANE AGENTS
ANTIPSORIATIC AGENTS)

PSYCHOSTIMULANTS
(*see under:*
CENTRAL NERVOUS SYSTEM STIMULANTS)

PSYCHOTHERAPEUTIC AGENTS

PSYCHOSTIMULANTS
(*see under:*
CENTRAL NERVOUS SYSTEM STIMULANTS)

R

RESPIRATORY AGENTS
(*see also under:*
ANTIHISTAMINES & COMBINATIONS
NASAL PREPARATIONS)

ANTITUSSIVES

NARCOTIC ANTITUSSIVES & COMBINATIONS
Ryna-C Liquid (Wallace) **525, 768**

NON-NARCOTIC ANTITUSSIVES & COMBINATIONS
Alka-Seltzer Plus Night-Time Cold Medicine Liqui-Gels (Bayer Consumer) **503, 604**
Alka-Seltzer Plus Cold & Cough Medicine Liqui-Gels (Bayer Consumer) **503, 604**
Alka-Seltzer Plus Cold & Flu Medicine Liqui-Gels (Bayer Consumer) **503, 604**
Benadryl Allergy Chewables (Pfizer Inc., Warner-Lambert Healthcare) **517, 689**
Benadryl Allergy Kapseal Capsules (Pfizer Inc., Warner-Lambert Healthcare) **516, 691**
Benadryl Allergy Liquid (Pfizer Inc., Warner-Lambert Healthcare) **517, 690**
Benadryl Allergy Ultratab Tablets (Pfizer Inc., Warner-Lambert Healthcare) **516, 691**
Benadryl Allergy/Cold Tablets (Pfizer Inc., Warner-Lambert Healthcare) **517, 691**
Benylin Adult Formula Cough Suppressant Liquid (Pfizer Inc., Warner-Lambert Healthcare) **518, 696**
Benylin Cough Suppressant/ Expectorant Liquid (Pfizer Inc., Warner-Lambert Healthcare) **518, 697**
Benylin Multi-Symptom Liquid (Pfizer Inc., Warner-Lambert Healthcare) **518, 697**
Benylin Pediatric Cough Suppressant Liquid (Pfizer Inc., Warner-Lambert Healthcare) **518, 698**
Comtrex Deep Chest Cold & Congestion Relief Softgels (Bristol-Myers) **506, 627**
Comtrex Maximum Strength Multi-Symptom Cold & Cough Relief Tablets and Caplets (Bristol-Myers) **506, 626**

Contac Severe Cold and Flu Caplets Maximum Strength (SmithKline Beecham Consumer) **523, 746**
Contac Severe Cold and Flu Caplets Non-Drowsy (SmithKline Beecham Consumer) **746**
Coricidin HBP Cough & Cold Tablets (Schering-Plough) **523, 738**
Coricidin HBP Maximum Strength Flu Tablets (Schering-Plough) **523, 738**
Delsym Extended-Release Suspension (Medeva) **664**
Dimetapp DM Cold & Cough Elixir (Whitehall-Robins) **775**
Dimetapp Nighttime Flu Liquid (Whitehall-Robins) **776**
Dimetapp Non-Drowsy Flu Syrup (Whitehall-Robins) **777**
Dimetapp Infant Drops Decongestant Plus Cough (Whitehall-Robins) **776**
Halls Mentho-Lyptus Drops (Pfizer Inc., Warner-Lambert Group) **516, 686**
Halls Sugar Free Mentho-Lyptus Drops (Pfizer Inc., Warner-Lambert Group) **516, 686**
Halls Sugar Free Squares (Pfizer Inc., Warner-Lambert Group) **516, 686**
Halls Plus Cough Drops (Pfizer Inc., Warner-Lambert Group) **516, 686**
PediaCare Cough-Cold Liquid (Pharmacia Consumer) **719**
PediaCare Infants' Drops Decongestant Plus Cough (Pharmacia Consumer) **719**
PediaCare NightRest Cough-Cold Liquid (Pharmacia Consumer) **719**
Robitussin Cold Caplets Cold & Congestion (Whitehall-Robins) **780**
Robitussin Cold Caplets Multi-Symptom Cold & Flu (Whitehall-Robins) **781**
Robitussin Cold Softgels Multi-Symptom Cold & Flu (Whitehall-Robins) **781**
Robitussin Cough Drops (Whitehall-Robins) **781**
Robitussin Honey Cough Drops (Whitehall-Robins) **784**
Robitussin Honey Cough Liquid (Whitehall-Robins) **784**
Robitussin Cough & Cold Infant Drops (Whitehall-Robins) **782**
Robitussin Maximum Strength Cough & Cold Liquid (Whitehall-Robins) **785**
Robitussin Pediatric Cough & Cold Formula Liquid (Whitehall-Robins) **785**
Robitussin Maximum Strength Cough Suppressant Liquid (Whitehall-Robins) **784**
Robitussin Pediatric Cough Suppressant Liquid (Whitehall-Robins) **784**
Robitussin Multi Symptom Honey Flu Liquid (Whitehall-Robins) **785**
Robitussin Nighttime Honey Flu Liquid (Whitehall-Robins) **786**

Robitussin Honey Calmers Throat Drops (Whitehall-Robins) **783**
Robitussin Sugar Free Throat Drops (Whitehall-Robins) **786**
Robitussin-CF Liquid (Whitehall-Robins) **783**
Robitussin DM Infant Drops (Whitehall-Robins) **783**
Robitussin-DM Liquid (Whitehall-Robins) **783**
Children's Sudafed Cold & Cough Liquid (Pfizer Inc., Warner-Lambert Healthcare) **520, 709**
Sudafed Cold & Cough Liquid Caps (Pfizer Inc., Warner-Lambert Healthcare) **520, 709**
Sudafed Severe Cold Formula Caplets (Pfizer Inc., Warner-Lambert Healthcare) **520, 711**
Sudafed Severe Cold Formula Tablets (Pfizer Inc., Warner-Lambert Healthcare) **520, 711**
TheraFlu Regular Strength Cold & Cough Night Time Hot Liquid (Novartis Consumer) **515, 676**
TheraFlu Maximum Strength Flu & Congestion Non-Drowsy Hot Liquid (Novartis Consumer) **515, 677**
TheraFlu Maximum Strength Flu & Cough Night Time Hot Liquid (Novartis Consumer) **515, 678**
TheraFlu Maximum Strength Severe Cold & Congestion Night Time Caplets (Novartis Consumer) **515, 678**
TheraFlu Maximum Strength Severe Cold & Congestion Night Time Hot Liquid (Novartis Consumer) **515, 678**
TheraFlu Maximum Strength Severe Cold & Congestion Non-Drowsy Caplets (Novartis Consumer) **515, 679**
TheraFlu Maximum Strength Severe Cold & Congestion Non-Drowsy Hot Liquid (Novartis Consumer) **515, 679**
Triaminic Cold & Cough Liquid (Novartis Consumer) **515, 681**
Triaminic Cold & Cough Softchews (Novartis Consumer) **515, 683**
Triaminic Cold & Night Time Cough Liquid (Novartis Consumer) **515, 681**
Triaminic Cold, Cough & Fever Liquid (Novartis Consumer) **515, 681**
Triaminic Cough Liquid (Novartis Consumer) **515, 682**
Triaminic Cough Softchews (Novartis Consumer) **515, 684**
Triaminic Cough & Congestion Liquid (Novartis Consumer) **515, 682**

RESPIRATORY AGENTS—cont.

ANTITUSSIVES—cont.

NON-NARCOTIC ANTITUSSIVES & COMBINATIONS—cont.

Triaminic Cough & Sore Throat Liquid (Novartis Consumer) **515, 682**

Triaminic Cough & Sore Throat Softchews (Novartis Consumer)........ **515, 684**

Triaminic Vapor Patch-Cherry Scent (Novartis Consumer) **515, 684**

Triaminic Vapor Patch-Menthol Scent (Novartis Consumer)........ **515, 684**

Children's Tylenol Cold Plus Cough Suspension Liquid and Chewable Tablets (McNeil Consumer) **510, 659**

Children's Tylenol Flu Suspension Liquid (McNeil Consumer) **511, 663**

Infants' Tylenol Cold Decongestant & Fever Reducer Concentrated Drops Plus Cough (McNeil Consumer) **511, 659**

Multi-Symptom Tylenol Cold Complete Formula Caplets (McNeil Consumer) **512, 651**

Multi-Symptom Tylenol Cold Non-Drowsy Caplets and Gelcaps (McNeil Consumer) **512, 651**

Multi-Symptom Tylenol Cold Severe Congestion Non-Drowsy Caplets (McNeil Consumer) **512, 652**

Maximum Strength Tylenol Flu NightTime Liquid (McNeil Consumer) **512, 653**

Maximum Strength Tylenol Flu Non-Drowsy Gelcaps (McNeil Consumer) **512, 653**

Vicks 44 Cough Relief Liquid (Procter & Gamble) **724**

Vicks 44D Cough & Head Congestion Relief Liquid (Procter & Gamble) **724**

Vicks 44E Cough & Chest Congestion Relief Liquid (Procter & Gamble) **725**

Pediatric Vicks 44e Cough & Chest Congestion Relief Liquid (Procter & Gamble) **728**

Vicks 44M Cough, Cold & Flu Relief Liquid (Procter & Gamble)............................. **725**

Pediatric Vicks 44m Cough & Cold Relief (Procter & Gamble)............................. **728**

Vicks Cough Drops, Menthol and Cherry Flavors (Procter & Gamble)............................. **726**

Vicks DayQuil LiquiCaps/Liquid Multi-Symptom Cold/Flu Relief (Procter & Gamble) **727**

Children's Vicks NyQuil Cold/ Cough Relief (Procter & Gamble)............................. **726**

Vicks NyQuil LiquiCaps/Liquid Multi-Symptom Cold/Flu Relief, Original and Cherry Flavors (Procter & Gamble)........ **727**

Vicks VapoRub Cream (Procter & Gamble)............................. **730**

Vicks VapoRub Ointment (Procter & Gamble) **730**

Vicks VapoSteam (Procter & Gamble)............................... **730**

BRONCHODILATORS

SYMPATHOMIMETICS & COMBINATIONS

Primatene Mist (Whitehall-Robins) **779**

Primatene Tablets (Whitehall-Robins) **780**

DECONGESTANTS & COMBINATIONS

Actifed Cold & Allergy Tablets (Pfizer Inc., Warner-Lambert Healthcare) **516, 688**

Actifed Cold & Sinus Caplets and Tablets (Pfizer Inc., Warner-Lambert Healthcare)... **516, 688**

Advil Cold and Sinus Caplets (Whitehall-Robins) **771**

Advil Cold and Sinus Tablets (Whitehall-Robins) **771**

Advil Flu & Body Ache Caplets (Whitehall-Robins) **772**

Aleve Cold & Sinus Caplets (Bayer Consumer)............. **503, 603**

Alka-Seltzer Plus Cold Medicine Liqui-Gels (Bayer Consumer)... **503, 604**

Alka-Seltzer Plus Night-Time Cold Medicine Liqui-Gels (Bayer Consumer)............. **503, 604**

Alka-Seltzer Plus Cold & Cough Medicine Liqui-Gels (Bayer Consumer) **503, 604**

Alka-Seltzer Plus Cold & Flu Medicine Liqui-Gels (Bayer Consumer) **503, 604**

Alka-Seltzer Plus Cold & Sinus Medicine Liqui-Gels (Bayer Consumer) **503, 604**

BC Allergy Sinus Cold Powder (Block) ... **619**

BC Sinus Cold Powder (Block)........... **619**

Benadryl Allergy/Cold Tablets (Pfizer Inc., Warner-Lambert Healthcare) **517, 691**

Benadryl Allergy/Congestion Tablets (Pfizer Inc., Warner-Lambert Healthcare)... **517, 692**

Benadryl Allergy & Sinus Liquid (Pfizer Inc., Warner-Lambert Healthcare) **693**

Benadryl Allergy & Sinus Fastmelt Tablets (Pfizer Inc., Warner-Lambert Healthcare)... **517, 693**

Benadryl Severe Allergy & Sinus Headache Caplets (Pfizer Inc., Warner-Lambert Healthcare) **517, 694**

Benadryl Children's Allergy/ Cold Fastmelt Tablets (Pfizer Inc., Warner-Lambert Healthcare) **517, 692**

Benylin Multi-Symptom Liquid (Pfizer Inc., Warner-Lambert Healthcare) **518, 697**

Children's Cēpacol Sore Throat Formula, Cherry Flavor Liquid (Williams) **788**

Children's Cēpacol Sore Throat Formula, Grape Flavor Liquid (Williams) **788**

Chlor-Trimeton Allergy/ Decongestant Tablets (Schering-Plough) **522, 736**

Comtrex Acute Head Cold & Sinus Pressure Relief Tablets (Bristol-Myers) **506, 627**

Comtrex Flu Therapy & Fever Relief Daytime Caplets (Bristol-Myers) **506, 628**

Comtrex Flu Therapy & Fever Relief Nighttime Tablets (Bristol-Myers) **506, 628**

Comtrex Maximum Strength Multi-Symptom Cold & Cough Relief Tablets and Caplets (Bristol-Myers)........ **506, 626**

Contac Non-Drowsy 12 Hour Cold Caplets (SmithKline Beecham Consumer) **523, 745**

Contac Non-Drowsy Timed Release 12 Hour Cold Caplets (SmithKline Beecham Consumer) **523, 746**

Contac Severe Cold and Flu Caplets Maximum Strength (SmithKline Beecham Consumer) **523, 746**

Contac Severe Cold and Flu Caplets Non-Drowsy (SmithKline Beecham Consumer) **746**

Coricidin 'D' Cold, Flu & Sinus Tablets (Schering-Plough) **522, 737**

Dimetapp Elixir (Whitehall-Robins)....... **777**

Dimetapp Cold and Fever Suspension (Whitehall-Robins) **775**

Dimetapp DM Cold & Cough Elixir (Whitehall-Robins) **775**

Dimetapp Nighttime Flu Liquid (Whitehall-Robins) **776**

Dimetapp Non-Drowsy Flu Syrup (Whitehall-Robins) **777**

Dimetapp Infant Drops Decongestant (Whitehall-Robins) **775**

Dimetapp Infant Drops Decongestant Plus Cough (Whitehall-Robins)....... **776**

Drixoral Allergy/Sinus Extended-Release Tablets (Schering-Plough) **523, 741**

Drixoral Cold & Allergy Sustained-Action Tablets (Schering-Plough) **523, 740**

Drixoral Cold & Flu Extended-Release Tablets (Schering-Plough) **523, 740**

Drixoral Nasal Decongestant Long-Acting Non-Drowsy Tablets (Schering-Plough) **523, 740**

Children's Motrin Cold Oral Suspension (McNeil Consumer) **509, 646**

Motrin Sinus/Headache Caplets (McNeil Consumer) **510, 643**

PediaCare Cough-Cold Liquid (Pharmacia Consumer) **719**

PediaCare Infants' Drops Decongestant (Pharmacia Consumer)............... **719**

PediaCare Infants' Drops Decongestant Plus Cough (Pharmacia Consumer) **719**

PediaCare NightRest Cough-Cold Liquid (Pharmacia Consumer) **719**

Robitussin Cold Softgels Severe Congestion (Whitehall-Robins)....... **782**

Robitussin Maximum Strength Cough & Cold Liquid (Whitehall-Robins) **785**

Robitussin Pediatric Cough & Cold Formula Liquid (Whitehall-Robins) ... **785**

Robitussin Multi Symptom Honey Flu Liquid (Whitehall-Robins) **785**

Robitussin Nighttime Honey Flu Liquid (Whitehall-Robins) **786**

Robitussin-PE Liquid (Whitehall-Robins) **782**

Ryna Liquid (Wallace).................... **768**

Ryna-C Liquid (Wallace)........... **525, 768**

Singlet Caplets (SmithKline Beecham Consumer).............................**761**

Sinutab Sinus Allergy Medication, Maximum Strength Formula, Tablets & Caplets (Pfizer Inc., Warner-Lambert Healthcare)...**520, 707**

Sinutab Sinus Medication, Maximum Strength Without Drowsiness Formula, Tablets & Caplets (Pfizer Inc., Warner-Lambert Healthcare)....................**520, 707**

Sudafed 12 Hour Tablets (Pfizer Inc., Warner-Lambert Healthcare)....................**520, 708**

Sudafed 24 Hour Tablets (Pfizer Inc., Warner-Lambert Healthcare)....................**520, 708**

Children's Sudafed Cold & Cough Liquid (Pfizer Inc., Warner-Lambert Healthcare)...**520, 709**

Children's Sudafed Nasal Decongestant Chewables (Pfizer Inc., Warner-Lambert Healthcare)....................**520, 711**

Children's Sudafed Nasal Decongestant Liquid Medication (Pfizer Inc., Warner-Lambert Healthcare)...**521, 711**

Sudafed Cold & Allergy Tablets (Pfizer Inc., Warner-Lambert Healthcare)....................**520, 708**

Sudafed Cold & Cough Liquid Caps (Pfizer Inc., Warner-Lambert Healthcare)...**520, 709**

Sudafed Cold & Sinus Liquid Caps (Pfizer Inc., Warner-Lambert Healthcare)...**520, 710**

Sudafed Nasal Decongestant Tablets (Pfizer Inc., Warner-Lambert Healthcare)...**520, 710**

Sudafed Severe Cold Formula Caplets (Pfizer Inc., Warner-Lambert Healthcare)...**520, 711**

Sudafed Severe Cold Formula Tablets (Pfizer Inc., Warner-Lambert Healthcare)...**520, 711**

Sudafed Sinus Headache Caplets (Pfizer Inc., Warner-Lambert Healthcare)...**520, 712**

Sudafed Sinus Headache Tablets (Pfizer Inc., Warner-Lambert Healthcare)...**520, 712**

Tavist Sinus Non-Drowsy Coated Caplets (Novartis Consumer).................**514, 676**

TheraFlu Regular Strength Cold & Cough Night Time Hot Liquid (Novartis Consumer)....**515, 676**

TheraFlu Regular Strength Cold & Sore Throat Night Time Hot Liquid (Novartis Consumer).................**515, 676**

TheraFlu Maximum Strength Flu & Cough Night Time Hot Liquid (Novartis Consumer)....**515, 678**

TheraFlu Maximum Strength Flu & Sore Throat Night Time Hot Liquid (Novartis Consumer).................**515, 677**

TheraFlu Maximum Strength Severe Cold & Congestion Night Time Caplets (Novartis Consumer).................**515, 678**

TheraFlu Maximum Strength Severe Cold & Congestion Night Time Hot Liquid (Novartis Consumer).................**515, 678**

TheraFlu Maximum Strength Severe Cold & Congestion Non-Drowsy Caplets (Novartis Consumer).................**515, 679**

TheraFlu Maximum Strength Severe Cold & Congestion Non-Drowsy Hot Liquid (Novartis Consumer).................**515, 679**

Triaminic Allergy Congestion Liquid (Novartis Consumer)....**515, 680**

Triaminic Cold & Allergy Liquid (Novartis Consumer).................**515, 681**

Triaminic Cold & Allergy Softchews (Novartis Consumer).................**515, 683**

Triaminic Cold & Cough Liquid (Novartis Consumer).................**515, 681**

Triaminic Cold & Cough Softchews (Novartis Consumer).................**515, 683**

Triaminic Cold & Night Time Cough Liquid (Novartis Consumer).................**515, 681**

Triaminic Cold, Cough & Fever Liquid (Novartis Consumer)....**515, 681**

Triaminic Cough Liquid (Novartis Consumer).................**515, 682**

Triaminic Cough & Congestion Liquid (Novartis Consumer)....**515, 682**

Triaminic Cough & Sore Throat Softchews (Novartis Consumer).................**515, 684**

Children's Tylenol Allergy-D Liquid (McNeil Consumer).....**510, 658**

Children's Tylenol Cold Suspension Liquid and Chewable Tablets (McNeil Consumer).................**510, 659**

Children's Tylenol Cold Plus Cough Suspension Liquid and Chewable Tablets (McNeil Consumer)............**510, 659**

Children's Tylenol Flu Suspension Liquid (McNeil Consumer).................**511, 663**

Children's Tylenol Sinus Suspension Liquid (McNeil Consumer).................**511, 663**

Infants' Tylenol Cold Decongestant & Fever Reducer Concentrated Drops (McNeil Consumer).....**511, 659**

Infants' Tylenol Cold Decongestant & Fever Reducer Concentrated Drops Plus Cough (McNeil Consumer).................**511, 659**

Maximum Strength Tylenol Allergy Sinus Caplets, Gelcaps, and Geltabs (McNeil Consumer)............**511, 649**

Maximum Strength Tylenol Allergy Sinus NightTime Caplets (McNeil Consumer)....**511, 649**

Multi-Symptom Tylenol Cold Complete Formula Caplets (McNeil Consumer)............**512, 651**

Multi-Symptom Tylenol Cold Non-Drowsy Caplets and Gelcaps (McNeil Consumer)...**512, 651**

Maximum Strength Tylenol Flu NightTime Gelcaps (McNeil Consumer).................**512, 653**

Maximum Strength Tylenol Flu NightTime Liquid (McNeil Consumer).................**512, 653**

Maximum Strength Tylenol Flu Non-Drowsy Gelcaps (McNeil Consumer).................**512, 653**

Maximum Strength Tylenol Sinus NightTime Caplets (McNeil Consumer)............**512, 655**

Maximum Strength Tylenol Sinus Non-Drowsy Geltabs, Gelcaps, Caplets, and Tablets (McNeil Consumer)....**512, 655**

Vicks 44D Cough & Head Congestion Relief Liquid (Procter & Gamble)....**724**

Vicks 44M Cough, Cold & Flu Relief Liquid (Procter & Gamble)...........**725**

Pediatric Vicks 44m Cough & Cold Relief (Procter & Gamble)...........**728**

Vicks DayQuil LiquiCaps/Liquid Multi-Symptom Cold/Flu Relief (Procter & Gamble).................**727**

Children's Vicks NyQuil Cold/Cough Relief (Procter & Gamble)...........**726**

Vicks NyQuil LiquiCaps/Liquid Multi-Symptom Cold/Flu Relief, Original and Cherry Flavors (Procter & Gamble).................**727**

Vicks VapoRub Cream (Procter & Gamble)..............................**730**

Vicks VapoRub Ointment (Procter & Gamble)..............................**730**

DECONGESTANTS, EXPECTORANTS & COMBINATIONS

Comtrex Deep Chest Cold & Congestion Relief Softgels (Bristol-Myers).................**506, 627**

Robitussin Cold Caplets Cold & Congestion (Whitehall-Robins).......**780**

Robitussin Cold Caplets Multi-Symptom Cold & Flu (Whitehall-Robins)..................**781**

Robitussin Cold Softgels Multi-Symptom Cold & Flu (Whitehall-Robins)..................**781**

Robitussin Cough & Cold Infant Drops (Whitehall-Robins)............**782**

Robitussin-CF Liquid (Whitehall-Robins)..................**783**

Sinutab Non-Drying Liquid Caps (Pfizer Inc., Warner-Lambert Healthcare)....................**520, 706**

Sudafed Cold & Cough Liquid Caps (Pfizer Inc., Warner-Lambert Healthcare)...**520, 709**

Sudafed Non-Drying Sinus Liquid Caps (Pfizer Inc., Warner-Lambert Healthcare)...**520, 712**

TheraFlu Maximum Strength Flu & Congestion Non-Drowsy Hot Liquid (Novartis Consumer).................**515, 677**

Triaminic Chest Congestion Liquid (Novartis Consumer)....**515, 680**

Multi-Symptom Tylenol Cold Severe Congestion Non-Drowsy Caplets (McNeil Consumer).................**512, 652**

EXPECTORANTS & COMBINATIONS

Benylin Cough Suppressant/ Expectorant Liquid (Pfizer Inc., Warner-Lambert Healthcare)....................**518, 697**

Primatene Tablets (Whitehall-Robins)....**780**

Robitussin Liquid (Whitehall-Robins)....**782**

Robitussin Cold Softgels Severe Congestion (Whitehall-Robins).......**782**

Robitussin DM Infant Drops (Whitehall-Robins)..................**783**

Robitussin-DM Liquid (Whitehall-Robins)..................**783**

Robitussin-PE Liquid (Whitehall-Robins)..................**782**

RESPIRATORY AGENTS—cont.

EXPECTORANTS & COMBINATIONS—cont.
Vicks 44E Cough & Chest Congestion
Relief Liquid (Procter & Gamble) **725**
Pediatric Vicks 44e Cough & Chest
Congestion Relief Liquid (Procter
& Gamble) **728**

MISCELLANEOUS COLD & COUGH PRODUCTS
Coricidin HBP Cough & Cold
Tablets (Schering-Plough) **523, 738**
Robitussin Maximum Strength Cough
& Cold Liquid (Whitehall-Robins) **785**
Robitussin Pediatric Cough & Cold
Formula Liquid (Whitehall-Robins) ... **785**
Triaminic Cold & Cough Liquid
(Novartis Consumer)........... **515, 681**
Triaminic Cold & Cough
Softchews (Novartis
Consumer)....................... **515, 683**
Triaminic Cold & Night Time
Cough Liquid (Novartis
Consumer) **515, 681**
Triaminic Cough Liquid (Novartis
Consumer) **515, 682**
Triaminic Cough & Congestion
Liquid (Novartis Consumer).... **515, 682**

MISCELLANEOUS COLD & COUGH PRODUCTS WITH ANALGESICS
Alka-Seltzer Plus Night-Time Cold
Medicine Liqui-Gels (Bayer
Consumer)....................... **503, 604**
Alka-Seltzer Plus Cold & Cough
Medicine Liqui-Gels (Bayer
Consumer) **503, 604**
Alka-Seltzer Plus Cold & Flu
Medicine Liqui-Gels (Bayer
Consumer) **503, 604**
Benadryl Allergy Sinus
Headache Caplets &
Gelcaps (Pfizer Inc.,
Warner-Lambert Healthcare)... **517, 693**
Comtrex Deep Chest Cold &
Congestion Relief Softgels
(Bristol-Myers) **506, 627**
Comtrex Maximum Strength
Multi-Symptom Cold &
Cough Relief Tablets and
Caplets (Bristol-Myers)......... **506, 626**
Contac Severe Cold and Flu
Caplets Maximum Strength
(SmithKline Beecham
Consumer) **523, 746**
Contac Severe Cold and Flu Caplets
Non-Drowsy (SmithKline Beecham
Consumer) **746**
Coricidin HBP Maximum
Strength Flu Tablets
(Schering-Plough) **523, 738**
Dimetapp Cold and Fever Suspension
(Whitehall-Robins) **775**
Dimetapp Nighttime Flu Liquid
(Whitehall-Robins) **776**
Dimetapp Non-Drowsy Flu Syrup
(Whitehall-Robins) **777**
Drixoral Allergy/Sinus
Extended-Release Tablets
(Schering-Plough) **523, 741**
Drixoral Cold & Flu
Extended-Release Tablets
(Schering-Plough) **523, 740**
Robitussin Cold Caplets
Multi-Symptom Cold & Flu
(Whitehall-Robins) **781**
Robitussin Cold Softgels
Multi-Symptom Cold & Flu
(Whitehall-Robins) **781**
Robitussin Multi Symptom Honey Flu
Liquid (Whitehall-Robins) **785**

Robitussin Nighttime Honey Flu Liquid
(Whitehall-Robins) **786**
Singlet Caplets (SmithKline Beecham
Consumer)........................... **761**
Sudafed Cold & Sinus Liquid
Caps (Pfizer Inc.,
Warner-Lambert Healthcare)... **520, 710**
TheraFlu Regular Strength Cold
& Cough Night Time Hot
Liquid (Novartis Consumer).... **515, 676**
TheraFlu Maximum Strength Flu
& Congestion Non-Drowsy
Hot Liquid (Novartis
Consumer) **515, 677**
TheraFlu Maximum Strength Flu
& Cough Night Time Hot
Liquid (Novartis Consumer).... **515, 678**
TheraFlu Maximum Strength
Severe Cold & Congestion
Night Time Caplets
(Novartis Consumer)........... **515, 678**
TheraFlu Maximum Strength
Severe Cold & Congestion
Night Time Hot Liquid
(Novartis Consumer)........... **515, 678**
TheraFlu Maximum Strength
Severe Cold & Congestion
Non-Drowsy Caplets
(Novartis Consumer)........... **515, 679**
TheraFlu Maximum Strength
Severe Cold & Congestion
Non-Drowsy Hot Liquid
(Novartis Consumer)........... **515, 679**
Triaminic Cold, Cough & Fever
Liquid (Novartis Consumer).... **515, 681**
Triaminic Cough & Sore Throat
Liquid (Novartis Consumer).... **515, 682**
Triaminic Cough & Sore Throat
Softchews (Novartis
Consumer) **515, 684**
Children's Tylenol Cold Plus
Cough Suspension Liquid
and Chewable Tablets
(McNeil Consumer) **510, 659**
Children's Tylenol Flu
Suspension Liquid (McNeil
Consumer) **511, 663**
Infants' Tylenol Cold
Decongestant & Fever
Reducer Concentrated
Drops Plus Cough (McNeil
Consumer) **511, 659**
Multi-Symptom Tylenol Cold
Complete Formula Caplets
(McNeil Consumer) **512, 651**
Multi-Symptom Tylenol Cold
Non-Drowsy Caplets and
Gelcaps (McNeil Consumer)... **512, 651**
Multi-Symptom Tylenol Cold
Severe Congestion
Non-Drowsy Caplets (McNeil
Consumer) **512, 652**
Maximum Strength Tylenol Flu
NightTime Liquid (McNeil
Consumer) **512, 653**
Maximum Strength Tylenol Flu
Non-Drowsy Gelcaps (McNeil
Consumer) **512, 653**
Vicks 44M Cough, Cold & Flu Relief
Liquid (Procter & Gamble) **725**
Vicks DayQuil LiquiCaps/Liquid
Multi-Symptom Cold/Flu Relief
(Procter & Gamble) **727**
Vicks NyQuil LiquiCaps/Liquid
Multi-Symptom Cold/Flu Relief,
Original and Cherry Flavors
(Procter & Gamble) **727**

MISCELLANEOUS RESPIRATORY AGENTS
Robitussin Honey Calmers Throat
Drops (Whitehall-Robins) **783**
Robitussin Sugar Free Throat Drops
(Whitehall-Robins) **786**

S

SALT SUBSTITUTES
Chlor-3 Shaker (Fleming) **633**

SCABICIDES
(see under:
SKIN & MUCOUS MEMBRANE AGENTS
ANTI-INFECTIVES
SCABICIDES & PEDICULICIDES)

SEBORRHEA TREATMENT
(see under:
SKIN & MUCOUS MEMBRANE AGENTS
ANTISEBORRHEIC AGENTS)

SEDATIVES & HYPNOTICS

MISCELLANEOUS SEDATIVES & HYPNOTICS
Alka-Seltzer PM Effervescent
Tablets (Bayer Consumer) **503, 605**
Extra Strength Bayer PM
Caplets (Bayer Consumer).... **504, 611**
Excedrin PM Tablets, Caplets,
and Geltabs (Bristol-Myers).... **506, 631**
Goody's PM Powder (Block) **621**
Nytol QuickCaps Caplets (Block) .. **506, 622**
Maximum Strength Nytol
QuickGels Softgels (Block) **506, 621**
Simply Sleep Caplets (McNeil
Consumer) **510, 647**
Sominex Original Formula Tablets
(SmithKline Beecham Consumer) ... **761**
Unisom SleepTabs (Pfizer Inc.,
Warner-Lambert Healthcare)... **521, 713**
Unisom Maximum Strength
SleepGels (Pfizer Inc.,
Warner-Lambert Healthcare)... **521, 713**

SHAMPOOS
(see under:
SKIN & MUCOUS MEMBRANE AGENTS
SHAMPOOS)

SKIN & MUCOUS MEMBRANE AGENTS

ACNE PREPARATIONS
DDS-Acidophilus Capsules, Tablets,
and Powder (UAS Labs).............. **767**

ANALGESICS & COMBINATIONS
Benadryl Itch Stopping Cream
Original Strength (Pfizer Inc.,
Warner-Lambert Healthcare)... **517, 695**
Benadryl Itch Stopping Cream
Extra Strength (Pfizer Inc.,
Warner-Lambert Healthcare)... **517, 695**
Benadryl Itch Stopping Spray
Original Strength (Pfizer Inc.,
Warner-Lambert Healthcare)... **517, 696**
Benadryl Itch Stopping Spray
Extra Strength (Pfizer Inc.,
Warner-Lambert Healthcare)... **517, 696**
BenGay External Analgesic
Products (Pfizer Inc.,
Warner-Lambert Healthcare)... **518, 696**
Thera-Gesic Creme (Mission)............ **667**
Vicks VapoRub Cream (Procter &
Gamble).............................. **730**
Vicks VapoRub Ointment (Procter &
Gamble).............................. **730**

ANESTHETICS & COMBINATIONS
Baby Anbesol Gel (Whitehall-Robins) **774**
Junior Anbesol Gel (Whitehall-Robins) ... **774**
Maximum Strength Anbesol Gel
(Whitehall-Robins) **774**
Maximum Strength Anbesol Liquid
(Whitehall-Robins) **774**

Bactine First Aid Liquid (Bayer
Consumer) **503, 611**
Betadine Brand Plus First Aid
Antibiotics + Pain Reliever
Ointment (Purdue Frederick) ...**522, 731**
Cēpacol Maximum Strength Sore
Throat Spray, Cherry Flavor
(Williams) **787**
Cēpacol Maximum Strength Sore
Throat Spray, Cool Menthol Flavor
(Williams) **787**
Cēpacol Maximum Strength Sore
Throat Spray, Honey Lemon Flavor
(Williams) **787**
Dermoplast Antibacterial Spray,
Hospital Strength (Medtech) **666**
Dermoplast Hospital Strength Spray
(Medtech) **666**
Hurricaine Topical Anesthetic Gel, 1
oz. Fresh Mint, Wild Cherry, Pina
Colada, Watermelon, 1/6 oz. Wild
Cherry, Watermelon (Beutlich).......**618**
Hurricaine Topical Anesthetic Liquid,
1 oz. Wild Cherry, Pina Colada,
.25 ml Dry Handle Swab Wild
Cherry, 1/6 oz. Wild Cherry
(Beutlich) **618**
Hurricaine Topical Anesthetic Spray
Extension Tubes (200) (Beutlich)....**618**
Hurricaine Topical Anesthetic Spray
Kit, 2 oz. Wild Cherry (Beutlich).....**618**
Hurricaine Topical Anesthetic Spray, 2
oz. Wild Cherry (Beutlich)...........**618**
Neosporin + Pain Relief
Maximum Strength Cream
(Pfizer Inc., Warner-Lambert
Healthcare) **519, 704**
Neosporin + Pain Relief
Maximum Strength Ointment
(Pfizer Inc., Warner-Lambert
Healthcare) **519, 704**
Zilactin-B Gel (Zila Consumer) **790**
Zilactin-L Liquid (Zila Consumer) **790**

ANORECTAL PREPARATIONS
Anusol HC-1 Hydrocortisone
Anti-Itch Cream (Pfizer Inc.,
Warner-Lambert Healthcare)...**516, 689**
Anusol Ointment (Pfizer Inc.,
Warner-Lambert Healthcare)...**516, 688**
Anusol Suppositories (Pfizer
Inc., Warner-Lambert
Healthcare) **516, 689**
Cortaid Maximum Strength Cream
(Pharmacia Consumer) **717**
Cortaid Maximum Strength Ointment
(Pharmacia Consumer) **717**
Cortaid Sensitive Skin Cream
(Pharmacia Consumer) **717**
Hurricaine Topical Anesthetic Gel, 1
oz. Fresh Mint, Wild Cherry, Pina
Colada, Watermelon, 1/6 oz. Wild
Cherry, Watermelon (Beutlich).......**618**
Hurricaine Topical Anesthetic Liquid,
1 oz. Wild Cherry, Pina Colada,
.25 ml Dry Handle Swab Wild
Cherry, 1/6 oz. Wild Cherry
(Beutlich) **618**
Hurricaine Topical Anesthetic Spray
Extension Tubes (200) (Beutlich)...**618**
Hurricaine Topical Anesthetic Spray
Kit, 2 oz. Wild Cherry (Beutlich).....**618**
Hurricaine Topical Anesthetic Spray, 2
oz. Wild Cherry (Beutlich)...........**618**
Preparation H Cream
(Whitehall-Robins) **778**
Preparation H Cooling Gel
(Whitehall-Robins) **778**

Preparation H Ointment
(Whitehall-Robins) **778**
Preparation H Suppositories
(Whitehall-Robins) **778**
Preparation H Medicated Wipes
(Whitehall-Robins) **779**
Tucks Pre-moistened Pads
(Pfizer Inc., Warner-Lambert
Healthcare) **521, 713**

ANTIHISTAMINES & COMBINATIONS
Benadryl Itch Relief Stick Extra
Strength (Pfizer Inc.,
Warner-Lambert Healthcare)...**517, 695**
Benadryl Itch Stopping Cream
Original Strength (Pfizer Inc.,
Warner-Lambert Healthcare)...**517, 695**
Benadryl Itch Stopping Cream
Extra Strength (Pfizer Inc.,
Warner-Lambert Healthcare)...**517, 695**
Benadryl Itch Stopping Gel
Original Strength (Pfizer Inc.,
Warner-Lambert Healthcare)...**517, 695**
Benadryl Itch Stopping Gel Extra
Strength (Pfizer Inc.,
Warner-Lambert Healthcare)...**517, 695**
Benadryl Itch Stopping Spray
Original Strength (Pfizer Inc.,
Warner-Lambert Healthcare)...**517, 696**
Benadryl Itch Stopping Spray
Extra Strength (Pfizer Inc.,
Warner-Lambert Healthcare)...**517, 696**
Caladryl Clear Lotion (Pfizer
Inc., Warner-Lambert
Healthcare) **518, 698**
Caladryl Lotion (Pfizer Inc.,
Warner-Lambert Healthcare)...**518, 698**

ANTI-INFECTIVES

ANTIBIOTICS & COMBINATIONS
Betadine Brand First Aid
Antibiotics + Moisturizer
Ointment (Purdue
Frederick) **522, 731**
Betadine Brand Plus First
Aid Antibiotics + Pain
Reliever Ointment
(Purdue Frederick) **522, 731**
Neosporin Ointment (Pfizer
Inc., Warner-Lambert
Healthcare) **519, 704**
Neosporin + Pain Relief
Maximum Strength
Cream (Pfizer Inc.,
Warner-Lambert
Healthcare) **519, 704**
Neosporin + Pain Relief
Maximum Strength
Ointment (Pfizer Inc.,
Warner-Lambert
Healthcare) **519, 704**
Polysporin Ointment (Pfizer
Inc., Warner-Lambert
Healthcare) **519, 706**
Polysporin Powder (Pfizer
Inc., Warner-Lambert
Healthcare) **519, 706**

ANTIFUNGALS & COMBINATIONS
Desenex Liquid Spray (Novartis
Consumer) **668**
Desenex Shake Powder
(Novartis Consumer).........**512, 668**
Desenex Spray Powder
(Novartis Consumer).........**512, 668**
Desenex Jock Itch Spray Powder
(Novartis Consumer) **668**
Lamisil^AT Cream (Novartis
Consumer) **513, 672**
Lamisil^AT Solution (Novartis
Consumer) **513, 672**

Lotrimin AF Cream, Lotion,
Solution, and Jock Itch
Cream (Schering-Plough).....**523, 742**
Lotrimin AF Spray Powder,
Spray Liquid, Spray
Deodorant Powder,
Shaker Powder and Jock
Itch Spray Powder
(Schering-Plough) **523, 742**
Nizoral A-D Shampoo
(McNeil Consumer) **510, 647**

**MISCELLANEOUS ANTI-INFECTIVES &
COMBINATIONS**
Bactine First Aid Liquid (Bayer
Consumer) **503, 611**
Betadine Ointment (Purdue
Frederick) **522, 732**
Betadine PrepStick
Applicator (Purdue
Frederick) **522, 732**
Betadine Skin Cleanser (Purdue
Frederick) **732**
Betadine Solution (Purdue
Frederick) **522, 732**
Clinical Care Antimicrobial Wound
Cleanser (Care-Tech) **632**
Dermoplast Antibacterial Spray,
Hospital Strength (Medtech) **666**
Listerine Mouthrinse (Pfizer
Inc., Warner-Lambert
Healthcare) **518, 702**
Cool Mint Listerine
Mouthrinse (Pfizer Inc.,
Warner-Lambert
Healthcare) **518, 702**
FreshBurst Listerine
Mouthrinse (Pfizer Inc.,
Warner-Lambert
Healthcare) **519, 702**
Massengill Medicated
Disposable Douche
(SmithKline Beecham
Consumer) **524, 753**
Techni-Care Surgical Scrub, Prep
and Wound Decontaminant
(Care-Tech)......................**632**

SCABICIDES & PEDICULICIDES
(see also under:
**ANTI-INFECTIVES, NON-SYSTEMIC
SCABICIDES & PEDICULICIDES**)
Nix Creme Rinse (Pfizer Inc.,
Warner-Lambert
Healthcare) **519, 704**
Permethrin Lotion (Alpharma) **602**
Maximum Strength Rid
Mousse (Bayer
Consumer) **505, 617**
Maximum Strength Rid
Shampoo (Bayer
Consumer) **505, 616**

ANTIPRURITICS
Anusol HC-1 Hydrocortisone
Anti-Itch Cream (Pfizer Inc.,
Warner-Lambert Healthcare)...**516, 689**
Benadryl Itch Relief Stick Extra
Strength (Pfizer Inc.,
Warner-Lambert Healthcare)...**517, 695**
Benadryl Itch Stopping Cream
Original Strength (Pfizer Inc.,
Warner-Lambert Healthcare)...**517, 695**
Benadryl Itch Stopping Cream
Extra Strength (Pfizer Inc.,
Warner-Lambert Healthcare)...**517, 695**
Benadryl Itch Stopping Gel
Original Strength (Pfizer Inc.,
Warner-Lambert Healthcare)...**517, 695**
Benadryl Itch Stopping Gel Extra
Strength (Pfizer Inc.,
Warner-Lambert Healthcare)...**517, 695**

SKIN & MUCOUS MEMBRANE AGENTS—cont.

ANTIPRURITICS—cont.
Benadryl Itch Stopping Spray
  Original Strength (Pfizer Inc.,
  Warner-Lambert Healthcare)...**517, 696**
Benadryl Itch Stopping Spray
  Extra Strength (Pfizer Inc.,
  Warner-Lambert Healthcare)...**517, 696**
Caladryl Clear Lotion (Pfizer
  Inc., Warner-Lambert
  Healthcare) **518, 698**
Caladryl Lotion (Pfizer Inc.,
  Warner-Lambert Healthcare)...**518, 698**
Cortaid Intensive Therapy Cream
  (Pharmacia Consumer) **717**
Cortaid Maximum Strength Cream
  (Pharmacia Consumer) **717**
Cortaid Maximum Strength Ointment
  (Pharmacia Consumer) **717**
Cortaid Sensitive Skin Cream
  (Pharmacia Consumer) **717**
Cortizone•5 Creme (Pfizer Inc.,
  Warner-Lambert Healthcare)...**518, 699**
Cortizone•5 Ointment (Pfizer Inc.,
  Warner-Lambert Healthcare)........**699**
Cortizone•10 Creme (Pfizer
  Inc., Warner-Lambert
  Healthcare) **518, 699**
Cortizone•10 Ointment (Pfizer Inc.,
  Warner-Lambert Healthcare)........**699**
Cortizone•10 Plus Creme
  (Pfizer Inc., Warner-Lambert
  Healthcare) **518, 700**
Cortizone•10 Quick Shot Spray
  (Pfizer Inc., Warner-Lambert
  Healthcare) **518, 699**
Cortizone for Kids Creme (Pfizer
  Inc., Warner-Lambert
  Healthcare) **518, 699**
Dermoplast Hospital Strength Spray
  (Medtech) **666**
Massengill Medicated Soft Cloth
  Towelette (SmithKline Beecham
  Consumer)..........................**753**
Tucks Pre-moistened Pads
  (Pfizer Inc., Warner-Lambert
  Healthcare) **521, 713**

ANTIPSORIATIC AGENTS
Cortaid Intensive Therapy Cream
  (Pharmacia Consumer) **717**
Cortaid Maximum Strength Cream
  (Pharmacia Consumer) **717**
Cortaid Maximum Strength Ointment
  (Pharmacia Consumer) **717**
Cortaid Sensitive Skin Cream
  (Pharmacia Consumer) **717**
Cortizone•5 Creme (Pfizer Inc.,
  Warner-Lambert Healthcare)...**518, 699**
Cortizone•5 Ointment (Pfizer Inc.,
  Warner-Lambert Healthcare)........**699**
Cortizone•10 Creme (Pfizer
  Inc., Warner-Lambert
  Healthcare) **518, 699**
Cortizone•10 Ointment (Pfizer Inc.,
  Warner-Lambert Healthcare)........**699**
Cortizone•10 Plus Creme
  (Pfizer Inc., Warner-Lambert
  Healthcare) **518, 700**
Cortizone•10 Quick Shot Spray
  (Pfizer Inc., Warner-Lambert
  Healthcare) **518, 699**
Cortizone for Kids Creme (Pfizer
  Inc., Warner-Lambert
  Healthcare) **518, 699**
Tegrin Dandruff Shampoo - Extra
  Conditioning (Block) **623**

Tegrin Dandruff Shampoo -
  Fresh Herbal (Block) **506, 624**
Tegrin Skin Cream (Block) **506, 624**

ANTISEBORRHEIC AGENTS
Cortaid Intensive Therapy Cream
  (Pharmacia Consumer) **717**
Cortaid Maximum Strength Cream
  (Pharmacia Consumer) **717**
Cortaid Maximum Strength Ointment
  (Pharmacia Consumer) **717**
Cortaid Sensitive Skin Cream
  (Pharmacia Consumer) **717**
Cortizone•5 Creme (Pfizer Inc.,
  Warner-Lambert Healthcare)...**518, 699**
Cortizone•5 Ointment (Pfizer Inc.,
  Warner-Lambert Healthcare)........**699**
Cortizone•10 Creme (Pfizer
  Inc., Warner-Lambert
  Healthcare) **518, 699**
Cortizone•10 Ointment (Pfizer Inc.,
  Warner-Lambert Healthcare)........**699**
Cortizone•10 Plus Creme
  (Pfizer Inc., Warner-Lambert
  Healthcare) **518, 700**
Cortizone•10 Quick Shot Spray
  (Pfizer Inc., Warner-Lambert
  Healthcare) **518, 699**
Nizoral A-D Shampoo (McNeil
  Consumer) **510, 647**
Tegrin Dandruff Shampoo - Extra
  Conditioning (Block) **623**
Tegrin Dandruff Shampoo -
  Fresh Herbal (Block) **506, 624**
Tegrin Skin Cream (Block) **506, 624**

ASTRINGENTS
Domeboro Powder Packets
  (Bayer Consumer)..............**504, 611**
Domeboro Effervescent Tablets
  (Bayer Consumer)..............**504, 611**
Tucks Pre-moistened Pads
  (Pfizer Inc., Warner-Lambert
  Healthcare) **521, 713**

BURN PREPARATIONS
A + D Original Ointment
  (Schering-Plough) **522, 733**
Betadine Brand First Aid
  Antibiotics + Moisturizer
  Ointment (Purdue Frederick)...**522, 731**
Betadine Brand Plus First Aid
  Antibiotics + Pain Reliever
  Ointment (Purdue Frederick)...**522, 731**
Betadine Ointment (Purdue
  Frederick) **522, 732**
Betadine Solution (Purdue
  Frederick) **522, 732**
Desitin Ointment (Pfizer Inc.,
  Warner-Lambert Healthcare)...**518, 700**
Humatrix Microclysmic Burn/Wound
  Healing Gel (Care-Tech)..............**632**
Neosporin Ointment (Pfizer Inc.,
  Warner-Lambert Healthcare)...**519, 704**
Neosporin + Pain Relief
  Maximum Strength Cream
  (Pfizer Inc., Warner-Lambert
  Healthcare) **519, 704**
Neosporin + Pain Relief
  Maximum Strength Ointment
  (Pfizer Inc., Warner-Lambert
  Healthcare) **519, 704**
Polysporin Ointment (Pfizer Inc.,
  Warner-Lambert Healthcare)...**519, 706**
Polysporin Powder (Pfizer Inc.,
  Warner-Lambert Healthcare)...**519, 706**

CLEANSING AGENTS
Betadine Skin Cleanser (Purdue
  Frederick) **732**

Bio-Complex 5000 Gentle Foaming
  Cleanser (Wellness International) ...**769**
Massengill Baby Powder Scent Soft
  Cloth Towelette (SmithKline
  Beecham Consumer) **753**
Techni-Care Surgical Scrub, Prep and
  Wound Decontaminant
  (Care-Tech)..........................**632**
Zanfel Urushiol Wash (Zanfel) **526, 790**

CONDITIONING RINSES
Bio-Complex 5000 Revitalizing
  Conditioner (Wellness
  International) **769**

DIAPER RASH PRODUCTS
A + D Original Ointment
  (Schering-Plough) **522, 733**
A + D Ointment with Zinc Oxide
  (Schering-Plough) **522, 733**
Balmex Diaper Rash Ointment
  (Block) **505, 619**
Balmex Medicated Plus Baby
  Powder (Block) **505, 619**
Desitin Baby Powder (Pfizer Inc.,
  Warner-Lambert Healthcare)...**518, 700**
Desitin Creamy Ointment (Pfizer
  Inc., Warner-Lambert
  Healthcare) **518, 700**
Desitin Ointment (Pfizer Inc.,
  Warner-Lambert Healthcare)...**518, 700**

EMOLLIENTS & MOISTURIZERS
A + D Original Ointment
  (Schering-Plough) **522, 733**
Balmex Diaper Rash Ointment
  (Block) **505, 619**
Lubriderm Advanced Therapy
  Creamy Lotion (Pfizer Inc.,
  Warner-Lambert Healthcare)...**519, 703**
Lubriderm Daily UV Lotion
  (Pfizer Inc., Warner-Lambert
  Healthcare) **519, 703**
Lubriderm Seriously Sensitive
  Lotion (Pfizer Inc.,
  Warner-Lambert Healthcare)...**519, 703**
Lubriderm Skin Therapy
  Moisturizing Lotion (Pfizer
  Inc., Warner-Lambert
  Healthcare) **519, 703**
StePHan Bio-Nutritional Daytime
  Hydrating Creme (Wellness
  International) **770**
StePHan Bio-Nutritional Eye-Firming
  Concentrate (Wellness
  International) **770**
StePHan Bio-Nutritional Nightime
  Moisture Creme (Wellness
  International) **770**
StePHan Bio-Nutritional Refreshing
  Moisture Gel (Wellness
  International) **770**
StePHan Bio-Nutritional Ultra
  Hydrating Fluid (Wellness
  International) **770**

FOOT CARE PRODUCTS
Lotrimin AF Spray Powder, Spray
  Liquid, Spray Deodorant
  Powder, Shaker Powder and
  Jock Itch Spray Powder
  (Schering-Plough) **523, 742**

HAIR GROWTH STIMULANTS
Rogaine Extra Strength for Men
  Topical Solution (Pharmacia
  Consumer)..........................**721**
Rogaine for Women Topical Solution
  (Pharmacia Consumer) **721**

KERATOLYTICS
(*see also under:*
SKIN & MUCOUS MEMBRANE AGENTS
WART PREPARATIONS)
Clear Away Gel with Aloe Wart
   Remover System (Schering-Plough) . **736**
Clear Away Liquid Wart Remover
   System (Schering-Plough) **736**
Clear Away One Step Wart
   Remover (Schering-Plough) **522, 737**
Clear Away One Step Wart
   Remover for Kids
   (Schering-Plough) **522, 737**
Clear Away One Step Plantar Wart
   Remover (Schering-Plough) **737**
Wart-Off Liquid (Pfizer Inc.,
   Warner-Lambert Healthcare)......... **716**

**MISCELLANEOUS SKIN & MUCOUS MEMBRANE
AGENTS**
Massengill Baby Powder Scent Soft
   Cloth Towelette (SmithKline
   Beecham Consumer) **753**

MOUTH & THROAT PRODUCTS

ANTIFUNGALS
(*see under:*
SKIN & MUCOUS MEMBRANE AGENTS
ANTI-INFECTIVES
ANTIFUNGALS & COMBINATIONS)
CANKER SORE PREPARATIONS
Junior Anbesol Gel
   (Whitehall-Robins) **774**
Maximum Strength Anbesol Gel
   (Whitehall-Robins) **774**
Maximum Strength Anbesol Liquid
   (Whitehall-Robins) **774**
Gly-Oxide Liquid (SmithKline
   Beecham Consumer) **524, 751**
Hurricaine Topical Anesthetic Gel,
   1 oz. Fresh Mint, Wild Cherry,
   Pina Colada, Watermelon,
   1/6 oz. Wild Cherry,
   Watermelon (Beutlich) **618**
Hurricaine Topical Anesthetic
   Liquid, 1 oz. Wild Cherry, Pina
   Colada, .25 ml Dry Handle
   Swab Wild Cherry, 1/6 oz.
   Wild Cherry (Beutlich) **618**
Hurricaine Topical Anesthetic
   Spray Extension Tubes (200)
   (Beutlich) **618**
Hurricaine Topical Anesthetic
   Spray Kit, 2 oz. Wild Cherry
   (Beutlich) **618**
Hurricaine Topical Anesthetic
   Spray, 2 oz. Wild Cherry
   (Beutlich) **618**
Zilactin Gel (Zila Consumer) **790**
Zilactin-B Gel (Zila Consumer)......... **790**

COLD SORE PREPARATIONS
Abreva Cream (SmithKline
   Beecham Consumer) **744**
Cēpacol Viractin Cold Sore
   and Fever Blister
   Treatment, Cream
   (Williams) **526, 788**
Cēpacol Viractin Cold Sore
   and Fever Blister
   Treatment, Gel
   (Williams) **526, 788**
Zilactin Gel (Zila Consumer) **790**
Zilactin-L Liquid (Zila Consumer) **790**

DENTAL PREPARATIONS
Junior Anbesol Gel
   (Whitehall-Robins) **774**
Maximum Strength Anbesol Gel
   (Whitehall-Robins) **774**
Maximum Strength Anbesol Liquid
   (Whitehall-Robins) **774**

Hurricaine Topical Anesthetic Gel,
   1 oz. Fresh Mint, Wild Cherry,
   Pina Colada, Watermelon,
   1/6 oz. Wild Cherry,
   Watermelon (Beutlich) **618**
Hurricaine Topical Anesthetic
   Liquid, 1 oz. Wild Cherry, Pina
   Colada, .25 ml Dry Handle
   Swab Wild Cherry, 1/6 oz.
   Wild Cherry (Beutlich) **618**
Hurricaine Topical Anesthetic
   Spray Extension Tubes (200)
   (Beutlich) **618**
Hurricaine Topical Anesthetic
   Spray Kit, 2 oz. Wild Cherry
   (Beutlich) **618**
Hurricaine Topical Anesthetic
   Spray, 2 oz. Wild Cherry
   (Beutlich) **618**
Tartar Control Listerine
   Mouthrinse (Pfizer Inc.,
   Warner-Lambert
   Healthcare) **519, 702**
Sensodyne Original Flavor (Block) **623**
Sensodyne Cool Gel (Block) **623**
Sensodyne Extra Whitening
   (Block) **623**
Sensodyne Fresh Mint (Block)......... **623**
Sensodyne Tartar Control (Block) **623**
Sensodyne Tartar Control Plus
   Whitening (Block) **623**
Sensodyne with Baking Soda
   (Block) **623**
Trident Advantage Mints
   (Pfizer Inc.,
   Warner-Lambert Group)...... **516, 687**
Trident Advantage Sugarless
   Gum (Pfizer Inc.,
   Warner-Lambert Group)...... **516, 687**
Trident for Kids Sugarless
   Gum (Pfizer Inc.,
   Warner-Lambert Group)...... **516, 687**
Zilactin-B Gel (Zila Consumer) **790**

LOZENGES & SPRAYS
Cēpacol Maximum Strength Sugar
   Free Sore Throat Lozenges,
   Cherry Flavor (Williams) **787**
Cēpacol Maximum Strength Sugar
   Free Sore Throat Lozenges,
   Cool Mint Flavor (Williams) **787**
Cēpacol Maximum Strength
   Sore Throat Lozenges,
   Cherry Flavor (Williams) **526, 787**
Cēpacol Maximum Strength
   Sore Throat Lozenges,
   Mint Flavor (Williams)........ **526, 787**
Cēpacol Regular Strength Sore
   Throat Lozenges, Cherry
   Flavor (Williams) **787**
Cēpacol Regular Strength Sore
   Throat Lozenges, Original
   Mint Flavor (Williams).............. **787**
Cēpacol Maximum Strength Sore
   Throat Spray, Honey Lemon
   Flavor (Williams) **787**
Celestial Seasonings
   Soothers Throat Drops
   (Pfizer Inc.,
   Warner-Lambert Group)...... **515, 685**
Halls Mentho-Lyptus Drops
   (Pfizer Inc.,
   Warner-Lambert Group)...... **516, 686**
Halls Sugar Free
   Mentho-Lyptus Drops
   (Pfizer Inc.,
   Warner-Lambert Group)...... **516, 686**

Halls Sugar Free Squares
   (Pfizer Inc.,
   Warner-Lambert Group)...... **516, 686**
Halls Plus Cough Drops
   (Pfizer Inc.,
   Warner-Lambert Group)...... **516, 686**
Vicks Cough Drops, Menthol and
   Cherry Flavors (Procter &
   Gamble)............................ **726**

**MISCELLANEOUS MOUTH & THROAT
PRODUCTS**
Certs Cool Mint Drops (Pfizer
   Inc., Warner-Lambert
   Group) **515, 685**
Certs Powerful Mints (Pfizer
   Inc., Warner-Lambert
   Group) **516, 686**
Gly-Oxide Liquid (SmithKline
   Beecham Consumer) **524, 751**
Trident Advantage Mints
   (Pfizer Inc.,
   Warner-Lambert Group)...... **516, 687**

ORAL RINSES
Cēpacol Antiseptic
   Mouthwash/Gargle,
   Original (Williams) **526, 786**
Cēpacol Antiseptic
   Mouthwash/Gargle,
   Mint (Williams)............... **526, 786**
Listerine Mouthrinse (Pfizer
   Inc., Warner-Lambert
   Healthcare) **518, 702**
Cool Mint Listerine
   Mouthrinse (Pfizer Inc.,
   Warner-Lambert
   Healthcare) **518, 702**
FreshBurst Listerine
   Mouthrinse (Pfizer Inc.,
   Warner-Lambert
   Healthcare) **519, 702**
Tartar Control Listerine
   Mouthrinse (Pfizer Inc.,
   Warner-Lambert
   Healthcare) **519, 702**
Listermint Alcohol-Free
   Mouthrinse (Pfizer Inc.,
   Warner-Lambert
   Healthcare) **519, 703**

TEETHING REMEDIES
Baby Anbesol Gel
   (Whitehall-Robins) **774**
Zilactin Baby Gel (Zila Consumer) **791**

POISON IVY, OAK OR SUMAC PRODUCTS
Benadryl Itch Relief Stick Extra
   Strength (Pfizer Inc.,
   Warner-Lambert Healthcare)... **517, 695**
Benadryl Itch Stopping Cream
   Original Strength (Pfizer Inc.,
   Warner-Lambert Healthcare)... **517, 695**
Benadryl Itch Stopping Cream
   Extra Strength (Pfizer Inc.,
   Warner-Lambert Healthcare)... **517, 695**
Benadryl Itch Stopping Gel
   Original Strength (Pfizer Inc.,
   Warner-Lambert Healthcare)... **517, 695**
Benadryl Itch Stopping Gel Extra
   Strength (Pfizer Inc.,
   Warner-Lambert Healthcare)... **517, 695**
Benadryl Itch Stopping Spray
   Original Strength (Pfizer Inc.,
   Warner-Lambert Healthcare)... **517, 696**
Benadryl Itch Stopping Spray
   Extra Strength (Pfizer Inc.,
   Warner-Lambert Healthcare)... **517, 696**
Caladryl Clear Lotion (Pfizer
   Inc., Warner-Lambert
   Healthcare) **518, 698**

SKIN & MUCOUS MEMBRANE AGENTS—cont.

POISON IVY, OAK OR SUMAC PRODUCTS—cont.
Caladryl Lotion (Pfizer Inc.,
Warner-Lambert Healthcare)...**518, 698**
Cortaid Intensive Therapy Cream
(Pharmacia Consumer) **717**
Cortaid Maximum Strength Cream
(Pharmacia Consumer) **717**
Cortaid Maximum Strength Ointment
(Pharmacia Consumer) **717**
Cortaid Sensitive Skin Cream
(Pharmacia Consumer) **717**
Cortizone•5 Creme (Pfizer Inc.,
Warner-Lambert Healthcare)...**518, 699**
Cortizone•5 Ointment (Pfizer Inc.,
Warner-Lambert Healthcare)........**699**
Cortizone•10 Creme (Pfizer
Inc., Warner-Lambert
Healthcare) **518, 699**
Cortizone•10 Ointment (Pfizer Inc.,
Warner-Lambert Healthcare)........**699**
Cortizone•10 Plus Creme
(Pfizer Inc., Warner-Lambert
Healthcare) **518, 700**
Cortizone•10 Quick Shot Spray
(Pfizer Inc., Warner-Lambert
Healthcare) **518, 699**
Cortizone for Kids Creme (Pfizer
Inc., Warner-Lambert
Healthcare) **518, 699**
Domeboro Powder Packets
(Bayer Consumer)..............**504, 611**
Domeboro Effervescent Tablets
(Bayer Consumer)..............**504, 611**

SHAMPOOS
Bio-Complex 5000 Revitalizing
Shampoo (Wellness International) ..**770**
Maximum Strength Rid
Shampoo (Bayer Consumer)...**505, 616**
Tegrin Dandruff Shampoo - Extra
Conditioning (Block) **623**
Tegrin Dandruff Shampoo -
Fresh Herbal (Block) **506, 624**

SKIN PROTECTANTS
Desitin Creamy Ointment (Pfizer
Inc., Warner-Lambert
Healthcare) **518, 700**
Desitin Ointment (Pfizer Inc.,
Warner-Lambert Healthcare)...**518, 700**
New Skin Liquid Bandage (Medtech) **667**

STEROIDS & COMBINATIONS
Cortaid Intensive Therapy Cream
(Pharmacia Consumer) **717**
Cortaid Maximum Strength Cream
(Pharmacia Consumer) **717**
Cortaid Maximum Strength Ointment
(Pharmacia Consumer) **717**
Cortaid Sensitive Skin Cream
(Pharmacia Consumer) **717**
Cortizone•5 Creme (Pfizer Inc.,
Warner-Lambert Healthcare)...**518, 699**
Cortizone•5 Ointment (Pfizer Inc.,
Warner-Lambert Healthcare)........**699**
Cortizone•10 Creme (Pfizer
Inc., Warner-Lambert
Healthcare) **518, 699**
Cortizone•10 Ointment (Pfizer Inc.,
Warner-Lambert Healthcare)........**699**
Cortizone•10 Plus Creme
(Pfizer Inc., Warner-Lambert
Healthcare) **518, 700**
Cortizone•10 Quick Shot Spray
(Pfizer Inc., Warner-Lambert
Healthcare) **518, 699**

Cortizone for Kids Creme (Pfizer
Inc., Warner-Lambert
Healthcare) **518, 699**
Massengill Medicated Soft Cloth
Towelette (SmithKline Beecham
Consumer) **753**

SUNBURN PREPARATIONS
Dermoplast Antibacterial Spray,
Hospital Strength (Medtech) **666**
Dermoplast Hospital Strength Spray
(Medtech)...........................**666**

SUNSCREENS
Lubriderm Daily UV Lotion (Pfizer
Inc., Warner-Lambert
Healthcare) **519, 703**

TAR-CONTAINING PREPARATIONS
Tegrin Dandruff Shampoo - Extra
Conditioning (Block) **623**
Tegrin Dandruff Shampoo -
Fresh Herbal (Block) **506, 624**
Tegrin Skin Cream (Block) **506, 624**

VAGINAL PRODUCTS
(see under:
VAGINAL PREPARATIONS)

WART PREPARATIONS
Clear Away Gel with Aloe Wart
Remover System
(Schering-Plough) **736**
Clear Away Liquid Wart Remover
System (Schering-Plough) **736**
Clear Away One Step Wart
Remover (Schering-Plough) **522, 737**
Clear Away One Step Wart
Remover for Kids
(Schering-Plough) **522, 737**
Clear Away One Step Plantar Wart
Remover (Schering-Plough) **737**
Compound W One Step Pads for Kids
(Medtech)...........................**664**
Compound W One Step Plantar Pads
(Medtech)...........................**664**
Compound W One Step Wart
Remover Pads (Medtech)............**664**
Compound W Wart Remover Gel
(Medtech)...........................**665**
Compound W Wart Remover Liquid
(Medtech)...........................**665**
Wart-Off Liquid (Pfizer Inc.,
Warner-Lambert Healthcare)........**716**

WET DRESSINGS
Domeboro Powder Packets
(Bayer Consumer)..............**504, 611**
Domeboro Effervescent Tablets
(Bayer Consumer)..............**504, 611**
Tucks Pre-moistened Pads
(Pfizer Inc., Warner-Lambert
Healthcare) **521, 713**

WOUND CARE PRODUCTS
Betadine Brand First Aid
Antibiotics + Moisturizer
Ointment (Purdue Frederick)...**522, 731**
Betadine Brand Plus First Aid
Antibiotics + Pain Reliever
Ointment (Purdue Frederick)...**522, 731**
Betadine Ointment (Purdue
Frederick) **522, 732**
Betadine Solution (Purdue
Frederick) **522, 732**
Clinical Care Antimicrobial Wound
Cleanser (Care-Tech).................**632**
Humatrix Microclysmic Burn/Wound
Healing Gel (Care-Tech)..............**632**
Techni-Care Surgical Scrub, Prep and
Wound Decontaminant
(Care-Tech)..........................**632**

SKIN CARE PRODUCTS
(see under:
SKIN & MUCOUS MEMBRANE AGENTS)

SKIN PROTECTANTS
(see under:
SKIN & MUCOUS MEMBRANE AGENTS
SKIN PROTECTANTS)

SLEEP AIDS
(see under:
SEDATIVES & HYPNOTICS)

SMOKING CESSATION AIDS
NicoDerm CQ Patch (SmithKline
Beecham Consumer) **524, 754**
Nicorette Gum (SmithKline
Beecham Consumer) **524, 758**

STEROIDS
(see under:
SKIN & MUCOUS MEMBRANE AGENTS
STEROIDS & COMBINATIONS)

SUNSCREENS
(see under:
SKIN & MUCOUS MEMBRANE AGENTS
SUNSCREENS)

SUPPLEMENTS
(see under:
DIETARY SUPPLEMENTS)

SYMPATHOMIMETICS
(see under:
NASAL PREPARATIONS
SYMPATHOMIMETICS & COMBINATIONS
OPHTHALMIC PREPARATIONS
SYMPATHOMIMETICS & COMBINATIONS
RESPIRATORY AGENTS
BRONCHODILATORS
SYMPATHOMIMETICS & COMBINATIONS
DECONGESTANTS & COMBINATIONS
DECONGESTANTS, EXPECTORANTS & COMBINATIONS)

T

TEETHING REMEDIES
(see under:
HOMEOPATHIC REMEDIES
TEETHING REMEDIES
SKIN & MUCOUS MEMBRANE AGENTS
MOUTH & THROAT PRODUCTS
TEETHING REMEDIES)

THROAT LOZENGES
(see under:
SKIN & MUCOUS MEMBRANE AGENTS
MOUTH & THROAT PRODUCTS
LOZENGES & SPRAYS)

TOPICAL PREPARATIONS
(see under:
NASAL PREPARATIONS
OPHTHALMIC PREPARATIONS
OTIC PREPARATIONS
SKIN & MUCOUS MEMBRANE AGENTS
VAGINAL PREPARATIONS)

V

VAGINAL PREPARATIONS

ANTI-INFECTIVES

ANTIFUNGALS & COMBINATIONS
Gyne-Lotrimin 3, 3-Day Cream
(Schering-Plough) **523, 741**
Mycelex-3 Vaginal Cream with 3
Disposable Applicators (Bayer
Consumer)..........................**613**
Mycelex-3 Vaginal Cream in 3
Pre-filled Applicators (Bayer
Consumer)..........................**613**
Mycelex-7 Combination-Pack
Vaginal Inserts & External
Vulvar Cream (Bayer
Consumer)..........................**614**
Mycelex-7 Vaginal Cream (Bayer
Consumer)..........................**614**

Mycelex-7 Vaginal Cream with 7
  Disposable Applicators (Bayer
  Consumer) **614**

CLEANSERS AND DOUCHES
Massengill Feminine Cleansing Wash
  (SmithKline Beecham Consumer) ... **753**
Massengill Disposable Douches
  (SmithKline Beecham Consumer) ... **752**
Massengill Baby Powder Scent Soft
  Cloth Towelette (SmithKline
  Beecham Consumer) **753**
Massengill Medicated
  Disposable Douche
  (SmithKline Beecham
  Consumer) **524, 753**

Massengill Medicated Soft Cloth
  Towelette (SmithKline Beecham
  Consumer) **753**
Preparation H Medicated Wipes
  (Whitehall-Robins) **779**
Tucks Pre-moistened Pads
  (Pfizer Inc., Warner-Lambert
  Healthcare) **521, 713**

MISCELLANEOUS VAGINAL PREPARATIONS
Vitara Cream (Products on
  Demand) **522, 731**

VITAMINS
(*see under:*
DIETARY SUPPLEMENTS
  VITAMINS & COMBINATIONS)

W

WART PREPARATIONS
(*see under:*
SKIN & MUCOUS MEMBRANE AGENTS
  WART PREPARATIONS)

WET DRESSINGS
(*see under:*
SKIN & MUCOUS MEMBRANE AGENTS
  WET DRESSINGS)

WOUND CARE
(*see under:*
SKIN & MUCOUS MEMBRANE AGENTS
  WOUND CARE PRODUCTS)

SECTION 4

ACTIVE INGREDIENTS INDEX

This index cross-references each brand by its generic ingredients. All entries in the Product Information sections are included. Under each generic heading, all fully described products are listed first, followed by those with only partial descriptions.

If an entry in the index lists multiple page numbers, the first one shown refers to the photograph of the product, the last one to its prescribing information.

- **Bold page numbers** indicate full product information.

- *Italic page numbers* signify partial information.

Classification of products under these headings has been determined in cooperation with the products' manufacturers or, if necessary, by the publisher alone.

A

ACETAMINOPHEN

Actifed Cold & Sinus Caplets and Tablets (Pfizer Inc., Warner-Lambert Healthcare).....................**516, 688**

Alka-Seltzer Plus Cold Medicine Liqui-Gels (Bayer Consumer).....................**503, 604**

Alka-Seltzer Plus Night-Time Cold Medicine Liqui-Gels (Bayer Consumer).............**503, 604**

Alka-Seltzer Plus Cold & Cough Medicine Liqui-Gels (Bayer Consumer) **503, 604**

Alka-Seltzer Plus Cold & Flu Medicine Liqui-Gels (Bayer Consumer) **503, 604**

Alka-Seltzer Plus Cold & Sinus Medicine Liqui-Gels (Bayer Consumer) **503, 604**

Benadryl Allergy/Cold Tablets (Pfizer Inc., Warner-Lambert Healthcare).....................**517, 691**

Benadryl Allergy Sinus Headache Caplets & Gelcaps (Pfizer Inc., Warner-Lambert Healthcare).....................**517, 693**

Benadryl Severe Allergy & Sinus Headache Caplets (Pfizer Inc., Warner-Lambert Healthcare).....................**517, 694**

Children's Cēpacol Sore Throat Formula, Cherry Flavor Liquid (Williams)..........................**788**

Children's Cēpacol Sore Throat Formula, Grape Flavor Liquid (Williams)..........................**788**

Comtrex Acute Head Cold & Sinus Pressure Relief Tablets (Bristol-Myers) **506, 627**

Comtrex Deep Chest Cold & Congestion Relief Softgels (Bristol-Myers)................**506, 627**

Comtrex Flu Therapy & Fever Relief Daytime Caplets (Bristol-Myers)................**506, 628**

Comtrex Flu Therapy & Fever Relief Nighttime Tablets (Bristol-Myers)................**506, 628**

Comtrex Maximum Strength Multi-Symptom Cold & Cough Relief Tablets and Caplets (Bristol-Myers)........**506, 626**

Contac Severe Cold and Flu Caplets Maximum Strength (SmithKline Beecham Consumer) **523, 746**

Contac Severe Cold and Flu Caplets Non-Drowsy (SmithKline Beecham Consumer) **746**

Coricidin 'D' Cold, Flu & Sinus Tablets (Schering-Plough) **522, 737**

Coricidin HBP Cold & Flu Tablets (Schering-Plough) **523, 738**

Coricidin HBP Maximum Strength Flu Tablets (Schering-Plough) **523, 738**

Coricidin HBP Night-Time Cold & Flu Tablets (Schering-Plough) **523, 738**

Dimetapp Cold and Fever Suspension (Whitehall-Robins) **775**

Dimetapp Nighttime Flu Liquid (Whitehall-Robins)....................**776**

Dimetapp Non-Drowsy Flu Syrup (Whitehall-Robins)....................**777**

Drixoral Allergy/Sinus Extended-Release Tablets (Schering-Plough) **523, 741**

Drixoral Cold & Flu Extended-Release Tablets (Schering-Plough)..............**523, 740**

Aspirin Free Excedrin Caplets and Geltabs (Bristol-Myers)...**507, 628**

Excedrin Extra-Strength Tablets, Caplets, and Geltabs (Bristol-Myers)........**507, 629**

Excedrin Migraine Tablets, Caplets, and Geltabs (Bristol-Myers)................**507, 630**

Excedrin PM Tablets, Caplets, and Geltabs (Bristol-Myers)...**506, 631**

Goody's Body Pain Formula Powder (Block)................................**620**

Goody's Extra Strength Headache Powder (Block) **620**

Goody's Extra Strength Pain Relief Tablets (Block) **620**

Goody's PM Powder (Block) **621**

Maximum Strength Midol Menstrual Caplets and Gelcaps (Bayer Consumer) ...**504, 612**

Maximum Strength Midol PMS Caplets and Gelcaps (Bayer Consumer)............**504, 613**

Maximum Strength Midol Teen Caplets (Bayer Consumer)....**504, 612**

Percogesic Aspirin-Free Coated Tablets (Medtech)...................**667**

Extra Strength Percogesic Aspirin-Free Coated Caplets (Medtech) **665**

Robitussin Cold Caplets Multi-Symptom Cold & Flu (Whitehall-Robins)...................**781**

ACETAMINOPHEN—cont.
Robitussin Cold Softgels
Multi-Symptom Cold & Flu
(Whitehall-Robins)...................**781**
Robitussin Multi Symptom Honey Flu
Liquid (Whitehall-Robins) **785**
Robitussin Nighttime Honey Flu
Liquid (Whitehall-Robins) **786**
Singlet Caplets (SmithKline
Beecham Consumer) **761**
Sinutab Sinus Allergy
Medication, Maximum
Strength Formula, Tablets
& Caplets (Pfizer Inc.,
Warner-Lambert
Healthcare)....................**520, 707**
Sinutab Sinus Medication,
Maximum Strength Without
Drowsiness Formula,
Tablets & Caplets (Pfizer
Inc., Warner-Lambert
Healthcare)....................**520, 707**
Sudafed Cold & Cough Liquid
Caps (Pfizer Inc.,
Warner-Lambert
Healthcare)....................**520, 709**
Sudafed Cold & Sinus Liquid
Caps (Pfizer Inc.,
Warner-Lambert
Healthcare)....................**520, 710**
Sudafed Severe Cold Formula
Caplets (Pfizer Inc.,
Warner-Lambert
Healthcare)....................**520, 711**
Sudafed Severe Cold Formula
Tablets (Pfizer Inc.,
Warner-Lambert
Healthcare)....................**520, 711**
Sudafed Sinus Headache
Caplets (Pfizer Inc.,
Warner-Lambert
Healthcare)....................**520, 712**
Sudafed Sinus Headache
Tablets (Pfizer Inc.,
Warner-Lambert
Healthcare)....................**520, 712**
Tavist Sinus Non-Drowsy
Coated Caplets (Novartis
Consumer) **514, 676**
TheraFlu Regular Strength Cold
& Cough Night Time Hot
Liquid (Novartis Consumer) ..**515, 676**
TheraFlu Regular Strength Cold
& Sore Throat Night Time
Hot Liquid (Novartis
Consumer) **515, 676**
TheraFlu Maximum Strength
Flu & Congestion
Non-Drowsy Hot Liquid
(Novartis Consumer)..........**515, 677**
TheraFlu Maximum Strength
Flu & Cough Night Time Hot
Liquid (Novartis Consumer) ..**515, 678**
TheraFlu Maximum Strength
Flu & Sore Throat Night
Time Hot Liquid (Novartis
Consumer) **515, 677**
TheraFlu Maximum Strength
Severe Cold & Congestion
Night Time Caplets
(Novartis Consumer)..........**515, 678**
TheraFlu Maximum Strength
Severe Cold & Congestion
Night Time Hot Liquid
(Novartis Consumer)..........**515, 678**
TheraFlu Maximum Strength
Severe Cold & Congestion
Non-Drowsy Caplets
(Novartis Consumer)..........**515, 679**

TheraFlu Maximum Strength
Severe Cold & Congestion
Non-Drowsy Hot Liquid
(Novartis Consumer)..........**515, 679**
Triaminic Cold, Cough & Fever
Liquid (Novartis Consumer) ..**515, 681**
Triaminic Cough & Sore Throat
Liquid (Novartis Consumer) ..**515, 682**
Triaminic Cough & Sore Throat
Softchews (Novartis
Consumer) **515, 684**
Children's Tylenol
Suspension Liquid
and Soft Chews
Chewable Tablets
(McNeil Consumer) **510, 511, 657**
Children's Tylenol Allergy-D
Liquid (McNeil Consumer) **510, 658**
Children's Tylenol Cold
Suspension Liquid and
Chewable Tablets (McNeil
Consumer) **510, 659**
Children's Tylenol Cold Plus
Cough Suspension Liquid
and Chewable Tablets
(McNeil Consumer) **510, 659**
Children's Tylenol Flu
Suspension Liquid (McNeil
Consumer) **511, 663**
Children's Tylenol Sinus
Suspension Liquid (McNeil
Consumer) **511, 663**
Infants' Tylenol Cold
Decongestant & Fever
Reducer Concentrated
Drops (McNeil Consumer) **511, 659**
Infants' Tylenol Cold
Decongestant & Fever
Reducer Concentrated
Drops Plus Cough (McNeil
Consumer) **511, 659**
Infants' Tylenol Concentrated
Drops (McNeil Consumer) **511, 657**
Junior Strength Tylenol
Soft Chews Chewable
Tablets (McNeil
Consumer) **511, 512, 657**
Extra Strength Tylenol Adult Liquid
Pain Reliever (McNeil Consumer)...**647**
Extra Strength Tylenol Gelcaps,
Geltabs, Caplets, and
Tablets (McNeil Consumer) ...**511, 647**
Regular Strength Tylenol
Tablets (McNeil Consumer) ...**511, 647**
Maximum Strength Tylenol
Allergy Sinus Caplets,
Gelcaps, and Geltabs
(McNeil Consumer) **511, 649**
Maximum Strength Tylenol
Allergy Sinus NightTime
Caplets (McNeil Consumer) ..**511, 649**
Tylenol Severe Allergy Caplets
(McNeil Consumer) **511, 649**
Tylenol Arthritis Pain Extended
Relief Caplets (McNeil
Consumer) **511, 647**
Multi-Symptom Tylenol Cold
Complete Formula Caplets
(McNeil Consumer) **512, 651**
Multi-Symptom Tylenol Cold
Non-Drowsy Caplets and
Gelcaps (McNeil
Consumer) **512, 651**
Multi-Symptom Tylenol Cold
Severe Congestion
Non-Drowsy Caplets
(McNeil Consumer) **512, 652**

Maximum Strength Tylenol Flu
NightTime Gelcaps (McNeil
Consumer) **512, 653**
Maximum Strength Tylenol Flu
NightTime Liquid (McNeil
Consumer) **512, 653**
Maximum Strength Tylenol Flu
Non-Drowsy Gelcaps
(McNeil Consumer) **512, 653**
Extra Strength Tylenol PM
Caplets, Geltabs, and
Gelcaps (McNeil
Consumer) **512, 654**
Maximum Strength Tylenol
Sinus NightTime Caplets
(McNeil Consumer) **512, 655**
Maximum Strength Tylenol
Sinus Non-Drowsy Geltabs,
Gelcaps, Caplets, and
Tablets (McNeil Consumer) ...**512, 655**
Maximum Strength Tylenol
Sore Throat Adult Liquid
(McNeil Consumer) **512, 656**
Women's Tylenol Menstrual
Relief Caplets (McNeil
Consumer) **512, 656**
Vanquish Caplets (Bayer
Consumer) **505, 617**
Vicks 44M Cough, Cold & Flu Relief
Liquid (Procter & Gamble) **725**
Vicks DayQuil LiquiCaps/Liquid
Multi-Symptom Cold/Flu Relief
(Procter & Gamble) **727**
Vicks NyQuil LiquiCaps/Liquid
Multi-Symptom Cold/Flu Relief,
Original and Cherry Flavors
(Procter & Gamble) **727**
ACETYL-L-CARNITINE HYDROCHLORIDE
Proxeed Powder (Sigma-Tau)......**523, 835**
ACETYLSALICYLIC ACID
(*see under:* **ASPIRIN**)
ACONITE
Nytol Natural Tablets (Block) **506, 622**
ALLIUM SATIVUM
Beta-C Tablets (Body Wise) **811**
Centrum Focused Formulas Heart
Tablets (Lederle Consumer) **816**
CorePlex Capsules (AdvoCare) **796**
One-A-Day Cholesterol Health
Tablets (Bayer Consumer) **505, 805**
Phyto-Vite Tablets (Wellness
International)......................**849**
System 3-4-3 Capsules (AdvoCare) **800**
Vitality Immunity Anti-Oxidant
Complex Capsules (Youngevity) *854*
ALOE
Desitin Creamy Ointment
(Pfizer Inc., Warner-Lambert
Healthcare)....................**518, 700**
ALOE VERA
Bio-Complex 5000 Gentle Foaming
Cleanser (Wellness
International)......................**769**
ProBiotic Restore Capsules
(AdvoCare) **799**
System 3-4-3 Capsules (AdvoCare) **800**
ALPHA GALACTOSIDASE ENZYME
Beano Liquid (Block)....................**809**
Beano Tablets (Block)...................**809**
ALPHA TOCOPHERAL ACETATE
(*see under:* **VITAMIN E**)
ALUMINUM HYDROXIDE
Amphojel Suspension (Mint
Flavor) (Wyeth-Ayerst).............**526, 789**
Gaviscon Extra Strength Liquid
(SmithKline Beecham
Consumer) **524, 751**

Gaviscon Extra Strength Tablets (SmithKline Beecham Consumer) **524, 751**
Gaviscon Regular Strength Liquid (SmithKline Beecham Consumer) **524, 751**
Gaviscon Regular Strength Tablets (SmithKline Beecham Consumer) **524, 750**
Maalox Antacid/Anti-Gas Oral Suspension (Novartis Consumer) **514, 673**
Maalox Max Maximum Strength Antacid/Anti-Gas Liquid (Novartis Consumer) ..**514, 673**
Mylanta Liquid (J&J • Merck)...........**634**
Mylanta Extra Strength Liquid (J&J • Merck) **507, 634**
Vanquish Caplets (Bayer Consumer) **505, 617**

ALUMINUM SULFATE
Domeboro Powder Packets (Bayer Consumer)............**504, 611**
Domeboro Effervescent Tablets (Bayer Consumer) **504, 611**

AMINO ACID PREPARATIONS
BioLean Capsules and Tablets (Wellness International) **842**
BioLean Accelerator Tablets (Wellness International) **842**
BioLean Free Tablets (Wellness International) **843**
BodyLean Powder (AdvoCare) **795**
CardiOptima Drink Mix Packets (AdvoCare) **795**
Catalyst Capsules (AdvoCare)..........**796**
Coffeccino Beverage Mix (AdvoCare)...**796**
Food for Thought Drink Mix (Wellness International) **844**
HeartBar (Cooke) **812**
HGH-Turn Back the Hands of Time Capsules (Youngevity)................**854**
IntelleQ Capsules (AdvoCare) **797**
LipoTrol Caplets (AdvoCare) **797**
Mass Appeal Tablets (Wellness International)..........................**845**
Metabolic Nutrition System (AdvoCare) **798**
Perfect Meal (AdvoCare)................**798**
Performance Optimizer System (AdvoCare) **798**
Plus Caplets (Mannatech) **508, 820**
ProForm Bars (AdvoCare)...............**799**
Pro-Xtreme Drink Mix (Wellness International)..........................**845**
Satiete Tablets (Wellness International)..........................**846**
Spark! Beverage Mix (AdvoCare) **800**
StePHan Clarity Capsules (Wellness International)..........................**844**
StePHan Elasticity Capsules (Wellness International) **847**
StePHan Elixir Capsules (Wellness International)..........................**848**
StePHan Essential Capsules (Wellness International) **848**
StePHan Feminine Capsules (Wellness International) **848**
StePHan Flexibility Capsules (Wellness International) **848**
StePHan Lovpil Capsules (Wellness International)..........................**849**
StePHan Masculine Capsules (Wellness International) **849**
StePHan Protector Capsules (Wellness International) **850**

StePHan Relief Capsules (Wellness International)..........................**850**
StePHan Tranquility Capsules (Wellness International) **851**
Super Food Soy Shake (Youngevity)....**854**
System 3-4-3 Capsules (AdvoCare) **800**
Vitamist Intra-Oral Spray (Mayor).......**821**
CardioCare (Mayor) *821*
C+Zinc (Mayor).........................*821*
Revitalizer (Mayor) *821*
Slender-Mist (Mayor)...................*821*
Winrgy Drink Mix (Wellness International)..........................**852**

ANAS BARBARIAE HEPATIS ET CORDIS EXTRACTUM
Oscillococcinum Pellets (Boiron) **625**

ANTIOXIDANTS
Super Anti-Oxidant Cell Protector Capsules (Youngevity)..............**854**

ASCORBIC ACID
(*see under:* **VITAMIN C**)

ASPIRIN
Alka-Seltzer Original Antacid and Pain Reliever Effervescent Tablets (Bayer Consumer) **503, 603**
Alka-Seltzer Cherry Antacid and Pain Reliever Effervescent Tablets (Bayer Consumer) **503, 603**
Alka-Seltzer Lemon Lime Antacid and Pain Reliever Effervescent Tablets (Bayer Consumer) **503, 603**
Alka-Seltzer Extra Strength Antacid and Pain Reliever Effervescent Tablets (Bayer Consumer) **503, 603**
Alka-Seltzer PM Effervescent Tablets (Bayer Consumer) **503, 605**
Genuine Bayer Tablets, Caplets and Gelcaps (Bayer Consumer) **503, 606**
Extra Strength Bayer Caplets and Gelcaps (Bayer Consumer) **504, 610**
Aspirin Regimen Bayer Children's Chewable Tablets (Orange or Cherry Flavored) (Bayer Consumer) ..**504, 607**
Aspirin Regimen Bayer Adult Low Strength 81 mg Tablets (Bayer Consumer) **503, 606**
Aspirin Regimen Bayer 81 mg Caplets with Calcium (Bayer Consumer) **607**
Aspirin Regimen Bayer Regular Strength 325 mg Caplets (Bayer Consumer).............**503, 606**
Extra Strength Bayer Arthritis Caplets (Bayer Consumer)....**504, 610**
Extra Strength Bayer Plus Caplets (Bayer Consumer)....**504, 610**
Extra Strength Bayer PM Caplets (Bayer Consumer)....**504, 611**
BC Powder (Block) **619**
BC Allergy Sinus Cold Powder (Block)................................**619**
Arthritis Strength BC Powder (Block)...**619**
BC Sinus Cold Powder (Block).........**619**
Ecotrin Enteric Coated Aspirin Low Strength Tablets (SmithKline Beecham Consumer) **524, 747**

Ecotrin Enteric Coated Aspirin Maximum Strength Tablets (SmithKline Beecham Consumer) **524, 747**
Ecotrin Enteric Coated Aspirin Regular Strength Tablets (SmithKline Beecham Consumer) **524, 747**
Excedrin Extra-Strength Tablets, Caplets, and Geltabs (Bristol-Myers)........**507, 629**
Excedrin Migraine Tablets, Caplets, and Geltabs (Bristol-Myers)........**507, 630**
Goody's Body Pain Formula Powder (Block)................................**620**
Goody's Extra Strength Headache Powder (Block) **620**
Goody's Extra Strength Pain Relief Tablets (Block) **620**
Vanquish Caplets (Bayer Consumer) **505, 617**

ASTRAGALUS
Biomune OSF Plus Capsules (Matol)........................**508, 820**
Cold Season Nutrition Booster Capsules (AdvoCare)...............**796**
StePHan Protector Capsules (Wellness International) **850**
System 3-4-3 Capsules (AdvoCare) **800**

ATTAPULGITE
Donnagel Liquid (Wyeth-Ayerst)...**526, 789**

B

BACITRACIN ZINC
Betadine Brand First Aid Antibiotics + Moisturizer Ointment (Purdue Frederick)....................**522, 731**
Betadine Brand Plus First Aid Antibiotics + Pain Reliever Ointment (Purdue Frederick)....................**522, 731**
Neosporin Ointment (Pfizer Inc., Warner-Lambert Healthcare)...................**519, 704**
Neosporin + Pain Relief Maximum Strength Ointment (Pfizer Inc., Warner-Lambert Healthcare)...................**519, 704**
Polysporin Ointment (Pfizer Inc., Warner-Lambert Healthcare)...................**519, 706**
Polysporin Powder (Pfizer Inc., Warner-Lambert Healthcare)...................**519, 706**

BELLADONNA ALKALOIDS
Hyland's Earache Tablets (Standard Homeopathic) **765**
Hyland's Teething Gel (Standard Homeopathic).......................**766**
Hyland's Teething Tablets (Standard Homeopathic).......................**766**

BENZALKONIUM CHLORIDE
Bactine First Aid Liquid (Bayer Consumer) **503, 611**

BENZETHONIUM CHLORIDE
Clinical Care Antimicrobial Wound Cleanser (Care-Tech)................**632**
Dermoplast Antibacterial Spray, Hospital Strength (Medtech)........**666**

BENZOCAINE
Baby Anbesol Gel (Whitehall-Robins)...**774**
Junior Anbesol Gel (Whitehall-Robins)....................**774**

BENZOCAINE—*cont.*
Maximum Strength Anbesol Gel
(Whitehall-Robins)...................**774**
Maximum Strength Anbesol Liquid
(Whitehall-Robins)...................**774**
Cēpacol Maximum Strength Sugar
Free Sore Throat Lozenges,
Cherry Flavor (Williams) **787**
Cēpacol Maximum Strength Sugar
Free Sore Throat Lozenges, Cool
Mint Flavor (Williams)..............**787**
Cēpacol Maximum Strength
Sore Throat Lozenges,
Cherry Flavor (Williams) **526, 787**
Cēpacol Maximum Strength
Sore Throat Lozenges, Mint
Flavor (Williams) **526, 787**
Dermoplast Antibacterial Spray,
Hospital Strength (Medtech)........**666**
Dermoplast Hospital Strength Spray
(Medtech) **666**
Hurricaine Topical Anesthetic Gel, 1
oz. Fresh Mint, Wild Cherry, Pina
Colada, Watermelon, 1/6 oz.
Wild Cherry, Watermelon
(Beutlich)...........................**618**
Hurricaine Topical Anesthetic Liquid,
1 oz. Wild Cherry, Pina Colada,
.25 ml Dry Handle Swab Wild
Cherry, 1/6 oz. Wild Cherry
(Beutlich) **618**
Hurricaine Topical Anesthetic Spray
Extension Tubes (200) (Beutlich)...**618**
Hurricaine Topical Anesthetic Spray
Kit, 2 oz. Wild Cherry (Beutlich) **618**
Hurricaine Topical Anesthetic Spray,
2 oz. Wild Cherry (Beutlich) **618**
Zilactin Baby Gel (Zila Consumer) **791**
Zilactin-B Gel (Zila Consumer) **790**

BENZYL ALCOHOL
Zilactin Gel (Zila Consumer) **790**

BETA SITOSTEROL
LipoTrol Caplets (AdvoCare) **797**

BIOFLAVONOIDS
Beta-C Tablets (Body Wise) **811**
C-Grams Caplets (AdvoCare) **795**
CorePlex Capsules (AdvoCare) **796**
Lipoflavonoid Caplets (Numark) **828**
Peridin-C Tablets (Beutlich) **618**
Phyto-Vite Tablets (Wellness
International).......................**849**
Right Choice A.M. Multi Formula
Caplets (Body Wise) **811**

BISACODYL
Correctol Laxative Tablets and
Caplets (Schering-Plough) **523, 739**
Dulcolax Suppositories
(Novartis Consumer)..........**513, 668**
Dulcolax Tablets (Novartis
Consumer) **513, 668**

BISMUTH SUBGALLATE
Devrom Chewable Tablets
(Parthenon) **685**

BISMUTH SUBSALICYLATE
Pepto-Bismol Original Liquid,
Original and Cherry
Chewable Tablets &
Caplets (Procter & Gamble) ..**521, 723**
Pepto-Bismol Maximum Strength
Liquid (Procter & Gamble) **724**

BLACK COHOSH
One-A-Day Menopause Health
Tablets (Bayer Consumer) **505, 808**
Remifemin Menopause Tablets
(SmithKline Beecham Consumer) ..**839**

BROMPHENIRAMINE MALEATE
Comtrex Acute Head Cold &
Sinus Pressure Relief
Tablets (Bristol-Myers) **506, 627**
Dimetapp Elixir (Whitehall-Robins)......**777**
Dimetapp Cold and Fever
Suspension (Whitehall-Robins) **775**
Dimetapp DM Cold & Cough Elixir
(Whitehall-Robins)..................**775**
Dimetapp Nighttime Flu Liquid
(Whitehall-Robins)..................**776**

BUTOCONAZOLE NITRATE
Mycelex-3 Vaginal Cream with 3
Disposable Applicators (Bayer
Consumer) **613**
Mycelex-3 Vaginal Cream in 3
Pre-filled Applicators (Bayer
Consumer) **613**

C

CAFFEINE
BC Powder (Block) **619**
Arthritis Strength BC Powder (Block)...**619**
BioLean Capsules and Tablets
(Wellness International) **842**
Aspirin Free Excedrin Caplets
and Geltabs (Bristol-Myers)...**507, 628**
Excedrin Extra-Strength
Tablets, Caplets, and
Geltabs (Bristol-Myers)........**507, 629**
Excedrin Migraine Tablets,
Caplets, and Geltabs
(Bristol-Myers)................**507, 630**
Goody's Extra Strength Headache
Powder (Block) **620**
Goody's Extra Strength Pain Relief
Tablets (Block).......................**620**
Maximum Strength Midol
Menstrual Caplets and
Gelcaps (Bayer Consumer) ...**504, 612**
Vanquish Caplets (Bayer
Consumer) **505, 617**
Vivarin Caplets (SmithKline
Beecham Consumer) **525, 763**
Vivarin Tablets (SmithKline
Beecham Consumer) **525, 763**

CALAMINE
Caladryl Lotion (Pfizer Inc.,
Warner-Lambert
Healthcare)...................**518, 698**

CALCIUM
One-A-Day Bedtime & Rest
Tablets (Bayer Consumer) **505, 805**
Os-Cal 250 + D Tablets
(SmithKline Beecham
Consumer) **525, 838**
Os-Cal 500 Tablets (SmithKline
Beecham Consumer) **525, 839**
Os-Cal 500 + D Tablets
(SmithKline Beecham
Consumer) **525, 839**
ReSource Wellness ForSight
Caplets (Novartis
Consumer) **514, 825**

CALCIUM CARBONATE
Aspirin Regimen Bayer 81 mg
Caplets with Calcium (Bayer
Consumer) **607**
Extra Strength Bayer Plus
Caplets (Bayer Consumer)....**504, 610**
Caltrate 600 Tablets (Lederle
Consumer) **814**
Caltrate 600 PLUS Chewables
(Lederle Consumer)................**815**
Caltrate 600 PLUS Tablets (Lederle
Consumer) **815**

Caltrate 600 + D Tablets (Lederle
Consumer)..........................**814**
Caltrate 600 + Soy Tablets (Lederle
Consumer)..........................**814**
D-Cal Chewable Caplets (A & Z
Pharm)........................**503, 794**
Quick Dissolve Maalox Antacid
Chewable Tablets (Novartis
Consumer) **514, 674**
Quick Dissolve Maalox Max
Maximum Strength
Antacid/Antigas Chewable
Tablets (Novartis
Consumer) **514, 674**
Marblen Suspension (Fleming) **633**
Children's Mylanta Upset
Stomach Relief Liquid
(J&J • Merck) **508, 634**
Children's Mylanta Upset
Stomach Relief Tablets
(J&J • Merck) **508, 634**
Mylanta Gelcaps (J&J • Merck)...**507, 637**
Mylanta Supreme Liquid (J&J •
Merck)........................**507, 636**
Mylanta Ultra Tabs Tablets
(J&J• Merck)..................**507, 637**
Extra Strength Mylanta Calci
Tabs Tablets (J&J • Merck) ...**507, 636**
Ultra Mylanta Calci Tabs
Tablets (J&J • Merck)........**507, 636**
One-A-Day Calcium Plus
Chewable Tablets (Bayer
Consumer) **505, 805**
Os-Cal Chewable Tablets
(SmithKline Beecham
Consumer) **525, 838**
Pepcid Complete Chewable
Tablets (J&J • Merck)........**508, 638**
ReSource Wellness CalciWise
Soft Chews (Novartis
Consumer) **514, 824**
Rolaids Tablets (Pfizer Inc.,
Warner-Lambert
Healthcare)...................**519, 706**
Extra Strength Rolaids Tablets
(Pfizer Inc., Warner-Lambert
Healthcare)...................**519, 706**
Slow-Mag Tablets (Shire) **835**
3M Titralac Antacid Tablets
(3M) **508, 640**
3M Titralac Extra Strength
Antacid Tablets (3M) **508, 640**
3M Titralac Plus Antacid
Tablets (3M)..................**508, 640**
Tums E-X Antacid/Calcium
Tablets (SmithKline
Beecham Consumer) **525, 763**
Tums E-X Sugar Free Antacid/
Calcium Tablets
(SmithKline Beecham
Consumer) **525, 763**
Tums Regular Antacid/Calcium
Tablets (SmithKline
Beecham Consumer) **525, 763**
Tums ULTRA Antacid/Calcium
Tablets (SmithKline
Beecham Consumer) **525, 763**

CALCIUM CITRATE
Citracal Liquitab Tablets (Mission) **823**
Citracal Tablets (Mission)...............**823**
Citracal Caplets + D (Mission)..........**823**
Citracal 250 MG + D Tablets
(Mission) **823**
Citracal Plus Tablets (Mission) **824**

CALCIUM GLYCEROPHOSPHATE
Prelief Tablets and Granulate
(AK Pharma)...................**503, 801**

CALCIUM POLYCARBOPHIL

FiberCon Caplets (Lederle
Consumer) **639**

Mitrolan Chewable Tablets
(Wyeth-Ayerst) **526, 789**

Phillips' FiberCaps Caplets
(Bayer Consumer) **505, 615**

CAMPHOR

Afrin Saline Aromatic Mist
(Schering-Plough) **734**

BenGay External Analgesic
Products (Pfizer Inc.,
Warner-Lambert
Healthcare)......................**518, 696**

Triaminic Vapor Patch-Cherry
Scent (Novartis Consumer)...**515, 684**

Triaminic Vapor Patch-Menthol
Scent (Novartis Consumer)...**515, 684**

Vicks VapoRub Cream (Procter &
Gamble) **730**

Vicks VapoRub Ointment (Procter &
Gamble) **730**

Vicks VapoSteam (Procter &
Gamble) **730**

CARBAMIDE PEROXIDE

Debrox Drops (SmithKline
Beecham Consumer) **523, 747**

Gly-Oxide Liquid (SmithKline
Beecham Consumer) **524, 751**

CARBOXYMETHYLCELLULOSE SODIUM

Fiber 10 Packets (AdvoCare) **797**

CASTOR OIL

Purge Liquid (Fleming) **633**

CETYLPYRIDINIUM CHLORIDE

Cēpacol Antiseptic
Mouthwash/Gargle,
Original (Williams)............**526, 786**

Cēpacol Antiseptic
Mouthwash/Gargle, Mint
(Williams).......................**526, 786**

CHLOROXYLENOL

Techni-Care Surgical Scrub, Prep
and Wound Decontaminant
(Care-Tech) **632**

CHLORPHENIRAMINE MALEATE

Actifed Cold & Sinus Caplets
and Tablets (Pfizer Inc.,
Warner-Lambert
Healthcare).....................**516, 688**

Alka-Seltzer Plus Cold
Medicine Liqui-Gels (Bayer
Consumer) **503, 604**

Alka-Seltzer Plus Cold & Cough
Medicine Liqui-Gels (Bayer
Consumer) **503, 604**

BC Allergy Sinus Cold Powder
(Block)...............................**619**

Chlor-Trimeton Allergy Tablets
(Schering-Plough) **522, 735**

Chlor-Trimeton Allergy/
Decongestant Tablets
(Schering-Plough) **522, 736**

Comtrex Flu Therapy & Fever
Relief Nighttime Tablets
(Bristol-Myers).................**506, 628**

Comtrex Maximum Strength
Multi-Symptom Cold &
Cough Relief Tablets and
Caplets (Bristol-Myers)........**506, 626**

Contac Severe Cold and Flu
Caplets Maximum Strength
(SmithKline Beecham
Consumer) **523, 746**

Coricidin 'D' Cold, Flu & Sinus
Tablets (Schering-Plough) **522, 737**

Coricidin HBP Cold & Flu
Tablets (Schering-Plough) **523, 738**

Coricidin HBP Cough & Cold
Tablets (Schering-Plough) **523, 738**

Coricidin HBP Maximum
Strength Flu Tablets
(Schering-Plough) **523, 738**

PediaCare Cough-Cold Liquid
(Pharmacia Consumer) **719**

PediaCare NightRest Cough-Cold
Liquid (Pharmacia Consumer) **719**

Robitussin Nighttime Honey Flu
Liquid (Whitehall-Robins) **786**

Ryna Liquid (Wallace) **768**

Ryna-C Liquid (Wallace)...........**525, 768**

Singlet Caplets (SmithKline
Beecham Consumer) **761**

Sinutab Sinus Allergy
Medication, Maximum
Strength Formula, Tablets
& Caplets (Pfizer Inc.,
Warner-Lambert
Healthcare)......................**520, 707**

Sudafed Cold & Allergy Tablets
(Pfizer Inc., Warner-Lambert
Healthcare)......................**520, 708**

TheraFlu Regular Strength Cold
& Cough Night Time Hot
Liquid (Novartis Consumer) ..**515, 676**

TheraFlu Regular Strength Cold
& Sore Throat Night Time
Hot Liquid (Novartis
Consumer) **515, 676**

TheraFlu Maximum Strength
Flu & Cough Night Time Hot
Liquid (Novartis Consumer) ..**515, 678**

TheraFlu Maximum Strength
Flu & Sore Throat Night
Time Hot Liquid (Novartis
Consumer) **515, 677**

TheraFlu Maximum Strength
Severe Cold & Congestion
Night Time Caplets
(Novartis Consumer).........**515, 678**

TheraFlu Maximum Strength
Severe Cold & Congestion
Night Time Hot Liquid
(Novartis Consumer).........**515, 678**

Triaminic Cold & Allergy Liquid
(Novartis Consumer)..........**515, 681**

Triaminic Cold & Allergy
Softchews (Novartis
Consumer) **515, 683**

Triaminic Cold & Cough Liquid
(Novartis Consumer)..........**515, 681**

Triaminic Cold & Cough
Softchews (Novartis
Consumer) **515, 683**

Triaminic Cold & Night Time
Cough Liquid (Novartis
Consumer) **515, 681**

Triaminic Cold, Cough & Fever
PediaCare Liquid (Novartis Consumer) ..**515, 681**

Children's Tylenol Cold
Suspension Liquid and
Chewable Tablets (McNeil
Consumer) **510, 659**

Children's Tylenol Cold Plus
Cough Suspension Liquid
and Chewable Tablets
(McNeil Consumer) **510, 659**

Children's Tylenol Flu
Suspension Liquid (McNeil
Consumer) **511, 663**

Maximum Strength Tylenol
Allergy Sinus Caplets,
Gelcaps, and Geltabs
(McNeil Consumer) **511, 649**

Multi-Symptom Tylenol Cold
Complete Formula Caplets
(McNeil Consumer) **512, 651**

Vicks 44M Cough, Cold & Flu Relief
Liquid (Procter & Gamble) **725**

Pediatric Vicks 44m Cough & Cold
Relief (Procter & Gamble)...........**728**

Children's Vicks NyQuil Cold/Cough
Relief (Procter & Gamble)...........**726**

CHOLINE

One-A-Day Memory &
Concentration Tablets
(Bayer Consumer) **505, 807**

CHONDROITIN SULFATE

Humatrix Microclysmic Burn/Wound
Healing Gel (Care-Tech) **632**

Second Look Capsules (AdvoCare).....**800**

Vitamist Intra-Oral Spray (Mayor) **821**

ArthriFlex (Mayor)......................*821*

Sun Joint Tablets (Sunpower)..........*841*

CHROMIUM PICOLINATE

One-A-Day Energy Formula
Tablets (Bayer Consumer) **505, 806**

CIMETIDINE

Tagamet HB 200 Suspension
(SmithKline Beecham
Consumer) **525, 762**

Tagamet HB 200 Tablets
(SmithKline Beecham
Consumer) **525, 761**

CITRIC ACID

Alka-Seltzer Original Antacid
and Pain Reliever
Effervescent Tablets (Bayer
Consumer) **503, 603**

Alka-Seltzer Cherry Antacid
and Pain Reliever
Effervescent Tablets (Bayer
Consumer) **503, 603**

Alka-Seltzer Lemon Lime
Antacid and Pain Reliever
Effervescent Tablets (Bayer
Consumer) **503, 603**

Alka-Seltzer Extra Strength
Antacid and Pain Reliever
Effervescent Tablets (Bayer
Consumer) **503, 603**

Alka-Seltzer Heartburn Relief
Tablets (Bayer Consumer) **503, 604**

Proceed Powder (Sigma-Tau)......**523, 835**

CLEMASTINE FUMARATE

Tavist 12 Hour Allergy Tablets
(Novartis Consumer)..........**514, 676**

CLOTRIMAZOLE

Gyne-Lotrimin 3, 3-Day Cream
(Schering-Plough) **523, 741**

Lotrimin AF Cream, Lotion,
Solution, and Jock Itch
Cream (Schering-Plough)......**523, 742**

Mycelex-7 Combination-Pack Vaginal
Inserts & External Vulvar Cream
(Bayer Consumer)...................**614**

Mycelex-7 Vaginal Cream (Bayer
Consumer) **614**

Mycelex-7 Vaginal Cream with 7
Disposable Applicators (Bayer
Consumer) **614**

COAL TAR

Tegrin Dandruff Shampoo - Extra
Conditioning (Block)..................**623**

Tegrin Dandruff Shampoo -
Fresh Herbal (Block) **506, 624**

Tegrin Skin Cream (Block) **506, 624**

COCAMIDOPROPYL PG-DIMONIUM CHLORIDE PHOSPHATE

Techni-Care Surgical Scrub, Prep
and Wound Decontaminant
(Care-Tech) **632**

COCOA BUTTER
Preparation H Suppositories
(Whitehall-Robins).................**778**

COD LIVER OIL
Desitin Ointment (Pfizer Inc.,
Warner-Lambert
Healthcare)...................**518, 700**

CODEINE PHOSPHATE
Ryna-C Liquid (Wallace)..........**525, 768**

COENZYME Q-10
CardiOptima Drink Mix Packets
(AdvoCare) **795**
Centrum Focused Formulas Heart
Tablets (Lederle Consumer) **816**
CorePlex Capsules (AdvoCare) **796**
Performance Optimizer System
(AdvoCare) **798**
Vitamist Intra-Oral Spray (Mayor) **821**
CardioCare (Mayor) *821*

COLLAGEN
Humatrix Microclysmic Burn/Wound
Healing Gel (Care-Tech) **632**

COLOSTRUM
Biomune OSF Plus Capsules
(Matol).....................**508, 820**
Transfer Factor Capsules
(4Life) **526, 814**

CORNSTARCH
Balmex Medicated Plus Baby
Powder (Block) **505, 619**
Desitin Baby Powder (Pfizer
Inc., Warner-Lambert
Healthcare)...................**518, 700**

CORTISOL
(*see under:* **HYDROCORTISONE**)

CROMOLYN SODIUM
NasalCrom Nasal Spray (Pharmacia
Consumer) **719**

CYANOCOBALAMIN
(*see under:* **VITAMIN B₁₂**)

D

DEHYDROEPIANDROSTERONE (DHEA)
DHEA Plus Capsules (Wellness
International)....................**844**
Vitamist Intra-Oral Spray (Mayor) **821**
DHEA (Mayor) *821*
Vitara Cream (Products on
Demand) **522, 731**

DEXBROMPHENIRAMINE MALEATE
Drixoral Allergy/Sinus
Extended-Release Tablets
(Schering-Plough) **523, 741**
Drixoral Cold & Allergy
Sustained-Action Tablets
(Schering-Plough) **523, 740**
Drixoral Cold & Flu
Extended-Release Tablets
(Schering-Plough) **523, 740**

DEXTROMETHORPHAN HYDROBROMIDE
Alka-Seltzer Plus Night-Time
Cold Medicine Liqui-Gels
(Bayer Consumer)...........**503, 604**
Alka-Seltzer Plus Cold & Cough
Medicine Liqui-Gels (Bayer
Consumer)..................**503, 604**
Alka-Seltzer Plus Cold & Flu
Medicine Liqui-Gels (Bayer
Consumer)..................**503, 604**
Benylin Adult Formula Cough
Suppressant Liquid (Pfizer
Inc., Warner-Lambert
Healthcare)...................**518, 696**

Benylin Cough Suppressant/
Expectorant Liquid (Pfizer
Inc., Warner-Lambert
Healthcare)...................**518, 697**
Benylin Multi-Symptom Liquid
(Pfizer Inc., Warner-Lambert
Healthcare)...................**518, 697**
Benylin Pediatric Cough
Suppressant Liquid (Pfizer
Inc., Warner-Lambert
Healthcare)...................**518, 698**
Comtrex Deep Chest Cold &
Congestion Relief Softgels
(Bristol-Myers)..............**506, 627**
Comtrex Maximum Strength
Multi-Symptom Cold &
Cough Relief Tablets and
Caplets (Bristol-Myers)........**506, 626**
Contac Severe Cold and Flu
Caplets Maximum Strength
(SmithKline Beecham
Consumer) **523, 746**
Contac Severe Cold and Flu Caplets
Non-Drowsy (SmithKline
Beecham Consumer) **746**
Coricidin HBP Cough & Cold
Tablets (Schering-Plough).....**523, 738**
Coricidin HBP Maximum
Strength Flu Tablets
(Schering-Plough) **523, 738**
Dimetapp DM Cold & Cough Elixir
(Whitehall-Robins)..................**775**
Dimetapp Nighttime Flu Liquid
(Whitehall-Robins)..................**776**
Dimetapp Non-Drowsy Flu Syrup
(Whitehall-Robins)..................**777**
Dimetapp Infant Drops
Decongestant Plus Cough
(Whitehall-Robins)..................**776**
PediaCare Cough-Cold Liquid
(Pharmacia Consumer) **719**
PediaCare Infants' Drops
Decongestant Plus Cough
(Pharmacia Consumer) **719**
PediaCare NightRest Cough-Cold
Liquid (Pharmacia Consumer) **719**
Robitussin Cold Caplets Cold &
Congestion (Whitehall-Robins)......**780**
Robitussin Cold Softgels Cold &
Congestion (Whitehall-Robins)......**780**
Robitussin Cold Caplets
Multi-Symptom Cold & Flu
(Whitehall-Robins)..................**781**
Robitussin Cold Softgels
Multi-Symptom Cold & Flu
(Whitehall-Robins)..................**781**
Robitussin Honey Cough Liquid
(Whitehall-Robins)..................**784**
Robitussin Cough & Cold Infant
Drops (Whitehall-Robins) **782**
Robitussin Maximum Strength
Cough & Cold Liquid
(Whitehall-Robins)..................**785**
Robitussin Pediatric Cough & Cold
Formula Liquid
(Whitehall-Robins)..................**785**
Robitussin Maximum Strength
Cough Suppressant Liquid
(Whitehall-Robins)..................**784**
Robitussin Pediatric Cough
Suppressant Liquid
(Whitehall-Robins)..................**784**
Robitussin Multi Symptom Honey Flu
Liquid (Whitehall-Robins) **785**
Robitussin Nighttime Honey Flu
Liquid (Whitehall-Robins) **786**
Robitussin-CF Liquid
(Whitehall-Robins)..................**783**

Robitussin DM Infant Drops
(Whitehall-Robins).................**783**
Robitussin-DM Liquid
(Whitehall-Robins).................**783**
Children's Sudafed Cold &
Cough Liquid (Pfizer Inc.,
Warner-Lambert
Healthcare)...................**520, 709**
Sudafed Cold & Cough Liquid
Caps (Pfizer Inc.,
Warner-Lambert
Healthcare)...................**520, 709**
Sudafed Severe Cold Formula
Caplets (Pfizer Inc.,
Warner-Lambert
Healthcare)...................**520, 711**
Sudafed Severe Cold Formula
Tablets (Pfizer Inc.,
Warner-Lambert
Healthcare)...................**520, 711**
TheraFlu Regular Strength Cold
& Cough Night Time Hot
Liquid (Novartis Consumer) ..**515, 676**
TheraFlu Maximum Strength
Flu & Congestion
Non-Drowsy Hot Liquid
(Novartis Consumer).........**515, 677**
TheraFlu Maximum Strength
Flu & Cough Night Time Hot
Liquid (Novartis Consumer) ..**515, 678**
TheraFlu Maximum Strength
Severe Cold & Congestion
Night Time Caplets
(Novartis Consumer).........**515, 678**
TheraFlu Maximum Strength
Severe Cold & Congestion
Night Time Hot Liquid
(Novartis Consumer).........**515, 678**
TheraFlu Maximum Strength
Severe Cold & Congestion
Non-Drowsy Caplets
(Novartis Consumer).........**515, 679**
TheraFlu Maximum Strength
Severe Cold & Congestion
Non-Drowsy Hot Liquid
(Novartis Consumer).........**515, 679**
Triaminic Cold & Cough Liquid
(Novartis Consumer).........**515, 681**
Triaminic Cold & Cough
Softchews (Novartis
Consumer) **515, 683**
Triaminic Cold & Night Time
Cough Liquid (Novartis
Consumer) **515, 681**
Triaminic Cold, Cough & Fever
Liquid (Novartis Consumer) ..**515, 681**
Triaminic Cough Liquid
(Novartis Consumer).........**515, 682**
Triaminic Cough Softchews
(Novartis Consumer).........**515, 684**
Triaminic Cough & Congestion
Liquid (Novartis Consumer) ..**515, 682**
Triaminic Cough & Sore Throat
Liquid (Novartis Consumer) ..**515, 682**
Triaminic Cough & Sore Throat
Softchews (Novartis
Consumer) **515, 684**
Children's Tylenol Cold Plus
Cough Suspension Liquid
and Chewable Tablets
(McNeil Consumer) **510, 659**
Children's Tylenol Flu
Suspension Liquid (McNeil
Consumer) **511, 663**
Infants' Tylenol Cold
Decongestant & Fever
Reducer Concentrated
Drops Plus Cough (McNeil
Consumer) **511, 659**

Multi-Symptom Tylenol Cold
Complete Formula Caplets
(McNeil Consumer) **512, 651**
Multi-Symptom Tylenol Cold
Non-Drowsy Caplets and
Gelcaps (McNeil
Consumer) **512, 651**
Multi-Symptom Tylenol Cold
Severe Congestion
Non-Drowsy Caplets
(McNeil Consumer) **512, 652**
Maximum Strength Tylenol Flu
NightTime Liquid (McNeil
Consumer) **512, 653**
Maximum Strength Tylenol Flu
Non-Drowsy Gelcaps
(McNeil Consumer) **512, 653**
Vicks 44 Cough Relief Liquid
(Procter & Gamble) **724**
Vicks 44D Cough & Head
Congestion Relief Liquid (Procter
& Gamble)......................... **724**
Vicks 44E Cough & Chest
Congestion Relief Liquid (Procter
& Gamble)......................... **725**
Pediatric Vicks 44e Cough & Chest
Congestion Relief Liquid (Procter
& Gamble)......................... **728**
Vicks 44M Cough, Cold & Flu Relief
Liquid (Procter & Gamble) **725**
Pediatric Vicks 44m Cough & Cold
Relief (Procter & Gamble)........... **728**
Vicks DayQuil LiquiCaps/Liquid
Multi-Symptom Cold/Flu Relief
(Procter & Gamble) **727**
Children's Vicks NyQuil Cold/Cough
Relief (Procter & Gamble)........... **726**
Vicks NyQuil LiquiCaps/Liquid
Multi-Symptom Cold/Flu Relief,
Original and Cherry Flavors
(Procter & Gamble) **727**

DEXTROMETHORPHAN POLISTIREX
Delsym Extended-Release
Suspension (Medeva)............... **664**

DEXTROSE
Emetrol Oral Solution (Lemon-Mint &
Cherry Flavors) (Pharmacia
Consumer) **718**

DHEA
(*see under:* **DEHYDROEPIANDROSTERONE**)

DIMENHYDRINATE
Dramamine Original Formula Tablets
(Pharmacia Consumer) **718**
Dramamine Chewable Formula
Tablets (Pharmacia Consumer)..... **718**
Vitamist Intra-Oral Spray (Mayor) **821**
VitaMotion-S (Mayor).................. *821*

DIMETHICONE
A + D Ointment with Zinc Oxide
(Schering-Plough) **522, 733**

DIOCTYL SODIUM SULFOSUCCINATE
(*see under:* **DOCUSATE SODIUM**)

DIPHENHYDRAMINE CITRATE
Alka-Seltzer PM Effervescent
Tablets (Bayer Consumer) **503, 605**
Benadryl Allergy & Sinus
Fastmelt Tablets (Pfizer
Inc., Warner-Lambert
Healthcare).................... **517, 693**
Benadryl Children's Allergy/
Cold Fastmelt Tablets
(Pfizer Inc., Warner-Lambert
Healthcare).................... **517, 692**
Excedrin PM Tablets, Caplets,
and Geltabs (Bristol-Myers)... **506, 631**
Goody's PM Powder (Block) **621**

DIPHENHYDRAMINE HYDROCHLORIDE
Extra Strength Bayer PM
Caplets (Bayer Consumer).... **504, 611**
Benadryl Allergy Chewables
(Pfizer Inc., Warner-Lambert
Healthcare)................... **517, 689**
Benadryl Allergy Kapseal
Capsules (Pfizer Inc.,
Warner-Lambert
Healthcare)................... **516, 691**
Benadryl Allergy Liquid (Pfizer
Inc., Warner-Lambert
Healthcare)................... **517, 690**
Benadryl Allergy Ultratab
Tablets (Pfizer Inc.,
Warner-Lambert
Healthcare)................... **516, 691**
Benadryl Allergy/Cold Tablets
(Pfizer Inc., Warner-Lambert
Healthcare)................... **517, 691**
Benadryl Allergy/Congestion
Tablets (Pfizer Inc.,
Warner-Lambert
Healthcare)................... **517, 692**
Benadryl Allergy & Sinus Liquid
(Pfizer Inc., Warner-Lambert
Healthcare)....................... **693**
Benadryl Allergy Sinus
Headache Caplets &
Gelcaps (Pfizer Inc.,
Warner-Lambert
Healthcare)................... **517, 693**
Benadryl Severe Allergy &
Sinus Headache Caplets
(Pfizer Inc., Warner-Lambert
Healthcare)................... **517, 694**
Benadryl Dye-Free Allergy
Liquid (Pfizer Inc.,
Warner-Lambert
Healthcare)................... **517, 690**
Benadryl Dye-Free Allergy
Liqui-Gels Softgels (Pfizer
Inc., Warner-Lambert
Healthcare)................... **517, 690**
Benadryl Itch Relief Stick Extra
Strength (Pfizer Inc.,
Warner-Lambert
Healthcare)................... **517, 695**
Benadryl Itch Stopping Cream
Original Strength (Pfizer
Inc., Warner-Lambert
Healthcare)................... **517, 695**
Benadryl Itch Stopping Cream
Extra Strength (Pfizer Inc.,
Warner-Lambert
Healthcare)................... **517, 695**
Benadryl Itch Stopping Gel
Original Strength (Pfizer
Inc., Warner-Lambert
Healthcare)................... **517, 695**
Benadryl Itch Stopping Gel
Extra Strength (Pfizer Inc.,
Warner-Lambert
Healthcare)................... **517, 695**
Benadryl Itch Stopping Spray
Original Strength (Pfizer
Inc., Warner-Lambert
Healthcare)................... **517, 696**
Benadryl Itch Stopping Spray
Extra Strength (Pfizer Inc.,
Warner-Lambert
Healthcare)................... **517, 696**
Coricidin HBP Night-Time Cold
& Flu Tablets
(Schering-Plough) **523, 738**
Nytol QuickCaps Caplets
(Block)....................... **506, 622**
Maximum Strength Nytol
QuickGels Softgels (Block) ... **506, 621**

Extra Strength Percogesic
Aspirin-Free Coated Caplets
(Medtech) **665**
Simply Sleep Caplets (McNeil
Consumer) **510, 647**
Sominex Original Formula Tablets
(SmithKline Beecham Consumer) .. **761**
Children's Tylenol Allergy-D
Liquid (McNeil Consumer) **510, 658**
Maximum Strength Tylenol
Allergy Sinus NightTime
Caplets (McNeil Consumer) .. **511, 649**
Tylenol Severe Allergy Caplets
(McNeil Consumer) **511, 649**
Maximum Strength Tylenol Flu
NightTime Gelcaps (McNeil
Consumer) **512, 653**
Extra Strength Tylenol PM
Caplets, Geltabs, and
Gelcaps (McNeil
Consumer) **512, 654**
Unisom Maximum Strength
SleepGels (Pfizer Inc.,
Warner-Lambert
Healthcare)................... **521, 713**

DISOCOREA
Hyland's Colic Tablets (Standard
Homeopathic) **765**

DOCOSANOL
Abreva Cream (SmithKline Beecham
Consumer) **744**

DOCUSATE CALCIUM
Surfak Liqui-Gels (Pharmacia
Consumer) **721**

DOCUSATE SODIUM
Ex•Lax Gentle Strength
Caplets (Novartis
Consumer) **513, 670**
Ex•Lax Stool Softener Caplets
(Novartis Consumer).......... **513, 671**
Phillips' Liqui-Gels (Bayer Consumer) .. **616**
Senokot-S Tablets (Purdue
Frederick).................... **522, 732**

DONG QUAI
Vitamist Intra-Oral Spray (Mayor) **821**
ArthriFlex (Mayor) *821*

DOXYLAMINE SUCCINATE
Alka-Seltzer Plus Night-Time
Cold Medicine Liqui-Gels
(Bayer Consumer)............. **503, 604**
Maximum Strength Tylenol Flu
NightTime Liquid (McNeil
Consumer) **512, 653**
Maximum Strength Tylenol
Sinus NightTime Caplets
(McNeil Consumer) **512, 655**
Unisom SleepTabs (Pfizer Inc.,
Warner-Lambert
Healthcare)................... **521, 713**
Vicks NyQuil LiquiCaps/Liquid
Multi-Symptom Cold/Flu Relief,
Original and Cherry Flavors
(Procter & Gamble) **727**

DYCLONINE HYDROCHLORIDE
Cēpacol Maximum Strength Sore
Throat Spray, Cherry Flavor
(Williams)......................... **787**
Cēpacol Maximum Strength Sore
Throat Spray, Cool Menthol
Flavor (Williams) **787**
Cēpacol Maximum Strength Sore
Throat Spray, Honey Lemon
Flavor (Williams) **787**

E

ECHINACEA
Cold Season Nutrition Booster
Capsules (AdvoCare)................**796**
ReSource Wellness ResistEx
Capsules (Novartis
Consumer) **514, 826**
System 3-4-3 Capsules (AdvoCare) **800**

ECHINACEA ANGUSTIFOLIA
Centrum Echinacea Softgels
(Whitehall-Robins)...................**852**
Vitamist Intra-Oral Spray (Mayor).......**821**
Echinacea + G (Mayor)................*821*

EGG PRODUCT
BioChoice Immune[26] Powder
and Capsules (Legacy for
Life)...........................**508, 818**
BioChoice Immune Support Powder
(Legacy for Life)....................**818**

EPHEDRA
BioLean Capsules and Tablets
(Wellness International) **842**
Fat Metabolizer + Capsules
(Youngevity) **854**
Metabolic Nutrition System
(AdvoCare) **798**
Thermo-E Caplets (AdvoCare)...........**801**

EPHEDRINE HYDROCHLORIDE
Primatene Tablets (Whitehall-Robins) ..**780**

EPINEPHRINE
Primatene Mist (Whitehall-Robins) **779**

ETHYL AMINOBENZOATE
(*see under:* BENZOCAINE)

EUCALYPTOL
Afrin Saline Aromatic Mist
(Schering-Plough) **734**
Listerine Mouthrinse (Pfizer
Inc., Warner-Lambert
Healthcare)....................**518, 702**
Cool Mint Listerine Mouthrinse
(Pfizer Inc., Warner-Lambert
Healthcare)....................**518, 702**
FreshBurst Listerine
Mouthrinse (Pfizer Inc.,
Warner-Lambert
Healthcare)....................**519, 702**
Tartar Control Listerine
Mouthrinse (Pfizer Inc.,
Warner-Lambert
Healthcare)....................**519, 702**

EUCALYPTUS, OIL OF
Vicks VapoRub Cream (Procter &
Gamble) **730**
Vicks VapoRub Ointment (Procter &
Gamble) **730**

F

FAMOTIDINE
Pepcid AC Tablets, Chewable
Tablets, and Gelcaps
(J&J • Merck) **508, 638**
Pepcid Complete Chewable
Tablets (J&J • Merck).........**508, 638**

FATTY ACIDS
Metabolic Nutrition System
(AdvoCare) **798**
StePHan Essential Capsules
(Wellness International) **848**
Vitamist Intra-Oral Spray (Mayor).......**821**
Blue-Green Sea Spray (Mayor)........*821*

FERROUS GLUCONATE
Fergon Iron Tablets (Bayer
Consumer) **504, 802**

FERROUS SULFATE
Feosol Tablets (SmithKline
Beecham Consumer) **524, 838**
Slow Fe Tablets (Novartis
Consumer) **514, 827**
Slow Fe with Folic Acid Tablets
(Novartis Consumer)..........**514, 828**

FOLIC ACID
Slow Fe with Folic Acid Tablets
(Novartis Consumer)..........**514, 828**

G

GARLIC
(*see under:* ALLIUM SATIVUM)

GARLIC EXTRACT
Vitamist Intra-Oral Spray (Mayor) **821**
Echinacea + G (Mayor)................*821*

GARLIC OIL
One-A-Day Garlic Softgels
(Bayer Consumer).............**505, 806**

GINKGO BILOBA
BioLean Free Tablets (Wellness
International)........................**843**
Centrum Focused Formulas Mental
Clarity Tablets (Lederle
Consumer)..........................**816**
Centrum Ginkgo Biloba Softgels
(Whitehall-Robins)...................**852**
Centrum Performance
Multivitamin-Multimineral Tablets
(Lederle Consumer).................**817**
CorePlex Capsules (AdvoCare) **796**
DHEA Plus Capsules (Wellness
International)........................**844**
FemEssence Capsules (AdvoCare) **796**
Ginkoba M/E Suppli-Cap
Capsules (Pharmaton) **521, 829**
Ginkoba Tablets (Pharmaton)...........**828**
IntelleQ Capsules (AdvoCare) **797**
One-A-Day Memory &
Concentration Tablets
(Bayer Consumer)............**505, 807**
Phyto-Vite Tablets (Wellness
International)........................**849**
ProForm Bars (AdvoCare) **799**
ReSource Wellness EnVigor
Caplets (Novartis
Consumer) **514, 824**
ReSource Wellness
MemorAble Softgels
(Novartis Consumer)..........**514, 825**
Right Choice A.M. Multi Formula
Caplets (Body Wise) **811**
Satiete Tablets (Wellness
International)........................**846**
StePHan Clarity Capsules (Wellness
International)........................**844**
StePHan Elixir Capsules (Wellness
International)........................**848**
Vitamist Intra-Oral Spray (Mayor) **821**
GinkgoMist (Mayor) *821*
St. John's Wort (Mayor)................*821*
VitaSight (Mayor).....................*821*
Power Circulation Tablets
(Sunpower) *841*
Sun Cardio Tablets (Sunpower)........*841*
Vitality Immunity Anti-Oxidant
Complex Capsules (Youngevity) *854*

GINSENG
BioLean Free Tablets (Wellness
International)........................**843**
Centrum Focused Formulas Energy
Tablets (Lederle Consumer) **816**
Centrum Ginseng Softgels
(Whitehall-Robins)...................**853**

Centrum Performance
Multivitamin-Multimineral Tablets
(Lederle Consumer)..................**817**
Ginkoba M/E Suppli-Cap
Capsules (Pharmaton)........**521, 829**
Ginsana Capsules (Pharmaton) **830**
Ginsana Chewy Squares
(Pharmaton) **521, 830**
Ginsana Sport Capsules
(Pharmaton)..................**521, 831**
Metabolic Nutrition System
(AdvoCare) **798**
MetaBoost Caplets (AdvoCare).........**798**
One-A-Day Energy Formula
Tablets (Bayer Consumer) **505, 806**
Performance Gold Caplets
(AdvoCare) **798**
Performance Optimizer System
(AdvoCare) **798**
ReSource Wellness EnVigor
Caplets (Novartis
Consumer) **514, 824**
ReSource Wellness ResistEx
Capsules (Novartis
Consumer) **514, 826**
ReSource Wellness 2[nd]Wind
Capsules (Novartis
Consumer) **514, 826**
Vitasana Gelcaps (Pharmaton) ...**521, 834**

GLUCOSAMINE
Aflexa Tablets (McNeil
Consumer) **508, 821**
Sun Joint Tablets (Sunpower)...........*841*

GLUCOSAMINE HYDROCHLORIDE
Ambrotose Powder
(Mannatech)..................**508, 819**
FemEssence Capsules (AdvoCare) **796**
ProMotion Capsules (AdvoCare)........**800**
Sure2Endure Tablets (Wellness
International)........................**851**

GLUCOSAMINE SULFATE
One-A-Day Joint Health Tablets
(Bayer Consumer) **505, 806**
ReSource Wellness FlexTend
Caplets (Novartis
Consumer) **514, 825**
Vitamist Intra-Oral Spray (Mayor).......**821**
ArthriFlex (Mayor) *821*

GLYCERIN
Preparation H Cream
(Whitehall-Robins)...................**778**
Visine Tears Eye Drops (Pfizer
Inc., Warner-Lambert
Healthcare)...................**521, 716**
Visine Tears Preservative Free
Eye Drops (Pfizer Inc.,
Warner-Lambert
Healthcare)...................**521, 716**

GLYCERYL GUAIACOLATE
(*see under:* GUAIFENESIN)

GOAT MILK
Meyenberg Goat Milk (Meyenberg).....**823**

GOLDEN ROOT
Performance Gold Caplets
(AdvoCare) **798**

GUAIFENESIN
Benylin Cough Suppressant/
Expectorant Liquid (Pfizer
Inc., Warner-Lambert
Healthcare)...................**518, 697**
Benylin Multi-Symptom Liquid
(Pfizer Inc., Warner-Lambert
Healthcare)...................**518, 697**
Comtrex Deep Chest Cold &
Congestion Relief Softgels
(Bristol-Myers).................**506, 627**

Primatene Tablets (Whitehall-Robins) .. **780**
Robitussin Liquid (Whitehall-Robins) ... **782**
Robitussin Cold Caplets Cold &
  Congestion (Whitehall-Robins)...... **780**
Robitussin Cold Softgels Cold &
  Congestion (Whitehall-Robins)...... **780**
Robitussin Cold Caplets
  Multi-Symptom Cold & Flu
  (Whitehall-Robins).................. **781**
Robitussin Cold Softgels
  Multi-Symptom Cold & Flu
  (Whitehall-Robins).................. **781**
Robitussin Cold Softgels Severe
  Congestion (Whitehall-Robins)...... **782**
Robitussin Cough & Cold Infant
  Drops (Whitehall-Robins) **782**
Robitussin-CF Liquid
  (Whitehall-Robins).................. **783**
Robitussin DM Infant Drops
  (Whitehall-Robins).................. **783**
Robitussin-DM Liquid
  (Whitehall-Robins).................. **783**
Robitussin-PE Liquid
  (Whitehall-Robins).................. **782**
Sinutab Non-Drying Liquid
  Caps (Pfizer Inc.,
  Warner-Lambert
  Healthcare).................. **520, 706**
Sudafed Cold & Cough Liquid
  Caps (Pfizer Inc.,
  Warner-Lambert
  Healthcare).................. **520, 709**
Sudafed Non-Drying Sinus
  Liquid Caps (Pfizer Inc.,
  Warner-Lambert
  Healthcare).................. **520, 712**
TheraFlu Maximum Strength
  Flu & Congestion
  Non-Drowsy Hot Liquid
  (Novartis Consumer).......... **515, 677**
Triaminic Chest Congestion
  Liquid (Novartis Consumer) .. **515, 680**
Multi-Symptom Tylenol Cold
  Severe Congestion
  Non-Drowsy Caplets
  (McNeil Consumer) **512, 652**
Vicks 44E Cough & Chest
  Congestion Relief Liquid (Procter
  & Gamble)........................ **725**
Pediatric Vicks 44e Cough & Chest
  Congestion Relief Liquid (Procter
  & Gamble)........................ **728**

H

HCG MONOCLONAL ANTIBODY TEST
e.p.t. Pregnancy Test (Pfizer
  Inc., Warner-Lambert
  Healthcare)................... **518, 701**

HERBALS, MULTIPLE
Advantin Capsules (AdvoCare)......... **794**
Ag-Immune Tablets (Body Wise) **810**
BioLean Capsules and Tablets
  (Wellness International) **842**
BioLean Accelerator Tablets
  (Wellness International) **842**
Cold Season Nutrition Booster
  Capsules (AdvoCare)............... **796**
Fiber 10 Packets (AdvoCare) **797**
Performance Optimizer System
  (AdvoCare) **798**
PhytAloe Capsules
  (Mannatech)................ **508, 819**
PhytAloe Powder (Mannatech).... **508, 819**
Prostatonin Softgel Capsules
  (Pharmaton).................. **521, 832**

ReSource Wellness AllerPro
  Capsules (Novartis
  Consumer) **514, 824**
Sleep-Tite Caplets (Wellness
  International)..................... **850**
Vitamist Intra-Oral Spray (Mayor) **821**
  CardioCare (Mayor) *821*
  Echinacea + G (Mayor)............... *821*
  Ex. O (Mayor)....................... *821*
  Re-Leaf (Mayor) *821*
  Smoke-Less (Mayor) *821*
Power Circulation Tablets
  (Sunpower)......................... *841*
Power Lasting Tablets (Sunpower)...... *841*
Sun Beauty 1 Tablets (Sunpower) *841*
Sun Beauty 2 Tablets (Sunpower) *841*
Sun Beauty 3 Tablets (Sunpower) *841*
Sun Cardio Tablets (Sunpower)........ *841*
Sun Joint Tablets (Sunpower).......... *841*

HERBALS WITH MINERALS
BioLean LipoTrim Capsules
  (Wellness International) **843**
Fat Metabolizer + Capsules
  (Youngevity) **854**
LipoTrol Caplets (AdvoCare) **797**
MetaBoost Caplets (AdvoCare)....... **798**
One-A-Day Bedtime & Rest
  Tablets (Bayer Consumer) **505, 805**
ProMotion Capsules (AdvoCare)....... **800**
Second Look Capsules (AdvoCare)..... **800**
StePHan Masculine Capsules
  (Wellness International) **849**

HERBALS WITH VITAMINS
FemEssence Capsules (AdvoCare) **796**
IntelleQ Capsules (AdvoCare) **797**
One-A-Day Cholesterol Health
  Tablets (Bayer Consumer) **505, 805**
One-A-Day Joint Health Tablets
  (Bayer Consumer)............. **505, 806**
ProForm Bars (AdvoCare) **799**
ReSource Wellness
  MemorAble Softgels
  (Novartis Consumer).......... **514, 825**
Right Choice A.M. Multi Formula
  Caplets (Body Wise) **811**
StePHan Clarity Capsules (Wellness
  International)..................... **844**
StePHan Relief Capsules (Wellness
  International)..................... **850**
Vitamist Intra-Oral Spray (Mayor) **821**
  GinkgoMist (Mayor) *821*
  Pine Bark and Grape Seed
    (Mayor) *821*
  St. John's Wort (Mayor)............. *821*
  Stress (Mayor) *821*
  VitaMotion-S (Mayor)................ *821*

HERBALS WITH VITAMINS & MINERALS
ActoTherm Caplets (AdvoCare) **794**
Antioxidant Booster Caplets
  (AdvoCare) **794**
CardiOptima Drink Mix Packets
  (AdvoCare) **795**
Centrum Performance
  Multivitamin-Multimineral Tablets
  (Lederle Consumer)................ **817**
Coffeccino Beverage Mix (AdvoCare)... **796**
CorePlex Capsules (AdvoCare) **796**
Macro-Mineral Complex Caplets
  (AdvoCare) **797**
Metabolic Nutrition System
  (AdvoCare) **798**
Performance Optimizer System
  (AdvoCare) **798**
Phyto-Vite Tablets (Wellness
  International)..................... **849**

ReSource Wellness EnVigor
  Caplets (Novartis
  Consumer) **514, 824**
ReSource Wellness StayCalm
  Caplets (Novartis
  Consumer) **514, 826**
ReSource Wellness VeinTain
  Caplets (Novartis
  Consumer) **514, 827**
Satiete Tablets (Wellness
  International)..................... **846**
StePHan Elasticity Capsules
  (Wellness International) **847**
StePHan Elixir Capsules (Wellness
  International)..................... **848**
StePHan Lovpil Capsules (Wellness
  International)..................... **849**
StePHan Tranquility Capsules
  (Wellness International) **851**
Super Food Soy Shake (Youngevity) **854**
Sure2Endure Tablets (Wellness
  International)..................... **851**
System 3-4-3 Capsules (AdvoCare) **800**
Thermo-E Caplets (AdvoCare).......... **801**
Thermo-G Caplets (AdvoCare) **801**
Vitamist Intra-Oral Spray (Mayor) **821**
  Osteo-CalMag (Mayor) *821*
  VitaSight (Mayor).................... *821*
Vitasana Gelcaps (Pharmaton) ... **521, 834**
ZZZ Spray Liquid (AdvoCare)........... **801**
Sun Liver Tablets (Sunpower)..... *525, 841*
Vitality Immunity Anti-Oxidant
  Complex Capsules (Youngevity) **854**

HESPERIDIN COMPLEX
Beta-C Tablets (Body Wise)............. **811**
Peridin-C Tablets (Beutlich) **618**

HESPERIDIN METHYL CHALCONE
Peridin-C Tablets (Beutlich) **618**

HOMEOPATHIC FORMULATIONS
Biomune OSF Express Spray
  (Matol)...................... **508, 640**
Hyland's Arnisport Tablets (Standard
  Homeopathic) **764**
Hyland's Back Ache with Arnica
  Caplets (Standard Homeopathic)... **764**
Hyland's Bumps 'n Bruises Tablets
  (Standard Homeopathic)........... **764**
Hyland's Calms Forté Tablets and
  Caplets (Standard Homeopathic)... **764**
Hyland's Cold Tablets with Zinc
  (Standard Homeopathic)........... **765**
Hyland's Colic Tablets (Standard
  Homeopathic) **765**
Hyland's Earache Tablets (Standard
  Homeopathic) **765**
Hyland's Leg Cramps with Quinine
  Tablets (Standard Homeopathic) ... **765**
Hyland's MenoCalm Tablets
  (Standard Homeopathic)........... **765**
Hyland's Nerve Tonic Tablets and
  Caplets (Standard Homeopathic)... **766**
Hyland's Teething Gel (Standard
  Homeopathic) **766**
Hyland's Teething Tablets (Standard
  Homeopathic) **766**
Relief Nasal & Throat Spray (Body
  Wise) **811**
Smile's Prid Salve (Standard
  Homeopathic) **766**

HORSE CHESTNUT SEED EXTRACT
Venastat Suppli-Cap Capsules
  (Pharmaton).................. **521, 833**

HYDROCORTISONE
Cortaid Intensive Therapy Cream
  (Pharmacia Consumer) **717**

HYDROCORTISONE—cont.
Cortaid Maximum Strength Cream
   (Pharmacia Consumer) **717**
Cortizone•5 Creme (Pfizer Inc.,
   Warner-Lambert
   Healthcare)....................**518, 699**
Cortizone•5 Ointment (Pfizer Inc.,
   Warner-Lambert Healthcare)........**699**
Cortizone•10 Creme (Pfizer
   Inc., Warner-Lambert
   Healthcare)....................**518, 699**
Cortizone•10 Ointment (Pfizer Inc.,
   Warner-Lambert Healthcare)........**699**
Cortizone•10 Plus Creme
   (Pfizer Inc., Warner-Lambert
   Healthcare)....................**518, 700**
Cortizone•10 Quick Shot
   Spray (Pfizer Inc.,
   Warner-Lambert
   Healthcare)....................**518, 699**
Cortizone for Kids Creme
   (Pfizer Inc., Warner-Lambert
   Healthcare)....................**518, 699**
Massengill Medicated Soft Cloth
   Towelette (SmithKline Beecham
   Consumer) **753**

HYDROCORTISONE ACETATE
Anusol HC-1 Hydrocortisone
   Anti-Itch Cream (Pfizer Inc.,
   Warner-Lambert
   Healthcare)....................**516, 689**
Cortaid Maximum Strength Ointment
   (Pharmacia Consumer) **717**
Cortaid Sensitive Skin Cream
   (Pharmacia Consumer) **717**

HYDROXYPROPYL METHYLCELLULOSE
Visine Tears Eye Drops (Pfizer
   Inc., Warner-Lambert
   Healthcare)....................**521, 716**
Visine Tears Preservative Free
   Eye Drops (Pfizer Inc.,
   Warner-Lambert
   Healthcare)....................**521, 716**

HYDROXYTRYPTOPHAN
ZZZ Spray Liquid (AdvoCare)............**801**

HYPERICUM
Brite-Life Caplets (AdvoCare) **795**
Centrum St. John's Wort Softgels
   (Whitehall-Robins)...................**853**
Movana Tablets (Pharmaton) **521, 832**
One-A-Day Tension & Mood
   Softgels (Bayer Consumer) ...**505, 808**
ReSource Wellness StayCalm
   Caplets (Novartis
   Consumer) **514, 826**
Satiete Tablets (Wellness
   International).........................**846**
Vitamist Intra-Oral Spray (Mayor).......**821**
   St. John's Wort (Mayor)..............*821*
Sun Beauty 1 Tablets (Sunpower) *841*

I

IBUPROFEN
Advil Caplets (Whitehall-Robins)........**771**
Advil Gel Caplets (Whitehall-Robins) ...**771**
Advil Liqui-Gels (Whitehall-Robins)......**771**
Advil Tablets (Whitehall-Robins) **771**
Children's Advil Oral Suspension
   (Whitehall-Robins)...................**773**
Children's Advil Chewable Tablets
   (Whitehall-Robins)...................**773**
Advil Cold and Sinus Caplets
   (Whitehall-Robins)...................**771**
Advil Cold and Sinus Tablets
   (Whitehall-Robins)...................**771**
Advil Flu & Body Ache Caplets
   (Whitehall-Robins)...................**772**

Infants' Advil Drops
   (Whitehall-Robins)...................**773**
Junior Strength Advil Tablets
   (Whitehall-Robins)...................**773**
Junior Strength Advil Chewable
   Tablets (Whitehall-Robins) **773**
Advil Migraine Liquigels
   (Whitehall-Robins)...................**772**
Children's Motrin Oral
   Suspension and Chewable
   Tablets (McNeil Consumer)...**509, 643**
Children's Motrin Cold Oral
   Suspension (McNeil
   Consumer) **509, 646**
Infants' Motrin Concentrated
   Drops (McNeil Consumer) **509, 643**
Junior Strength Motrin Caplets
   and Chewable Tablets
   (McNeil Consumer) **509, 643**
Motrin IB Tablets, Caplets, and
   Gelcaps (McNeil
   Consumer) **510, 642**
Motrin Migraine Pain Caplets
   (McNeil Consumer) **510, 646**
Motrin Sinus/Headache
   Caplets (McNeil Consumer) ..**510, 643**

IGNATIUS BEANS
Nytol Natural Tablets (Block) **506, 622**

IRON
(*see under:* **FERROUS GLUCONATE; FERROUS
SULFATE**)

IRON CARBONYL
Feosol Caplets (SmithKline
   Beecham Consumer) **524, 837**

K

KAVA-KAVA
One-A-Day Bedtime & Rest
   Tablets (Bayer Consumer) **505, 805**
One-A-Day Tension & Mood
   Softgels (Bayer Consumer) ...**505, 808**
Sleep-Tite Caplets (Wellness
   International)........................**850**
Vitamist Intra-Oral Spray (Mayor) **821**
   St. John's Wort (Mayor)..............*821*

KETOCONAZOLE
Nizoral A-D Shampoo (McNeil
   Consumer) **510, 647**

KETOPROFEN
Orudis KT Tablets (Whitehall-Robins)...**778**

L

LACTASE (BETA-D-GALACTOSIDASE)
Lactaid Original Strength
   Caplets (McNeil Consumer) ..**509, 822**
Lactaid Extra Strength Caplets
   (McNeil Consumer) **509, 822**
Lactaid Ultra Caplets and
   Chewable Tablets (McNeil
   Consumer) **509, 822**
Lactaid Drops (McNeil
   Consumer) **509, 822**

LACTIC ACID
Amlactin 12% Moisturizing Lotion
   and Cream (Upsher-Smith) *767*

LACTOBACILLUS ACIDOPHILUS
DDS-Acidophilus Capsules, Tablets,
   and Powder (UAS Labs).............**767**
FemEssence Capsules (AdvoCare) **796**
Fiber 10 Packets (AdvoCare) **797**
Perfect Meal (AdvoCare)...............**798**
ProBiotic Restore Capsules
   (AdvoCare) **799**
Super Food Soy Shake (Youngevity) **854**
System 3-4-3 Capsules (AdvoCare) **800**

LACTOBACILLUS REUTERI
Probiotica Tablets (McNeil
   Consumer) **510, 822**

LANOLIN
A + D Original Ointment
   (Schering-Plough) **522, 733**
Lubriderm Skin Therapy
   Moisturizing Lotion (Pfizer
   Inc., Warner-Lambert
   Healthcare)....................**519, 703**

L-ARGININE
Natural Arousal Cream
   (Strategic Science)............**525, 840**
Natural Sensation Cream
   (Strategic Science)................**841**
Nature's Own Pain Expeller Cream
   (Strategic Science)................**841**
Warm Cream (Strategic
   Science)...........................**525, 841**

LECITHIN
Ambrotose with Lecithin Capsules
   (Mannatech)........................**819**
One-A-Day Menopause Health
   Tablets (Bayer Consumer) **505, 808**
ReSource Wellness
   MemorAble Softgels
   (Novartis Consumer) **514, 825**

LEVMETAMFETAMINE
Vicks Vapor Inhaler (Procter &
   Gamble) **730**

LEVOCARNITINE FUMARATE
Proceed Powder (Sigma-Tau)......**523, 835**

LEVULOSE
Emetrol Oral Solution (Lemon-Mint &
   Cherry Flavors) (Pharmacia
   Consumer) **718**

LIDOCAINE
Zilactin-L Liquid (Zila Consumer) **790**

LIDOCAINE HYDROCHLORIDE
Bactine First Aid Liquid (Bayer
   Consumer) **503, 611**

LOPERAMIDE HYDROCHLORIDE
Imodium A-D Liquid and
   Caplets (McNeil Consumer) ..**509, 641**
Imodium Advanced Chewable
   Tablets (McNeil Consumer)...**509, 641**

M

MAGNESIUM CARBONATE
Gaviscon Extra Strength Liquid
   (SmithKline Beecham
   Consumer) **524, 751**
Gaviscon Extra Strength
   Tablets (SmithKline
   Beecham Consumer) **524, 751**
Gaviscon Regular Strength
   Liquid (SmithKline
   Beecham Consumer) **524, 751**
Marblen Suspension (Fleming) **633**
One-A-Day Calcium Plus
   Chewable Tablets (Bayer
   Consumer) **505, 805**

MAGNESIUM CHLORIDE
Chlor-3 Shaker (Fleming)...............**633**
Slow-Mag Tablets (Shire) **835**

MAGNESIUM GLUCONATE
Magonate Liquid (Fleming)..............**814**
Magonate Natal Liquid (Fleming) **814**
Magonate Tablets (Fleming) **814**

MAGNESIUM HYDROXIDE
Ex•Lax Milk of Magnesia
   Liquid (Novartis Consumer) ..**513, 670**
Maalox Antacid/Anti-Gas Oral
   Suspension (Novartis
   Consumer) **514, 673**

Maalox Max Maximum
Strength Antacid/Anti-Gas
Liquid (Novartis Consumer) ..**514, 673**
Mylanta Gelcaps (J&J • Merck)...**507, 637**
Mylanta Liquid (J&J • Merck)...........**634**
Mylanta Extra Strength Liquid
(J&J • Merck) **507, 634**
Mylanta Supreme Liquid (J&J •
Merck)......................**507, 636**
Mylanta Ultra Tabs Tablets
(J&J • Merck) **507, 637**
Pepcid Complete Chewable
Tablets (J&J • Merck).........**508, 638**
Phillips' Chewable Tablets (Bayer
Consumer) **615**
Phillips' Milk of Magnesia
Liquid (Original, Cherry, &
Mint) (Bayer Consumer).......**505, 616**
Rolaids Tablets (Pfizer Inc.,
Warner-Lambert
Healthcare)...................**519, 706**
Extra Strength Rolaids Tablets
(Pfizer Inc., Warner-Lambert
Healthcare)...................**519, 706**
Vanquish Caplets (Bayer
Consumer) **505, 617**

MAGNESIUM OXIDE
Beelith Tablets (Beach) **809**

MAGNESIUM SALICYLATE
Momentum Backache Relief Extra
Strength Caplets (Medtech) **666**

MAGNESIUM TRISILICATE
Gaviscon Regular Strength
Tablets (SmithKline
Beecham Consumer) **524, 750**

MALT SOUP EXTRACT
Maltsupex Powder, Liquid,
Tablets (Wallace)..............**525, 767**

MECLIZINE HYDROCHLORIDE
Bonine Chewable Tablets
(Pfizer Inc., Warner-Lambert
Healthcare)...................**518, 698**
Dramamine Less Drowsy Tablets
(Pharmacia Consumer) **718**

MELATONIN
Vitamist Intra-Oral Spray (Mayor) **821**
Melatonin (Mayor)...................*821*
ZZZ Spray Liquid (AdvoCare)...........**801**

MENTHOL
Afrin Saline Aromatic Mist
(Schering-Plough) **734**
BenGay External Analgesic
Products (Pfizer Inc.,
Warner-Lambert
Healthcare)...................**518, 696**
Cēpacol Maximum Strength Sugar
Free Sore Throat Lozenges,
Cherry Flavor (Williams) **787**
Cēpacol Maximum Strength Sugar
Free Sore Throat Lozenges, Cool
Mint Flavor (Williams)..............**787**
Cēpacol Maximum Strength
Sore Throat Lozenges,
Cherry Flavor (Williams) **526, 787**
Cēpacol Maximum Strength
Sore Throat Lozenges, Mint
Flavor (Williams) **526, 787**
Cēpacol Regular Strength Sore
Throat Lozenges, Cherry Flavor
(Williams)........................**787**
Cēpacol Regular Strength Sore
Throat Lozenges, Original Mint
Flavor (Williams) **787**
Celestial Seasonings Soothers
Throat Drops (Pfizer Inc.,
Warner-Lambert Group).......**515, 685**
Dermoplast Hospital Strength Spray
(Medtech) **666**
Halls Mentho-Lyptus Drops
(Pfizer Inc., Warner-Lambert
Group)......................**516, 686**

Halls Sugar Free
Mentho-Lyptus Drops
(Pfizer Inc., Warner-Lambert
Group) **516, 686**
Halls Sugar Free Squares
(Pfizer Inc., Warner-Lambert
Group)......................**516, 686**
Halls Plus Cough Drops (Pfizer
Inc., Warner-Lambert
Group).......................**516, 686**
Listerine Mouthrinse (Pfizer
Inc., Warner-Lambert
Healthcare)...................**518, 702**
Cool Mint Listerine Mouthrinse
(Pfizer Inc., Warner-Lambert
Healthcare)...................**518, 702**
FreshBurst Listerine
Mouthrinse (Pfizer Inc.,
Warner-Lambert
Healthcare)...................**519, 702**
Tartar Control Listerine
Mouthrinse (Pfizer Inc.,
Warner-Lambert
Healthcare)...................**519, 702**
Robitussin Cough Drops
(Whitehall-Robins)...................**781**
Robitussin Honey Cough Drops
(Whitehall-Robins)...................**784**
Robitussin Honey Calmers Throat
Drops (Whitehall-Robins) **783**
Robitussin Sugar Free Throat Drops
(Whitehall-Robins)...................**786**
Thera-Gesic Creme (Mission)...........**667**
Triaminic Vapor Patch-Cherry
Scent (Novartis Consumer)...**515, 684**
Triaminic Vapor Patch-Menthol
Scent (Novartis Consumer)...**515, 684**
Vicks Cough Drops, Menthol and
Cherry Flavors (Procter &
Gamble) **726**
Vicks VapoRub Cream (Procter &
Gamble) **730**
Vicks VapoRub Ointment (Procter &
Gamble) **730**

METHYL SALICYLATE
BenGay External Analgesic
Products (Pfizer Inc.,
Warner-Lambert
Healthcare)...................**518, 696**
Listerine Mouthrinse (Pfizer
Inc., Warner-Lambert
Healthcare)...................**518, 702**
Cool Mint Listerine Mouthrinse
(Pfizer Inc., Warner-Lambert
Healthcare)...................**518, 702**
FreshBurst Listerine
Mouthrinse (Pfizer Inc.,
Warner-Lambert
Healthcare)...................**519, 702**
Tartar Control Listerine
Mouthrinse (Pfizer Inc.,
Warner-Lambert
Healthcare)...................**519, 702**
Thera-Gesic Creme (Mission)...........**667**

METHYLCELLULOSE
Citrucel Caplets (SmithKline
Beecham Consumer) **745**
Citrucel Orange Flavor Powder
(SmithKline Beecham
Consumer) **523, 744**
Citrucel Sugar Free Orange
Flavor Powder (SmithKline
Beecham Consumer) **523, 745**

MICONAZOLE NITRATE
Desenex Liquid Spray (Novartis
Consumer) **668**
Desenex Shake Powder
(Novartis Consumer).........**512, 668**
Desenex Spray Powder
(Novartis Consumer).........**512, 668**

Desenex Jock Itch Spray Powder
(Novartis Consumer)..............**668**
Lotrimin AF Spray Powder,
Spray Liquid, Spray
Deodorant Powder, Shaker
Powder and Jock Itch Spray
Powder (Schering-Plough).....**523, 742**

MILK OF MAGNESIA
(*see under:* **MAGNESIUM HYDROXIDE**)

MINERAL OIL
Anusol Ointment (Pfizer Inc.,
Warner-Lambert
Healthcare)...................**516, 688**
Lubriderm Skin Therapy
Moisturizing Lotion (Pfizer
Inc., Warner-Lambert
Healthcare)...................**519, 703**
Preparation H Ointment
(Whitehall-Robins)...................**778**

MINERALS, MULTIPLE
Caltrate 600 PLUS Chewables
(Lederle Consumer).................**815**
Caltrate 600 PLUS Tablets (Lederle
Consumer) **815**
Centrum Focused Formulas Bone
Health Tablets (Lederle
Consumer).......................**815**
HGH-Turn Back the Hands of Time
Capsules (Youngevity)..............**854**
Right Choice P.M. Multi Formula
Caplets (Body Wise).............**812**
Super Anti-Oxidant Cell Protector
Capsules (Youngevity)..............**854**
Vitamist Intra-Oral Spray (Mayor) **821**
Colloidal Minerals (Mayor)............*821*
Chitosan Fat Snatcher Capsules
(Youngevity) *853*

MINOXIDIL
Rogaine Extra Strength for Men
Topical Solution (Pharmacia
Consumer) **721**
Rogaine for Women Topical Solution
(Pharmacia Consumer) **721**

MULTIMINERALS
(*see under:* **VITAMINS WITH MINERALS**)

MULTIVITAMINS
(*see under:* **VITAMINS, MULTIPLE**)

MULTIVITAMINS WITH MINERALS
(*see under:* **VITAMINS WITH MINERALS**)

N

N-METHYLNICOTINATE
Vitara Cream (Products on
Demand) **522, 731**

NAPHAZOLINE HYDROCHLORIDE
Visine-A Eye Drops (Pfizer Inc.,
Warner-Lambert
Healthcare)...................**521, 714**

NAPROXEN SODIUM
Aleve Tablets, Caplets and
Gelcaps (Bayer Consumer) ...**503, 602**
Aleve Cold & Sinus Caplets
(Bayer Consumer)............**503, 603**

NEOMYCIN
Neosporin Ointment (Pfizer
Inc., Warner-Lambert
Healthcare)...................**519, 704**
Neosporin + Pain Relief
Maximum Strength Cream
(Pfizer Inc., Warner-Lambert
Healthcare)...................**519, 704**
Neosporin + Pain Relief
Maximum Strength
Ointment (Pfizer Inc.,
Warner-Lambert
Healthcare)...................**519, 704**

NIACIN
Nicotinex Elixir (Fleming)...............**633**

NICOTINE
NicoDerm CQ Patch
(SmithKline Beecham
Consumer) **524, 754**

NICOTINE POLACRILEX
Nicorette Gum (SmithKline
Beecham Consumer) **524, 758**

NICOTINIC ACID
(*see under:* NIACIN)

O

OCTYL METHOXYCINNAMATE
Bio-Complex 5000 Revitalizing
Conditioner (Wellness
International)......................**769**
Bio-Complex 5000 Revitalizing
Shampoo (Wellness
International)......................**770**
Lubriderm Daily UV Lotion
(Pfizer Inc., Warner-Lambert
Healthcare)....................**519, 703**

OCTYL SALICYLATE
Lubriderm Daily UV Lotion
(Pfizer Inc., Warner-Lambert
Healthcare)....................**519, 703**

OLEORESIN CAPSICUM
Nature's Own Pain Expeller Cream
(Strategic Science)..................**841**

OMEGA-3 POLYUNSATURATES
(*see under:* FATTY ACIDS)

OXYBENZONE
Lubriderm Daily UV Lotion
(Pfizer Inc., Warner-Lambert
Healthcare)....................**519, 703**

OXYMETAZOLINE HYDROCHLORIDE
Afrin Original Nasal Spray
(Schering-Plough) **522, 733**
Afrin Extra Moisturizing Nasal Spray
(Schering-Plough) **733**
Afrin Severe Congestion Nasal Spray
(Schering-Plough) **733**
Afrin Sinus Nasal Spray
(Schering-Plough) **733**
Afrin No Drip Original Nasal
Spray (Schering-Plough).......**522, 735**
Afrin No Drip Extra Moisturizing
Nasal Spray (Schering-Plough)......**735**
Afrin No Drip Severe Congestion
Nasal Spray (Schering-Plough)......**735**
Afrin No Drip Sinus Nasal Spray
(Schering-Plough) **735**
Afrin Original Pump Mist
(Schering-Plough) **733**
Neo-Synephrine 12 Hour Nasal
Spray (Bayer Consumer)......**504, 615**
Neo-Synephrine 12 Hour Extra
Moisturizing Nasal Spray (Bayer
Consumer) **615**
Vicks Sinex 12-Hour Nasal Spray
and Ultra Fine Mist (Procter &
Gamble) **729**
Visine L.R. Eye Drops (Pfizer
Inc., Warner-Lambert
Healthcare)....................**521, 715**

P

PAMABROM
Maximum Strength Midol PMS
Caplets and Gelcaps
(Bayer Consumer).............**504, 613**
Maximum Strength Midol Teen
Caplets (Bayer Consumer)....**504, 612**
Women's Tylenol Menstrual
Relief Caplets (McNeil
Consumer) **512, 656**

PAUSINYSTALIA YOHIMBE
Power Lasting Tablets (Sunpower)......*841*

PECTIN
Celestial Seasonings Soothers
Throat Drops (Pfizer Inc.,
Warner-Lambert Group)....**515, 685**
Halls Plus Cough Drops (Pfizer
Inc., Warner-Lambert
Group) **516, 686**

PERMETHRIN
Nix Creme Rinse (Pfizer Inc.,
Warner-Lambert
Healthcare)....................**519, 704**
Permethrin Lotion (Alpharma) **602**

PETROLATUM
A + D Original Ointment
(Schering-Plough) **522, 733**
Desitin Creamy Ointment
(Pfizer Inc., Warner-Lambert
Healthcare)....................**518, 700**
Lubriderm Skin Therapy
Moisturizing Lotion (Pfizer
Inc., Warner-Lambert
Healthcare)....................**519, 703**
Preparation H Cream
(Whitehall-Robins)...................**778**
Preparation H Ointment
(Whitehall-Robins)...................**778**

PHENIRAMINE MALEATE
Visine-A Eye Drops (Pfizer Inc.,
Warner-Lambert
Healthcare)....................**521, 714**

PHENYLEPHRINE HYDROCHLORIDE
Afrin Nasal Decongestant Children's
Pump Mist (Schering-Plough) **734**
Neo-Synephrine Nasal Drops,
Regular and Extra Strength
(Bayer Consumer).......**504, 614**
Neo-Synephrine Nasal Sprays,
Mild, Regular and Extra
Strength (Bayer Consumer)...**504, 614**
Preparation H Cream
(Whitehall-Robins)...................**778**
Preparation H Cooling Gel
(Whitehall-Robins)...................**778**
Preparation H Ointment
(Whitehall-Robins)...................**778**
Preparation H Suppositories
(Whitehall-Robins)...................**778**
Vicks Sinex Nasal Spray and Ultra
Fine Mist (Procter & Gamble).......**729**

PHENYLTOLOXAMINE CITRATE
Percogesic Aspirin-Free Coated
Tablets (Medtech)...................**667**

PHOSPHORIC ACID
Emetrol Oral Solution (Lemon-Mint &
Cherry Flavors) (Pharmacia
Consumer) **718**

PIPERONYL BUTOXIDE
Maximum Strength Rid
Mousse (Bayer Consumer) ...**505, 617**

POLYETHYLENE GLYCOL
Advanced Relief Visine Eye
Drops (Pfizer Inc.,
Warner-Lambert
Healthcare)....................**521, 714**
Visine Tears Eye Drops (Pfizer
Inc., Warner-Lambert
Healthcare)....................**521, 716**
Visine Tears Preservative Free
Eye Drops (Pfizer Inc.,
Warner-Lambert
Healthcare)....................**521, 716**

POLYMYXIN B SULFATE
Betadine Brand First Aid
Antibiotics + Moisturizer
Ointment (Purdue
Frederick)....................**522, 731**
Betadine Brand Plus First Aid
Antibiotics + Pain Reliever
Ointment (Purdue
Frederick)....................**522, 731**

Neosporin Ointment (Pfizer
Inc., Warner-Lambert
Healthcare)....................**519, 704**
Neosporin + Pain Relief
Maximum Strength Cream
(Pfizer Inc., Warner-Lambert
Healthcare)....................**519, 704**
Neosporin + Pain Relief
Maximum Strength
Ointment (Pfizer Inc.,
Warner-Lambert
Healthcare)....................**519, 704**
Polysporin Ointment (Pfizer
Inc., Warner-Lambert
Healthcare)....................**519, 706**
Polysporin Powder (Pfizer Inc.,
Warner-Lambert
Healthcare)....................**519, 706**

POTASSIUM BITARTRATE
Ceo-Two Evacuant Suppository
(Beutlich)..........................**618**

POTASSIUM CHLORIDE
Chlor-3 Shaker (Fleming)................**633**

POTASSIUM NITRATE
Sensodyne Original Flavor (Block)......**623**
Sensodyne Cool Gel (Block) **623**
Sensodyne Extra Whitening (Block) **623**
Sensodyne Fresh Mint (Block)..........**623**
Sensodyne Tartar Control (Block) **623**
Sensodyne Tartar Control Plus
Whitening (Block) **623**
Sensodyne with Baking Soda (Block) ..**623**

POVIDONE IODINE
Betadine Ointment (Purdue
Frederick)....................**522, 732**
Betadine PrepStick Applicator
(Purdue Frederick) **522, 732**
Betadine Skin Cleanser (Purdue
Frederick)..........................**732**
Betadine Solution (Purdue
Frederick)....................**522, 732**
Massengill Medicated
Disposable Douche
(SmithKline Beecham
Consumer) **524, 753**

PRAMOXINE HYDROCHLORIDE
Anusol Ointment (Pfizer Inc.,
Warner-Lambert
Healthcare)....................**516, 688**
Betadine Brand Plus First Aid
Antibiotics + Pain Reliever
Ointment (Purdue
Frederick)....................**522, 731**
Caladryl Clear Lotion (Pfizer
Inc., Warner-Lambert
Healthcare)....................**518, 698**
Caladryl Lotion (Pfizer Inc.,
Warner-Lambert
Healthcare)....................**518, 698**
Neosporin + Pain Relief
Maximum Strength Cream
(Pfizer Inc., Warner-Lambert
Healthcare)....................**519, 704**
Neosporin + Pain Relief
Maximum Strength
Ointment (Pfizer Inc.,
Warner-Lambert
Healthcare)....................**519, 704**

PSEUDOEPHEDRINE HYDROCHLORIDE
Actifed Cold & Allergy Tablets
(Pfizer Inc., Warner-Lambert
Healthcare)....................**516, 688**
Actifed Cold & Sinus Caplets
and Tablets (Pfizer Inc.,
Warner-Lambert
Healthcare)....................**516, 688**
Advil Cold and Sinus Caplets
(Whitehall-Robins)...................**771**
Advil Cold and Sinus Tablets
(Whitehall-Robins)...................**771**

Advil Flu & Body Ache Caplets
(Whitehall-Robins)..................**772**
Aleve Cold & Sinus Caplets
(Bayer Consumer)............**503, 603**
Alka-Seltzer Plus Cold
Medicine Liqui-Gels (Bayer
Consumer) **503, 604**
Alka-Seltzer Plus Night-Time
Cold Medicine Liqui-Gels
(Bayer Consumer)...........**503, 604**
Alka-Seltzer Plus Cold & Cough
Medicine Liqui-Gels (Bayer
Consumer) **503, 604**
Alka-Seltzer Plus Cold & Flu
Medicine Liqui-Gels (Bayer
Consumer) **503, 604**
Alka-Seltzer Plus Cold & Sinus
Medicine Liqui-Gels (Bayer
Consumer) **503, 604**
BC Allergy Sinus Cold Powder
(Block)..........................**619**
BC Sinus Cold Powder (Block)..........**619**
Benadryl Allergy/Cold Tablets
(Pfizer Inc., Warner-Lambert
Healthcare)...................**517, 691**
Benadryl Allergy/Congestion
Tablets (Pfizer Inc.,
Warner-Lambert
Healthcare)...................**517, 692**
Benadryl Allergy & Sinus Liquid
(Pfizer Inc., Warner-Lambert
Healthcare)...........................**693**
Benadryl Allergy & Sinus
Fastmelt Tablets (Pfizer
Inc., Warner-Lambert
Healthcare)...................**517, 693**
Benadryl Allergy Sinus
Headache Caplets &
Gelcaps (Pfizer Inc.,
Warner-Lambert
Healthcare)...................**517, 693**
Benadryl Severe Allergy &
Sinus Headache Caplets
(Pfizer Inc., Warner-Lambert
Healthcare)...................**517, 694**
Benadryl Children's Allergy/
Cold Fastmelt Tablets
(Pfizer Inc., Warner-Lambert
Healthcare)...................**517, 692**
Benylin Multi-Symptom Liquid
(Pfizer Inc., Warner-Lambert
Healthcare)...................**518, 697**
Children's Cēpacol Sore Throat
Formula, Cherry Flavor Liquid
(Williams)............................**788**
Children's Cēpacol Sore Throat
Formula, Grape Flavor Liquid
(Williams)............................**788**
Comtrex Acute Head Cold &
Sinus Pressure Relief
Tablets (Bristol-Myers) **506, 627**
Comtrex Deep Chest Cold &
Congestion Relief Softgels
(Bristol-Myers).................**506, 627**
Comtrex Flu Therapy & Fever
Relief Daytime Caplets
(Bristol-Myers)................**506, 628**
Comtrex Flu Therapy & Fever
Relief Nighttime Tablets
(Bristol-Myers)................**506, 628**
Comtrex Maximum Strength
Multi-Symptom Cold &
Cough Relief Tablets and
Caplets (Bristol-Myers)........**506, 626**
Contac Non-Drowsy 12 Hour
Cold Caplets (SmithKline
Beecham Consumer) **523, 745**

Contac Non-Drowsy Timed
Release 12 Hour Cold
Caplets (SmithKline
Beecham Consumer) **523, 746**
Contac Severe Cold and Flu
Caplets Maximum Strength
(SmithKline Beecham
Consumer)...................**523, 746**
Contac Severe Cold and Flu Caplets
Non-Drowsy (SmithKline
Beecham Consumer) **746**
Dimetapp Elixir (Whitehall-Robins)......**777**
Dimetapp Cold and Fever
Suspension (Whitehall-Robins) **775**
Dimetapp DM Cold & Cough Elixir
(Whitehall-Robins)...................**775**
Dimetapp Nighttime Flu Liquid
(Whitehall-Robins)...................**776**
Dimetapp Non-Drowsy Flu Syrup
(Whitehall-Robins)...................**777**
Dimetapp Infant Drops
Decongestant (Whitehall-Robins)...**775**
Dimetapp Infant Drops
Decongestant Plus Cough
(Whitehall-Robins)...................**776**
Children's Motrin Cold Oral
Suspension (McNeil
Consumer) **509, 646**
Motrin Sinus/Headache
Caplets (McNeil Consumer) ..**510, 643**
PediaCare Cough-Cold Liquid
(Pharmacia Consumer) **719**
PediaCare Infants' Drops
Decongestant (Pharmacia
Consumer)...........................**719**
PediaCare Infants' Drops
Decongestant Plus Cough
(Pharmacia Consumer) **719**
PediaCare NightRest Cough-Cold
Liquid (Pharmacia Consumer) **719**
Robitussin Cold Caplets Cold &
Congestion (Whitehall-Robins)......**780**
Robitussin Cold Softgels Cold &
Congestion (Whitehall-Robins)......**780**
Robitussin Cold Caplets
Multi-Symptom Cold & Flu
(Whitehall-Robins)...................**781**
Robitussin Cold Softgels
Multi-Symptom Cold & Flu
(Whitehall-Robins)...................**781**
Robitussin Cold Softgels Severe
Congestion (Whitehall-Robins)......**782**
Robitussin Cough & Cold Infant
Drops (Whitehall-Robins) **782**
Robitussin Maximum Strength
Cough & Cold Liquid
(Whitehall-Robins)...................**785**
Robitussin Pediatric Cough & Cold
Formula Liquid
(Whitehall-Robins)...................**785**
Robitussin Multi Symptom Honey Flu
Liquid (Whitehall-Robins) **785**
Robitussin Nighttime Honey Flu
Liquid (Whitehall-Robins) **786**
Robitussin-CF Liquid
(Whitehall-Robins)...................**783**
Robitussin-PE Liquid
(Whitehall-Robins)...................**782**
Ryna Liquid (Wallace)..................**768**
Ryna-C Liquid (Wallace)...........**525, 768**
Singlet Caplets (SmithKline
Beecham Consumer) **761**
Sinutab Non-Drying Liquid
Caps (Pfizer Inc.,
Warner-Lambert
Healthcare)...................**520, 706**

Sinutab Sinus Allergy
Medication, Maximum
Strength Formula, Tablets
& Caplets (Pfizer Inc.,
Warner-Lambert
Healthcare)...................**520, 707**
Sinutab Sinus Medication,
Maximum Strength Without
Drowsiness Formula,
Tablets & Caplets (Pfizer
Inc., Warner-Lambert
Healthcare)...................**520, 707**
Sudafed 12 Hour Tablets
(Pfizer Inc., Warner-Lambert
Healthcare)...................**520, 708**
Sudafed 24 Hour Tablets
(Pfizer Inc., Warner-Lambert
Healthcare)...................**520, 708**
Children's Sudafed Cold &
Cough Liquid (Pfizer Inc.,
Warner-Lambert
Healthcare)...................**520, 709**
Children's Sudafed Nasal
Decongestant Chewables
(Pfizer Inc., Warner-Lambert
Healthcare)...................**520, 711**
Children's Sudafed Nasal
Decongestant Liquid
Medication (Pfizer Inc.,
Warner-Lambert
Healthcare)...................**521, 711**
Sudafed Cold & Allergy Tablets
(Pfizer Inc., Warner-Lambert
Healthcare)...................**520, 708**
Sudafed Cold & Cough Liquid
Caps (Pfizer Inc.,
Warner-Lambert
Healthcare)...................**520, 709**
Sudafed Cold & Sinus Liquid
Caps (Pfizer Inc.,
Warner-Lambert
Healthcare)...................**520, 710**
Sudafed Nasal Decongestant
Tablets (Pfizer Inc.,
Warner-Lambert
Healthcare)...................**520, 710**
Sudafed Non-Drying Sinus
Liquid Caps (Pfizer Inc.,
Warner-Lambert
Healthcare)...................**520, 712**
Sudafed Severe Cold Formula
Caplets (Pfizer Inc.,
Warner-Lambert
Healthcare)...................**520, 711**
Sudafed Severe Cold Formula
Tablets (Pfizer Inc.,
Warner-Lambert
Healthcare)...................**520, 711**
Sudafed Sinus Headache
Caplets (Pfizer Inc.,
Warner-Lambert
Healthcare)...................**520, 712**
Sudafed Sinus Headache
Tablets (Pfizer Inc.,
Warner-Lambert
Healthcare)...................**520, 712**
Tavist Sinus Non-Drowsy
Coated Caplets (Novartis
Consumer) **514, 676**
TheraFlu Regular Strength Cold
& Cough Night Time Hot
Liquid (Novartis Consumer) ..**515, 676**
TheraFlu Regular Strength Cold
& Sore Throat Night Time
Hot Liquid (Novartis
Consumer) **515, 676**
TheraFlu Maximum Strength
Flu & Congestion
Non-Drowsy Hot Liquid
(Novartis Consumer)..........**515, 677**
TheraFlu Maximum Strength
Flu & Cough Night Time Hot
Liquid (Novartis Consumer) ..**515, 678**

PSEUDOEPHEDRINE HYDROCHLORIDE—
cont.
TheraFlu Maximum Strength
Flu & Sore Throat Night
Time Hot Liquid (Novartis
Consumer) **515, 677**
TheraFlu Maximum Strength
Severe Cold & Congestion
Night Time Caplets
(Novartis Consumer)..........**515, 678**
TheraFlu Maximum Strength
Severe Cold & Congestion
Night Time Hot Liquid
(Novartis Consumer)..........**515, 678**
TheraFlu Maximum Strength
Severe Cold & Congestion
Non-Drowsy Caplets
(Novartis Consumer)..........**515, 679**
TheraFlu Maximum Strength
Severe Cold & Congestion
Non-Drowsy Hot Liquid
(Novartis Consumer)..........**515, 679**
Triaminic Allergy Congestion
Liquid (Novartis Consumer) ..**515, 680**
Triaminic Chest Congestion
Liquid (Novartis Consumer) ..**515, 680**
Triaminic Cold & Allergy Liquid
(Novartis Consumer)..........**515, 681**
Triaminic Cold & Allergy
Softchews (Novartis
Consumer) **515, 683**
Triaminic Cold & Cough Liquid
(Novartis Consumer)..........**515, 681**
Triaminic Cold & Cough
Softchews (Novartis
Consumer) **515, 683**
Triaminic Cold & Night Time
Cough Liquid (Novartis
Consumer) **515, 681**
Triaminic Cold, Cough & Fever
Liquid (Novartis Consumer) ..**515, 681**
Triaminic Cough Liquid
(Novartis Consumer)..........**515, 682**
Triaminic Cough & Congestion
Liquid (Novartis Consumer) ..**515, 682**
Triaminic Cough & Sore Throat
Liquid (Novartis Consumer) ..**515, 682**
Triaminic Cough & Sore Throat
Softchews (Novartis
Consumer) **515, 684**
Children's Tylenol Allergy-D
Liquid (McNeil Consumer) **510, 658**
Children's Tylenol Cold
Suspension Liquid and
Chewable Tablets (McNeil
Consumer) **510, 659**
Children's Tylenol Cold Plus
Cough Suspension Liquid
and Chewable Tablets
(McNeil Consumer) **510, 659**
Children's Tylenol Flu
Suspension Liquid (McNeil
Consumer) **511, 663**
Children's Tylenol Sinus
Suspension Liquid (McNeil
Consumer) **511, 663**
Infants' Tylenol Cold
Decongestant & Fever
Reducer Concentrated
Drops (McNeil Consumer) **511, 659**
Infants' Tylenol Cold
Decongestant & Fever
Reducer Concentrated
Drops Plus Cough (McNeil
Consumer) **511, 659**
Maximum Strength Tylenol
Allergy Sinus Caplets,
Gelcaps, and Geltabs
(McNeil Consumer) **511, 649**

Maximum Strength Tylenol
Allergy Sinus NightTime
Caplets (McNeil Consumer) ..**511, 649**
Multi-Symptom Tylenol Cold
Complete Formula Caplets
(McNeil Consumer) **512, 651**
Multi-Symptom Tylenol Cold
Non-Drowsy Caplets and
Gelcaps (McNeil
Consumer) **512, 651**
Multi-Symptom Tylenol Cold
Severe Congestion
Non-Drowsy Caplets
(McNeil Consumer) **512, 652**
Maximum Strength Tylenol Flu
NightTime Gelcaps (McNeil
Consumer) **512, 653**
Maximum Strength Tylenol Flu
NightTime Liquid (McNeil
Consumer) **512, 653**
Maximum Strength Tylenol Flu
Non-Drowsy Gelcaps
(McNeil Consumer) **512, 653**
Maximum Strength Tylenol
Sinus NightTime Caplets
(McNeil Consumer) **512, 655**
Maximum Strength Tylenol
Sinus Non-Drowsy Geltabs,
Gelcaps, Caplets, and
Tablets (McNeil Consumer) ...**512, 655**
Vicks 44D Cough & Head
Congestion Relief Liquid (Procter
& Gamble)........................**724**
Vicks 44M Cough, Cold & Flu Relief
Liquid (Procter & Gamble) **725**
Pediatric Vicks 44m Cough & Cold
Relief (Procter & Gamble)...........**728**
Vicks DayQuil LiquiCaps/Liquid
Multi-Symptom Cold/Flu Relief
(Procter & Gamble) **727**
Children's Vicks NyQuil Cold/Cough
Relief (Procter & Gamble).........**726**
Vicks NyQuil LiquiCaps/Liquid
Multi-Symptom Cold/Flu Relief,
Original and Cherry Flavors
(Procter & Gamble) **727**

PSEUDOEPHEDRINE SULFATE
Chlor-Trimeton Allergy/
Decongestant Tablets
(Schering-Plough)..........**522, 736**
Coricidin 'D' Cold, Flu & Sinus
Tablets (Schering-Plough).....**522, 737**
Drixoral Allergy/Sinus
Extended-Release Tablets
(Schering-Plough)..........**523, 741**
Drixoral Cold & Allergy
Sustained-Action Tablets
(Schering-Plough) **523, 740**
Drixoral Cold & Flu
Extended-Release Tablets
(Schering-Plough) **523, 740**
Drixoral Nasal Decongestant
Long-Acting Non-Drowsy
Tablets (Schering-Plough).....**523, 740**

PSYLLIUM PREPARATIONS
Fiber 10 Packets (AdvoCare) **797**
Metamucil Dietary Fiber Supplement
(Procter & Gamble) **834**
Metamucil Powder, Original Texture
Orange Flavor (Procter &
Gamble) **722**
Metamucil Powder, Original Texture
Regular Flavor (Procter &
Gamble) **722**
Metamucil Smooth Texture
Powder, Orange Flavor
(Procter & Gamble) **521, 722**

Metamucil Smooth Texture Powder,
Sugar-Free, Orange Flavor
(Procter & Gamble) **722**
Metamucil Smooth Texture Powder,
Sugar-Free, Regular Flavor
(Procter & Gamble) **722**
Metamucil Wafers, Apple Crisp
& Cinnamon Spice Flavors
(Procter & Gamble) **521, 722**
Perdiem Fiber Therapy
Granules (Novartis
Consumer) **514, 675**
Perdiem Overnight Relief
Granules (Novartis
Consumer) **514, 674**
StePHan Relief Capsules (Wellness
International)........................**850**
System 3-4-3 Capsules (AdvoCare) **800**
PUMPKIN
One-A-Day Prostate Health
Softgels (Bayer Consumer) ...**505, 808**
PYRANTEL PAMOATE
Pin-X Pinworm Treatment
(Effcon)......................**507, 632**
PYRETHRUM EXTRACT
Maximum Strength Rid
Mousse (Bayer Consumer) ...**505, 617**
PYRIDOXINE HYDROCHLORIDE
(*see under:* **VITAMIN B₆**)
PYRILAMINE MALEATE
Maximum Strength Midol
Menstrual Caplets and
Gelcaps (Bayer Consumer) ...**504, 612**
Maximum Strength Midol PMS
Caplets and Gelcaps
(Bayer Consumer)............**504, 613**
PYROXYLIN
New Skin Liquid Bandage (Medtech)...**667**

Q
QUININE
Hyland's Leg Cramps with Quinine
Tablets (Standard Homeopathic) ...**765**

R
RANITIDINE HYDROCHLORIDE
Zantac 75 Tablets (Pfizer Inc.,
Warner-Lambert
Healthcare)....................**528, 717**

S
SALICYLAMIDE
BC Powder (Block) **619**
Arthritis Strength BC Powder (Block)...**619**
SALICYLIC ACID
Clear Away Gel with Aloe Wart
Remover System
(Schering-Plough) **736**
Clear Away Liquid Wart Remover
System (Schering-Plough)...........**736**
Clear Away One Step Wart
Remover (Schering-Plough) ...**522, 737**
Clear Away One Step Wart
Remover for Kids
(Schering-Plough) **522, 737**
Clear Away One Step Plantar Wart
Remover (Schering-Plough) **737**
Compound W One Step Pads for
Kids (Medtech)......................**664**
Compound W One Step Plantar Pads
(Medtech)..........................**664**
Compound W One Step Wart
Remover Pads (Medtech)..........**664**
Compound W Wart Remover Gel
(Medtech)..........................**665**
Compound W Wart Remover Liquid
(Medtech)..........................**665**
Wart-Off Liquid (Pfizer Inc.,
Warner-Lambert Healthcare)........**716**
SAW PALMETTO
(*see under:* **SERENOA REPENS**)

SENNA
Perdiem Overnight Relief
Granules (Novartis
Consumer) **514, 674**
Senokot Children's Syrup
(Purdue Frederick) **522, 732**
Senokot Granules (Purdue
Frederick)........................**522, 732**
Senokot Syrup (Purdue
Frederick).........................**522, 732**
Senokot Tablets (Purdue
Frederick).........................**522, 732**
Senokot-S Tablets (Purdue
Frederick).........................**522, 732**
SenokotXTRA Tablets (Purdue
Frederick).........................**732**
System 3-4-3 Capsules (AdvoCare) **800**

SENNOSIDES
Ex•Lax Gentle Strength
Caplets (Novartis
Consumer) **513, 670**
Ex•Lax Regular Strength Pills
(Novartis Consumer) **513, 670**
Ex•Lax Regular Strength
Chocolated Pieces
(Novartis Consumer)..........**513, 669**
Ex•Lax Maximum Strength
Pills (Novartis Consumer) **513, 670**
Nature's Remedy Tablets
(Block)............................**506, 621**

SERENOA REPENS
Centrum Focused Formulas Prostate
Softgels (Lederle Consumer) **816**
Centrum Saw Palmetto Softgels
(Whitehall-Robins)....................**853**
FemEssence Capsules (AdvoCare) **796**
One-A-Day Prostate Health
Softgels (Bayer Consumer) ...**505, 808**
Performance Optimizer System
(AdvoCare) **798**
Power Lasting Tablets (Sunpower)......*841*

SHARK CARTILAGE
Second Look Capsules (AdvoCare).....**800**

SHARK LIVER OIL
Preparation H Cream
(Whitehall-Robins)....................**778**
Preparation H Ointment
(Whitehall-Robins)....................**778**
Preparation H Suppositories
(Whitehall-Robins)....................**778**

SIMETHICONE
Maximum Strength Gas Aid
Softgels (McNeil
Consumer) **509, 640**
Gas-X Chewable Tablets
(Novartis Consumer)..........**513, 671**
Extra Strength Gas-X Liquid
(Novartis Consumer)..........**513, 671**
Extra Strength Gas-X Softgels
(Novartis Consumer)..........**513, 671**
Extra Strength Gas-X Chewable
Tablets (Novartis
Consumer) **513, 671**
Maximum Strength Gas-X
Softgels (Novartis
Consumer) **513, 671**
Imodium Advanced Chewable
Tablets (McNeil Consumer) ...**509, 641**
Maalox Antacid/Anti-Gas Oral
Suspension (Novartis
Consumer) **514, 673**
Maalox Max Maximum
Strength Antacid/Anti-Gas
Liquid (Novartis Consumer) ..**514, 673**
Quick Dissolve Maalox Max
Maximum Strength
Antacid/Antigas Chewable
Tablets (Novartis
Consumer) **514, 674**
Mylanta Liquid (J&J • Merck)...........**634**

Mylanta Extra Strength Liquid
(J&J • Merck) **507, 634**
Mylanta Gas Softgels (J&J •
Merck)...........................**507, 637**
Mylanta Gas Tablets (J&J • Merck) **637**
Maximum Strength Mylanta
Gas Tablets (J&J • Merck)....**507, 637**
Infants' Mylicon Drops (J&J •
Merck)...........................**508, 634**
Phazyme-125 mg Quick
Dissolve Chewable Tablets
(Block)...........................**506, 622**
Phazyme-180 mg Ultra
Strength Softgels (Block) **506, 622**
3M Titralac Plus Antacid
Tablets (3M)....................**508, 640**

SODIUM BICARBONATE
Alka-Seltzer Original Antacid
and Pain Reliever
Effervescent Tablets (Bayer
Consumer) **503, 603**
Alka-Seltzer Cherry Antacid
and Pain Reliever
Effervescent Tablets (Bayer
Consumer) **503, 603**
Alka-Seltzer Lemon Lime
Antacid and Pain Reliever
Effervescent Tablets (Bayer
Consumer) **503, 603**
Alka-Seltzer Extra Strength
Antacid and Pain Reliever
Effervescent Tablets (Bayer
Consumer) **503, 603**
Alka-Seltzer Heartburn Relief
Tablets (Bayer Consumer) **503, 604**
Ceo-Two Evacuant Suppository
(Beutlich) **618**

SODIUM CHLORIDE
Afrin Saline Aromatic Mist
(Schering-Plough) **734**
Afrin Extra Moisturizing Saline
Mist (Schering-Plough) **522, 734**
Chlor-3 Shaker (Fleming)...............**633**
Natru-Vent Saline Nasal Spray
(Boehringer Ingelheim)........**506, 625**
Ocean Nasal Mist (Fleming) **633**

SODIUM FLUORIDE
Sensodyne Original Flavor (Block)......**623**
Sensodyne Cool Gel (Block) **623**
Sensodyne Fresh Mint (Block).........**623**
Sensodyne Tartar Control (Block) **623**
Sensodyne Tartar Control Plus
Whitening (Block) **623**
Sensodyne with Baking Soda (Block) ..**623**

SODIUM MONOFLUOROPHOSPHATE
Sensodyne Extra Whitening (Block) ...**623**

SOY ISOFLAVONES
Caltrate 600 + Soy Tablets (Lederle
Consumer) **814**

ST. JOHN'S WORT
(*see under:* **HYPERICUM**)

STARCH
Anusol Suppositories (Pfizer
Inc., Warner-Lambert
Healthcare)....................**516, 689**

T

TERBINAFINE HYDROCHLORIDE
Lamisil^AT Cream (Novartis
Consumer) **513, 672**
Lamisil^AT Solution (Novartis
Consumer) **513, 672**

TETRACAINE
Cēpacol Viractin Cold Sore and
Fever Blister Treatment,
Cream (Williams) **526, 788**

TETRACAINE HYDROCHLORIDE
Cēpacol Viractin Cold Sore and
Fever Blister Treatment,
Gel (Williams) **526, 788**

TETRAHYDROZOLINE HYDROCHLORIDE
Visine Original Eye Drops
(Pfizer Inc., Warner-Lambert
Healthcare)....................**521, 715**
Visine A.C. Eye Drops (Pfizer
Inc., Warner-Lambert
Healthcare)....................**521, 715**
Advanced Relief Visine Eye
Drops (Pfizer Inc.,
Warner-Lambert
Healthcare)....................**521, 714**

THYMOL
Listerine Mouthrinse (Pfizer
Inc., Warner-Lambert
Healthcare)....................**518, 702**
Cool Mint Listerine Mouthrinse
(Pfizer Inc., Warner-Lambert
Healthcare)....................**518, 702**
FreshBurst Listerine
Mouthrinse (Pfizer Inc.,
Warner-Lambert
Healthcare)....................**519, 702**
Tartar Control Listerine
Mouthrinse (Pfizer Inc.,
Warner-Lambert
Healthcare)....................**519, 702**

TRIPROLIDINE HYDROCHLORIDE
Actifed Cold & Allergy Tablets
(Pfizer Inc., Warner-Lambert
Healthcare)....................**516, 688**

V

VALERIANA OFFICINALIS
Alluna Sleep Tablets (SmithKline
Beecham Consumer) **837**
One-A-Day Bedtime & Rest
Tablets (Bayer Consumer) ...**505, 805**
ReSource Wellness StayCalm
Caplets (Novartis
Consumer) **514, 826**
Sleep-Tite Caplets (Wellness
International) **850**
StePHan Tranquility Capsules
(Wellness International) **851**

VINEGAR
Massengill Disposable Douches
(SmithKline Beecham Consumer) ..**752**

VINPOCETINE
Intelectol Tablets (Covex) **507, 813**

VITAMIN A
Beta-C Tablets (Body Wise).............**811**
Centrum Focused Formulas Prostate
Softgels (Lederle Consumer) **816**
ReSource Wellness ForSight
Caplets (Novartis
Consumer) **514, 825**

VITAMIN B$_3$
(*see under:* **NIACIN**)

VITAMIN B$_6$
Beelith Tablets (Beach) **809**
Brite-Life Caplets (AdvoCare) **795**
One-A-Day Memory &
Concentration Tablets
(Bayer Consumer)............**505, 807**

VITAMIN B$_{12}$
One-A-Day Memory &
Concentration Tablets
(Bayer Consumer)............**505, 807**
Vitamist Intra-Oral Spray (Mayor) **821**
B12 (Mayor)............................*821*

VITAMIN B COMPLEX
One-A-Day Energy Formula
Tablets (Bayer Consumer) **505, 806**

VITAMIN B COMPLEX WITH VITAMIN C
One-A-Day Tension & Mood
Softgels (Bayer Consumer) ...**505, 808**

VITAMIN C

Beta-C Tablets (Body Wise) **811**
C-Grams Caplets (AdvoCare) **795**
Halls Defense Drops (Pfizer
   Inc., Warner-Lambert
   Group) **516, 687**
Peridin-C Tablets (Beutlich) **618**

VITAMIN D

Caltrate 600 PLUS Chewables
   (Lederle Consumer) **815**
Caltrate 600 PLUS Tablets (Lederle
   Consumer) **815**
Caltrate 600 + D Tablets (Lederle
   Consumer) **814**
Caltrate 600 + Soy Tablets (Lederle
   Consumer) **814**
Centrum Focused Formulas Bone
   Health Tablets (Lederle
   Consumer) **815**
Citracal Caplets + D (Mission).........**823**
Citracal 250 MG + D Tablets
   (Mission) **823**
Citracal Plus Tablets (Mission) **824**
D-Cal Chewable Caplets (A & Z
   Pharm) **503, 794**
One-A-Day Calcium Plus
   Chewable Tablets (Bayer
   Consumer).................**505, 805**
Os-Cal 250 + D Tablets
   (SmithKline Beecham
   Consumer) **525, 838**
Os-Cal 500 + D Tablets
   (SmithKline Beecham
   Consumer) **525, 839**

VITAMIN E

One-A-Day Cholesterol Health
   Tablets (Bayer Consumer) **505, 805**
One-A-Day Menopause Health
   Tablets (Bayer Consumer) **505, 808**
StePHan Bio-Nutritional Daytime
   Hydrating Creme (Wellness
   International).......................**770**

VITAMINS, MULTIPLE

Bugs Bunny Children's
   Multivitamin Plus Extra C
   Chewable Tablets (Sugar
   Free) (Bayer Consumer).......**504, 804**
Centrum Focused Formulas Energy
   Tablets (Lederle Consumer) **816**
Flintstones Original Children's
   Multivitamin Chewable
   Tablets (Bayer Consumer) **504, 802**
Flintstones Children's
   Multivitamin Plus Extra C
   Chewable Tablets (Bayer
   Consumer) **504, 804**
HeartBar (Cooke) **812**
Lipoflavonoid Caplets (Numark) **828**
One-A-Day Essential Tablets
   (Bayer Consumer).............**504, 806**
ReSource Wellness CalciWise
   Soft Chews (Novartis
   Consumer) **514, 824**
Right Choice A.M. Multi Formula
   Caplets (Body Wise) **811**
Vitamist Intra-Oral Spray (Mayor) **821**
   Anti-Oxidant (Mayor)...................*821*
   CardioCare (Mayor) *821*
   Folacin (Mayor) *821*

VITAMINS WITH IRON

Bugs Bunny Children's
   Multivitamin Plus Iron
   Chewable Tablets (Bayer
   Consumer) **504, 802**

Flintstones Children's
   Multivitamin Plus Iron
   Chewable Tablets (Bayer
   Consumer) **504, 802**

VITAMINS WITH MINERALS

BioChoice Immune Support Powder
   (Legacy for Life) **818**
BodyLean Powder (AdvoCare) **795**
Bugs Bunny Complete
   Children's Multivitamin/
   Multimineral Chewable
   Tablets (Sugar Free) (Bayer
   Consumer) **504, 803**
Centrum Focused Formulas Heart
   Tablets (Lederle Consumer) **816**
Centrum Focused Formulas Mental
   Clarity Tablets (Lederle
   Consumer) **816**
Centrum Kids Complete Children's
   Chewables (Lederle Consumer) **817**
Centrum Performance
   Multivitamin-Multimineral Tablets
   (Lederle Consumer).................**817**
Centrum Tablets (Lederle Consumer) ..**815**
Centrum Silver Tablets (Lederle
   Consumer) **818**
Flintstones Children's
   Multivitamin Plus Calcium
   Chewable Tablets (Bayer
   Consumer) **504, 804**
Flintstones Complete
   Children's Mutivitamin/
   Multimineral Chewable
   Tablets (Bayer Consumer) **504, 803**
Food for Thought Drink Mix
   (Wellness International) **844**
One-A-Day Antioxidant Softgels
   (Bayer Consumer).............**504, 805**
One-A-Day 50 Plus Tablets
   (Bayer Consumer).............**504, 804**
One-A-Day Kids Complete
   Tablets (Bayer Consumer) **505, 806**
One-A-Day Maximum Tablets
   (Bayer Consumer).............**504, 807**
One-A-Day Men's Tablets
   (Bayer Consumer).............**504, 808**
One-A-Day Women's Tablets
   (Bayer Consumer).............**504, 809**
Perfect Meal (AdvoCare)................**798**
ReSource Wellness FlexTend
   Caplets (Novartis
   Consumer) **514, 825**
ReSource Wellness ForSight
   Caplets (Novartis
   Consumer) **514, 825**
Spark! Beverage Mix (AdvoCare) **800**
StePHan Essential Capsules
   (Wellness International) **848**
StePHan Feminine Capsules
   (Wellness International) **848**
StePHan Flexibility Capsules
   (Wellness International) **848**
Vitamist Intra-Oral Spray (Mayor) **821**
   ArthriFlex (Mayor) *821*
   C+Zinc (Mayor).......................*821*
   E+Selenium (Mayor) *821*
   Multiple (Mayor) *821*
   Revitalizer (Mayor) *821*
   Slender-Mist (Mayor)..................*821*
Winrgy Drink Mix (Wellness
   International).......................**852**

W

WHEY

Biomune OSF Plus Capsules
   (Matol)......................**508, 820**
BodyLean Powder (AdvoCare) **795**

Perfect Meal (AdvoCare)...............**798**
Performance Gold Caplets
   (AdvoCare) **798**
ProForm Bars (AdvoCare) **799**
Pro-Xtreme Drink Mix (Wellness
   International).......................**845**

WITCH HAZEL

Preparation H Cooling Gel
   (Whitehall-Robins)................**778**
Preparation H Medicated Wipes
   (Whitehall-Robins)................**779**
Tucks Pre-moistened Pads
   (Pfizer Inc., Warner-Lambert
   Healthcare)..................**521, 713**

X

XYLOMETAZOLINE HYDROCHLORIDE

Natru-Vent Nasal Spray, Adult
   Strength (Boehringer
   Ingelheim) **506, 624**
Natru-Vent Nasal Spray,
   Pediatric Strength
   (Boehringer Ingelheim)........**506, 625**

Y

YOHIMBE
(see under: **PAUSINYSTALIA YOHIMBE**)

Z

ZINC

One-A-Day Prostate Health
   Softgels (Bayer Consumer) ...**505, 808**

ZINC ACETATE

Benadryl Itch Relief Stick Extra
   Strength (Pfizer Inc.,
   Warner-Lambert
   Healthcare)..................**517, 695**
Benadryl Itch Stopping Cream
   Original Strength (Pfizer
   Inc., Warner-Lambert
   Healthcare)..................**517, 695**
Benadryl Itch Stopping Cream
   Extra Strength (Pfizer Inc.,
   Warner-Lambert
   Healthcare)..................**517, 695**
Benadryl Itch Stopping Spray
   Original Strength (Pfizer
   Inc., Warner-Lambert
   Healthcare)..................**517, 696**
Benadryl Itch Stopping Spray
   Extra Strength (Pfizer Inc.,
   Warner-Lambert
   Healthcare)..................**517, 696**
Caladryl Clear Lotion (Pfizer
   Inc., Warner-Lambert
   Healthcare)..................**518, 698**

ZINC OXIDE

A + D Ointment with Zinc Oxide
   (Schering-Plough) **522, 733**
Anusol Ointment (Pfizer Inc.,
   Warner-Lambert
   Healthcare)..................**516, 688**
Balmex Diaper Rash Ointment
   (Block)......................**505, 619**
Balmex Medicated Plus Baby
   Powder (Block) **505, 619**
Desitin Baby Powder (Pfizer
   Inc., Warner-Lambert
   Healthcare)..................**518, 700**
Desitin Creamy Ointment
   (Pfizer Inc., Warner-Lambert
   Healthcare)..................**518, 700**
Desitin Ointment (Pfizer Inc.,
   Warner-Lambert
   Healthcare)..................**518, 700**

ZINC SULFATE

Visine A.C. Eye Drops (Pfizer
   Inc., Warner-Lambert
   Healthcare)..................**521, 715**

SECTION 5

COMPANION DRUG INDEX

This index provides you with a quick-reference guide to over-the-counter products that may be used, in conjunction with prescription drug therapy, to reverse drug-induced side effects, relieve symptoms of the illness itself, or treat sequelae of the initial disease. All entries are derived from the FDA-approved prescribing information published by *PDR*.

The products listed are generally considered effective for temporary symptomatic relief. Please bear in mind, however, that they may not be appropriate for sustained therapy, and that certain common side effects may be harbingers of more serious reactions. Remember, too, that each case must be approached on an individual basis. When making a recommendation, be sure to adjust for the patient's age, concurrent medical conditions, and complete drug regimen. Consider timing as well, since simultaneous ingestion may not be recommended in all instances.

Please note that only products fully described in *Physicians' Desk Reference* and its companion volumes are included in this index. The publisher therefore cannot guarantee that all entries are totally accurate or complete. Keep in mind, too, that although a given over-the-counter product is usually an appropriate companion for an entire class of prescription medications, certain drugs within the class may be exceptions. If you have any doubt about the suitability of a particular OTC product in a given situation, be sure to check the underlying *PDR* prescribing information and the relevant medical literature.

ACUTE MOUNTAIN SICKNESS, HEADACHE SECONDARY TO

Acute mountain sickness may be treated with acetazolamide. The following products may be recommended for relief of headache:

Advil Caplets 771
Advil Gel Caplets 771
Advil Liqui-Gels 771
Advil Tablets 771
Children's Advil
 Oral Suspension 773
Children's Advil Chewable
 Tablets.....................................773
Junior Strength Advil Tablets........773
Junior Strength Advil Chewable
 Tablets.....................................773
Aleve Tablets, Caplets
 and Gelcaps............................602
Alka-Seltzer Original Antacid
 and Pain Reliever
 Effervescent Tablets 603
Alka-Seltzer Cherry Antacid
 and Pain Reliever
 Effervescent Tablets 603
Alka-Seltzer
 Lemon Lime Antacid and
 Pain Reliever
 Effervescent Tablets 603
Alka-Seltzer Extra Strength
 Antacid and Pain Reliever
 Effervescent Tablets 603
Alka-Seltzer PM
 Effervescent Tablets 605
Genuine Bayer Tablets,
 Caplets and Gelcaps.................606

Extra Strength Bayer
 Caplets and Gelcaps................610
Aspirin Regimen Bayer
 Adult Low Strength
 81 mg Tablets 606
Aspirin Regimen Bayer
 Regular Strength 325 mg
 Caplets 606
Genuine Bayer
 Professional Labeling
 (Aspirin Regimen Bayer) 608
Extra Strength Bayer Arthritis
 Caplets 610
Extra Strength Bayer Plus
 Caplets 610
Extra Strength Bayer PM
 Caplets 611
Ecotrin Enteric Coated Aspirin
 Low Strength Tablets 747
Ecotrin Enteric Coated Aspirin
 Maximum Strength Tablets 747
Ecotrin Enteric Coated Aspirin
 Regular Strength Tablets 747
Aspirin Free Excedrin
 Caplets and Geltabs 628
Excedrin Extra-Strength Tablets,
 Caplets, and Geltabs 629
Excedrin PM Tablets,
 Caplets, and Geltabs 631
Goody's Body Pain Formula
 Powder....................................620
Goody's Extra Strength
 Headache Powder....................620
Goody's PM Powder 621
Momentum Backache Relief
 Extra Strength Caplets 666

Children's Motrin
 Oral Suspension and
 Chewable Tablets.....................643
Infants' Motrin
 Concentrated Drops.................643
Junior Strength Motrin
 Caplets and Chewable Tablets..643
Motrin IB Tablets,
 Caplets, and Gelcaps...............642
Orudis KT Tablets 778
Percogesic
 Aspirin-Free Coated Tablets 667
Extra Strength Percogesic
 Aspirin-Free Coated Caplets......665
Children's Tylenol Suspension
 Liquid and Soft Chews
 Chewable Tablets.....................657
Infants' Tylenol
 Concentrated Drops.................657
Junior Strength Tylenol
 Soft Chews Chewable Tablets...657
Extra Strength Tylenol
 Adult Liquid Pain Reliever.........647
Extra Strength Tylenol Gelcaps,
 Geltabs, Caplets,
 and Tablets 647
Regular Strength Tylenol
 Tablets.....................................647
Tylenol Arthritis Pain
 Extended Relief Caplets 647
Extra Strength Tylenol PM
 Caplets, Geltabs,
 and Gelcaps............................654
Maximum Strength Tylenol
 Sore Throat Adult Liquid...........656
Vanquish Caplets........................617

ALCOHOLISM, HYPOCALCEMIA SECONDARY TO

Alcoholism may be treated with disulfiram or naltrexone hydrochloride. The following products may be recommended for relief of hypocalcemia:

Caltrate 600 Tablets **814**
Caltrate 600 PLUS Chewables.....**815**
Caltrate 600 PLUS Tablets **815**
Caltrate 600 + D Tablets..............**814**
Caltrate 600 + Soy Tablets..........**814**
Citracal Liquitab Tablets **823**
Citracal Tablets............................**823**
Citracal Caplets + D....................**823**
D-Cal Chewable Caplets **794**
Extra Strength Mylanta
   Calci Tabs Tablets....................**636**
One-A-Day Calcium Plus
   Chewable Tablets.....................**805**
Os-Cal Chewable Tablets **838**
Os-Cal 250 + D Tablets...............**838**
Os-Cal 500 Tablets......................**839**
Os-Cal 500 + D Tablets...............**839**
Tums E-X Antacid/
   Calcium Tablets **763**
Tums E-X Sugar Free
   Antacid/Calcium Tablets **763**
Tums Regular Antacid/
   Calcium Tablets **763**
Tums ULTRA Antacid/
   Calcium Tablets **763**

ALCOHOLISM, HYPOMAGNESEMIA SECONDARY TO

Alcoholism may be treated with disulfiram or naltrexone hydrochloride. The following products may be recommended for relief of hypomagnesemia:

Beelith Tablets............................**809**
Magonate Liquid **814**
Magonate Natal Liquid **814**
Magonate Tablets **814**
Slow-Mag Tablets **835**

ALCOHOLISM, VITAMINS AND MINERALS DEFICIENCY SECONDARY TO

Alcoholism may be treated with disulfiram or naltrexone hydrochloride. The following products may be recommended for relief of vitamins and minerals deficiency:

Centrum Performance
   Multivitamin-Multimineral
   Tablets....................................**817**
Centrum Tablets **815**
Centrum Silver Tablets **818**
One-A-Day Essential Tablets.........**806**
One-A-Day 50 Plus Tablets...........**804**
One-A-Day Maximum Tablets **807**
One-A-Day Men's Tablets **808**
One-A-Day Women's Tablets..........**809**

ANCYLOSTOMIASIS, IRON-DEFICIENCY ANEMIA SECONDARY TO

Ancylostomiasis may be treated with mebendazole or thiabendazole. The following products may be recommended for relief of iron-deficiency anemia:

Feosol Caplets.............................**837**
Feosol Tablets **838**
Fergon Iron Tablets **802**
Slow Fe Tablets **827**
Slow Fe with Folic Acid
   Tablets....................................**828**

ANEMIA, IRON-DEFICIENCY

May result from the use of chronic salicylate therapy or nonsteroidal anti-inflammatory drugs. The following products may be recommended:

Feosol Caplets.............................**837**
Feosol Tablets **838**
Fergon Iron Tablets **802**
Slow Fe Tablets **827**
Slow Fe with Folic Acid
   Tablets....................................**828**

ANGINA, UNSTABLE

May be treated with beta blockers, calcium channel blockers or nitrates. The following products may be recommended for relief of symptoms:

Genuine Bayer
   Professional Labeling
   (Aspirin Regimen Bayer) **608**
Ecotrin Enteric Coated
   Aspirin Low Strength Tablets **747**
Ecotrin Enteric Coated Aspirin
   Maximum Strength Tablets **747**
Ecotrin Enteric Coated
   Aspirin Regular Strength
   Tablets....................................**747**

ARTHRITIS

May be treated with corticosteroids or nonsteroidal anti-inflammatory drugs. The following products may be recommended for relief of symptoms:

BenGay External Analgesic
   Products **696**
Nature's Own Pain Expeller
   Cream......................................**841**
Thera-Gesic Creme......................**667**
Vicks VapoRub Cream **730**
Vicks VapoRub Ointment **730**

BRONCHITIS, CHRONIC, ACUTE EXACERBATION OF

May be treated with quinolones, sulfamethoxazole-trimethoprim, cefixime, cefpodoxime proxetil, cefprozil, ceftibuten dihydrate, cefuroxime axetil, cilastatin, clarithromycin, imipenem or loracarbef. The following products may be recommended for relief of symptoms:

Benylin Cough Suppressant/
   Expectorant Liquid **697**
Benylin Multi-Symptom Liquid **697**
Comtrex Deep Chest Cold &
   Congestion Relief Softgels **627**
Delsym Extended-Release
   Suspension **664**

PediaCare Infants' Drops
   Decongestant Plus Cough **719**
Primatene Tablets **780**
Robitussin Liquid **782**
Robitussin Cold Caplets
   Cold & Congestion...................**780**
Robitussin Cold Softgels
   Cold & Congestion...................**780**
Robitussin Cold Caplets
   Multi-Symptom Cold & Flu **781**
Robitussin Cold Softgels
   Multi-Symptom Cold & Flu **781**
Robitussin Cold Softgels
   Severe Congestion...................**782**
Robitussin Cough & Cold
   Infant Drops.............................**782**
Robitussin Maximum Strength
   Cough & Cold Liquid **785**
Robitussin DM Infant Drops.........**783**
Robitussin-DM Liquid **783**
Robitussin-PE Liquid....................**782**
Sinutab Non-Drying
   Liquid Caps.............................**706**
Sudafed Cold & Cough
   Liquid Caps.............................**709**
Sudafed Non-Drying Sinus
   Liquid Caps.............................**712**
Triaminic Chest Congestion
   Liquid **680**
Triaminic Vapor Patch
   Cherry Scent...........................**684**
Triaminic Vapor Patch-Menthol
   Scent......................................**684**
Vicks 44E Cough & Chest
   Congestion Relief Liquid...........**725**
Pediatric Vicks 44e
   Cough & Chest Congestion
   Relief Liquid **728**
Vicks VapoRub Cream **730**
Vicks VapoRub Ointment **730**
Vicks VapoSteam **730**

BURN INFECTIONS, SEVERE, NUTRIENTS DEFICIENCY SECONDARY TO

Severe burn infections may be treated with anti-infectives. The following products may be recommended for relief of nutrients deficiency:

Bugs Bunny Children's
   Multivitamin Plus Iron
   Chewable Tablets.....................**802**
Bugs Bunny Children's
   Multivitamin Plus Extra C
   Chewable Tablets
   (Sugar Free) **804**
Bugs Bunny Complete Children's
   Multivitamin/Multimineral
   Chewable Tablets
   (Sugar Free) **803**
Centrum Kids Complete
   Children's Chewables **817**
Centrum Performance
   Multivitamin-Multimineral
   Tablets....................................**817**

Centrum Tablets **815**
Centrum Silver Tablets **818**
Flintstones Original Children's
    Multivitamin Chewable
    Tablets.................................**802**
Flintstones Children's
    Multivitamin Plus Calcium
    Chewable Tablets....................**804**
Flintstones Children's
    Multivitamin Plus Extra C
    Chewable Tablets....................**804**
Flintstones Children's
    Multivitamin Plus Iron
    Chewable Tablets....................**802**
Flintstones Complete
    Children's Mutivitamin/
    Multimineral Chewable
    Tablets.................................**803**
One-A-Day Essential Tablets........**806**
One-A-Day 50 Plus Tablets...........**804**
One-A-Day Kids Complete
    Tablets.................................**806**
One-A-Day Maximum Tablets **807**
One-A-Day Men's Tablets **808**
One-A-Day Women's Tablets........**809**
Pro-Xtreme Drink Mix...................**845**

CANCER, NUTRIENTS DEFICIENCY SECONDARY TO

Cancer may be treated with chemotherapeutic agents. The following products may be recommended for relief of nutrients deficiency:

Bugs Bunny Children's
    Multivitamin Plus Iron
    Chewable Tablets....................**802**
Bugs Bunny Children's
    Multivitamin Plus Extra C
    Chewable Tablets
    (Sugar Free) **804**
Bugs Bunny Complete Children's
    Multivitamin/Multimineral
    Chewable Tablets
    (Sugar Free) **803**
Centrum Kids Complete
    Children's Chewables **817**
Centrum Performance
    Multivitamin-Multimineral
    Tablets.................................**817**
Centrum Tablets **815**
Centrum Silver Tablets **818**
Flintstones Original Children's
    Multivitamin Chewable
    Tablets.................................**802**
Flintstones Children's
    Multivitamin Plus Calcium
    Chewable Tablets....................**804**
Flintstones Children's
    Multivitamin Plus Extra C
    Chewable Tablets....................**804**
Flintstones Children's
    Multivitamin Plus Iron
    Chewable Tablets....................**802**
Flintstones Complete Children's
    Mutivitamin/Multimineral
    Chewable Tablets....................**803**

One-A-Day Essential Tablets.........**806**
One-A-Day 50 Plus Tablets...........**804**
One-A-Day Kids Complete Tablets.**806**
One-A-Day Maximum Tablets **807**
One-A-Day Men's Tablets **808**
One-A-Day Women's Tablets.........**809**
Pro-Xtreme Drink Mix...................**845**

CANDIDIASIS, VAGINAL

May be treated with antifungal agents The following products may be recommended for relief of symptoms:

Massengill
    Feminine Cleansing Wash **753**
Massengill
    Disposable Douches................**752**
Massengill
    Baby Powder Scent
    Soft Cloth Towelette.................**753**
Massengill Medicated
    Disposable Douche..................**753**

CONGESTIVE HEART FAILURE, NUTRIENTS DEFICIENCY SECONDARY TO

Congestive heart failure may be treated with ACE inhibitors, cardiac glycosides or diuretics. The following products may be recommended for relief of nutrients deficiency:

Centrum Performance
    Multivitamin-Multimineral
    Tablets.................................**817**
Centrum Tablets **815**
Centrum Silver Tablets **818**
One-A-Day Essential Tablets.........**806**
One-A-Day 50 Plus Tablets...........**804**
One-A-Day Maximum Tablets **807**
One-A-Day Men's Tablets **808**
One-A-Day Women's Tablets.........**809**
Pro-Xtreme Drink Mix...................**845**

CONSTIPATION

May result from the use of ACE inhibitors, HMG-CoA reductase inhibitors, anticholinergics, anticonvulsants, antidepressants, beta blockers, bile acid sequestrants, butyrophenones, calcium and aluminum-containing antacids, calcium channel blockers, ganglionic blockers, hematinics, monoamine oxidase inhibitors, narcotic analgesics, nonsteroidal anti-inflammatory drugs or phenothiazines. The following products may be recommended:

Ceo-Two Evacuant Suppository **618**
Citrucel Caplets **745**
Citrucel Orange Flavor Powder **744**
Citrucel Sugar Free
    Orange Flavor Powder **745**
Colace Capsules,
    Syrup and Drops......................**743**
Correctol Laxative
    Tablets and Caplets **739**
Dulcolax Suppositories................**668**
Dulcolax Tablets..........................**668**
Ex·Lax Gentle Strength Caplets...**670**
Ex·Lax Regular Strength Pills **670**

Ex·Lax Regular Strength
    Chocolated Pieces **669**
Ex·Lax Maximum Strength Pills ...**670**
Ex·Lax Stool Softener Caplets.....**671**
FiberCon Caplets **639**
Maltsupex Powder, Liquid,
    Tablets.................................**767**
Metamucil Powder, Original
    Texture Orange Flavor...............**722**
Metamucil Powder, Original
    Texture Regular Flavor..............**722**
Metamucil Smooth Texture
    Powder, Orange Flavor..............**722**
Metamucil Smooth Texture
    Powder, Sugar-Free,
    Orange Flavor **722**
Metamucil Smooth Texture
    Powder, Sugar-Free,
    Regulár Flavor **722**
Metamucil Wafers, Apple Crisp
    & Cinnamon Spice Flavors........**722**
Mitrolan Chewable Tablets...........**789**
Nature's Remedy Tablets.............**621**
Perdiem Fiber Therapy
    Granules **675**
Perdiem Overnight Relief
    Granules **674**
Peri-Colace Capsules and Syrup...**743**
Phillips' FiberCaps Caplets **615**
Phillips' Liqui-Gels......................**616**
Purge Liquid **633**
Senokot Children's Syrup **732**
Senokot Granules **732**
Senokot Syrup **732**
Senokot Tablets...........................**732**
Senokot-S Tablets **732**
SenokotXTRA Tablets **732**
Surfak Liqui-Gels **721**

CYSTIC FIBROSIS, NUTRIENTS DEFICIENCY SECONDARY TO

Cystic fibrosis may be treated with dornase alfa. The following products may be recommended for relief of nutrients deficiency:

Centrum Performance
    Multivitamin-Multimineral
    Tablets.................................**817**
Centrum Tablets **815**
Centrum Silver Tablets **818**
One-A-Day Essential Tablets.........**806**
One-A-Day 50 Plus Tablets...........**804**
One-A-Day Kids Complete
    Tablets.................................**806**
One-A-Day Maximum Tablets **807**
One-A-Day Men's Tablets **808**
One-A-Day Women's Tablets.........**809**

DENTAL CARIES

May be treated with fluoride preparations or vitamin and fluoride supplements. The following products may be recommended for relief of symptoms:

Sensodyne Original Flavor............**623**

DENTAL CARIES —cont.

Sensodyne Cool Gel....................**623**
Sensodyne Extra Whitening..........**623**
Sensodyne Fresh Mint.................**623**
Sensodyne Tartar Control **623**
Sensodyne Tartar Control Plus
    Whitening................................**623**
Sensodyne with Baking Soda.......**623**

**DIABETES MELLITUS, CONSTIPATION
SECONDARY TO**

Diabetes mellitus may be treated with
insulins or oral hypoglycemic agents. The
following products may be recommended
for relief of constipation:

Ceo-Two Evacuant Suppository **618**
Citrucel Caplets...........................**745**
Citrucel Orange Flavor Powder **744**
Citrucel Sugar Free
    Orange Flavor Powder **745**
Colace Capsules, Syrup and
    Drops **743**
Correctol Laxative Tablets and
    Caplets **739**
Dulcolax Suppositories................**668**
Dulcolax Tablets.........................**668**
Ex·Lax Gentle Strength Caplets...**670**
Ex·Lax Regular Strength Pills **670**
Ex·Lax Regular Strength
    Chocolated Pieces **669**
Ex·Lax Maximum Strength Pills ...**670**
Ex·Lax Stool Softener Caplets.....**671**
FiberCon Caplets **639**
Maltsupex Powder, Liquid,
    Tablets....................................**767**
Metamucil Powder, Original
    Texture Orange Flavor...............**722**
Metamucil Powder, Original
    Texture Regular Flavor..............**722**
Metamucil Smooth Texture
    Powder, Orange Flavor..............**722**
Metamucil Smooth Texture
    Powder, Sugar-Free,
    Orange Flavor **722**
Metamucil Smooth Texture
    Powder, Sugar-Free,
    Flavor **722**
Metamucil Wafers, Apple Crisp
    & Cinnamon Spice Flavors........**722**
Mitrolan Chewable Tablets...........**789**
Nature's Remedy Tablets.............**621**
Perdiem Fiber Therapy Granules...**675**
Perdiem Overnight Relief
    Granules **674**
Peri-Colace Capsules and
    Syrup......................................**743**
Phillips' FiberCaps Caplets **615**
Phillips' Liqui-Gels......................**616**
Senokot Children's Syrup **732**
Senokot Granules **732**

Senokot Syrup.............................**732**
Senokot Tablets..........................**732**
Senokot-S Tablets.......................**732**
SenokotXTRA Tablets **732**
Surfak Liqui-Gels **721**

**DIABETES MELLITUS, POORLY CON-
TROLLED, CANDIDAL VULVOVAGINITIS
SECONDARY TO**

Diabetes mellitus may be treated with
insulins or oral hypoglycemic agents. The
following products may be recommended
for relief of candidal vulvovaginitis:

Gyne-Lotrimin 3, 3-Day Cream......**741**
Mycelex-3 Vaginal Cream with
    3 Disposable Applicators **613**
Mycelex-3 Vaginal Cream in
    3 Pre-filled Applicators **613**
Mycelex-7 Combination-Pack
    Vaginal Inserts &
    External Vulvar Cream..............**614**
Mycelex-7 Vaginal Cream............**614**
Mycelex-7 Vaginal Cream with
    7 Disposable Applicators **614**

**DIABETES MELLITUS, POORLY CON-
TROLLED, GINGIVITIS SECONDARY TO**

Diabetes mellitus may be treated with
insulins or oral hypoglycemic agents. The
following products may be recommended
for relief of gingivitis:

Listerine Mouthrinse **702**
Cool Mint Listerine Mouthrinse **702**
FreshBurst Listerine Mouthrinse ..**702**
Tartar Control Listerine
    Mouthrinse..............................**702**
Sensodyne Original Flavor............**623**
Sensodyne Cool Gel....................**623**
Sensodyne Extra Whitening..........**623**
Sensodyne Fresh Mint.................**623**
Sensodyne Tartar Control **623**
Sensodyne Tartar Control Plus
    Whitening................................**623**
Sensodyne with Baking Soda.......**623**

**DIABETES MELLITUS, POORLY CON-
TROLLED, VITAMINS AND MINERALS
DEFICIENCY SECONDARY TO**

Diabetes mellitus may be treated with
insulins or oral hypoglycemic agents. The
following products may be recommended
for relief of vitamins and minerals deficiency:

Centrum Performance
    Multivitamin-Multimineral
    Tablets....................................**817**
Centrum Tablets **815**
Centrum Silver Tablets **818**
One-A-Day Essential Tablets........**806**
One-A-Day 50 Plus Tablets..........**804**
One-A-Day Kids Complete
    Tablets....................................**806**
One-A-Day Maximum Tablets **807**
One-A-Day Men's Tablets **808**
One-A-Day Women's Tablets........**809**

**DIABETES MELLITUS, PRURITUS
SECONDARY TO**

Diabetes mellitus may be treated with
insulins or oral hypoglycemic agents. The
following products may be recommended
for relief of pruritus:

Lubriderm Advanced Therapy
    Creamy Lotion **703**
Lubriderm Seriously Sensitive
    Lotion **703**
Lubriderm Skin Therapy
    Moisturizing Lotion...................**703**
StePHan Bio-Nutritional
    Daytime Hydrating Creme **770**
StePHan Bio-Nutritional
    Nightime Moisture Creme..........**770**
StePHan Bio-Nutritional
    Ultra Hydrating Fluid.................**770**

DIAPER DERMATITIS

May result from the use of cefpodoxime
proxetil, cefprozil, cefuroxime axetil or
varicella virus vaccine, live. The following
products may be recommended:

A + D Original Ointment...............**733**
A + D Ointment with Zinc Oxide ...**733**
Balmex Diaper Rash Ointment **619**
Balmex Medicated Plus
    Baby Powder **619**
Desitin Baby Powder **700**
Desitin Creamy Ointment.............**700**
Desitin Ointment.........................**700**

DIARRHEA

May result from the use of ACE
inhibitors, beta blockers, cardiac glycosides, chemotherapeutic agents, diuretics, magnesium-containing antacids, nonsteroidal anti-inflammatory drugs, potassium supplements, acarbose, alprazolam, colchicine, divalproex sodium, etho-
suximide, fluoxetine hydrochloride,
guanethidine monosulfate, hydralazine
hydrochloride, levodopa, lithium carbonate, lithium citrate, mesna, metformin
hydrochloride, misoprostol, olsalazine
sodium, pancrelipase, procainamide
hydrochloride, reserpine, succimer,
ticlopidine hydrochloride or valproic acid.
The following products may be
recommended:

Donnagel Liquid..........................**789**
Imodium A-D Liquid and
    Caplets **641**
Imodium Advanced Chewable
    Tablets....................................**641**
Pepto-Bismol Original Liquid,
    Original and Cherry
    Chewable Tablets & Caplets **723**
Pepto-Bismol Maximum
    Strength Liquid.........................**724**

DIARRHEA, INFECTIOUS

May be treated with sulfamethoxazole-trimethoprim, ciprofloxacin or furazolidone. The following products may be recommended for relief of symptoms:

Donnagel Liquid **789**

Imodium A-D Liquid and
Caplets **641**

Imodium Advanced Chewable
Tablets **641**

Pepto-Bismol Original Liquid,
Original and Cherry
Chewable Tablets & Caplets **723**

Pepto-Bismol Maximum Strength
Liquid **724**

DYSPEPSIA

May result from the use of chronic systemic corticosteroid therapy, nonsteroidal anti-inflammatory drugs, ulcerogenic medications or mexiletine hydrochloride. The following products may be recommended:

Alka-Seltzer Heartburn Relief
Tablets **604**

Amphojel Suspension
(Mint Flavor) **789**

Ex · Lax Milk of Magnesia
Liquid **670**

Gaviscon Extra Strength
Liquid **751**

Gaviscon Extra Strength
Tablets **751**

Gaviscon Regular Strength
Liquid **751**

Maalox Antacid/Anti-Gas Oral
Suspension **673**

Maalox Max Maximum Strength
Antacid/Anti-Gas Liquid **673**

Quick Dissolve Maalox Antacid
Chewable Tablets **674**

Quick Dissolve Maalox Max
Maximum Strength
Antacid/Antigas
Chewable Tablets **674**

Marblen Suspension **633**

Mylanta Gelcaps **637**

Mylanta Liquid **634**

Mylanta Extra Strength Liquid **634**

Mylanta Supreme Liquid **636**

Mylanta Ultra Tabs Tablets **637**

Extra Strength Mylanta
Calci Tabs Tablets **636**

Phillips' Chewable Tablets **615**

Phillips' Milk of Magnesia Liquid
(Original, Cherry, & Mint).......... **616**

Rolaids Tablets **706**

Extra Strength Rolaids Tablets **706**

3M Titralac Antacid Tablets **640**

3M Titralac Extra Strength
Antacid Tablets **640**

3M Titralac Plus Antacid
Tablets **640**

Tums E-X Antacid/Calcium
Tablets **763**

Tums E-X Sugar Free
Antacid/Calcium Tablets **763**

Tums Regular Antacid/
Calcium Tablets **763**

Tums ULTRA Antacid/
Calcium Tablets **763**

EMESIS, UNPLEASANT TASTE SECONDARY TO

Emesis may be treated with antiemetics. The following products may be recommended for relief of unpleasant taste:

Cēpacol Antiseptic
Mouthwash/Gargle, Original **786**

Cēpacol Antiseptic
Mouthwash/Gargle, Mint.......... **786**

Certs Cool Mint Drops **685**

Certs Powerful Mints **686**

Listerine Mouthrinse **702**

Cool Mint Listerine
Mouthrinse **702**

FreshBurst Listerine
Mouthrinse **702**

Tartar Control Listerine
Mouthrinse **702**

Listermint Alcohol-Free
Mouthrinse **703**

Trident Advantage Mints **687**

Trident Advantage
Sugarless Gum......................... **687**

ENTEROBIASIS, PERIANAL PRURITUS SECONDARY TO

Enterobiasis may be treated with mebendazole. The following products may be recommended for relief of perianal pruritus:

Anusol HC-1 Hydrocortisone
Anti-Itch Cream **689**

Benadryl Itch Relief Stick
Extra Strength **695**

Cortaid Intensive Therapy
Cream...................................... **717**

Cortaid Maximum Strength
Cream...................................... **717**

Cortaid Maximum Strength
Ointment.................................. **717**

Cortaid Sensitive Skin Cream **717**

Cortizone · 5 Creme..................... **699**

Cortizone · 5 Ointment **699**

Cortizone · 10 Creme................... **699**

Cortizone · 10 Ointment **699**

Cortizone · 10 Plus Creme **700**

Cortizone for Kids Creme **699**

Massengill Medicated Soft
Cloth Towelette **753**

FEVER

May result from the use of immunization. The following products may be recommended:

Advil Caplets **771**

Advil Gel Caplets **771**

Advil Liqui-Gels **771**

Advil Tablets **771**

Children's Advil
Oral Suspension **773**

Children's Advil
Chewable Tablets..................... **773**

Junior Strength Advil
Tablets.................................... **773**

Junior Strength Advil
Chewable Tablets..................... **773**

Aleve Tablets, Caplets and
Gelcaps **602**

Alka-Seltzer PM
Effervescent Tablets **605**

Genuine Bayer Tablets,
Caplets and Gelcaps................ **606**

Extra Strength Bayer
Caplets and Gelcaps................ **610**

Aspirin Regimen Bayer
Adult Low Strength
81 mg Tablets **606**

Aspirin Regimen Bayer
Regular Strength
325 mg Caplets **606**

Genuine Bayer
Professional Labeling
(Aspirin Regimen Bayer) **608**

Extra Strength Bayer Arthritis
Caplets **610**

Extra Strength Bayer Plus
Caplets **610**

Extra Strength Bayer PM
Caplets **611**

BC Powder **619**

BC Allergy Sinus Cold Powder **619**

Arthritis Strength BC Powder **619**

BC Sinus Cold Powder................. **619**

Ecotrin Enteric Coated
Aspirin Low Strength Tablets **747**

Ecotrin Enteric Coated
Aspirin Maximum Strength
Tablets.................................... **747**

Ecotrin Enteric Coated
Aspirin Regular Strength
Tablets.................................... **747**

Aspirin Free Excedrin Caplets
and Geltabs **628**

Excedrin Extra-Strength Tablets,
Caplets, and Geltabs **629**

Excedrin PM Tablets,
Caplets, and Geltabs **631**

Goody's Body Pain Formula
Powder.................................... **620**

Goody's Extra Strength
Headache Powder..................... **620**

Goody's Extra Strength
Pain Relief Tablets **620**

Goody's PM Powder **621**

Momentum Backache Relief
Extra Strength Caplets **666**

Children's Motrin
Oral Suspension and
Chewable Tablets..................... **643**

Infants' Motrin Concentrated
Drops **643**

Fever —cont.

Junior Strength Motrin Caplets
and Chewable Tablets 643

Motrin IB Tablets, Caplets, and
Gelcaps 642

Orudis KT Tablets 778

Percogesic Aspirin-Free Coated
Tablets...667

Extra Strength Percogesic
Aspirin-Free Coated Caplets......665

Children's Tylenol Suspension
Liquid and Soft Chews
Chewable Tablets.......................657

Infants' Tylenol Concentrated
Drops 657

Junior Strength Tylenol
Soft Chews Chewable Tablets...657

Extra Strength Tylenol Adult
Liquid Pain Reliever 647

Extra Strength Tylenol
Gelcaps, Geltabs, Caplets,
and Tablets 647

Regular Strength Tylenol
Tablets...647

Tylenol Arthritis Pain
Extended Relief Caplets 647

Extra Strength Tylenol PM
Caplets, Geltabs, and
Gelcaps 654

Maximum Strength Tylenol
Sore Throat Adult Liquid...........656

Vanquish Caplets.........................617

FLATULENCE

May result from the use of nonsteroidal anti-inflammatory drugs, potassium supplements, acarbose, cisapride, guanadrel sulfate, mesalamine, metformin hydrochloride, methyldopa, octreotide acetate or ursodiol. The following products may be recommended:

Beano Liquid 809

Beano Tablets...............................809

Maximum Strength Gas Aid
Softgels 640

Gas-X Chewable Tablets 671

Extra Strength Gas-X Liquid 671

Extra Strength Gas-X Softgels 671

Extra Strength Gas-X
Chewable Tablets.......................671

Maximum Strength Gas-X
Softgels 671

Mylanta Gas Softgels 637

Mylanta Gas Tablets.....................637

Maximum Strength Mylanta
Gas Tablets.................................637

Infants' Mylicon Drops 634

Phazyme-125 mg Quick
Dissolve Chewable Tablets 622

Phazyme-180 mg
Ultra Strength Softgels..............622

FLU-LIKE SYNDROME

May result from the use of gemcitabine hydrochloride, interferon alfa-2B, recombinant, interferon alfa-N3 (human leukocyte derived), interferon beta-1B, interferon gamma-1B or succimer. The following products may be recommended:

Advil Caplets 771

Advil Gel Caplets 771

Advil Liqui-Gels 771

Advil Tablets 771

Children's Advil
Oral Suspension 773

Children's Advil
Chewable Tablets.....................773

Junior Strength Advil Tablets........773

Junior Strength Advil
Chewable Tablets.....................773

Aleve Tablets, Caplets
and Gelcaps.............................602

Alka-Seltzer Original Antacid
and Pain Reliever
Effervescent Tablets 603

Alka-Seltzer Cherry Antacid
and Pain Reliever
Effervescent Tablets 603

Alka-Seltzer Lemon Lime
Antacid and Pain Reliever
Effervescent Tablets 603

Alka-Seltzer Extra Strength
Antacid and Pain Reliever
Effervescent Tablets 603

Alka-Seltzer PM
Effervescent Tablets 605

Genuine Bayer Tablets,
Caplets and Gelcaps................606

Extra Strength Bayer
Caplets and Gelcaps................610

Aspirin Regimen Bayer
Adult Low Strength
81 mg Tablets 606

Aspirin Regimen Bayer
Regular Strength
325 mg Caplets 606

Genuine Bayer
Professional Labeling
(Aspirin Regimen Bayer) 608

Extra Strength Bayer
Arthritis Caplets 610

Extra Strength Bayer Plus
Caplets 610

Extra Strength Bayer PM
Caplets 611

BC Powder 619

BC Allergy Sinus Cold Powder 619

Arthritis Strength BC Powder 619

BC Sinus Cold Powder.................619

Ecotrin Enteric Coated
Aspirin Low Strength Tablets 747

Ecotrin Enteric Coated
Aspirin Maximum Strength
Tablets..747

Ecotrin Enteric Coated
Aspirin Regular Strength
Tablets..747

Aspirin Free Excedrin
Caplets and Geltabs 628

Excedrin Extra-Strength Tablets,
Caplets, and Geltabs 629

Excedrin PM Tablets,
Caplets, and Geltabs 631

Goody's Body Pain Formula
Powder.......................................620

Goody's Extra Strength
Headache Powder....................620

Goody's Extra Strength
Pain Relief Tablets 620

Goody's PM Powder 621

Momentum Backache Relief
Extra Strength Caplets 666

Children's Motrin
Oral Suspension and
Chewable Tablets.....................643

Infants' Motrin
Concentrated Drops.................643

Junior Strength Motrin
Caplets and Chewable Tablets..643

Motrin IB Tablets,
Caplets, and Gelcaps...............642

Orudis KT Tablets 778

Oscillococcinum Pellets...............625

Percogesic Aspirin-Free
Coated Tablets 667

Extra Strength Percogesic
Aspirin-Free Coated Caplets......665

Children's Tylenol Suspension
Liquid and Soft Chews
Chewable Tablets.....................657

Infants' Tylenol
Concentrated Drops.................657

Junior Strength Tylenol
Soft Chews Chewable Tablets...657

Extra Strength Tylenol
Adult Liquid Pain Reliever.........647

Extra Strength Tylenol
Gelcaps, Geltabs,
Caplets, and Tablets 647

Regular Strength Tylenol
Tablets...647

Tylenol Arthritis Pain
Extended Relief Caplets 647

Extra Strength Tylenol PM
Caplets, Geltabs, and Gelcaps .654

Maximum Strength Tylenol
Sore Throat Adult Liquid...........656

Vanquish Caplets.........................617

FLUSHING EPISODES

May result from the use of lipid lowering doses of niacin. The following products may be recommended:

Advil Caplets 771

Advil Gel Caplets 771

Advil Liqui-Gels 771

Advil Tablets 771

Alka-Seltzer PM
Effervescent Tablets 605

Genuine Bayer Tablets,
    Caplets and Gelcaps.................**606**
Extra Strength Bayer
    Caplets and Gelcaps................**610**
Aspirin Regimen Bayer Children's
    Chewable Tablets
    (Orange or Cherry Flavored)......**607**
Aspirin Regimen Bayer Adult
    Low Strength
    81 mg Tablets **606**
Aspirin Regimen Bayer
    Regular Strength
    325 mg Caplets **606**
Extra Strength Bayer Arthritis
    Caplets **610**
Ecotrin Enteric Coated Aspirin
    Low Strength Tablets **747**
Ecotrin Enteric Coated Aspirin
    Maximum Strength Tablets **747**
Ecotrin Enteric Coated Aspirin
    Regular Strength Tablets **747**
Motrin IB Tablets, Caplets, and
    Gelcaps **642**

GASTRITIS, IRON-DEFICIENCY SECONDARY TO

Gastritis may be treated with histamine H_2 receptor antagonists, proton pump inhibitors or sucralfate. The following products may be recommended for relief of iron deficiency:

Feosol Caplets...........................**837**
Feosol Tablets **838**
Fergon Iron Tablets **802**
Slow Fe Tablets **827**
Slow Fe with Folic Acid Tablets.....**828**

GASTROESOPHAGEAL REFLUX DISEASE

May be treated with histamine H_2 antagonists, proton pump inhibitors or sucralfate. The following products may be recommended for relief of symptoms:

Alka-Seltzer Heartburn Relief
    Tablets...................................**604**
Amphojel Suspension
    (Mint Flavor)...........................**789**
Ex·Lax Milk of Magnesia Liquid ...**670**
Gaviscon Extra Strength Liquid **751**
Gaviscon Extra Strength
    Tablets...................................**751**
Gaviscon Regular Strength
    Liquid **751**
Maalox Antacid/Anti-Gas Oral
    Suspension **673**
Maalox Max Maximum Strength
    Antacid/Anti-Gas Liquid............**673**
Quick Dissolve Maalox Antacid
    Chewable Tablets.....................**674**
Quick Dissolve Maalox Max
    Maximum Strength
    Antacid/Antigas
    Chewable Tablets.....................**674**
Marblen Suspension **633**
Mylanta Gelcaps **637**
Mylanta Liquid **634**
Mylanta Extra Strength Liquid **634**
Mylanta Supreme Liquid..............**636**
Mylanta Ultra Tabs Tablets...........**637**
Extra Strength Mylanta
    Calci Tabs Tablets....................**636**
Pepto-Bismol Original Liquid,
    Original and Cherry
    Chewable Tablets & Caplets **723**
Pepto-Bismol
    Maximum Strength Liquid.........**724**
Phillips' Chewable Tablets **615**
Phillips' Milk of Magnesia
    Liquid (Original, Cherry,
    & Mint) **616**
Rolaids Tablets...........................**706**
Extra Strength Rolaids Tablets **706**
3M Titralac Antacid Tablets **640**
3M Titralac Extra Strength
    Antacid Tablets.......................**640**
3M Titralac Plus Antacid
    Tablets...................................**640**
Tums E-X Antacid/Calcium
    Tablets...................................**763**
Tums E-X Sugar Free
    Antacid/Calcium Tablets **763**
Tums Regular Antacid/Calcium
    Tablets...................................**763**
Tums ULTRA Antacid/Calcium
    Tablets...................................**763**

GINGIVAL HYPERPLASIA

May result from the use of calcium channel blockers, cyclosporine, fosphenytoin sodium or phenytoin. The following products may be recommended:

Listerine Mouthrinse **702**
Cool Mint Listerine Mouthrinse **702**
FreshBurst Listerine Mouthrinse ..**702**
Tartar Control Listerine
    Mouthrinse..............................**702**
Sensodyne Original Flavor............**623**
Sensodyne Cool Gel....................**623**
Sensodyne Extra Whitening..........**623**
Sensodyne Fresh Mint.................**623**
Sensodyne Tartar Control **623**
Sensodyne Tartar Control Plus
    Whitening................................**623**
Sensodyne with Baking Soda.......**623**

HUMAN IMMUNODEFICIENCY VIRUS (HIV) INFECTIONS, NUTRIENTS DEFICIENCY SECONDARY TO

HIV infections may be treated with non-nucleoside reverse transcriptase inhibitors, nucleoside reverse transcriptase inhibitors or protease inhibitors. The following products may be recommended for relief of nutrients deficiency:

Bugs Bunny Children's
    Multivitamin Plus Iron
    Chewable Tablets.....................**802**
Bugs Bunny Children's
    Multivitamin Plus Extra C
    Chewable Tablets
    (Sugar Free) **804**
Bugs Bunny Complete
    Children's Multivitamin/
    Multimineral Chewable
    Tablets (Sugar Free).................**803**
Centrum Kids Complete
    Children's Chewables **817**
Centrum Performance
    Multivitamin-Multimineral
    Tablets...................................**817**
Centrum Tablets **815**
Centrum Silver Tablets **818**
Flintstones Original Children's
    Multivitamin Chewable
    Tablets...................................**802**
Flintstones Children's
    Multivitamin Plus Calcium
    Chewable Tablets.....................**804**
Flintstones Children's
    Multivitamin Plus Extra C
    Chewable Tablets.....................**804**
Flintstones Children's
    Multivitamin Plus Iron
    Chewable Tablets.....................**802**
Flintstones Complete Children's
    Mutivitamin/Multimineral
    Chewable Tablets.....................**803**
One-A-Day Essential Tablets.........**806**
One-A-Day 50 Plus Tablets...........**804**
One-A-Day Kids Complete
    Tablets...................................**806**
One-A-Day Maximum Tablets **807**
One-A-Day Men's Tablets **808**
One-A-Day Women's Tablets.........**809**
Pro-Xtreme Drink Mix...................**845**

HUMAN IMMUNODEFICIENCY VIRUS (HIV) INFECTIONS, SEBORRHEIC DERMATITIS SECONDARY TO

HIV infections may be treated with non-nucleoside reverse transcriptase inhibitors, nucleoside reverse transcriptase inhibitors or protease inhibitors. The following products may be recommended for relief of seborrheic dermatitis:

Cortaid Intensive Therapy
    Cream.....................................**717**
Cortaid Maximum Strength
    Cream.....................................**717**
Cortaid Maximum Strength
    Ointment.................................**717**
Cortaid Sensitive Skin Cream **717**
Nizoral A-D Shampoo...................**647**
Tegrin Dandruff Shampoo -
    Extra Conditioning...................**623**
Tegrin Dandruff Shampoo -
    Fresh Herbal **624**
Tegrin Skin Cream......................**624**

HUMAN IMMUNODEFICIENCY VIRUS (HIV) INFECTIONS, XERODERMA SECONDARY TO

HIV infections may be treated with non-nucleoside reverse transcriptase inhibitors, nucleoside reverse transcriptase inhibitors or protease inhibitors. The following products may be recommended for relief of xeroderma:

Lubriderm Advanced Therapy
Creamy Lotion **703**
Lubriderm Seriously Sensitive
Lotion **703**
Lubriderm Skin Therapy
Moisturizing Lotion...................**703**
StePHan Bio-Nutritional
Daytime Hydrating Creme **770**
StePHan Bio-Nutritional
Nightime Moisture Creme.........**770**
StePHan Bio-Nutritional
Ultra Hydrating Fluid.................**770**

HYPERTHYROIDISM, NUTRIENTS DEFICIENCY SECONDARY TO

Hyperthyroidism may be treated with methimazole. The following products may be recommended for relief of nutrients deficiency:

Bugs Bunny Children's
Multivitamin Plus Iron
Chewable Tablets.....................**802**
Bugs Bunny Children's
Multivitamin Plus Extra C
Chewable Tablets
(Sugar Free) **804**
Bugs Bunny Complete Children's
Multivitamin/Multimineral
Chewable Tablets
(Sugar Free) **803**
Centrum Kids Complete
Children's Chewables **817**
Centrum Performance
Multivitamin-Multimineral
Tablets.....................................**817**
Centrum Tablets **815**
Centrum Silver Tablets **818**
Flintstones Original Children's
Multivitamin Chewable
Tablets.....................................**802**
Flintstones Children's
Multivitamin Plus Calcium
Chewable Tablets.....................**804**
Flintstones Children's
Multivitamin Plus Extra C
Chewable Tablets.....................**804**
Flintstones Children's
Multivitamin Plus Iron
Chewable Tablets.....................**802**
Flintstones Complete Children's
Mutivitamin/Multimineral
Chewable Tablets.....................**803**
One-A-Day Essential Tablets.........**806**
One-A-Day 50 Plus Tablets...........**804**
One-A-Day Maximum Tablets **807**
One-A-Day Men's Tablets **808**
One-A-Day Women's Tablets.........**809**
Pro-Xtreme Drink Mix...................**845**

HYPOKALEMIA

May result from the use of thiazides, thiazides, corticosteroids, diuretics, diuretics, aldesleukin, amphotericin B, carboplatin, etretinate, foscarnet sodium, mycophenolate mofetil, pamidronate disodium or tacrolimus. The following products may be recommended:

Chlor-3 Shaker.............................**633**

HYPOMAGNESEMIA

May result from the use of aldesleukin, aminoglycosides, amphotericin B, caroboplatin, cisplatin, cyclosporine, diuretics, foscarnet, pamidronate, sargramostim or tacrolimus. The following products may be recommended:

Beelith Tablets............................**809**
Chlor-3 Shaker............................**633**
Magonate Liquid **814**
Magonate Natal Liquid **814**
Magonate Tablets **814**
Slow-Mag Tablets **835**

HYPOPARATHYROIDISM

May be treated with vitamin D sterols. The following products may be recommended for relief of symptoms:

Caltrate 600 Tablets **814**
Caltrate 600 PLUS Chewables.....**815**
Caltrate 600 PLUS Tablets **815**
Caltrate 600 + D Tablets.............**814**
Caltrate 600 + Soy Tablets..........**814**
Citracal Liquitab Tablets **823**
Citracal Tablets............................**823**
Citracal Caplets + D....................**823**
D-Cal Chewable Caplets **794**
Extra Strength Mylanta
Calci Tabs Tablets....................**636**
One-A-Day Calcium Plus
Chewable Tablets.....................**805**
Os-Cal Chewable Tablets **838**
Os-Cal 250 + D Tablets...............**838**
Os-Cal 500 Tablets **839**
Os-Cal 500 + D Tablets...............**839**
Tums E-X Antacid/Calcium
Tablets.....................................**763**
Tums E-X Sugar Free
Antacid/Calcium Tablets **763**
Tums Regular Antacid/Calcium
Tablets.....................................**763**
Tums ULTRA Antacid/Calcium
Tablets.....................................**763**

HYPOTHYROIDISM, CONSTIPATION SECONDARY TO

Hypothyroidism may be treated with thyroid hormones. The following products may be recommended for relief of constipation:

Ceo-Two Evacuant Suppository **618**
Citrucel Caplets **745**
Citrucel Orange Flavor Powder **744**
Citrucel Sugar Free
Orange Flavor Powder **745**
Colace Capsules, Syrup
and Drops **743**
Correctol Laxative Tablets
and Caplets **739**
Dulcolax Suppositories................**668**
Dulcolax Tablets..........................**668**
Ex·Lax Gentle Strength Caplets...**670**
Ex·Lax Regular Strength Pills **670**
Ex·Lax Regular Strength
Chocolated Pieces **669**
Ex·Lax Maximum Strength Pills ...**670**
Ex·Lax Stool Softener Caplets.....**671**
FiberCon Caplets **639**
Maltsupex Powder, Liquid,
Tablets.....................................**767**
Metamucil Powder, Original
Texture Orange Flavor.................**722**
Metamucil Powder, Original
Texture Regular Flavor...............**722**
Metamucil Smooth Texture
Powder, Orange Flavor...............**722**
Metamucil Smooth Texture
Powder, Sugar-Free,
Orange Flavor **722**
Metamucil Smooth Texture
Powder, Sugar-Free,
Regular Flavor **722**
Metamucil Wafers,
Apple Crisp &
Cinnamon Spice Flavors...........**722**
Mitrolan Chewable Tablets...........**789**
Nature's Remedy Tablets **621**
Perdiem Fiber Therapy Granules...**675**
Perdiem Overnight Relief
Granules **674**
Peri-Colace Capsules and Syrup...**743**
Phillips' FiberCaps Caplets **615**
Phillips' Liqui-Gels......................**616**
Purge Liquid **633**
Senokot Children's Syrup **732**
Senokot Granules **732**
Senokot Syrup.............................**732**
Senokot Tablets...........................**732**
Senokot-S Tablets **732**
SenokotXTRA Tablets **732**
Surfak Liqui-Gels **721**

HYPOTHYROIDISM, XERODERMA SECONDARY TO

Hypothyroidism may be treated with thyroid hormones. The following products may be recommended for relief of xeroderma:

Lubriderm Advanced Therapy
Creamy Lotion **703**
Lubriderm Seriously Sensitive
Lotion **703**
Lubriderm Skin Therapy
Moisturizing Lotion...................**703**

StePHan Bio-Nutritional
Daytime Hydrating Creme **770**
StePHan Bio-Nutritional
Nightime Moisture Creme.........**770**
StePHan Bio-Nutritional Ultra
Hydrating Fluid.........................**770**

INFECTIONS, BACTERIAL, UPPER RESPIRATORY TRACT

May be treated with amoxicillin-clavulanate, cephalosporins, doxycycline, erythromycin, macrolide antibiotics, penicillins, amoxicillin trihydrate or minocycline hydrochloride. The following products may be recommended for relief of symptoms:

Actifed Cold & Allergy Tablets **688**
Actifed Cold & Sinus
Caplets and Tablets **688**
Advil Caplets **771**
Advil Gel Caplets **771**
Advil Liqui-Gels **771**
Advil Tablets **771**
Children's Advil
Oral Suspension **773**
Children's Advil
Chewable Tablets.....................**773**
Advil Cold and Sinus Caplets **771**
Advil Cold and Sinus Tablets........**771**
Advil Flu & Body Ache Caplets **772**
Infants' Advil Drops.....................**773**
Junior Strength Advil Tablets........**773**
Junior Strength Advil Chewable
Tablets...................................**773**
Afrin Nasal Decongestant
Children's Pump Mist...............**734**
Afrin Original Nasal Spray **733**
Afrin Extra Moisturizing
Nasal Spray **733**
Afrin Severe Congestion
Nasal Spray **733**
Afrin Sinus Nasal Spray...............**733**
Afrin No Drip Original
Nasal Spray **735**
Afrin No Drip Extra Moisturizing
Nasal Spray **735**
Afrin No Drip Severe Congestion
Nasal Spray **735**
Afrin No Drip Sinus Nasal Spray...**735**
Afrin Original Pump Mist..............**733**
Afrin Saline Aromatic Mist **734**
Aleve Tablets, Caplets
and Gelcaps...........................**602**
Aleve Cold & Sinus Caplets **603**
Alka-Seltzer Original Antacid
and Pain Reliever
Effervescent Tablets **603**
Alka-Seltzer Cherry Antacid
and Pain Reliever
Effervescent Tablets **603**
Alka-Seltzer Lemon Lime
Antacid and Pain Reliever
Effervescent Tablets **603**

Alka-Seltzer Extra Strength
Antacid and Pain Reliever
Effervescent Tablets **603**
Alka-Seltzer Plus Cold Medicine
Liqui-Gels..............................**604**
Alka-Seltzer Plus Night-Time
Cold Medicine Liqui-Gels **604**
Alka-Seltzer Plus Cold & Cough
Medicine Liqui-Gels.................**604**
Alka-Seltzer Plus Cold & Flu
Medicine Liqui-Gels..................**604**
Alka-Seltzer Plus Cold & Sinus
Medicine Liqui-Gels..................**604**
Alka-Seltzer PM
Effervescent Tablets **605**
Genuine Bayer Tablets,
Caplets and Gelcaps.................**606**
Extra Strength Bayer
Caplets and Gelcaps.................**610**
Aspirin Regimen Bayer Adult
Low Strength
81 mg Tablets **606**
Aspirin Regimen Bayer Regular
Strength 325 mg Caplets **606**
Genuine Bayer
Professional Labeling
(Aspirin Regimen Bayer) **608**
Extra Strength Bayer Arthritis
Caplets **610**
Extra Strength Bayer Plus
Caplets **610**
Extra Strength Bayer PM
Caplets **611**
BC Powder **619**
BC Allergy Sinus Cold Powder **619**
Arthritis Strength BC Powder **619**
BC Sinus Cold Powder.................**619**
Benadryl Allergy Chewables **689**
Benadryl Allergy Kapseal
Capsules................................**691**
Benadryl Allergy Liquid **690**
Benadryl Allergy Ultratab
Tablets...................................**691**
Benadryl Allergy/Cold Tablets **691**
Benadryl Allergy/Congestion
Tablets...................................**692**
Benadryl Allergy & Sinus Liquid ...**693**
Benadryl Allergy & Sinus
Fastmelt Tablets **693**
Benadryl Allergy Sinus
Headache Caplets & Gelcaps ...**693**
Benadryl Severe Allergy &
Sinus Headache Caplets..........**694**
Benadryl Children's Allergy/
Cold Fastmelt Tablets **692**
Benadryl Dye-Free Allergy Liquid ..**690**
Benadryl Dye-Free Allergy
Liqui-Gels Softgels...................**690**
Benylin Adult Formula Cough
Suppressant Liquid..................**696**
Benylin Cough
Suppressant/Expectorant
Liquid **697**
Benylin Multi-Symptom Liquid **697**

Benylin Pediatric Cough
Suppressant Liquid..................**698**
Celestial Seasonings Soothers
Throat Drops **685**
Children's Cēpacol Sore
Throat Formula,
Cherry Flavor Liquid **788**
Children's Cēpacol Sore Throat
Formula, Grape Flavor Liquid **788**
Cēpacol Maximum Strength
Sugar Free Sore Throat
Lozenges, Cherry Flavor **787**
Cēpacol Maximum Strength
Sugar Free Sore Throat
Lozenges, Cool Mint Flavor.......**787**
Cēpacol Maximum Strength
Sore Throat Lozenges,
Cherry Flavor...........................**787**
Cēpacol Maximum Strength
Sore Throat Lozenges,
Mint Flavor **787**
Cēpacol Regular Strength
Sore Throat Lozenges,
Cherry Flavor...........................**787**
Cēpacol Regular Strength
Sore Throat Lozenges,
Original Mint Flavor **787**
Cēpacol Maximum Strength
Sore Throat Spray,
Cherry Flavor...........................**787**
Cēpacol Maximum Strength
Sore Throat Spray,
Cool Menthol Flavor **787**
Cēpacol Maximum Strength
Sore Throat Spray,
Honey Lemon Flavor.................**787**
Chlor-Trimeton Allergy Tablets **735**
Chlor-Trimeton Allergy/
Decongestant Tablets **736**
Comtrex Acute Head Cold &
Sinus Pressure Relief Tablets ...**627**
Comtrex Deep Chest
Cold & Congestion Relief
Softgels **627**
Comtrex Flu Therapy & Fever
Relief Daytime Caplets.............**628**
Comtrex Flu Therapy & Fever
Relief Nighttime Tablets **628**
Comtrex Maximum Strength
Multi-Symptom Cold &
Cough Relief Tablets and
Caplets **626**
Contac Non-Drowsy 12 Hour
Cold Caplets **745**
Contac Non-Drowsy Timed
Release 12 Hour Cold
Caplets **746**
Contac Severe Cold and Flu
Caplets Maximum Strength **746**
Contac Severe Cold and Flu
Caplets Non-Drowsy.................**746**
Coricidin 'D' Cold, Flu & Sinus
Tablets...................................**737**

**INFECTIONS, BACTERIAL, UPPER RES-
PIRATORY TRACT —cont.**

Coricidin HBP Cold & Flu
Tablets....................................**738**
Coricidin HBP Cough & Cold
Tablets....................................**738**
Coricidin HBP Maximum
Strength Flu Tablets.................**738**
Coricidin HBP Night-Time
Cold & Flu Tablets **738**
Delsym Extended-Release
Suspension.............................**664**
Dimetapp Elixir **777**
Dimetapp Cold and Fever
Suspension.............................**775**
Dimetapp DM Cold & Cough
Elixir **775**
Dimetapp Nighttime Flu Liquid **776**
Dimetapp Non-Drowsy Flu Syrup ..**777**
Dimetapp Infant Drops
Decongestant...........................**775**
Dimetapp Infant Drops
Decongestant Plus Cough **776**
Drixoral Allergy/Sinus
Extended-Release Tablets..........**741**
Drixoral Cold & Allergy
Sustained-Action Tablets **740**
Drixoral Cold & Flu
Extended-Release Tablets..........**740**
Drixoral Nasal Decongestant
Long-Acting Non-Drowsy
Tablets....................................**740**
Ecotrin Enteric Coated Aspirin
Low Strength Tablets **747**
Ecotrin Enteric Coated Aspirin
Maximum Strength Tablets.......**747**
Ecotrin Enteric Coated Aspirin
Regular Strength Tablets **747**
Aspirin Free Excedrin Caplets
and Geltabs **628**
Excedrin Extra-Strength Tablets,
Caplets, and Geltabs **629**
Excedrin PM Tablets, Caplets,
and Geltabs **631**
Goody's Extra Strength
Headache Powder....................**620**
Goody's Extra Strength
Pain Relief Tablets...................**620**
Goody's PM Powder **621**
Halls Mentho-Lyptus Drops..........**686**
Halls Sugar Free Mentho-Lyptus
Drops **686**
Halls Sugar Free Squares............**686**
Halls Plus Cough Drops...............**686**
Momentum Backache Relief
Extra Strength Caplets **666**
Children's Motrin Oral Suspension
and Chewable Tablets..............**643**
Children's Motrin Cold
Oral Suspension **646**
Infants' Motrin
Concentrated Drops.................**643**
Junior Strength Motrin Caplets
and Chewable Tablets **643**

Motrin IB Tablets, Caplets,
and Gelcaps............................**642**
Motrin Sinus/Headache
Caplets **643**
Natru-Vent Nasal Spray,
Adult Strength **624**
Natru-Vent Nasal Spray,
Pediatric Strength **625**
Neo-Synephrine Nasal Drops,
Regular and Extra Strength.......**614**
Neo-Synephrine Nasal Sprays,
Mild, Regular and
Extra Strength **614**
Neo-Synephrine 12 Hour
Nasal Spray **615**
Orudis KT Tablets **778**
PediaCare Cough-Cold Liquid **719**
PediaCare Infants' Drops
Decongestant...........................**719**
PediaCare Infants' Drops
Decongestant Plus Cough **719**
PediaCare NightRest
Cough-Cold Liquid **719**
Percogesic Aspirin-Free Coated
Tablets....................................**667**
Extra Strength Percogesic
Aspirin-Free Coated Caplets......**665**
Relief Nasal & Throat Spray.........**811**
Robitussin Cold Caplets
Cold & Congestion...................**780**
Robitussin Cold Softgels
Cold & Congestion...................**780**
Robitussin Cold Caplets
Multi-Symptom Cold & Flu **781**
Robitussin Cold Softgels
Multi-Symptom Cold & Flu **781**
Robitussin Cold Softgels
Severe Congestion...................**782**
Robitussin Cough Drops.............**781**
Robitussin Honey Cough Drops....**784**
Robitussin Honey Cough Liquid....**784**
Robitussin Cough & Cold
Infant Drops **782**
Robitussin Maximum Strength
Cough & Cold Liquid **785**
Robitussin Pediatric
Cough & Cold Formula Liquid ...**785**
Robitussin Maximum Strength
Cough Suppressant Liquid........**784**
Robitussin Pediatric Cough
Suppressant Liquid...................**784**
Robitussin Multi Symptom
Honey Flu Liquid **785**
Robitussin Nighttime
Honey Flu Liquid **786**
Robitussin Honey Calmers
Throat Drops **783**
Robitussin Sugar Free
Throat Drops **786**
Robitussin-CF Liquid....................**783**
Robitussin DM Infant Drops.........**783**
Robitussin-DM Liquid **783**
Robitussin-PE Liquid....................**782**

Ryna Liquid **768**
Ryna-C Liquid **768**
Singlet Caplets **761**
Sinutab Non-Drying Liquid Caps ...**706**
Sinutab Sinus Allergy
Medication, Maximum
Strength Formula,
Tablets & Caplets **707**
Sinutab Sinus Medication,
Maximum Strength
Without Drowsiness Formula,
Tablets & Caplets **707**
Sudafed 12 Hour Tablets.............**708**
Sudafed 24 Hour Tablets.............**708**
Children's Sudafed
Cold & Cough Liquid **709**
Children's Sudafed Nasal
Decongestant Chewables **711**
Children's Sudafed
Nasal Decongestant
Liquid Medication **711**
Sudafed Cold & Allergy Tablets **708**
Sudafed Cold & Cough
Liquid Caps **709**
Sudafed Cold & Sinus
Liquid Caps **710**
Sudafed Nasal Decongestant
Tablets....................................**710**
Sudafed Non-Drying Sinus
Liquid Caps **712**
Sudafed Severe Cold Formula
Caplets **711**
Sudafed Severe Cold Formula
Tablets....................................**711**
Sudafed Sinus Headache
Caplets **712**
Sudafed Sinus Headache
Tablets....................................**712**
Tavist 12 Hour Allergy Tablets......**676**
Tavist Sinus Non-Drowsy
Coated Caplets........................**676**
TheraFlu Regular Strength
Cold & Cough Night Time
Hot Liquid **676**
TheraFlu Regular Strength
Cold & Sore Throat
Night Time Hot Liquid **676**
TheraFlu Maximum Strength
Flu & Congestion
Non-Drowsy Hot Liquid **677**
TheraFlu Maximum Strength
Flu & Cough Night Time
Hot Liquid **678**
TheraFlu Maximum Strength
Flu & Sore Throat
Night Time Hot Liquid **677**
TheraFlu Maximum Strength
Severe Cold & Congestion
Night Time Caplets **678**
TheraFlu Maximum Strength
Severe Cold & Congestion
Night Time Hot Liquid **678**

TheraFlu Maximum Strength
Severe Cold & Congestion
Non-Drowsy Caplets **679**
TheraFlu Maximum Strength
Severe Cold & Congestion
Non-Drowsy Hot Liquid **679**
Triaminic Allergy Congestion
Liquid **680**
Triaminic Chest Congestion
Liquid **680**
Triaminic Cold & Allergy Liquid **681**
Triaminic Cold & Allergy
Softchews **683**
Triaminic Cold & Cough Liquid **681**
Triaminic Cold & Cough
Softchews **683**
Triaminic Cold & Night Time
Cough Liquid **681**
Triaminic Cold, Cough & Fever
Liquid **681**
Triaminic Cough Liquid **682**
Triaminic Cough Softchews **684**
Triaminic Cough & Congestion
Liquid **682**
Triaminic Cough & Sore Throat
Liquid **682**
Triaminic Cough & Sore Throat
Softchews **684**
Triaminic Vapor Patch-Cherry
Scent...................................**684**
Triaminic Vapor Patch-Menthol
Scent...................................**684**
Children's Tylenol Suspension
Liquid and Soft Chews
Chewable Tablets....................**657**
Children's Tylenol Allergy-D
Liquid **658**
Children's Tylenol Cold
Suspension Liquid and
Chewable Tablets....................**659**
Children's Tylenol Cold Plus
Cough Suspension Liquid
and Chewable Tablets **659**
Children's Tylenol Flu
Suspension Liquid **663**
Children's Tylenol Sinus
Suspension Liquid **663**
Infants' Tylenol Cold
Decongestant &
Fever Reducer
Concentrated Drops.................**659**
Infants' Tylenol Cold
Decongestant &
Fever Reducer Concentrated
Drops Plus Cough....................**659**
Infants' Tylenol Concentrated
Drops **657**
Junior Strength Tylenol
Soft Chews Chewable Tablets...**657**
Extra Strength Tylenol Adult
Liquid Pain Reliever **647**
Extra Strength Tylenol Gelcaps,
Geltabs, Caplets, and
Tablets.................................**647**

Regular Strength Tylenol
Tablets.................................**647**
Maximum Strength Tylenol
Allergy Sinus Caplets,
Gelcaps, and Geltabs...............**649**
Maximum Strength Tylenol
Allergy Sinus NightTime
Caplets **649**
Tylenol Severe Allergy Caplets **649**
Tylenol Arthritis Pain
Extended Relief Caplets **647**
Multi-Symptom Tylenol Cold
Complete Formula Caplets **651**
Multi-Symptom Tylenol Cold
Non-Drowsy Caplets and
Gelcaps **651**
Multi-Symptom Tylenol Cold
Severe Congestion
Non-Drowsy Caplets **652**
Maximum Strength Tylenol Flu
NightTime Gelcaps...................**653**
Maximum Strength Tylenol Flu
NightTime Liquid.....................**653**
Maximum Strength Tylenol Flu
Non-Drowsy Gelcaps **653**
Extra Strength Tylenol PM
Caplets, Geltabs,
and Gelcaps...........................**654**
Maximum Strength Tylenol
Sinus NightTime Caplets **655**
Maximum Strength Tylenol
Sinus Non-Drowsy Geltabs,
Gelcaps, Caplets, and
Tablets.................................**655**
Maximum Strength Tylenol
Sore Throat Adult Liquid...........**656**
Unisom Maximum Strength
SleepGels **713**
Vanquish Caplets **617**
Vicks 44 Cough Relief Liquid **724**
Vicks 44D Cough & Head
Congestion Relief Liquid...........**724**
Vicks 44E Cough & Chest
Congestion Relief Liquid...........**725**
Pediatric Vicks 44e Cough &
Chest Congestion Relief
Liquid **728**
Vicks 44M Cough, Cold & Flu
Relief Liquid **725**
Pediatric Vicks 44m
Cough & Cold Relief.................**728**
Vicks Cough Drops, Menthol
and Cherry Flavors...................**726**
Vicks DayQuil LiquiCaps/
Liquid Multi-Symptom
Cold/Flu Relief **727**
Children's Vicks NyQuil
Cold/Cough Relief **726**
Vicks NyQuil LiquiCaps/
Liquid Multi-Symptom
Cold/Flu Relief, Original
and Cherry Flavors...................**727**

Vicks Sinex Nasal Spray
and Ultra Fine Mist **729**
Vicks Sinex 12-Hour
Nasal Spray and
Ultra Fine Mist.......................**729**
Vicks Vapor Inhaler **730**
Vicks VapoRub Cream **730**
Vicks VapoRub Ointment **730**
Vicks VapoSteam **730**

INFECTIONS, SKIN AND SKIN STRUCTURE

May be treated with aminoglycosides, amoxicillin, amoxicillin-clavulanate, cephalosporins, doxycycline, erythromycin, macrolide antibiotics, penicillins or quinolones. The following products may be recommended for relief of symptoms:

Bactine First Aid Liquid...............**611**
Betadine Brand First Aid
Antibiotics + Moisturizer
Ointment...............................**731**
Betadine Brand Plus First Aid
Antibiotics + Pain Reliever
Ointment...............................**731**
Betadine Ointment......................**732**
Betadine Skin Cleanser...............**732**
Betadine Solution **732**
Neosporin Ointment **704**
Neosporin + Pain Relief
Maximum Strength Cream........**704**
Neosporin + Pain Relief
Maximum Strength Ointment **704**
Polysporin Ointment....................**706**
Polysporin Powder......................**706**

IRRITABLE BOWEL SYNDROME

May be treated with anticholinergic combinations, dicyclomine hydrochloride or hyoscyamine sulfate. The following products may be recommended for relief of symptoms:

Beano Liquid **809**
Beano Tablets............................**809**
Citrucel Caplets **745**
Citrucel Orange Flavor Powder **744**
Citrucel Sugar Free
Orange Flavor Powder **745**
FiberCon Caplets **639**
Maximum Strength Gas Aid
Softgels.................................**640**
Gas-X Chewable Tablets **671**
Extra Strength Gas-X Liquid **671**
Extra Strength Gas-X Softgels **671**
Extra Strength Gas-X Chewable
Tablets.................................**671**
Maximum Strength Gas-X
Softgels **671**
Metamucil Powder, Original
Texture Orange Flavor..............**722**
Metamucil Powder, Original
Texture Regular Flavor.............**722**
Metamucil Smooth Texture
Powder, Orange Flavor..............**722**

IRRITABLE BOWEL SYNDROME —cont.

Metamucil Smooth Texture
Powder, Sugar-Free,
Orange Flavor **722**
Metamucil Smooth Texture
Powder, Sugar-Free,
Regular Flavor **722**
Metamucil Wafers, Apple Crisp &
Cinnamon Spice Flavors **722**
Mitrolan Chewable Tablets...........**789**
Mylanta Gas Softgels **637**
Mylanta Gas Tablets....................**637**
Maximum Strength
Mylanta Gas Tablets **637**
Perdiem Fiber Therapy Granules...**675**
Phazyme-125 mg Quick Dissolve
Chewable Tablets.....................**622**
Phazyme-180 mg
Ultra Strength Softgels.............**622**
Phillips' FiberCaps Caplets **615**

ISCHEMIC HEART DISEASE

May be treated with beta blockers, calci-
um channel blockers, isosorbide dini-
trate, isosorbide mononitrate or nitroglyc-
erin. The following products may be rec-
ommended for relief of symptoms:
Genuine Bayer
Professional Labeling
(Aspirin Regimen Bayer) **608**
Ecotrin Enteric Coated Aspirin
Low Strength Tablets **747**
Ecotrin Enteric Coated Aspirin
Maximum Strength Tablets **747**
Ecotrin Enteric Coated Aspirin
Regular Strength Tablets **747**

KERATOCONJUNCTIVITIS, VERNAL

May be treated with ophthalmic mast cell
stabilizers. The following products may
be recommended for relief of symptoms:
Benadryl Allergy Chewables **689**
Benadryl Allergy Kapseal
Capsules..................................**691**
Benadryl Allergy Liquid **690**
Benadryl Allergy Ultratab
Tablets.....................................**691**
Benadryl Dye-Free Allergy
Liquid **690**
Benadryl Dye-Free Allergy
Liqui-Gels Softgels...................**690**
Chlor-Trimeton Allergy Tablets **735**
Tavist 12 Hour Allergy Tablets......**676**
Tylenol Severe Allergy Caplets **649**
Unisom Maximum Strength
SleepGels **713**

MYOCARDIAL INFARCTION, ACUTE

May be treated with ACE inhibitors, anticoagulants, beta blockers, thrombolytic
agents or nitroglycerin. The following
products may be recommended for relief
of symptoms:
Genuine Bayer
Professional Labeling
(Aspirin Regimen Bayer) **608**

Ecotrin Enteric Coated Aspirin
Low Strength Tablets **747**
Ecotrin Enteric Coated Aspirin
Maximum Strength Tablets **747**
Ecotrin Enteric Coated Aspirin
Regular Strength Tablets **747**

**NASAL POLYPS, RHINORRHEA
SECONDARY TO**

Nasal polyps may be treated with nasal
steroidal anti-inflammatory agents. The
following products may be recommended
for relief of rhinorrhea:
Actifed Cold & Allergy Tablets **688**
Benadryl Allergy Chewables **689**
Benadryl Allergy Kapseal
Capsules..................................**691**
Benadryl Allergy Liquid **690**
Benadryl Allergy Ultratab
Tablets.....................................**691**
Benadryl Allergy/Congestion
Tablets.....................................**692**
Benadryl Allergy & Sinus
Liquid **693**
Benadryl Allergy & Sinus
Fastmelt Tablets **693**
Benadryl Allergy Sinus
Headache Caplets
& Gelcaps **693**
Benadryl Dye-Free Allergy
Liquid **690**
Benadryl Dye-Free Allergy
Liqui-Gels Softgels...................**690**
Chlor-Trimeton Allergy Tablets **735**
Chlor-Trimeton
Allergy/Decongestant Tablets ...**736**
Contac Non-Drowsy 12 Hour
Cold Caplets **745**
Contac Non-Drowsy
Timed Release
12 Hour Cold Caplets **746**
Dimetapp Elixir **777**
Drixoral Cold & Allergy
Sustained-Action Tablets **740**
Ryna Liquid **768**
Sudafed Cold & Allergy Tablets **708**
Tavist 12 Hour Allergy Tablets......**676**
TheraFlu Regular Strength
Cold & Sore Throat
Night Time Hot Liquid **676**
Triaminic Cold & Allergy Liquid **681**
Triaminic Cold & Allergy
Softchews **683**
Maximum Strength Tylenol
Allergy Sinus Caplets,
Gelcaps, and Geltabs...............**649**
Maximum Strength Tylenol
Allergy Sinus NightTime
Caplets **649**
Tylenol Severe Allergy Caplets **649**
Unisom Maximum Strength
SleepGels **713**

**NECATORIASIS, IRON-DEFICIENCY
ANEMIA SECONDARY TO**

Necatoriasis may be treated with meben-
dazole or thiabendazole. The following
products may be recommended for relief
of iron-deficiency anemia:
Feosol Caplets............................**837**
Feosol Tablets **838**
Fergon Iron Tablets **802**
Slow Fe Tablets **827**
Slow Fe with Folic Acid Tablets.....**828**

OSTEOPOROSIS

May be treated with bisphosphonates,
calcitonin or estrogens. The following
products may be recommended for relief
of symptoms:
Caltrate 600 Tablets **814**
Caltrate 600 PLUS Chewables **815**
Caltrate 600 PLUS Tablets **815**
Caltrate 600 + D Tablets.............**814**
Caltrate 600 + Soy Tablets..........**814**
Citracal Liquitab Tablets **823**
Citracal Tablets...........................**823**
Citracal Caplets + D....................**823**
D-Cal Chewable Caplets **794**
Extra Strength Mylanta
Calci Tabs Tablets....................**636**
One-A-Day Calcium Plus
Chewable Tablets.....................**805**
Os-Cal Chewable Tablets **838**
Os-Cal 250 + D Tablets...............**838**
Os-Cal 500 Tablets **839**
Os-Cal 500 + D Tablets...............**839**
Tums E-X Antacid/Calcium
Tablets....................................**763**
Tums E-X Sugar Free
Antacid/Calcium Tablets **763**
Tums Regular Antacid/Calcium
Tablets....................................**763**
Tums ULTRA
Antacid/Calcium Tablets **763**

OSTEOPOROSIS, SECONDARY

May result from the use of chemothera-
peutic agents, phenytoin, prolonged glu-
cocorticoid therapy, thyroid hormones,
carbamazepine or methotrexate sodium.
The following products may be recom-
mended:
Caltrate 600 Tablets **814**
Caltrate 600 PLUS Chewables **815**
Caltrate 600 PLUS Tablets **815**
Caltrate 600 + D Tablets............**814**
Caltrate 600 + Soy Tablets..........**814**
Citracal Liquitab Tablets **823**
Citracal Tablets...........................**823**
Citracal Caplets + D....................**823**
D-Cal Chewable Caplets **794**
Extra Strength Mylanta
Calci Tabs Tablets....................**636**
One-A-Day Calcium Plus
Chewable Tablets.....................**805**
Os-Cal Chewable Tablets **838**
Os-Cal 250 + D Tablets...............**838**

Os-Cal 500 Tablets **839**

Os-Cal 500 + D Tablets **839**

Tums E-X Antacid/Calcium
  Tablets.....................................**763**

Tums E-X Sugar Free
  Antacid/Calcium Tablets **763**

Tums Regular Antacid/Calcium
  Tablets.....................................**763**

Tums ULTRA Antacid/Calcium
  Tablets.....................................**763**

OTITIS MEDIA, ACUTE

May be treated with amoxicillin, amoxi-cillin-clavulanate, cephalosporins, eryth-romycin-sulfisoxazole, macrolide antibi-otics or sulfamethoxazole-trimethoprim. The following products may be recom-mended for relief of symptoms:

Actifed Cold & Allergy Tablets **688**

Advil Caplets **771**

Advil Gel Caplets **771**

Advil Liqui-Gels **771**

Advil Tablets **771**

Children's Advil
  Oral Suspension **773**

Children's Advil
  Chewable Tablets.....................**773**

Advil Cold and Sinus Caplets **771**

Advil Cold and Sinus Tablets **771**

Advil Flu & Body Ache Caplets **772**

Infants' Advil Drops.....................**773**

Junior Strength Advil Tablets **773**

Junior Strength Advil
  Chewable Tablets.....................**773**

Aleve Tablets, Caplets
  and Gelcaps.............................**602**

Aleve Cold & Sinus Caplets **603**

Alka-Seltzer Plus Cold & Cough
  Medicine Liqui-Gels..................**604**

Alka-Seltzer Plus Cold & Sinus
  Medicine Liqui-Gels..................**604**

Benadryl Allergy/Cold Tablets **691**

Benadryl Allergy/Congestion
  Tablets.....................................**692**

Benadryl Allergy & Sinus Liquid ...**693**

Benadryl Allergy & Sinus
  Fastmelt Tablets **693**

Benadryl Allergy Sinus Headache
  Caplets & Gelcaps...................**693**

Chlor-Trimeton
  Allergy/Decongestant Tablets ...**736**

Comtrex Acute Head Cold &
  Sinus Pressure Relief Tablets ...**627**

Contac Non-Drowsy 12 Hour
  Cold Caplets **745**

Contac Non-Drowsy
  Timed Release
  12 Hour Cold Caplets **746**

Dimetapp Elixir **777**

Dimetapp Cold and Fever
  Suspension..............................**775**

Dimetapp Infant Drops
  Decongestant...........................**775**

Drixoral Allergy/Sinus
  Extended-Release Tablets..........**741**

Drixoral Cold & Allergy
  Sustained-Action Tablets **740**

Drixoral Cold & Flu
  Extended-Release Tablets..........**740**

Drixoral Nasal Decongestant
  Long-Acting Non-Drowsy
  Tablets.....................................**740**

Excedrin PM Tablets,
  Caplets, and Geltabs **631**

Goody's PM Powder **621**

Hyland's Earache Tablets **765**

Children's Motrin
  Oral Suspension and
  Chewable Tablets.....................**643**

Children's Motrin Cold
  Oral Suspension **646**

Infants' Motrin
  Concentrated Drops.................**643**

Junior Strength Motrin Caplets
  and Chewable Tablets **643**

Motrin IB Tablets, Caplets, and
  Gelcaps **642**

Orudis KT Tablets **778**

PediaCare Infants' Drops
  Decongestant...........................**719**

Percogesic Aspirin-Free Coated
  Tablets.....................................**667**

Extra Strength Percogesic
  Aspirin-Free Coated Caplets......**665**

Ryna Liquid **768**

Ryna-C Liquid **768**

Sudafed 12 Hour Tablets.............**708**

Sudafed 24 Hour Tablets.............**708**

Children's Sudafed Nasal
  Decongestant Chewables **711**

Children's Sudafed Nasal
  Decongestant Liquid
  Medication **711**

Sudafed Cold & Allergy Tablets **708**

Sudafed Cold & Sinus
  Liquid Caps **710**

Sudafed Nasal Decongestant
  Tablets.....................................**710**

Sudafed Sinus Headache
  Caplets **712**

Sudafed Sinus Headache
  Tablets.....................................**712**

TheraFlu Regular Strength
  Cold & Sore Throat
  Night Time Hot Liquid **676**

TheraFlu Maximum Strength
  Flu & Sore Throat
  Night Time Hot Liquid **677**

Triaminic Allergy Congestion
  Liquid **680**

Triaminic Cold & Allergy Liquid **681**

Triaminic Cold & Allergy
  Softchews **683**

Children's Tylenol
  Suspension Liquid and
  Soft Chews Chewable Tablets...**657**

Children's Tylenol Cold
  Suspension Liquid and
  Chewable Tablets.....................**659**

Children's Tylenol Sinus
  Suspension Liquid **663**

Infants' Tylenol Cold
  Decongestant &
  Fever Reducer
  Concentrated Drops.................**659**

Infants' Tylenol
  Concentrated Drops.................**657**

Junior Strength Tylenol
  Soft Chews Chewable Tablets...**657**

Extra Strength Tylenol Adult
  Liquid Pain Reliever **647**

Extra Strength Tylenol Gelcaps,
  Geltabs, Caplets, and
  Tablets.....................................**647**

Regular Strength Tylenol
  Tablets.....................................**647**

Maximum Strength Tylenol
  Allergy Sinus Caplets,
  Gelcaps, and Geltabs...............**649**

Maximum Strength Tylenol
  Allergy Sinus NightTime
  Caplets **649**

Tylenol Arthritis Pain
  Extended Relief Caplets **647**

Maximum Strength Tylenol
  Flu NightTime Gelcaps **653**

Maximum Strength Tylenol
  Flu NightTime Liquid **653**

Extra Strength Tylenol PM
  Caplets, Geltabs,
  and Gelcaps.............................**654**

Maximum Strength Tylenol
  Sinus NightTime Caplets **655**

Maximum Strength Tylenol
  Sinus Non-Drowsy Geltabs,
  Gelcaps, Caplets, and
  Tablets.....................................**655**

Maximum Strength Tylenol
  Sore Throat Adult Liquid...........**656**

Vanquish Caplets **617**

PANCREATIC INSUFFICIENCY, NUTRIENTS DEFICIENCY SECONDARY TO

Pancreatic insufficiency may be treated with pancrelipase. The following products may be recommended for relief of nutrients deficiency:

Centrum Performance
  Multivitamin-Multimineral
  Tablets.....................................**817**

Centrum Tablets **815**

Centrum Silver Tablets **818**

One-A-Day Essential Tablets.........**806**

One-A-Day 50 Plus Tablets...........**804**

One-A-Day Kids Complete
  Tablets.....................................**806**

One-A-Day Maximum Tablets **807**

One-A-Day Men's Tablets **808**

One-A-Day Women's Tablets.........**809**

PARKINSON'S DISEASE, CONSTIPATION SECONDARY TO

Parkinson's disease may be treated with centrally active anticholinergic agents, dopaminergic agents or selective inhibitor of MAO type B. The following products may be recommended for relief of constipation:

Ceo-Two Evacuant Suppository **618**
Citrucel Caplets **745**
Citrucel Orange Flavor Powder **744**
Citrucel Sugar Free
    Orange Flavor Powder **745**
Colace Capsules, Syrup
    and Drops **743**
Correctol Laxative Tablets
    and Caplets **739**
Dulcolax Suppositories................**668**
Dulcolax Tablets.........................**668**
Ex·Lax Gentle Strength Caplets...**670**
Ex·Lax Regular Strength Pills **670**
Ex·Lax Regular Strength
    Chocolated Pieces **669**
Ex·Lax Maximum Strength Pills ...**670**
Ex·Lax Stool Softener Caplets.....**671**
FiberCon Caplets **639**
Maltsupex Powder, Liquid,
    Tablets...................................**767**
Metamucil Powder, Original
    Texture Orange Flavor...............**722**
Metamucil Powder, Original
    Texture Regular Flavor..............**722**
Metamucil Smooth Texture
    Powder, Orange Flavor...............**722**
Metamucil Smooth Texture
    Powder, Sugar-Free,
    Orange Flavor **722**
Metamucil Smooth Texture
    Powder, Sugar-Free,
    Regular Flavor **722**
Metamucil Wafers,
    Apple Crisp &
    Cinnamon Spice Flavors...........**722**
Mitrolan Chewable Tablets...........**789**
Nature's Remedy Tablets.............**621**
Perdiem Overnight Relief
    Granules **674**
Phillips' FiberCaps Caplets **615**
Phillips' Liqui-Gels......................**616**
Purge Liquid **633**
Senokot Children's Syrup **732**
Senokot Granules **732**
Senokot Syrup............................**732**
Senokot Tablets..........................**732**
Senokot-S Tablets.......................**732**
SenokotXTRA Tablets **732**
Surfak Liqui-Gels **721**

PARKINSON'S DISEASE, SEBORRHEIC DERMATITIS SECONDARY TO

Parkinson's disease may be treated with centrally active anticholinergic agents, dopaminergic agents or selective inhibitor of MAO type B. The following products may be recommended for relief of seborrheic dermatitis:

Cortaid Intensive Therapy
    Cream.....................................**717**
Cortaid Maximum Strength
    Cream.....................................**717**
Cortaid Maximum Strength
    Ointment.................................**717**
Cortaid Sensitive Skin Cream **717**
Tegrin Dandruff Shampoo -
    Extra Conditioning....................**623**
Tegrin Dandruff Shampoo -
    Fresh Herbal **624**
Tegrin Skin Cream......................**624**

PEPTIC ULCER DISEASE

May be treated with histamine H_2 receptor antagonists, proton pump inhibitors or sucralfate. The following products may be recommended for relief of symptoms:

Alka-Seltzer Heartburn Relief
    Tablets...................................**604**
Amphojel Suspension
    (Mint Flavor)...........................**789**
Ex·Lax Milk of Magnesia Liquid...**670**
Gaviscon Extra Strength Liquid **751**
Gaviscon Extra Strength
    Tablets...................................**751**
Gaviscon Regular Strength
    Liquid **751**
Maalox Antacid/Anti-Gas
    Oral Suspension **673**
Maalox Max Maximum Strength
    Antacid/Anti-Gas Liquid............**673**
Quick Dissolve Maalox Antacid
    Chewable Tablets.....................**674**
Quick Dissolve Maalox Max
    Maximum Strength
    Antacid/Antigas
    Chewable Tablets.....................**674**
Mylanta Gelcaps **637**
Mylanta Liquid **634**
Mylanta Extra Strength Liquid **634**
Mylanta Supreme Liquid..............**636**
Mylanta Ultra Tabs Tablets..........**637**
Extra Strength Mylanta
    Calci Tabs Tablets....................**636**
Pepto-Bismol Original Liquid,
    Original and Cherry
    Chewable Tablets & Caplets **723**
Pepto-Bismol Maximum Strength
    Liquid **724**
Phillips' Chewable Tablets **615**
Phillips' Milk of Magnesia
    Liquid (Original, Cherry,
    & Mint) **616**
Rolaids Tablets **706**
Extra Strength Rolaids Tablets **706**
3M Titralac Antacid Tablets **640**
3M Titralac Extra Strength
    Antacid Tablets........................**640**
3M Titralac Plus Antacid
    Tablets...................................**640**
Tums E-X Antacid/Calcium
    Tablets...................................**763**
Tums E-X Sugar Free
    Antacid/Calcium Tablets **763**
Tums Regular
    Antacid/Calcium Tablets **763**
Tums ULTRA
    Antacid/Calcium Tablets **763**

PEPTIC ULCER DISEASE, IRON DEFICIENCY SECONDARY TO

Peptic ulcer disease may be treated with histamine H_2 receptor antagonists, proton pump inhibitors or sucralfate. The following products may be recommended for relief of iron deficiency:

Feosol Caplets............................**837**
Feosol Tablets **838**
Fergon Iron Tablets **802**
Slow Fe Tablets **827**
Slow Fe with Folic Acid Tablets.....**828**

PHARYNGITIS

May be treated with cephalosporins, macrolide antibiotics or penicillins. The following products may be recommended for relief of symptoms:

Advil Caplets **771**
Advil Gel Caplets **771**
Advil Liqui-Gels **771**
Advil Tablets **771**
Children's Advil
    Oral Suspension **773**
Children's Advil
    Chewable Tablets.....................**773**
Infants' Advil Drops.....................**773**
Junior Strength Advil Tablets........**773**
Junior Strength Advil
    Chewable Tablets.....................**773**
Aleve Tablets, Caplets
    and Gelcaps............................**602**
Alka-Seltzer Plus Night-Time
    Cold Medicine Liqui-Gels **604**
Alka-Seltzer Plus Cold & Flu
    Medicine Liqui-Gels..................**604**
Alka-Seltzer PM
    Effervescent Tablets **605**
Genuine Bayer Tablets,
    Caplets and Gelcaps................**606**
Extra Strength Bayer
    Caplets and Gelcaps................**610**
Aspirin Regimen Bayer Adult
    Low Strength 81 mg Tablets.....**606**
Aspirin Regimen Bayer
    Regular Strength
    325 mg Caplets **606**
Genuine Bayer
    Professional Labeling
    (Aspirin Regimen Bayer) **608**
Extra Strength Bayer
    Arthritis Caplets **610**
Extra Strength Bayer Plus
    Caplets **610**
Extra Strength Bayer PM
    Caplets **611**

BC Powder **619**
BC Allergy Sinus Cold Powder......**619**
Arthritis Strength BC Powder **619**
BC Sinus Cold Powder.................**619**
Benadryl Children's
    Allergy/Cold Fastmelt Tablets ...**692**
Benylin Adult Formula Cough
    Suppressant Liquid.................**696**
Benylin Cough
    Suppressant/Expectorant
    Liquid **697**
Benylin Multi-Symptom Liquid **697**
Benylin Pediatric Cough
    Suppressant Liquid.................**698**
Celestial Seasonings
    Soothers Throat Drops.............**685**
Children's Cēpacol Sore Throat
    Formula, Cherry Flavor Liquid ...**788**
Children's Cēpacol Sore Throat
    Formula, Grape Flavor Liquid **788**
Cēpacol Maximum Strength
    Sugar Free Sore Throat
    Lozenges, Cherry Flavor...........**787**
Cēpacol Maximum Strength
    Sugar Free Sore Throat
    Lozenges, Cool Mint Flavor.......**787**
Cēpacol Maximum Strength
    Sore Throat Lozenges,
    Cherry Flavor.......................**787**
Cēpacol Maximum Strength
    Sore Throat Lozenges,
    Mint Flavor..........................**787**
Cēpacol Regular Strength
    Sore Throat Lozenges,
    Cherry Flavor.......................**787**
Cēpacol Regular Strength
    Sore Throat Lozenges,
    Original Mint Flavor.................**787**
Cēpacol Maximum Strength
    Sore Throat Spray,
    Cherry Flavor.......................**787**
Cēpacol Maximum Strength
    Sore Throat Spray, Cool
    Menthol Flavor......................**787**
Cēpacol Maximum Strength
    Sore Throat Spray, Honey
    Lemon Flavor.........................**787**
Comtrex Acute Head
    Cold & Sinus
    Pressure Relief Tablets **627**
Comtrex Deep Chest
    Cold & Congestion Relief
    Softgels **627**
Comtrex Flu Therapy & Fever
    Relief Nighttime Tablets **628**
Comtrex Maximum Strength
    Multi-Symptom Cold & Cough
    Relief Tablets and Caplets........**626**
Contac Severe Cold and Flu
    Caplets Maximum Strength **746**
Contac Severe Cold and Flu
    Caplets Non-Drowsy.................**746**

Coricidin 'D' Cold, Flu & Sinus
    Tablets................................**737**
Coricidin HBP Cold & Flu
    Tablets................................**738**
Coricidin HBP Cough & Cold
    Tablets................................**738**
Coricidin HBP Maximum
    Strength Flu Tablets **738**
Coricidin HBP Night-Time
    Cold & Flu Tablets **738**
Delsym Extended-Release
    Suspension **664**
Dimetapp Cold and Fever
    Suspension **775**
Dimetapp DM Cold & Cough
    Elixir **775**
Dimetapp Nighttime Flu
    Liquid **776**
Dimetapp Non-Drowsy Flu
    Syrup.................................**777**
Dimetapp Infant Drops
    Decongestant Plus Cough **776**
Ecotrin Enteric Coated Aspirin
    Low Strength Tablets **747**
Ecotrin Enteric Coated Aspirin
    Maximum Strength Tablets **747**
Ecotrin Enteric Coated Aspirin
    Regular Strength Tablets **747**
Aspirin Free Excedrin
    Caplets and Geltabs **628**
Excedrin Extra-Strength Tablets,
    Caplets, and Geltabs **629**
Excedrin PM Tablets, Caplets,
    and Geltabs **631**
Goody's Extra Strength
    Headache Powder...................**620**
Goody's Extra Strength
    Pain Relief Tablets **620**
Goody's PM Powder **621**
Halls Mentho-Lyptus Drops..........**686**
Halls Sugar Free
    Mentho-Lyptus Drops **686**
Halls Sugar Free Squares............**686**
Halls Plus Cough Drops..............**686**
Hurricaine Topical
    Anesthetic Spray
    Extension Tubes (200).............**618**
Hurricaine Topical
    Anesthetic Spray Kit,
    2 oz. Wild Cherry....................**618**
Hurricaine Topical
    Anesthetic Spray, 2 oz.
    Wild Cherry **618**
Momentum Backache Relief
    Extra Strength Caplets **666**
Children's Motrin
    Oral Suspension and
    Chewable Tablets....................**643**
Infants' Motrin
    Concentrated Drops.................**643**
Junior Strength Motrin Caplets
    and Chewable Tablets..............**643**
Motrin IB Tablets, Caplets,
    and Gelcaps **642**

Orudis KT Tablets **778**
PediaCare Cough-Cold Liquid **719**
PediaCare Infants' Drops
    Decongestant Plus Cough **719**
PediaCare NightRest
    Cough-Cold Liquid...................**719**
Percogesic Aspirin-Free Coated
    Tablets................................**667**
Extra Strength Percogesic
    Aspirin-Free Coated Caplets......**665**
Relief Nasal & Throat Spray.........**811**
Robitussin Cold Caplets
    Cold & Congestion...................**780**
Robitussin Cold Softgels
    Cold & Congestion...................**780**
Robitussin Cold Caplets
    Multi-Symptom Cold & Flu **781**
Robitussin Cold Softgels
    Multi-Symptom Cold & Flu **781**
Robitussin Cough Drops.............**781**
Robitussin Honey Cough
    Drops **784**
Robitussin Honey Cough
    Liquid **784**
Robitussin Cough & Cold
    Infant Drops **782**
Robitussin Maximum Strength
    Cough & Cold Liquid **785**
Robitussin Pediatric
    Cough & Cold Formula Liquid ...**785**
Robitussin Maximum Strength
    Cough Suppressant Liquid........**784**
Robitussin Pediatric Cough
    Suppressant Liquid..................**784**
Robitussin Multi Symptom
    Honey Flu Liquid **785**
Robitussin Nighttime
    Honey Flu Liquid **786**
Robitussin Honey Calmers
    Throat Drops **783**
Robitussin Sugar Free
    Throat Drops **786**
Robitussin-CF Liquid.................**783**
Robitussin DM Infant Drops.........**783**
Robitussin-DM Liquid **783**
Ryna-C Liquid **768**
Children's Sudafed
    Cold & Cough Liquid **709**
Sudafed Cold & Cough
    Liquid Caps...........................**709**
Sudafed Severe Cold Formula
    Caplets **711**
Sudafed Severe Cold Formula
    Tablets................................**711**
TheraFlu Regular Strength
    Cold & Cough Night Time
    Hot Liquid **676**
TheraFlu Maximum Strength
    Flu & Congestion
    Non-Drowsy Hot Liquid **677**
TheraFlu Maximum Strength
    Flu & Cough Night Time
    Hot Liquid **678**

PHARYNGITIS —cont.

TheraFlu Maximum Strength
Flu & Sore Throat
Night Time Hot Liquid **677**
TheraFlu Maximum Strength
Severe Cold & Congestion
Night Time Caplets **678**
TheraFlu Maximum Strength
Severe Cold & Congestion
Night Time Hot Liquid **678**
TheraFlu Maximum Strength
Severe Cold & Congestion
Non-Drowsy Caplets..................**679**
TheraFlu Maximum Strength
Severe Cold & Congestion
Non-Drowsy Hot Liquid **679**
Triaminic Cold & Cough
Softchews **683**
Triaminic Cough Liquid **682**
Triaminic Cough Softchews **684**
Triaminic Cough & Congestion
Liquid **682**
Triaminic Cough & Sore Throat
Liquid **682**
Triaminic Cough & Sore Throat
Softchews **684**
Triaminic Vapor Patch-Cherry
Scent......................................**684**
Triaminic Vapor Patch-Menthol
Scent......................................**684**
Children's Tylenol
Suspension Liquid and
Soft Chews Chewable Tablets...**657**
Children's Tylenol Cold Plus
Cough Suspension Liquid
and Chewable Tablets **659**
Children's Tylenol Flu
Suspension Liquid **663**
Infants' Tylenol Cold
Decongestant & Fever
Reducer Concentrated
Drops Plus Cough.....................**659**
Infants' Tylenol
Concentrated Drops.................**657**
Junior Strength Tylenol
Soft Chews Chewable
Tablets...................................**657**
Extra Strength Tylenol Adult
Liquid Pain Reliever **647**
Extra Strength Tylenol Gelcaps,
Geltabs, Caplets, and
Tablets...................................**647**
Regular Strength Tylenol
Tablets...................................**647**
Tylenol Arthritis Pain
Extended Relief Caplets **647**
Multi-Symptom Tylenol Cold
Complete Formula Caplets **651**
Multi-Symptom Tylenol Cold
Non-Drowsy Caplets and
Gelcaps **651**

Multi-Symptom Tylenol Cold
Severe Congestion
Non-Drowsy Caplets **652**
Maximum Strength Tylenol
Flu NightTime Gelcaps **653**
Extra Strength Tylenol PM
Caplets, Geltabs, and
Gelcaps **654**
Maximum Strength Tylenol
Sore Throat Adult Liquid..........**656**
Vanquish Caplets **617**
Vicks 44 Cough Relief Liquid **724**
Vicks 44D Cough & Head
Congestion Relief Liquid...........**724**
Vicks 44E Cough & Chest
Congestion Relief Liquid...........**725**
Pediatric Vicks 44e Cough &
Chest Congestion Relief
Liquid **728**
Vicks 44M Cough, Cold & Flu
Relief Liquid **725**
Pediatric Vicks 44m Cough &
Cold Relief **728**
Vicks Cough Drops, Menthol
and Cherry Flavors...................**726**
Vicks DayQuil LiquiCaps/
Liquid Multi-Symptom
Cold/Flu Relief **727**
Children's Vicks NyQuil
Cold/Cough Relief **726**
Vicks NyQuil LiquiCaps/Liquid
Multi-Symptom Cold/Flu
Relief, Original and
Cherry Flavors **727**
Vicks VapoRub Cream **730**
Vicks VapoRub Ointment **730**
Vicks VapoSteam **730**

PHOTOSENSITIVITY REACTIONS

May result from the use of thiazides, antidepressants, antihistamines, estrogens, nonsteroidal anti-inflammatory drugs, phenothiazines, quinolones, sulfonamides, sulfonylurea hypoglycemic agents, tetracyclines, topical retinoids, captopril, diltiazem hydrochloride, enalapril maleate, fluorouracil, griseofulvin, labetalol hydrochloride, lisinopril, methoxsalen, methyldopa, minoxidil, nalidixic acid or nifedipine. The following products may be recommended:

Lubriderm Daily UV Lotion **703**

PRURITUS, PERIANAL

May result from the use of broad-spectrum antibiotics. The following products may be recommended:

Anusol HC-1 Hydrocortisone
Anti-Itch Cream.......................**689**
Benadryl Itch Relief Stick
Extra Strength **695**
Cortaid Intensive Therapy
Cream....................................**717**
Cortaid Maximum Strength
Cream....................................**717**

Cortaid Maximum Strength
Ointment................................**717**
Cortaid Sensitive Skin Cream **717**
Cortizone·5 Creme....................**699**
Cortizone·5 Ointment.................**699**
Cortizone·10 Creme...................**699**
Cortizone·10 Ointment..............**699**
Cortizone·10 Plus Creme **700**
Cortizone for Kids Creme **699**
Massengill Medicated Soft
Cloth Towelette.......................**753**

PSORALEN WITH UV-A LIGHT (PUVA) THERAPY

May be treated with methoxsalen. The following products may be recommended for relief of symptoms:

Lubriderm Daily UV Lotion **703**

RENAL OSTEODYSTROPHY, HYPOCAL-CEMIA SECONDARY TO

Renal osteodystrophy may be treated with vitamin D sterols. The following products may be recommended for relief of hypocalcemia:

Caltrate 600 Tablets **814**
Caltrate 600 PLUS Chewables.....**815**
Caltrate 600 PLUS Tablets **815**
Caltrate 600 + D Tablets.............**814**
Caltrate 600 + Soy Tablets.........**814**
Citracal Liquitab Tablets **823**
Citracal Tablets.........................**823**
Citracal Caplets + D....................**823**
D-Cal Chewable Caplets **794**
Extra Strength Mylanta
Calci Tabs Tablets....................**636**
One-A-Day Calcium Plus
Chewable Tablets.....................**805**
Os-Cal Chewable Tablets **838**
Os-Cal 250 + D Tablets...............**838**
Os-Cal 500 Tablets **839**
Os-Cal 500 + D Tablets...............**839**
Tums E-X Antacid/
Calcium Tablets **763**
Tums E-X Sugar Free
Antacid/Calcium Tablets **763**
Tums Regular Antacid/Calcium
Tablets...................................**763**
Tums ULTRA Antacid/Calcium
Tablets...................................**763**

RESPIRATORY TRACT ILLNESS, INFLUENZA A VIRUS-INDUCED

May be treated with amantadine hydrochloride or rimantadine hydrochloride. The following products may be recommended for relief of symptoms:

Actifed Cold & Allergy Tablets **688**
Actifed Cold & Sinus
Caplets and Tablets **688**
Advil Caplets **771**
Advil Gel Caplets **771**
Advil Liqui-Gels **771**
Advil Tablets **771**
Children's Advil
Oral Suspension......................**773**

Children's Advil Chewable
 Tablets.....................................**773**
Advil Cold and Sinus Caplets.......**771**
Advil Cold and Sinus Tablets........**771**
Advil Flu & Body Ache Caplets **772**
Infants' Advil Drops....................**773**
Junior Strength Advil Tablets........**773**
Junior Strength Advil
 Chewable Tablets.....................**773**
Afrin Nasal Decongestant
 Children's Pump Mist...............**734**
Afrin Original Nasal Spray............**733**
Afrin Extra Moisturizing
 Nasal Spray **733**
Afrin Severe Congestion
 Nasal Spray **733**
Afrin Sinus Nasal Spray...............**733**
Afrin No Drip Original
 Nasal Spray **735**
Afrin No Drip Extra Moisturizing
 Nasal Spray **735**
Afrin No Drip Severe Congestion
 Nasal Spray **735**
Afrin No Drip Sinus
 Nasal Spray **735**
Afrin Original Pump Mist..............**733**
Afrin Saline Aromatic Mist **734**
Aleve Tablets, Caplets and
 Gelcaps **602**
Aleve Cold & Sinus Caplets **603**
Alka-Seltzer Original Antacid
 and Pain Reliever
 Effervescent Tablets **603**
Alka-Seltzer Cherry Antacid
 and Pain Reliever
 Effervescent Tablets **603**
Alka-Seltzer Lemon Lime
 Antacid and Pain Reliever
 Effervescent Tablets **603**
Alka-Seltzer Extra Strength
 Antacid and Pain Reliever
 Effervescent Tablets **603**
Alka-Seltzer Plus Cold
 Medicine Liqui-Gels.................**604**
Alka-Seltzer Plus Night-Time
 Cold Medicine Liqui-Gels **604**
Alka-Seltzer Plus Cold & Cough
 Medicine Liqui-Gels.................**604**
Alka-Seltzer Plus Cold & Flu
 Medicine Liqui-Gels.................**604**
Alka-Seltzer Plus Cold & Sinus
 Medicine Liqui-Gels.................**604**
Alka-Seltzer PM Effervescent
 Tablets..................................**605**
Genuine Bayer Tablets,
 Caplets and Gelcaps................**606**
Extra Strength Bayer
 Caplets and Gelcaps................**610**
Aspirin Regimen Bayer Adult
 Low Strength 81 mg Tablets.....**606**
Aspirin Regimen Bayer Regular
 Strength 325 mg Caplets **606**

Genuine Bayer Professional
 Labeling (Aspirin Regimen
 Bayer)...................................**608**
Extra Strength Bayer Arthritis
 Caplets **610**
Extra Strength Bayer Plus
 Caplets **610**
Extra Strength Bayer PM
 Caplets **611**
BC Powder **619**
BC Allergy Sinus Cold Powder......**619**
Arthritis Strength BC Powder **619**
BC Sinus Cold Powder.................**619**
Benadryl Allergy Chewables.........**689**
Benadryl Allergy Kapseal
 Capsules................................**691**
Benadryl Allergy Liquid **690**
Benadryl Allergy Ultratab
 Tablets..................................**691**
Benadryl Allergy/Cold Tablets **691**
Benadryl Allergy/Congestion
 Tablets..................................**692**
Benadryl Allergy & Sinus
 Liquid **693**
Benadryl Allergy & Sinus
 Fastmelt Tablets......................**693**
Benadryl Allergy Sinus
 Headache Caplets &
 Gelcaps **693**
Benadryl Severe Allergy &
 Sinus Headache Caplets..........**694**
Benadryl Children's
 Allergy/Cold Fastmelt
 Tablets..................................**692**
Benadryl Dye-Free Allergy
 Liquid **690**
Benadryl Dye-Free Allergy
 Liqui-Gels Softgels...................**690**
Benylin Adult Formula Cough
 Suppressant Liquid...................**696**
Benylin Cough Suppressant/
 Expectorant Liquid **697**
Benylin Multi-Symptom Liquid **697**
Benylin Pediatric Cough
 Suppressant Liquid...................**698**
Celestial Seasonings
 Soothers Throat Drops.............**685**
Children's Cēpacol
 Sore Throat Formula,
 Cherry Flavor Liquid **788**
Children's Cēpacol
 Sore Throat Formula,
 Grape Flavor Liquid **788**
Cēpacol Maximum Strength
 Sugar Free Sore Throat
 Lozenges, Cherry Flavor...........**787**
Cēpacol Maximum Strength
 Sugar Free Sore Throat
 Lozenges, Cool Mint Flavor.......**787**
Cēpacol Maximum Strength
 Sore Throat Lozenges,
 Cherry Flavor..........................**787**

Cēpacol Maximum Strength
 Sore Throat Lozenges,
 Mint Flavor.............................**787**
Cēpacol Regular Strength
 Sore Throat Lozenges,
 Cherry Flavor..........................**787**
Cēpacol Regular Strength
 Sore Throat Lozenges,
 Original Mint Flavor **787**
Cēpacol Maximum Strength
 Sore Throat Spray,
 Cherry Flavor..........................**787**
Cēpacol Maximum Strength
 Sore Throat Spray,
 Cool Menthol Flavor **787**
Cēpacol Maximum Strength
 Sore Throat Spray,
 Honey Lemon Flavor.................**787**
Chlor-Trimeton Allergy Tablets **735**
Chlor-Trimeton Allergy/
 Decongestant Tablets **736**
Comtrex Acute Head Cold &
 Sinus Pressure Relief
 Tablets..................................**627**
Comtrex Deep Chest Cold &
 Congestion Relief Softgels **627**
Comtrex Flu Therapy & Fever
 Relief Daytime Caplets.............**628**
Comtrex Flu Therapy & Fever
 Relief Nighttime Tablets **628**
Comtrex Maximum Strength
 Multi-Symptom Cold &
 Cough Relief Tablets and
 Caplets **626**
Contac Non-Drowsy 12 Hour
 Cold Caplets **745**
Contac Non-Drowsy Timed
 Release 12 Hour Cold
 Caplets **746**
Contac Severe Cold and Flu
 Caplets Maximum Strength **746**
Contac Severe Cold and Flu
 Caplets Non-Drowsy.................**746**
Coricidin 'D' Cold, Flu & Sinus
 Tablets..................................**737**
Coricidin HBP Cold & Flu
 Tablets..................................**738**
Coricidin HBP Cough & Cold
 Tablets..................................**738**
Coricidin HBP Maximum
 Strength Flu Tablets.................**738**
Coricidin HBP Night-Time
 Cold & Flu Tablets **738**
Delsym Extended-Release
 Suspension **664**
Dimetapp Elixir **777**
Dimetapp Cold and Fever
 Suspension **775**
Dimetapp DM Cold & Cough
 Elixir **775**
Dimetapp Nighttime Flu
 Liquid **776**
Dimetapp Non-Drowsy Flu
 Syrup....................................**777**

RESPIRATORY TRACT ILLNESS,
INFLUENZA A VIRUS-INDUCED —*cont.*

Dimetapp Infant Drops
Decongestant Plus Cough **776**
Drixoral Allergy/Sinus
Extended-Release Tablets.........**741**
Drixoral Cold & Allergy
Sustained-Action Tablets **740**
Drixoral Cold & Flu
Extended-Release Tablets **740**
Ecotrin Enteric Coated Aspirin
Low Strength Tablets **747**
Ecotrin Enteric Coated Aspirin
Maximum Strength Tablets **747**
Ecotrin Enteric Coated Aspirin
Regular Strength Tablets **747**
Aspirin Free Excedrin Caplets
and Geltabs **628**
Excedrin Extra-Strength Tablets,
Caplets, and Geltabs **629**
Excedrin PM Tablets, Caplets,
and Geltabs **631**
Goody's Body Pain Formula
Powder....................................**620**
Goody's Extra Strength
Headache Powder....................**620**
Goody's Extra Strength
Pain Relief Tablets **620**
Goody's PM Powder **621**
Halls Mentho-Lyptus Drops..........**686**
Halls Sugar Free
Mentho-Lyptus Drops **686**
Halls Sugar Free Squares............**686**
Halls Plus Cough Drops...............**686**
Momentum Backache Relief
Extra Strength Caplets **666**
Children's Motrin
Oral Suspension and
Chewable Tablets.....................**643**
Children's Motrin Cold Oral
Suspension **646**
Infants' Motrin
Concentrated Drops.................**643**
Junior Strength Motrin
Caplets and Chewable
Tablets....................................**643**
Motrin IB Tablets, Caplets,
and Gelcaps............................**642**
Motrin Sinus/Headache
Caplets **643**
Natru-Vent Nasal Spray, Adult
Strength...................................**624**
Natru-Vent Nasal Spray,
Pediatric Strength **625**
Neo-Synephrine Nasal Drops,
Regular and Extra Strength.......**614**
Neo-Synephrine Nasal Sprays,
Mild, Regular and
Extra Strength **614**
Neo-Synephrine 12 Hour
Nasal Spray **615**
Orudis KT Tablets **778**
PediaCare Cough-Cold Liquid **719**

PediaCare Infants' Drops
Decongestant.........................**719**
PediaCare Infants' Drops
Decongestant Plus Cough **719**
PediaCare NightRest
Cough-Cold Liquid **719**
Percogesic Aspirin-Free Coated
Tablets....................................**667**
Extra Strength Percogesic
Aspirin-Free Coated Caplets......**665**
Relief Nasal & Throat Spray.........**811**
Robitussin Cold Caplets
Cold & Congestion...................**780**
Robitussin Cold Softgels
Cold & Congestion...................**780**
Robitussin Cold Caplets
Multi-Symptom Cold & Flu **781**
Robitussin Cold Softgels
Multi-Symptom Cold & Flu **781**
Robitussin Cold Softgels
Severe Congestion...................**782**
Robitussin Cough Drops..............**781**
Robitussin Honey Cough Drops....**784**
Robitussin Honey Cough Liquid....**784**
Robitussin Cough & Cold
Infant Drops **782**
Robitussin Maximum Strength
Cough & Cold Liquid **785**
Robitussin Pediatric
Cough & Cold Formula Liquid ...**785**
Robitussin Maximum Strength
Cough Suppressant Liquid........**784**
Robitussin Pediatric Cough
Suppressant Liquid...................**784**
Robitussin Multi Symptom
Honey Flu Liquid......................**785**
Robitussin Nighttime
Honey Flu Liquid **786**
Robitussin Honey Calmers
Throat Drops **783**
Robitussin Sugar Free
Throat Drops **786**
Robitussin-CF Liquid....................**783**
Robitussin DM Infant Drops.........**783**
Robitussin-DM Liquid **783**
Robitussin-PE Liquid....................**782**
Ryna Liquid **768**
Ryna-C Liquid **768**
Singlet Caplets **761**
Sinutab Non-Drying Liquid
Caps.......................................**706**
Sinutab Sinus Allergy
Medication, Maximum
Strength Formula,
Tablets & Caplets **707**
Sinutab Sinus Medication,
Maximum Strength
Without Drowsiness Formula,
Tablets & Caplets **707**
Children's Sudafed
Cold & Cough Liquid **709**
Sudafed Cold & Allergy
Tablets....................................**708**

Sudafed Cold & Cough
Liquid Caps.............................**709**
Sudafed Cold & Sinus
Liquid Caps.............................**710**
Sudafed Non-Drying Sinus
Liquid Caps.............................**712**
Sudafed Severe Cold Formula
Caplets **711**
Sudafed Severe Cold Formula
Tablets....................................**711**
Sudafed Sinus Headache
Caplets **712**
Sudafed Sinus Headache
Tablets....................................**712**
Tavist 12 Hour Allergy Tablets......**676**
Tavist Sinus Non-Drowsy
Coated Caplets........................**676**
TheraFlu Regular Strength
Cold & Cough Night Time
Hot Liquid **676**
TheraFlu Regular Strength
Cold & Sore Throat
Night Time Hot Liquid **676**
TheraFlu Maximum Strength
Flu & Congestion
Non-Drowsy Hot Liquid **677**
TheraFlu Maximum Strength
Flu & Cough Night Time
Hot Liquid **678**
TheraFlu Maximum Strength
Flu & Sore Throat
Night Time Hot Liquid **677**
TheraFlu Maximum Strength
Severe Cold & Congestion
Night Time Caplets **678**
TheraFlu Maximum Strength
Severe Cold & Congestion
Night Time Hot Liquid **678**
TheraFlu Maximum Strength
Severe Cold & Congestion
Non-Drowsy Caplets.................**679**
TheraFlu Maximum Strength
Severe Cold & Congestion
Non-Drowsy Hot Liquid **679**
Triaminic Chest Congestion
Liquid **680**
Triaminic Cold & Allergy
Liquid **681**
Triaminic Cold & Allergy
Softchews **683**
Triaminic Cold & Cough Liquid **681**
Triaminic Cold & Cough
Softchews **683**
Triaminic Cold & Night Time
Cough Liquid **681**
Triaminic Cold, Cough & Fever
Liquid **681**
Triaminic Cough Liquid **682**
Triaminic Cough Softchews..........**684**
Triaminic Cough & Congestion
Liquid **682**
Triaminic Cough &
Sore Throat Liquid **682**

Triaminic Cough & Sore Throat
Softchews **684**
Triaminic Vapor Patch-
Cherry Scent **684**
Triaminic Vapor Patch-
Menthol Scent..............................**684**
Children's Tylenol
Suspension Liquid and
Soft Chews Chewable Tablets...**657**
Children's Tylenol Allergy-D
Liquid **658**
Children's Tylenol Cold
Suspension Liquid and
Chewable Tablets........................**659**
Children's Tylenol Cold Plus
Cough Suspension Liquid
and Chewable Tablets **659**
Children's Tylenol Flu
Suspension Liquid **663**
Children's Tylenol Sinus
Suspension Liquid **663**
Infants' Tylenol Cold
Decongestant & Fever
Reducer Concentrated Drops....**659**
Infants' Tylenol Cold
Decongestant & Fever
Reducer Concentrated
Drops Plus Cough **659**
Infants' Tylenol
Concentrated Drops **657**
Junior Strength Tylenol
Soft Chews Chewable Tablets...**657**
Extra Strength Tylenol Adult
Liquid Pain Reliever **647**
Extra Strength Tylenol
Gelcaps, Geltabs,
Caplets, and Tablets **647**
Regular Strength Tylenol
Tablets...**647**
Maximum Strength Tylenol
Allergy Sinus Caplets,
Gelcaps, and Geltabs................**649**
Maximum Strength Tylenol
Allergy Sinus NightTime
Caplets **649**
Tylenol Severe Allergy Caplets **649**
Tylenol Arthritis Pain
Extended Relief Caplets **647**
Multi-Symptom Tylenol Cold
Complete Formula Caplets **651**
Multi-Symptom Tylenol Cold
Non-Drowsy Caplets
and Gelcaps...............................**651**
Multi-Symptom Tylenol Cold
Severe Congestion
Non-Drowsy Caplets.................**652**
Maximum Strength Tylenol
Flu NightTime Gelcaps **653**
Maximum Strength Tylenol
Flu NightTime Liquid **653**
Maximum Strength Tylenol
Flu Non-Drowsy Gelcaps...........**653**
Extra Strength Tylenol PM
Caplets, Geltabs, and
Gelcaps **654**

Maximum Strength Tylenol
Sinus NightTime Caplets **655**
Maximum Strength Tylenol
Sinus Non-Drowsy Geltabs,
Gelcaps, Caplets, and
Tablets...**655**
Maximum Strength Tylenol
Sore Throat Adult Liquid...........**656**
Unisom Maximum Strength
SleepGels **713**
Vanquish Caplets **617**
Vicks 44 Cough Relief Liquid **724**
Vicks 44D Cough & Head
Congestion Relief Liquid............**724**
Vicks 44E Cough & Chest
Congestion Relief Liquid............**725**
Pediatric Vicks 44e
Cough & Chest Congestion
Relief Liquid **728**
Vicks 44M Cough, Cold & Flu
Relief Liquid **725**
Pediatric Vicks 44m
Cough & Cold Relief..................**728**
Vicks Cough Drops, Menthol
and Cherry Flavors....................**726**
Vicks DayQuil
LiquiCaps/Liquid
Multi-Symptom
Cold/Flu Relief **727**
Children's Vicks NyQuil
Cold/Cough Relief **726**
Vicks NyQuil
LiquiCaps/Liquid
Multi-Symptom
Cold/Flu Relief,
Original and Cherry Flavors.......**727**
Vicks Sinex Nasal Spray
and Ultra Fine Mist **729**
Vicks Sinex 12-Hour
Nasal Spray and
Ultra Fine Mist...........................**729**
Vicks Vapor Inhaler **730**
Vicks VapoRub Cream **730**
Vicks VapoRub Ointment **730**
Vicks VapoSteam **730**

RHINITIS, NONALLERGIC

May be treated with nasal steroids or ipratropium bromide. The following products may be recommended for relief of symptoms:

Benadryl Allergy Chewables **689**
Benadryl Allergy Kapseal
Capsules....................................**691**
Benadryl Allergy Liquid **690**
Benadryl Allergy Ultratab
Tablets...**691**
Benadryl Dye-Free Allergy
Liquid **690**
Benadryl Dye-Free Allergy
Liqui-Gels Softgels **690**
Chlor-Trimeton Allergy Tablets **735**
Tavist 12 Hour Allergy Tablets......**676**
Tylenol Severe Allergy Caplets **649**
Unisom Maximum Strength
SleepGels **713**

RHINITIS, NONALLERGIC VASOMOTOR

May be treated with nasal steroids or ipratropium bromide. The following products may be recommended for relief of symptoms:

Actifed Cold & Allergy Tablets **688**
Benadryl Allergy/Congestion
Tablets.....................................**692**
Benadryl Allergy & Sinus Liquid ...**693**
Benadryl Allergy & Sinus
Fastmelt Tablets......................**693**
Benadryl Allergy Sinus
Headache Caplets & Gelcaps ...**693**
Chlor-Trimeton Allergy/
Decongestant Tablets **736**
Contac Non-Drowsy 12 Hour
Cold Caplets **745**
Contac Non-Drowsy
Timed Release
12 Hour Cold Caplets **746**
Dimetapp Elixir **777**
Drixoral Cold & Allergy
Sustained-Action Tablets **740**
NasalCrom Nasal Spray...............**719**
Ryna Liquid **768**
Sudafed Cold & Allergy
Tablets......................................**708**
TheraFlu Regular Strength
Cold & Sore Throat
Night Time Hot Liquid **676**
Triaminic Cold & Allergy Liquid **681**
Triaminic Cold & Allergy
Softchews **683**
Maximum Strength Tylenol
Allergy Sinus Caplets,
Gelcaps, and Geltabs...............**649**
Maximum Strength Tylenol
Allergy Sinus NightTime
Caplets **649**

SERUM-SICKNESSLIKE REACTIONS

May result from the use of amoxicillin, amoxicillin-clavulanate, penicillins, sulfamethoxazole-trimethoprim, antivenin (crotalidae) polyvalent, antivenin (micrurus fulvius), metronidazole, ofloxacin, streptomycin sulfate, sulfadoxine, sulfamethoxazole or sulfasalazine. The following products may be recommended:

Benadryl Allergy Chewables **689**
Benadryl Allergy Kapseal
Capsules...................................**691**
Benadryl Allergy Liquid **690**
Benadryl Allergy Ultratab
Tablets......................................**691**
Benadryl Dye-Free Allergy
Liquid **690**
Benadryl Dye-Free Allergy
Liqui-Gels Softgels **690**
Chlor-Trimeton Allergy Tablets **735**
Tavist 12 Hour Allergy Tablets......**676**
Tylenol Severe Allergy Caplets **649**
Unisom Maximum Strength
SleepGels **713**

SINUSITIS

May be treated with amoxicillin, amoxicillin-clavulanate, cefprozil, cefuroxime axetil, clarithromycin or loracarbef. The following products may be recommended for relief of symptoms:

Actifed Cold & Allergy Tablets **688**
Actifed Cold & Sinus
    Caplets and Tablets **688**
Advil Caplets **771**
Advil Gel Caplets **771**
Advil Liqui-Gels **771**
Advil Tablets **771**
Children's Advil
    Oral Suspension **773**
Children's Advil
    Chewable Tablets **773**
Advil Cold and Sinus Caplets **771**
Advil Cold and Sinus Tablets........**771**
Advil Flu & Body Ache Caplets **772**
Infants' Advil Drops.....................**773**
Junior Strength Advil Tablets........**773**
Junior Strength Advil
    Chewable Tablets.....................**773**
Afrin Original Nasal Spray **733**
Afrin Extra Moisturizing
    Nasal Spray **733**
Afrin Severe Congestion
    Nasal Spray **733**
Afrin Sinus Nasal Spray...............**733**
Afrin No Drip Original
    Nasal Spray **735**
Afrin No Drip
    Extra Moisturizing
    Nasal Spray **735**
Afrin No Drip Severe
    Congestion Nasal Spray **735**
Afrin No Drip Sinus
    Nasal Spray **735**
Afrin Original Pump Mist..............**733**
Afrin Saline Aromatic Mist **734**
Aleve Tablets, Caplets
    and Gelcaps...........................**602**
Aleve Cold & Sinus Caplets **603**
Alka-Seltzer Plus Cold
    Medicine Liqui-Gels.................**604**
Alka-Seltzer Plus Cold &
    Cough Medicine Liqui-Gels **604**
Alka-Seltzer Plus Cold & Sinus
    Medicine Liqui-Gels.................**604**
Alka-Seltzer PM
    Effervescent Tablets **605**
Genuine Bayer Tablets,
    Caplets and Gelcaps...............**606**
Extra Strength Bayer
    Caplets and Gelcaps...............**610**
Aspirin Regimen Bayer Adult
    Low Strength 81 mg Tablets.....**606**
Aspirin Regimen Bayer Regular
    Strength 325 mg Caplets.........**606**
Genuine Bayer
    Professional Labeling
    (Aspirin Regimen Bayer) **608**

Extra Strength Bayer Arthritis
    Caplets **610**
Extra Strength Bayer Plus
    Caplets **610**
Extra Strength Bayer PM
    Caplets **611**
BC Powder **619**
BC Allergy Sinus Cold Powder......**619**
Arthritis Strength BC Powder **619**
BC Sinus Cold Powder.................**619**
Benadryl Allergy/Cold Tablets......**691**
Benadryl Allergy/Congestion
    Tablets..................................**692**
Benadryl Allergy & Sinus Liquid ...**693**
Benadryl Allergy Sinus
    Headache Caplets & Gelcaps ...**693**
Benadryl Severe Allergy &
    Sinus Headache Caplets **694**
Children's Cēpacol
    Sore Throat Formula,
    Cherry Flavor Liquid **788**
Children's Cēpacol
    Sore Throat Formula,
    Grape Flavor Liquid **788**
Chlor-Trimeton Allergy/
    Decongestant Tablets **736**
Comtrex Acute Head Cold &
    Sinus Pressure Relief
    Tablets..................................**627**
Comtrex Flu Therapy & Fever
    Relief Daytime Caplets.............**628**
Contac Non-Drowsy 12 Hour
    Cold Caplets **745**
Contac Non-Drowsy
    Timed Release
    12 Hour Cold Caplets **746**
Dimetapp Elixir **777**
Dimetapp Cold and Fever
    Suspension............................**775**
Dimetapp Infant Drops
    Decongestant.........................**775**
Drixoral Allergy/Sinus
    Extended-Release Tablets.........**741**
Drixoral Cold & Allergy
    Sustained-Action Tablets **740**
Drixoral Cold & Flu
    Extended-Release Tablets.........**740**
Drixoral Nasal Decongestant
    Long-Acting Non-Drowsy
    Tablets..................................**740**
Ecotrin Enteric Coated Aspirin
    Low Strength Tablets **747**
Ecotrin Enteric Coated Aspirin
    Maximum Strength Tablets **747**
Ecotrin Enteric Coated Aspirin
    Regular Strength Tablets **747**
Aspirin Free Excedrin Caplets
    and Geltabs **628**
Excedrin Extra-Strength
    Tablets, Caplets, and
    Geltabs **629**
Excedrin PM Tablets,
    Caplets, and Geltabs **631**

Goody's Extra Strength
    Headache Powder...................**620**
Goody's Extra Strength
    Pain Relief Tablets..................**620**
Goody's PM Powder **621**
Momentum Backache Relief
    Extra Strength Caplets **666**
Children's Motrin
    Oral Suspension and
    Chewable Tablets....................**643**
Children's Motrin Cold
    Oral Suspension **646**
Infants' Motrin
    Concentrated Drops.................**643**
Junior Strength Motrin
    Caplets and Chewable
    Tablets..................................**643**
Motrin IB Tablets,
    Caplets, and Gelcaps...............**642**
Motrin Sinus/Headache
    Caplets **643**
Natru-Vent Nasal Spray,
    Adult Strength **624**
Natru-Vent Nasal Spray,
    Pediatric Strength **625**
Neo-Synephrine Nasal Drops,
    Regular and Extra Strength.......**614**
Neo-Synephrine Nasal Sprays,
    Mild, Regular and
    Extra Strength **614**
Neo-Synephrine 12 Hour
    Nasal Spray **615**
Orudis KT Tablets **778**
PediaCare Infants' Drops
    Decongestant.........................**719**
Percogesic Aspirin-Free Coated
    Tablets..................................**667**
Extra Strength Percogesic
    Aspirin-Free Coated Caplets......**665**
Ryna Liquid **768**
Singlet Caplets **761**
Sinutab Non-Drying Liquid Caps ...**706**
Sinutab Sinus Allergy
    Medication, Maximum
    Strength Formula, Tablets
    & Caplets..............................**707**
Sinutab Sinus Medication,
    Maximum Strength Without
    Drowsiness Formula,
    Tablets & Caplets **707**
Sudafed 12 Hour Tablets.............**708**
Sudafed 24 Hour Tablets.............**708**
Children's Sudafed Nasal
    Decongestant Chewables.........**711**
Children's Sudafed Nasal
    Decongestant Liquid
    Medication **711**
Sudafed Cold & Allergy Tablets **708**
Sudafed Cold & Sinus
    Liquid Caps...........................**710**
Sudafed Nasal Decongestant
    Tablets..................................**710**
Sudafed Non-Drying Sinus
    Liquid Caps **712**
Sudafed Sinus Headache
    Caplets **712**

Sudafed Sinus Headache
Tablets.....................................**712**
Tavist Sinus Non-Drowsy
Coated Caplets.........................**676**
TheraFlu Regular Strength
Cold & Sore Throat
Night Time Hot Liquid **676**
TheraFlu Maximum Strength
Flu & Sore Throat
Night Time Hot Liquid **677**
Triaminic Allergy Congestion
Liquid **680**
Triaminic Chest Congestion
Liquid **680**
Triaminic Cold & Allergy Liquid **681**
Triaminic Cold & Allergy
Softchews **683**
Triaminic Cold & Cough Liquid **681**
Triaminic Cold & Night Time
Cough Liquid **681**
Triaminic Cold, Cough &
Fever Liquid............................**681**
Triaminic Cough &
Sore Throat Liquid **682**
Triaminic Cough &
Sore Throat Softchews.............**684**
Children's Tylenol
Suspension Liquid and
Soft Chews Chewable Tablets...**657**
Children's Tylenol Allergy-D
Liquid **658**
Children's Tylenol Cold
Suspension Liquid and
Chewable Tablets.....................**659**
Children's Tylenol Sinus
Suspension Liquid **663**
Infants' Tylenol Cold
Decongestant &
Fever Reducer
Concentrated Drops.................**659**
Infants' Tylenol
Concentrated Drops.................**657**
Junior Strength Tylenol
Soft Chews Chewable Tablets...**657**
Extra Strength Tylenol Adult
Liquid Pain Reliever **647**
Extra Strength Tylenol
Geltabs, Caplets,
and Tablets.............................**647**
Regular Strength Tylenol
Tablets...................................**647**
Maximum Strength Tylenol
Allergy Sinus Caplets,
Gelcaps, and Geltabs...............**649**
Maximum Strength Tylenol
Allergy Sinus NightTime
Caplets **649**
Tylenol Arthritis Pain
Extended Relief Caplets **647**
Multi-Symptom Tylenol Cold
Severe Congestion
Non-Drowsy Caplets **652**
Maximum Strength Tylenol Flu
NightTime Gelcaps....................**653**
Maximum Strength Tylenol Flu
NightTime Liquid......................**653**

Extra Strength Tylenol PM
Caplets, Geltabs,
and Gelcaps............................**654**
Maximum Strength Tylenol
Sinus NightTime Caplets **655**
Maximum Strength Tylenol
Sinus Non-Drowsy Geltabs,
Gelcaps, Caplets,
and Tablets **655**
Maximum Strength Tylenol
Sore Throat Adult Liquid...........**656**
Vanquish Caplets **617**
Vicks Sinex Nasal Spray
and Ultra Fine Mist **729**
Vicks Sinex 12-Hour
Nasal Spray and
Ultra Fine Mist........................**729**
Vicks Vapor Inhaler **730**

SINUSITIS, HALITOSIS SECONDARY TO
Sinusitis may be treated with amoxicillin,
amoxicillin-clavulanate, cefprozil, cefuroxime axetil, clarithromycin or loracarbef.
The following products may be recommended for relief of halitosis:

Cēpacol Antiseptic
Mouthwash/Gargle, Original **786**
Cēpacol Antiseptic
Mouthwash/Gargle, Mint..........**786**
Certs Cool Mint Drops **685**
Certs Powerful Mints **686**
Listerine Mouthrinse....................**702**
Cool Mint Listerine
Mouthrinse..............................**702**
FreshBurst Listerine
Mouthrinse..............................**702**
Tartar Control Listerine
Mouthrinse..............................**702**
Listermint Alcohol-Free
Mouthrinse..............................**703**
Trident Advantage Mints **687**
Trident Advantage
Sugarless Gum.........................**687**

SKIN IRRITATION
May result from the use of transdermal
drug delivery systems. The following
products may be recommended:

Anusol HC-1 Hydrocortisone
Anti-Itch Cream.......................**689**
Benadryl Itch Relief Stick
Extra Strength **695**
Benadryl Itch Stopping Cream
Original Strength......................**695**
Benadryl Itch Stopping Cream
Extra Strength **695**
Benadryl Itch Stopping Gel
Original Strength......................**695**
Benadryl Itch Stopping Gel
Extra Strength **695**
Cortaid Intensive Therapy
Cream.....................................**717**
Cortaid Maximum Strength
Cream.....................................**717**
Cortaid Maximum Strength
Ointment.................................**717**
Cortaid Sensitive Skin Cream **717**

Cortizone·5 Creme.....................**699**
Cortizone·5 Ointment.................**699**
Cortizone·10 Creme...................**699**
Cortizone·10 Ointment...............**699**
Cortizone·10 Plus Creme **700**
Cortizone·10 Quick Shot Spray ...**699**
Cortizone for Kids Creme **699**

STOMATITIS, APHTHOUS
May result from the use of selective
serotonin reuptake inhibitors,
aldesleukin, clomipramine hydrochloride,
didanosine, foscarnet sodium, indinavir
sulfate, indomethacin, interferon alfa-2B,
recombinant, methotrexate sodium,
naproxen, naproxen sodium, nicotine
polacrilex or stavudine. The following
products may be recommended:

Cēpacol Maximum Strength
Sugar Free Sore Throat
Lozenges, Cherry Flavor..........**787**
Cēpacol Maximum Strength
Sugar Free Sore Throat
Lozenges, Cool Mint Flavor.......**787**
Cēpacol Maximum Strength
Sore Throat Lozenges,
Cherry Flavor...........................**787**
Cēpacol Maximum Strength
Sore Throat Lozenges,
Mint Flavor **787**
Cēpacol Regular Strength
Sore Throat Lozenges,
Cherry Flavor...........................**787**
Cēpacol Regular Strength
Sore Throat Lozenges,
Original Mint Flavor **787**
Cēpacol Maximum Strength
Sore Throat Spray,
Cherry Flavor...........................**787**
Cēpacol Viractin Cold Sore
and Fever Blister
Treatment, Cream....................**788**
Cēpacol Viractin Cold Sore
and Fever Blister Treatment,
Gel **788**
Gly-Oxide Liquid **751**
Zilactin Gel **790**
Zilactin-B Gel **790**
Zilactin-L Liquid..........................**790**

TASTE DISTURBANCES
May result from the use of biguanides,
acetazolamide, butorphanol tartrate, captopril, cefuroxime axetil, clarithromycin,
etidronate disodium, felbamate, flu-
nisolide, gemfibrozil, griseofulvin, interferon alfa-2B, recombinant, lithium carbonate, lithium citrate, mesna, metron-
idazole, nedocromil sodium, penicil-
lamine, rifampin or succimer. The following products may be recommended:

Cēpacol Antiseptic
Mouthwash/Gargle, Original **786**
Cēpacol Antiseptic
Mouthwash/Gargle, Mint..........**786**

TASTE DISTURBANCES —cont.

Certs Cool Mint Drops **685**
Certs Powerful Mints **686**
Listerine Mouthrinse **702**
Cool Mint Listerine
   Mouthrinse..............................**702**
FreshBurst Listerine
   Mouthrinse..............................**702**
Tartar Control Listerine
   Mouthrinse..............................**702**
Listermint Alcohol-Free
   Mouthrinse..............................**703**
Trident Advantage Mints **687**
Trident Advantage
   Sugarless Gum........................**687**

TONSILITIS, HALITOSIS SECONDARY TO

Tonsilitis may be treated with erythro-mycin, macrolide antibiotics, cefaclor, cefadroxil, cefixime, cefpodoxime prox-etil, cefprozil, ceftibuten dihydrate or cefuroxime axetil. The following products may be recommended for relief of halitosis:

Cēpacol Antiseptic
   Mouthwash/Gargle, Original **786**
Cēpacol Antiseptic
   Mouthwash/Gargle, Mint..........**786**
Certs Cool Mint Drops **685**
Certs Powerful Mints **686**
Listerine Mouthrinse **702**
Cool Mint Listerine
   Mouthrinse..............................**702**
FreshBurst Listerine
   Mouthrinse..............................**702**
Tartar Control Listerine
   Mouthrinse..............................**702**
Listermint Alcohol-Free
   Mouthrinse..............................**703**
Trident Advantage Mints **687**
Trident Advantage
   Sugarless Gum........................**687**

TUBERCULOSIS, NUTRIENTS DEFICIENCY SECONDARY TO

Tuberculosis may be treated with capreo-mycin sulfate, ethambutol hydrochloride, ethionamide, isoniazid, pyrazinamide, rifampin or streptomycin sulfate. The fol-lowing products may be recommended for relief of nutrients deficiency:

Bugs Bunny Children's
   Multivitamin Plus Iron
   Chewable Tablets.....................**802**
Bugs Bunny Children's
   Multivitamin Plus Extra C
   Chewable Tablets
   (Sugar Free) **804**
Bugs Bunny Complete
   Children's Multivitamin/
   Multimineral Chewable
   Tablets (Sugar Free).................**803**

Centrum Kids Complete
   Children's Chewables **817**
Centrum Performance
   Multivitamin-Multimineral
   Tablets...................................**817**
Centrum Tablets **815**
Centrum Silver Tablets **818**
Flintstones Original Children's
   Multivitamin Chewable
   Tablets...................................**802**
Flintstones Children's
   Multivitamin Plus Calcium
   Chewable Tablets.....................**804**
Flintstones Children's
   Multivitamin Plus Extra C
   Chewable Tablets.....................**804**
Flintstones Children's
   Multivitamin Plus Iron
   Chewable Tablets.....................**802**
Flintstones Complete
   Children's Mutivitamin/
   Multimineral Chewable
   Tablets...................................**803**
One-A-Day Essential Tablets........**806**
One-A-Day 50 Plus Tablets...........**804**
One-A-Day Kids Complete
   Tablets...................................**806**
One-A-Day Maximum Tablets **807**
One-A-Day Men's Tablets **808**
One-A-Day Women's Tablets........**809**
Pro-Xtreme Drink Mix..................**845**

VAGINOSIS, BACTERIAL

May be treated with sulfabenzamide/ sulfacetamide/sulfathiozole or metron-idazole. The following products may be recommended for relief of symptoms:

Massengill Feminine
   Cleansing Wash.......................**753**
Massengill Disposable Douches ..**752**
Massengill Baby Powder
   Scent Soft Cloth Towelette **753**
Massengill Medicated
   Disposable Douche...................**753**

VULVOVAGINITIS, CANDIDAL

May result from the use of estrogen-con-taining oral contraceptives, immunosup-pressants or recent broad-spectrum antibiotic therapy. The following products may be recommended:

Gyne-Lotrimin 3, 3-Day Cream......**741**
Mycelex-3 Vaginal Cream with
   3 Disposable Applicators **613**
Mycelex-3 Vaginal Cream in
   3 Pre-filled Applicators **613**
Mycelex-7 Combination-Pack
   Vaginal Inserts & External
   Vulvar Cream...........................**614**
Mycelex-7 Vaginal Cream.............**614**
Mycelex-7 Vaginal Cream with
   7 Disposable Applicators **614**

XERODERMA

May result from the use of aldesleukin, protease inhibitors, retinoids, topical acne preparations, topical corticos-teroids, topical retinoids, benzoyl perox-ide, clofazimine, interferon alfa-2A, recombinant, interferon alfa-2B, recombi-nant or pentostatin. The following prod-ucts may be recommended:

Lubriderm Advanced Therapy
   Creamy Lotion **703**
Lubriderm Seriously Sensitive
   Lotion **703**
Lubriderm Skin Therapy
   Moisturizing Lotion...................**703**
StePHan Bio-Nutritional
   Daytime Hydrating Creme.........**770**
StePHan Bio-Nutritional
   Nightime Moisture Creme.........**770**
StePHan Bio-Nutritional
   Ultra Hydrating Fluid.................**770**

XEROMYCTERIA

May result from the use of anticholiner-gics, antihistamines, retinoids, apracloni-dine hydrochloride, clonidine, etretinate, ipratropium bromide, isotretinoin or lodoxamide tromethamine.The following products may be recommended:

Afrin Extra Moisturizing
   Saline Mist...............................**734**
Natru-Vent Saline Nasal Spray **625**
Ocean Nasal Mist **633**

XEROSTOMIA

May result from the use of anticholinergics, antidepressants, diuretics, phenothiazines, alprazolam, bromocriptine mesylate, buspirone hydrochloride, butorphanol tartrate, clomipramine hydrochloride, clonidine, clozapine, dexfenfluramine hydrochloride, didanosine, disopyramide phosphate, etretinate, flumazenil, fluvoxamine maleate, guanfacine hydrochloride, isotretinoin, leuprolide acetate, pergolide mesylate, selegiline hydrochloride, tramadol hydrochloride or zolpidem tartrate. The following products may be recommended:

Cēpacol Antiseptic
   Mouthwash/Gargle, Original **786**
Cēpacol Antiseptic
   Mouthwash/Gargle, Mint..........**786**
Listerine Mouthrinse **702**
Cool Mint Listerine Mouthrinse **702**
FreshBurst Listerine
   Mouthrinse..............................**702**
Tartar Control Listerine
   Mouthrinse..............................**702**
Listermint Alcohol-Free
   Mouthrinse..............................**703**

DRUG INFORMATION CENTERS

For additional information on overdosage, adverse reactions, drug interactions, and any other medication problem, specialized drug information centers are strategically located throughout the nation. Use the directory that follows to find the center nearest you. Listings are alphabetical by state and city.

ALABAMA

BIRMINGHAM

Drug Information Service
University of Alabama
Hospital
619 S. 20th St.
1720 Jefferson Tower
Birmingham, AL 35249-6860
Mon.-Fri. 8 AM-5 PM
205-934-2162
Fax: 205-934-3501

Global Drug Information Center
Samford University
McWhorter School of Pharmacy
800 Lakeshore Dr.
Birmingham, AL 35229-7027
Mon.-Fri. 8 AM-4:30 PM
205-870-2659
Fax: 205-726-4012
samford. edu.schools/
pharmacy/dic/index.html

HUNTSVILLE

Huntsville Hospital Drug Information Center
101 Sivley Rd.
Huntsville, AL 35801
Mon.-Fri. 8 AM-5 PM
256-517-8284
Fax: 256-517-6558

ARIZONA

TUCSON

Arizona Poison and Drug Information Center
Arizona Health Sciences Center
University Medical Center
1501 N. Campbell Ave.
Room 1156
Tucson, AZ 85724
7 days/week, 24 hours
520-626-6016
800-362-0101 (AZ)
Fax: 520-626-2720

ARKANSAS

LITTLE ROCK

Arkansas Poison and Drug Information Center
4301 W. Markham St.,
Slot 522-2
Little Rock, AK 72205
7 days/week, 7 AM-Midnight
501-686-5540
Fax: 501-686-7357

CALIFORNIA

LOS ANGELES

Los Angeles Regional Drug Information Center
LAC & USC Medical Center
1200 N. State St.
Room 1107 A & B
Los Angeles, CA 90033
Mon.-Fri. 8AM-4:30PM
323-226-7741
Fax: 323-226-4194

SAN DIEGO

Drug Information Center
U.S. Naval Hospital
34800 Bob Wilson Dr.
San Diego, CA 92134-5000
Mon.-Fri. 8 AM-4 PM
619-532-8417
Fax: 619-352-5898

Drug Information Service
University of California
San Diego Medical Center
135 Dickinson St.
San Diego, CA 92103-8925
Mon.-Fri. 9 AM-5 PM
900-288-8273
Fax: 858-715-6323

STANFORD

Drug Information Center
Stanford Hospital and Clinics Department of Pharmacy
300 Pasteur Dr.
Room H-0301
Stanford, CA 94305
Mon.-Fri. 8 AM-4 PM
650-723-6422
Fax: 650-725-5028

COLORADO

DENVER

Rocky Mountain Poison and Drug Consultation Center
1010 Yosemite Circle
Denver, CO 80230
Mon.-Fri. 8 AM-4:30 PM
303-893-3784
(For Denver County residents only)
Fax: 303-739-1119

Drug Information Center
University of Colorado
Health Science Center
4200 E. 9th Ave., Box C239
Denver, CO 80262
Mon.-Fri. 8:30 AM-4:30 PM
303-315-8489
Fax: 303-315-3353

CONNECTICUT

FARMINGTON

Drug Information Service
University of Connecticut
Health Center
263 Farmington Ave.
Farmington, CT 06030
Mon.-Fri. 7 AM-4 PM
860-679-2783
Fax: 860-679-1231
wnelson@nso.uchc.edu

HARTFORD

Drug Information Center
Hartford Hospital
P.O. Box 5037
80 Seymour St.
Hartford, CT 06102
Mon.-Fri. 8:30 AM-5 PM
860-545-2221
860-545-2961
Fax: 860-545-4371

NEW HAVEN

Drug Information Center
Yale-New Haven Hospital
20 York St.
New Haven, CT 06504
Mon.-Fri. 12 PM-4:30 PM
203-688-2248
Fax: 203-688-3691

DISTRICT OF COLUMBIA

Drug Information Service
Howard University Hospital
Room BB06
2041 Georgia Ave. NW
Washington, DC 20060
7 days/week, 24 hours
202-865-1325
Fax: 202-865-7410

FLORIDA

GAINESVILLE

Drug Information & Pharmacy Resource Center
SHANDS Hospital at University of Florida
P.O. Box 100316
Gainesville, FL 32610-0316
Mon.-Fri. 9 AM-5 PM
352-395-0408
(for healthcare professionals only)
Fax: 352-338-9860

JACKSONVILLE

Drug Information Service
SHANDS Jacksonville
655 W. 8th St.
Jacksonville, FL 32209
Mon.-Fri. 8 AM-5 PM
904-244-4185
Fax: 904-244-4272

MIAMI

Drug Information Center (119)
Miami VA Medical Center
1201 NW 16th St.
Pharmacy 119
Miami, FL 33125
Mon.-Fri. 7:00 AM-3:30 PM
305-324-3237
(for healthcare professionals only)
Fax: 305-324-3394

ORLANDO

Orlando Regional Drug Information Service Orlando Regional Healthcare System
1414 Kuhl Ave., MP 192
Orlando, FL 32806
Mon.-Fri. 8 AM-5 PM
    407-841-5111,
      ext. 8717
Fax: 407-650-9052

TALLAHASSEE

Drug Information Education Center Florida Agricultural and Mechanical University College of Pharmacy
Honor House, Room 200
Tallahassee, FL 32307
Mon.-Fri. 9 AM-5 PM
    850-488-5239
    850-599-3064
    800-451-3181
Fax: 850-412-7020

GEORGIA

ATLANTA

Emory University Hospital Dept. of Pharmaceutical Services-Drug Information
1364 Clifton Rd. NE
Atlanta, GA 30322
Mon.-Fri. 8:30 AM-5 PM
    404-712-4640
Fax: 404-712-7577

Drug Information Service Northside Hospital
1000 Johnson Ferry Rd. NE
Atlanta, GA 30342
Mon.-Fri. 9 AM-4 PM
    404-851-8676 (GA)
Fax: 404-851-8682

AUGUSTA

Drug Information Center University of Georgia Medical College of GA
Room BIW201
1120 15th St.
Augusta, GA 30912-5600
Mon.-Fri. 8:30 AM-5 PM
    706-721-2887
Fax: 706-721-3827

IDAHO

POCATELLO

Idaho Drug Information Service
Campus Box 8092
Pocatello, ID 83209
Mon.-Fri. 8 AM-5 PM
    208-282-4689
Fax: 208-282-3003

ILLINOIS

CHICAGO

Drug Information Center Northwestern Memorial Hospital
251 E. Huron
Feinberg LC-700B
Chicago, IL 60611
Mon.-Fri. 8 AM-5 PM
    312-926-7573
Fax: 312-926-7956

Saint Joseph Hospital Pharmacy
2900 N. Lake Shore Dr.
Chicago, IL 60657
7 days/week, 24 hours
    773-665-3140
Fax: 773-665-3462

Drug Information Services University of Chicago
5841 S. Maryland Ave.
MC 0010
Chicago, IL 60637
Mon.-Fri. 8 AM-5 PM
    773-702-1388
Fax: 773-702-6631

Drug Information Center University of Illinois at Chicago
833 S. Wood St.
Chicago, IL 60612
Mon.-Fri. 8 AM-4 PM
    312-996-0209
Fax: 312-996-0448

HARVEY

Drug Information Center Ingalls Memorial Hospital
1 Ingalls Dr.
Harvey, IL 60426
Mon.-Fri. 8 AM-4:30 PM
    708-915-6413
    800-543-6543 (IL)
Fax: 708-915-4609

HINES

Drug Information Service Hines Veterans Administration Hospital
Inpatient Pharmacy (119B)
P.O. Box 5000
Hines, IL 60141-5000
Mon.-Fri. 8 AM-4:30 PM
    708-202-8387
Fax: 708-202-2201

PARK RIDGE

Drug Information Center Lutheran General Hospital
1775 Dempster St.
Park Ridge, IL 60068
Mon.-Fri. 7:30 AM-4 PM
    847-723-8128
Fax: 847-723-2326

INDIANA

INDIANAPOLIS

Drug Information Center St. Vincent Hospital and Health Services
2001 W. 86th St.
P.O. Box 40970
Indianapolis, IN 46240
Mon.-Fri. 8 AM-4 PM
    317-338-3200
(for healthcare professionals only)
Fax: 317-338-3041

IOWA

DES MOINES

Regional Drug Information Center Mercy Medical Center-Des Moines
1111 Sixth Ave.
Des Moines, IA 50314
Mon.-Fri. 8 AM-4:30 PM
    515-247-3286
    (answered 7 days/week, 24 hours)
Fax: 515-247-3966

IOWA CITY

Drug Information Center University of Iowa Hospitals and Clinics
200 Hawkins Dr.
Iowa City, IA 52242
Mon.-Fri. 8 AM-5 PM
    319-356-2600
(for healthcare professionals only)
Fax: 319-384-8840

SIOUX CITY

Iowa Statewide Poison Center
2720 Stone Park Blvd.
Sioux City, IA 51104
7 days/week, 24 hours
    712-277-2222
    800-352-2222 (IA)
Fax: 712-234-8775

KANSAS

KANSAS CITY

Drug Information Center University of Kansas Medical Center
3901 Rainbow Blvd.
Kansas City, KS 66160
Mon.-Fri. 8 AM-6 PM
    913-588-2328
(for healthcare professionals only)
Fax: 913-588-2350

KENTUCKY

LEXINGTON

Drug Information Center Chandler Medical Center College of Pharmacy University of Kentucky
800 Rose St., C-117
Lexington, KY 40536-0293
Mon.-Fri. 8 AM-5 PM
    606-323-5320
Fax: 606-323-2049

LOUISIANA

NEW ORLEANS

Xavier University Drug Information Center Tulane University Hospital and Clinic
Box HC12
1415 Tulane Ave.
New Orleans, LA 70112
Mon.-Fri. 9 AM-5 PM
    504-588-5670
Fax: 504-588-5862
mharris@tulane.edu

MARYLAND

ANDREWS AFB

Drug Information Services
89 MDTS/SGQP
1050 W. Perimeter Rd.
Suite D1-119
Andrews AFB, MD 20762-6660
Mon.-Fri. 7:30 AM-6 PM
    240-857-4565
Fax: 240-857-8892

ANNAPOLIS

The Anne Arundel Medical Center Dept. of Pharmacy
P.O. Box 64
Franklin St.
Annapolis, MD 21401
7 days/week, 24 hours
    410-267-1126
    410-267-1000
    (switchboard)
Fax: 410-267-1628

BALTIMORE

Drug Information Service Johns Hopkins Hospital
600 N. Wolfe St.,
Halsted 503
Baltimore, MD 21287-6180
Mon.-Fri. 8:30 AM-5 PM
    410-955-6348
Fax: 410-955-8283

Drug Information Service University of Maryland at Baltimore School of Pharmacy
506 W. Fayette, 3rd Floor
Baltimore, MD 21201
Mon.-Fri. 8:30 AM-5 PM
    410-706-7568
Fax: 410-706-0897

BETHESDA

**Drug Information Center
National Institutes of
Health**
Building 10, Room 1S-259
10 Center Drive (MSC1196)
Bethesda, MD 20892-1196
Mon.-Fri. 8:30 AM-5 PM
  301-496-2407
Fax: 301-496-0210

EASTON

**Drug Information Pharmacy
Dept.
Memorial Hospital**
219 S. Washington St.
Easton, MD 21601
Mon.-Fri. 7 AM-Midnight
Sat.-Sun. 7 AM-5:30 PM
  410-822-1000
Fax: 410-820-9489

MASSACHUSETTS

BOSTON

**Drug Information Services
Brigham and Women's
Hospital**
75 Frances St.
Boston, MA 02115
Mon.-Fri. 7 AM-3:30 PM
  617-732-7166
Fax: 617-732-7497

**Drug Information Center
New England Medical
Center Pharmacy**
750 Washington St.,
Box 420
Boston, MA 02111
Mon.-Fri. 9 AM-5 PM
  617-636-8985
Fax: 617-636-4567

WORCESTER

**Drug Information Center
U.M.M.H.C. Hospital**
55 Lake Ave. North
Worcester, MA 01655
Mon.-Fri. 8:30 AM-5 PM
  508-856-3456
  508-856-2775
Fax: 508-856-1850

MICHIGAN

ANN ARBOR

**Drug Information and
Pharmacy Services
University of Michigan
Medical Center**
1500 East Medical Center Dr.
UHB2 D301 Box 0008
Ann Arbor, MI 48109/0008
Mon.-Fri. 8 AM-5 PM
  734-936-8200
  734-936-8251
Fax: 734-936-7027

DETROIT

**Drug Information Services
Harper Hospital**
3990 John R. St.
Detroit, MI 48201
Mon.-Fri. 8 AM-5 PM
  313-745-4556
  313-745-2006
Fax: 313-745-1628

PONTIAC

**Drug Information Center
St. Joseph Mercy Hospital**
900 Woodward
Pontiac, MI 48341
Mon.-Fri. 8 AM-4:30 PM
  248-858-3055
Fax: 248-858-3010

ROYAL OAK

**Drug Information Services
William Beaumont Hospital**
3601 West 13 Mile Rd.
Royal Oak, MI 48073-6769
Mon.-Fri. 8 AM-4:30 PM
  248-551-4077
Fax: 248-551-3301

SOUTHFIELD

**Drug Information Service
Providence Hospital**
16001 West 9 Mile Rd.
Southfield, MI 48075
Mon.-Fri. 8 AM-4 PM
  248-424-3125
Fax: 248-424-5364

MISSISSIPPI

JACKSON

**Drug Information Center
University of Mississippi
Medical Center**
2500 N. State St.
Jackson, MS 39216
Mon.-Fri. 8 AM-4:30 PM
  601-984-2060
Fax: 601-984-2064

MISSOURI

KANSAS CITY

**University of Missouri-
Kansas City
Drug Information Center**
2411 Holmes St., MG-200
Kansas City, MO 64108-2792
Mon.-Fri. 8 AM-5 PM
  816-235-5490
Fax: 816-235-5491

SPRINGFIELD

**Drug Information
St. Johns Regional
Health Center**
1235 E. Cherokee
Springfield, MO 65804
Mon.-Fri. 7:30 AM-4:30 PM
  417-885-3488
Fax: 417-888-7788

ST. JOSEPH

**Drug Information Service
Heartland Hospital West**
801 Faraon St.
St. Joseph, MO 64501
Mon.-Fri. 9 AM-5:30 PM
  816-271-7582
Fax: 816-271-7590

MONTANA

MISSOULA

**Drug Information Service
University of Montana
School of Pharmacy
and Allied Health Sciences**
Missoula, MT 59812-1077
Mon.-Fri. 8 AM-5 PM
  406-243-5254
Fax: 406-243-4353

NEBRASKA

OMAHA

**Drug Information Service
School of Pharmacy
Creighton University**
2500 California Plaza
Omaha, NE 68178
Mon.-Fri. 8:30 AM-5:00 PM
  402-280-5101
Fax: 402-280-5149

NEW JERSEY

NEW BRUNSWICK

**Drug Information Service
Robert Wood Johnson
University Hospital
Pharmacy Department**
1 Robert Wood Johnson
Place
New Brunswick, NJ 08901
Mon.-Fri. 8:30 AM-4:30 PM
  732-937-8842
Fax: 732-937-8584

NEWARK

**New Jersey Poison
Information and Education
System**
201 Lyons Ave.
Newark, NJ 07112
7 days/week, 24 hours
  973-926-7443
Fax: 973-926-0013

NEW MEXICO

ALBUQUERQUE

**New Mexico Poison &
Drug Information Center
University of New Mexico**
Albuquerque, NM 87131
7 days/week, 24 hours
  505-272-2222
  800-432-6866 (NM)
Fax: 505-272-5892

NEW YORK

BROOKLYN

**International Drug
Information Center
Long Island University
Arnold & Marie Schwartz
College of Pharmacy &
Health Sciences**
1 University Plaza
RM-HS509
75 Dekalb Ave.
Brooklyn, NY 11201
Mon.-Fri. 9 AM-5 PM
  718-488-1064
Fax: 718-780-4056

**Drug Information Center
Brookdale University
Hospital and Medical
Center**
1 Brookdale Plaza
Brooklyn, NY 11212
Mon.-Fri. 8 AM-4:30 PM
  718-240-5983
Fax: 718-240-5987

COOPERSTOWN

**Drug Information Center
Bassett Healthcare**
1 Atwell Rd.
Cooperstown, NY 13326
Mon.-Fri. 8:30 AM-5 PM
  607-547-3686
Fax: 607-547-3629

JAMAICA

**Drug Information Center
St. John's University
College of Pharmacy and
Allied Health Professions**
8000 Utopia Pkwy.
Jamaica, NY 11439
Mon.-Fri. 8:30 AM-3:30 PM
  718-990-2149
Fax: 718-990-2151

NEW YORK CITY

**Drug Information Center
Bellevue Hospital Center**
462 1st Ave.
New York, NY 10016
7 days/week, 24 hours
  212-562-6501
Fax: 212-562-2949

Drug Information Center
Memorial Sloan-Kettering
Cancer Center
1275 York Ave.
RM S-712
New York, NY 10021
Mon.-Fri. 9 AM-5 PM
212-639-7552
Fax: 212-639-2171

Drug Information Center
Mount Sinai Medical
Center
1 Gustave Levy Pl.
New York, NY 10029
Mon.-Fri. 9 AM-5 PM
212-241-6619
Fax: 212-348-7927

Drug Information Service
New York Presbyterian
Hospital
Room K04
525 E. 68th St.
New York, NY 10021
Mon.-Fri. 9 AM-5 PM
212-746-0741
Fax: 212-746-8506

ROCHESTER
Poison and Drug
Information Center
University of Rochester
601 Elmwood Ave.
Rochester, NY 14642
7 days/week, 24 hours
716-275-3718
716-275-3232
(after 5 PM)
Fax: 716-244-1677

STONY BROOK
Suffolk Drug Information
Center
University Hospital
S.U.N.Y. - Stony Brook
Stony Brook, NY 11794
Mon.-Fri. 8 AM-3:00 PM
631-444-2675
631-444-2680
(after hours)
Fax: 631-444-7935

NORTH CAROLINA
BUIES CREEK
Drug Information Center
School of Pharmacy
Campbell University
P.O. Box 1090
Buies Creek, NC 27506
Mon.-Fri. 8:30 AM-4:30 PM
910-893-1478
800-327-5467 (NC)
Fax: 910-893-1476

CHAPEL HILL
Drug Information Center
University of North
Carolina Hospitals
101 Manning Dr.
Chapel Hill, NC 27514
Mon.-Fri. 8 AM-4:30 PM
919-966-2373
Fax: 919-966-1791

GREENVILLE
Eastern Carolina Drug
Information Center
Pitt County
Memorial Hospital
Dept. of Pharmacy Service
2100 Stantonsburg Rd.
Greenville, NC 27834
Mon.-Fri. 8 AM-5 PM
252-816-4257
Fax: 252-816-7425

WINSTON-SALEM
Drug Information
Service Center
Wake-Forest University
Baptist Medical Center
Medical Center Blvd.
Winston-Salem, NC 27157
Mon.-Fri. 8 AM-5 PM
336-716-2037
Fax: 336-716-2186

NORTH DAKOTA
FARGO
North Dakota Institute for
Pharmaceutical Care
North Dakota State
University
College of Pharmacy
110 Sudro Hall
Fargo, ND 58105-5055
Mon.-Fri. 8:30 AM-4:30 PM
701-231-7939
Fax: 701-231-7606

OHIO
ADA
Drug Information Center
Raabe College of
Pharmacy
Ohio Northern University
Ada, OH 45810
Mon.-Fri. 9 AM-5 PM
419-772-2307
Fax: 419-772-2289

CLEVELAND
Drug Information Center
Cleveland Clinic
Foundation
9500 Euclid Ave.
Cleveland, OH 44195
Mon.-Fri. 8:30 AM-4:30 PM
216-444-6456
Fax: 216-444-6157

COLUMBUS
Drug Information Center
Ohio State University
Hospital
Dept. of Pharmacy
Doan Hall 368
410 W. 10th Ave.
Columbus, OH 43210-1228
Mon.-Fri. 8 AM-4 PM
614-293-8679
Fax: 614-293-3264

Drug Information Center
Riverside Methodist
Hospital
3535 Olentangy River Rd.
Columbus, OH 43214
Mon.-Fri. 8 AM-5 PM
614-566-5425
Fax: 614-566-5447

TOLEDO
Drug Information Services
St. Vincent Mercy Medical
Center
2213 Cherry St.
Toledo, Ohio 43608-2691
Mon.-Fri. 8 AM-4 PM
419-251-4227
Fax: 419-251-3662

OKLAHOMA
OKLAHOMA CITY
Drug Information Service
Integris Health
3300 Northwest
Expressway
Oklahoma City, OK 73112
Mon.-Fri. 8 AM-4:30 PM
405-949-3660
Fax: 405-951-8274

Drug Information Center
Presbyterian Hospital
700 NE 13th St.
Oklahoma City, OK 73104
Mon.-Fri. 8 AM-4:30 PM
405-271-6226
Fax: 405-271-6281

TULSA
Drug Information Service
St. Francis Hospital
6161 S. Yale Ave.
Tulsa, OK 74136
Mon.-Fri. 7 AM-4:30 PM
918-494-6339
(for healthcare
professionals only)
Fax: 918-494-1893

PENNSYLVANIA
PHILADELPHIA
Drug Information Center
Temple University Hospital
Dept. of Pharmacy
3401 N. Broad St.
Philadelphia, PA 19140
Mon.-Fri. 8 AM-4:30 PM
215-707-4644
Fax: 215-707-3463

Drug Information Service
Dept. of Pharmacy
Thomas Jefferson
University Hospital
111 S. 11th St.
Philadelphia, PA 19107-5098
Mon.-Fri. 8 AM-5 PM
215-955-8877
Fax: 215-923-3316

PITTSBURGH
The Christopher and
Nicole Browett
Pharmaceutical
Information Center
Mylan School of Pharmacy
Duquesne University
431 Mellon Hall
Pittsburgh, PA 15282
Mon.-Fri. 8 AM-4 PM
412-396-4600
Fax: 412-396-4488

Drug Information and
Pharmacoepidemiology
Center
University of Pittsburgh
Medical Center
137 Victoria Hall
Pittsburgh, PA 15261
Mon.-Fri. 8:30 AM-4:30 PM
412-624-3784
Fax: 412-624-6350

UPLAND
Drug Information Center
Crozer-Chester Medical
Center
Dept. of Pharmacy
1 Medical Center Blvd.
Upland, PA 19013
Mon.-Fri. 8 AM-4:30 PM
610-447-2851
610-447-2862
(after hours)
(both numbers are
for healthcare
professionals only)
Fax: 610-447-2820

WILKES-BARRE
Drug Information Center
Nesbitt School of
Pharmacy Wilkes
University
150-180 S. River St.
Stark Learning Center,
Room 1060
Wilkes-Barre, PA 18766
Mon.-Fri. 9 AM- 3 PM
    570-408-3295
Fax: 570-408-7828
dicenter@wilkes.edu

WILLIAMSPORT
Drug Information
Pharmacy Dept.
Susquehanna Health
System
Rural Avenue Campus
Williamsport, PA 17701
24 hours/7 days a week
    570-321-3083
Fax: 570-321-3230

PUERTO RICO

PONCE
Centro Informacion
Medicamentos
Escuela de Medicina de
Ponce
P.O. Box 7004
Ponce, PR 00732
Mon.-Fri. 8 AM-4:30 PM
    787-259-7085
    (Spanish and
    English)
    787-840-2575
    (switchboard)
Fax: 787-259-7085

RHODE ISLAND

PROVIDENCE
Rhode Island
Poison Control Center
Rhode Island Hospital,
Dept. of Pharmacy
593 Eddy St.
Providence, RI 02903
7 days/week, 24 hours
    401-444-5547
Fax: 401-444-8062

SOUTH CAROLINA

CHARLESTON
Drug Information Service
Medical University of
South Carolina
150 Ashley Ave.
Rutledge Tower Annex,
Room 604
P.O. Box 25058
Charleston, SC 29425-0810
Mon.-Fri. 9 AM-5:30 PM
    843-792-3896
    800-922-5250
Fax: 843-792-5532

SPARTANBURG
Drug Information Center
Spartanburg Regional
Medical Center
101 E. Wood St.
Spartanburg, SC 29303
Mon.-Fri. 8 AM-5 PM
    864-560-6910
Fax: 864-560-7323

TENNESSEE

MEMPHIS
South East Regional Drug
Information Center
VA Medical Center
1030 Jefferson Ave.
Memphis, TN 38104
Mon.-Fri. 7:30 AM-4 PM
    901-523-8990,
    ext. 6720
Fax: 901-577-7306

Drug Information Center
University of Tennessee
875 Monroe Ave.
Suite 116
Memphis, TN 38163
Mon.-Fri. 8 AM-5 PM
    901-448-5555
Fax: 901-448-5419

TEXAS

GALVESTON
Drug Information Center
University of Texas
Medical Branch
301 University Blvd. - G01
Galveston, TX 77555-0701
Mon.-Fri. 8 AM-5 PM
    409-772-2734
Fax: 409-747-5222

HOUSTON
Drug Information Center
Ben Taub General Hospital
Texas Southern
University/HCHD
1504 Taub Loop
Houston, TX 77030
Mon.-Fri. 8 AM-5 PM
    713-793-2917
Fax: 713-793-2998

Drug Information Center
Methodist Hospital
6565 Fannin (MSDB109)
Houston, TX 77030
Mon.-Fri. 8 AM-5 PM
    713-790-4190
Fax: 713-793-1224

LACKLAND A.F.B.
Drug Information Center
Dept. of Pharmacy
Wilford Hall Medical
Center
2200 Berquist Dr., Suite 1
Lackland A.F.B., TX 78236
7 days/week, 24 hours
    210-292-5418
Fax: 210-292-3722

LUBBOCK
Drug Information and
Consultation Service
Covenant Medical Center
3615 19th St.
Lubbock, TX 79410
Mon.-Fri. 8 AM-5 PM
    806-725-0419
Fax: 806-725-0305

TEMPLE
Drug Information Center
Scott and White
Memorial Hospital
2401 S. 31st St.
Temple, TX 76508
Mon.-Fri. 8 AM-6 PM
    254-724-4636
Fax: 254-724-1731

UTAH

SALT LAKE CITY
Drug Information Service
University of Utah Hospital
Dept. of Pharmacy
Services
Room A-050
50 N. Medical Dr.
Salt Lake City, UT 84132
Mon.-Fri. 8:30 AM-4:30 PM
    801-581-2073
Fax: 801-585-6688

VIRGINIA

CHARLOTTESVILLE
Drug Information Service
University of Virginia
Health System
Dept. of Pharmacy
Services
P.O. Box 10002
Charlottesville, VA 22906
Mon.-Fri. 8 AM-4:30 PM
    804-924-8034
Fax: 804-982-1682

RICHMOND
Drug Information Service
Medical College of Virginia
Hospitals
Dept. of Pharmacy
Virginia Commonwealth
University
401 N. 12th St.,
Room B306
Richmond, VA 23298
Mon.-Fri. 8 AM-5 PM
    804-828-4636
Fax: 804-225-3919

WASHINGTON

SPOKANE
Washington State
University
College of Pharmacy
601 W. First Ave.
Spokane, WA 99201-3899
Mon.-Fri. 8 AM-4 PM
    509-358-7662
Fax: 509-358-7627

WEST VIRGINIA

MORGANTOWN
West Virginia Drug
Information Center
WV University-
Robert C. Byrd
Health Sciences Center
1124 HSN, P.O. Box 9550
Morgantown, WV 26506
Mon.-Fri. 8:30 AM-5 PM
    304-293-6640
    800-352-2501 (WV)
Fax: 304-293-7672

WISCONSIN

MADISON
University of Wisconsin
Hospital & Clinics
Poison Control Center
600 Highland Ave.
Madison, WI 53792
    800-815-8855 (WI)
drug.info@hosp.wisc.edu
(for healthcare
professionals only)

WYOMING

LARAMIE
Drug Information Center
University of Wyoming
P.O. Box 3375
Laramie, WY 82071
Mon.-Fri. 8 AM-5 PM
    307-766-6988
Fax: 307-766-2953

POISON CONTROL CENTERS

Most of the centers listed below are certified by the American Association of Poison Control Centers. **Certified centers are marked by an asterisk after the name**. Each has to meet certain criteria. It must, for example, serve a large geographic area; it must be open 24 hours a day and provide direct-dial or toll-free access; it must be supervised by a med- ical director; and it must have registered pharmacists or nurses available to answer questions from the public.

Within each state, centers are listed alphabetically by city. Telephone numbers designated "TTY" are teletype lines for the hearing-impaired. "TDD" numbers reach a telecommunication device for the deaf.

ALABAMA

BIRMINGHAM

Regional Poison Control Center, The Children's Hospital of Alabama (*)

1600 7th Ave. South
Birmingham, AL 35233
Business: 205-939-9720
Emergency: 205-933-4050
             205-939-9201
             800-292-6678
             (AL)
Fax: 205-939-9245

TUSCALOOSA

Alabama Poison Center (*)

2503 Phoenix Dr.
Tuscaloosa, AL 35405
Business: 205-345-0600
Emergency: 205-345-0600
             800-462-0800
             (AL)
Fax: 205-343-7410

ALASKA

ANCHORAGE

Anchorage Poison Control Center, Providence Hospital

P.O. Box 196604
3200 Providence Dr.
Anchorage, AK 99519-6604
Business: 907-562-2211,
             ext. 3193
Emergency: 907-261-3193
             800-478-3193
             (AK)
Fax: 907-261-3684

FAIRBANKS

Fairbanks Poison Control Center

1650 Cowles St.
Fairbanks, AK 99701
Business and
Emergency: 907-456-7182
Fax: 907-458-5553

ARIZONA

PHOENIX

Samaritan Regional Poison Center (*)
Good Samaritan Regional Medical Center

Ancillary-1
1111 East McDowell Rd.
Phoenix, AZ 85006
Business: 602-495-4884
Emergency: 602-253-3334
             800-362-0101
             (AZ)
Fax: 602-256-7579

TUCSON

Arizona Poison and Drug Information Center (*)
Arizona Health Sciences Center

1501 North Campbell Ave.
Room. 1156
Tucson, AZ 85724
Emergency: 520-626-6016
             800-362-0101
             (AZ)
Fax: 520-626-2720

ARKANSAS

LITTLE ROCK

Arkansas Poison and Drug Information Center College of Pharmacy - UAMS

4301 West Markham St.
Mail Slot 522/2
Little Rock, AR 72205-7122
Business: 501-686-6161
Emergency: 800-376-4766
TDD/TTY: 800-641-3805

CALIFORNIA

FRESNO

California Poison Control System-Fresno/Madera (*)
Valley Children's Hospital

9300 Valley Children's Place
Madera, CA 93638-8762
Business: 559-353-3000
Emergency: 800-876-4766
             (CA)

SACRAMENTO

California Poison Control System-Sacramento (*)

UCDMC-HSF Room 1024
2315 Stockton Blvd.
Sacramento, CA 95817
Business: 916-227-1400
Emergency: 800-876-4766
             (CA)
TDD/TTY: 800-972-3323
Fax: 916-227-1414

SAN DIEGO

California Poison Control System-San Diego (*)
UCSD Medical Center

200 West Arbor Dr.
San Diego, CA 92103-8925
Emergency: 800-876-4766
             (CA)
TDD/TTY: 800-972-3323

SAN FRANCISCO (*)

California Poison Control System-San Francisco
San Francisco General Hospital

1001 Potrero Ave.,
Room 1E86
San Francisco, CA 94110
Emergency: 800-876-4766
             (CA)
TDD/TTY: 800-876-4766

COLORADO

DENVER

Rocky Mountain Poison and Drug Center (*)

1010 Yosemite Circle,
Bldg 752, Suite B
Denver, CO 80230-6800
Business: 303-739-1100
Emergency: 303-739-1123
             800-332-3073
             (CO)
TTY: 303-739-1127
             (CO)
Fax: 303-739-1119

CONNECTICUT

FARMINGTON

Connecticut Regional Poison Control Center (*)
University of Connecticut Health Center

263 Farmington Ave.
Farmington, CT 06030-5365
Business: 860-679-3056
Emergency: 800-343-2722
             (CT)
TDD/TTY: 860-679-4346
Fax: 860-679-1623

DELAWARE

PHILADELPHIA, PA

The Poison Control Center of Philadelphia (*)

3535 Market St.
Suite 985
Philadelphia, PA 19104-3309
Business: 215-590-2003
Emergency: 800-722-7112
             215-386-2100
Fax: 215-590-4419

DISTRICT OF COLUMBIA

WASHINGTON, DC

National Capital Poison Center (*)

3201 New Mexico Ave., NW
Suite 310
Washington, DC 20016
Business: 202-362-3867
Emergency: 202-625-3333
TTY: 202-362-8563
Fax: 202-362-8377

FLORIDA

JACKSONVILLE

**Florida Poison Information Center-Jacksonville (*)
SHANDS Jacksonville Medical Center**

655 W. 8th St.
Jacksonville, FL 32209
Emergency: 904-244-4480
800-282-3171
(FL)
TDD/TTY: 800-282-3171
(FL)
Fax: 904-244-4063

MIAMI

**Florida Poison Information Center-Miami (*)
University of Miami, School of Medicine Department of Pediatrics**

P.O. Box 016960 (R-131)
Miami, FL 33101
Business: 305-585-5253
Emergency: 305-585-8417
800-282-3171
(FL)
Fax: 305-545-9762

TAMPA

**Florida Poison Information Center-Tampa (*)
Tampa General Hospital**

P.O. Box 1289
Tampa, FL 33601
Emergency: 813-253-4444
800-282-3171
(FL)
Fax: 813-253-4443

GEORGIA

ATLANTA

**Georgia Poison Center (*)
Hughes Spalding Children's Hospital, Grady Health System**

80 Butler St., SE
P.O. Box 26066
Atlanta, GA 30335-3801
Emergency: 404-616-9000
800-282-5846
(GA)
TDD: 404-616-9287
Fax: 404-616-6657

HAWAII

HONOLULU

Hawaii Poison Center

1319 Punahou St.
Honolulu, HI 96826
Emergency: 808-941-4411
800-362-3585
(outer islands only)
Fax: 808-535-7922

IDAHO

(DENVER, CO)

Rocky Mountain Poison & Drug Center (*)

1010 Yosemite Circle,
Bldg 752, Suite B
Denver, CO 80230-6800
Emergency: 800-860-0620
(ID)
208-334-4570
TTY: 303-739-1127
(ID)
Fax: 303-739-1119

ILLINOIS

CHICAGO

Illinois Poison Center (*)

222 South Riverside Plaza
Suite 1900
Chicago, IL 60606
Business: 312-906-6136
Emergency: 800-942-5969
(IL)
TDD/TTY: 312-906-6185
Fax: 312-803-5400

URBANA

ASPCA/National Animal Poison Control Center

1717 S. Philo Rd., Suite 36
Urbana, IL 61802
Business: 217-337-5030
Emergency: 888-426-4435
Fax: 217-337-0599

INDIANA

INDIANAPOLIS

Indiana Poison Center (*)

I-65 at 21st St.
P.O. Box 1367
Indianapolis, IN 46206
Emergency: 317-929-2323
800-382-9097
(IN)
TTY: 317-929-2336
Fax: 317-929-2337

IOWA

SIOUX CITY

Iowa Statewide Poison Control Center

2720 Stone Park Blvd.
Sioux City, IA 51104
Business: 712-279-3710
Emergency: 800-352-2222
(IA)
712-277-2222
Fax: 712-234-8775

KANSAS

KANSAS CITY

Mid-America Poison Control Center, University of Kansas Medical Center

3901 Rainbow Blvd.
Room B-400
Kansas City, KS 66160-7231
Business & 913-588-6638
Emergency: 800-332-6633
(KS)
TDD/TTY: 913-588-6639
Fax: 913-588-2350

TOPEKA

Stormont-Vail Regional Medical Center Emergency Department

1500 S.W. 10th
Topeka, KS 66604-1353
Business: 785-354-6000
Emergency: 785-354-6100
Fax: 785-354-5004

KENTUCKY

LOUISVILLE

Kentucky Regional Poison Center (*)

Medical Towers South
Suite 572
234 E. Gray St.
Louisville, KY 40202
Business: 502-629-7264
Emergency: 502-589-8222
800-722-5725
(Louisville only)
Fax: 502-629-7277

LOUISIANA

MONROE

**Louisiana Drug and Poison Information Center (*)
University of Louisiana at Monroe College of Pharmacy**

Sugar Hall
Monroe, LA 71209-6430
Business: 318-342-1710
Emergency: 800-256-9822
(LA)
Fax: 318-342-1744

MAINE

PORTLAND

**Maine Poison Center
Maine Medical Center**

22 Bramhall St.
Portland, ME 04102
Emergency: 207-871-2950
800-442-6305
(ME)
TDD/TTY: 207-871-2879
Fax: 207-871-6226

MARYLAND

BALTIMORE

**Maryland Poison Center (*)
University of Maryland at Baltimore School of Pharmacy**

20 North Pine St., PH 230
Baltimore, MD 21201
Business: 410-706-7604
Emergency: 410-706-7701
800-492-2414
(MD)
TDD: 410-706-1858
Fax: 410-706-7184

MASSACHUSETTS

BOSTON

Regional Center for Poison Control and Prevention (*)

300 Longwood Ave.
Boston, MA 02115
Emergency: 617-232-2120
          800-682-9211
                (MA, RI)
TDD/TTY: 888-244-5313
Fax: 617-738-0032

MICHIGAN

DETROIT

**Regional Poison Control Center (*)
Children's Hospital of Michigan**

4160 John R. Harper Prof.
Office Bldg.
Suite 616
Detroit, MI 48201
Business: 313-745-5335
Emergency: 313-745-5711
          800-764-7661
                (MI)
TDD/TTY: 800-356-3232
Fax: 313-745-5493

GRAND RAPIDS

Spectrum Health Regional Poison Center (*)

1840 Wealthy SE
Grand Rapids, MI 49506-2968
Business: 616-774-7851
Emergency: 800-764-7661
                (MI)
TDD/TTY: 800-356-3232
Fax: 616-774-7204

MINNESOTA

MINNEAPOLIS

**Hennepin Regional Poison Center (*)
Hennepin County Medical Center**

701 Park Ave.
Minneapolis, MN 55415
Business: 612-347-3144
Emergency: 800-764-7661
                (MN, SD)
          612-347-3141
TTY: 612-904-4691
Fax: 612-904-4289

ST. PAUL

PROSAR International Poison Center

1295 Bandana Blvd.
Suite 335
St. Paul, MN 55108
Business: 651-917-6100
Emergency: 888-779-7921
Fax: 651-641-0341

MISSISSIPPI

HATTIESBURG

Poison Center, Forrest General Hospital

P. O. Box 16389
400 South 28th Ave.
Hattiesburg, MS 39404
Emergency: 601-288-2100
          601-288-2197
          601-288-2199
Fax: 601-288-2125

JACKSON

Mississippi Regional Poison Control Center, University of Mississippi Medical Center

2500 North State St.
Jackson, MS 39216
Business: 601-984-1675
Emergency: 601-354-7660
Fax: 601-984-1676

MISSOURI

ST. LOUIS

Cardinal Glennon Children's Hospital Regional Poison Center (*)

1465 South Grand Blvd.
St. Louis, MO 63104
Emergency: 800-366-8888
                (MO)
          314-772-5200
TTY: 314-577-5336
Fax: 314-577-5355

MONTANA

(DENVER, CO)

Rocky Mountain Poison and Drug Center (*)

1010 Yosemite Circle,
Bldg 752, Suite B
Denver, CO 80230-6800
Emergency: 800-525-5042
                (MT)
          303-739-1123
Fax: 303-739-1119

NEBRASKA

OMAHA

**The Poison Center (*)
Children's Hospital**

8301 Dodge St.
Omaha, NE 68114
Emergency: 402-354-5555
                (Omaha)
          800-955-9119
                (NE, WY)

NEVADA

(DENVER, CO)

Rocky Mountain Poison and Drug Center (*)

1010 Yosemite Circle,
Bldg 752, Suite B
Denver, CO 80230-6800
Emergency: 800-446-6179
                (NV)
          303-739-1123
Fax: 303-739-1119

(PORTLAND, OR)

**Oregon Poison Center (*)
Oregon Health Sciences University**

3181 SW Sam Jackson
Park Rd, CB550
Portland, OR 97201
Emergency: 503-494-8968
Fax: 503-494-4980

NEW HAMPSHIRE

LEBANON

New Hampshire Poison Information Center, Dartmouth-Hitchcock Medical Center

1 Medical Center Dr.
Lebanon, NH 03756
Emergency: 603-650-8000
          800-562-8236
                (NH)
Fax: 603-650-8986

NEW JERSEY

NEWARK

New Jersey Poison Information and Education System (*)

201 Lyons Ave.
Newark, NJ 07112
Business: 973-926-7443
Emergency: 800-764-7661
                (NJ)
TDD/TTY: 973-926-8008
Fax: 973-926-0013

NEW MEXICO

ALBUQUERQUE

**New Mexico Poison and Drug Information Center (*)
University of New Mexico**

Health Science Center
Library, Room 130
Albuquerque, NM 87131-1076
Emergency: 505-272-2222
          800-432-6866
                (NM)
Fax: 505-272-5892

NEW YORK

BUFFALO

**Western New York Regional Poison Control Center (*)
Children's Hospital of Buffalo**

219 Bryant St.
Buffalo, NY 14222
Business: 716-878-7657
Emergency: 716-878-7654
          800-888-7655
(NY Western Regions Only)

MINEOLA

**Long Island Regional Poison and Drug Information Center (*)
Winthrop University Hospital**

259 First St.
Mineola, NY 11501
Emergency: 516-542-2323
          516-663-2650
TDD: 516-747-3323
                (Nassau)
          516-924-8811
                (Suffolk)
Fax: 516-739-2070

NEW YORK CITY

**New York City Poison Control Center (*)
NYC Dept. of Health**

455 First Ave., Room 123
New York, NY 10016
Business: 212-447-8152
Emergency: 800-210-3985
(English)   212-340-4494
          212-POISONS
          (212-764-7667)
Emergency: 212-VENENOS
(Spanish)   (212-836-3667)
TDD: 212-689-9014
Fax: 212-447-8223

ROCHESTER

Finger Lakes Regional Poison and Drug Information Center (*) University of Rochester Medical Center

601 Elmwood Ave.
Box 321
Rochester, NY 14642
Business: 716-273-4155
Emergency: 716-275-3232
                   800-333-0542
                              (NY)
TTY: 716-273-3854
Fax: 716-244-1677

SLEEPY HOLLOW

Hudson Valley Regional Poison Center (*) Phelps Memorial Hospital Center

701 N. Broadway
Sleepy Hollow, NY 10591
Emergency: 914-366-3030
                   800-336-6997
                              (NY)
Fax: 914-366-1400

SYRACUSE

Central New York Poison Center (*) SUNY Health Science Center

750 East Adams St.
Syracuse, NY 13210
Business: 315-464-7078
Emergency: 315-476-4766
                   800-252-5655
                              (NY)
Fax: 315-464-7077

NORTH CAROLINA

CHARLOTTE

Carolinas Poison Center (*) Carolinas Medical Center

5000 Airport Center Pkwy.
Suite B
P.O. Box 32861
Charlotte, NC 28232
Business: 704-395-3795
Emergency: 704-355-4000
                   800-848-6946

NORTH DAKOTA

FARGO

North Dakota Poison Information Center, Meritcare Medical Center

720 4th St. North
Fargo, ND 58122
Business: 701-234-6062
Emergency: 701-234-5575
                   800-732-2200
                   (ND, MN, SD)
Fax: 701-234-5090

OHIO

CINCINNATI

Cincinnati Drug & Poison Information Center and Regional Poison Control System (*)

3333 Burnet Ave.
Vernon Place, 3rd floor
Cincinnati, OH 45229
Emergency: 513-558-5111
                   800-872-5111
                              (OH)
TDD/TTY: 800-253-7955
Fax: 513-636-5069

CLEVELAND

Greater Cleveland Poison Control Center

11100 Euclid Ave.
Cleveland, OH 44106-6010
Emergency: 216-231-4455
                   888-231-4455
                              (OH)
Fax: 216-844-3242

COLUMBUS

Central Ohio Poison Center (*)

700 Children's Dr.
Room L032
Columbus, OH 43205-2696
Business: 614-722-2635
Emergency: 614-228-1323
                   800-682-7625
                              (OH)
                   800-762-0727
                              (OH)
                   937-222-2227
                   (Dayton Region)
TTY: 614-222-2272
Fax: 614-221-2672

TOLEDO

Poison Information Center of NW Ohio, Medical College of Ohio Hospital

3000 Arlington Ave.
Toledo, OH 43614
Emergency: 419-383-3897
                   800-589-3897
                              (OH)
Fax: 419-383-6066

OKLAHOMA

OKLAHOMA CITY

Oklahoma Poison Control Center, University of Oklahoma

940 Northeast 13th St.
Room 3512
Oklahoma City, OK 73104
Business: 405-271-5062
Emergency: 800-764-7661
                              (OK)
                   405-271-5454
TDD: 405-271-1122
Fax: 405-271-1816

OREGON

PORTLAND

Oregon Poison Center, CB 550 (*) Oregon Health Sciences University

3181 S.W. Sam Jackson
Park Rd.
Portland, OR 97201
Emergency: 503-494-8968
                   800-452-7165
                              (OR)
Fax: 503-494-4980

PENNSYLVANIA

HERSHEY

Central Pennsylvania Poison Center (*) Pennsylvania State University Milton S. Hershey Medical Center

MC H043, P.O. Box 850
500 University Dr.
Hershey, PA 17033-0850
Emergency: 800-521-6110
                   717-531-6111
TTY: 717-531-8335
Fax: 717-531-6932

PHILADELPHIA

The Poison Control Center (*)

3535 Market St., Suite 985
Philadelphia, PA 19104-3309
Business: 215-590-2003
Emergency: 215-386-2100
                   800-722-7112
Fax: 215-590-4419

PITTSBURGH

Pittsburgh Poison Center (*) Children's Hospital of Pittsburgh

3705 Fifth Ave.
Pittsburgh, PA 15213
Business: 412-692-5600
Emergency: 412-681-6669
Fax: 412-692-7497

PUERTO RICO

SANTURCE

San Jorge Children's Hospital Poison Center

258 San Jorge St.
Santurce, PR 00912
Emergency: 787-726-5674

RHODE ISLAND

(BOSTON, MA)

Regional Center for Poison Control and Prevention Serving Massachusetts and Rhode Island (*)

300 Longwood Ave.
Boston, MA 02115
Emergency: 800-682-9211
                              (MA, RI)
                   617-232-2120
TDD/TTY: 888-244-5313

SOUTH CAROLINA

COLUMBIA

Palmetto Poison Center, College of Pharmacy, University of South Carolina

Columbia, SC 29208
Business: 803-777-7909
Emergency: 803-777-1117
                   800-922-1117
                              (SC)
Fax: 803-777-6127

SOUTH DAKOTA

(FARGO, ND)

North Dakota Poison Information Center Meritcare Medical Center

720 4th St. North
Fargo, ND 58122
Business: 701-234-6062
Emergency: 701-234-5575
                   800-732-2200
                   (SD, MN, ND)
Fax: 701-234-5090

(MINNEAPOLIS, MN)

Hennepin Regional Poison Center (*) Hennepin County Medical Center

701 Park Ave.
Minneapolis, MN 55415
Business: 612-347-3144
Emergency: 800-764-7661
              (MN, SD)
              612-904-4691
TTY: 612-904-4289

TENNESSEE

MEMPHIS

Southern Poison Center

875 Monroe Ave.
Suite 104
Memphis, TN 38163
Business: 901-448-6800
Emergency: 901-528-6048
              800-288-9999
                      (TN)
Fax: 901-448-5419

NASHVILLE

Middle Tennessee Poison Center (*)

1161 21st Ave. South
501 Oxford House
Nashville, TN 37232-4632
Business: 615-936-0760
Emergency: 615-936-2034
              (Greater Nashville)
              800-288-9999
                      (TN)
Fax: 615-936-0756

TEXAS

AMARILLO

Texas Panhandle Poison Center Northwest Texas Hospital

1501 S. Coulter Dr.
Amarillo, TX 79106
Emergency: 806-354-1100
              800-764-7661
                      (TX)

DALLAS

North Texas Poison Center (*) Texas Poison Center Network Parkland Health and Hospital System

5201 Harry Hines Blvd.
P.O. Box 35926
Dallas, TX 75235
Business: 214-589-0911
Emergency: 800-764-7661
                      (TX)
Fax: 214-590-5008

EL PASO

West Texas Regional Poison Center (*)

4815 Alameda Ave.
El Paso, TX 79905
Business: 915-534-3800
Emergency: 800-764-7661
                      (TX)

GALVESTON

Southeast Texas Poison Center (*) The University of Texas Medical Branch

3112 Trauma Bldg.
301 University Ave.
Galveston, TX 77555-1175
Business: 409-766-4403
Emergency: 800-764-7661
                      (TX)
              409-765-1420
Fax: 409-772-3917

SAN ANTONIO

South Texas Poison Center (*) The University of Texas Health Science Center–San Antonio

7703 Floyd Curl Dr., MC 7849
San Antonio, TX 78229-3900
Emergency: 210-567-5762
              800-764-7661
                      (TX)
TDD/TTY: 800-764-7661
                      (TX)
Fax: 210-567-5718

TEMPLE

Central Texas Poison Center (*) Scott & White Memorial Hospital

2401 South 31st St.
Temple, TX 76508
Emergency: 800-764-7661
                      (TX)
              254-724-7401
Fax: 254-724-1731

UTAH

SALT LAKE CITY

Utah Poison Control Center (*)

410 Chipeta Way
Suite 230
Salt Lake City, UT 84108
Emergency: 801-581-2151
              800-456-7707
                      (UT)
Fax: 801-581-4199

VERMONT

BURLINGTON

Vermont Poison Center, Fletcher Allen Health Care

111 Colchester Ave.
Burlington, VT 05401
Business: 802-847-2721
Emergency: 802-658-3456
              877-658-3456
              (toll-free)
Fax: 802-847-4802

VIRGINIA

CHARLOTTESVILLE

Blue Ridge Poison Center (*) University of Virginia Health System

PO Box 800774
Charlottesville, VA 22908-0774
Emergency: 804-924-5543
              800-451-1428
                      (VA)
Fax: 804-971-8657

RICHMOND

Virginia Poison Center (*) Virginia Commonwealth University

P.O. Box 980522
Richmond, VA 23298-0522
Emergency: 800-552-6337
                      (VA)
              804-828-9123
TDD/TTY: 800-828-1120
Fax: 804-828-5291

WASHINGTON

SEATTLE

Washington Poison Center (*)

155 NE 100th St.
Suite 400
Seattle, WA 98125-8012
Business: 206-517-2351
Emergency: 206-526-2121
              800-732-6985
                      (WA)
TDD: 800-572-0638
                      (WA)
              206-517-2394
Fax: 206-526-8490

WEST VIRGINIA

CHARLESTON

West Virginia Poison Center (*)

3110 MacCorkle Ave. SE
Charleston, WV 25304
Business: 304-347-1212
Emergency: 304-348-4211
              800-642-3625
                      (WV)
Fax: 304-348-9560

WISCONSIN

MADISON

Poison Control Center, University of Wisconsin Hospital and Clinics

600 Highland Ave.
F6-133
Madison, WI 53792
Business: 608-262-7537
Emergency: 800-815-8855
                      (WI)

MILWAUKEE

Children's Hospital of Wisconsin Poison Center

9000 W. Wisconsin Ave.
P.O. Box 1997
Milwaukee, WI 53201
Business: 414-266-2000
Emergency: 414-266-2222
              800-815-8855
                      (WI)
Fax: 414-266-2820

WYOMING

(OMAHA, NE)

The Poison Center (*) Children's Hospital

8301 Dodge St.
Omaha, NE 68114
Emergency: 800-955-9119
                      (WY, NE)

PRODUCT IDENTIFICATION GUIDE

To aid in quick identification, this section provides full-color, actual-size photographs of tablets and capsules. A variety of other dosage forms and packages are shown at less than actual size. In all, the section contains a total of nearly 800 photos.

Products in this section are arranged alphabetically by manufacturer. In some instances, not all dosage forms and sizes are pictured. For more information on any of the products in this section, please turn to the page indicated above the product's photo or check directly with the product's manufacturer.

While every effort has been made to guarantee faithful reproduction of the photos in this section, changes in size, color, and design are always a possibility. Be sure to confirm a product's identity with the manufacturer or your pharmacist.

MANUFACTURER'S INDEX

A & Z Pharmaceutical Inc. 503

AkPharma Inc. 503

Bayer Corporation Consumer Care Division 503

Block Drug 505

Boehringer Ingelheim Consumer H.C. 506

Bristol-Myers Products 506

Covex 507

Effcon Laboratories 507

J&J-Merck Consumer 507

Legacy for Life 508

4Life Research™, LC 526

3M 508

Mannatech, Inc. 508

Matol Botanical International, LTD 508

McNeil Consumer Healthcare 508

Novartis Consumer Health, Inc. 512

Pfizer Inc., Warner-Lambert
  Consumer Group 515

Pfizer Inc., Warner-Lambert
  Consumer Healthcare 516

Pharmaton 521

Procter & Gamble 521

Products On Demand 522

The Purdue Frederick Company 522

Schering-Plough HealthCare Products............522

Sigma-Tau Pharmaceuticals, Inc. 523

SmithKline Beecham Consumer
  Healthcare, L.P. 523

Strategic Science and Technologies, Inc.........525

Sunpower Nutraceutical Inc. 525

Wallace Laboratories 525

J.B. Williams Co. 526

Wyeth-Ayerst Pharmaceuticals 526

Zanfel Laboratories Inc. 526

A & Z PHARMACEUTICAL INC.

A & Z Pharmaceutical Inc.
P. 794

Calcium Supplement with Fruit Flavor
Packages of 30 and 60 caplets
D-Cal™

AKPHARMA INC.

AkPharma Inc.
P. 801

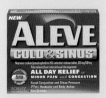

Dietary Supplement
Granulate and Tablets

Prelief®

BAYER CORPORATION

Bayer Corporation
Consumer Care Division
P. 603

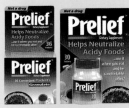

Aleve® Cold & Sinus

**SEEKING AN
ALTERNATIVE?**

Check the
Product Category Index,
where you'll find
alphabetical listings of
all the products in each
therapeutic class.

Bayer Corporation
Consumer Care Division
P. 602

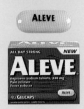

Aleve®

Bayer Corporation
Consumer Care Division
P. 603

Original, Extra Strength,
Lemon Lime and Cherry
Effervescent Antacid and
Pain Reliever
Alka-Seltzer®

Bayer Corporation
Consumer Care Division
P. 604

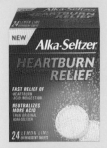

**Alka-Seltzer®
Heartburn Relief**

Bayer Corporation
Consumer Care Division
P. 605

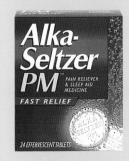

Alka-Seltzer PM®

Bayer Corporation
Consumer Care Division
P. 604

Cold, Cold & Cough, Cold & Flu,
Cold & Sinus and Night-Time.
**Alka-Seltzer Plus®
Cold Medicine Liqui-Gels®**

Bayer Corporation
Consumer Care Division
P. 611

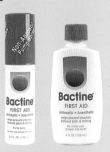

Antiseptic/Anesthetic
First Aid Spray and Liquid
Bactine®

Bayer Corporation
Consumer Care Division
P. 606

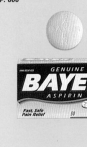

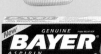

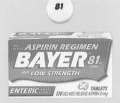

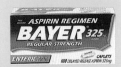

Genuine Bayer Tablets and Gelcaps,
Aspirin Regimen 81 mg,
Aspirin Regimen 325 mg

BAYER® Aspirin

Bayer Corporation
Consumer Care Division
P. 607

Low Strength, Chewable Aspirin
Orange and Cherry Flavors

Aspirin Regimen
BAYER® Children's

Bayer Corporation
Consumer Care Division
P. 610

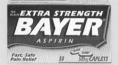

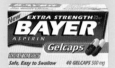

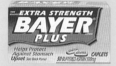

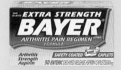

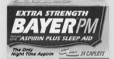

Extra Strength Caplets and Gelcaps,
Plus, Arthritis Pain Regimen and PM

Extra Strength
BAYER® Aspirin

Bayer Corporation
Consumer Care Division
P. 802

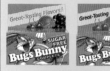

Sugar Free Children's
Chewable Vitamins
Complete, with Extra C and Plus Iron

Bugs Bunny™ Vitamins

Bayer Corporation
Consumer Care Division
P. 611

Astringent Solution
Effervescent Tablets and
Powder Packets

Domeboro®

Bayer Corporation
Consumer Care Division
P. 802

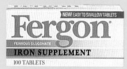

Ferrous Gluconate
Iron Supplement

Fergon®

Bayer Corporation
Consumer Care Division
P. 802

Complete, Plus Extra C,
Plus Iron, Original
and Plus Calcium

Flintstones® Children's
Chewable Vitamins

Bayer Corporation
Consumer Care Division
P. 612

Maximum Strength
Caplets and Gelcaps

Midol® Menstrual

Bayer Corporation
Consumer Care Division
P. 613

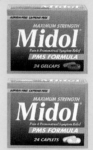

Maximum Strength
Gelcaps and Caplets

Midol® PMS

Bayer Corporation
Consumer Care Division
P. 612

Maximum Strength Caplets

Midol® Teen

Bayer Corporation
Consumer Care Division
P. 614

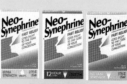

Nasal Decongestant
Spray and Drops
Available in Mild, Regular, Extra
Strength and Max 12-Hour Formula

Neo-Synephrine®

Bayer Corporation
Consumer Care Division
P. 804

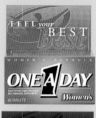

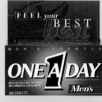

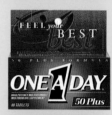

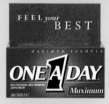

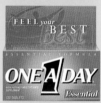

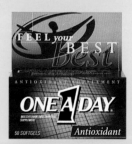

Women's, Men's, 50 Plus, Maximum
and Essential.

One-A-Day® Vitamins

Bayer Corporation
Consumer Care Division
P. 805

One-A-Day®
Antioxidant Plus

Bayer Corporation
Consumer Care Division
P. 805

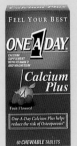

500 mg Calcium Carbonate
Plus Vitamin D and Magnesium

One-A-Day® Calcium Plus

Bayer Corporation
Consumer Care Division
P. 806

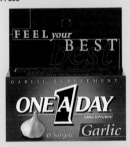

One-A-Day®
Garlic Softgels

Bayer Corporation
Consumer Care Division
P. 806

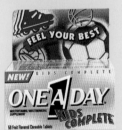

One-A-Day®
Kids Complete

**LOOKING FOR
A PARTICULAR
COMPOUND?**

In the
Active Ingredients Index
(Yellow Pages),
you'll find all the
brands that contain it.

Bayer Corporation
Consumer Care Division
P. 805

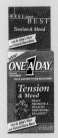 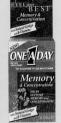

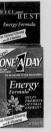 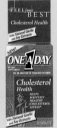

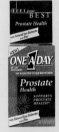 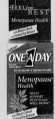

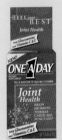 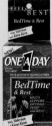

Specialized Nutritional Supplements

Tension & Mood,
Memory & Concentration,
Energy Formula, Cholesterol Health,
Prostate Health, Menopause Health,
Joint Health, Bed Time and Rest

One-A-Day®

Bayer Corporation
Consumer Care Division
P. 615

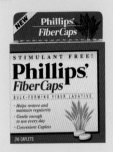

Phillips'® Fiber Caps

Bayer Corporation
Consumer Care Division
P. 616

Available in Mint, Original,
and Cherry Flavors
4 oz, 12 oz and 26 oz Bottles

Phillips'®
Milk of Magnesia

Bayer Corporation
Consumer Care Division
P. 616

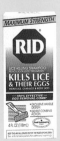

Rid® Lice Killing
Shampoo

Bayer Corporation
Consumer Care Division
P. 617

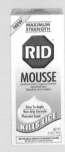

Rid® Mousse

Bayer Corporation
Consumer Care Division
P. 617

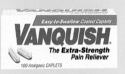

Extra-Strength Pain Formula

Vanquish®

BLOCK DRUG

Block Drug
P. 619

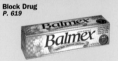

Available in 2 oz. and 4 oz. tubes
and 16 oz. jar

Balmex®
Diaper Rash Ointment

Block Drug
P. 619

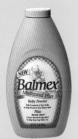

Available in 13 oz. bottle.

Balmex® Medicated Plus
Baby Powder

Block Drug
P. 621

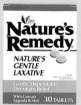

Available in packages of
15, 30 and 60 tablets.
A stimulant laxative with
natural active ingredients.

**Nature's Remedy®
Nature's Gentle Laxative**

Block Drug
P. 621

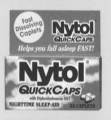

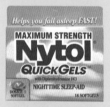

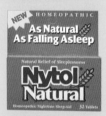

QuickCaps®, QuickGels™
and Natural

Nytol®

Block Drug
P. 622

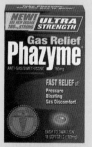

180 mg Softgels

Gas Relief Phazyme®

Block Drug
P. 622

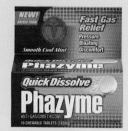

125 mg Chewable tablets

**Quick Dissolve
Phazyme®**

Block Drug
P. 623

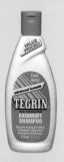

**Tegrin®
Dandruff Shampoo**

Block Drug
P. 624

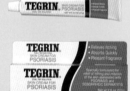

**Tegrin® Skin Cream
for Psoriasis**

**FACED WITH AN
Rx SIDE EFFECT?**

Turn to the
Companion Drug Index
(Green Pages)
for products that provide
symptomatic relief.

Boehringer Ingelheim Consumer H.C.
P. 624

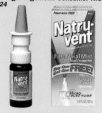

Adult Strength

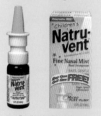

Pediatric Strength

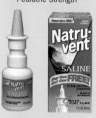

Saline Nasal Spray

Natru-Vent™

Bristol-Myers Products
P. 628

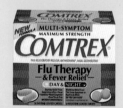

**Comtrex®
Multi-Symptom
Flu Therapy & Fever Relief**

Bristol-Myers Products
P. 626

Available in blister packages
of 24 tablets and caplets.
Also available:
Allergy-Sinus Treatment, Day/Night;
Flu Therapy & Fever Relief, Day/Night;
and Non-Drowsy formulations.

**Comtrex® Multi-Symptom
Cold & Cough Relief**

Bristol-Myers Products
P. 627

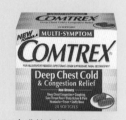

Available in blister packages
of 24 softgels

**Comtrex® Deep Chest
Cold & Congestion Relief**

Bristol-Myers Products
P. 627

Available in blister package
of 24 tablets

**Comtrex® Acute
Head Cold & Sinus
Pressure Relief**

Bristol-Myers Products
P. 631

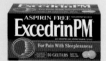

Tablets in bottles of 10
Tablets and Caplets in bottles of
24, 50 and 100
Geltabs in bottles of 24, 50 and 100

Excedrin PM®

Bristol-Myers Products
P. 628

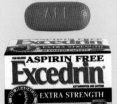

Bottles of 24, 50
and 100 caplets and geltabs

Aspirin Free Excedrin®

Bristol-Myers Products
P. 628

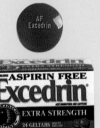

Bottles of 12, 24, 50, 100, 175
and 275, metal tins of 12 tablets
Bottles of 24, 50, 100, 175, 275
caplets and 24, 50 and 100 geltabs
(2 bottles of 50 each)

Extra Strength Excedrin®

Bristol-Myers Products
P. 630

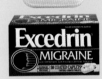
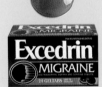

Bottles of 24, 50, 100, 175
and 275 tablets.
Bottles of 24, 50, 100 and 175 caplets.
Bottles of 24, 50 and 100 geltabs
(2 bottles of 50 each)

Excedrin® Migraine

COVEX

Covex
P. 813

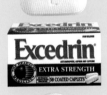

Powerful Memory Enhancer

Intelectol™

EFFCON

Effcon Laboratories
P. 632

Oral Suspension available
in 60 mL and 30 mL.
For the treatment of
pinworm infections.

Pin-X®
(pyrantel pamoate)

J&J-MERCK CONSUMER

J&J-Merck Consumer
P. 634

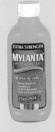

Extra Strength
Fast-Acting Mylanta®

J&J-Merck Consumer
P. 636

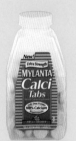

Extra Strength

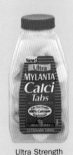

Ultra Strength

Mylanta® Calci-Tabs

J&J-Merck Consumer
P. 637

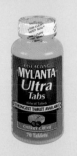

Mylanta® Fast-Acting
Ultra Tabs

J&J-Merck Consumer
P. 637

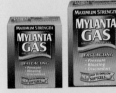

Mylanta® Gas
Maximum Strength

J&J-Merck Consumer
P. 637

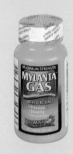

Mylanta® Gas
Maximum Strength

J&J-Merck Consumer
P. 637

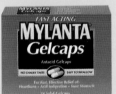

Mylanta® Fast Acting
Gelcaps Antacid

J&J-Merck Consumer
P. 636

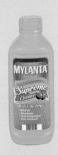

Fast-Acting Mylanta®
Supreme Tasting Antacid

J&J-Merck Consumer
P. 634

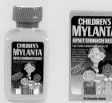

400 mg/5 mL   400 mg/tablet

**Children's Mylanta®
Upset Stomach Relief
Liquid and Tablets**

J&J-Merck Consumer
P. 634

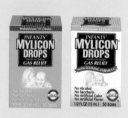

Infants Mylicon® Drops

J&J-Merck Consumer
P. 638

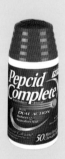

Pepcid Complete®

J&J-Merck Consumer
P. 638

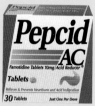

Tablets

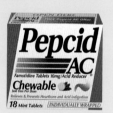

Chewable Tablets

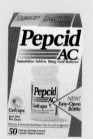

Gelcaps

Pepcid AC®

Legacy for Life™
P. 818

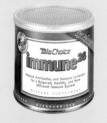

BioChoice® immune²⁶

3M

3M
P. 640

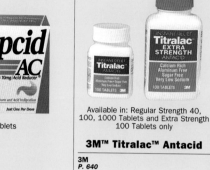

Available in: Regular Strength 40,
100, 1000 Tablets and Extra Strength
100 Tablets only

3M™ Titralac™ Antacid

3M
P. 640

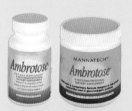

Antacid with Simethicone
Available in 100 Tablets

**3M™ Titralac™
Plus Antacid**

MANNATECH, INC.

Mannatech, Inc.
P. 819

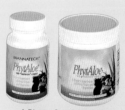

A Glyconutritional Dietary Supplement

Ambrotose®

Mannatech, Inc.
P. 819

A Dietary Supplement of
Dried Fruits and Vegetables

Phyt•Aloe®

Mannatech, Inc.
P. 820

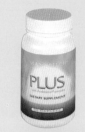

Dietary Supplement

**PLUS with
Ambrotose® complex**

**MATOL BOTANICAL
INTERNATIONAL, LTD.**

Matol Botanical International, Ltd.
P. 640

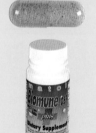

.75 fl oz

**Biomune OSF™
EXPRESS**

Matol Botanical International, Ltd.
P. 820

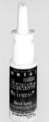

**Biomune OSF™
Plus**

MCNEIL

McNeil Consumer Healthcare
P. 821

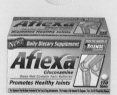

Tablets available in bottles of
50, 110 and 250.

Aflexa™ Tablets

McNeil Consumer Healthcare
P. 640

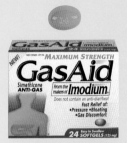

Softgels available in blister packs of 12, 24 and 48.

Maximum Strength GasAid®

McNeil Consumer Healthcare
P. 641

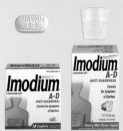

Available in 2 and 4 fl. oz. bottles with a convenient dosage cup, and caplets in 6's, 12's, 18's, 24's and 48's

Imodium® A-D

McNeil Consumer Healthcare
P. 641

Vanilla mint chewable tablets available in 6's, 12's, 18's, 30's and 42's

Imodium® Advanced

Lactaid Inc. Marketed By
McNeil Consumer Healthcare
P. 822

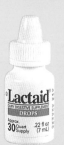

Available in 30 qt. supply

Lactaid® Drops

Lactaid Inc. Marketed By
McNeil Consumer Healthcare
P. 821

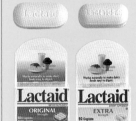

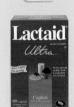

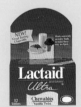

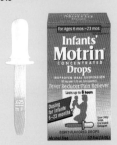

ORIGINAL STRENGTH available in bottles of 120
EXTRA STRENGTH available in bottles of 50
ULTRA CAPLETS available in single serve packets of 12, 32, 60 and 90 counts
ULTRA CHEWABLE TABLETS available in bottles of 12 and 32 counts

Lactaid® Caplets and Chewable Tablets

McNeil Consumer Healthcare
P. 643

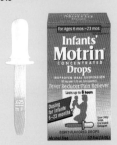

50 mg/1.25 mL
Available in 1/2 fl. oz. bottle

Infants' Motrin® Concentrated Drops

McNeil Consumer Healthcare
P. 643

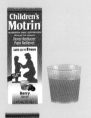

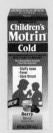

Available in Berry, Bubble Gum and Grape flavors in 4 fl. oz. with child-resistant safety cap and convenient dosage cup.

Children's Motrin® Oral Suspension

McNeil Consumer Healthcare
P. 643

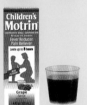

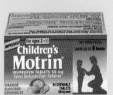

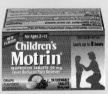

Available in Orange and Grape-Flavored Chewable Tablets of 50 mg. Available in bottles of 24 with child-resistant safety cap.

Children's Motrin® Chewable Tablets

McNeil Consumer Healthcare
P. 646

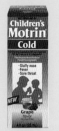

Available in Berry and Grape flavors in 4 fl. oz. with child-resistant safety cap and convenient dosage cup.

Children's Motrin® Cold Oral Suspension

McNeil Consumer Healthcare
P. 643

Available in bottles of 24 with child-resistant safety cap.

Junior Strength Motrin® Caplets

McNeil Consumer Healthcare
P. 643

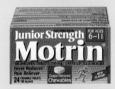

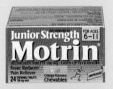

Available in Orange and Grape-flavored Chewable Tablets of 100 mg. Available in bottles of 24 with child-resistant safety cap.

Junior Strength Motrin® Chewable Tablets

McNeil Consumer Healthcare
P. 645

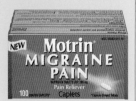

Caplets available in tamper-evident packaging of 24, 50 and 100.

Motrin® Migraine Pain

McNeil Consumer Healthcare
P. 642

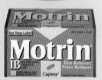

Gelcaps available in tamper evident packaging of 24 and 50. Caplets available in tamper evident packaging of 24, 50, 60, 100, 135, 165, 250 and 500. Tablets available in tamper evident packaging of 24, 50, 100, 130, 135 and 165.

Motrin® IB

McNeil Consumer Healthcare
P. 643

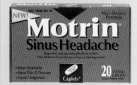

Caplets available in blister packs of 20's and 40's

Motrin® Sinus Headache

McNeil Consumer Healthcare
P. 647

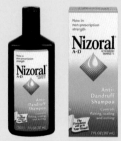

Available in 4 and 7 fl. oz. bottles.

Nizoral® A-D

McNeil Consumer Healthcare
P. 822

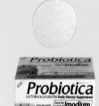

Tablets available in bottles of 60 and 90.

Probiotica

McNeil Consumer Healthcare
P. 647

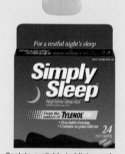

Caplets available in blister packs of 24, 48 and 72.

Simply Sleep™

McNeil Consumer Healthcare
P. 658

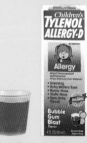

Available in Bubble Gum Blast flavor in child-resistant 4 fl. oz. bottles.

**Children's TYLENOL®
Allergy-D Liquid**

McNeil Consumer Healthcare
P. 657

Fruit flavor: bottles of 30 with child-resistant safety cap and blister packs of 60 and 96

Bubble Gum and Grape flavor bottles: of 30 with child-resistant safety cap

**Children's TYLENOL®
Soft Chews
Chewable Tablets**

McNeil Consumer Healthcare
P. 657

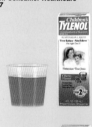

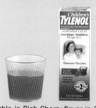

Available in Rich Cherry flavor in 2 and 4 fl. oz. bottles. Bubble Gum and Grape flavors in 4 fl. oz. with child-resistant safety cap and convenient dosage cup. Alcohol Free, 80 mg per 1/2 teaspoon

**Children's TYLENOL®
Suspension Liquid**

McNeil Consumer Healthcare
P. 659

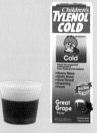

Available in 4 fl. oz. bottle with child-resistant safety cap and convenient dosage cup. Great Grape flavor.

**Children's TYLENOL®
Cold Liquid**

McNeil Consumer Healthcare
P. 659

Available in blister pack of 24 chewable tablets. Great Grape flavor.

**Children's TYLENOL® Cold
Chewable Tablets**

McNeil Consumer Healthcare
P. 659

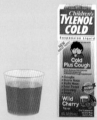

Available in 4 fl. oz. bottle with child-resistant safety cap and convenient dosage cup. Wild Cherry flavor.

**Children's TYLENOL®
Cold Plus Cough
Suspension Liquid**

McNeil Consumer Healthcare
P. 659

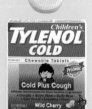

Available in blister pack of 24 chewable tablets. Wild Cherry flavor.

**Children's TYLENOL®
Cold Plus Cough
Chewable Tablets**

McNeil Consumer Healthcare
P. 663

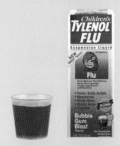

Available in Bubble Gum Blast flavor in child-resistant 4 fl. oz. bottles.

Children's TYLENOL® Flu Suspension Liquid

McNeil Consumer Healthcare
P. 663

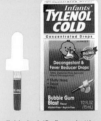

Available in Fruit Burst flavor in child-resistant 4 fl. oz. bottles.

Children's TYLENOL® Sinus Liquid

McNeil Consumer Healthcare
P. 659

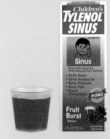

Available in 1/2 fl. oz. bottle with child-resistant safety cap and calibrated dropper. Bubble Gum flavor, Alcohol-free.

Infant's TYLENOL® Cold Decongestant and Fever Reducer Concentrated Drops

---

McNeil Consumer Healthcare
P. 659

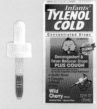

Available in 1/2 fl. oz. bottle with child-resistant safety cap and calibrated dropper. Wild Cherry flavor, Alcohol-free.

Infants' TYLENOL® Cold Decongestant and Fever Reducer Concentrated Drops Plus Cough

---

McNeil Consumer Healthcare
P. 657

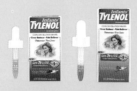

Available in Rich Cherry flavor and Rich Grape flavor 1/2 oz. bottle with child-resistant safety cap and calibrated dropper. Rich Grape Flavor, Alcohol Free, 80 mg per 0.8 mL. Cherry flavor also available in 1 oz. bottle.

Infants' TYLENOL® Concentrated Drops

McNeil Consumer Healthcare
P. 657

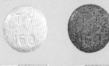

Available in blister pack of 24 chewable tablets. Fruit flavor and Grape flavor.

Junior Strength TYLENOL® Soft Chews Chewable Tablets

McNeil Consumer Healthcare
P. 647

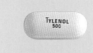

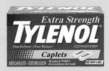

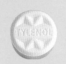

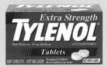

Caplets: tamper-resistant vials of 10 and bottles of 24's, 50's, 100's, 150's and 250's

Tablets: tamper-resistant vials of 10 and bottles of 30's, 60's and 200's

Liquid: tamper-evident bottles of 8 fl. oz.

Extra Strength TYLENOL®

McNeil Consumer Healthcare
P. 647

Tablets available in 100's.

Regular Strength TYLENOL®

McNeil Consumer Healthcare
P. 649

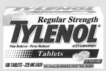

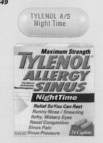

Caplets available in blister packs of 24's

Maximum Strength TYLENOL® Allergy Sinus NightTime

McNeil Consumer Healthcare
P. 649

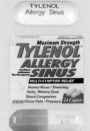

Caplets in blister packs of 24 & 48
Gelcaps in blister packs of 24 & 48
Geltabs in blister packs of 24 & 48

Maximum Strength TYLENOL® Allergy Sinus

McNeil Consumer Healthcare
P. 649

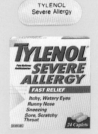

Caplets available in blister packs of 12's and 24's

TYLENOL® Severe Allergy

McNeil Consumer Healthcare
P. 647

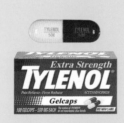

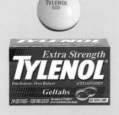

Gelcaps available in tamper-resistant bottles of 24's, 50's, 100's, 150's and 225's

Geltabs available in tamper-resistant bottles of 24's, 50's, 100's and 150's

Extra Strength TYLENOL®

McNeil Consumer Healthcare
P. 647

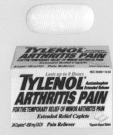

Caplets available in 24's, 50's, 100's, 150's and 290's

TYLENOL® Arthritis Pain Extended Relief

McNeil Consumer Healthcare
P. 651

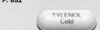

Caplets available in
blister packs of 24

**Multi-Symptom
TYLENOL® Cold
Complete Formula**

McNeil Consumer Healthcare
P. 651

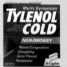

Caplets available in
blister packs of 24
Gelcaps available in
blister packs of 24

**Multi-Symptom TYLENOL®
Cold Non-Drowsy**

McNeil Consumer Healthcare
P. 652

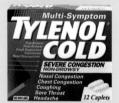

Available in blister
packs of 24

**TYLENOL® Cold Severe
Congestion Non-Drowsy**

McNeil Consumer Healthcare
P. 653

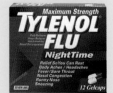

Gelcaps Available in
blister packs of 12's and 24's

**Maximum Strength
TYLENOL® Flu NightTime**

McNeil Consumer Healthcare
P. 653

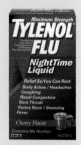

Available in 8 oz. bottles

**Maximum Strength
TYLENOL® Flu
NightTime Liquid**

McNeil Consumer Healthcare
P. 653

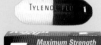

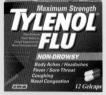

Gelcaps available in blister
packs of 24

**Maximum Strength
TYLENOL® Flu
Non-Drowsy**

McNeil Consumer Healthcare
P. 654

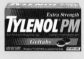

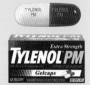

Geltabs available in tamper-resistant
bottles of 24, 50 and 100

Caplets available in tamper-resistant
bottles of 24, 50, 100 and 150

Gelcaps available in tamper-resistant
bottles of 24 and 50

Geltabs, Caplets and Gelcaps
available in bottles of 50 for
households without children

**Extra Strength
TYLENOL® PM**

McNeil Consumer Healthcare
P. 655

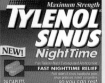

Available in blister packs of 24.

**Maximum Strength
TYLENOL® Sinus
NightTime Caplets**

McNeil Consumer Healthcare
P. 655

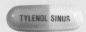

Caplets, Gelcaps and Geltabs
in blister packs of 24 and 48

**Maximum Strength
TYLENOL® Sinus**

McNeil Consumer Healthcare
P. 656

Cherry and Honey Lemon flavors
available in 8 fl. oz.

**Maximum Strength
TYLENOL® Sore Throat**

McNeil Consumer Healthcare
P. 656

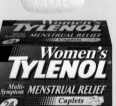

Caplets available in tamper-evident
bottles of 24 and 40.

**Women's TYLENOL®
Menstrual Relief**

NOVARTIS CONSUMER HEALTH

Novartis Consumer Health, Inc.
P. 668

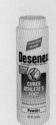

Powder   Spray Powder

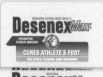

Antifungal Cream
Available in 12 g and 24 g

Desenex®

Novartis Consumer Health, Inc.
P. 668

Tablets 10's, 25's, 50's, 100's
Suppositories 4's, 8's, 16's, 50's

Dulcolax® Laxative

Novartis Consumer Health, Inc.
P. 670

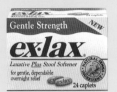

Gentle Strength 24's

Ex•Lax®

Novartis Consumer Health, Inc.
P. 671

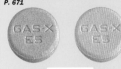

Extra Strength Cherry 18's, 48's
Extra Strength Peppermint 18's, 48's
(125 mg simethicone)

Gas-X®

Novartis Consumer Health, Inc.
P. 671

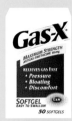

Maximum Strength Softgels
in packs of 50's
(166 mg simethicone)

Gas-X®

Novartis Consumer Health, Inc.
P. 669

Regular Strength 8's, 30's, 60's
Maximum Relief Formula 24's, 48's, 90's
Chocolated Laxative 6's, 18's and 48's

Ex•Lax®

Novartis Consumer Health, Inc.
P. 670

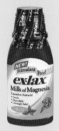

Mint Flavor
12 and 26 oz.

**Ex•Lax®
Milk of Magnesia**

Novartis Consumer Health, Inc.
P. 671

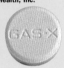

Cherry 12's, 36's
Peppermint 12's, 36's
(80 mg simethicone)

Gas-X®

Novartis Consumer Health, Inc.
P. 672

Athlete's Foot available in
12 g and 24 g
Jock Itch available in 12 g

Lamisil® AT™ Cream

Novartis Consumer Health, Inc.
P. 671

Stimulant-Free Stool
Softener Caplets 40's

Ex•Lax®

Novartis Consumer Health, Inc.
P. 670

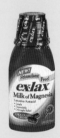

Chocolate Creme
12 and 26 oz.

**Ex•Lax®
Milk of Magnesia**

Novartis Consumer Health, Inc.
P. 671

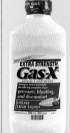
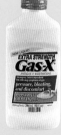

Extra Strength Cherry
and Peppermint Liquid
(50 mg per 5 mL simethicone)

Gas-X®

Novartis Consumer Health, Inc.
P. 672

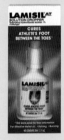

30 mL (1 oz)

**Lamisil® AT™
Athlete's Foot
Solution Dropper**

Novartis Consumer Health, Inc.
P. 671

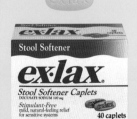

Stimulant-Free Stool
Softener Caplets 40's

Ex•Lax®

Novartis Consumer Health, Inc.
P. 670

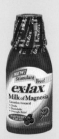

Raspberry Creme
12 and 26 oz.

**Ex•Lax®
Milk of Magnesia**

Novartis Consumer Health, Inc.
P. 671

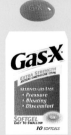

Extra Strength Softgels
in packs of 10's, 30's, 50's, 60's
(125 mg simethicone)

Gas-X®

Novartis Consumer Health, Inc.
P. 672

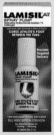

30 mL (1 oz)

**Lamisil® AT™
Athlete's Foot
Spray Pump**

Novartis Consumer Health, Inc.
P. 672

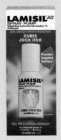

30 mL (1 oz)

**Lamisil® AT™
Jock Itch
Spray Pump**

Novartis Consumer Health, Inc.
P. 674

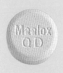

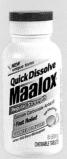

Assorted 45, 85 and 145 ct
Wild Berry 45 ct
Lemon 45, 85 ct
Wintergreen 85 ct

**Maalox® Quick Dissolve
Tablets Antacid/Calcium
Supplement**

Novartis Consumer Health, Inc.
P. 674

Assorted 35, 65, 90 ct
Wild Berry 35, 65 ct
Lemon 35, 65 ct

**Maximum Strength
Maalox® Quick Dissolve
Tablets Antacid/Calcium
Supplement**

Novartis Consumer Health, Inc.
P. 673

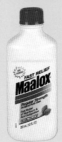

Cooling Mint Liquid
Also available in Smooth Cherry and
Refreshing Lemon
Bottles of 5 (Mint Only), 12 & 26 oz.

Maalox® Antacid

Novartis Consumer Health, Inc.
P. 673

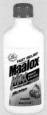

Cherry Liquid

Also available in Lemon, Mint,
Vanilla Creme, Peaches & Creme,
and Wild Berry

**Maximum Strength
Maalox® Antacid/Anti-Gas**

Novartis Consumer Health, Inc.
P. 674

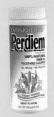

100% Natural Fiber Plus
Vegetable Laxative
Available in 250 gm,
400 gm and 600 gm

**Perdiem®
Overnight Relief**

Novartis Consumer Health, Inc.
P. 675

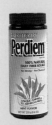

100% Natural
Daily Fiber Source
available in 250 gm

Perdiem® Fiber Therapy

Novartis Consumer Health, Inc.
P. 824

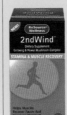
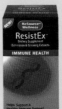

Stamina &   Eye Health
Muscle Recovery

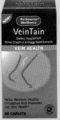
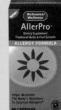

Immune Health   Stress Management

Vein Health   Allergy Formula

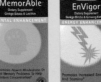

Mental   Energy
Enhancement   Enhancement

Novartis Consumer Health, Inc.
P. 675

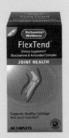

Joint Health

ReSource® Wellness

Novartis Consumer Health, Inc.
P. 824

600 mg

**ReSource Wellness®
CalciWise™
Dietary Supplement**
Calcium chew

Novartis Consumer Health, Inc.
P. 827

Slow Release Iron available
in 30, 60 and 90 ct.
Slow Release Iron & Folic Acid
available in 20 ct.

Slow Fe®

Novartis Consumer Health, Inc.
P. 676

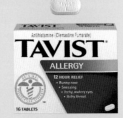

8, 16 count

Tavist® Allergy

Novartis Consumer Health, Inc.
P. 676

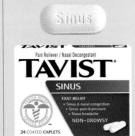

24, 48 count

Tavist® Sinus

Novartis Consumer Health, Inc.
P. 679

Available in 12 ct and 24 ct.
Severe Cold & Congestion Non-Drowsy

**TheraFlu®
Maximum Strength**

Novartis Consumer Health, Inc.
P. 678

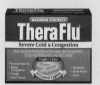

Available in 12 ct and 24 ct.
Severe Cold & Congestion Night Time

**TheraFlu®
Maximum Strength**

Novartis Consumer Health, Inc.
P. 677

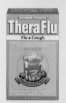
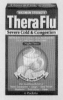

Flu & Congestion Non-Drowsy
Flu & Cough Night Time
Flu & Sore Throat Night Time
Severe Cold & Congestion Non-Drowsy
Formulas above available in 6 ct
Severe Cold & Congestion Night Time
Available in 6 ct and 12 ct.

**TheraFlu®
Maximum Strength**

Novartis Consumer Health, Inc.
P. 676

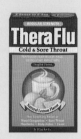

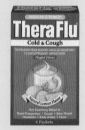

Cold & Sore Throat Night Time
Available in 6 ct
Cold & Cough Night Time
Available in 6 ct and 12 ct.

**TheraFlu®
Regular Strength**

Novartis Consumer Health, Inc.
P. 683

Cough   Cold & Allergy

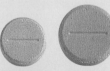

Cold & Cough   Cough &
                      Sore Throat

Triaminic® Softchews®

Novartis Consumer Health, Inc.
P. 680

Allergy Congestion

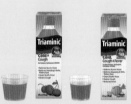

Chest Congestion   Cold & Allergy

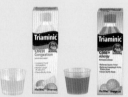

Cold & Cough   Cold, Cough & Fever

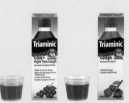

Cold & Night Time   Cough
Cough

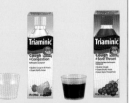

Cough & Congestion   Cough & Sore
                     Throat

Triaminic®

Novartis Consumer Health, Inc.
P. 684

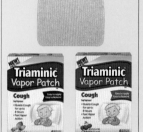

Menthol and
Mentholated Cherry Scents

Triaminic® Vapor Patch

Novartis Consumer Health, Inc.

Triaminicin®
Cold, Allergy, Sinus Medicine

12's, 24's, 48's

Triaminicin®

**PFIZER INC.,
WARNER-LAMBERT
CONSUMER GROUP**

Pfizer Inc., Warner-Lambert Consumer Group
P. 685

Herbal Throat Drops
Available in Honey-Lemon Chamomile,
Harvest Cherry and Sunshine Citrus

**Celestial Seasonings®
Soothers™**

Pfizer Inc., Warner-Lambert Consumer Group
P. 685

Breath drops available in Peppermint,
Freshmint and Cinnamint flavors in
slide top cartons of about 27 each.

**Certs® Cool Mint Drops®
with a Retsyn® Center**

Pfizer Inc., Warner-Lambert Consumer Group
P. 686

Tablets available in a credit card size
vial of 50 tablets each.
Available in Spearmint
and Peppermint flavors.

**Certs® Powerful Mints
with Retsyn® Crystals**

Pfizer Inc., Warner-Lambert Consumer Group
P. 687

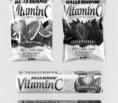

100% Daily Value
Vitamin C in each drop.
Available in Assorted Citrus, Strawberry
and Harvest Cherry flavors.

Halls® Defense

Pfizer Inc., Warner-Lambert Consumer Group
P. 686

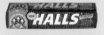

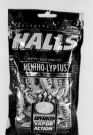

Cough Suppressant Drops
Spearmint, Mentho-Lyptus®,
Ice Blue, Honey-Lemon,
Cherry and Strawberry Flavors

Halls® Mentho-Lyptus®

Pfizer Inc., Warner-Lambert Consumer Group
P. 686

Honey-Lemon, Mentho-Lyptus® & Cherry

**Halls® Plus
Cough Suppressant
Throat Drops
with Medicine Center**

Pfizer Inc., Warner-Lambert Consumer Group
P. 686

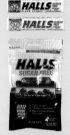

Cough Suppressant Drops
Black Cherry, Citrus Blend
and Mountain Menthol

**Halls® Sugar Free
Squares Mentho-Lyptus®**

Pfizer Inc., Warner-Lambert Consumer Group
P. 687

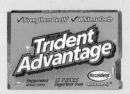

Sugarless Dental Gum available in
Peppermint and Coolmint® flavors in
12-pellet blister foil

**Trident Advantage™
with Recaldent™**

Pfizer Inc., Warner-Lambert Consumer Group
P. 687

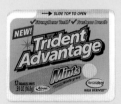

Sugarless Mints available in
Peppermint and Wintergreen flavors
in a 12-mint plastic vial.

**Trident Advantage™
Mints with Recaldent™**

Pfizer Inc., Warner-Lambert Consumer Group
P. 687

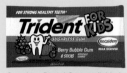

Sugarless Dental Gum available in
Berry Gum Flavor in a 8-stick pack.

**Trident for Kids™
with Recaldent™**

PFIZER INC, WARNER-LAMBERT CONSUMER HEALTHCARE

Pfizer Inc, Warner-Lambert Consumer
Healthcare
P. 688

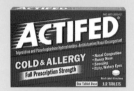

Available in boxes
of 12 and 24 tablets

Actifed® Cold & Allergy

Pfizer Inc, Warner-Lambert Consumer
Healthcare
P. 688

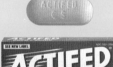
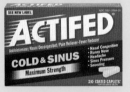

Available in boxes
of 24 caplets and tablets

Actifed® Cold & Sinus

Pfizer Inc, Warner-Lambert Consumer
Healthcare
P. 691

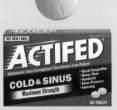

Pfizer Inc, Warner-Lambert Consumer
Healthcare
P. 688

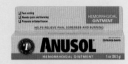

Ointment available in 1 oz. tubes

Anusol®

Pfizer Inc, Warner-Lambert Consumer
Healthcare
P. 689

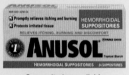

Suppositories available
in boxes of 12 and 24

Anusol®

Pfizer Inc, Warner-Lambert Consumer
Healthcare
P. 689

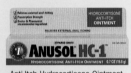

Anti-Itch Hydrocortisone Ointment
Available in 0.7 oz. tube

Anusol HC-1™

Pfizer Inc, Warner-Lambert Consumer
Healthcare
P. 691

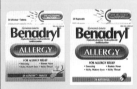

Capsules and Tablets
Available in boxes of 24 and 48
Tablets also available in
bottles of 100

Benadryl® Allergy

Pfizer Inc, Warner-Lambert Consumer Healthcare
P. 690

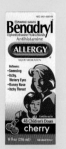

Available in 4 oz. and 8 oz. bottles

Benadryl® Allergy Liquid Medication

Pfizer Inc, Warner-Lambert Consumer Healthcare
P. 693

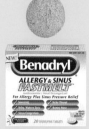

Available in boxes of 20 dissolving tablets

Benadryl® Allergy and Sinus FASTMELT

Pfizer Inc, Warner-Lambert Consumer Healthcare
P. 690

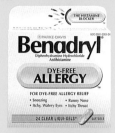

Available in Boxes of 24

Benadryl® Dye-Free Allergy Liqui-Gels® Softgels

Pfizer Inc, Warner-Lambert Consumer Healthcare
P. 696

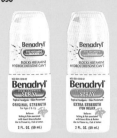

Original and Extra Strength

Benadryl® Itch Stopping Spray

Pfizer Inc, Warner-Lambert Consumer Healthcare
P. 689

Available in boxes of 24 chewable Tablets

Benadryl® Allergy Chewables

Pfizer Inc, Warner-Lambert Consumer Healthcare
P. 693

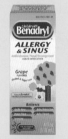

Available in 4 oz. bottles

Children's Benadryl® Allergy and Sinus Liquid Medication

Pfizer Inc, Warner-Lambert Consumer Healthcare
P. 693

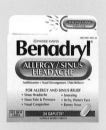

Benadryl® Allergy/ Sinus Headache

Pfizer Inc, Warner-Lambert Consumer Healthcare
P. 695

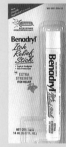

Extra Strength

Benadryl® Itch Relief Stick

Pfizer Inc, Warner-Lambert Consumer Healthcare
P. 691

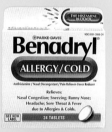

Available in boxes of 24 Tablets

Benadryl® Allergy/Cold

Pfizer Inc, Warner-Lambert Consumer Healthcare
P. 692

Available in boxes of 20 dissolving tablets

Benadryl® Children's Allergy/Cold FASTMELT

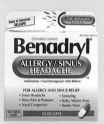

Available in boxes of 24 and 48 Caplets, box of 24 Gelcaps

Benadryl® Allergy/ Sinus Headache

Pfizer Inc, Warner-Lambert Consumer Healthcare
P. 695

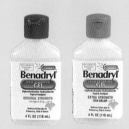

Original and Extra Strength

Benadryl® Itch Stopping Gel

Pfizer Inc, Warner-Lambert Consumer Healthcare
P. 692

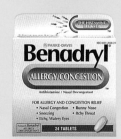

Available in boxes of 24 Tablets

Benadryl® Allergy/ Congestion

Pfizer Inc, Warner-Lambert Consumer Healthcare
P. 690

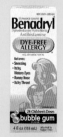

Available in 4 fl. oz. bottles

Benadryl® Dye-Free Allergy Liquid Medication

Pfizer Inc, Warner-Lambert Consumer Healthcare
P. 695

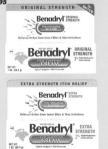

Original and Extra Strength

Benadryl® Itch Stopping Cream

Pfizer Inc, Warner-Lambert Consumer Healthcare
P. 694

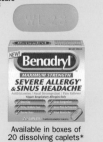

Available in boxes of 20 dissolving caplets*

†Benadryl® Severe Allergy and Sinus Headache Maximum Strength

* Capsule-shaped tablets † Upper Respiratory allergies only

Pfizer Inc, Warner-Lambert Consumer
Healthcare
P. 696

Arthritis Formula, Greaseless,
Original Formula, Ultra Strength
and Vanishing Scent.

BENGAY®

Pfizer Inc, Warner-Lambert Consumer
Healthcare
P. 696

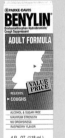

Available in 4 oz. bottles

**Benylin® Adult
Cough Suppressant**

Pfizer Inc, Warner-Lambert Consumer
Healthcare
P. 697

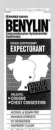

Available in 4 oz. bottles

**Benylin® Cough
Suppressant Expectorant**

Pfizer Inc, Warner-Lambert Consumer
Healthcare
P. 697

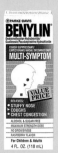

Available in 4 oz. bottles

Benylin® Multi-Symptom

Pfizer Inc, Warner-Lambert Consumer
Healthcare
P. 698

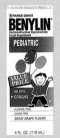

Available in 4 oz. bottles

**Benylin® Pediatric
Cough Suppressant**

Pfizer Inc, Warner-Lambert Consumer
Healthcare
P. 698

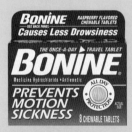

8 and 16 Chewable Tablets

Bonine®

Pfizer Inc, Warner-Lambert Consumer
Healthcare
P. 698

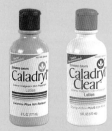

Itch Relief Plus Drying Action.
Available in Lotion, Clear Lotion

Caladryl®

Pfizer Inc, Warner-Lambert Consumer
Healthcare
P. 699

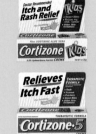

Kids available in 1/2 oz.
and 1 oz. Creme
Cortizone•5 available in 1 oz.
and 2 oz. Creme and 1 oz. Ointment

Cortizone•5®

Pfizer Inc, Warner-Lambert Consumer
Healthcare
P. 699

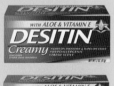

Cortizone•10 available in 1/2 oz.,
1 oz., and 2 oz. Creme and 1 oz.
and 2 oz. Ointment.
Cortizone•10 Plus available in
1 oz. and 2 oz. Creme.
Cortizone•10 Quick Shot Spray
available in 1.5 oz.

Cortizone•10®

Pfizer Inc, Warner-Lambert Consumer
Healthcare
P. 700

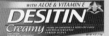

Diaper Rash Ointment

DESITIN® Creamy

Pfizer Inc, Warner-Lambert Consumer
Healthcare
P. 700

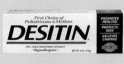
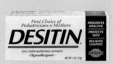

Diaper Rash Ointment

DESITIN®

Pfizer Inc, Warner-Lambert Consumer
Healthcare
P. 700

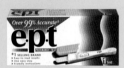

**DESITIN® Cornstarch
Baby Powder**

Pfizer Inc, Warner-Lambert Consumer
Healthcare
P. 701

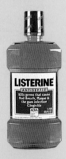

1 and 2 Pregnancy Test Kits Available
One Step. Easy to read.
Over 99% accurate in
Laboratory Tests.

e.p.t®

Pfizer Inc, Warner-Lambert Consumer
Healthcare
P. 702

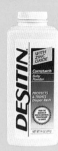

Listerine® Antiseptic

Pfizer Inc, Warner-Lambert Consumer
Healthcare
P. 702

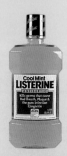

**Cool Mint
Listerine® Antiseptic**

Pfizer Inc, Warner-Lambert Consumer
Healthcare
P. 702

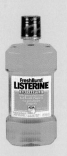

FreshBurst Listerine®

Pfizer Inc, Warner-Lambert Consumer
Healthcare
P. 702

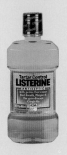

Tartar Control Listerine®

Pfizer Inc, Warner-Lambert Consumer
Healthcare
P. 703

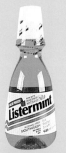

**Listermint®
Alcohol-Free Mouthwash**

Pfizer Inc, Warner-Lambert Consumer
Healthcare
P. 703

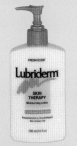

Available in Scented and
Fragrance Free

Lubriderm® Lotion

Pfizer Inc, Warner-Lambert Consumer
Healthcare
P. 703

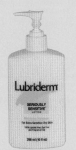

**Lubriderm® Seriously
Sensitive® Lotion**

Pfizer Inc, Warner-Lambert Consumer
Healthcare
P. 703

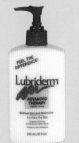

**Lubriderm® Advanced
Therapy Creamy Lotion**

Pfizer Inc, Warner-Lambert Consumer
Healthcare
P. 703

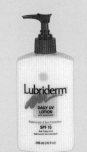

**Lubriderm® Daily UV
Lotion with Sunscreen**

Pfizer Inc, Warner-Lambert Consumer
Healthcare
P. 704

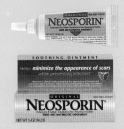

First Aid Antibiotic Ointment
Available in 1/2 oz. (14.2g) or 1 oz.
(28.3g) tubes; 1/32 oz. (0.9 g)
foil packets

Neosporin®

Pfizer Inc, Warner-Lambert Consumer
Healthcare
P. 704

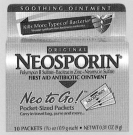

First Aid Antibiotic Ointment.
Available in Individual Foil Packets.
1/32 oz. (0.9 g) 10 packets per Box

Neosporin® Neo to Go!™

Pfizer Inc, Warner-Lambert Consumer
Healthcare
P. 704

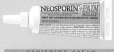
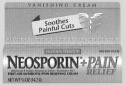

First Aid Antibiotic
Pain Relieving Cream
Available in 1/2 oz. (14.2g) tubes

Neosporin®+Pain Relief

Pfizer Inc, Warner-Lambert Consumer
Healthcare
P. 704

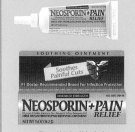

First Aid Antibiotic/
Pain Relieving Ointment
Available in 1/2 oz. (14.2g)
and 1 oz. (28.3g) tubes

Neosporin® Plus

Pfizer Inc, Warner-Lambert Consumer
Healthcare
P. 704

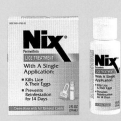

Lice Treatment Creme Rinse
2 fl. oz. (59 mL)
Also available in:
2-bottle family pack

Nix®

Pfizer Inc, Warner-Lambert Consumer
Healthcare
P. 705

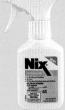

Lice Control Spray for
Bedding and Furniture
*NOT FOR HUMAN USE

Nix®

Pfizer Inc, Warner-Lambert Consumer
Healthcare
P. 706

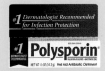

First Aid Antibiotic Powder & Ointment
Powder, 0.35 oz. (10g) Ointment,
1/2 oz. (14.2g) and 1 oz. tubes and
1/32 oz (28.3g) (0.9g) foil packets

Polysporin®

Pfizer Inc, Warner-Lambert Consumer
Healthcare
P. 706

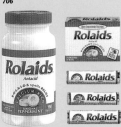

Fast, Effective Relief from
Heartburn, Acid Indigestion or
Sour Stomach
Original Peppermint,
Spearmint, and Cherry Flavors

Rolaids®

Pfizer Inc, Warner-Lambert Consumer
Healthcare
P. 706

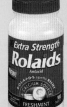

Freshmint and fruit

Extra Stength Rolaids®

Pfizer Inc, Warner-Lambert Consumer
Healthcare
P. 706

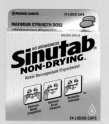

Available in Boxes of 24

**Sinutab® Non-Drying
Liquid Caps**

Pfizer Inc, Warner-Lambert Consumer
Healthcare
P. 707

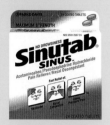

Maximum Strength
Without Drowsiness Formula
Available in 24 Caplets or Tablets

Sinutab® Sinus

Pfizer Inc, Warner-Lambert Consumer
Healthcare
P. 707

Maximum Strength Formula
Available in 24 Caplets or Tablets

Sinutab® Sinus Allergy

Pfizer Inc, Warner-Lambert Consumer
Healthcare
P. 708

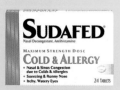

Available in boxes of 24

**Sudafed® Cold
and Allergy**

Pfizer Inc, Warner-Lambert Consumer
Healthcare
P. 709

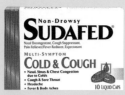

Available in 10's or 20's Liquid Caps

Sudafed® Cold & Cough

Pfizer Inc, Warner-Lambert Consumer
Healthcare
P. 710

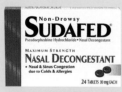

Available in boxes of
10 and 20 liquid caps

**Sudafed®
Cold and Sinus**

Pfizer Inc, Warner-Lambert Consumer
Healthcare
P. 710

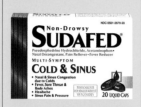

30 mg Tablets
Available in 24, 48 and 96

**Sudafed®
Nasal Decongestant**

Pfizer Inc, Warner-Lambert Consumer
Healthcare
P. 712

Available in 24 Liquid Caps

**Sudafed® Non-Drying
Sinus Liquid Caps**

Pfizer Inc, Warner-Lambert Consumer
Healthcare
P. 711

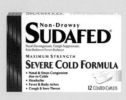

Pfizer Inc, Warner-Lambert Consumer
Healthcare
P. 711

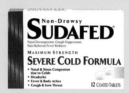

Available in 12's or 24's
caplets, 12's in tablets

**Sudafed®
Severe Cold Formula**

Pfizer Inc, Warner-Lambert Consumer
Healthcare
P. 708

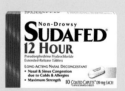

12 Hour Caplets
Available in 10 and 20 caplets

Sudafed® 12 Hour

Pfizer Inc, Warner-Lambert Consumer
Healthcare
P. 708

Available in boxes of 5 and 10 tablets.

Sudafed® 24 Hour

Pfizer Inc, Warner-Lambert Consumer
Healthcare
P. 712

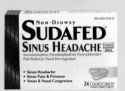

Pfizer Inc, Warner-Lambert Consumer
Healthcare
P. 709

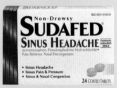

Available in 24's or 48's caplets;
24's tablets

**Sudafed® Sinus
Headache**

Pfizer Inc, Warner-Lambert Consumer
Healthcare
P. 709

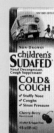

Available in 4 fl. oz. bottles

**Children's Sudafed®
Cold & Cough
Liquid Medication**

Pfizer Inc, Warner-Lambert Consumer
Healthcare
P. 711

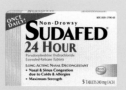

Available in boxes of
24 chewable tablets

**Children's Sudafed®
Nasal Decongestant**

Pfizer Inc, Warner-Lambert Consumer Healthcare
P. 711

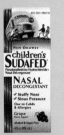

Available in 4 fl. oz. bottles

**Children's Sudafed®
Nasal Decongestant
Liquid Medication**

Pfizer Inc, Warner-Lambert Consumer Healthcare
P. 714

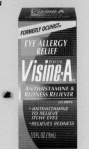

Itching and Redness
Reliever Eye Drops

Visine®-A™

Pharmaton
P. 831

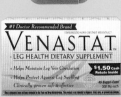

100 mg
Capsules

Ginsana® Sport

Pharmaton
P. 833

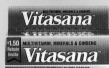

Dietary Supplement for Leg Health

Venastat™

Pfizer Inc, Warner-Lambert Consumer Healthcare
P. 713

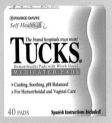

Pre-Moistened Pads
Available in 40 and 100 pad packages
Tucks® Take Alongs available in 12
individually packed towelettes.

Tucks®

Pfizer Inc, Warner-Lambert Consumer Healthcare
P. 716

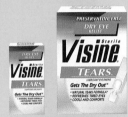

Dry Eye Relief

Visine® Tears™

Pharmaton
P. 830

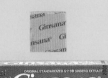

50 mg
Chewy Squares

Ginsana®

Pharmaton
P. 834

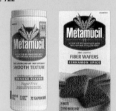

Daily Dietary Supplement

Vitasana™

Pfizer Inc, Warner-Lambert Consumer Healthcare
P. 713

Nighttime Sleep Aid

SleepGels available in
8, 16 and 32 softgels

SleepTabs available in
8, 16, 32 and 48 tablets

Unisom®

Pfizer Inc, Warner-Lambert Consumer Healthcare
P. 717

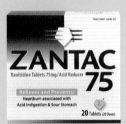

Available in boxes of
4, 10, 20, 30, 60, 80 and 90 tablets

Zantac® 75

Pharmaton
P. 832

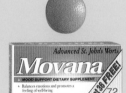

300 mg
Dietary Supplement for Mood Support

Movana™

Procter & Gamble
P. 722

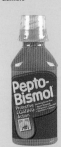

Available in 30, 48, 72, 114 and 180
dose canisters and cartons of 30
one-dose packets.
Also available in sugar free.
Cinnamon Spice and Apple Crisp
Wafers available in 12-dose cartons.

Metamucil®

Pfizer Inc, Warner-Lambert Consumer Healthcare
P. 714

Advanced Relief, Original,
L.R. Long Lasting and
A.C. Seasonal Relief.

Visine®

Pharmaton
P. 829

Mental Performance
Dietary Supplement

Ginkoba M/E™

Pharmaton
P. 832

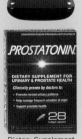

Dietary Supplement
for Urinary and
Prostate Health

Prostatonin®

Procter & Gamble
P. 723

Also available in Maximum Strength
Liquid, Chewable Tablets and
Swallowable Caplets

Pepto-Bismol®

PRODUCTS ON DEMAND

Products On Demand
P. 731

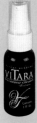

1 oz

**Vitara™
Feminine Cream**

PURDUE FREDERICK

The Purdue Frederick Company
P. 732

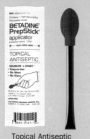

Topical Antiseptic

Betadine® PrepStick®

The Purdue Frederick Company
P. 731

Maximum Strength Ointment

Antibiotics plus Moisturizer

Antibiotics plus Pain Reliever

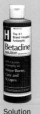

Solution

Betadine®

The Purdue Frederick Company
P. 732

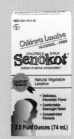

Natural Vegetable Laxative
Children's Syrup

Senokot®

The Purdue Frederick Company
P. 732

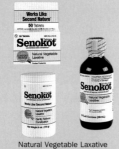

Natural Vegetable Laxative
Available in Tablets, Granules,
and Syrup.

Senokot®

The Purdue Frederick Company
P. 732

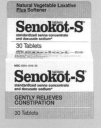

Natural Vegetable Laxative
Plus Softener Tablets

Senokot-S®

SCHERING-PLOUGH

Schering-Plough HealthCare Products
P. 733

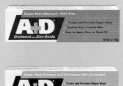

Original Ointment and
Ointment with Zinc Oxide

A and D® Ointment

Schering-Plough HealthCare Products
P. 733

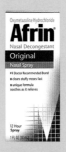

**Afrin® Original 12 Hour
Nasal Spray**

Schering-Plough HealthCare Products
P. 735

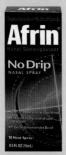

**Afrin® No Drip
12 Hour Nasal Spray**

Schering-Plough HealthCare Products
P. 734

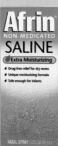

Non-medicated

**Afrin® Saline
Extra Moisturizing**

Schering-Plough HealthCare Products
P. 737

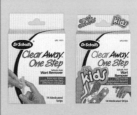

**Clear Away® One Step
Wart Removers**

Schering-Plough HealthCare Products
P. 735

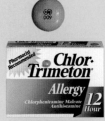

12 Hour Allergy Tablets

Schering-Plough HealthCare Products
P. 735

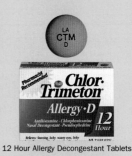

12 Hour Allergy Decongestant Tablets

Chlor-Trimeton®

Schering-Plough HealthCare Products
P. 737

For Relief Of Cold,
Flu & Sinus Symptoms

Coricidin´D´®

Schering-Plough HealthCare Products
P. 738

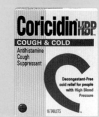

Cough and Cold Relief for people with
High Blood Pressure

Coricidin HBP®

Schering-Plough HealthCare Products
P. 738

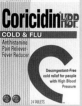

Cold and Flu Relief for people with
High Blood Pressure

Coricidin HBP®

Schering-Plough HealthCare Products
P. 738

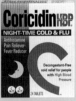

Night-Time Cold and Flu Relief
for people with High Blood Pressure

Coricidin HBP®

Schering-Plough HealthCare Products
P. 738

Maximum Strength Flu Relief
for people with High Blood Pressure

Coricidin HBP®

Schering-Plough HealthCare Products
P. 739

Available in
Laxative Tablets and Caplets,
Combination Vegetable Laxative
Plus Stool Softener and
Stool Softener Gelcaps.

Correctol®

Schering-Plough HealthCare Products
P. 740

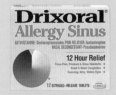

12 Hour Sustained-Action Tablets

Drixoral® Cold & Allergy

Schering-Plough HealthCare Products
P. 741

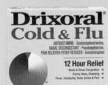

12 Hour Extended-Release Tablets

Drixoral® Allergy Sinus

Schering-Plough HealthCare Products
P. 740

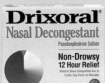

12 Hour Extended-Release Tablets

Drixoral® Cold & Flu

Schering-Plough HealthCare Products
P. 740

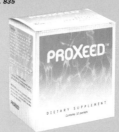

12 Hour Extended-Release Tablets

Drixoral® Nasal Decongestant

Schering-Plough HealthCare Products
P. 741

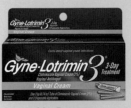

3-Day Treatment
Vaginal Cream

Gyne-Lotrimin 3®

Schering-Plough HealthCare Products
P. 742

Antifungal for Athlete's Foot
and Jock Itch

Lotrimin® AF

Schering-Plough HealthCare Products
P. 742

Spray Powder, Spray Liquid, Spray
Deodorant Powder, Shaker Powder,
Jock Itch Spray Powder

Lotrimin® AF
(2% miconazole nitrate)

Sigma–Tau Pharmaceuticals, Inc.
P. 835

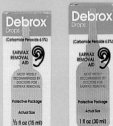

Dietary Supplement
Promotes optimum sperm quality

Proxeed™

SmithKline Beecham
Consumer Healthcare, L.P.
P. 744

Fiber Therapy for Regularity
Sugar Free Orange available in:
8.6 oz., 16.9 oz., and 32 oz.
Regular Orange available in:
16 oz., 30 oz., and 50 oz. containers

Citrucel®

SmithKline Beecham
Consumer Healthcare, L.P.
P. 745

Nasal Decongestant/Antihistamine
Packages of 10 and 20
Maximum Strength Caplets or
Regular Strength Capsules

Contac® 12 Hour Cold

SmithKline Beecham
Consumer Healthcare, L.P.
P. 746

Multisymptom Cold & Flu Relief
Maximum Strength Formula:
Packages of 16 and 30 caplets
Non-Drowsy Formula:
Packages of 16 caplets

Contac® Severe Cold & Flu

SmithKline Beecham
Consumer Healthcare, L.P.
P. 747

Drops
1/2 Fl. oz. 1 Fl. oz.

Debrox®

SmithKline Beecham
Consumer Healthcare, L.P.
P. 747

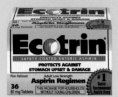

Adult Low Strength Tablets
in Bottles of 36

Ecotrin®

SmithKline Beecham
Consumer Healthcare, L.P.
P. 747

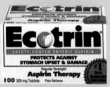

Regular Strength Tablets
in bottles of 100, 250

Ecotrin®

SmithKline Beecham
Consumer Healthcare, L.P.
P. 747

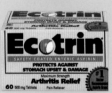

Maximum Strength Tablets
in bottles of 60, 150.

Ecotrin®

**SEEKING AN
ALTERNATIVE?**

Check the
Product Category Index,
where you'll find
alphabetical listings of
all the products in each
therapeutic class.

SmithKline Beecham
Consumer Healthcare, L.P.
P. 837

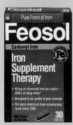

Packages of 30 caplets

SmithKline Beecham
Consumer Healthcare, L.P.
P. 751

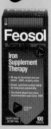

Packages of 100 tablets

Feosol®

SmithKline Beecham
Consumer Healthcare, L.P.
P. 751

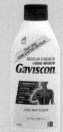

12 Fl. oz.

**Gaviscon® Regular
Strength Liquid Antacid**

SmithKline Beecham
Consumer Healthcare, L.P.
P. 750

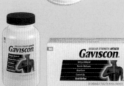

100-Tablet bottles
30-Tablet box (foil-wrapped 2s)
**Gaviscon® Regular
Strength Antacid**

SmithKline Beecham
Consumer Healthcare, L.P.
P. 751

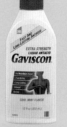

Extra Strength Formula
12 Fl. Oz.

**Gaviscon® Extra Strength
Liquid Antacid**

SmithKline Beecham
Consumer Healthcare, L.P.
P. 750

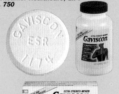

Extra Strength Formula
100-Tablet bottles
6 and 30-Tablet box
(foil-wrapped 2's)

**Gaviscon® Extra
Strength Antacid**

SmithKline Beecham
Consumer Healthcare, L.P.
P. 751

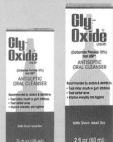

1/2 Fl. oz.   2 Fl. oz.

Gly-Oxide® Liquid

SmithKline Beecham
Consumer Healthcare, L.P.
P. 753

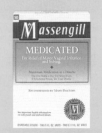

Medicated Disposable Douche
With Povidone-iodine
Available in single or twin packs

Massengill®

SmithKline Beecham
Consumer Healthcare, L.P.
P. 754

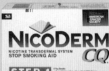

Step 1
Also available in 2 week kit

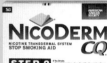

Step 2
Also available in 2 week kit

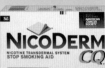

Step 3
Also available in 2 week kit

Includes User's Guide, Audio Tape and
Child Resistant Disposal Tray
Stop Smoking Aid
Nicotine Transdermal System

NicoDerm® CQ™

SmithKline Beecham
Consumer Healthcare, L.P.
P. 758

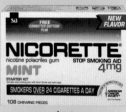

4 mg
For Smokers over 24
Cigarettes a day
Refill pack available
Stop Smoking Aid
Nicotine Polacrilex Gum

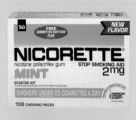

2 mg
For Smokers under 25
Cigarettes a day
Refill pack available
Stop Smoking Aid
Nicotine Polacrilex Gum

Nicorette®

**SmithKline Beecham
Consumer Healthcare, L.P.
P. 838**

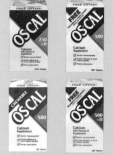

Calcium Supplement
Os-Cal®

**SmithKline Beecham
Consumer Healthcare, L.P.
P. 761**

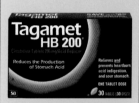

Acid Reducer
Packages of 6, 12, 18,
30, 50, 70 and 80

Tagamet HB 200®

**SmithKline Beecham
Consumer Healthcare, L.P.
P. 762**

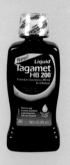

Liquid Tagamet HB 200®

**SmithKline Beecham
Consumer Healthcare, L.P.
P. 763**

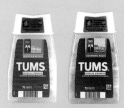

Peppermint and
Assorted Flavors

Tums®

**SmithKline Beecham
Consumer Healthcare, L.P.
P. 763**

Tropical Fruit, Wintergreen,
Assorted Flavors, Assorted Berry
and SugarFree Orange Cream
Tums E-X®

**SmithKline Beecham
Consumer Healthcare, L.P.
P. 763**

Assorted Mint and Fruit Flavors.
Also available in Tropical Fruit,
Assorted Berries and
Spearmint flavors

Tums® Ultra™

**SmithKline Beecham
Consumer Healthcare, L.P.
P. 763**

Alertness Aid with Caffeine
Available in tablets and caplets

Vivarin®

**LOOKING FOR
A PARTICULAR
COMPOUND?**

In the
Active Ingredients Index
(Yellow Pages),
you'll find all the
brands that contain it.

STRATEGIC SCIENCE AND TECHNOLOGIES, INC.

**Strategic Science and Technologies, Inc.
P. 840**

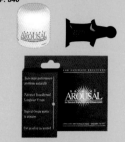

Natural Arousal™

**Strategic Science and Technologies, Inc.
P. 840**

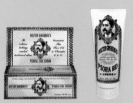

Psoria Rid Cream

**Strategic Science and Technologies, Inc.
P. 841**

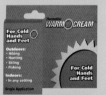

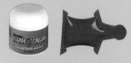

Warm Cream™

SUNPOWER

**Sunpower Nutraceutical Inc.
P. 841**

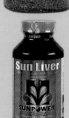

Sun Liver™

WALLACE

**Wallace Laboratories
P. 767**

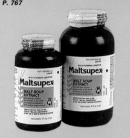

8 fl. oz. (1/2 pt) and 16 fl. oz. (1 pt)
Maltsupex® Liquid
(malt soup extract)

**Wallace Laboratories
P. 767**

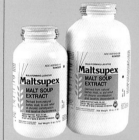

8 oz. (1/2 lb) and 16 oz. (1 lb)
Maltsupex® Powder
(malt soup extract)

**Wallace Laboratories
P. 767**

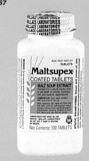

100 Tablets
Maltsupex® Tablets
(malt soup extract)

**Wallace Laboratories
P. 768**

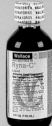

1 Pint (473 mL)
Also available: 4 fl. oz. (118 mL)
Ryna-C® Liquid
(antitussive/antihistamine/
decongestant)

J.B. WILLIAMS CO.

J.B. Williams Co.
P. 786

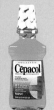

Original and Mint Antiseptic
Mouthwash/Gargle
Available in 4, 12, 24
and 32 Fl. oz. bottles

Cepacol®

J.B. Williams Co.
P. 787

Maximum Strength Sore Throat Lozenges
Mint and Cherry Flavors
also available in Regular Strength
18 Lozenges per pack
Also available in
Sugar Free Maximum Strength
16 Lozenges per pack

Cepacol®

J.B. Williams Co.
P. 788

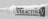

Cold Sore Treatment
Available in a gel and a cream
0.25 oz. tubes.

Cepacol® Viractin®

WYETH-AYERST

Tamper-Resistant/ Evident Packaging

Statements alerting consumers to
the specific type of Tamper-
Resistant/Evident Packaging
appear on the bottle labels and
cartons of all over-the-counter
products of Wyeth-Ayerst. This
includes plastic cap seals on bottles, individually wrapped tablets
or suppositories, and sealed
cartons. This packaging has been
developed to better
protect the consumer.

Wyeth-Ayerst Pharmaceuticals
P. 789

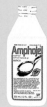

12 Fl. oz. bottle Suspension Antacid

Amphojel®

Wyeth-Ayerst Pharmaceuticals
P. 789

Available in bottles of 4 and 8 Fl. oz.

Donnagel®

Wyeth-Ayerst Pharmaceuticals
P. 789

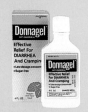

500 mg. Chewable Tablet in Cartons
of 36 individually packaged blister units
Also available in bottles of 100 tablets.

Mitrolan®

ZANFEL

Zanfel Laboratories Inc.
P. 790

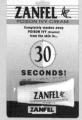

Poison Ivy Cream

Zanfel™

4LIFE RESEARCH™, LC

4LIFE
P. 814

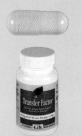

Dietary Supplement

Transfer Factor™

4LIFE
P. 814

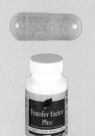

Dietary Supplement

Transfer Factor Plus™

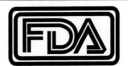

U.S. FOOD AND DRUG ADMINISTRATION

Professional and Consumer Information Numbers

Medical Product Reporting Programs

MedWatch (24 hour service) 800-332-1088
Reporting of problems with drugs, devices, biologics (except vaccines), medical foods, dietary supplements.

Vaccine Adverse Event Reporting System (24 hour service) 800-822-7967
Reporting of vaccine-related problems.

Mandatory Medical Device Reporting 301-827-0360
Reporting required from user facilities regarding device-related deaths and serious injuries.

Veterinary Adverse Drug Reaction Program 888-332-8387
Reporting of adverse drug events in animals.

Medical Advertising Information 301-827-2828
Inquiries from health professionals regarding product promotion.

USP Medication Errors 800-233-7767
Reporting of medication errors or near-errors to help avoid future problems through improvement in product names and packaging.

Information for Health Professionals

Center for Drugs Information Branch 301-827-4573
Information on human drugs including hormones.

Center for Biologics Office of Communication 301-827-2000
Information on biological products including vaccines and blood.

Center for Devices and Radiological Health 301-443-4190
Automated request for information on medical devices and radiation-emitting products.

Emergency Operations 301-443-1240
Emergencies involving FDA-regulated products, tampering reports, and emergency Investigational New Drug requests.

Office of Orphan Products Development 301-827-3666
Information on products for rare diseases.

General Information

General Consumer Inquiries 888-463-6332
Consumer information on regulated products/issues.

Freedom of Information 301-827-6500
Requests for publicly available FDA documents.

Office of Public Affairs 301-827-6250
Interviews/press inquiries on FDA activities.

Center for Food Safety and Applied Nutrition 888-723-3366
Information on food safety, seafood, dietary supplements, women's nutrition, and cosmetics.

SECTION 7

NONPRESCRIPTION DRUG INFORMATION

This section presents information on nonprescription drugs, self-testing kits, and other medical products marketed for home use by consumers. It is made possible through the courtesy of the manufacturers whose products appear on the following pages. The information concerning each product has been prepared, edited, and approved by professional staff of the manufacturer.

Pharmaceutical product descriptions in this section must be in compliance with the Code of Federal Regulations labeling requirements for over-the-counter drugs. The descriptions are designed to provide all information necessary for informed use, including, when applicable, active ingredients, inactive ingredients, indications, actions, warnings, cautions, drug interactions, symptoms and treatment of oral overdosage, dosage and directions for use, professional labeling, and how supplied. In some cases, additional information has been supplied to complement the standard labeling.

In compiling this section, the publisher has emphasized the necessity of describing products comprehensively. The descriptions seen here include all information made available by the manufacturer. The publisher does not warrant or guarantee any product described here, and does not perform any independent analysis of the information provided. Inclusion of a product in this book does not represent an endorsement, and the publisher does not necessarily advocate the use of any product listed.

Alpharma
U.S. Pharmaceuticals Division

**7205 WINDSOR BOULEVARD
BALTIMORE, MD 21244**

For General Inquiries Contact:
Customer Service
(800) 638-9096

PERMETHRIN LOTION 1%
Lice Treatment

Description:
EACH FLUID OUNCE CONTAINS: Active Ingredient: Permethrin 280 mg (1%). Inactive Ingredients: Balsam fir canada, cetyl alcohol, citric acid, FD&C Yellow No. 6, fragrance, hydrolyzed animal protein, hydroxyethyl cellulose, polyoxyethylene 10 cetyl ether, propylene glycol, stearalkonium chloride, water, isopropyl alcohol 5.6 g (20%), methylparaben 56 mg (0.2%), and propylparaben 22 mg (0.08%).

Permethrin Lotion 1% kills lice and their unhatched eggs with usually only one application. Permethrin Lotion 1% protects against head lice reinfestation for 14 days. The creme rinse formula leaves hair manageable and easy to comb.

Indications: For the treatment of head lice. For prophylactic use during head lice epidemics.

Warnings: For external use only. Keep out of eyes when rinsing hair. Adults and children: Close eyes and do not open eyes until product is rinsed out. If product gets into the eyes, immediately flush with water. Do not use near the eyes or permit contact with mucous membranes, such as inside the nose, mouth, or vagina, as irritation may occur. Children: Also protect children's eyes with a washcloth, towel or other suitable material or method. This product should not be used on pediatric patients less than 2 months of age. Itching, redness, or swelling of the scalp may occur. If skin irritation persists or infection is present or develops, discontinue use and consult a doctor. Consult a doctor if infestation of eyebrows or eyelashes occurs. This product may cause breathing difficulty or an asthmatic episode in susceptible persons. As with any drug, if you are pregnant or nursing a baby, seek the advice of a health professional before using this product. Keep this and all drugs out of the reach of children. In case of accidental ingestion, seek professional assistance or contact a Poison Control Center immediately.

Dosage and Administration:
Treatment: Permethrin Lotion 1% should be used after hair has been washed with patient's regular shampoo, rinsed with water and towel dried. A sufficient amount should be applied to saturate hair and scalp (especially behind the ears and on the nape of the neck). Leave on hair for 10 minutes but not longer. Rinse with water. A single application is usually sufficient. If live lice are observed seven days or more after the first application of this product, a second treatment should be given. For proper head lice management, remove nits with the nit comb provided.

Head lice live on the scalp and lay small white eggs (nits) on the hair shaft close to the scalp. The nits are most easily found on the nape of the neck or behind the ears. All personal headgear, scarfs, coats, and bed linen should be disinfected by machine washing in hot water and drying, using the hot cycle of a dryer for at least 20 minutes. Personal articles of clothing or bedding that cannot be washed may be dry-cleaned, sealed in a plastic bag for a period of about 2 weeks, or sprayed with a product specifically designed for this purpose. Personal combs and brushes may be disinfected by soaking in hot water (above 130°F) for 5 to 10 minutes. Thorough vacuuming of rooms inhabited by infected patients is recommended.

Prophylaxis: Prophylactic use of Permethrin Lotion 1% is only recommended for individuals exposed to head lice epidemics in which at least 20% of the population at an institution are infested and for immediate household members of infested individuals. Causal use is strongly discouraged.

The method of application of Permethrin Lotion 1% for prophylaxis is identical to that described above for treatment of a lice infestation except nit removal is not required.

Directions For Use: One application of Permethrin Lotion 1% has been shown to protect greater than 95% of patients against reinfestation for at least two weeks. In epidemic settings, a second prophylactic application is recommended two weeks after the first because the life cycle of a head louse is approximately four weeks.

How Supplied: Bottles of 2 fl. oz. (59 mL) with nit removal comb and Family Pack of 2 bottles, 2 fl. oz. (59 mL) each, with 2 nit removal combs.
Store at 15° to 25°C (59° to 77°F).
Manufactured by
Alpharma USPD Inc.
Baltimore, MD 21244
FORM NO. 5242   Rev. 9/99
VC1587

**IF YOU SUSPECT
AN INTERACTION. . .**
The 1,800-page
PDR Companion Guide™ can help.
Use the order form
in the front of this book.

Bayer Corporation Consumer Care Division

**36 Columbia Road
P.O. Box 1910
Morristown, NJ 07962-1910**

Direct Inquiries to:
Consumer Relations
(800) 331-4536
www.bayercare.com

For Medical Emergency Contact:
Bayer Corporation
Consumer Care Division
(800) 331-4536

ALEVE®
Naproxen Sodium Tablets, 220 mg
Pain reliever/fever reducer

ALEVE Tablets, Caplets* or Gelcaps**
Naproxen Sodium Tablets, USP

Active Ingredient:
naproxen sodium
(in each tablet, caplet*, gelcap)**
220 mg (naproxen 200 mg)
Inactive Ingredients (Tablets/Caplets*): magnesium stearate, microcrystalline cellulose, opadry YS-1-4215, povidone, talc.
Inactive Ingredients (Gelcaps):** D&C yellow #10 lake, edetate disodium, edible ink, FD&C blue #1, FD&C yellow #6 lake, gelatin, glycerin, hydroxypropyl methylcellulose, magnesium stearate, microcrystalline cellulose, polyethylene glycol, povidone, stearic acid, talc, titanium dioxide, and triacetin.
Purpose:
Pain reliever/fever reducer

Uses: Temporarily relieves minor aches and pains due to:
- common cold
- backache
- headache
- menstrual cramps
- toothache
- minor pain of arthritis
- muscular aches

Temporarily reduces fever

Warnings:
Allergy Alert: naproxen sodium may cause a severe allergic reaction which may include: • hives • facial swelling • asthma (wheezing) • shock
Alcohol Warning: If you consume 3 or more alcoholic drinks every day, ask your doctor whether you should take naproxen sodium or other pain relievers/fever reducers. Naproxen sodium may cause stomach bleeding.
Do not use:
- if you have ever had an allergic reaction to any other pain reliever/fever reducer
- with any other pain reliever/fever reducer
- for more than 10 days for pain
- for more than 3 days for fever
Ask a doctor before use if:
- the painful area is red or swollen
- you take other drugs on a regular basis
- you are under a doctor's care for any continuing condition

- you have had serious side effects from any pain reliever

Stop use and ask a doctor if:

- an allergic reaction occurs, seek medical help right away
- any new or unexpected symptoms occur
- symptoms continue or worsen
- you have difficulty swallowing
- it feels like the pill is stuck in your throat
- you develop heartburn
- stomach pain occurs with use of this product or if even mild symptoms persist

If pregnant or breast-feeding, ask a health professional before use. **IT IS ESPECIALLY IMPORTANT NOT TO USE NAPROXEN SODIUM DURING THE LAST 3 MONTHS OF PREGNANCY UNLESS SPECIFICALLY DIRECTED TO DO SO BY A DOCTOR BECAUSE IT MAY CAUSE PROBLEMS IN THE UNBORN CHILD OR COMPLICATIONS DURING DELIVERY.**

Keep out of reach of children. In case of accidental overdose, seek professional assistance or contact a Poison Control Center immediately.

Dietary information: (in each tablet, caplet*, gelcap**)

- sodium 20 mg

Directions: Drink a full glass of water with each dose.

Adults: • Take 1 tablet (caplet*, gelcap**) every 8 to 12 hours while symptoms persist. For the first dose you may take 2 tablets (caplets*, gelcaps**) within the first hour. The smallest effective dose should be used.

Do not take more than:

- 2 tablets (caplets*, gelcaps**) in any 8 to 12 hour period
- 3 tablets (caplets*, gelcaps**) in a 24 hour period.

Over age 65: • Do not take more than 1 tablet (caplet*, gelcap**) every 12 hours unless directed by a doctor.

Children under 12 years of age: • Do not give this product to children under 12 unless directed by a doctor.

*capsule-shaped tablet(s)
**gelatin coated capsule-shaped tablet(s)

Store at room temperature: Avoid high humidity and excessive heat 104°F (40°C).

How Supplied: Aleve tablets in boxes of 24, 50, 100, 150. Caplets of 8, 24, 50, 100, 150, 200. Gelcaps of 20, 40, 80.

Shown in Product Identification Guide, page 503

Aleve® Cold & Sinus
Pain reliever/fever reducer/nasal decongestant

Active Ingredients:
(in each caplet)　　　　　　**Purpose:**
Naproxen sodium 220 mg Pain reliever/
(naproxen 200 mg) .... Fever reducer
Pseudoephedrine HCl 120 mg,
extended-release .. Nasal decongestant

Inactive Ingredients: colloidal silicon dioxide, FD&C blue #1 lake, hydroxypropyl methylcellulose, lactose, magnesium stearate, microcrystalline cellulose, pharmaceutical glaze, polyethylene glycol, povidone, propylene glycol, talc, titanium dioxide

Uses: temporarily relieves these cold, sinus and flu symptoms:

- sinus pressure
- minor body aches and pains
- headache
- nasal and sinus congestion (promotes sinus drainage and restores freer breathing through the nose)
- fever

Warnings:

Allergy Alert: Naproxen sodium may cause a severe allergic reaction which may include:

- hives
- facial swelling
- asthma (wheezing)
- shock

Alcohol Warning: If you consume 3 or more alcoholic drinks every day, ask your doctor whether you should take naproxen sodium or other pain relievers/fever reducers. Naproxen sodium may cause stomach bleeding.

Do not use if you:

- have ever had an allergic reaction to any other pain reliever/fever reducer
- are now taking a prescription monoamine oxidase inhibitor (MAOI) (certain drugs for depression, psychiatric or emotional conditions, or Parkinson's disease), or for 2 weeks after stopping the MAOI drug. If you do not know if your prescription drug contains an MAOI, ask a doctor or pharmacist before taking this product.

Ask a doctor before use if you have:

- heart disease
- high blood pressure
- thyroid disease
- diabetes
- trouble urinating due to an enlarged prostate gland
- had serious side effects from any pain reliever/fever reducer

Ask a doctor or pharmacist before use if you are:

- using any other product containing naproxen or pseudoephedrine
- taking any other pain reliever/fever reducer or nasal decongestant
- under a doctor's care for any continuing medical condition
- taking other drugs on a regular basis

When using this product • do not use more than directed

Stop use and ask a doctor if:

- an allergic reaction occurs. Seek medical help right away.
- you get nervous, dizzy, or sleepless
- you develop heartburn
- nasal congestion lasts more than 7 days
- symptoms continue or get worse
- you have trouble swallowing or the caplet feels stuck in your thoat
- new or unexpected symptoms occur
- stomach pain occurs with use of this product or if even mild symptoms persist
- fever lasts for more than 3 days

If pregnant or breast-feeding, ask a health professional before use.

It is especially important not to use naproxen sodium during the last 3 months of pregnancy unless definitely directed to do so by a doctor because it may cause problems in the unborn child or complications during delivery.

Keep out of reach of children. In case of overdose, get medical help or contact a Poison Control Center right away.

Directions:

- **swallow whole;** do not crush or chew
- **drink a full glass of water with each dose**
- adults and children 12 years and older: **1 caplet every 12 hours;** do not take more than 2 caplets in 24 hours
- children under 12 years: ask a doctor

Other information:

- **each caplet contains:** sodium 20 mg
- store at 20 to 25° C (68–77°F)
- store in a dry place

Questions or Comments? call **1-800-395-0689**

Distributed by: Bayer Corporation Consumer Care Division Morristown, NJ 07960 USA　　B-R LLC

Shown in Product Identification Guide, page 503

ALKA-SELTZER® Original
ALKA-SELTZER® Extra Strength
ALKA-SELTZER® Lemon Lime
ALKA-SELTZER® Cherry
Effervescent Antacid Pain Reliever

Active ingredients:
ALKA-SELTZER® Original:
Aspirin 325 mg, Citric acid 1000 mg, Heat Treated Sodium Bicarbonate 1916 mg.
ALKA-SELTZER® Extra Strength:
Aspirin 500 mg, Citric acid 1000 mg, Heat Treated Sodium Bicarbonate 1985 mg.
ALKA-SELTZER® Lemon Lime and Cherry:
Aspirin 325 mg, Citric acid 1000 mg, Heat Treated Sodium Bicarbonate 1700 mg.

Inactive Ingredients:
ALKA-SELTZER® Original:
none.
ALKA-SELTZER® Extra Strength:
Artificial and Natural Flavors.
ALKA-SELTZER® Lemon Lime:
Artificial Flavor, Aspartame, Tableting Aids.
ALKA-SELTZER Cherry:
Artificial Flavor, Aspartame, Tableting Aids.
Phenylketonurics:
Each tablet contains 9 mg (Lemon Lime) or 12.3 mg (Cherry) of Phenylalanine.
Sodium Content per tablet:
Alka-Seltzer® Original: 567 mg
Alka-Seltzer® Extra Strength: 588 mg
Alka-Seltzer® Lemon Lime and Cherry: 503 mg.

Indications: For fast relief of heartburn, acid indigestion, sour stomach with headache, or body aches and pains. Also

Continued on next page

Alka-Seltzer—Cont.

for fast relief of upset stomach with headache from overindulgence in food and drink—especially recommended for taking before bed and again on arising. Effective for pain relief alone: headache, or body and muscular aches and pains.

Directions:

Alka-Seltzer® Original, Cherry and Lemon Lime.

Adults: Dissolve 2 tablets in 4 oz. of water every 4 hours not to exceed 8 tablets in 24 hours (60 years or older, 4 tablets in a 24-hour period).

Alka-Seltzer® Extra Strength.

Adults: Dissolve 2 tablets in 4 oz. of water every 6 hours not to exceed 7 tablets in 24 hours (60 years or older, 4 tablets in a 24-hour period).

CAUTION: If symptoms persist or recur frequently, or if you are under treatment for ulcer, consult your doctor.

Warnings: Children and teenagers should not use this medicine for chicken pox or flu symptoms before a doctor is consulted about Reye's syndrome, a rare but serious illness reported to be associated with aspirin. As with any drug, if you are pregnant or nursing a baby, seek the advice of a health professional before using this product. **IT IS ESPECIALLY IMPORTANT NOT TO USE ASPIRIN DURING THE LAST 3 MONTHS OF PREGNANCY UNLESS SPECIFICALLY DIRECTED TO DO SO BY A DOCTOR BECAUSE IT MAY CAUSE PROBLEMS IN THE UNBORN CHILD OR COMPLICATIONS DURING DELIVERY.**

Do not use the daily maximum dosage for more than 10 days except under the advice and supervision of a doctor. Do not take this product if you are allergic to aspirin or have asthma, if you have bleeding problems, or if you are on a sodium restricted diet. If ringing in the ears or a loss of hearing occurs, consult a doctor before taking any more of this product.

Do not take this product for pain for more than 10 days unless directed by a doctor. If pain persists or gets worse, if new symptoms occur, or if redness or swelling is present, consult a doctor because these could be signs of a serious condition. Keep this and all drugs out of the reach of children.

Alcohol Warning: If you consume 3 or more alcoholic drinks every day, ask your doctor whether you should take aspirin or other pain relievers/fever reducers. Aspirin may cause stomach bleeding.

Drug Interaction Precaution: Do not take this product if you are taking a prescription drug for anticoagulation (thinning the blood), diabetes, gout, or arthritis unless directed by a doctor. Antacids may interact with certain prescription drugs. If you are presently taking a prescription drug, do not take this product without checking with your doctor or other health professional.

How Supplied: Foil sealed effervescent tablets in cartons of 12's in 6 foil twin packs; 24's in 12 foil twin packs; 36's in 18 foil twin packs.

Original Alka-Seltzer also available in cartons of 72 and 100.

Shown in Product Identification Guide, page 503

ALKA-SELTZER® HEARTBURN RELIEF

Antacid Medicine

Active Ingredients (In each tablet)

	Purpose
Citric Acid 1000 mg	Antacid
Sodium Bicarbonate (heat-treated) 1940 mg	Antacid

Inactive Ingredients: Amiflex, Aspartame, Flavors, Mannitol, Potassium Acesulfame

Uses:

Provides relief of: •heartburn •acid indigestion •upset stomach associated with the above conditions

Warnings: Do not exceed recommended dosage.

Do not use this product if you are on a sodium-restricted diet unless directed by a doctor.

Do not take more than the maximum recommended daily dosage (See **Directions**) in a 24-hour period, or use the maximum dosage of this product for more than 2 weeks, except under the advice and supervision of a physician.

Ask a doctor or pharmacist before use if you are presently taking a prescription drug. Antacids may interact with certain prescription drugs.

Stop use and ask a doctor if symptoms last for more than 2 weeks.

If pregnant or breast-feeding, ask a health professional before use.

Keep out of reach of children.

Directions: Fully dissolve Alka-Seltzer Heartburn Relief tablets in 4 ounces of water before taking.

[See table below]

Other information: Each 2 tablet dose contains: **Sodium 1150 mg.**

Phenylketonurics: Contains Phenylalanine 11 mg per 2 tablet dose.

Alka-Seltzer Heartburn Relief in water contains the antacid Sodium Citrate as the principal active ingredient.

How Supplied: Alka-Seltzer Heartburn Relief is available in packages of 24 lemon lime effervescent tablets or 36 lemon lime effervescent tablets.

Questions or comments: 1-800-800-4793 or www.alka-seltzer.com

Bayer Corporation
Consumer Care Division
Morristown, NJ 07960
USA

Shown in Product Identification Guide, page 503

ALKA-SELTZER PLUS® NIGHT-TIME COLD MEDICINE LIQUI-GELS®

ALKA-SELTZER PLUS® COLD & COUGH MEDICINE LIQUI-GELS®

ALKA-SELTZER PLUS® COLD MEDICINE LIQUI-GELS®

ALKA-SELTZER PLUS® COLD & SINUS MEDICINE LIQUI-GELS®

ALKA-SELTZER PLUS® COLD & FLU MEDICINE LIQUI-GELS®

Active Ingredients:
[See first table on next page]

Inactive Ingredients:
[See second table on next page]

Indications: Provides temporary relief of these major symptoms of cold and flu: [See third table on next page]

Directions for Use: ALKA-SELTZER PLUS® COLD MEDICINE, COLD & COUGH MEDICINE, COLD & FLU MEDICINE, AND COLD & SINUS MEDICINE

ADULTS: Swallow 2 softgels with water. CHILDREN (6–12 years): Swallow 1 softgel with water. CHILDREN (under 6 years): Consult a doctor. Repeat every 4 hours, not to exceed 4 doses per day, or as directed by a doctor.

ALKA-SELTZER PLUS® NIGHT-TIME COLD MEDICINE:

ADULTS AND CHILDREN 12 YEARS AND OLDER: Swallow 2 softgels with water at bedtime. May repeat every 6 hours, not to exceed 8 softgels in a 24-hour period or as directed by a doctor. CHILDREN under 12 years of age consult a doctor.

Warnings: Do not exceed recommended dosage. If nervousness, dizziness or sleeplessness occur, discontinue

Adults and children 12 years and older	2 tablets every 4 hours as needed, or as directed by a doctor.	Do not exceed 8 tablets in 24 hours.
Adult 60 years of age and older	2 tablets every 4 hours as needed, or as directed by a doctor.	Do not exceed 4 tablets in 24 hours.
Children under 12 years	Ask a doctor.	

use and call a doctor. (If symptoms do not improve within 7 days or are accompanied by a fever, consult a doctor.)**
If sore throat is severe, persists for more than 2 days, is accompanied by or followed by fever, rash, headache, nausea or vomiting, consult a doctor promptly. May cause excitability especially in children.*
Do not take this product, unless directed by a doctor, if you have a breathing problem such as emphysema or chronic bron-

chitis*, or glaucoma, difficulty in urination due to enlargement of the prostate gland or heart disease, high blood pressure, diabetes, or thyroid disease. [May cause drowsiness; alcohol, sedatives and tranquilizers may increase drowsiness effect. Avoid alcoholic beverages while taking this product. Do not take this product if you are taking sedatives or tranquilizers without first consulting your doctor. Use caution when driving a motor vehicle or operating machinery.]*

Alka-Seltzer Plus Liqui-Gels

per softgel	Night-Time	Cold & Cough	Cold	Cold & Sinus	Cold & Flu
Acetaminophen 325 mg	✔	✔	✔	✔	✔
Chlorpheniramine Maleate 2 mg		✔	✔		
Dextromethorphan Hydrobromide 10 mg	✔	✔			✔
Doxylamine Succinate 6.25 mg	✔				
Pseudoephedrine HCl 30 mg.	✔	✔	✔	✔	✔

Alka-Seltzer Plus Liqui-Gels

per softgel	Night-Time	Cold & Cough	Cold	Cold & Sinus	Cold & Flu
Artificial Color(s)	✔	✔	✔	✔	✔
Gelatin	✔	✔	✔	✔	✔
Glycerin	✔	✔	✔	✔	✔
Polyethylene Glycol	✔	✔	✔	✔	✔
Potassium Acetate	✔	✔	✔	✔	✔
Povidone	✔	✔	✔	✔	✔
Purified Water	✔	✔	✔	✔	✔
Sorbitol	✔	✔	✔	✔	✔
Titanium Dioxide	✔	✔	✔	✔	✔

Alka-Seltzer Plus Liqui-Gels

per softgel	Night-Time	Cold & Cough	Cold	Cold & Sinus	Cold & Flu
Body Aches & Pains	✔	✔	✔	✔	✔
Coughing	✔	✔			✔
Fever	✔	✔	✔	✔	✔
Headache	✔	✔	✔	✔	✔
Nasal & Sinus Congestion	✔	✔	✔	Nasal	✔
Runny Nose	✔	✔	✔		
Sinus Pain & Pressure				✔	
Sneezing	✔	✔	✔		
Sore Throat	✔	✔	✔	✔	✔

As with any drug, if you are pregnant or nursing a baby seek the advice of a health professional before using this product. Keep this and all medication out of the reach of children. In case of accidental overdose, contact a physician or Poison Control Center immediately. Prompt medical attention is critical for adults as well as children even if you do not notice any signs or symptoms. (A persistent cough may be a sign of a serious condition. If cough persists for more than 1 week, tends to recur or is accompanied by fever, rash or persistent headache, consult a doctor. Do not take this product for persistent or chronic cough such as occurs with smoking, asthma, emphysema or if cough is accompanied by excessive phlegm (mucus) unless directed by a doctor.)***
Do not take this product for more than 7 days or for fever for more than 3 days unless directed by a doctor. If symptoms, including pain or fever persist, do not improve or get worse, if new symptoms occur or if redness or swelling is present, consult a doctor because these could be signs of a serious condition.**
Alcohol Warning: If you consume 3 or more alcoholic drinks every day, ask your doctor whether you should take acetaminophen or other pain relievers/fever reducers. Acetaminophen may cause liver damage.
Drug Interaction Precaution: Do not take this product if you are now taking a prescription monoamine oxidase inhibitor (MAOI) (certain drugs for depression, psychiatric or emotional conditions, or Parkinson's disease), or for 2 weeks after stopping the MAOI drug. If you are uncertain whether your prescription drug contains an MAOI, consult a health professional before taking this product.
*Does not apply to Alka-Seltzer Plus Cold & Sinus Medicine or Cold & Flu Medicine.
**Does not apply to Alka-Seltzer Plus Cold & Sinus Medicine.
***Does not apply to Alka-Seltzer Plus Cold Medicine or Cold & Sinus Medicine.

How Supplied: Carton of 12 and 20 softgels.
Liqui-Gels® is a trademark of R.P. Scherer Corp.
Shown in Product Identification Guide, page 503

ALKA-SELTZER PM™
[ə-ka sēl-sur]
PAIN RELIEVER &
SLEEP AID MEDICINE

Indications: For the temporary relief of occasional headaches and minor aches and pains with accompanying sleeplessness.

Active Ingredients: Each effervescent tablet contains 325 mg aspirin and 38 mg diphenhydramine citrate.

Continued on next page

Alka-Seltzer PM—Cont.

Inactive Ingredients: Acesulfame Potassium, Artificial and Natural Flavors, Aspartame, Citric acid, Sodium bicarbonate, Tableting aids.

Directions: Adults: Dissolve 2 tablets in 4 oz. of water and take at bedtime, if needed, or as directed by a doctor.

Warnings: Do not give to children under 12 years of age. **Children and teenagers should not use this medicine for chicken pox or flu symptoms before a doctor is consulted about Reye's syndrome, a rare but serious illness reported to be associated with aspirin.** Do not take this product for pain for more than 10 days or for fever for more than 3 days unless directed by a doctor. If pain or fever persists or gets worse, if new symptoms occur, or if redness or swelling is present, consult a doctor because these could be signs of a serious condition. Do not take this product if you are allergic to aspirin or if you have asthma unless directed by a doctor. Each tablet contains 503 mg of sodium. If ringing in the ears or a loss of hearing occurs, consult a doctor before taking any more of this product. Unless directed by a doctor, do not take this product if you have ulcers or bleeding problems, or if you have stomach problems that persist or recur frequently, such as persistent stomach pain, heartburn, or upset stomach. If sleeplessness persists continuously for more than 2 weeks, consult your doctor. Insomnia may be a symptom of serious underlying medical illness. Do not take this product, unless directed by a doctor, if you have a breathing problem such as emphysema or chronic bronchitis, or if you have glaucoma or difficulty in urination due to enlargement of the prostate gland. Avoid alcoholic beverages while taking this product. Do not take this product if you are taking sedatives or tranquilizers, without first consulting your doctor. Keep this and all drugs out of the reach of children. In case of accidental overdose, seek professional assistance or contact a poison control center immediately. As with any drug, if you are pregnant or nursing a baby, seek the advice of a health professional before using this product. **IT IS ESPECIALLY IMPORTANT NOT TO USE ASPIRIN DURING THE LAST 3 MONTHS OF PREGNANCY UNLESS SPECIFICALLY DIRECTED TO DO SO BY A DOCTOR BECAUSE IT MAY CAUSE PROBLEMS IN THE UNBORN CHILD OR COMPLICATIONS DURING DELIVERY.**

Alcohol Warning: If you consume 3 or more alcoholic drinks every day, ask your doctor whether you should take aspirin or other pain relievers/fever reducers. Aspirin may cause stomach bleeding.

Phenylketonurics: CONTAINS PHENYLALANINE 4.04 mg per tablet.

Drug Interaction Precaution: Do not take this product if you are taking a prescription drug for anticoagulation (thinning the blood), diabetes, gout, or arthritis unless directed by a doctor. Helps protect against the stomach upset aspirin users may sometimes experience.

For more information or a free sample, visit our web site at www.alka-seltzer.com

How Supplied: 24 Effervescent tablets.

Shown in Product Identification Guide, page 503

Genuine BAYER® Aspirin Tablets, Caplets and Gelcaps

Active Ingredient: 325 mg aspirin per tablet, caplet, or gelcap, coated for easy swallowing.

Inactive Ingredients: Caplets & Tablets—Hydroxypropyl Methylcellulose, Starch and Triacetin. Gelcaps—Butylparaben, D&C Yellow #10, Gelatin, Glycerin, Hydroxypropyl Methylcellulose, Methylparaben, Propylparaben, Sodium Lauryl Sulfate, Sorbitan Trioleate, Starch, Titanium Dioxide, Triacetin.

Indications: For the temporary relief of: headache, pain and fever of colds, muscle aches and pains, menstrual pain, toothache pain, minor aches and pains of arthritis.

Directions: Adults and Children 12 years and over: One or two tablets/caplets/gelcaps with water every 4 hours, as needed, up to a maximum of 12 tablets/caplets/gelcaps per 24 hours or as directed by a doctor. Do not give to children under 12 unless directed by a doctor.

Warnings: **Children and teenagers should not use this medicine for chicken pox or flu symptoms before a doctor is consulted about Reye's syndrome, a rare but serious illness reported to be associated with aspirin.** Do not take this product for pain for more than 10 days or for fever for more than 3 days unless directed by a doctor. If pain or fever persists or gets worse, if new symptoms occur, or if redness or swelling is present consult a doctor because these could be signs of a serious condition. Do not take this product if you are allergic to aspirin, have asthma, have stomach problems (such as heartburn, upset stomach or stomach pain) that persist or recur, gastric ulcers or bleeding problems unless directed by a doctor. If ringing in the ears or loss of hearing occurs, consult a doctor before taking any more of this product. Keep this and all drugs out of the reach of children. In case of accidental overdose, seek professional assistance or contact a poison control center immediately. As with any drug, if you are pregnant or nursing a baby, seek the advice of a health professional before using this product. **IT IS ESPECIALLY IMPORTANT NOT TO USE ASPIRIN DURING THE LAST 3 MONTHS OF PREGNANCY UNLESS SPECIFICALLY DIRECTED TO DO SO BY A DOCTOR BECAUSE IT MAY CAUSE PROBLEMS IN THE UNBORN CHILD OR COMPLICATIONS DURING DELIVERY.**

Alcohol Warning: If you consume 3 or more alcoholic drinks every day, ask your doctor whether you should take aspirin or other pain relievers/fever reducers. Aspirin may cause stomach bleeding.

Drug Interaction Precaution: Do not take this product if you are taking a prescription drug for anticoagulation (thinning the blood), diabetes, gout or arthritis unless directed by doctor. See "Professional Labeling" listing on page xxx.

How Supplied:
Genuine Bayer Aspirin 325 mg (5 grains) is supplied in packs of 12 tablets, bottles of 24, 50, 100, 200, 300, bottles of 50 and 100 caplets, and bottles of 40 and 80 gelcaps.

Shown in Product Identification Guide, page 503

ASPIRIN REGIMEN BAYER® 81 mg
ASPIRIN REGIMEN BAYER® 325 mg
Delayed Release Enteric Aspirin Adult Low Strength 81 mg Tablets and Regular Strength 325 mg Caplets

Enteric Coated Tablets and Caplets

The enteric coating on Aspirin Regimen Bayer allows the tablet/caplet to pass through the stomach to the intestine before it dissolves, helping to protect against stomach upset.

Active Ingredient: Aspirin Regimen Bayer 81 mg — 81 mg aspirin per tablet Aspirin Regimen Bayer 325 mg — 325 mg aspirin per caplet

Inactive Ingredients:
Regular Strength 325mg—D&C Yellow #10, FD&C Yellow #6, Hydroxypropyl Methylcellulose, Iron Oxides, Methacrylic Acid Copolymer, Starch, Titanium Dioxide, Triacetin.

Adult Low Strength 81mg—Croscarmellose Sodium, D&C Yellow #10, FD&C Yellow #6, Hydroxypropyl Methylcellulose, Iron Oxides, Lactose, Methacrylic Acid, Microcrystalline Cellulose, Polysorbate 80, Sodium Lauryl Sulfate, Starch, Titanium Dioxide, Triacetin.

Indications: For the temporary relief of minor aches and pains or as recommended by your doctor. Ask your doctor about new uses for Aspirin Regimen Bayer Adult low strength 81 mg. Aspirin. Because of its delayed action, ASPIRIN REGIMEN BAYER will not provide fast relief of headaches, fever or other symptoms needing immediate relief.

See **PROFESSIONAL LABELING**

Directions: For nonprescription analgesic indications: Adults & children 12 years and older: Take one or two 325 mg caplets or four to eight 81 mg tablets every 4 hours with water.

Do not exceed 4000 mg in 24 hours. Dosage may be modified as directed by a doctor.

Warnings: Children and teenagers should not use this medicine for chicken pox or flu symptoms before a doctor is consulted about Reye's syndrome, a rare but serious illness reported to be associated with aspirin. Do not take for pain for more than 10 days or for fever for more than 3 days unless directed by a doctor. If pain or fever persists or gets worse, if new symptoms occur, or if redness or swelling is present, consult a doctor because these could be signs of a serious illness. Do not take this product if you are allergic to aspirin, have asthma, have stomach problems (such as heartburn, upset stomach or stomach pain) that persist or recur, gastric ulcers or bleeding problems unless directed by a doctor. If ringing in the ears or loss of hearing occurs, consult a doctor before taking any more of this product. Keep this and all drugs out of the reach of children. In case of accidental overdose, seek professional assistance or contact a poison control center immediately. As with any drug, if you are pregnant or nursing a baby, seek the advice of a health professional before using this product. **IT IS ESPECIALLY IMPORTANT NOT TO USE ASPIRIN DURING THE LAST 3 MONTHS OF PREGNANCY UNLESS SPECIFICALLY DIRECTED TO DO SO BY A DOCTOR BECAUSE IT MAY CAUSE PROBLEMS IN THE UNBORN CHILD OR COMPLICATIONS DURING DELIVERY.**

Alcohol Warning: If you consume 3 or more alcoholic drinks every day, ask your doctor whether you should take aspirin or other pain relievers/fever reducers. Aspirin may cause stomach bleeding.

Drug Interaction Precaution: Do not take this product if you are taking a prescription drug for anticoagulation (thinning the blood), diabetes, gout or arthritis unless directed by a doctor.
See "Professional Labeling" listing on page 608.

Safety: The safety of enteric-coated aspirin has been demonstrated in a number of endoscopic studies comparing enteric-coated aspirin and plain aspirin, as well as buffered aspirin and "arthritis strength" doses. In these studies, endoscopies were performed in healthy volunteers either before and/or during, and/or after administration of various aspirin doses. Compared to all the other preparations, the enteric-coated aspirin produced significantly less damage to the gastric mucosa.

Bioavailability: Dissolution of the enteric coating occurs at a neutral to basic pH and is therefore dependent on gastric emptying into the duodenum. With continued dosing, appropriate therapeutic plasma levels are maintained.

How Supplied: Aspirin Regimen Bayer 325 mg (5 grains) is supplied in bottles of 100 caplets.
Aspirin Regimen Bayer 81 mg (1.25 grains) is supplied in bottles of 32, 120, 180 tablets.
Shown in Product Identification Guide, page 503

ASPIRIN REGIMEN BAYER®
81 mg WITH CALCIUM
Caplets

Each caplet provides 81 mg of aspirin and 10% (100 mg) of the Daily Value of Calcium as part of the buffered base of Calcium Carbonate.

Active Ingredient: 81 mg Aspirin per caplet in a buffered base of Calcium Carbonate (250 mg = 100 mg of elemental calcium).

Inactive Ingredients: Colloidal Silicon Dioxide, FD&C Blue #2 Lake, Hydroxypropyl Methylcellulose, Microcrystalline Cellulose, Propylene Glycol, Sodium Starch Glycolate, Starch, Titanium Dioxide, Zinc Stearate.

Indications. For the temporary relief of minor aches and pains or as recommended by your doctor.

Directions: Adults and Children 12 years and over, take 4 to 8 caplets with water every 4 hours, as needed, up to a maximum of 32 caplets per 24 hours or as directed by a doctor.

Warnings: Children and teenagers should not use this medicine for chicken pox or flu symptoms before a doctor is consulted about Reye's syndrome, a rare but serious illness reported to be associated with aspirin. Do not take for pain for more than 10 days or for fever for more than 3 days unless directed by a doctor. If pain or fever persists or gets worse, if new symptoms occur or if redness or swelling is present, consult a doctor because these could be signs of a serious condition. Do not take this product if you are allergic to aspirin, have asthma, have stomach problems (such as heartburn, upset stomach or stomach pain) that persist or recur, gastric ulcers or bleeding problems unless directed by a doctor. If ringing in the ears or loss of hearing occurs, consult a doctor before taking any more of this product. Keep this and all drugs out of the reach of children. In case of accidental overdose, seek professional assistance or contact a poison control center immediately. As with any drug, if you are pregnant or nursing a baby, seek the advice of a health professional before using this product. **IT IS ESPECIALLY IMPORTANT NOT TO USE ASPIRIN DURING THE LAST 3 MONTHS OF PREGNANCY UNLESS DIRECTED TO DO SO BY A DOCTOR BECAUSE IT MAY CAUSE PROBLEMS IN THE UNBORN CHILD OR COMPLICATIONS DURING DELIVERY.**

Alcohol Warning: If you consume 3 or more alcoholic drinks every day, ask your doctor whether you should take aspirin or other pain relievers/fever reducers. Aspirin may cause stomach bleeding.

Drug Interaction Precaution: Do not take this product if you are taking any prescription drug including those for anticoagulation (thinning the blood), diabetes, gout or arthritis unless directed by a doctor.
See "Professional Labeling" listing on page 608.

How Supplied: Aspirin Regimen Bayer 81 mg with Calcium (1.25 grains) is supplied in bottles of 60 caplets.

Aspirin Regimen
BAYER® Children's Chewable
Tablets
Orange & Cherry Flavored

Active Ingredients: 81 mg Aspirin per tablet

Inactive Ingredients: Orange Flavored: Dextrose Excipient, FD&C Yellow #6, Flavor, Saccharin Sodium, Starch.
Cherry Flavored: D&C Red #27 Lake, Dextrose Excipient, FD&C Red #40 Lake, Flavor, Saccharin Sodium, Starch.

Indications: For the temporary relief of minor aches, pains and headaches, and to reduce fever associated with colds, sore throats and teething.

Directions:
To be administered only under adult supervision.

Age (Years)	Weight (lbs)	Dosage
2 to under 4	32 to 35	2 tablets
4 to under 6	36 to 45	3 tablets
6 to under 9	46 to 65	4 tablets
9 to under 11	66 to 76	4–5 tablets
11 to under 12	77 to 83	4–6 tablets
Adults and Children 12 yrs and over		5–8 tablets

Repeat every four hours, while symptoms persist, up to a maximum of five doses in 24 hours or as directed by a doctor. Drink water with each dose. Children under 2 years: consult a doctor.

Warnings: Children and teenagers should not use this medicine for chicken pox or flu symptoms before a doctor is consulted about Reye's syndrome, a rare but serious illness reported to be associated with aspirin. Do not take for pain for more than 10 days (for adults) or 5 days (for children), and do not take for fever for more than 3 days unless directed by a doctor. If pain or fever persists or gets worse, if new symptoms occur, or if redness or swelling is present, consult a doctor because

Continued on next page

Aspirin Regimen Bayer—Cont.

these could be signs of a serious condition. Do not give this product to children for the pain of arthritis unless directed by a doctor. If sore throat is severe, persists for more than 2 days, is accompanied or followed by fever, headache, rash, nausea, or vomiting, consult a doctor promptly. Do not take this product for at least 7 days after tonsillectomy or oral surgery unless directed by a doctor. Do not take this product if you are allergic to aspirin, have asthma, have stomach problems (such as heartburn, upset stomach or stomach pain) that persist or recur or have gastric ulcers or bleeding problems unless directed by a doctor. If ringing in the ears or loss of hearing occurs, consult a doctor before taking any more of this product.

Keep this and all drugs out of the reach of children. In case of accidental overdose, contact a doctor immediately. As with any drug, if you are pregnant or nursing a baby, seek the advice of a health professional before using this product. **IT IS ESPECIALLY IMPORTANT NOT TO USE ASPIRIN DURING THE LAST 3 MONTHS OF PREGNANCY UNLESS SPECIFICALLY DIRECTED TO DO SO BY A DOCTOR BECAUSE IT MAY CAUSE PROBLEMS IN THE UNBORN CHILD OR COMPLICATIONS DURING DELIVERY.**

Alcohol Warning: If you consume 3 or more alcoholic drinks every day, ask your doctor whether you should take aspirin or other pain relievers/fever reducers. Aspirin may cause stomach bleeding.

Drug Interaction Precaution: Do not take this product if taking a prescription drug for anticoagulation (thinning the blood), diabetes, gout or arthritis unless directed by a doctor.

See "Professional labeling" below.

How Supplied: Aspirin Regimen Bayer Children's chewable 81 mg (1.25 grains) is supplied in bottles of 36 tablets.

Store at room temperature.

Shown in Product Identification Guide, page 504

PROFESSIONAL LABELING

Genuine Bayer Aspirin
Aspirin Regimen Bayer 325 mg
Aspirin Regimen Bayer 81 mg
Aspirin Regimen Bayer 81 mg with Calcium
Aspirin Regimen Bayer Childrens Chewable 81 mg

Professional Labeling:

Indications And Usage: Vascular Indications (Ischemic Stroke, TIA, Acute MI, Prevention of Recurrent MI, Unstable Angina Pectoris, and Chronic Stable Angina Pectoris): Aspirin is indicated to:

(1) Reduce the combined risk of death and nonfatal stroke in patients who have had ischemic stroke or transient ischemia of the brain due to fibrin platelet emboli, (2) reduce the risk of vascular mortality in patients with a suspected acute MI, (3) reduce the combined risk of death and nonfatal MI in patients with a previous MI or unstable angina pectoris, and (4) reduce the combined risk of MI and sudden death in patients with chronic stable angina pectoris.

Revascularization Procedures (Coronary Artery Bypass Graft (CABG), Percutaneous Transluminal Coronary Angioplasty (PTCA), and Carotid Endarterectomy): Aspirin is indicated in patients who have undergone revascularization procedures (i.e., CABG, PTCA, or carotid endarterectomy) when there is a preexisting condition for which aspirin is already indicated.

Rheumatologic Disease Indications (Rheumatoid Arthritis, Juvenile Rheumatoid Arthritis, Spondyloarthropathies, Osteoarthritis, and the Arthritis and Pleurisy of Systemic Lupus Erythematosus (SLE)): Aspirin is indicated for the relief of the signs and symptoms of rheumatoid arthritis, juvenile rheumatoid arthritis, osteoarthritis, spondyloarthropathies, and arthritis and pleurisy associated with SLE.

Contraindications: Allergy: Aspirin is contraindicated in patients with known allergy to nonsteroidal anti-inflammatory drug products and in patients with the syndrome of asthma, rhinitis, and nasal polyps. Aspirin may cause severe urticaria, angioedema, or bronchospasm (asthma).

Reye's syndrome: Aspirin should not be used in children or teenagers for viral infections, with or without fever, because of the risk of Reye's syndrome with concomitant use of aspirin in certain viral illnesses.

Warnings: Alcohol Warning: Patients who consume three or more alcoholic drinks every day should be counseled about the bleeding risks involved with chronic, heavy alcohol use while taking aspirin.

Coagulation Abnormalities: Even low doses of aspirin can inhibit platelet function leading to an increase in bleeding time. This can adversely affect patients with inherited (hemophilia) or acquired (liver disease or vitamin K deficiency) bleeding disorders.

GI Side Effects: GI side effects include stomach pain, heartburn, nausea, vomiting, and gross GI bleeding. Although minor upper GI symptoms, such as dyspepsia, are common and can occur anytime during therapy, physicians should remain alert for signs of ulceration and bleeding, even in the absence of previous GI symptoms. Physicians should inform patients about the signs and symptoms of GI side effects and what steps to take if they occur.

Peptic Ulcer Disease: Patients with a history of active peptic ulcer disease should avoid using aspirin, which can cause gastric mucosal irritation and bleeding.

Precautions:

General: Renal Failure: Avoid aspirin in patients with severe renal failure (glomerular filtration rate less than 10 mL/minute).

Hepatic Insufficiency: Avoid aspirin in patients with severe hepatic insufficiency.

Sodium Restricted Diets: Patients with sodium-retaining states, such as congestive heart failure or renal failure, should avoid sodium-containing buffered aspirin preparations because of their high sodium content.

Laboratory Tests: Aspirin has been associated with elevated hepatic enzymes, blood urea nitrogen and serum creatinine, hyperkalemia, proteinuria, and prolonged bleeding time.

Drug Interactions: Angiotensin Converting Enzyme (ACE) Inhibitors: The hyponatremic and hypotensive effects of ACE inhibitors may be diminished by the concomitant administration of aspirin due to its indirect effect on the renin-angiotensin conversion pathway.

Acetazolamide: Concurrent use of aspirin and acetazolamide can lead to high serum concentrations of acetazolamide (and toxicity) due to competition at the renal tubule for secretion.

Anticoagulant Therapy (Heparin and Warfarin): Patients on anticoagulation therapy are at increased risk for bleeding because of drug-drug interactions and the effect on platelets. Aspirin can displace warfarin from protein binding sites, leading to prolongation of both the prothrombin time and the bleeding time. Aspirin can increase the anticoagulant activity of heparin, increasing bleeding risk.

Anticonvulsants: Salicylate can displace protein-bound phenytoin and valproic acid, leading to a decrease in the total concentration of phenytoin and an increase in serum valproic acid levels.

Beta Blockers: The hypotensive effects of beta blockers may be diminished by the concomitant administration of aspirin due to inhibition of renal prostaglandins, leading to decreased renal blood flow, and salt and fluid retention.

Diuretics: The effectiveness of diuretics in patients with underlying renal or cardiovascular disease may be diminished by the concomitant administration of aspirin due to inhibition of renal prostaglandins, leading to decreased renal blood flow and salt and fluid retention.

Methotrexate: Salicylate can inhibit renal clearance of methotrexate, leading to bone marrow toxicity, especially in the elderly or renal impaired.

Nonsteroidal Anti-inflammatory Drugs (NSAID's): The concurrent use of aspirin with other NSAID's should be avoided because this may increase bleeding or lead to decreased renal function.

Oral Hypoglycemics: Moderate doses of aspirin may increase the effectiveness of oral hypoglycemic drugs, leading to hypoglycemia.

Uricosuric Agents (Probenecid and Sulfinpyrazone): Salicylates antagonize the uricosuric action of uricosuric agents.

Carcinogenesis, Mutagenesis, Impairment of Fertility: Administration of aspirin for 68 weeks at 0.5 percent in the feed of rats was not carcinogenic. In the Ames Salmonella assay, aspirin was not mutagenic; however, aspirin did induce chromosome aberrations in cultured human fibroblasts. Aspirin inhibits ovulation in rats. (See Pregnancy.)

Pregnancy: Pregnant women should only take aspirin if clearly needed. Because of the known effects of NSAID's on the fetal cardiovascular system (closure of the ductus arteriosus), use during the third trimester of pregnancy should be avoided. Salicylate products have also been associated with alterations in maternal and neonatal hemostasis mechanisms, decreased birth weight, and with perinatal mortality.

Labor and Delivery: Aspirin should be avoided 1 week prior to and during labor and delivery because it can result in excessive blood loss at delivery. Prolonged gestation and prolonged labor due to prostaglandin inhibition have been reported.

Nursing Mothers: Nursing mothers should avoid using aspirin because salicylate is excreted in breast milk. Use of high doses may lead to rashes, platelet abnormalities, and bleeding in nursing infants.

Pediatric Use: Pediatric dosing recommendations for juvenile rheumatoid arthritis are based on well-controlled clinical studies. An initial dose of 90–130 mg/kg/day in divided doses, with an increase as needed for anti-inflammatory efficacy (target plasma salicylate levels of 150–300 mcg/mL) are effective. At high doses (i.e., plasma levels of greater than 200 mcg/mL), the incidence of toxicity increases.

Adverse Reactions: Many adverse reactions due to aspirin ingestion are dose-related. The following is a list of adverse reactions that have been reported in the literature. (See **Warnings.**)

Body as a Whole: Fever, hypothermia, thirst.

Cardiovascular: Dysrhythmias, hypotension, tachycardia.

Central Nervous System: Agitation, cerebral edema, coma, confusion, dizziness, headache, subdural or intracranial hemorrhage, lethargy, seizures.

Fluid and Electrolyte: Dehydration, hyperkalemia, metabolic acidosis, respiratory alkalosis.

Gastrointestinal: Dyspepsia, GI bleeding, ulceration and perforation, nausea, vomiting, transient elevations of hepatic enzymes, hepatitis, Reye's Syndrome, pancreatitis.

Hematologic: Prolongation of the prothrombin time, disseminated intravascular coagulation, coagulopathy, thrombocytopenia.

Hypersensitivity: Acute anaphylaxis, angioedema, asthma, bronchospasm, laryngeal edema, urticaria.

Musculoskeletal: Rhabdomyolysis.

Metabolism: Hypoglycemia (in children), hyperglycemia.

Reproductive: Prolonged pregnancy and labor, stillbirths, lower birth weight infants, antepartum and postpartum bleeding.

Respiratory: Hyperpnea, pulmonary edema, tachypnea.

Special Senses: Hearing loss, tinnitus. Patients with high frequency hearing loss may have difficulty perceiving tinnitus. In these patients, tinnitus cannot be used as a clinical indicator of salicylism.

Urogenital: Interstitial nephritis, papillary necrosis, proteinuria, renal insufficiency and failure.

Drug Abuse And Dependence: Aspirin is nonnarcotic. There is no known potential for addiction associated with the use of aspirin.

Overdosage: Salicylate toxicity may result from acute ingestion (overdose) or chronic intoxication. The early signs of salicylic overdose (salicylism), including tinnitus (ringing in the ears), occur at plasma concentrations approaching 200 mcg/mL. Plasma concentrations of aspirin above 300 mcg/mL are clearly toxic. Severe toxic effects are associated with levels above 400 mcg/mL. (See **Clinical Pharmacology.**) A single lethal dose of aspirin in adults is not known with certainty but death may be expected at 30 g. For real or suspected overdose, a Poison Control Center should be contacted immediately. Careful medical management is essential.

Signs and Symptoms: In acute overdose, severe acid-base and electrolyte disturbances may occur and are complicated by hyperthermia and dehydration. Respiratory alkalosis occurs early while hyperventilation is present, but is quickly followed by metabolic acidosis.

Treatment: Treatment consists primarily of supporting vital functions, increasing salicylate elimination, and correcting the acid-base disturbance. Gastric emptying and/or lavage is recommended as soon as possible after ingestion, even if the patient has vomited spontaneously. After lavage and/or emesis, administration of activated charcoal, as a slurry, is beneficial, if less than 3 hours have passed since ingestion. Charcoal adsorption should not be employed prior to emesis and lavage.

Severity of aspirin intoxication is determined by measuring the blood salicylate level. Acid-base status should be closely followed with serial blood gas and serum pH measurements. Fluid and electrolyte balance should aslo be maintained.

In severe cases, hyperthermia and hypovolemia are the major immediate threats to life. Children should be sponged with tepid water. Replacement fluid should be administered intravenously and augmented with correction of acidosis. Plasma electrolytes and pH should be monitored to promote alkaline diuresis of salicylate if renal function is normal. Infusion of glucose may be required to control hypoglycemia.

Hemodialysis and peritoneal dialysis can be performed to reduce the body drug content. In patients with renal insufficiency or in cases of life-threatening intoxication, dialysis is usually required. Exchange transfusion may be indicated in infants and young children.

Dosage and Administration: Each dose of aspirin should be taken with a full glass of water unless patient is fluid restricted. Anti-inflammatory and analgesic dosages should be individualized. When aspirin is used in high doses, the development of tinnitus may be used as a clinical sign of elevated plasma salicylate levels except in patients with high frequency hearing loss.

Ischemic Stroke and TIA: 50–325 mg once a day. Continue therapy indefinitely.

Suspected Acute MI: The initial dose of 160–162.5 mg is administered as soon as an MI is suspected. The maintenance dose of 160–162.5 mg a day is continued for 30 days post-infaction. After 30 days, consider further therapy based on dosage and administration for prevention of recurrent MI.

Prevention of Recurrent MI: 75–325 mg once a day. Continue therapy indefinitely.

Unstable Angina Pectoris: 75–325 mg once a day. Continue therapy indefinitely.

Chronic Stable Angina Pectoris: 75–325 mg once a day. Continue therapy indefinitely.

CABG: 325 mg daily starting 6 hours post-procedure. Continue therapy for 1 year post-procedure.

PTCA: The initial dose of 325 mg should be given 2 hours presurgery. Maintenance dose is 160–325 mg daily. Continue therapy indefinitely.

Carotid Endarterectomy: Doses of 80 mg once daily to 650 mg twice daily, started presurgery, are recommended. Continue therapy indefinitely.

Rheumatoid Arthritis: The initial dose is 3 g a day in divided doses. Increase as needed for anti-inflammatory efficacy with target plasma salicylate levels of 150–300 mcg/mL. At high doses (i.e., plasma levels of greater than 200 mcg/mL), the incidence of toxicity increases.

Juvenile Rheumatoid Arthritis: Initial dose is 90–130 mg/kg/day in divided doses. Increase as needed for anti-inflammatory efficacy with target plasma salicylate levels of 150–300 mcg/mL. At high doses (i.e., plasma levels of greater than 200 mcg/mL), the incidence of toxicity increases.

Continued on next page

Bayer Prof. Labeling—Cont.

Spondyloarthropathies: Up to 4 g per day in divided doses.
Osteoarthritis: Up to 3 g per day in divided doses.
Arthritis and Pleurisy of SLE: The initial dose is 3 g a day in divided doses. Increase as needed for anti-inflammatory efficacy with target plasma salicylate levels of 150–300 mcg/mL. At high doses (i.e., plasma levels of greater than 200 mcg/mL, the incidence of toxicity increases.

Extra Strength BAYER® Aspirin Arthritis Pain Regimen Formula Caplets

Enteric Coated Caplets
The enteric coating on BAYER® Aspirin Arthritis Pain Regimen Formula is designed to allow the caplet to pass through the stomach to the intestine before it dissolves, helping to protect against stomach upset.

Active Ingredient: 500 mg Aspirin per caplet.

Inactive Ingredients: D&C Yellow #10, FD&C Yellow #6, Hydroxypropyl Methylcellulose, Iron Oxide, Methacrylic Acid Copolymer, Starch, Titanium Dioxide, Triacetin.

Indications: For the temporary relief of minor aches and pains of arthritis or as recommended by your doctor.
Because of its delayed action, BAYER® Aspirin Arthritis Pain Regimen Formula will not provide fast relief of headaches, fever or other symptoms needing immediate relief.

Directions: Adults and Children 12 years and over, take 2 caplets with water every 6 hours, as needed, up to a maximum of 8 caplets per 24 hours. Ask your doctor about recommended dosages for other indications.

Warnings: Children and teenagers should not use this medicine for chicken pox or flu symptoms before a doctor is consulted about Reye's syndrome, a rare but serious illness reported to be associated with aspirin. Do not take for pain for more than 10 days or for fever for more than 3 days unless directed by a doctor. If pain or fever persists or gets worse, if new symptoms occur or if redness or swelling is present, consult a doctor because these could be signs of a serious condition. Do not take this product if you are allergic to aspirin, have asthma, have stomach problems (such as heartburn, upset stomach or stomach pain) that persist or recur, gastric ulcers or bleeding problems unless directed by a doctor. If ringing in the ears or loss of hearing occurs, consult a doctor before taking any more of this product. Keep this and all drugs out of the reach of children. In case of acciden-tal overdose, seek professional assistance or contact a poison control center immediately. As with any drug, if you are pregnant or nursing a baby, seek the advice of a health professional before using this product. **IT IS ESPECIALLY IMPORTANT NOT TO USE ASPIRIN DURING THE LAST 3 MONTHS OF PREGNANCY UNLESS SPECIFICALLY DIRECTED TO DO SO BY A DOCTOR BECAUSE IT MAY CAUSE PROBLEMS IN THE UNBORN CHILD OR COMPLICATIONS DURING DELIVERY.**

Alcohol Warning: If you consume 3 or more alcoholic drinks every day, ask your doctor whether you should take aspirin or other pain relievers/fever reducers. Aspirin may cause stomach bleeding.

Drug Interaction Precaution: Do not take this product if you are taking a prescription drug for anticoagulation (thinning the blood), diabetes, gout or arthritis unless directed by a doctor.

How Supplied: Extra Strength Bayer aspirin 500 mg (7.7 grains) is supplied in bottles of 50 caplets. Store at room temperature.
Shown in Product Identification Guide, page 504

Extra Strength BAYER® Aspirin Caplets and Gelcaps

Active Ingredient: Extra Strength Bayer Aspirin—Aspirin 500 mg per caplet or gelcap contains a thin, inert, coated for easier swallowing.

Inactive Ingredients: Caplets—Hydroxypropyl Methylcellulose, Starch and Triacetin.
Gelcaps—Butylparaben, FD&C Red #40, Gelatin, Glycerin, Hydroxypropyl Methylcellulose, Methylparaben, Propylparaben, Sodium Lauryl Sulfate, Sorbitan Trioleate, Starch, Titanium Dioxide, Triacetin.

Indications: For temporary relief of: Headache, pain and fever of colds, muscle aches and pains, menstrual pain, toothache pain, minor aches and pains of arthritis.

Directions: Adults and Children 12 years and over: Take 1 or 2 caplets/gelcaps with water every 4 to 6 hours, as needed, up to a maximum of 8 caplets/gelcaps per 24 hours or as directed by a doctor. Do not give to children under 12 unless directed by a doctor.

Warnings: Children and teenagers should not use this medicine for chicken pox or flu symptoms before a doctor is consulted about Reye's syndrome, a rare but serious illness reported to be associated with aspirin. Do not take for pain for more than 10 days or for fever for more than 3 days unless directed by a doctor. If pain or fever persists or gets worse, if new symptoms occur or if redness or swelling is present consult a doctor because these could be signs of a serious condition. Do not take this product if you are allergic to aspirin, have asthma, have stomach problems (such as heartburn, upset stomach or stomach pain) that persist or recur, gastric ulcers or bleeding problems unless directed by a doctor. If ringing in the ears or loss of hearing occurs, consult a doctor before taking any more of this product. Keep this and all drugs out of the reach of children. In case of accidental overdose, seek professional assistance or contact a poison control center immediately. As with any drug, if you are pregnant or nursing a baby, seek the advice of a health professional before using this product. **IT IS ESPECIALLY IMPORTANT NOT TO USE ASPIRIN DURING THE LAST 3 MONTHS OF PREGNANCY UNLESS SPECIFICALLY DIRECTED TO DO SO BY A DOCTOR BECAUSE IT MAY CAUSE PROBLEMS IN THE UNBORN CHILD OR COMPLICATIONS DURING DELIVERY.**

Alcohol Warning: If you consume 3 or more alcoholic drinks every day, ask your doctor whether you should take aspirin or other pain relievers/fever reducers. Aspirin may cause stomach bleeding.

Drug Interaction Precaution: Do not take this product if you are taking a prescription drug for anticoagulation (thinning the blood), diabetes, gout or arthritis unless directed by a doctor.

How Supplied: Extra Strength Bayer Aspirin 500 mg (7.7 grains) is available in bottles of 50 caplets and bottles of 40 and 80 gelcaps.
Shown in Product Identification Guide, page 504

Extra Strength BAYER® PLUS Buffered Aspirin Caplets

Active Ingredient: 500 mg Aspirin per caplet, in a buffered base of Calcium Carbonate.

Inactive Ingredients Colloidal Silicon Dioxide, D&C Red #7 Lake, FD&C Blue #2 Lake, FD&C Red #40 Lake, Hydroxypropyl Methylcellulose, Microcrystalline Cellulose, Propylene Glycol, Sodium Starch Glycolate, Starch, Titanium Dioxide, Zinc Stearate.

Indications: Provides effective, temporary relief of: headache, pain and fever of colds, muscle aches and pains, menstrual pain, toothache pain, minor aches and pains of arthritis.

Directions: Adults and Children 12 years and over: Take 1 or 2 caplets with water every 4 to 6 hours, as needed, up to a maximum of 8 caplets per 24 hours or as directed by a doctor. Do not give to children under 12 unless directed by a doctor.

Warnings: Children and teenagers should not use this medicine for

chicken pox or flu symptoms before a doctor is consulted about Reye's syndrome, a rare but serious illness reported to be associated with aspirin. Do not take for pain for more than 10 days or for fever for more than 3 days unless directed by a doctor. If pain or fever persists or gets worse, if new symptoms occur or if redness or swelling is present consult a doctor because these could be signs of a serious condition. Do not take this product if you are allergic to aspirin, have asthma, have stomach problems (such as heartburn, upset stomach or stomach pain) that persist or recur, gastric ulcers or bleeding problems unless directed by a doctor. If ringing in the ears or loss of hearing occurs, consult a doctor before taking any more of this product. Keep this and all drugs out of the reach of children. In case of accidental overdose, seek professional assistance or contact a poison control center immediately. As with any drug, if you are pregnant or nursing a baby, seek the advice of a health professional before using this product. **IT IS ESPECIALLY IMPORTANT NOT TO USE ASPIRIN DURING THE LAST 3 MONTHS OF PREGNANCY UNLESS SPECIFICALLY DIRECTED TO DO SO BY A DOCTOR BECAUSE IT MAY CAUSE PROBLEMS IN THE UNBORN CHILD OR COMPLICATIONS DURING DELIVERY.**

Alcohol Warning: If you consume 3 or more alcoholic drinks every day, ask your doctor whether you should take aspirin or other pain relievers/fever reducers. Aspirin may cause stomach bleeding.

Drug Interaction Precaution: Do not take this product if you are taking a prescription drug for anticoagulation (thinning the blood), diabetes, gout or arthritis unless directed by a doctor.

How Supplied: Extra Strength Bayer Plus Aspirin 500 mg (7.7 grains) is supplied in bottles of 50 caplets.

Shown in Product Identification Guide, page 504

Extra Strength BAYER® PM Aspirin Plus Sleep Aid Caplets

Indications: For the temporary relief of occasional headaches and minor aches and pains with accompanying sleeplessness.

Active Ingredients: 500 mg Aspirin, 25 mg Diphenhydramine Hydrochloride per caplet.

Inactive Ingredients: Colloidal Silicon Dioxide, Dibasic Calcium Phosphate, Dibutyl Sebacate, Ethylcellulose, FD&C Blue #1 Lake, FD&C Blue #2 Lake, Hydroxypropyl Methylcellulose, Microcrystalline Cellulose, Oleic Acid, Propylene Glycol, Starch, Titanium Dioxide, Zinc Stearate.

Directions: Adults and Children 12 years of age and over, take 2 caplets with water at bedtime, if needed, or as directed by a doctor.

Warnings: Do not give to children under 12 years of age. **Children and teenagers should not use this medicine for chicken pox or flu symptoms before a doctor is consulted about Reye's syndrome, a rare but serious illness reported to be associated with aspirin.** Do not take this product for pain for more than 10 days or for fever for more than 3 days unless directed by a doctor. If pain or fever persists or gets worse, if new symptoms occur, or if redness or swelling is present, consult a doctor because these could be signs of a serious condition. Do not take this product if you are allergic to aspirin or if you have asthma unless directed by a doctor. If ringing in the ears or a loss of hearing occurs, consult a doctor before taking any more of this product. Do not take this product if you have stomach problems (such as heartburn, upset stomach, or stomach pain) that persist or recur, or if you have ulcers or bleeding problems, unless directed by a doctor. If sleeplessness persists continuously for more than 2 weeks, consult your doctor. Insomnia may be a symptom of serious underlying medical illness. Do not take this product, unless directed by a doctor, if you have a breathing problem such as emphysema or chronic bronchitis, or if you have glaucoma or difficulty in urination due to enlargement of the prostate gland. Avoid alcoholic beverages while taking this product. Do not take this product if you are taking sedatives or tranquilizers, without first consulting your doctor. Keep this and all drugs out of the reach of children. In case of accidental overdose, seek professional assistance or contact a poison control center immediately. As with any drug, if you are pregnant or nursing a baby, seek the advice of a health professional before using this product. **IT IS ESPECIALLY IMPORTANT NOT TO USE ASPIRIN DURING THE LAST 3 MONTHS OF PREGNANCY UNLESS SPECIFICALLY DIRECTED TO DO SO BY A DOCTOR BECAUSE IT MAY CAUSE PROBLEMS IN THE UNBORN CHILD OR COMPLICATIONS DURING DELIVERY.**

Alcohol Warning: If you consume 3 or more alcoholic drinks every day, ask your doctor whether you should take aspirin or other pain relievers/fever reducers. Aspirin may cause stomach bleeding.

Drug Interaction Precaution: Do not take this product if you are taking a prescription drug for anticoagulation (thinning the blood), diabetes, gout, or arthritis unless directed by a doctor.

How Supplied: Bottles of 40 caplets.

Store at room temperature.

Shown in Product Identification Guide, page 504

BACTINE® Antiseptic-Anesthetic First Aid Liquid

Product Information

Active Ingredients: Benzalkonium chloride 0.13% w/w, and lidocaine Hydrochloride 2.5% w/w.

Inactive Ingredients: Edetate disodium, fragrances, octoxynol 9, propylene glycol, purified water.

Indications: First aid to help prevent bacterial contamination or skin infection and for the temporary relief of pain and itching in minor cuts, scrapes, and burns.

Directions: For adults and children 2 years of age and older. Clean the affected area. Apply a small amount of this product on the area 1 to 3 times daily. May be covered with a sterile bandage. If bandaged, let dry first. Children under 2 years of age: consult a doctor.

Warnings: For External Use Only. Do not use in the eyes or apply over large areas of the body. In case of deep or puncture wounds, animal bites, or serious burns, consult a doctor. Stop use and consult a doctor if the condition worsens or if symptoms persist for more than seven days or clear up and occur again within a few days. Do not use for longer than one week unless directed by a doctor. Do not use in large quantities, particularly over raw surfaces or blistered areas. Keep this and all drugs out of the reach of children. In case of accidental ingestion, seek professional assistance or contact a Poison Control Center immediately.

Caution: Keep from freezing.

How Supplied: Bactine Antiseptic-Anesthetic First Aid Liquid is available as 2 oz, 4 oz, and 16 oz. liquid with child resistant closures and 3.5 oz. pump spray.

Shown in Product Identification Guide, page 503

DOMEBORO® Astringent SOLUTION (Powder Packets)

DOMEBORO® Astringent SOLUTION (Effervescent Tablets)

Uses: Temporarily relieves minor skin irritation due to poison ivy, poison oak, poison sumac, insect bites, athlete's foot or rashes caused by soaps, detergents, cosmetics or jewelry.

Active Ingredients:
Domeboro® Astringent Powder Packets:

                               Purpose:

Aluminum Acetate .... Astringent (Each powder packet, when dissolved in water and ready for use, provides the active ingredient Aluminum Acetate resulting from the reaction of Calcium Acetate 938 mg, and Aluminum Sulfate

Continued on next page

Domeboro—Cont.

1191 mg. The resulting astringent solution is buffered to an acid pH.)
Domeboro® Astringent Tablets:
(In each tablet)*   **Purpose:**
Aluminum Acetate 525 mg .. Astringent

Inactive Ingredients:
Domeboro® Astringent Powder Packets: Dextrin.
Domeboro® Astringent Tablets: Dextrin, Polyethylene Glycol, Sodium Bicarbonate.

Directions:
Domeboro® Astringent Powder Packets:

Dissolve one, two, or three packets of Domeboro® powder in 16 ounces of water to obtain the following modified Burow's Solution:

Number of Packets	Dilution	% Aluminum acetate
one packet	1:40 dilution	0.16%
two packets	1:20 dilution	0.32%
three packets	1:13 diluton	0.48%

- Do not strain or filter the solution.
- Can be used as a compress, wet dressing, or as a soak.

AS A COMPRESS OR WET DRESSING:
- Saturate a clean, soft, white cloth (such as a diaper or torn sheet) in the solution.
- Gently squeeze and apply loosely to the affected area.
- Saturate the cloth in the solution every 15 to 30 minutes and apply to the affected area.
- Discard the solution after each use.
- Repeat as often as necessary.
AS A SOAK:
- Soak affected area in the solution for 15 to 30 minutes.
- Discard solution after each use.
- Repeat 3 times a day.
Domeboro® Astringent Tablets
- Dissolve one, two, or three tablets in 12 ounces of water and stir the solution until fully dissolved to obtain the following modified Burow's Solution.

Number of Tablets	Dilution	% Aluminum Acetate
one tablet	1:40 dilution	0.16%
two tablets	1:20 dilution	0.32%
three tablets	1:13 diluton	0.48%

- Do not strain or filter the solution.
- Can be used as a compress, wet dressing, or as a soak.

AS A COMPRESS OR WET DRESSING:
- Saturate a clean, soft, white cloth (such as a diaper or torn sheet) in the solution.
- Gently squeeze and apply loosely to the affected area.
- Saturate the cloth in the solution every 15 minutes and apply to the affected area.
- Discard the solution after each use.
- Repeat as often as necessary.
AS A SOAK:
- Soak affected area in the solution for 15 to 30 minutes.
- Discard solution after each use.
- Repeat 3 times a day.

Warnings:
Domeboro® Astringent Powder Packets:
For external use only. Avoid contact with the eyes.
When using this product, do not cover compress or wet dressing with plastic to prevent evaporation.
Stop use and ask a doctor if conditions worsen or symptoms persist more than 7 days.
Keep out of reach of children. If swallowed, get medical help or contact a Poison Control Center right away.
Domeboro® Astringent Tablets:
For external use only. Avoid contact with the eyes.
When using this product, do not cover compress or wet dressing with plastic to prevent evaporation.
Stop use and ask a doctor if condition worsens or symptoms persist for more than 7 days. These could be signs of a serious condition.
Keep out of reach of children. If swallowed, get medical help or contact a Poison Control Center right away.
Other information: * Each tablet, when dissolved in water and ready for use, provides the active ingredient Aluminum Acetate, resulting from the reaction of Calcium Acetate 606 mg and Aluminum Sulfate 879 mg. The resulting astringent solution is buffered to an acid pH.

How Supplied:
Domeboro® Astringent Powder Packets: Boxes of 12 powder packets.
Domeboro® Astringent Tablets: Boxes of 100 Effervescent Tablets.
Questions or comments? 1-800-800-4793 or www.bayercare.com
Shown in Product Identification Guide, page 504

Maximum Strength
MIDOL® Teen
Pain & Multi-Symptom Menstrual Relief
Aspirin Free/Caffeine Free
Caplet

Active Ingredients: Each caplet contains Acetaminophen 500 mg and Pamabrom 25 mg.

Inactive Ingredients: Croscarmellose Sodium, D&C Red #7 Lake, FD&C Blue #2 Lake, Hydroxpropyl Methylcellulose, Magnesium Stearate, Microcrystalline Cellulose, Starch, Titanium Dioxide and Triacetin.

Indication: Provides maximum strength relief of: cramps, bloating, water-weight gain, headaches, backaches, and muscular aches and pains.

Directions: Adults and children 12 years and over: Take 2 caplets with water. Repeat every 4 hours, as needed, up to a maximum of 8 caplets per day. Under age 12: Consult your doctor.

Warnings: Do not use for more than 10 days unless directed by a doctor. If pain persists for more than 10 days, consult a doctor immediately. Keep this and all drugs out of the reach of children. In case of accidental overdose, immediate medical attention is essential for adults as well as for children even if you do not notice any signs or symptoms. As with any drug, if you are pregnant or nursing a baby, seek the advice of a health professional before using this product.

Alcohol Warning: If you consume 3 or more alcoholic drinks every day, ask your doctor whether you should take acetaminophen or other pain relievers/fever reducers. Acetaminophen may cause liver damage.

How Supplied: Caplets-White capsule-shaped caplets available in packages of 24 caplets containing 3 blisters of 8 caplets each.
Shown in Product Identification Guide, page 504

Maximum Strength
MIDOL® Menstrual
Pain & Multi-Symptom Menstrual Relief
Aspirin Free
Caplets and Gelcaps
[See table at top of next page]

Inactive Ingredients: *Caplets:* Carnauba Wax, Croscarmellose Sodium, FD&C Blue #2, Hydroxypropyl Methylcellulose, Magnesium Stearate, Microcrystalline Cellulose, Pregelatinized Starch, Propylene Glycol, Shellac, Titanium Dioxide, Triacetin.
Gelcaps: Croscarmellose Sodium, D&C Red #33 Lake, EDTA Sodium, FD&C Blue #1 Lake, Gelatin, Glycerin, Hydroxypropyl Methylcellulose, Iron Oxide, Magnesium Stearate, Microcrystalline Cellulose, Starch, Stearic Acid, Titanium Dioxide, Triacetin.

Uses: For the temporary relief of these symptoms associated with menstrual periods:
- cramps
- bloating
- water-weight gain
- headaches
- backaches
- muscle aches
- fatigue

Directions: Adults and children 12 years and older: take 2 caplets with water. Repeat every 4 hours, as needed. Do not exceed 8 caplets per day. Children 12 years of age and under: consult a doctor.

Active ingredients (in each caplet and gelcap):   **Purpose:**
Acetaminophen 500 mg .... Pain Reliever
Caffeine 60 mg .... Diuretic, Stimulant
Pyrilamine Maleate 15 mg .... Diuretic

Warnings:
Alcohol warning: If you consume 3 or more alcoholic drinks every day, ask your doctor whether you should take acetaminophen or other pain relievers/fever reducers. Acetaminophen may cause liver damage.
Caffeine warning: The recommended dose of this product contains about as much caffeine as a cup of coffee. Limit the use of caffeine-containing medications, foods, or beverages while taking this product because too much caffeine may cause nervousness, irritability, sleeplessness, and occasionally, rapid heartbeat.
Ask a doctor before use if you have
• a breathing problem such as emphysema or chronic bronchitis
• glaucoma
• difficulty in urination due to enlargement of the prostate gland
Ask a doctor or pharmacist before use if you are taking sedatives or tranquilizers.
When using this product
• do not take for more than 10 days, unless directed by a doctor
• you may get drowsy
• avoid alcoholic drinks
• alcohol, sedatives, and tranquilizers may increase drowsiness
• be careful when driving a motor vehicle or operating machinery
• excitability may occur, especially in children
Stop use and ask a doctor if pain persists for more than 10 days. This may be the sign of a serious condition.
If pregnant or breast-feeding, ask a health professional before use.
Keep out of reach of children. In case of overdose, get medical help or contact a Poison Control Center right away. Prompt medical help is critical for adults as well as for children even if you do not notice any signs or symptoms.
Other Information: Store at room temperature.
How Supplied: *Caplets:* White capsule-shaped caplets available in packages of 24 caplets containing 3 blisters of 8 caplets each, and 8 caplet containing 1 blister of 8 caplets each. Also: 16 and 40 caplets
Gelcaps: Dark/light blue capsule-shaped gelcaps available in packages of 24 gelcaps containing 3 blisters of 8 gelcaps.
Shown in Product Identification Guide, page 504

**Maximum Strength
MIDOL® PMS
Pain & Premenstrual Symptom Relief
Aspirin Free/Caffeine Free
Caplets and Gelcaps**

Active Ingredients: Each caplet or gelcap contains Acetaminophen 500 mg, Pamabrom 25 mg and Pyrilamine Maleate 15 mg.

Inactive Ingredients: Caplets—Croscarmellose Sodium, D&C Red #30, D&C Yellow #10, Hydroxypropyl Methylcellulose, Magnesium Stearate, Microcrystalline Cellulose, Pregelatinized Starch and Triacetin.

Gelcaps—Croscarmellose Sodium, D&C Red #27 Lake, EDTA Disodium, FD&C Blue #1, FD&C Red #40 Lake, Gelatin, Glycerin, Hydroxypropyl Methylcellulose, Iron Oxides, Magnesium Stearate, Microcrystalline Cellulose, Starch, Stearic Acid, Titanium Dioxide, Triacetin.

Indications: Provides maximum strength relief of: bloating, water-weight gain, cramps, headaches and backaches.

Directions: Adults and children 12 years and over: Take 2 caplets or gelcaps with water. Repeat every 4 hours, as needed, up to a maximum of 8 caplets or gelcaps per day. Under age 12: Consult your doctor.

Warnings: Do not take this product for more than 10 days unless directed by a doctor. If pain persists for more than 10 days, consult a doctor immediately. May cause drowsiness; alcohol, sedatives and tranquilizers may increase drowsiness. Avoid alcoholic beverages while taking this product. Do not take this product if you are taking sedatives or tranquilizers without first consulting your doctor. Use caution when driving or operating machinery. May cause excitability especially in children. Do not take this product, unless directed by a doctor, if you have a breathing problem such as emphysema or chronic bronchitis or if you have glaucoma or difficulty in urination due to enlargement of the prostate gland. Keep this and all drugs out of the reach of children. In case of accidental overdose, immediate medical attention is essential for adults as well as for children even if you do not notice any signs or symptoms. As with any drug, if you are pregnant or nursing a baby, seek the advice of a health professional before using this product.

Alcohol Warning: If you consume 3 or more alcoholic drinks every day, ask your doctor whether you should take acetaminophen or other pain relievers/fever reducers. Acetaminophen may cause liver damage.

How Supplied: Caplets-White capsule-shaped caplets available in packages of 24 caplets containing 3 blisters of 8 caplets each, and 8 caplets containing 1 blister of 8 caplets each.

Gelcaps—Dark/light pink capsule-shaped gelcaps available in packages of 24 gelcaps containing 3 blisters of 8 gelcaps.

Shown in Product Identification Guide, page 504

**MYCELEX®-3
3 Day Treatment in Pre-filled Applicators
Tube of Vaginal Cream and 3 Disposable Applicators**

Indications: For the treatment of vaginal yeast (Candida) infection.
Active Ingredient: Butoconazole Nitrate (2%).
Note: The active ingredient in this product (butoconazole nitrate 2%) is not the same active ingredient found in Mycelex®-7.

Inactive Ingredients: Cetyl Alcohol, Glyceryl Stearate and PEG-100 Stearate, Methylparaben and Propylparaben (preservatives), Mineral Oil, Polysorbate 60, Propylene Glycol, Sorbitan Monostearate, Stearyl Alcohol and Water (purified).

Precautions: IF THIS IS THE FIRST TIME YOU HAVE HAD VAGINAL ITCH AND DISCOMFORT, CONSULT YOUR DOCTOR. IF YOU HAVE HAD A DOCTOR DIAGNOSE A VAGINAL YEAST INFECTION BEFORE AND HAVE THE SAME SYMPTOMS NOW, USE MYCELEX®-3 AS DIRECTED FOR 3 CONSECUTIVE DAYS.

Directions: *Antifungal Vaginal Cream with 3 Disposable Applicators:* Fill the applicator and insert one applicator of cream into vagina for three days in a row, preferably at bedtime. Dispose of applicator after use.
Antifungal Vaginal Cream in 3 Pre-filled Applicators: Insert one applicator of cream into the vagina for three days in a row, preferably at bedtime. Dispose of applicator after use.

Warnings:
• Do not use if you have abdominal pain, fever, or foul-smelling discharge. Contact your doctor immediately.
• If your infection isn't gone in three days, you may have a condition other than a yeast infection or you may need to use more medication. Consult your doctor. If your symptoms return within two months or if you think you have been exposed to the human immunodeficiency virus (HIV) that causes AIDS, consult your doctor immediately. Recurring infections may be a sign of pregnancy or a serious condition, such as AIDS or diabetes.
• Do not use this product if you are pregnant or think you may be pregnant, have diabetes, a positive HIV test or AIDS. Consult Your Doctor.
• Do not rely on condoms or diaphragms to prevent sexually transmitted disease or pregnancy while using this product. This product may damage condoms and diaphragms and may cause them to fail. Use another method of birth control to prevent pregnancy while using this product.
• Do not use tampons while using this medicine.

Continued on next page

Mycelex-3—Cont.

- Do not use in girls under 12 years of age.
- Keep this and all drugs out of the reach of children.
- For vaginal use only. Do not use in eyes or take by mouth. In case of accidental ingestion, seek professional assistance or contact a Poison Control Center immediately.

How Supplied: *Antifungal Vaginal Cream with 3 Disposable Applicators:* One 20g (0.7 oz) tube of vaginal cream and 3 disposable applicators. *Antifungal Vaginal Cream in 3 Pre-filled Applicators:* Three disposable applicators pre-filled to deliver 5g vaginal cream (butoconazole nitrate 2%).
Avoid excessive heat above 30°C (86°F) and avoid freezing.

MYCELEX®-7
- **Antifungal Vaginal Cream with Applicator**
- **Antifungal Cream with 7 Disposable Applicators**
- **Combination-Pack: Vaginal Inserts and External Vulvar Cream**

Indications: For the treatment of vaginal yeast (*Candida*) infection.
Combination Pack: For treatment of vaginal yeast (*Candida*) infection and the relief of external vulvar itching and irritation associated with vaginal yeast infections

Active Ingredient:
Cream: Clotrimazole 1%
Vaginal Inserts: each insert contains 100 mg clotrimazole

Inactive Ingredients:
Cream: Benzyl alcohol, cetostearyl alcohol, cetyl esters wax, octyldodecanol, polysorbate 60, purified water, sorbitan monostearate
Inserts: Corn starch, lactose, magnesium stearate, povidone

Precautions: IF THIS IS THE FIRST TIME YOU HAVE HAD VAGINAL ITCH (OR VULVAR ITCH—RELATES ONLY TO COMBINATION PACK) AND DISCOMFORT, CONSULT YOUR DOCTOR. IF YOU HAVE HAD A DOCTOR DIAGNOSE A VAGINAL YEAST INFECTION BEFORE AND HAVE THE SAME SYMPTOMS NOW, USE MYCELEX®-7 AS DIRECTED FOR 7 CONSECUTIVE DAYS.
Before using, read the enclosed educational pamphlet.

Directions:
Antifungal Vaginal Cream with Applicator: Fill the applicator and insert one applicator full of cream into the vagina, preferably at bedtime. Repeat this procedure daily for 7 consecutive days.
Antifungal Vaginal Cream with Disposable Applicators: Fill the applicator and insert one applicator full of cream into the vagina, preferably at bedtime.

Dispose of each applicator after use. Do not flush in toilet. Repeat this procedure daily with a new applicator for 7 consecutive days.
Combination Pack Inserts: Unwrap one insert, place it in the applicator, and use the applicator to place the insert into the vagina, preferably at bedtime. Repeat this procedure daily for 7 consecutive days.
Cream: Squeeze a small amount of cream onto your finger and gently spread the cream onto the irritated area of the vulva. Use once or twice daily for up to 7 days as needed to relieve external vulvar itching. THE CREAM SHOULD NOT BE USED FOR VULVAR ITCHING DUE TO CAUSES OTHER THAN A YEAST INFECTION.

Warning: DO NOT USE IF YOU HAVE ABDOMINAL PAIN, FEVER, OR FOUL-SMELLING DISCHARGE. CONTACT YOUR DOCTOR IMMEDIATELY.
IF YOU DO NOT IMPROVE IN 3 DAYS OR IF YOU DO NOT GET WELL IN 7 DAYS, YOU MAY HAVE A CONDITION OTHER THAN A YEAST INFECTION. CONSULT YOUR DOCTOR. If your symptoms return within two months or if you have infections that do not clear up easily with proper treatment, consult your doctor. You could be pregnant or there could be a serious underlying medical cause for your infections, including diabetes or a damaged immune system (including damage from infection with HIV—the virus that causes AIDS). (PLEASE READ PATIENT PACKAGE PAMPHLET.)
Mycelex®-7 may reduce the effectiveness of condoms, diaphragms, or vaginal spermicides. This effect is temporary and occurs only during treatment.
Do not use during pregnancy except under the advice and supervision of a doctor. Do not use tampons while using this medication. Keep this and all drugs out of the reach of children. In case of accidental ingestion, seek professional assistance or contact a Poison Control Center immediately. NOT FOR USE IN CHILDREN LESS THAN 12 YEARS OF AGE.
If you have any questions about MYCELEX®-7 or vaginal yeast infection, contact your physician.

How Supplied:
Antifungal Vaginal Cream with Applicator: 1.5 oz. (45g) tube of vaginal cream and applicator. (7-day therapy).
Antifungal Vaginal Cream with 7 Disposable Applicators: One 45g (1.5 oz.) tube of vaginal cream and 7 applicators (7-day therapy).
Combination-Pack: 7 vaginal inserts and applicator (7-day therapy) and one 7g (0.25 oz) tube of external vulvar cream.

Store at room temperature between 2° and 30°C (36° and 86°F).

NEO-SYNEPHRINE®
Mild Formula, Regular Strength, Extra Strength

Active Ingredients:
Mild Formula: 0.25% phenylephrine hydrochloride
Regular Strength: 0.5% phenylephrine hydrochloride
Extra Strength: 1% phenylephrine hydrochloride

Inactive Ingredients: Benzalkonium Chloride, Thimerosal, Citric Acid, Purified Water, Sodium Chloride, Sodium Citrate.

Uses: Temporarily relieves nasal congestion due to common cold, hay fever, or other respiratory allergies or association with sinusitis.
Temporary relieves stuffy nose and restores freer breathing through the nose. Helps clear nasal passages; shrinks swollen membranes. Helps decongest sinus openings and passages; temporary relieves sinus congestion and pressure.

Directions: For a 0.25% solution (Mild): Adults and children 6 to under 12 years of age (with adult supervision): 2 or 3 sprays in each nostril not more often than every 4 hours. Children under 6 years of age: consult a doctor.
For a 0.5% solution (Regular) or for a 1.0% solution (Extra):
Adults and children 12 years of age and over: 2 or 3 drops or sprays in each nostril not more often than every 4 hours. Children under 12 years ask a doctor.

Warnings:
Do not exceed recommended dosage. This product may cause temporary discomfort such as burning, stinging, sneezing, or an increase in nasal discharge. The use of this container by more than one person may spread infection. Do not use this product for more than 3 days. Use only as directed. Frequent or prolonged use may cause nasal congestion to recur or worsen. If symptoms persist, consult a doctor. Do not use this product if you have (or give this product to a child who has) heart disease, high blood pressure, thyroid disease, diabetes, or difficulty in urination due to enlargement of the prostate gland unless directed by a doctor.
Keep this and all drugs out of the reach of children. As with any drug if you are pregnant or nursing a baby seek the advice of a health professional before using this product.
In case of accidental ingestion, seek professional assistance or contact a poison control center immediately.

Storage:
Store at room temperature. Protect from light. Do not use if solution is brown or contains a precipitate.

How Supplied: Mild Formula (0.25%) in 15 mL spray. Regular Strength (0.5%) in 15 mL drops and spray. Extra Strength (1.0%) in 15 mL drops and spray.

Shown in Product Identification Guide, page 504

NEO-SYNEPHRINE®
12 Hour
(nasal spray)
12 Hour Extra Moisturizing
(nasal spray)

Active Ingredient: Oxymetazoline Hydrochloride 0.05%.

Inactive Ingredients: Benzalkonium Chloride, Phenylmercuric Acetate, Glycerin, Glycine, Purified Water, Sorbitol and may also contain Sodium Chloride.

Uses: Temporarily relieves nasal congestion due to a common cold, hay fever, or other upper respiratory allergies or associated with sinusitis. Temporarily relieves stuffy nose and restores freer breathing through the nose. Helps clear nasal passages; shrinks swollen membranes. Helps decongest sinus openings and passages; temporarily relieves sinus congestion and pressure.

Directions: Adults and children 6 to under 12 years of age (with adult supervision): 2 or 3 sprays in each nostril not more often than every 10 to 12 hours. Do not exceed 2 doses in any 24-hour period. Children under 6 years of age: ask a doctor.

Warnings: Do not exceed recommended dosage. This product may cause temporary discomfort such as burning, stinging, sneezing, or an increase in nasal discharge. The use of the container by more than one person may spread infection. Do not use this product for more than 3 days. Use only as directed. Frequent or prolonged use may cause nasal congestion to recur or worsen. If symptoms persist, consult a doctor. Ask a doctor before use if you have: heart disease, high blood pressure, thyroid disease, diabetes, or difficulty in urination due to enlargement of the prostate gland.
Keep this and all drugs out of the reach of children. If swallowed, get medical help or contact a Poison Control Center right away. If pregnant or breast-feeding, ask a health professional before use.

Storage:
Store at room temperature. Protect from light.

How Supplied: *Nasal Spray 12 Hour* — plastic squeeze bottles of 15 ml (¹/₂ fl. oz.); *12 Hour Extra Moisturizing Nasal Spray* — 15 ml (¹/₂ fl. oz).

Shown in Product Identification Guide, page 504

Age	Recommended Dose	Daily Maximum
Adults & children 12 and over	2 caplets once a day	Up to 4 times a day
Children (6 to under 12 years)	1 caplet once a day	Up to 4 times a day
Children under 6 years	Consult a physician	

PHILLIPS'® CHEWABLE TABLETS ANTACID-LAXATIVE STIMULANT FREE

As A Laxative:
Indications: To relieve occasional constipation (irregularity). This product generally produces bowel movement in 1/2 to 6 hours.
As An Antacid:
Indications: To relieve acid indigestion, sour stomach, and heartburn.

Active Ingredient: per tablet: Magnesium Hydroxide 311 mg.

Inactive Ingredients: Colloidal Silicon Dioxide, Dextrates, Magnesium Stearate, Maltodextrin, Natural Flavor, Starch, Sucrose.
Sodium Content: 0.92 mg per tablet.

Directions: Adults and Children 12 years and older, Chew 6–8 tablets. **Children 6–11 years,** Chew 3–4 tablets; **2–5 years,** Chew 1–2 tablets; **Under 2,** Consult a doctor. Take preferably before bedtime, followed with a full glass (8 oz.) of liquid.

Warnings: Do not take any laxative if abdominal pain, nausea, vomiting or kidney disease are present unless directed by a doctor. If you have noticed a sudden change in bowel habits persisting for over 2 weeks, consult a doctor before using a laxative. Laxative products should not be used for a period longer than 1 week, unless directed by a doctor. Rectal bleeding or failure to have a bowel movement after use of a laxative may indicate a serious condition. Discontinue use and consult your doctor.
Do not take more than the maximum recommended daily dosage in a 24-hour period, or use the maximum dosage of this product for more than 2 weeks, or use this product if you have kidney disease, except under the advice and supervision of a doctor. May have a laxative effect.

Drug Interaction Precaution: May interact with certain prescription drugs. If you are presently taking a prescription drug, do not take this product without checking with your doctor or other healthcare professional.
Keep this and all drugs out of the reach of children. In case of accidental overdose, seek professional assistance or contact a Poison Control Center immediately. As with any drug, if you are pregnant or nursing a baby, seek the advice of a healthcare professional before using this product.

How Supplied: Bottles of 100 Tablets
Questions? Comments?
Please call 1-800-331-4536.
Visit our website at
www.bayercare.com

PHILLIPS'® FIBERCAPS
BULK-FORMING FIBER LAXATIVE

Active Ingredient: Each caplet contains 625 mg calcium polycarbophil equivalent to 500 mg polycarbophil.

Inactive Ingredients: Acacia, Calcium Carbonate, Caramel, Colloidal Silicon Dioxide, Croscarmellose Sodium, Crospovidone, Gelatin, Hydroxypropyl Cellulose, Hydroxypropyl Methylcellulose, Magnesium Stearate, Maltodextrin, Microcrystalline Cellulose, Mineral Oil, Polyethylene Glycol, Povidone, Stearic Acid.

Uses: Helps restore and maintain regularity and relieve constipation. This product generally produces bowel movement in 12 to 72 hours.

Directions:
[See table above]
PHILLIPS' FIBERCAPS work naturally so continued use for one to three days is normally required to provide full benefit. PHILLIPS' FIBERCAPS dosage may vary according to diet, exercise, previous laxative use or severity of constipation. TAKE THIS PRODUCT ACCORDING TO THE DOSAGE CHART ABOVE WITH AT LEAST A FULL GLASS (8 OUNCES) OF LIQUID. TAKING THIS PRODUCT WITHOUT ENOUGH LIQUID MAY CAUSE CHOKING. SEE WARNINGS. Do not take more than the maximum daily dose.

Warnings: Do not use laxative products when abdominal pain, nausea or vomiting are present unless directed by a doctor. If you have noticed a sudden change in bowel habits that persists over a period of 2 weeks, consult a doctor before using a laxative. Laxative products should not be used for a period longer than 1 week unless directed by a doctor. Rectal bleeding or failure to have a bowel movement after use of a laxative may indicate a serious condition. Discontinue use and consult your doctor. **TAKING THIS PRODUCT WITHOUT ADEQUATE FLUID MAY CAUSE IT TO SWELL AND BLOCK YOUR THROAT OR ESOPHAGUS AND MAY CAUSE CHOKING. DO NOT TAKE THIS PRODUCT IF YOU HAVE DIFFICULTY IN SWALLOWING. IF YOU EXPERIENCE CHEST PAIN, VOMITING OR DIFFICULTY IN SWALLOWING OR BREATHING AFTER TAKING THIS PRODUCT, SEEK IMMEDIATE MEDICAL ATTENTION.** Keep this and all drugs out of the reach of children. In case of accidental overdose, seek professional assistance or consult a poison control center immediately.

Drug Interaction Precaution: Contains calcium. If you are taking any form

Continued on next page

Phillips' Fibercaps—Cont.

of tetracycline antibiotic, PHILLIPS' FIBERCAPS should be taken at least 1 hour before or 2 hours after you have taken the antibiotic.

How Supplied: 36 and 60 Caplets
Shown in Product Identification Guide, page 505

PHILLIP'S® LIQUI-GELS®

Uses:
• For the relief of occasional constipation (irregularity).
• This product generally produces a bowel movement in 12–72 hours.

**Active ingredient
(in each dosage unit):   Purpose:**
Docusate Sodium
100 mg .... Stool Softener Laxative

Inactive ingredients: FD&C Blue #2 Aluminum Lake, Gelatin, Glycerin, Methylparaben, Polyethylene Glycol, Propylene Glycol, Propylparaben, Sorbitol, Titanium Dioxide

Phillips' Liqui-Gels are a very low sodium product. Each Liqui-Gel contains 5 mg of sodium.

Directions:
Take Phillips' Liqui-Gels with a full glass (8 oz) of water.

Adults and children 12 years and over	Take 1 to 3 Liqui-Gels daily. This dose may be taken as a single daily dose or in divided doses.
Children 6 to under 12 years	Take 1 Liqui-Gel daily.
Children under 6 years of age	Consult a doctor.

Warnings: Ask a doctor before use if you have abdominal pain, nausea, vomiting or if you have noticed a sudden change in bowel habits that persists over a period of 2 weeks. **Ask a doctor or pharmacist before use if you are** presently taking mineral oil. **Stop use and ask a doctor if** you have rectal bleeding or failure to have a bowel movement after use. These could be signs of a serious condition. **Do not use** laxative products for a period longer than 1 week unless directed by a doctor. **If pregnant or breast-feeding,** ask a health professional before use. KEEP OUT OF THE REACH OF CHILDREN. In case of overdosage, get medical help or contact a Poison Control Center right away.
Storage: Store at controlled room temperature (59°–86°F) in a dry place.
Liqui-Gels is a registered trademark of R.P. Scherer Corp.

How Supplied: Blister packs of 10, 30 Liqui-Gels.

PHILLIPS'® MILK OF MAGNESIA
Original Formula
Cherry Formula
Mint Formula

Active Ingredients:
Original Formula: Magnesium Hydroxide 400 mg per teaspoon (5 ml).
Cherry Formula: Magnesium Hydroxide 400 mg per teaspoon (5 ml).
Mint Formula: Magnesium Hydroxide 400 mg per teaspoon (5 ml).

Inactive Ingredients:
Original Formula: Purified Water.
Cherry Formula: Carboxymethylcellulose Sodium, Citric Acid, D&C Red #28, Flavor, Glycerin, Microcrystalline Cellulose, Purified Water, Sodium Citrate, Sodium Hypochlorite, Sucrose, Xanthan Gum.
Mint Formula: Artifical and Natural Flavors, Mineral Oil, Purified Water, Sodium Saccarin.

Indications: AS A LAXATIVE—To relieve occasional constipation (irregularity). This product generally produces bowel movement in $1/2$ to 6 hours.

AS AN ANTACID—To relieve acid indigestion, sour stomach and heartburn.

Directions: For Laxative Use - Adults and Children 12 years & older: 2–4 tablespoonsful at bedtime or upon arising, followed by a full glass (8 oz.) of liquid. Children 6–11 years: 1–2 tablespoonsful, followed by a full glass (8 oz.) of liquid. Children 2–5 years: 1–3 teaspoonsful, followed by a full glass (8 oz.) of liquid. Children under 2 years: Consult a doctor. SHAKE WELL BEFORE USING.

Directions: For Antacid Use - Adults and Children 12 years & older: 1–3 teaspoonsful with a little water, up to four times a day or as directed by a doctor. SHAKE WELL BEFORE USING.

Drug Interaction Precaution: Antacids may interact with certain prescription drugs. If you are presently taking a prescription drug, do not take this product without checking with your doctor or other health professional.

Laxative Warnings: Do not use laxative products when abdominal pain, nausea, vomiting or kidney disease are present unless directed by a doctor. If you have noticed a sudden change in bowel habits persisting for over 2 weeks, consult a doctor before using a laxative. Laxative products should not be used for a period longer than 1 week, unless directed by a doctor. Rectal bleeding or failure to have a bowel movement after use of a laxative may indicate a serious condition. Discontinue use and consult your doctor.

Phillips' Milk of Magnesia is a saline laxative.

Antacid Warnings: Do not take more than the maximum recommended daily dosage in a 24 hour period (See Directions), or use the maximum dosage of this product for more than two weeks, or use this product if you have kidney disease, except under the advice and supervision of a doctor. May have laxative effect.

If pregnant or breast-feeding, ask a health professional before use. Keep this and all drugs out of the reach of children. In case of accidental overdose, seek professional assistance or contact a poison control center immediately.

Storage: Keep tightly closed and avoid freezing.

How Supplied: Phillips' Milk of Magnesia is available in Original, Mint, and Cherry formulas and comes in 4 oz., 12 oz., and 26 oz. bottles. Also available in chewable tablets and concentrated liquid formulas.
Shown in Product Identification Guide, page 505

MAXIMUM STRENGTH RID®
LICE KILLING SHAMPOO
Pediculicide (Lice Treatment)

Product Description: Kills lice and their eggs (head lice, crab lice and body lice).

Active Ingredients: Piperonyl Butoxide 4%, Pyrethrum Extract equivalent to 0.33% Pyrethrins.

Inactive Ingredients: C_{13}–C_{14} Isoparaffin, Fragrance, Isopropyl Alcohol, PEG-25 Hydrogenated Castor Oil, Water, Xanthan Gum.

Indications: For the treatment of head, pubic (crab) and body lice.

Warnings:
☐ Use with caution on persons allergic to ragweed.
☐ For external use only. Do not use near the eyes or permit contact with mucous membranes, such as inside the nose, mouth, or vagina, as irritation may occur. Keep out of eyes when rinsing hair. Adults and children: Close eyes tightly and do not open eyes until product is rinsed out. Also, protect children's eyes with washcloth, towel or other suitable material, or by a similar method. If product gets into the eyes, immediately flush with water.
☐ If skin irritation or infection is present or develops, discontinue use and consult a doctor. Consult a doctor if infestation of eyebrows or eyelashes occurs.
☐ In case of accidental ingestion, seek professional assistance or contact a Poison Control Center immediately.

☐ Keep this and all drugs out of the reach of children.

Application:
A. Helpful Hints
1. Use RID® on <u>dry</u> hair. Hair should not be wet prior to applying RID® because it may dilute the active ingredients and reduce its effectiveness.
2. You must thoroughly comb out the lice eggs in order to prevent reinfestation. This will take time, but is <u>very</u> important. RID® Egg & Nit Comb Out Gel can make this process faster and easier. Carefully read the package insert.

Directions:
IMPORTANT: READ WARNINGS BEFORE USING.
1. Apply to affected area until all the hair is thoroughly wet with product.
2. Allow product to remain on area for 10 minutes but no longer.
3. Add sufficient warm water to form a lather and shampoo as usual. Rinse thoroughly.
4. A fine-toothed comb or special lice/nit removing comb may be used to help remove dead lice or their eggs (nits) from hair.
5. A second treatment must be done in 7 to 10 days to kill any newly hatched lice.
☐ Store at room temperature 59°–86°F (15°–30°C).
☐ Do not reuse original container.
☐ Securely wrap original container in several layers of newspaper and discard in trash.

Head lice: Head lice live on the scalp and lay small white eggs (nits) on the hair shaft close to the scalp. The nits are most easily found on the nape of the neck or behind the ears. All personal headgear, scarfs, coats, and bed linen should be disinfected by machine washing in hot water and drying, using the hot cycle of a dryer for at least 20 minutes. Personal articles of clothing or bedding that cannot be washed may be dry-cleaned, sealed in a plastic bag for a period of about 2 weeks, or sprayed with a product specifically designed for this purpose. Personal combs and brushes may be disinfected by soaking in hot water (above 130°F, 54°C) for 5 to 10 minutes. Thorough vacuuming of rooms inhabited by infected patients is recommended.

Additional Information:
Call 1-800-RID-LICE (1-800-743-5423) or visit www.licerid.com for further information. Comprehensive patient education materials are available free of charge through 1-800-RID-LICE.

How Supplied: Sizes Available: 2 FL OZ (59mL), 4 FL OZ (118mL), 8 FL OZ (236mL), and Lice Elimination Kit containing 4 FL OZ (118mL) Lice Killing Shampoo and 5 OZ (141.8g) Lice Control Spray For Bedding & Furniture.

Shown in Product Identification Guide, page 505

MAXIMUM STRENGTH RID® MOUSSE
Pyrethrum extract/Piperonyl Butoxide Aerosolized Foam Pediculicide (Lice Treatment)

Active Ingredients (calculated without propellant)
Piperonyl butoxide (4%)
Pyrethrum extract* (equivalent to 0.33% pyrethrins)

*50% extract (not USP)

Inactive Ingredients: cetearyl alcohol, isobutane, PEG-20 stearate, propane, propylene glycol, purified water, quaternium-52, SD Alcohol 3-C (26.5% w/w)

Uses: treats head, public (crab), and body lice

Warnings:
- **For external use only**
- **Flammable:** Keep away from fire or flame
Do not use near the eyes
Ask a doctor before use if you have an allergy to ragweed
When using this product:
- keep out of eyes when rising hair
- close eyes tightly and do not open eyes until product is rinsed out
- protect eyes with washcloth, towel or other suitable method
- if product gets into the eyes, immediately flush with water
- do not use inside the nose, mouth, or vagina. Irritation may occur.
- do not inhale; use in a well ventilated area
- do not puncture or incinerate. Contents under pressure.
Stop use and ask a doctor if:
- skin irritation or infection is present or develops
- infestation of eyebrows or eyelashes occurs
Keep out of reach of children. If swallowed, get medical help or contact a Poison Control Center right away.

Directions:
- **Important: Read warnings before using:**
- shake well before using
- holding the can upside down, apply RID® Mousse to **dry hair** or other affected area. Massage until all the hair is thoroughly wet with product. For best results against head lice, see complete Directions in the Consumer Information Insert.
- allow product to remain on the hair for 10 minutes but no longer
- wash area thoroughly with warm water and soap or shampoo
- a fine-toothed comb or a special lice/nit removing comb may be used to help remove dead lice or their eggs (nits) from hair
- a second treatment must be done in 7 to 10 days to kill any newly hatched lice

Other Information:
- store at 20°–25°C (68°–77°F)
- do not store at temperature above 43°C (110°F)
- keep in a cool place out of the sun
Questions? call **1-800-RID LICE (1-800-743-5423)**

Distributed By
Bayer Corporation
Consumer Care Division
Morristown, N.J. 07960 USA
Shown in Product Identification Guide, page 505

VANQUISH®
Extra Strength Pain Reliever Analgesic Caplets

Vanquish Caplets, the extra-strength pain formula with two buffers, is specially shaped for easy swallowing.

Active Ingredients: 227 mg Aspirin, 194 mg Acetaminophen and 33 mg Caffeine per caplet, in a formulation buffered with Aluminum Hydroxide and Magnesium Hydroxide.

Inactive Ingredients: Hydroxypropyl Methylcellulose, Microcrystalline Cellulose, Polyethylene Glycol, Silicon Dioxide, Starch, Titanium Dioxide, Zinc Stearate.

Store at room temperature.

Indications: Fast, safe, temporary relief of minor aches and pains associated with headaches, colds and flu, backaches, muscle aches, menstrual pain and minor pain of arthritis.

Directions: Adults (12 years and over), take 2 caplets with water every 4 hours, as needed, up to a maximum of 12 caplets in 24 hours or as directed by a doctor. **Children under 12 years,** consult a doctor.

Warnings: Children and teenagers should not use this medicine for chicken pox or flu symptoms before a doctor is consulted about Reye's syndrome, a rare but serious illness reported to be associated with aspirin. Do not take for pain for more than 10 days or for fever for more than 3 days unless directed by a doctor. If pain or fever persists or gets worse, if new symptoms occur or if redness or swelling is present, consult a doctor because these could be signs of a serious condition. Do not take this product if you are allergic to aspirin, have asthma, have stomach problems (such as heartburn, upset stomach or stomach pain) that persist or recur or if you have gastric ulcers or bleeding problems unless directed by a doctor. If ringing in the ears or loss of hearing occurs, consult a doctor before taking any more of this product. Keep this and all drugs out of the reach of children. In case of accidental overdose, immediate medical attention is essential for adults as well as for children even if you do not notice any signs or symptoms. As with any drug, if you are pregnant or nursing a baby, seek the advice of a health professional before using this product. **IT IS ESPECIALLY IMPORTANT NOT TO USE ASPIRIN DURING THE LAST 3 MONTHS OF PREGNANCY UNLESS SPECIFICALLY DIRECTED TO DO SO BY A DOCTOR**

Continued on next page

Vanquish—Cont.

BECAUSE IT MAY CAUSE PROB-
LEMS IN THE UNBORN CHILD OR
COMPLICATIONS DURING DELIV-
ERY.

Alcohol Warning: If you consume 3 or
more alcoholic drinks every day, ask your
doctor whether you should take acetaminophen and aspirin or other pain re-
lievers/fever reducers. Acetaminophen
and aspirin may cause liver damage and
stomach bleeding.

Drug Interaction Precaution: Do
not take this product if you are taking a
prescription drug for anticoagulation
(thinning of the blood), diabetes, gout, or
arthritis unless directed by a doctor.

How Supplied: Bottles of 60 and 100 caplets.

*Shown in Product Identification
Guide, page 505*

Beutlich LP
Pharmaceuticals

**1541 SHIELDS DRIVE
WAUKEGAN, IL 60085-8304**

Direct Inquiries to:
847-473-1100
800-238-8542 in US & Canada
FAX 847–473-1122
www.beutlich.com
e-mail fjb1541@worldnet.att.net

CEO–TWO® Evacuant
Laxative Adult Rectal Suppository

NDC #0283-0763-09

Composition: Each suppository contains sodium bicarbonate and potassium
bitartrate in a special blend of water-
soluble polyethylene glycols.

Indications: For relief of occasional
constipation, irregularity or for bowel
training programs. CEO-TWO generally
produces a bowel movement in 5–30 minutes. The lubrication provided by the
emollient base combined with the gentle
pressure of the released carbon dioxide
slowly distends the rectal ampulla stimulating peristalsis. CEO-TWO does not
interfere with normal digestion, is not
habit forming, won't cause cramping or
irritation or alter the normal peristaltic
reflex, and it leaves no residue.

Administration and Dosage: Adults
and children over 12 years of age. Rectal
dosage is one suppository containing 0.6
gram of sodium bicarbonate and 0.9
gram potassium bitartrate in a single
daily dose. For children under 12 years of
age: consult a doctor. For most effective
results and ease of insertion, moisten a
CEO-TWO suppository by placing it under a warm water tap for 30 seconds or in
a cup of water for 10 seconds before insertion. Insert rectally past the largest
diameter of the suppository. Patient
should retain in the rectum as long as
possible (usually about 5–30 minutes).

Warnings: For rectal use only. Do not
use this product if you are on a low salt
diet unless directed by a doctor. (172 milligrams of sodium per suppository) Do
not lubricate with mineral oil or petrolatum prior to use. Do not use when abdominal pain, nausea or vomiting are
present unless directed by a doctor. Laxative products should not be used for
longer than one week unless directed by
a doctor. If you have noticed a sudden
change of bowel habits that persists over
a period of 2 weeks, consult a doctor before using a laxative. Rectal bleeding or
failure to have a bowel movement after
use of a laxative may indicate a serious
problem. Discontinue use and consult
your doctor.

How Supplied: In box of 10 individually foil wrapped white opaque suppositories. Keep in cool dry place. **DO NOT
REFRIGERATE**

HURRICAINE® TOPICAL
ANESTHETIC

Composition: HURRICAINE contains
20% benzocaine in a flavored, water soluble polyethylene glycol base.

Action and Indications: HURRIC-
AINE is a topical anesthetic that provides rapid anesthesia on all accessible
mucous membrane in 15 to 30 seconds,
short duration of 15 minutes, has virtually no systemic absorption, and tastes
good. Hurricaine is used as a lubricant
and topical anesthetic to facilitate passage of fiberoptic gastroscopes, laryngo-
scopes, proctoscopes and sigmoidoscopes.
In addition, Hurricaine is effective in
suppressing the pharyngeal and tracheal
gag reflex during the placement of nasogastric tubes. Hurricaine is used to control pain and discomfort during certain
gynecological procedures such as IUD insertion, vaginal speculum placement,
and as a preinjection anesthesia prior to
LEEP procedures and paracervical
blocks. Hurricaine is also effective for the
temporary relief of pain due to sore
throat, stomatitis and mucositis. It is
also effective in controlling various types
of pain associated with dental procedures
and the temporary relief of minor mouth
irritations, canker sores and irritation to
the mouth and gums caused by dentures
or orthodontic appliances.

Contraindications: Patients with a
known hypersensitivity to benzocaine
should not use HURRICAINE. True allergic reactions are rare.

Adverse Reactions: Methemoglobine-
mia has been reported following the use
of benzocaine on extremely rare occasions. Intravenous methylene blue is the
specific therapy for this condition.

**Cautions: DO NOT USE IN THE
EYES.
NOT FOR INJECTION.
KEEP THIS AND ALL DRUGS OUT OF
THE REACH OF CHILDREN.**

Packaging Available
GEL
1 oz. Jar Fresh Mint NDC #0283-
0998-31
1 oz. Jar Wild Cherry NDC #0283-
0871-31
1 oz. Jar Pina Colada NDC #0283-
0886-31
1 oz. Jar Watermelon NDC #0283-
0293-31
1/6 oz. Tube Wild Cherry NDC #0283-
0871-75
1/6 oz. Tube Watermelon NDC #0283-
0293-75
LIQUID
1 fl. oz. Jar Wild Cherry NDC #0283-
0569-31
1 fl. oz. Jar Pina Colada NDC #0283-
1886-31
1/6 oz. Tube Wild Cherry NDC #0283-
0569-75
.25 ml Dry Handle Swab Wild Cherry
100 Each Per Box NDC #0283-0693-01
.25 ml Dry Handle Swab Wild Cherry
6 Each Per Travel Pack NDC #0283-
0693-36
SPRAY
2 oz. Aerosol Wild Cherry NDC #0283-
0679-02
SPRAY KIT
2 oz. Aerosol Wild Cherry NDC #0283-
0183-02 with 200 Disposable Extension
Tubes

PERIDIN-C®

Composition: Each orange colored
tablet contains 2 popular antioxidants;
Vitamin C and Bioflavonoids.
Ascorbic Acid 200 mg.
Hesperidin Complex 150 mg.
Hesperidin Methyl Chalcone 50 mg. F.D.
& C. #6. Sugar Free.

Dosage: 1 tablet daily or as directed.

How Supplied: In bottles of:
100 tablets NDC #0283-0597-01
500 tablets NDC #0283-0597-05

UNKNOWN DRUG?
Consult the
Product Identification Guide
(Gray Pages)
for full-color photos of
leading over-the-counter
medications

Block Drug Company, Inc.

257 CORNELISON AVENUE
JERSEY CITY, NJ 07302

Direct Inquiries to:
Consumer Affairs/Block
(201) 434-3000 Ext. 1308

For Medical Emergencies Contact:
Consumer Affairs/Block
(201) 434-3000 Ext. 1308

BALMEX®
Medicated Plus™ Baby Powder

Description: Balmex® Medicated Plus™ Baby Powder helps prevent and treat diaper rash with cornstarch (86.9%) and zinc oxide (10%), plus it contains WATER LOCK®, a patented, safe, super absorbing ingredient that helps keep your baby dry.

Indications and Uses: Balmex Medicated Plus Baby Powder helps treat and prevent diaper rash, protects chafed skin associated with diaper rash and helps protect from wetness. The cornstarch and zinc oxide based formulation provides a protective barrier on the skin against the natural causes of irritation, a super absorbing starch copolymer which allows our formula to absorb 2 times more moisture than cornstarch alone.

Directions: Change wet and soiled diapers promptly, cleanse the diaper area, and allow to dry. Apply powder liberally as often as necessary, with each diaper change, especially at bedtime or anytime when exposure to wet diapers may be prolonged. Apply powder close to the body away from the child's face. Carefully shake the powder into the diaper or into the hand and apply to diaper area.

Warnings: Avoid contact with eyes. Keep powder away from child's face to avoid inhalation, which can cause breathing problems. For external use only. Do not use on broken skin. If condition worsens or does not improve within 7 days, contact a physician. Keep out of reach of children. If swallowed, get medical help or contact a Poison Control Center right away.

Active Ingredients: Topical starch (cornstarch) 86.9%, zinc oxide 10%.

Inactive Ingredients: Fragrance, Starch Copolymer (WATER LOCK®), Tribasic Calcium Phosphate

How Supplied: 13 oz. (368g.) Bottle
WATER LOCK® is a registered trademark of Grain Processing Corporation
Shown in Product Identification Guide, page 505

BALMEX®
Diaper Rash Ointment (Zinc Oxide)
With Aloe & Vitamin E

Description: Balmex® Diaper Rash Ointment with Aloe & Vitamin E contains Zinc Oxide (11.3%) in a unique formulation including Peruvian Balsam suitable for topical application for the treatment and prevention of diaper rash.

Indications and Uses: Balmex helps treat and prevent diaper rash while it moisturizes and nourishes the skin. The zinc oxide based formulation provides a protective barrier on the skin against the natural causes of irritation. Balmex spreads on smooth and wipes off the baby easily, without causing irritation to the affected area. Balmex tactile properties promote compliance amongst mothers.

Directions: Change wet and soiled diapers promptly, cleanse the diaper area, and allow to dry. Apply ointment liberally as often as necessary, with each diaper change, especially at bedtime or anytime when exposure to wet diapers may be prolonged.

Warnings: Avoid contact with the eyes. For external use only. If condition worsens or does not improve within 7 days, contact a physician. Keep out of reach of children. If swallowed, get medical help or contact a Poison Control Center right away.

Active Ingredient: Zinc Oxide (11.3%).

Inactive Ingredients: Aloe Vera Gel, Balsan (Specially Purified Balsam Peru), Beeswax, Benzoic Acid, Dimethicone, Methylparaben, Mineral Oil, Propylparaben, Purified Water, Sodium Borate, Tocopheryl (Vitamin E Acetate).

How Supplied: 2 oz. (57g.) and 4 oz. (113g.) tubes and 16 oz. (454g.) jar.
Shown in Product Identification Guide, page 505

BC® POWDER
ARTHRITIS STRENGTH BC® POWDER
BC® COLD POWDER LINE

Description: BC® POWDER: Active Ingredients: Each powder contains Aspirin 650 mg, Salicylamide 195 mg and Caffeine 33.3 mg. Inactive Ingredients: Dioctylsodium Sulfosuccinate, Fumaric Acid, Lactose and Potassium Chloride. ARTHRITIS STRENGTH BC® POWDER: Active Ingredients: Each powder contains Aspirin 742 mg, Salicylamide 222 mg and Caffeine 38 mg. Inactive Ingredients: Dioctylsodium Sulfosuccinate, Fumaric Acid, Lactose and Potassium Chloride.
BC® ALLERGY SINUS COLD POWDER

Active Ingredients: Aspirin 650 mg, and Chlorpheniramine Maleate 4 mg per powder. Inactive Ingredients: Fumaric Acid, Glycine, Lactose, Potassium Chloride, Silica, Sodium Lauryl Sulfate. BC® SINUS COLD POWDER. **Active Ingredients:** Aspirin 650 mg and Phenylpropanolamine Hydrochloride 25 mg per powder, Pseudoephedrine Hydrochloride 60 mg. Inactive Ingredients: Fumaric Acid, Glycine, Lactose, Potassium Chloride, Silica, Sodium Lauryl Sulfate.

Indications: BC Powder is for relief of simple headache; for temporary relief of minor arthritic pain, neuralgia, neuritis and sciatica; for relief of muscular aches, discomfort and fever of colds; and for relief of normal menstrual pain and pain of tooth extraction.
Arthritis Strength BC Powder is specially formulated to fight occasional minor pain and inflammation of arthritis. Like Original Formula BC, Arthritis Strength BC provides fast temporary relief of minor arthritis pain and inflammation, neuralgia, neuritis and sciatica; relief of muscular aches, discomfort and fever of colds; and pain of tooth extraction.
BC Allergy Sinus Cold Powder is for relief of multiple symptoms such as body aches, fever, nasal congestion, sneezing, running nose, and watery itchy eyes associated with allergy and sinus attacks and the onset of colds. BC Sinus Cold Powder is for relief of such symptoms as body aches, fever, and nasal congestion.

BC® Powder, Arthritis
Strength BC® Powder:

Warnings: Children and teenagers should not use this medicine for chicken pox or flu symptoms before a doctor is consulted about Reye's Syndrome, a rare but serious illness reported to be associated with aspirin. Keep this and all medicines out of children's reach. In case of accidental overdose, contact a physician or poison control center immediately.
As with any drug, if you are pregnant or nursing a baby seek the advice of a health professional before using this product.
IT IS ESPECIALLY IMPORTANT NOT TO USE ASPIRIN DURING THE LAST 3 MONTHS OF PREGNANCY UNLESS SPECIFICALLY DIRECTED TO DO SO BY A DOCTOR BECAUSE IT MAY CAUSE PROBLEMS IN THE UNBORN CHILD OR COMPLICATIONS DURING DELIVERY.

Alcohol Warning: If you consume 3 or more alcoholic drinks every day, ask your doctor whether you should take aspirin or other pain relievers/fever reducers. Aspirin may cause stomach bleeding.
This product contains aspirin and should not be taken by individuals who are sensitive to aspirin. If pain persists for more than 10 days, or redness is present, consult a physician immediately.
BC Cold Powder Line:

Warnings: Children and teenagers should not use BC for chicken pox

Continued on next page

BC Powders—Cont.

or flu symptoms before a doctor is consulted about Reye's Syndrome, a rare but serious illness reported to be associated with aspirin. Keep BC and all medicines out of children's reach. In case of accidental overdose, contact a physician or poison control center immediately. As with any drug, if you are pregnant or nursing a baby seek the advice of a health professional before using BC.

Alcohol Warning: If you consume 3 or more alcoholic drinks every day, ask your doctor whether you should take aspirin or other pain relievers/fever reducers. Aspirin may cause stomach bleeding.

IT IS ESPECIALLY IMPORTANT NOT TO USE ASPIRIN DURING THE LAST 3 MONTHS OF PREGNANCY UNLESS SPECIFICALLY DIRECTED TO DO SO BY A DOCTOR BECAUSE IT MAY CAUSE PROBLEMS IN THE UNBORN CHILD OR COMPLICATIONS DURING DELIVERY.
Do not exceed recommended dosage.
If nervousness, dizziness, or sleeplessness occur, discontinue use and consult a doctor. If symptoms do not improve within 7 days, or are accompanied by fever that lasts more than 3 days, or if new symptoms occur, consult a physician before continuing use. Do not take BC if you are sensitive to aspirin, or have heart disease, high blood pressure, thyroid disease, diabetes, asthma, glaucoma, emphysema, chronic pulmonary disease, shortness of breath, difficulty in breathing or difficulty in urination due to enlargement of the prostate gland, or if you are presently taking a prescription antihypertensive or antidepressant drug unless directed by a doctor. *"Drug interaction precaution.* Do not use this product if you are now taking a prescription monoamine oxidase inhibitor (MAOI) (certain drugs for depression, psychiatric or emotional conditions, or Parkinson's disease), or for 2 weeks after stopping the MAOI drug. If you are uncertain whether your prescription drug contains an MAOI, consult a health professional before taking this product." BC Allergy Sinus Cold Powder with antihistamine may cause drowsiness. Avoid alcoholic beverages when taking this product because it may increase drowsiness. Use caution when driving a motor vehicle or operating machinery. May cause excitability, especially in children.

Overdosage: In case of accidental overdosage, contact a physician or poison control center immediately.

Dosage and Administration: BC® Powder, Arthritis Strength BC® Powder, BC® Cold Powder Line:
Place one powder on tongue and follow with liquid. If you prefer, stir powder into glass of water or other liquid. May be used every three to four hours, (every 4–6 hours for BC® Cold Powder Line, (up to 3 powders each 24 hours.) For BC® Powder and Arthritis Strength BC® up to 4 powders each 24 hours. For children under 12, consult a physician.

How Supplied: BC Powder: Available in tamper evident overwrapped envelopes of 2 or 6 powders, as well as tamper evident boxes of 24 and 50 powders.
Arthritis Strength BC Powder: Available in tamper evident over wrapped envelopes of 6 powders, and tamper evident overwrapped boxes of 24 and 50 powders.
BC Cold Powder Line:
Available in tamper-evident overwrapped envelopes of 6 powders, as well as tamper-evident boxes of 12 powders.

GOODY'S
Body Pain Formula Powder

Indications: FOR TEMPORARY RELIEF OF MINOR BODY ACHES & PAINS DUE TO MUSCULAR ACHES, ARTHRITIS & HEADACHES.

Directions: Adults: Place one powder on tongue and follow with liquid, or stir powder into a glass of water or other liquid. May be repeated in 4 to 6 hours. Do not take more than 4 powders in any 24-hour period. Children under 12 years of age: Consult a doctor.

Warnings: Children and teenagers should not use this medicine for chicken pox or flu symptoms before a doctor is consulted about Reye's Syndrome, a rare but serious illness reported to be associated with aspirin. As with any drug, if you are pregnant, or nursing a baby, seek the advice of a health professional before using this product.
IT IS ESPECIALLY IMPORTANT NOT TO USE ASPIRIN DURING THE LAST 3 MONTHS OF PREGNANCY UNLESS SPECIFICALLY DIRECTED TO DO SO BY A DOCTOR BECAUSE IT MAY CAUSE PROBLEMS IN THE UNBORN CHILD OR COMPLICATIONS DURING DELIVERY.
Alcohol Warning: If you consume 3 or more alcoholic drinks every day, ask your doctor whether you should take acetaminophen and aspirin or other pain relievers/fever reducers. Acetaminophen and aspirin may cause liver damage and stomach bleeding.
Keep this and all medicines out of the reach of children. In case of accidental overdose, contact a doctor or poison control center immediately.
This product contains aspirin and should not be taken by individuals who are sensitive to aspirin. If pain persists for more than 10 days, or redness is present, consult a physician immediately.

Active Ingredients: Each powder contains: 500 mg. aspirin and 325 mg. acetaminophen.

Inactive Ingredients: Each powder contains: Lactose and Potassium Chloride.

DIST. BY: GOODY'S PHARMACEUTICALS
Memphis, TN 38113

GOODY'S®
Extra Strength Headache Powder

Indications: For Temporary Relief of Minor Aches & Pains Due to Headaches, Arthritis, Colds & Fever

Directions: Adults: Place one powder on tongue and follow with liquid or stir powder into a glass of water or other liquid. May be repeated in 4 to 6 hours. Do not take more than 4 powders in any 24-hour period. Children under 12 years of age: Consult a doctor.

Warnings: Children and teenagers should not use this medicine for chicken pox or flu symptoms before a doctor is consulted about Reye's Syndrome, a rare but serious illness reported to be associated with aspirin. As with any drug, if you are pregnant, or nursing a baby, seek the advice of a health professional before using this product.
IT IS ESPECIALLY IMPORTANT NOT TO USE ASPIRIN DURING THE LAST 3 MONTHS OF PREGNANCY UNLESS SPECIFICALLY DIRECTED TO DO SO BY A DOCTOR BECAUSE IT MAY CAUSE PROBLEMS IN THE UNBORN CHILD OR COMPLICATIONS DURING DELIVERY.
Alcohol Warning: If you consume 3 or more alcoholic drinks every day, ask your doctor whether you should take acetaminophen and aspirin or other pain relievers/fever reducers. Acetaminophen and aspirin may cause liver damage and stomach bleeding. **Keep this and all medicines out of the reach of children. In case of accidental overdose, contact a doctor or poison control center immediately.**
This product contains aspirin and should not be taken by individuals who are sensitive to aspirin. If pain persists for more than 10 days or redness is present, consult a physician immediately.

Active Ingredients: Each Powder contains 520 mg. aspirin in combination with 260 mg. acetaminophen and 32.5 mg. caffeine.

Inactive Ingredients: Lactose and Potassium Chloride.
Dist. By: GOODY'S PHARMACEUTICALS
Memphis, TN 38113

GOODY'S®
Extra Strength Pain Relief Tablets

Indications: Goody's EXTRA STRENGTH tablets are a specially developed pain reliever that provide fast & effective temporary relief from minor aches & pain due to headaches, arthritis, colds or "flu," muscle strain, backache &

menstrual discomfort. It is recommended for temporary relief of toothaches and to reduce fever.

Dosage: Adults: Two tablets with water or other liquid. May be repeated in 4 to 6 hours. Do not take more than 8 tablets in any 24-hour period. Children under 12 years of age: Consult a doctor.

Warnings: Children and teenagers should not use this medicine for chicken pox or flu symptoms before a doctor is consulted about Reye's Syndrome, a rare but serious illness reported to be associated with aspirin. As with any drug, if you are pregnant, or nursing a baby, seek the advice of a health professional before using this product. IT IS ESPECIALLY IMPORTANT NOT TO USE ASPIRIN DURING THE LAST 3 MONTHS OF PREGNANCY UNLESS SPECIFICALLY DIRECTED TO DO SO BY A DOCTOR BECAUSE IT MAY CAUSE PROBLEMS IN THE UNBORN CHILD OR COMPLICATIONS DURING DELIVERY. **Alcohol Warning:** If you consume 3 or more alcoholic drinks every day, ask your doctor whether you should take acetaminophen and aspirin or other pain relievers/fever reducers. Acetaminophen and aspirin may cause liver damage and stomach bleeding. **Keep this and all medicines out of the reach of children. In case of accidental overdose, contact a doctor or poison control center immediately.** This product contains aspirin and should not be taken by individuals who are sensitive to aspirin. If pain persists for more than 10 days, or redness is present, consult a physician immediately.

Active Ingredients: Each tablet contains 260 mg. aspirin in combination with 130 mg. acetaminophen and 16.25 mg. caffeine. **Inactive Ingredients:** Corn Starch, Crospovidone, Povidone, Pregelatinized Starch and Stearic Acid. Dist. By: GOODY'S PHARMACEUTICALS Memphis, TN 38113

GOODY'S PM® POWDER
For Pain with Sleeplessness

Indications: For temporary relief of occasional headaches and minor aches and pains with accompanying sleeplessness.

Directions: Adults and children 12 years of age and older: One dose (2 powders). Take both powders at bedtime, if needed, or as directed by a doctor. Place powders on tongue and follow with liquid. If you prefer, stir powders into glass of water or other liquid.

Warnings: KEEP THIS AND ALL MEDICINES OUT OF THE REACH OF CHILDREN. IN CASE OF ACCIDENTAL OVERDOSE, CONTACT A DOCTOR OR POISON CONTROL CENTER IMMEDIATELY. PROMPT MEDICAL

Adults and children 12 years of age and over	2 Tablets once or twice daily with water, not to exceed 4 tablets twice a day
Children 6 to under 12 years of age	1 Tablet once or twice daily with water, not to exceed 2 tablets twice a day
Children 2 to under 6 years of age	1/2 Tablet once or twice daily with water, not to exceed 1 tablet twice a day
Children under 2 years of age	Consult a doctor

ATTENTION IS CRITICAL FOR ADULTS AS WELL AS FOR CHILDREN EVEN IF YOU DO NOT NOTICE ANY SIGNS OR SYMPTOMS. As with any drug, if you are pregnant or nursing a baby, seek the advice of a health professional before using this product. Do not give this product to children under 12 years of age. Do not use for more than 10 days or for fever for more than 3 days unless directed by a doctor. Consult your doctor if symptoms persist or get worse or new ones occur. If sleeplessness persists continuously for more than 2 weeks consult your doctor. Insomnia may be a symptom of serious underlying medical illness. Do not take this product, unless directed by a doctor, if you have a breathing problem such as emphysema or chronic bronchitis or if you have glaucoma or difficulty in urination due to enlargement of the prostate gland. **Do Not Use** with any other product containing diphenhydramine, including one applied topically. Avoid alcoholic beverages while taking this product. Do not use this product if you are taking sedatives or tranquilizers without first consulting your doctor. **Alcohol Warning:** If you consume 3 or more alcoholic drinks every day, ask your doctor whether you should take acetaminophen or other pain relievers/fever reducers. Acetaminophen may cause liver damage.

Caution: This product will cause drowsiness. Do not drive a motor vehicle or operate machinery after use.

Active Ingredients: Each powder contains 500 mg. Acetaminophen and 38 mg. Diphenhydramine Citrate.

Inactive Ingredients: Citric Acid, Docusate Sodium, Fumaric Acid, Glycine, Lactose, Magnesium Stearate, Potassium Chloride, Silica Gel, Sodium Citrate Dihydrate. Dist. by: Goody's Pharmaceuticals, Memphis, TN 38113

NATURE'S REMEDY®
Nature's Gentle Laxative

Description: Nature's Remedy® is a stimulant laxative with an active ingredient, Sennosides, that gently stimulates the body's natural function.

Indication: For relief of occasional constipation. Nature's Remedy tablets generally produce bowel movement in 6 to 12 hours.

Active Ingredients:
(in each tablet): **Purpose:**
Sennosides, USP,
8.6 mg .... Stimulant laxative

Inactive Ingredients: FD&C blue #2 aluminum lake, FD&C yellow #6 aluminum lake, hydroxypropyl cellulose, hydroxypropyl methylcellulose, lactose, microcrystalline cellulose, polyethylene glycol, pregelatinized starch, silicon dioxide stearic acid, titanium dioxide

Directions:
[See table above]

Warnings: Keep out of reach of children. Do not use laxative products when abdominal pain, nausea, or vomiting are present unless directed by a doctor. If you have noticed a sudden change in bowel habits that persists over a period of 2 weeks, consult a doctor before using a laxative. Laxative products should not be used for a period longer than 1 week unless directed by a doctor. Rectal bleeding or failure to have a bowel movement after use of a laxative may indicate a serious condition. Discontinue use and consult your doctor. In case of accidental overdose, seek professional assistance or contact a Poison Control Center immediately. As with any drug, if you are pregnant or nursing a baby, seek the advice of a health professional before using this product.

Store at room temperature, avoid excessive heat (greater than 100°F) or high humidity.

How Supplied: Beige, film-coated tablets with foil-backed blister packaging in boxes of 15, 30 and 60.
Shown in Product Identification Guide, page 506

Maximum Strength
NYTOL® QUICKGELS® SOFTGELS

Indication: For relief of occasional sleeplessness.

Directions: Adults and children 12 years of age and over: oral dosage is one softgel (50 mg) at bedtime if needed, or as directed by a doctor.

Warnings: Do not give to children under 12 years of age. If sleeplessness persists continuously for more than two weeks, consult your doctor. Insomnia may be a symptom of serious underlying

Continued on next page

Nytol Softgels—Cont.

medical illness. **Do not take this product, unless directed by a doctor, if you have a breathing problem such as emphysema or chronic bronchitis, or if you have glaucoma or difficulty in urination due to enlargement of the prostate gland. Do not use** with any other product containing diphenhydramine, including one applied topically. Avoid alcoholic beverages while taking this product. Do not take this product if you are taking sedatives or tranquilizers, without first consulting your doctor. In case of accidental overdose, seek professional assistance or contact a Poison Control Center immediately. As with any drug, if you are pregnant or nursing a baby, seek the advice of a health professional before using this product. Keep out of reach of children.

Drug Interactions: Alcohol and other drugs which cause CNS depression will heighten the depressant effect of this product. Monoamine oxidase (MAO) inhibitors will prolong and intensify the anticholinergic effects of antihistamines.

Symptoms and Treatment of Oral Overdosage: In adults overdose may cause CNS depression resulting in hypnosis and coma. In children CNS hyperexcitability may follow sedation; the stimulant phase may bring tremor, delirium and convulsions. Gastrointestinal reactions may include dry mouth, appetite loss, nausea and/or vomiting. Respiratory distress and cardiovascular complications (hypotension) may be evident. Treatment includes inducing emesis and controlling symptoms.

Active Ingredient: Diphenhydramine Hydrochloride 50 mg per softgel.

Inactive Ingredients: Edible Ink, Gelatin, Glycerin, Polyethylene Glycol, Purified Water, Sorbitol.

How Supplied: Available in packages of 8 and 16 softgels.
Shown in Product Identification Guide, page 506

NYTOL® NATURAL
Homeopathic Nighttime Sleep-Aid

Indication: Temporary relief of occasional sleeplessness.

Dosage and Administration: Adults and children 12 years of age and over: Chew 2–3 tablets ½ hour before bedtime if needed, or as directed by a doctor.

Warnings: Do not give to children under 12 years of age. If sleeplessness persists continuously for more than two weeks, consult your doctor. Insomnia may be a symptom of serious underlying medical illness. As with any drug, if you are pregnant or nursing a baby, seek the advice of a health care professional before using this product. In case of accidental overdose, seek professional assis-

tance or contact a Poison Control Center immediately. Keep out of reach of children. Avoid alcoholic beverages while taking this product. Do not take this product if you are taking sedatives or tranquilizers without first consulting your doctor.

Active Ingredients: Each tablet contains equal parts of Ignatia amara 3X (St. Ignatius' Bean); Aconitum radix 6X (Aconite Root).

Inactive Ingredients: Lactose, Magnesium Stearate.

How Supplied: Available in tamper-evident packages of 16 and 32 tablets.
Shown in Product Identification Guide, page 506

NYTOL® QUICK CAPS® CAPLETS

Indication: For relief of occasional sleeplessness.

Directions: Adults and children 12 years of age and over: oral dosage is two caplets (50 mg) at bedtime if needed, or as directed by a doctor.

Warnings: Do not give to children under 12 years of age. If sleeplessness persists continuously for more than two weeks, consult your doctor. Insomnia may be a symptom of serious underlying medical illness. **Do not take this product, unless directed by a doctor, if you have a breathing problem such as emphysema or chronic bronchitis, or if you have glaucoma or difficulty in urination due to enlargement of the prostate gland. Do not use** with any other product containing diphenhydramine, including one applied topically. Avoid alcoholic beverages while taking this product. Do not take this product if you are taking sedatives or tranquilizers, without first consulting your doctor. In case of accidental overdose, seek professional assistance or contact a Poison Control Center immediately. As with any drug, if you are pregnant or nursing a baby, seek the advice of a health professional before using this product. Keep out of reach of children.

Drug Interactions: Alcohol and other drugs which cause CNS depression will heighten the depressant effect of this product. Monoamine oxidase (MAO) inhibitors will prolong and intensify the anticholinergic effects of antihistamines.

Symptoms and Treatment of Oral Overdosage: In adults, overdose may cause CNS depression resulting in hypnosis and coma. In children, CNS hyperexcitability may follow sedation; the stimulant phase may bring tremor, delirium and convulsions. Gastrointestinal reactions may include dry mouth, appetite loss, nausea and/or vomiting. Respiratory distress and cardiovascular complications (hypotension) may be evident. Treatment includes inducing emesis and controlling symptoms.

Active Ingredient: Diphenhydramine Hydrochloride 25 mg per caplet.

Inactive Ingredients: Corn Starch, Lactose, Microcrystalline Cellulose, Silica, Stearic Acid.

How Supplied: Available in tamper-evident packages of 16, 32 and 72 caplets.
Shown in Product Identification Guide, page 506

Quick Dissolve
PHAZYME®–125 MG Chewable Tablets
[fay-zime]

Description: A great tasting, smooth cool mint chewable tablet containing simethicone, an antiflatulent to alleviate or relieve the symptoms referred to as gas. Uniquely formulated to dissolve quickly and completely in your mouth. It has no known side effects or drug interactions.

Active Ingredient: Each tablet contains simethicone 125 mg.

Inactive Ingredients: Aspartame, citricacid, colloidal silicon dioxide, crospovidone, dextrates, maltodextrin, mannitol, peppermint flavor, pregelatinized starch, sodium bicarbonate, sorbitol, talc, tribasic calcium phosphate.

Actions: Simethicone minimizes gas formation and relieves gas entrapment in both the stomach and the lower G.I. tract. This action combats the distress due to gastrointestinal gas.

Other Information: Each tablet contains sodium 8 mg. Phenylketonurics: contains phenylalanine 0.4 mg per tablet.

Indication: Relieves pressure, bloating or fullness commonly referred to as gas.

Warnings: Keep this and all drugs out of the reach of children. If condition persists, consult your physician.
Store at room temperature 59°–86°F (15°–30°C).

Dosage: Directions: Chew one or two tablets thoroughly, as needed after a meal. Do not exceed four tablets per day except under the advice and supervision of a physician.

How Supplied: White, bevel-edged tablets imprinted with "Phazyme 125" in 18 count and 48 count bottles.
Shown in Product Identification Guide, page 506

Ultra Strength
PHAZYME®–180 MG Softgels
[fay-zime]

Description: An orange, easy to swallow softgel, containing simethicone, an antiflatulent to alleviate or relieve the symptoms referred to as gas. It has no known side effects or drug interactions.

Active Ingredient: Each softgel contains simethicone 180 mg.

Inactive Ingredients: FD&C Yellow No. 6, gelatin, glycerin, and white edible ink.

Actions: Simethicone minimizes gas formation and relieves gas entrapment in both the stomach and the lower G.I. tract. This action combats the distress due to gastrointestinal gas.

Indication: Relieves pressure, bloating or fullness commonly referred to as gas.

Warnings: Keep this and all drugs out of the reach of children. If condition persists, consult your physician. Store at room temperature 59°–86°F (15°–30°C).

Dosage: Directions: Swallow one or two softgels as needed after a meal. Do not exceed two softgels per day except under the advice and supervision of a physician.

How Supplied: Orange softgel imprinted with "PZ 180" in 12 count and 36 count blister pack, 60 count and 100 count bottles.

Shown in Product Identification Guide, page 506

**SENSODYNE® FRESH MINT
SENSODYNE® COOL GEL
SENSODYNE® WITH BAKING SODA
SENSODYNE® TARTAR CONTROL
SENSODYNE® TARTAR CONTROL PLUS WHITENING
SENSODYNE® ORIGINAL FLAVOR
SENSODYNE® EXTRA WHITENING
Anticavity toothpaste for sensitive teeth**

Active Ingredients: 5% Potassium Nitrate and 0.15% w/v Sodium Monofluorophosphate (Extra Whitening) or Sodium Fluoride (Fresh Mint, 0.15% w/v; Baking Soda, 0.15% w/v; Cool Gel, 0.13% w/v; Tartar Control, 0.13% w/v; Tartar Control Plus Whitening 0.145% w/v; Original Flavor, 0.13% w/v). Sensodyne Fresh Mint, Sensodyne Cool Gel, Sensodyne with Baking Soda, Sensodyne Tartar Control, Sensodyne Tartar Control Plus Whitening, Sensodyne Original Flavor and Sensodyne Extra Whitening contain fluoride for cavity prevention and Potassium Nitrate clinically proven to reduce pain sensitivity for relief of dentinal hypersensitivity resulting from the exposure of tooth dentin due to periodontal surgery, cervical (gum line) erosion, abrasion or recession which causes pain on contact with hot, cold, or tactile stimuli.

Inactive Ingredients: *Baking Soda:* Flavor, Glycerin, Hydrated Silica, Hydroxyethylcellulose, Methylparaben, Propylparaben, Silica, Sodium Bicarbonate, Sodium Lauryl Sulfate, Sodium Saccharin, Titanium Dioxide, Water.
Extra Whitening: Calcium Peroxide, Flavor, Glycerin, Hydrated Silica, PEG-12, PEG-75, Silica, Sodium Carbonate, Sodium Lauryl Sulfate, Sodium Saccharin, Titanium Dioxide, Water.

Tartar Control: Cellulose Gum, Cocamidopropyl Betaine, Flavor, Glycerin, Hydrated Silica, Silica, Sodium Bicarbonate, Sodium Saccharin, Tetrapotassium Pyrophosphate, Titanium Dioxide, Water.
Tartar Control Plus Whitening: Cellulose Gum, Flavor, Glycerin, Polyethylene Glycol, Silica, Sodium Lauryl Sulfate, Sodium Saccharin, Tetrapotassium Pyrophosphate, Titanium Dioxide, Water.
Cool Gel: Cellulose Gum, FD&C Blue #1, Flavor, Glycerin, Hydrated Silica, Silica, Sodium Methyl Cocoyl Taurate, Sodium Saccharin, Sorbitol, Trisodium Phosphate, Water.
Fresh Mint: D&C Yellow #10, FD&C Blue #1, Flavor, Glycerin, Hydrated Silica, Sodium Lauryl Sulfate, Sodium Saccharin, Sorbitol, Titanium Dioxide, Trisodium Phosphate, Water, Xanthan Gum.
Original Flavor: Cellulose Gum, D&C Red No. 28, Glycerin, Hydrated Silica, Peppermint Oil, Silica, Sodium Methyl Cocoyl Taurate, Sodium Saccharin, Sorbitol, Titanium Dioxide, Trisodium Phosphate, Water.

Actions: All Sensodyne Formulas significantly reduce tooth hypersensitivity, with response to therapy evident after two weeks of use. Controlled double-blind clinical studies provide substantial evidence of the safety and effectiveness of Potassium Nitrate. The current theory on mechanism of action is that potassium nitrate has an effect on neural transmission, interrupting the signal which would result in the sensation of pain. Fluorides are anticariogenic, forming fluoroapatite in the outer surface of the dental enamel which is resistant to acids and caries.

Warnings: Sensitive teeth may indicate a serious problem that may need prompt care by a dentist. See your dentist if the problem persists or worsens. Do not use this product longer than 4 weeks unless recommended by a dentist or physician. Keep this and all drugs out of the reach of children. If you accidentally swallow more than used for brushing, seek professional assistance or contact a Poison Control Center immediately.

Dosage and Administration: Adults and children 12 years of age and older: Apply a 1-inch strip of the product onto a soft bristle toothbrush. Brush teeth thoroughly for at least 1 minute twice a day (morning and evening) or as recommended by a dentist or physician. Make sure to brush all sensitive areas of the teeth. Children under 12 years of age: consult a dentist or physician.

How Supplied: All Sensodyne formulas are supplied in 2.1 oz. (60g), 4.0 oz. (113g) and 6.0 oz. (170g) tubes. Sensodyne Cool Gel is supplied in 4.0 oz. only. Sensodyne Baking Soda is supplied in 4.0 oz and 6.0 oz. only.

TEGRIN® DANDRUFF SHAMPOO – EXTRA CONDITIONING

Description: Tegrin® Dandruff Shampoo contains 7% Coal Tar Solution, USP, equivalent to 1.1% coal tar, in a pleasantly scented, high-foaming, cleansing shampoo base with emollients, conditioners and other formula components.

Indications: Tegrin® Dandruff Shampoo controls the flaking and itching of the scalp associated with dandruff, seborrheic dermatitis, and psoriasis.

Directions: Shake well. Wet hair. Lather, rinse, repeat. For best results use at least twice a week or as directed by a doctor.

Warnings: For external use only. Avoid contact with eyes. If contact occurs, rinse eyes thoroughly with water. If condition worsens or does not improve after regular use of this product as directed, consult a doctor. Use caution in exposing skin to sunlight after applying this product. It may increase tendency to sunburn for up to 24 hours after application. Do not use for prolonged periods without consulting a doctor. Do not use this product with other forms of psoriasis therapy, such as ultraviolet radiation or prescription drugs, unless directed by a doctor. Keep out of reach of children. In case of accidental ingestion, seek professional assistance or contact a Poison Control Center immediately.

Active Ingredient: 7% Coal Tar Solution, USP, Equivalent to 1.1% Coal Tar. Coal Tar is obtained in the destructive distillation of bituminous coal and is a highly effective agent for controlling the flaking and itching of the scalp associated with dandruff, seborrheic dermatitis, and psoriasis. The action of coal tar is believed to be keratolytic, antiseptic, antipruritic, and astringent. The coal tar solution used in Tegrin® Dandruff Shampoo is prepared in such a way as to reduce the pitch and other irritant components found in crude coal tar without reduction in therapeutic potency.

Coal Tar Solution has been used clinically for many years as a remedy for dandruff and for scaling associated with scalp disorders such as seborrhea and psoriasis. Its mechanism of action has not been fully established, but it is believed to retard the rate of turnover of epidermal cells with regular use. A number of clinical studies have demonstrated the performance attributes of Tegrin® Dandruff Shampoo against dandruff and seborrheic dermatitis. In addition to relieving the above symptoms, Tegrin® Dandruff Shampoo, used regularly, maintains scalp and hair cleanliness and leaves the hair lustrous and manageable.

Inactive Ingredients for:
Tegrin® Dandruff Shampoo – Extra Conditioning

Continued on next page

Tegrin—Cont.

Alcohol (7.0%), Ammonium Lauryl Sulfate, Citric Acid, FD&C Blue #1, Fragrance, Glycol Stearate (and) Sodium Laureth Sulfate (and) Hexylene Glycol, Guar Hydroxypropyltrimonium Chloride, Hydroxypropyl Methylcellulose, Lauramide DEA, Methylparaben, Propylparaben, Sodium Lauryl Sulfate, Water.

How supplied: Tegrin® Dandruff Shampoo is available in Extra Conditioning and Fresh Herbal formulas and supplied in 7 fl. oz. (207 ml) plastic bottles.
Shown in Product Identification Guide, page 506

TEGRIN® DANDRUFF SHAMPOO-FRESH HERBAL

Description: Tegrin® Dandruff Shampoo contains 7% Coal Tar Solution, USP, equivalent to 1.1% coal tar, in a pleasantly scented, high-foaming, cleansing shampoo base with emollients, conditioners and other formula components.

Indications: Tegrin® Dandruff Shampoo controls the flaking and itching of the scalp associated with dandruff, seborrheic dermatitis, and psoriasis.

Directions: Shake well. Wet hair. Lather, rinse, repeat. For best results use at least twice a week or as directed by a doctor.

Warnings: For external use only. Avoid contact with eyes. If contact occurs, rinse eyes thoroughly with water. If condition worsens or does not improve after regular use of this product as directed, consult a doctor. Use caution in exposing skin to sunlight after applying this product. It may increase tendency to sunburn for up to 24 hours after application. Do not use for prolonged periods without consulting a doctor. Do not use this product with other forms of psoriasis therapy, such as ultraviolet radiation or prescription drugs, unless directed by a doctor. Keep out of reach of children. In case of accidental ingestion, seek professional assistance or contact a Poison Control Center immediately.

Active Ingredient: 7% Coal Tar Solution, USP, Equivalent to 1.1% Coal Tar. Coal Tar is obtained in the destructive distillation of bituminous coal and is a highly effective agent for controlling the flaking and itching of the scalp associated with dandruff, seborrheic dermatitis and psoriasis. The action of coal tar is believed to be keratolytic, antiseptic, antipruritic, and astringent. The coal tar solution used in Tegrin® Dandruff Shampoo is prepared in such a way as to reduce the pitch and other irritant components found in crude coal tar without reduction in therapeutic potency. Coal Tar Solution has been used clinically for many years as a remedy for dandruff and for scaling associated with scalp disorders such as seborrhea and psoriasis. Its mechanism of action has not been fully established, but it is believed to retard the rate of turnover of epidermal cells with regular use. A number of clinical studies have demonstrated the performance attributes of Tegrin® Dandruff Shampoo against dandruff and seborrheic dermatitis. In addition to relieving the above symptoms, Tegrin® Dandruff Shampoo, used regularly, maintains scalp and hair cleanliness and leaves the hair lustrous and manageable.

Inactive Ingredients For:
Tegrin® Dandruff Shampoo–Fresh Herbal
Alcohol (7.0%), Citric Acid, Cocamide DEA, FD&C Blue #1, Fragrance, Glycol Stearate (and) Sodium Laureth Sulfate (and) Hexylene Glycol, Hydroxypropyl Methylcellulose, Methylparaben, Propylparaben, Sodium Lauryl Sulfate, Water.

How Supplied: Tegrin® Dandruff Shampoo is available in Extra Conditioning and Fresh Herbal formulas and supplied in 7 fl. oz. (207 ml) plastic bottles.

TEGRIN® SKIN CREAM FOR PSORIASIS

Description: Tegrin® Skin Cream for Psoriasis contains 5% Coal Tar Solution, USP, equivalent to 0.8% Coal Tar and alcohol of 4.7%.

Indications: For relief of itching, flaking and irritation of the skin associated with psoriasis and seborrheic dermatitis.

Directions: Apply to affected areas one to four times daily or as directed by a doctor.

Warnings: For external use only. Avoid contact with eyes. If contact occurs, rinse eyes thoroughly with water. If condition worsens or does not improve after regular use of this product as directed, consult a doctor. Use caution in exposing skin to sunlight after applying this product. It may increase tendency to sunburn for up to 24 hours after application. Do not use for prolonged periods without consulting a doctor. Do not use this product with other forms of psoriasis therapy, such as ultra-violet radiation or prescription drugs, unless directed by a doctor. If the condition covers a large area of the body, consult your doctor before using this product. Keep out of reach of children. In case of accidental ingestion, seek professional assistance or contact a Poison Control Center immediately.

Active Ingredient: 5% Coal Tar Solution, USP, equivalent to 0.8% Coal Tar.

Inactive Ingredients: Acetylated Lanolin Alcohol, Alcohol (4.7%), Carbomer-934P, Ceteth-2, Ceteth-16, Cetyl Acetate, Cetyl Alcohol, D&C Red No. 28, Fragrance, Glyceryl Tribehenate, Laneth-16, Lanolin Alcohol, Laureth-23, Methyl Gluceth-20, Methylchloroisothiazolinone, Methylisothiazolinone, Mineral Oil, Octyldodecanol, Oleth-16, Petrolatum, Potassium Hydroxide, Purified Water, Steareth-16, Stearyl Alcohol, Titanium Dioxide.

How Supplied: Tegrin® Skin Cream for Psoriasis is available in a 2 oz (57g) tube.
Shown in Product Identification Guide, page 506

Boehringer Ingelheim Consumer Healthcare Products Division of Boehringer Ingelheim Pharmceuticals Inc.

900 RIDGEBURY ROAD
P.O. BOX 368
RIDGEFIELD, CT 06877

For direct inquiries contact:
1-888-285-9159

NATRU-VENT™
Nasal Decongestant Spray
(Xylometazoline HCl 0.1%)
Adult Strength

Active Ingredient: Xylometazoline Hydrochloride 0.1%
Other Ingredients: Purified water, sorbitol, mono and dibasic sodium phosphates.
Contains No Preservatives such as Benzalkonium Chloride, Chlorhexidine Gluconate, Benzylalcohol, Edetate Disodium or Thimerisol.

Description:
Natru-Vent Nasal Decongestant Products are the first fast, long-lasting topical nasal decongestant sprays without preservatives

Natru-vent—
- Advanced silver filter technology in the unique MicroPure™ pump filtration system allows air and fluid to travel separate paths, preventing contamination and making harsh preservatives unnecessary. Prevents germs from entering the solution for up to 3 years, even after opening.
- Easy single spray per nostril dosing pump delivers the precise measured dose each time.
- Natru-vent starts to work immediately upon contact with the nasal membranes and provides up to 10 hours of relief without drowsiness.

Indications: For temporary relief of nasal congestion due to colds, hay fever or other upper respiratory allergies, or associated with sinusitis. Shrinks swollen nasal membranes so you can breathe more freely.

Warnings: Do not exceed recommended dosage. This product may cause

temporary discomfort such as burning, stinging, sneezing, or an increase in nasal discharge. The use of this container by more than one person may spread infection. Do not use this product for more than 3 days. Use only as directed. Frequent or prolonged use may cause nasal congestion to recur or worsen. If symptoms persist, consult a doctor. Do not use this product in a child who has heart disease, high blood pressure, thyroid disease, or diabetes, unless directed by a doctor. In case of accidental ingestion or overdose, seek professional assistance or contact a Poison Control Center immediately. **Keep this and all drugs out of the reach of children.**

Directions: Adults and children 12 years of age and over: One spray in each nostril not more than every 8 to 10 hours. Do not give to children under 12 years of age unless directed by a doctor.

How Supplied: Natru-Vent Adult Nasal Spray in 10 mL glass pump bottle. Distributed by Boehringer Ingelheim Consumer Healthcare Products. Division of Boehringer Ingelheim Pharmaceuticals Inc. Ridgefield CT 06877 Product of Germany ©Copyright Boehringer Ingelheim Pharmaceuticals Inc. 1999. All rights reserved. Patent pending
4059250 001
Shown in Product Identification Guide, page 506

NATRU-VENT™
Nasal Decongestant Spray
(Xylometazoline HCl 0.05%)
Pediatric Strength

Active Ingredient: Xylometazoline Hydrochloride 0.05%
Other Ingredients: Purified water, sorbitol, mono and dibasic sodium phosphates.
Contains No Preservatives such as Benzalkonium Chloride, Chlorhexidine Gluconate, Benzylalcohol, Edetate Disodium or Thimerisol.

Description: Natru-Vent Decongestant products are the first fast, long-lasting topical nasal decongestant sprays without preservatives.
Natru-vent—
• Advanced silver filter technology in the unique Micro Pure™ pump filtration system allows air and fluid to travel separate paths, preventing contamination and making harsh preservatives unnecessary. Prevents germs from entering the solution for up to 3 years, even after opening.
• Easy single spray per nostril dosing pump delivers the precise measured dose each time.
• Natru-vent starts to work immediately upon contact with the nasal membranes and provides up to 10 hours of relief without drowsiness.

Indications: For temporary relief of nasal congestion due to colds, hay fever or other upper respiratory allergies, or

associated with sinusitis. Shrinks swollen nasal membranes so you can breathe more freely.

Warnings: Do not exceed recommended dosage. This product may cause temporary discomfort such as burning, stinging, sneezing, or an increase in nasal discharge. The use of this container by more than one person may spread infection. Do not use this product for more than 3 days. Use only as directed. Frequent or prolonged use may cause nasal congestion to recur or worsen. If symptoms persist, consult a doctor. Do not use this product in a child who has heart disease, high blood pressure, thyroid disease, or diabetes, unless directed by a doctor. In case of accidental ingestion or overdose, seek professional assistance or contact a Poison Control Center immediately. **Keep this and all drugs out of the reach of children.**

Directions: Children 6 to under 12 years of age (with adult supervision): One spray in each nostril not more than every 8 to 10 hours. Children 2 to under 6 years of age (with adult supervision): one spray in each nostril not more often than every 8 to 10 hours. **Use only recommended amount. Do not exceed 3 doses in any 24-hour period.** Children under 2 years of age: consult a doctor.

How Supplied: Natru-vent Pediatric Nasal Spray in 10 mL glass pump bottle. Distributed by Boehringer Ingelheim Consumer Health Care Products. Division of Boehringer Ingelheim Pharmaceuticals Inc. Ridgefield CT 06877 Product of Germany. © Copyright Boehringer Ingelheim Pharmaceuticals Inc. 1999. All rights reserved. Patent Pending
4059250 001
Shown in Product Identification Guide, page 506

NATRU-VENT™
Saline Nasal Spray
Saline Moisturizing Mist

Ingredients: Purified Water, 0.9% Sodium Chloride.
Contains no alcohol. Contains no preservatives such as Benzalkonium Chloride, Chlorhepidine Gluconate, Benzylalcohol, Edetate Disodium or Thimerosol.

Description: Natru-Vent Saline Moisturizing Mist is the first preservative-free Saline Mist.
• Advanced Silver filter technology in the unique Micro Pure™ pump filtration system allows air and fluid to travel separate paths, preventing contamination and making harsh preservatives unnecessary. The Micro Pure™ pump prevents germs from entering the solution for up to 3 years, even after opening.
• Preservatives can cause the cilia to vibrate more slowly and therefore inhibit their cleansing function.
• Natru-Vent is so safe and gentle it can be used for infants.

• Easy single spray dosing pump delivers the precise measured dose each time.
• Natru-Vent Saline Moisturizing Mist is physiologically compatible with your nasal membranes to restore moisture naturally.

Indications: Relieves dry, irritated, inflamed or crusty nasal passages due to low humidity, heated environments, air travel, allergies or colds and the over use of nasal decongestant sprays (rebound congestion).

Warnings: The use of this metered dose pump by more than one person may spread infection. **Keep out of the reach of children.**

Directions: For infants, children or adults, one spray in each nostril as often as needed or as directed by a doctor.

How Supplied: Natru-Vent Saline Moisturizing Mist—30 mL plastic pump bottle. Distributed by Boehringer Ingelheim Consumer HealthCare Products. Division of Boehringer Ingelheim Pharmaceuticals Inc. Ridgefield CT 06877 Product of Germany. © Copyright Boehringer Ingelheim Pharmaceuticals Inc. 1999. All rights reserved. Patent pending Questions about NATRU-VENT? Call toll-free 1-888-285-9159
Shown in Product Identification Guide, page 506

BOIRON
6 CAMPUS BLVD.
NEWTOWN SQUARE, PA 19073

Direct Inquiries and Medical Emergencies:
Boiron Information Center
info@boiron.com
(800)264-7661

OSCILLOCOCCINUM®
[oh-sill'o-cox-see'num']

Active Ingredients: Anas barbariae hepatis et cordis extractum 200CK. *Made according to the Homeopathic Pharmacopeia of the United States.*

Inactive Ingredients: sucrose, lactose.

Use: For temporary relief of symptoms of flu such as fever, chills, body aches and pains.

Directions: (Adults and children 2 years of age and older):
Take 1 dose at the onset of symptoms (dissolve entire contents of one tube in the mouth).
Repeat for 2 more doses at 6 hour intervals.

Continued on next page

Oscillococcinum—Cont.

Warnings: Do not use if the label sealing the cap is broken.
Ask a doctor before use in children under 2 years of age.
Stop using this product and consult a doctor if symptoms persist for more than 3 days or worsen.
As with any drug, if pregnant or nursing a baby, ask a health professional before use.
Keep this and all medication out of reach of children.
Diabetics: this product contains sugar.

How Supplied: White pellets in unit dose containers of 0.04 oz. (1 gram) each. Supplied in boxes of 3 unit doses or 6 unit doses.
NDC #0220-9280-32 (3 doses) and NDC #0220-9280-33 (6 doses)
Made in France

Bristol-Myers Products

(A Bristol-Myers Squibb Company)
345 PARK AVENUE
NEW YORK, NY 10154

Direct Inquiries to:
Bristol-Myers Products Division
Consumer Affairs Department
1350 Liberty Avenue
Hillside, NJ 07207

Questions or Comments?
1-(800) 468-7746

COMTREX® PROFESSIONAL INFORMATION

All of the following listed Comtrex drug products contain acetaminophen. In case of overdose, please read the following Acetylcysteine information:

Overdose Information:
Acetylcysteine As An Antidote For Acetaminophen Overdose
Acetaminophen is rapidly absorbed from the upper gastrointestinal tract with peak plasma levels occurring between 30 and 60 minutes after therapeutic doses and usually within 4 hours following an overdose. The parent compound, which is nontoxic, is extensively metabolized in the liver to form principally the sulfate and glucuronide conjugates which are also nontoxic and are rapidly excreted in the urine. A small fraction of an ingested dose is metabolized in the liver by the cytochrome P-450 mixed function oxidase enzyme system to form a reactive, potentially toxic, intermediate metabolite which preferentially conjugates with hepatic glutathione to form the nontoxic cysteine and mercapturic acid derivatives which are then excreted by the kidney. Therapeutic doses of acetaminophen do not saturate the glucuronide and sulfate conjugation pathways and do not result in the formation of sufficient reactive metabolite to deplete glutathione stores. However, following ingestion of a large overdose (150 mg/kg or greater) the glucuronide and sulfate conjugation pathways are saturated resulting in a larger fraction of the drug being metabolized via the P-450 pathway. The increased formation of reactive metabolite may deplete the hepatic stores of glutathione with subsequent binding of the metabolite to protein molecules within the hepatocyte resulting in cellular necrosis. Acetylcysteine has been shown to reduce the extent of liver injury following acetaminophen overdose.
Early symptoms following a potentially hepatotoxic overdose may include: nausea, vomiting, diaphoresis and general malaise. Clinical and laboratory evidence of hepatic toxicity may not be apparent until 48 to 72 hours postingestion. In most adults and adolescents, regardless of the quantity of acetaminophen reported to have been ingested, administer acetylcysteine immediately. Acetylcysteine therapy should be initiated and continued for a full course of therapy. Its effectiveness depends on early administration, with benefit seen principally in patients treated within 16 hours of the overdose.
If acetaminophen plasma assay capability is not available, and the estimated acetaminophen ingestion exceeds 150 mg/kg., acetylcysteine therapy should be initiated and continued for a full course of therapy.
For full prescribing information, refer to the acetylcysteine package insert. Do not await the results of assays for acetaminophen level before initiating treatment with acetylcysteine. The following additional procedures are recommended: The stomach should be emptied promptly by lavage or by induction of emesis with syrup of ipecac.
A serum acetaminophen assay should be obtained as early as possible, but no sooner than four hours following ingestion. Liver function studies should be obtained initially and repeated at 24-hour intervals.
For additional emergency information call your regional poison center or toll-free (1-800-525-6115) to the Rocky Mountain Poison Center for assistance in diagnosis and for directions in the use of acetylcysteine as an antidote.

COMTREX® Maximum Strength
[cŏm 'trĕx]
Multi-Symptom Cold & Cough Relief

Composition: Each tablet or caplet contains: Acetaminophen 500 mg, Pseudoephedrine HCl 30 mg, Chlorpheniramine Maleate 2 mg, Dextromethorphan HBr 15 mg.
Other Ingredients: Tablet/Caplet: Benzoic Acid, Corn Starch, D&C Yellow No. 10 Lake, FD&C Red No. 40 Lake, Hydroxypropyl Methylcellulose, Magnesium Stearate, Methylparaben, Mineral Oil, Polysorbate 20, Povidone, Propylene Glycol, Propylparaben, Simethicone Emulsion, Sorbitan Monolaurate, Stearic Acid, Titanium Dioxide. May also contain: Carnauba wax, D&C Yellow No. 10, FD&C Red No. 40.

Indications: For the temporary relief of the following symptoms associated with the common cold and flu: minor aches, pains, headache, muscular aches, sore throat pain, and fever; cough; nasal congestion; runny nose and sneezing.

Directions: Adults and children 12 years of age and over: 2 tablets or caplets every 6 hours while symptoms persist, not to exceed 8 tablets or caplets in 24 hours, or as directed by a doctor. Children under 12 years of age: Consult a doctor.

Alcohol Warning: If you consume 3 or more alcoholic drinks every day, ask your doctor whether you should take acetaminophen or other pain relievers/fever reducers. Acetaminophen may cause liver damage.

Warnings: Keep out of reach of children. In case of overdose, get medical help, or contact a Poison Control Center right away. Prompt medical attention is critical for adults as well as children even if you do not notice any signs or symptoms. As with any drug, if you are pregnant or nursing a baby, seek the advice of a health professional before using this product. Do not take this product for more than 7 days. A persistent cough may be a sign of a serious condition. If cough persists for more than 7 days, tends to recur, or is accompanied by rash, persistent headache, fever that lasts for more than 3 days, or if new symptoms occur, consult a doctor. If sore throat is severe, persists for more than 2 days, is accompanied or followed by fever, headache, rash, nausea, or vomiting, consult a doctor promptly. Do not take this product for persistent or chronic cough such as occurs with smoking, asthma, emphysema, or if cough is accompanied by excessive phlegm (mucus) unless directed by a doctor. **Do not exceed recommended dosage.** If nervousness, dizziness, or sleeplessness occur, discontinue use and consult a doctor. If symptoms do not improve within 7 days or are accompanied by fever, consult a doctor. Do not take this product unless directed by a doctor, if you have a breathing problem such as emphysema or chronic bronchitis, heart disease, high blood pressure, thyroid disease, diabetes, glaucoma, or difficulty in urination due to enlargement of the prostate gland. May cause excitability especially in children. May cause marked drowsiness; alcohol, sedatives, and tranquilizers may increase the drowsiness effect. Avoid alcoholic beverages while taking this product. Do not take this product if you are taking sedatives or tranquilizers, without first con-

sulting your doctor. Use caution when driving a motor vehicle or operating machinery.

Drug Interaction Precaution: Do not use this product if you are now taking a prescription monoamine oxidase inhibitor (MAOI) (certain drugs for depression, psychiatric or emotional conditions, or Parkinson's disease), or for 2 weeks after stopping the MAOI drug. If you are uncertain whether your prescription drug contains an MAOI, consult a health professional before taking this product.

Overdose: Acetylcystine as an antidote for acetaminophen overdose. See COMTREX PROFESSIONAL INFORMATION section at the beginning of the Comtrex listing.

How Supplied:
Comtrex Multi-Symptom Cold and Cough Relief is supplied as:
Coated yellow tablet with letters "Cx" debossed on one surface.
Supplied in Blister packages of 24's
Coated yellow caplet with "Cx" debossed on one side.
Supplied in Blister packages of 24's
Store tablets and caplets at room temperature.
Other COMTREX products also available: Acute Head Cold & Sinus Pressure Relief, Deep Chest Cold and Congestion Relief, Sore Throat Relief, Allergy Sinus Treatment, Day/Night, Comtrex Flu Therapy & Fever Relief Day & Night and Non-Drowsy formulations.

Shown in Product Identification Guide, page 506

COMTREX® ACUTE HEAD COLD
Sinus Pressure Relief
[cŏm-trĕx]

Composition: Each tablet contains: Acetaminophen 500 mg, Brompheniramine maleate 2 mg, Pseudoephedrine hydrochloride 30 mg.

Other Ingredients: Benzoic Acid, Carnauba Wax, Corn Starch, Croscarmellose Sodium, FD&C Red No. 40 Lake, Hydroxypropyl Methylcellulose, Magnesium Stearate, Methylparaben, Microcrystalline Cellulose, Polyethylene Glycol, Polysorbate 80, Propylparaben, Stearic Acid, Titanium Dioxide.

Indications: For the temporary relief of the following symptoms associated with the common cold and flu: minor aches, pains, headache, muscular aches, sore throat pain, and fever; nasal congestion, and sinus pressure; runny nose and sneezing.

Directions: Adults and children 12 years of age and over: 2 tablets every 6 hours, while symptoms persist, not to exceed 8 tablets in 24 hours, or as directed by your doctor. Children under 12 years of age: consult a doctor.

Alcohol Warning: If you consume 3 or more alcoholic drinks every day, ask your doctor whether you should take acetaminophen or other pain relievers/fever reducers. Acetaminophen may cause liver damage.

Warnings: Keep out of reach of children. In case of overdose get medical help or contact a Poison Control Center right away. Prompt medical attention is critical for adults as well as children even if you do not notice any signs or symptoms. As with any drug, if you are pregnant or nursing a baby, seek the advice of a health professional before using this product. Do not take this product for more than 7 days. If symptoms do not improve or are accompanied by fever that lasts for more than 3 days, or if new symptoms occur, consult a doctor. If sore throat is severe, persists for more than 2 days, is accompanied or followed by fever, headache, rash, nausea, or vomiting, consult a doctor promptly. **Do not exceed recommended dosage.** If nervousness, dizziness, or sleeplessness occur, discontinue use and consult a doctor. If symptoms do not improve within 7 days or are accompanied by fever, consult a doctor. Do not take this product, unless directed by a doctor, if you have a breathing problem such as emphysema or chronic bronchitis, heart disease, high blood pressure, thyroid disease, diabetes, glaucoma, or difficulty in urination due to enlargement of the prostate gland. May cause excitability especially in children. May cause drowsiness; alcohol, sedatives, and tranquilizers may increase the drowsiness effect. Avoid alcoholic beverages while taking this product. Do not take this product if you are taking sedatives or tranquilizers, without first consulting your doctor. Use caution when driving a motor vehicle or operating machinery.

Drug Interaction Precaution: Do not use this product if you are now taking a prescription monoamine oxidase inhibitor (MAOI) (certain drugs for depression, psychiatric or emotional conditions, or Parkinson's disease), or for 2 weeks after stopping the MAOI drug. If you are uncertain whether your prescription drug contains an MAOI, consult a health professional before taking this product.

Overdose:
Acetylcysteine As An Antidote For Acetaminophen Overdose
See COMTREX PROFESSIONAL INFORMATION section at the beginning of Comtrex listing.

How Supplied:
Round, red coated tablets with "AHC" debossed on one side, supplied in blisters of 24's.

Other Comtrex products also available: Deep Chest Cold & Congestion Relief, Allergy Sinus Treatment, Day/Night, Sore Throat Relief, Comtrex Flu Therapy and Fever Relief, Day & Night and Non-Drowsy Formulations.

Shown in Product Identification Guide, page 506

COMTREX® DEEP CHEST COLD
& Congestion Relief

Composition: Each softgel contains: Acetaminophen 250 mg, Dextromethorphan HBr 10 mg, Guaifenesin 100 mg, and Pseudoephedrine HCl 30 mg.
OTHER INGREDIENTS: FD&C Yellow No. 6, Gelatin, Glycerin, Polyethylene Glycol, Povidone, Propylene Glycol, Sorbitol, Water

Uses: For the temporary relief of the following symptoms associated with the common cold and flu: minor aches, pains, headache, muscular aches, sore throat pain, and fever; cough; and nasal congestion. Helps loosen phlegm (mucus) and thin bronchial secretions to drain bronchial tubes and make coughs more productive.

Alcohol Warning: If you consume 3 or more alcoholic drinks every day, ask your doctor whether you should take acetaminophen or other pain relievers/fever reducers. Acetaminophen may cause liver damage.

Warnings: Keep out of reach of children. In case of overdose, get medical help or contact a Poison Control Center right away. Prompt medical attention is critical for adults as well as for children even if you do not notice any signs or symptoms. As with any drug, if you are pregnant or nursing a baby, seek the advice of a health professional before using this product. Do not take this product for more than 7 days or for fever for more than 3 days unless directed by a doctor. If pain or fever persists or gets worse, or if new symptoms occur, consult a doctor. A persistent cough may be a sign of a serious condition. If cough persists for more than 1 week, tends to recur, or is accompanied by fever, rash, or persistent headache, consult a doctor. Do not take this product for persistent or chronic cough such as occurs with smoking, asthma, chronic bronchitis, emphysema, or where cough is accompanied by excessive phlegm (mucus) unless directed by a doctor. If sore throat is severe, persists for more than 2 days, is accompanied or followed by fever, headache, rash, nausea, or vomiting, consult a doctor promptly. **Do not exceed recommended dosage.** If nervousness, dizziness, or sleeplessness occur, discontinue use and consult a doctor. If symptoms do not improve within 7 days or are accompanied by fever, consult a doctor. Do not take this product if you have heart disease, high blood pressure, thyroid disease, diabetes, or difficulty in urination due to enlargement of the prostate gland unless directed by a doctor.

Drug Interaction Precaution: Do not use if you are now taking a prescription monoamine oxidase inhibitor (MAOI) (certain drugs for depression, psychiatric, or emotional conditions, or Parkinson's disease), or for 2 weeks after

Continued on next page

Comtrex Deep Chest—Cont.

stopping the MAOI drug. If you do not know if your prescription drug contains an MAOI, ask a doctor or pharmacist before taking this product.

Overdose: Acetylcysteine as an antidote for acetaminophen overdose. See COMTREX PROFESSIONAL INFORMATION section at the beginning of this Comtrex listing.

Directions: Adults and children 12 years of age and over: 2 softgels every 4 hours, while symptoms persist, not to exceed 12 softgels in 24 hours, or as directed by your doctor. Children under 12 years of age: consult a doctor.

How Supplied: Orange oval shaped softgel imprinted with "Comtrex CC" in white, available in blister packs of 24's. Other Comtrex products available: Acute Head Cold & Sinus Pressure Relief, Allergy-Sinus Treatment, Flu Therapy & Fever Relief Day & Night, Sore Throat Relief, Cold & Cough Relief Day & Night and Non-Drowsy Formulations.

Store at Controlled Room Temperature 20°–25°C (68°–77°F)

Shown in Product Identification Guide, page 506

COMTREX® DAY & NIGHT
Flu Therapy & Fever Relief
18 DAYTIME CAPLETS
6 NIGHTTIME TABLETS

Description: Day & Night COMTREX® Flu Therapy and Fever Relief provides you with two different maximum strength formulas. COMTREX Daytime (orange caplets) is non-drowsy and contains the maximum levels of a non-aspirin analgesic and of a nasal decongestant allowed. COMTREX® Nighttime (green tablets), contains the same ingredients PLUS the maximum level of an antihistamine—so you can rest.

Composition: Each daytime orange caplet contains: Acetaminophen 500 mg and Pseudoephedrine HCl 30 mg. Each nighttime green tablet contains: Acetaminophen 500 mg, Chlorpheniramine Maleate 2 mg, and Pseudoephedrine HCl 30 mg. **Other Ingredients:** Each Daytime Caplet contains: Benzoic Acid, Carnauba Wax, Corn Starch, D&C Yellow No. 10 Aluminum Lake, D&C Yellow No. 10, FD&C Red No. 40 Aluminum Lake, FD&C Red No. 40, Hydroxypropyl Methylcellulose, Mineral Oil, Polysorbate 20, Povidone, Propylene Glycol, Simethicone Emulsion, Sorbitan Monolaurate, Stearic Acid, Titanium Dioxide. Each Nighttime Tablet contains: Benzoic Acid, Carnauba Wax, Corn Starch, D&C Yellow No. 10 Aluminum Lake, FD&C Blue No. 1 Aluminum Lake, FD&C Red No. 40 Aluminum Lake, Hydroxypropyl Methylcellulose, Magnesium Stearate, Methylpara-

ben, Mineral Oil, Polysorbate 20, Povidone, Propylene Glycol, Propylparaben, Simethicone Emulsion, Sodium Citrate, Sorbitan Monolaurate, Stearic Acid, Titanium Dioxide. Nighttime Tablets may also contain: FD&C Blue No. 1, D&C Yellow No. 10.

Uses: COMTREX DAYTIME CAPLETS: For the temporary relief of minor aches, and pains, associated with the common cold and flu, sore throat pain, muscular aches, headache, fever, and nasal congestion. COMTREX® NIGHTTIME TABLETS: Provide the same relief as the daytime caplets PLUS temporarily relieves runny nose and reduces sneezing.

Alcohol Warning: If you consume 3 or more alcoholic drinks every day, ask your doctor whether you should take acetaminophen or other pain relievers/fever reducers. Acetaminophen may cause liver damage.

Warnings For Daytime Caplets & Nighttime Tablets: Keep out of reach of children. In case of overdose, get medical help or contact a Poison Control Center right away. Prompt medical attention is critical for adults as well as children even if you do not notice any signs or symptoms. As with any drug, if you are pregnant or nursing a baby, seek the advice of a health professional before using this product. Do not take this product for more than 7 days. If symptoms do not improve or are accompanied by fever that lasts for more than 3 days, or if new symptoms occur, or if redness or swelling is present, consult a doctor. If sore throat is severe, persists for more than 2 days, is accompanied or followed by fever, headache, rash, nausea, or vomiting, consult a doctor promptly. **Do not exceed recommended dosage.** If nervousness, dizziness, or sleeplessness occur, discontinue use and consult a doctor. Do not take this product unless directed by a doctor, if you have a breathing problem such as emphysema or chronic bronchitis, heart disease, high blood pressure, thyroid disease, diabetes, glaucoma, or difficulty in urination due to enlargement of the prostate gland.

Additional Warnings For Nighttime Tablets: May cause excitability especially in children. May cause drowsiness; alcohol, sedatives, and tranquilizers may increase the drowsiness effect. Avoid alcoholic beverages while taking this product. Do not take this product if you are taking sedatives or tranquilizers, without first consulting your doctor. Use caution when driving a motor vehicle or operating machinery.

Drug Interaction Precaution: Do not use if you are now taking a prescription monoamine oxidase inhibitor (MAOI) (certain drugs for depression, psychiatric, or emotional conditions, or Parkinson's disease), or for 2 weeks after stopping the MAOI drug. If you do not know if your prescription drug contains an MAOI, ask a doctor or pharmacist before taking this product.

Overdose: Acetylcysteine as an antidote for acetaminophen overdose. See COMTREX PROFESSIONAL INFORMATION section at the beginning of this Comtrex listing.

Directions: Adults: 2 Daytime Caplets every 6 hours while symptoms persist, not to exceed 4 Daytime Caplets in 24 hours, or as directed by your doctor. 2 Nighttime Tablets at bedtime, if needed, to be taken no sooner than 6 hours after the last Daytime Caplets dose, or as directed by a doctor. Children under 12 years of age: consult a doctor.

How Supplied: 18 Daytime Caplets and 6 Nighttime Tablets
Other Comtrex products available: Acute Head Cold & Sinus Pressure Relief, Allergy-Sinus Treatment, Deep Chest Cold & Congestion Relief, Sore Throat Relief, Cold & Cough Relief Day & Night and Non-Drowsy Formulations.

Store at Room Temperature
Shown in Product Identification Guide, page 506

Aspirin Free EXCEDRIN®

Active Ingredients: Each caplet and geltab contains Acetaminophen 500 mg and Caffeine 65 mg.

Inactive Ingredients: (caplet) benzoic acid, carnauba wax, corn starch, D&C Red # 27 Lake, D&C Yellow # 10 Lake, FD&C Blue # 1 Lake, hydroxypropyl methylcellulose, magnesium stearate, methylparaben, microcrystalline cellulose, mineral oil, polysorbate 20, povidone, propylene glycol, propylparaben, simethicone emulsion, sorbitan monolaurate, stearic acid, titanium dioxide.
May also contain: croscarmellose sodium, FD&C Red # 40, saccharin sodium, sodium starch glycolate.
Inactive Ingredients: (geltab) benzoic acid, corn starch, FD&C Red # 40, FD&C Yellow # 6, gelatin, hydroxypropyl methylcellulose, magnesium stearate, methylparaben, microcrystalline cellulose, mineral oil, polysorbate 20, povidone, propylene glycol, propylparaben, simethicone emulsion, sorbitan monolaurate, stearic acid, titanium dioxide.
May also contain: croscarmellose sodium, sodium starch glycolate

Indications: For the temporary relief of minor aches and pains associated with headache, sinusitis, a cold, muscular aches, premenstrual and menstrual cramps, toothache, and for the minor pain from arthritis.

Directions: Adults: 2 caplets or geltabs every 6 hours while symptoms persist, not to exceed 8 caplets or geltabs in 24 hours, or as directed by a doctor. Children under 12 years of age: Consult a doctor.

Alcohol Warning: If you consume 3 or more alcoholic drinks every day, ask your doctor whether you should take aceta-

minophen or other pain relievers/fever reducers. Acetaminophen may cause liver damage.

Warnings: Keep out of reach of children. In case of overdose, get medical help or contact a Poison Control Center right away. Prompt medical attention is critical for adults as well as for children even if you do not notice any signs or symptoms. As with any drug, if you are pregnant or nursing a baby, seek the advice of a health professional before using this product. Do not take this product for pain for more than 10 days or for fever for more than 3 days unless directed by a doctor. If pain or fever persists or gets worse, if new symptoms occur, of if redness or swelling is present, consult a doctor because these could be signs of a serious condition. Consult a dentist promptly for toothache.

Overdose: Acetylcysteine As An Antidote For Acetaminophen Overdose

Acetaminophen is rapidly absorbed from the upper gastrointestinal tract with peak plasma levels occurring between 30 and 60 minutes after therapeutic doses and usually within 4 hours following an overdose. The parent compound, which is nontoxic, is extensively metabolized in the liver to form principally the sulfate and glucuronide conjugates which are also nontoxic and are rapidly excreted in the urine. A small fraction of an ingested dose is metabolized in the liver by the cytochrome P-450 mixed function oxidase enzyme system to form a reactive, potentially toxic, intermediate metabolite which preferentially conjugates with hepatic glutathione to form the nontoxic cysteine and mercapturic acid derivatives which are then excreted by the kidney. Therapeutic doses of acetaminophen do not saturate the glucuronide and sulfate conjugation pathways and do not result in the formation of sufficient reactive metabolite to deplete glutathione stores. However, following ingestion of a large overdose (150 mg/kg or greater) the glucuronide and sulfate conjugation pathways are saturated resulting in a larger fraction of the drug being metabolized via the P-450 pathway. The increased formation of reactive metabolite may deplete the hepatic stores of glutathione with subsequent binding of the metabolite to protein molecules within the hepatocyte resulting in cellular necrosis. Acetylcysteine has been shown to reduce the extent of liver injury following acetaminophen overdose. Early symptoms following a potentially hepatotoxic overdose may include: nausea, vomiting, diaphoresis and general malaise. Clinical and laboratory evidence of hepatic toxicity may not be apparent until 48 to 72 hours postingestion. In most adults and adolescents, regardless of the quantity of acetaminophen reported to have been ingested, administer acetylcysteine immediately. Acetylcysteine therapy should be initiated and continued for a full course of therapy. Its effec-

tiveness depends on early administration, with benefit seen principally in patients treated within 16 hours of the overdose.

If acetaminophen plasma assay capability is not available, and the estimated acetaminophen ingestion exceeds 150 mg/kg, acetylcysteine therapy should be initiated and continued for a full course of therapy.

For full prescribing information, refer to the acetylcysteine package insert. Do not await the results of assays for acetaminophen level before initiating treatment with acetylcysteine. The following additional procedures are recommended: The stomach should be emptied promptly by lavage or by induction of emesis with syrup of ipecac. A serum acetaminophen assay should be obtained as early as possible, but no sooner than four hours following ingestion. Liver function studies should be obtained initially and repeated at 24-hour intervals.

For additional emergency information call your regional poison center or toll-free (1-800-525-6115) to the Rocky Mountain Poison Center for assistance in diagnosis and for directions in the use of acetylcysteine as an antidote.

How Supplied: Aspirin Free EXCEDRIN® is supplied as: Coated red caplets with "AF Excedrin" printed in white on one side in bottles of 24's, 50's and 100's. Easy to swallow red geltabs with "AF Excedrin" printed in white on one side supplied in bottles of 24's, 50's, 100's (2 bottles of 50 each).

Store at room temperature.

Shown in Product Identification Guide, page 507

EXCEDRIN® Extra-Strength Analgesic

[ĕx "cĕd 'rin]

Active Ingredients: Each tablet, caplet, or geltab contains Acetaminophen 250 mg, Aspirin 250 mg, and Caffeine 65 mg.

Inactive Ingredients: (tablet, caplet) benzoic acid, carnauba wax, hydroxypropylcellulose, hydroxypropyl methylcellulose, microcrystalline cellulose, mineral oil, polysorbate 20, povidone, propylene glycol, simethicone emulsion, sorbitan monolaurate, stearic acid.

May also contain: FD&C blue # 1, titanium dioxide

Inactive Ingredients: (geltab) benzoic acid, D&C yellow #10 lake, disodium EDTA, FD&C blue #1 lake, FD&C red # 40 lake, ferric oxide, gelatin, glycerin, hydroxypropylcellulose, hydroxypropyl methylcellulose, maltitol solution, microcrystalline cellulose, mineral oil, pepsin, polysorbate 20, povidone, propylene glycol, propyl gallate, simethicone emulsion, sorbitan monolaurate, stearic acid, titanium dioxide.

Uses: For the temporary relief of minor aches and pains associated with head-

ache, sinusitis, a cold, muscular aches, premenstrual and menstrual cramps, toothache, and for the minor pain from arthritis.

Warnings: Children and teenagers should not use this medicine for chicken pox or flu symptoms before a doctor is consulted about Reye's syndrome, a rare but serious illness reported to be associated with aspirin.

Alcohol Warning: If you consume 3 or more alcoholic drinks every day, ask your doctor whether you should take acetaminophen and aspirin or other pain relievers/fever reducers. Acetaminophen and aspirin may cause liver damage and stomach bleeding.

Keep out of reach of children. In case of overdose, get medical help or contact a Poison Control Center right away. Prompt medical attention is critical for adults as well as for children even if you do not notice any signs or symptoms. As with any drug, if you are pregnant or nursing a baby, seek the advice of a health professional before using this product. IT IS ESPECIALLY IMPORTANT NOT TO USE ASPIRIN DURING THE LAST 3 MONTHS OF PREGNANCY UNLESS SPECIFICALLY DIRECTED TO DO SO BY A DOCTOR BECAUSE IT MAY CAUSE PROBLEMS IN THE UNBORN CHILD OR COMPLICATIONS DURING DELIVERY. Do not take this product for pain for more than 10 days or for fever for more than 3 days unless directed by a doctor. If pain or fever persists or gets worse, if new symptoms occur, or if redness or swelling is present, consult a doctor because these could be signs of a serious condition. Consult a dentist promptly for toothache. Do not take this product if you are allergic to aspirin, have asthma, have stomach problems (such as heartburn, upset stomach or stomach pain) that persist or recur, or if you have ulcers or bleeding problems, unless directed by a doctor. If ringing in the ears or loss of hearing occurs, consult a doctor before taking any more of this product.

Drug Interaction Precaution: Do not take this product if you are taking a prescription drug for anticoagulation (thinning the blood), diabetes, gout or arthritis unless directed by a doctor.

Directions: Adults: 2 tablets, caplets or geltabs with water every 6 hours while symptoms persist, not to exceed 8 tablets, caplets or geltabs in 24 hours, or as directed by a doctor. Children under 12 years of age: Consult a doctor.

Overdose: Acetylcysteine As An Antidote For Acetaminophen Overdose

Acetaminophen is rapidly absorbed from the upper gastrointestinal tract with peak plasma levels occurring between 30 and 60 minutes after therapeutic doses and usually within 4 hours following an overdose. The parent compound, which

Continued on next page

Excedrin Extra-Strength—Cont.

is nontoxic, is extensively metabolized in the liver to form principally the sulfate and glucuronide conjugates which are also nontoxic and are rapidly excreted in the urine. A small fraction of an ingested dose is metabolized in the liver by the cytochrome P-450 mixed function oxidase enzyme system to form a reactive, potentially toxic, intermediate metabolite which preferentially conjugates with hepatic glutathione to form the nontoxic cysteine and mercapturic acid derivatives which are then excreted by the kidney. Therapeutic doses of acetaminophen do not saturate the glucuronide and sulfate conjugation pathways and do not result in the formation of sufficient reactive metabolite to deplete glutathione stores. However, following ingestion of a large overdose (150 mg/kg or greater) the glucuronide and sulfate conjugation pathways are saturated resulting in a larger fraction of the drug being metabolized via the P-450 pathway. The increased formation of reactive metabolite may deplete the hepatic stores of glutathione with subsequent binding of the metabolite to protein molecules within the hepatocyte resulting in cellular necrosis. Acetylcysteine has been shown to reduce the extent of liver injury following acetaminophen overdose. Early symptoms following a potentially hepatotoxic overdose may include: nausea, vomiting, diaphoresis and general malaise. Clinical and laboratory evidence of hepatic toxicity may not be apparent until 48 to 72 hours postingestion. In most adults and adolescents, regardless of the quantity of acetaminophen reported to have been ingested, administer acetylcysteine immediately. Acetylcysteine therapy should be initiated and continued for a full course of therapy. Its effectiveness depends on early administration, with benefit seen principally in patients treated within 16 hours of the overdose.

If acetaminophen plasma assay capability is not available, and the estimated acetaminophen ingestion exceeds 150 mg/kg, acetylcysteine therapy should be initiated and continued for a full course of therapy.

For full prescribing information, refer to the acetylcysteine package insert. Do not await the results of assays for acetaminophen level before initiating treatment with acetylcysteine. The following additional procedures are recommended: The stomach should be emptied promptly by lavage or by induction of emesis with syrup of ipecac. A serum acetaminophen assay should be obtained as early as possible, but no sooner than four hours following ingestion. Liver function studies should be obtained initially and repeated at 24-hour intervals.

For additional emergency information call your regional poison center or toll-free (1-800-525-6115) to the Rocky Mountain Poison Center for assistance in diagnosis and for directions in the use of acetylcysteine as an antidote.

How Supplied: Extra Strength EXCEDRIN® is supplied as:
Coated white circular tablet with letter "E" debossed on one side. Supplied in bottles of 12's, 24's, 50's, 100's, 175's, 275's and metal tins of 12's.
Coated white caplets with "E" debossed on one side. Supplied in bottles of 24's, 50's, 100's, 175's, 275's.
Gel-coated round geltabs–green on one side, white on the other, printed with black "E" on one side. Supplied in bottles of 24's, 50's and 100's (2 bottles of 50 each).
Store at room temperature.
Shown in Product Identification Guide, page 507

EXCEDRIN® MIGRAINE
Pain Reliever/Pain Reliever Aid

Active Ingredients: Each tablet, caplet or geltab contains Acetaminophen 250mg, Aspirin 250mg and Caffeine 65mg.

Inactive Ingredients: (tablet and caplet) benzoic acid, carnauba wax, hydroxypropylcellulose, hydroxypropyl methylcellulose, microcrystalline cellulose, mineral oil, polysorbate 20, povidone, propylene glycol, simethicone emulsion, sorbitan monolaurate, stearic acid, may also contain: FD&C blue no. 1, titanium dioxide.

Inactive Ingredients: (geltab) benzoic acid, D&C yellow #10 lake, disodium EDTA, FD&C blue #1 lake, FD&C red #40 lake, ferric oxide, gelatin, glycerin, hydroxypropylcellulose, hydroxypropyl methylcellulose, maltitol solution, microcrystalline cellulose, mineral oil, pepsin, polysorbate 20, povidone, propylene glycol, propyl gallate, simethicone emulsion, sorbitan monolaurate, stearic acid, titanium dioxide.

Use: Treats migraine.

Warnings:

Reye's Syndrome: Children and teenagers should not use this drug for chicken pox, or flu symptoms before a doctor is consulted about Reye's syndrome, a rare but serious illness reported to be associated with aspirin.

Allergy alert: aspirin may cause a severe allergic reaction which may include: • hives • facial swelling • asthma (wheezing) • shock

Alcohol warning: If you consume 3 or more alcoholic drinks every day, ask your doctor whether you should take acetaminophen and aspirin or other pain relievers/fever reducers. Acetaminophen and aspirin may cause liver damage and stomach bleeding.

Caffeine warning: The recommended dose of this product contains about as much caffeine as a cup of coffee. Limit the use of caffeine-containing medications, foods, or beverages while taking this product because too much caffeine

may cause nervousness, irritability, sleeplessness, and, occasionally, rapid heart beat.

Do not use • if you have ever had an allergic reaction to any other pain reliever/fever reducer

Ask a doctor before use if you have
• never had migraines diagnosed by a health professional
• a headache that is different from your usual migraines
• the worst headache of your life
• fever and stiff neck
• headaches beginning after or caused by head injury, exertion, coughing or bending
• experienced your first headache after the age of 50
• daily headaches
• asthma
• bleeding problems
• ulcers
• stomach problems such as heartburn, upset stomach, or stomach pain that do not go away or recur
• a migraine so severe as to require bed rest
• problems or serious side effects from taking pain relievers or fever reducers

Ask a doctor or pharmacist before use if you are taking a prescription drug for:
• anticoagulation (thinning of the blood)
• diabetes
• gout
• arthritis

Stop use and ask a doctor if
• an allergic reaction occurs. Seek medical help right away.
• your migraine is not relieved or worsens after first dose
• new or unexpected symptoms occur
• ringing in the ears or loss of hearing occurs

If pregnant or breast-feeding, ask a health professional before use. It is especially important not to use aspirin during the last 3 months of pregnancy unless definitely directed to do so by a doctor because it may cause problems in the unborn child or complications during delivery.

Keep out of reach of children. In case of overdose, get medical help or contact a Poison Control Center right away. Quick medical attention is critical for adults as well as for children even if you do not notice any signs or symptoms.

Directions:
• adults: take 2 (tablets, caplets or geltabs) with a glass of water
• if symptoms persist or worsen, ask your doctor
• do not take more than 2 (tablets, caplets, or geltabs) in 24 hours, unless directed by a doctor
• under 18 years of age: ask a doctor

Overdose: Acetylcysteine As An Antidote For Acetaminophen Overdose
Acetaminophen is rapidly absorbed from the upper gastrointestinal tract with peak plasma levels occurring between 30 and 60 minutes after therapeutic doses and usually within 4 hours following an overdose. The parent compound, which is nontoxic, is extensively metabolized in the liver to form principally the sulfate and glucuronide conjugates which are

also nontoxic and are rapidly excreted in the urine. A small fraction of an ingested dose is metabolized in the liver by the cytochrome P-450 mixed function oxidase enzyme system to form a reactive, potentially toxic, intermediate metabolite which preferentially conjugates with hepatic glutathione to form the nontoxic cysteine and mercapturic acid derivatives which are then excreted by the kidney. Therapeutic doses of acetaminophen do not saturate the glucuronide and sulfate conjugation pathways and do not result in the formation of sufficient reactive metabolite to deplete glutathione stores. However, following ingestion of a large overdose (150 mg/kg or greater) the glucuronide and sulfate conjugation pathways are saturated resulting in a larger fraction of the drug being metabolized via the P-450 pathway. The increased formation of reactive metabolite may deplete the hepatic stores of glutathione with subsequent binding of the metabolite to protein molecules within the hepatocyte resulting in cellular necrosis. Acetylcysteine has been shown to reduce the extent of liver injury following acetaminophen overdose. Early symptoms following a potentially hepatotoxic overdose may include: nausea, vomiting, diaphoresis and general malaise. Clinical and laboratory evidence of hepatic toxicity may not be apparent until 48 to 72 hours postingestion. In most adults and adolescents, regardless of the quantity of acetaminophen reported to have been ingested, administer acetylcysteine immediately. Acetylcysteine therapy should be initiated and continued for a full course of therapy. Its effectiveness depends on early administration, with benefit seen principally in patients treated within 16 hours of the overdose. If acetaminophen plasma assay capability is not available, and the estimated acetaminophen ingestion exceeds 150 mg/kg, acetylcysteine therapy should be initiated and continued for a full course of therapy.

For full prescription information, refer to the acetylcysteine package insert. Do not await the results of assays for acetaminophen level before initiating treatment with acetylcysteine. The following additional procedures are recommended: The stomach should be emptied promptly by lavage or by induction of emesis with syrup of ipecac. A serum acetaminophen assay should be obtained as early as possible, but no sooner than four hours following ingestion. Liver function studies should be obtained initially and repeated at 24-hour intervals. For additional emergency information call your regional poison center or toll-free (1-800-525-6115) to the Rocky Mountain Poison Center for assistance in diagnosis and for directions in the use of acetylcysteine as an antidote.

How Supplied: EXCEDRIN® MIGRAINE is supplied as:

Coated white circular tablets or coated white caplets with letter "E" debossed on one side. Supplied in bottles of 24's, 50's, 100's, and 175's. 275's (tablets) are available in club store packages. Coated round geltabs–green on one side, white on the other, printed with black "E" on one side. Supplied in bottles of 24's, 50's and 100's (2 bottles of 50 each).
Store at 20–25°C (68–77°F).

Shown in Product Identification Guide, page 507

EXCEDRIN® PM
[ĕx "cĕd 'rĭn]
Pain Reliever/Nighttime Sleep-Aid

Active Ingredients: Each tablet, caplet or geltab contains: Acetaminophen 250 mg and Diphenhydramine Citrate 38 mg

Inactive Ingredients: (Tablet and Caplet) benzoic acid, carnauba wax, corn starch, D&C yellow #10 aluminum lake, FD&C blue #1 aluminum lake, hydroxypropyl methylcellulose, magnesium stearate, methylparaben, mineral oil, povidone, propylene glycol, propylparaben, simethicone emulsion, sodium citrate, stearic acid, titanium dioxide. May also contain: D&C Yellow #10, FD&C Blue #1, polysorbate 20, sorbitan monolaurate. (Geltab) benzoic acid, corn starch, D&C Red #33, edetate disodium, FD&C Blue #1, FD&C Blue #1 Lake, gelatin, glycerin, hydroxypropyl methylcellulose, magnesium stearate, methylparaben, mineral oil, polysorbate 20, pregelatinized starch, propylene glycol, propylparaben, simethicone emulsion, sorbitan monolaurate, stearic acid, titanium dioxide. May also contain: D&C Yellow #10, D&C Yellow #10 Lake.

Uses: For temporary relief of occasional headaches and minor aches and pains with accompanying sleeplessness.
Alcohol Warning: If you consume 3 or more alcoholic drinks every day, ask your doctor whether you should take acetaminophen or other pain relievers/fever reducers. Acetaminophen may cause liver damage.

Warnings: Keep out of reach of children. In case of overdose, get medical help or contact a Poison Control Center right away. Prompt medical attention is critical for adults as well as for children even if you do not notice any signs or symptoms. As with any drug, if you are pregnant or nursing a baby, seek the advice of a health professional before using this product. Do not give to children under 12 years of age or use for more than 10 days unless directed by a doctor. If symptoms persist or get worse, if new ones occur, or if sleeplessness persists continuously for more than 2 weeks, consult your doctor. Insomnia may be a symptom of serious underlying medical illness. Do not take this product, unless directed by a doctor, if you have a breathing problem such as emphysema or chronic bronchitis, or if you have glaucoma or difficulty in urination due to en-largement of the prostate gland. Avoid alcoholic beverages while taking this product. Do not take this product if you are taking sedatives or tranquilizers, without first consulting your doctor.

Directions:
Adults and children 12 years of age and over: 2 tablets, caplets, or geltabs at bedtime if needed or as directed by a doctor.

Overdose: Acetylcysteine As An Antidote For Acetaminophen Overdose
Acetaminophen is rapidly absorbed from the upper gastrointestinal tract with peak plasma levels occurring between 30 and 60 minutes after therapeutic doses and usually within 4 hours following an overdose. The parent compound, which is nontoxic, is extensively metabolized in the liver to form principally the sulfate and glucuronide conjugates which are also nontoxic and are rapidly excreted in the urine. A small fraction of an ingested dose is metabolized in the liver by the cytochrome P-450 mixed function oxidase enzyme system to form a reactive, potentially toxic, intermediate metabolite which preferentially conjugates with hepatic glutathione to form the nontoxic cysteine and mercapturic acid derivatives which are then excreted by the kidney. Therapeutic doses of acetaminophen do not saturate the glucuronide and sulfate conjugation pathways and do not result in the formation of sufficient reactive metabolite to deplete glutathione stores. However, following ingestion of a large overdose (150 mg/kg or greater) the glucuronide and sulfate conjugation pathways are saturated resulting in a larger fraction of the drug being metabolized via the P-450 pathway. The increased formation of reactive metabolite may deplete the hepatic stores of glutathione with subsequent binding of the metabolite to protein molecules within the hepatocyte resulting in cellular necrosis. Acetylcysteine has been shown to reduce the extent of liver injury following acetaminophen overdose. Early symptoms following a potentially hepatotoxic overdose may include: nausea, vomiting, diaphoresis and general malaise. Clinical and laboratory evidence of hepatic toxicity may not be apparent until 48 to 72 hours postingestion. In most adults and adolescents, regardless of the quantity of acetaminophen reported to have been ingested, administer acetylcysteine immediately. Acetylcysteine therapy should be initiated and continued for a full course of therapy. Its effectiveness depends on early administration, with benefit seen principally in patients treated within 16 hours of the overdose.

If acetaminophen plasma assay capability is not available, and the estimated acetaminophen ingestion exceeds 150 mg/kg, acetylcysteine therapy should be initiated and continued for a full course of therapy.

Continued on next page

Excedrin P.M.—Cont.

For full prescribing information, refer to the acetylcysteine package insert. Do not await the results of assays for acetaminophen level before initiating treatment with acetylcysteine. The following additional procedures are recommended: The stomach should be emptied promptly by lavage or by induction of emesis with syrup of ipecac. A serum acetaminophen assay should be obtained as early as possible, but no sooner than four hours following ingestion. Liver function studies should be obtained initially and repeated at 24-hour intervals.

For additional emergency information call your regional poison center or toll-free (1-800-525-6115) to the Rocky Mountain Poison Center for assistance in diagnosis and for directions in the use of acetylcysteine as an antidote.

How Supplied: EXCEDRIN PM® is supplied as:
Light blue circular coated tablets with "PM" debossed on one side. Supplied in bottles of 10's, 24's, 50's, 100's.
Light blue coated caplet with "PM" debossed on one side. Supplied in bottles of 24's, 50's, 100's.
Gel coated-light blue and white geltabs with "PM" printed in black on one side. Supplied in bottles of 24's, 50's, 100's. Store at room temperature.

Shown in Product Identification Guide, page 506

Care-Tech® Laboratories, Inc.

**Over-The-Counter Pharmaceuticals
3224 SOUTH KINGSHIGHWAY BOULEVARD
ST. LOUIS, MO 63139**

Direct Inquiries to:
Sherry L. Brereton
(314) 772-4610
FAX: (314) 772-4613

For Medical Emergencies Contact:
Customer Service
(800) 325-9681
FAX: (314) 772-4613

CLINICAL CARE® ANTIMICROBIAL WOUND CLEANSER

Composition: Active Ingredient: Benzethonium Chloride .1%
Inactive Ingredients: Water, Amphoteric 2, Aloe Vera Gel, DMDM Hydantoin, Citric Acid.

Actions and Uses: Clinical Care is an antimicrobial, emulsifying solution which aids in removing debris and particulate matter from open, dermal wounds. Clinical Care inhibits the growth of pathogenic organisms. Proven effective at eliminating S. aureus, P. aeruginosa, S. typhimurium, Aspergillus, E. coli, MRSA, S. pyogenes and K. pneumonia. Will not produce dermal irritation. Broad-spectrum action for decontamination of diabetic ulcers, vascular ulcers and emergency medical situations. Requires no water or rinsing.

Precautions: External Use Only. Non-Toxic. No contra-indicators.

Directions: Spray affected area as necessary to debride. Use sterile gauze to gently remove debris and necrotic tissue at dermal surface.

How Supplied: 4 oz. spray, 12 oz. spray NDC# 46706-226

HUMATRIX® MICROCLYSMIC GEL
Burn/Wound Healing Gel for Tissue Trauma

Composition: Water, Propylene Glycol, Glycerine, Hydrolyzed Collagen, Citric Acid, Carbomer, Triethanolamine, Chondroitin Sulfate, Preservatives.

Actions and Uses: Provides endothermic and biomimetic properties to cool traumatized tissue and aid in the homeostasis of healing. HUMATRIX® provides the ultimate moisturization for burns, autograft procedures, radiation irritation, glycolic acid peel irritation, mechanical injuries, laser treatment, and chronic wound therapy. Humatrix is almost pure protein in content and aids in rapid cellular regeneration. Reduces surface temperature of tissue 12–15° within 2 minutes of application.

Precautions: External use only. Non-toxic. No contra-indications.

Directions: Cleanse the area with Techni-Care® Surgical Scrub, Prep. and Wound Cleanser, Rinse thoroughly with Clinical Care® Antimicrobial Wound Cleanser. Do not pat dry. Apply a layer of HUMATRIX® Microclysmic Gel approximately 2–4mm. thick. Cover the wound with a non-occlusive dressing. Re-apply at every dressing change to maintain a moist wound environment. Use prior to lasing procedures to reduce pain, irritation, and laser burns.

How Supplied: 8.5 oz. Spray Bottle, 4 oz. tubes, NDC# 46706-440-03

TECHNI–CARE® SURGICAL SCRUB, Prep and Wound Decontaminant

Composition: Active Ingredient: U.S.P. Chloroxylenol 3% and Cocamidopropyl PG-Dimonium Chloride Phosphate 3%
Inactive Ingredients: Water, Sodium Lauryl Sulfate, Cocamide DEA, Propylene Glycol, Cocamidopropyl Betaine, Citric Acid, Tetrasodium EDTA, Aloe Vera Gel, Hydrolyzed Animal Protein, D&C Yellow #10.

Actions and Uses: Techni-Care represents entirerly new technology in a broad-spectrum, topical, antiseptic microbicide for skin degerming. 99.99% Bacterial reduction in 30 second contact usage. Techni-Care may be used for disinfection of wounds, for pre-op and post-op along with surgical scrub applications. Non-staining and non-irritating to dermal tissue. Techni-Care conditions dermal tissue and phospholipid promotes a more rapid rate of cellular regeneration. Use for treatment of acute, chronic wounds in replacement of topical, antibiotic therapy. Techni-Care is effective at eliminating MRSA and VREF in topical applications or infected wounds.

Precautions: Non-Toxic, Non-Irritating, External Use Only. Can be used safely around ears and eyes or as directed by a physician. No Contra-indications. Safe for mucous membranes.

Directions: Apply, lather and rinse well. For pre-op, apply and let dry, no rinsing required. Swab into wound bed for 2–3 minutes for decontamination and removal of organic materials. Rinse with Clinical Care or sterile saline solution.

How Supplied: 12 mL packets, 4 oz., 8 oz., 12 oz., 16 oz., 32 oz., Gallons and peel paks NDC #46706–222

Effcon™ Laboratories, Inc.

**P.O. BOX 7499
MARIETTA, GA 30065-1499**

Address inquiries to:
Brad Rivet
(800-722-2428)
Fax: (770-428-6811)

For Medical Emergency Contact:
Brad Rivet
(800-722-2428)
Fax: (770-428-6811)

PIN-X®
Pinworm Treatment

Description: Each 1 mL of liquid for oral administration contains:
    Pyrantel base .... 50 mg
      (as Pyrantel Pamoate)

Indication: For the treatment of pinworms.

Warnings: Keep this and all drugs out of the reach of children. In case of accidental overdose, seek professional assistance or contact a poison control center immediately.
If you are pregnant or have liver disease, do not take this product unless directed by a doctor.

Directions for Use: Adults and children 2 years to under 12 years of age: oral dosage is a single dose of 5 milli-

grams of pyrantel base per pound, or 11 milligrams per kilogram, of body weight not to exceed 1 gram. Dosage information is summarized on the following dosing schedule:

Weight		Dosage
	(taken as a single dose)	
25 to 37 lbs.	=	$^1/_2$ tsp.
38 to 62 lbs.	=	1 tsp.
63 to 87 lbs.	=	$1^1/_2$ tsp.
88 to 112 lbs.	=	2 tsp.
113 to 137 lbs.	=	$2^1/_2$ tsp.
138 to 162 lbs.	=	3 tsp. (1 tbsp.)
163 to 187 lbs.	=	$3^1/_2$ tsp.
188 lbs. & over	=	4 tsp.

SHAKE WELL BEFORE USING

How Supplied: Pin-X is supplied as a tan to yellowish, caramel-flavored suspension which contains 50 mg of pyrantel base (as pyrantel pamoate) per mL, in bottles of 30 mL (1 fl oz). NDC 55806-024-10 and in bottles of 60 mL (2 fl oz) NDC 55806-024-11
Store at controlled room temperature 15°–30°C (59°–86°F).
Manufactured for:
Effcon™ Laboratories Inc.
Marietta, GA 30065-1499
Rev. 1/89
Code 587A00
Shown in Product Identification Guide, page 507

EDUCATIONAL MATERIAL

Patient Education Brochures—Pin-X® Pinworm Treatment

Effcon Laboratories provides complimentary Patient Education Brochures for patient counseling regarding the treatment and prevention of pinworm infestation. Brochures are available for all healthcare professionals and may be requested by phone (800-722-2428); fax (770-428-6811); or through Effcon's web page (www.effcon.com).

UNKNOWN DRUG?
Consult the
Product Identification Guide
(Gray Pages)
for full-color photos of
leading over-the-counter
medications

Fleming & Company
1600 FENPARK DR.
FENTON, MO 63026

Direct Inquiries to:
Tom Fleming
636 343-8200
FAX (636) 343-9865
e-mail: info@flemingcompany.com

CHLOR-3
Medicinal Condiment

DESCRIPTION
Medical condiment containing sodium chloride 50%; potassium chloride 30%; magnesium chloride 20%.

Active Ingredients: A mixture of sodium chloride (50% 24.3 mEq/half tsp. iodized); potassium chloride (30% 11.5 mEq/half tsp.); magnesium chloride (20% 5.7 mEq/half tsp.).

Indications: The first medicinal condiment to restore needed K^+ & Mg^{++} lost during diuresis, at the expense of Na^+. To restore electrolytes lost by overcooking foods, or to add to diets that lack green vegetables, bananas, etc. And to replace conventional salting of foods in culinary and gourmet arts.

Symptoms and Treatment of Oral Overdosage: Hyperkalemia and hypermagnesemia are not end-stage results of usage.

How Supplied: In 8-oz plastic shaker, tamper-evident bottles.

MARBLEN Antacid

Description: A peach-apricot flavored antacid suspension in a non-sugar base. Each teaspoonful (5mL) contains:

Calcium Carbonate	**520 mg**
Magnesium Carbonate	**400 mg.**

Indications: To be used for temporary relief of heartburn, sour stomach, and/or acid indigestion.

Action: The peach/apricot (pink) antacid suspension is sugar-free and neutralizes 18 mEq acid per teaspoonful with a low sodium content of 18 mg per fl.oz.

Warnings: Do not take more than 12 teaspoonfuls (60mL) in a 24 hour period or use this maximum dosage for more than two weeks. Do not use this product if you have kidney disease except under the advice and supervision of a physician.

Drug Interaction Precautions: Antacids may interact with certain prescription drugs. If you are presently taking a prescription drug, do not take this product without checking with your physician or health care professional.

Dosage: 1 or 2 teaspoonfuls as symptoms occur. Repeat hourly if symptoms return, or as directed by physician.

How Supplied: Plastic pints. Keep tightly closed. SHAKE WELL BEFORE USING.

NICOTINEX Elixir
Niacin Dietary Supplement

Composition: Contains niacin 50 mg./ tsp. in a sherry wine base (amber color).

Action and Uses: Produces peripheral flushing. To increase micro-circulation of inner-ear in Meniere's, tinnitus and labyrinthine syndromes. For 'cold hands & feet', and as a vehicle for additives.

Administration and Dosage: One or two teaspoonsful on fasting stomach, or as directed by physician.

Side Effects: Patients should be warned of dermal flush. Ulcer and gout patients may be affected by 10% alcoholic content.

Contraindications: Severe hypotension and hemorrhage.

How Supplied: Plastic pints.

OCEAN® Nasal Mist
(buffered isotonic saline)

Description: A 0.65% special saline made isotonic by the addition of a dual preservative system and buffering excipients prevent nasal irritation.
Ingredients: 0.65% Sodium Chloride and Phenylcarbinol and Benzalkonium Chloride as preservatives.

Action and Uses: For dry nasal membranes including rhinitis medicamentosa, rhinitis sicca and atrophic rhinitis. For patients 'hooked on nose drops' and glaucoma patients on diuretics having dry nasal capillaries. OCEAN® may also be used as a mist or drop. Upright delivers a spray; horizontally a stream; upside down a drop.

Administration and Dosage: For dry nasal membranes, two squeezes in each nostril P.R.N.

Supplied: Plastic 45cc spray bottles and pints.

PURGE
(Flavored Castor Oil Stimulant Laxative)

Composition: Contains 95% castor oil (USP) in a sweetened lemon flavored base that completely masks the odor and taste of the oil.

Indications: Preparation of the bowel for x-ray, surgery and proctological procedures, IVPs, and constipation.

Continued on next page

Purge—Cont.

Dosage: Adults and children 12 years of age and over: 15–60 mL (1–4 tbsp) in a single dose. Children 2 to under 12 years of age: 5–15 mL (1–3 tsp) in a single dose. Children under 2 years: consult a physician.

Precaution: Not indicated when nausea, vomiting, abdominal pain or symptoms of appendicitis occur. Pregnancy, use only on advice of physician.

Supplied: Plastic 1 oz. & 2 oz. bottles.

Hyland's, Inc.

See Standard Homeopathic Company

Johnson & Johnson • MERCK

Consumer Pharmaceuticals Co.
7050 CAMP HILL ROAD
FORT WASHINGTON, PA 19034

Direct Inquiries to:
Consumer Affairs Department
Fort Washington, PA 19034
(215) 273-7000
For Medical Information Contact:
In Emergencies:
(215) 273-7000

INFANTS' MYLICON® Drops
[*my 'li-con*]
SIMETHICONE/ANTIGAS

Active Ingredients: Each 0.3 mL contains 20 mg of pure simethicone.

Inactive Ingredients: Carboxymethylcellulose sodium, citric acid, maltitol, microcrystalline cellulose, natural flavor, purified water, Red 22, Red 28, sodium benzoate, sodium citrate, xanthan gum. *Non-staining formula does not contain: Red 22 or Red 28.*

Indications: For relief of the symptoms of excess gas in the digestive tract. Such gas is frequently caused by excessive swallowing of air or by eating foods that disagree. The defoaming action of INFANTS' MYLICON® Drops relieves flatulence by dispersing and preventing the formation of mucus-surrounded gas pockets in the gastrointestinal tract. INFANTS' MYLICON® Drops act in the stomach and intestines to change the surface tension of gas bubbles enabling them to coalesce, thereby freeing and eliminating the gas more easily by belching or passing flatus.

Directions: Shake Well Before Using. All dosages may be repeated as needed, after meals and at bedtime or as directed by a physician. Do not exceed 12 doses per day. Fill the dropper to rec-ommended dosage level and dispense liquid slowly into baby's mouth, toward the inner cheek. Dosage can also be mixed with 1 oz. of cool water, infant formula or other suitable liquids. For best results, clean dropper after each use and replace original cap.

Warnings: Do not use if printed plastic overwrap or printed neck wrap is missing or broken. Do not exceed 12 doses per day unless directed by a physician. Keep this and all drugs out of the reach of children.

How Supplied: INFANTS' MYLICON® Drops are available in bottles of 15 mL (0.5 fl ox) and 30 mL (1.0 fl oz). NDC 16837-630 (Original Pink) and NDC 16837-911 (Non-Staining Formula).
Shown in Product Identification Guide, page 508

CHILDREN'S MYLANTA®
UPSET STOMACH RELIEF
CALCIUM CARBONATE/ANTACID
LIQUID AND TABLETS

Description: Children's Mylanta is a specially formulated antacid to quickly and effectively relieve the upset stomach kids sometime experience.

Active Ingredients: Each tablet or 5 ml teaspoonful contains 400 mg of calcium carbonate.

Inactive Ingredients: Tablets: Citric acid, confectioner's sugar, D&C Red #27, flavors, magnesium stearate, sorbitol, starch.
Liquid: Butylparaben, cellulose, flavor propylparaben, purified water, D&C Red #22, D&C Red #28, simethicone, sodium saccharin, sorbitol, xanthan gum. May contain tartaric acid.

Acid Neutralizing Capacity:

Tablet	Liquid
8 mEq	8 mEq

Indications: For the relief of acid indigestion, sour stomach, or heartburn and upset stomach associated with these conditions, or overindulgence in food and drink.

Directions: Find the right dose on the chart below. If possible use weight as your dosing guide; otherwise use age. Repeat dosing as needed. DO NOT USE MORE THAN THREE TIMES PER DAY.

WEIGHT (LB)	AGE (YR)	TABLET	LIQUID (TSP)
Under 24	Under 2	Consult	Physician
24–47	2–5	1	1
48–95	6–11	2	2

Warnings: Keep this and all drugs out of the reach of children. Do not take more than 3 tablets or 3 teaspoonfuls (2–5 years) or 6 tablets or 6 teaspoonfuls (6–11 years) in a 24-hour period, or use the maximum dosage of this product for more than two weeks, except under the advice and supervision of a physician.

Drug Interaction Precaution: Antacids may interact with certain prescription drugs. If your child is presently taking a prescription drug, do not give this product without checking with your physician or other health professional.

How Supplied: Children's Mylanta Upset Stomach Relief is supplied as a liquid and chewable tablets in bubble gum flavor.
NDC 16837-810   Bubble Gum tablets
NDC 16837-820   Bubble Gum liquid
Shown in Product Identification Guide, page 508

FAST-ACTING MYLANTA® AND EXTRA STRENGTH FAST-ACTING MYLANTA®
[*my-lan'ta*]
Aluminum, Magnesium and Simethicone
Liquid
Antacid/Anti-Gas

Description: Fast-acting MYLANTA® and Extra Strength Fast-Acting MYLANTA® are well-balanced, pleasant-tasting, antacid/anti-gas medications that provide consistent, effective relief of symptoms associated with gastric hyperacidity and excess gas. Non-constipating and very low sodium Fast-Acting MYLANTA® and Extra Strength Fast-Acting MYLANTA® contain two proven antacids, aluminum hydroxide and magnesium hydroxide, plus simethicone for gas relief.

Active Ingredients: Each 5 mL teaspoon contains:

	MYLANTA®	MYLANTA® Extra Strength
Aluminum Hydroxide (equiv. to dried gel, USP)	200 mg	400 mg
Magnesium Hydroxide	200 mg	400 mg
Simethicone	20 mg	40 mg

Inactive Ingredients:
LIQUIDS:
Butylparaben, carboxymethylcellulose sodium, flavors, hydroxypropyl methylcellulose, microcrystalline cellulose, propylparaben, purified water, saccharin sodium, and sorbitol.
The following flavors also contain the listed inactive ingredients:
(Cherry: FD&C Red #40; Mint D&C Yellow #10, FD&C Green #3; Lemon: D&C Yellow #10)

SODIUM CONTENT
Each 5 mL teaspoon contains the following amount of sodium:

	MYLANTA®	MYLANTA® Extra Strength
Liquid	0.6 mg	0.9 mg

Acid Neutralizing Capacity:

Two teaspoonfuls have the following acid neutralizing capacity:

	Fast Acting MYLANTA®	Extra Strength Fast Acting MYLANTA®
Liquid	25.5 mEq.	51.0 mEq.

Indications:

Fast-Acting MYLANTA® and Extra Strength Fast-Acting MYLANTA® are indicated for the relief of acid indigestion, heartburn, sour stomach, and symptoms of gas and upset stomach associated with those conditions. Fast-Acting MYLANTA® and Extra Strength Fast-Acting MYLANTA® are also indicated as antacids for the symptomatic relief of hyperacidity associated with the diagnosis of peptic ulcer, gastritis, peptic esophagitis, heartburn and hiatal hernia and as antiflatulents to alleviate the symptoms of mucus-entrapped gas, including postoperative gas pain.

Advantages:

Fast-Acting MYLANTA and Extra Strength Fast-Acting MYLANTA are homogenized for a smooth, creamy taste. The choice of three pleasant-tasting liquid flavors and the non-constipating formula encourage patient acceptance, thereby minimizing the skipping of prescribed doses. Fast-Acting MYLANTA and Extra Strength Fast-Acting MYLANTA liquid are very low in sodium. Fast-Acting MYLANTA and Extra Strength Fast-Acting MYLANTA provide consistent relief in patients suffering from distress associated with hyperacidity, mucus-entrapped gas, or swallowed air.

Directions: Liquid:

Shake well. 2-4 teaspoonfuls between meals and at bedtime, or as directed by a physician.

Warnings:

Keep this and all drugs out of the reach of children. Do not take more than 24 tsps of Fast-Acting MYLANTA® or 12 tsps of Extra Strength Fast-Acting MYLANTA® in a 24-hour period or use the maximum dose of this product for more than two weeks, except under the advice and supervison of a physician. Do not use this product if you have kidney disease.

Prolonged use of aluminum-containing antacids in patients with renal failure may result in or worsen dialysis osteomalacia. Elevated tissue aluminum levels contribute to the development of the dialysis encephalopathy and osteomalacia syndromes. Small amounts of aluminum are absorbed from the gastrointestinal tract and renal excretion of aluminum is impaired in renal failure. Aluminum is not well removed by dialysis because it is bound to albumin and transferrin, which do not cross dialysis membranes. As a result, aluminum is deposited in bone, and dialysis osteomalacia may develop when large amounts of aluminum are ingested orally by patients with impaired renal function.

Aluminum forms insoluble complexes with phosphate in the gastrointestinal tract, thus decreasing phosphate absorption. Prolonged use of aluminum-containing antacids by normophosphatemic patients may result in hypophosphatemia if phosphate intake is not adequate. In its more severe forms, hypophosphatemia can lead to anorexia, malaise, muscle weakness, and osteomalacia.

Drug Interaction Precaution:

Antacids may interact with certain prescription drugs. If you are presently taking a prescription drug, do not take this product without checking with your physician or other health professional.

How Supplied:

Fast-Acting MYLANTA® and Extra Strength Fast-Acting MYLANTA® are available as white liquid suspensions in pleasant-tasting flavors, Original, Cherry Creme and Cool Mint Creme. Liquids are supplied in bottles of 5 oz, 12 oz, and 24 oz. Also available for hospital use in liquid unit dose bottles of 1 oz and bottles of 5 oz.

MYLANTA®

NDC 16837-610 ORIGINAL LIQUID
NDC 16837-629 COOL MINT CREME LIQUID
NDC 16837-621 CHERRY CREME LIQUID
NDC 16837-817 Lemon Twist Liquid

MYLANTA® Extra Strength

NDC 16837-652 ORIGINAL LIQUID
NDC 16837-624 COOL MINT CREME LIQUID
NDC 16837-622 CHERRY CREME LIQUID
NDC 16837-818 Lemon Twist Liquid

PROFESSIONAL LABELING

Indications: Stress-induced upper gastrointestinal hemorrhage: Extra Strength Fast-Acting MYLANTA® is indicated for the prevention of stress-induced upper gastrointestinal hemorrhage. Hyperacidic conditions: As an antacid, for the symptomatic relief of hyperacidity associated with the diagnosis of peptic ulcer and other gastrointestinal conditions where a high degree of acid neutralization is desired.

Directions: Prevention of stress-induced upper gastrointestinal hemorrhage: 1) Aspirate stomach via nasogastric tube* and record pH. 2) Instill 10 mL of Extra Strength Fast-Acting MYLANTA® followed by 30 mL of water via nasogastric tube. Clamp tube. 3) Wait one hour. Aspirate stomach and record pH. 4a) If pH equals or exceeds 4.0, apply drainage or intermittent suction for one hour, then repeat the cycle. 4b) If pH is less than 4.0, instill double (20 mL) Extra Strength Fast-Acting MYLANTA® followed by 30 mL of water. Clamp tube. 5) Wait one hour. If pH equals or exceeds 4.0, see number 7, if pH is still less than 4.0, instill double (40 mL) Extra Strength Fast-Acting MYLANTA® followed by 30 mL of water. Clamp tube. 6) Wait one hour. If pH equals or exceeds 4.0, see number 7. If pH is still less than 4.0, instill double (80 mL)† Extra Strength Fast-Acting MYLANTA® followed by 30 mL of water. 7) Drain for one hour and repeat cycle with the effective dosage of Extra Strength Fast-Acting MYLANTA®.

*If nasogastric tube is not in place, administer 20 mL of Extra Strength Fast-Acting MYLANTA® orally q2h.

†In a recent clinical study[1] 20 mL of Extra Strength Fast-Acting MYLANTA®, q2h, was sufficient in more than 85 percent of the patients. No patient studied required more than 80 mL of Extra Strength Fast-Acting MYLANTA® q2h.

In hyperacid states for symptomatic relief: One or two teaspoonfuls as needed between meals and at bedtime or as directed by a physician. Higher dosage regimens may be employed under the direct supervision of a physician in the treatment of active peptic ulcer disease.

Precautions: Aluminum-magnesium hydroxide containing antacids should be used with caution in patients with renal impairment.

Adverse Effects: Occasional regurgitation and mild diarrhea have been reported with the dosage recommended for the prevention of stress-induced upper gastrointestinal hemorrhage.

References: 1. Zinner MJ, Zuidema GD, Smigh PL, Mignosa M: The prevention of upper gastrointestinal tract bleeding in patients in an intensive care unit. *Surg Gynecol Obster* 153:214–220, 1981. 2. Lucas CE, Sugawa C, Riddle J, et al.: Natural history and surgical dilemma of "stress" gastric bleeding. *Arch Surg* 102:266–273, 1971. 3. Hastings PR, Skillman JJ, Bushnell LS, Silen W: Antacid titration in the prevention of acute gastrointestinal bleeding: a controlled, randomized trial in 100 critically ill patients. *N Engl J Med* 298:1042–1045, 1978. 4. Day SB, MacMillan BG, Altemeier WA: *Curling's Ulcer, An Experience of Nature.* Springfield, IL, Charles C Thomas Co., 1972, p. 205. 5. Skillman JJ, Bushnell LS, Goldman H, Silen W: Respiratory failure, hypotension, sepsis, and jaundice. A clinical syndrome associated with lethal hemorrhage from acute stress ulceration of the stomach. *Am J Surg* 117:523–530, 1969. 6. Priebe HJ, Skillman J, Bushnell LS, et al. Antacid versus cimetidine in preventing acute gastrointestinal bleeding. *N Engl J Med* 302:426–430, 1980. 7. Silen W: The prevention and management of stress ulcers. *Hosp Pract* 15:93–97, 1980. 8. Hermann V, Kaminski DL: Evaluation of intragastric pH in acutely ill patients. *Arch Surg* 114:511–514, 1979. 9. Martin LF, Staloch DK, Simonowitz DA, et al.: Failure of cimetidine prophylaxis in the crit-

Continued on next page

Fast-Acting Mylanta—Cont.

ically ill. *Arch Surg* 114:492–496, 1979. 10. Zinner MJ, Turtinen L, Gurll NJ, Reynolds DG: The effect of metiamide on gastric mucosal injury in rat restraint. *Clin Res* 23:484A, 1975. 11. Zinner M, Turtinen BA, Gurll NJ: The role of acid and ischemia in production of stress ulcers during canine hemorrhagic shock. *Surgery* 77:807–816, 1975. 12. Winans CS: Prevention and treatment of stress ulcer bleeding: Antacids or cimetidine? *Drug Ther Bull* (hospital) 12:37–45, 1981.

Shown in Product Identification Guide, page 507

FAST ACTING MYLANTA SUPREME ANTACID LIQUID

Description: Fast acting Mylanta Supreme is a revolutionary liquid antacid that works fast and tastes great. It has a fresh smooth taste and texture that goes down easy and doesn't leave that chalky aftertaste. Plus, Mylanta Supreme is rich in calcium.

Active Ingredients: Each 5 ml teaspoon contains:

Calcium carbonate 400 mg
Magnesium hydroxide 135 mg

Inactive Ingredients: Flavors, hydroxyethyl cellulose, purified water, simethicone, sodium saccharin, sorbitol, xanthan gum. *Cool Mint Liquid Flavor* also contain: D&C Yellow #10, FD&C Blue #1.

Sodium Content: Each 5 ml teaspoon contains 0.7 mg of sodium.

ACID NEUTRALIZING CAPACITY: Two teaspoonfuls provide 25.2 MEq of acid neutralizing capacity.

Indications: Mylanta Supreme is indicated for the relief of heartburn, acid indigestion, sour stomach, upset stomach associated with these conditions and overindulgence in food and drink.

Directions: Shake Well. Take 2–4 teaspoonfuls between meals, at bedtime, or as directed by a physician.

Warnings: Keep this and all drugs out of the reach of children. Do not take more than 18 teaspoonfuls in a 24-hour period, or use the maximum dosage for more than two weeks, or use this product if you have kidney disease except under the advice and supervision of a physician.

Drug Interaction Precaution: Antacids may interact with certain prescription drugs. If you are presently taking a prescription drug, do not take this product without checking with your physician or other health professional.

How Supplied: Fast Acting Mylanta Supreme is available as white liquid suspensions in cherry, and cool mint flavors.

NDC 16837-825 Cherry
NDC 16837-819 Mint
Shown in Product Identification Guide, page 507

Ultra MYLANTA CALCI TABS
Antacid/Calcium Supplement
Extra Strength MYLANTA CALCI TABS
Antacid/Calcium Supplement

Indications: For fast relief of acid indigestion, heartburn, sour stomach and upset stomach associated with these symptoms. Can also be used as a daily source of extra calcium.

Active Ingredient: Ultra Mylanta Calci Tabs - Calcium Carbonate USP, 1,000 mg per tablet
Extra Strength Calci Tabs - Calcium Carbonate USP, 750 mg per tablet

Inactive Ingredients: Ultra Mylanta Calci Tabs: Fruit Medley and Cool Mint: Dextrose, Maltodextrin, Magnesium Stearate, Starch, Cellulose, Citric and Fumaric Acids, Natural and Artificial Flavors, Mineral Oil, Sucrose, Ethylmaltol, Crospovidone, Hydroxypropyl Methylcellulose and Stearic Acid and may contain (Cool Mint: FD&C Yellow #5 (tartrazine), FD&C Blue #1; Fruit Medley: FD&C Blue #1, D&C red #27, FD&C Yellow #6, FD&C Yellow #5 (Tartrazine).
Extra Strength Mylanta Calci Tabs: Fruit Medley and Cool Mint: Dextrose, Maltodextrin, Microcrystalline Cellulose, Magnesium Stearate, Starch, Cellulose, Citric and Fumaric Acids, Natural and Artificial Flavors, Mineral Oil, Sucrose, Ethylmaltol, Crospovidone, Hydroxypropyl Methylcellulose and Stearic Acid and may contain (Cool Mint: FD&C Yellow #5 (Tartrazine), FD&C Blue #1; Fruit Medley: FD&C Blue #1 D&C Red #27 FD&C Yellow #6, FD&C Yellow #5 (Tartrazine).

Actions: Mylanta Calci Tabs provide rapid neutralization of stomach acid. Each Ultra Mylanta Calci Tab tablet has an acid-neutralizing capacity (ANC) of 20 mEq and each Extra Strength Mylanta Calci Tab tablet has an ANC of 15 mEq per tablet.

Warnings: Ultra Mylanta Calci Tabs - Do not take more than 8 tablets in a 24-hour period or use the maximum dosage of this product for more than two weeks except under the advice and supervision of a physician. Keep this and all drugs out of the reach of children. **Extra Strength Calci Tabs -** Do not take more than 10 tablets in a 24-hour period or use the maximum dosage of this product for more than two weeks except under the advice and supervision of a physician. Keep this and all drugs out of the reach of children.

Drug Interaction Precaution: Antacids may interact with certain prescription drugs. If you are presently taking a prescription drug, do not take this product without checking with your physician or health professional.

Directions For Antacid Use: Ultra Mylanta Calci Tabs – Chew 2–3 tablets as symptoms occur. Repeat hourly if symptoms return or as directed by a physician. **Extra Strength Mylanta Calci Tabs –** Chew 2–4 talbets as symptoms occur. Repeat hourly if symptoms return or as directed by a physician.

Use As A Dietary Supplement: IMPORTANT INFORMATION ON OSTEOPOROSIS:
Research shows that certain ethnic, age and other groups are at a higher risk for developing osteoporosis, including Caucasian and Asian teen and young adult women, menopausal women, older persons and those persons with a family history of fragile bones. **A balanced diet with enough calcium and regular exercise will help you to build and maintain healthy bones and may reduce your risk of developing osteoporosis later in life.** Adequate calcium is important, but daily intakes above 2,000 mg are not likely to provide any additional benefit.

Directions For Calcium Supplement Use: Ultra Mylanta Calci Tabs – Chew 2 tablets twice daily. Average daily calcium intake should not exceed 6 tablets. *Other Information:* The 1,000 mg of calcium carbonate in each tablet provide 400 mg of elemental calcium. **Extra Strength Mylanta Calci Tabs –** Chew 2 tablets twice daily. Average daily calcium intake should not exceed 8 tablets. *Other Information:* The 750 mg of calcium carbonate in each tablet provide 300 mg of elemental calcium. [See table below]

Supplement Facts:

Serving Size	Ultra Mylanta Calci Tabs 2 Tablets		Extra Strength Mylanta Calci Tabs 2 Tablets	
Amount Per Serving		*% Daily Value*		*% Daily Value*
Calories	10		10	
Total Carbohydrates	2 g	less than 1%	2 g	less than 1%
Sugars	2 g		2 g	
Calcium	800 mg	80%	600	60%

How Supplied: Ultra and Extra Strength Mylanta Calci Tab are provided in chewable tablets in Fruit Medley and Cool Mint Flavors.

NDC 16837-059-96   96 Chewable Tablets Fruit Medley

NDC 16837-057-96   96 Chewable Tablets Cool Mint

NDC 16837-058-72   72 Chewable Tablets Fruit Medley

NDC 16837-056-72   72 Chewable Tablets Cool Mint

Shown in Product Identification Guide, page 507

MYLANTA® GAS Relief Tablets
Maximum Strength MYLANTA® GAS
Relief Tablets
[*My-lan '-ta*]
Maximum Strength MYLANTA® GAS Softgels

Active Ingredients:
Each tablet contains:

	Simethicone
MYLANTA® GAS Relief Maximum Strength	80 mg
MYLANTA® GAS Relief Maximum Strength	125 mg
MYLANTA® GAS Softgels	125 mg.

Inactive Ingredients: TABLETS: Dextrates, flavor, magnesium stearate, silicon dioxide, tribasic calcium phosphate. Cherry: D&C Red #7.

SOFTELGELS: FD&C blue #1, gelatin, glycerin, iron oxide black, peppermint oil, titanium dioxide.

Indications: For relief of the symptoms of excess gas in the digestive tract. Such gas is frequently caused by excessive swallowing of air or by eating foods that disagree. Maximum Strength MYLANTA® GAS Softgels, MYLANTA® GAS Relief, and Maximum Strength MYLANTA® GAS Relief Tablets are high capacity antiflatulents for adjunctive treatment of many conditions in which the retention of gas may be a problem, such as the following: air swallowing, postoperative gaseous distention, peptic ulcer, spastic or irritable colon, diverticulosis. If condition persists, consult your physician.

Maximum Strength MYLANTA® GAS Softgels, MYLANTA® GAS Relief, and Maximum Strength MYLANTA® GAS Relief Tablets have a defoaming action that relieves flatulence by dispersing and preventing the formation of mucus-surrounded gas pockets in the gastrointestinal tract. Maximum Strength MYLANTA® GAS Softgels, MYLANTA® GAS Relief, and Maximum Strength MYLANTA® GAS Relief Tablets act in the stomach and intestines to change the surface tension of gas bubbles enabling them to coalesce, thereby freeing and eliminating the gas more easily by belching or passing flatus.

Directions: MYLANTA® GAS Relief Tablets:
One tablet four times daily after meals and at bedtime. May also be taken as needed up to six tablets daily or as directed by a physician.

Maximum Strength MYLANTA® GAS Relief Tablets:
One tablet four times daily after meals and at bedtime or as directed by a physician.

Maximum Strength MYLANTA® GAS Softgels:
Take 1–2 softgels as needed after meals and at bedtime. Do not exceed 4 softgels per day unless directed by a physician.

Warnings: Keep this and all drugs out of the reach of children.

How Supplied: MYLANTA® GAS Relief Tablets are available as white (mint) or pink (cherry) scored, chewable tablets identified "MYL GAS 80." Mint NDC 16837-858. Cherry NDC 16837-859.

Maximum Strength MYLANTA® GAS Relief Tablets are available as white, scored, chewable tablets identified "MYL GAS 125." NDC 16837-455.

Maximum Strength MYLANTA® GAS Softgels are available as blue softgels. "MYL" NDC 16837-611.

Shown in Product Identification Guide, page 507

FAST-ACTING MYLANTA ULTRA TABS
AND FAST-ACTING MYLANTA ANTACID GELCAPS
[*mylan 'ta*]
Calcium Carbonate and Magnesium Hydroxide Tablets/Gelcaps Antacid

Description: Fast-Acting Mylanta Ultra Tabs and Fast-Acting Mylanta Antacid Gelcaps are well balanced, pleasant tasting antacid medications that provide consistent, effective relief of symptoms associated with gastric hyperacidity. Non-constipating and very low in sodium, Fast-Acting Mylanta Ultra Tabs and Fast-Acting Mylanta Antacid Gelcaps contain two proven antacids, calcium carbonate and magnesium hydroxide.

Active Ingredients
Each tablet/gelcap contains:

	Fast-Acting Mylanta Antacid Gelcaps	Fast-Acting Mylanta Ultra Tabs
Calcium Carbonate	550mg	700mg
Magnesium Hydroxide	125mg	300mg

Inactive Ingredients: Fast-Acting Mylanta Antacid Gelcaps: Benzyl alcohol, butylparaben, castor oil, crospovidone, D&C Red #28, D&C Yellow #10, disodium calcium edetate, FD&C Blue #1, FD&C, Red #40, gelatin, hydroxypropyl methylcellulose, magnesium stearate, methylparaben, microcrystalline cellulose, propylene glycol, propylparaben, sodium lauryl sulfate, sodium propionate, starch, titanium dioxide.

Fast-Acting Mylanta Ultra Tabs: Cherry: Citric Acid, confectioner's sugar, D&C Red #27, flavors, magnesium stearate, sodium lauryl sulfate, sorbitol, starch.

Mint: Confectioner's sugar, D&C Yellow #10, FD&C Blue #1, flavors, magnesium stearate, sodium lauryl sulfate, sorbitol, starch.

Each tablet/gelcap contains the following amount of sodium:

Fast-Acting Mylanta Ultra Tabs	Fast-Acting Mylanta Antacid Gelcaps
0.6mg	0.7mg

Acid Neutralizing Capacity
Two tablets/gelcaps have the following acid neutralizing capacity:

Fast-Acting Mylanta Ultra Tabs	Fast-Acting Mylanta Antacid Gelcaps
48.6mEq	23.0mEq

Indications: Fast-Acting Mylanta Ultra Tabs and Fast-Acting Mylanta Antacid Gelcaps are indicated for the relief of heartburn, acid indigestion, sour stomach and upset stomach associated with these conditions. Fast-Acting Mylanta Ultra Tabs and Fast-Acting Mylanta Antacid Gelcaps are also indicated as antacids for the symptomatic relief of hyperacidity associated with the diagnosis of peptic ulcer, gastritis, peptic esophagitis, heartburn and hiatal hernia.

Directions: Thoroughly chew 2–4 tablets between meals, at bedtime or as directed by a physician.

Swallow 2–4 gelcaps as needed or directed by physician.

Warnings: Keep this and all drugs out of the reach of children. Do not take more than 10 Tablets of Fast-Acting Mylanta Ultra Tabs or 12 Gelcaps of Fast-Acting Mylanta Antacid Gelcaps in a 24-hour period, or use the maximum dosage for more than two weeks. Do not use this product if you have kidney disease, except under the advise and supervision of a physician.

Drug Interaction Precaution: Antacids may interact with certain prescription drugs. If you are presently taking a prescription drug, do not take this product without checking with your physician or other health professional.

Continued on next page

Fast-Acting Mylanta—Cont.

How Supplied:

Fast-Acting Mylanta Antacid Gel-caps:
NDC: 16837-850-24   24 Gelcaps
NDC: 16837-850-50   50 Gelcaps
NDC: 16837-850-10   100 Gelcaps

Fast-Acting Mylanta Ultra Tabs:
NDC: 16837-849-36   3 Roll Mint Pack
NDC: 16837-849-35   35 Mint Tablets
NDC: 16837-849-70   70 Mint Tablets
NDC: 16837-869-35   35 Cherry Tablets
NDC: 16837-869-70   70 Cherry Tablets

Shown in Product Identification Guide, page 507

PEPCID AC®

TABLETS, Chewable Tablets and Gelcaps

Description:

Active Ingredient: Famotidine 10 mg per tablet.
Inactive Ingredients: TABLETS: Hydroxypropyl cellulose, hydroxypropyl methylcellulose, red iron oxide, magnesium stearate, microcrystalline cellulose, starch, talc, titanium dioxide.
CHEWABLE TABLETS: aspartame, cellulose acetate, flavors, hydroxypropyl cellulose, hydroxypropyl methylcellulose, lactose, magnesium stearate, mannitol, microcrystalline cellulose, red ferric oxide.
GELCAPS: benzyl alcohol, black iron oxide, butylparaben, castor oil, edetate calcium disodium, FD&C red #40, gelatin, hydroxypropyl methylcellulose, magnesium stearate, methylparaben, microcrystalline cellulose, pregelatinized corn starch, propylene glycol, propylparaben, sodium lauryl sulfate, sodium propionate, talc, titanium dioxide.

Product Benefits:

• **1 Tablet, Chewable Tablet or Gelcap** relieves heartburn and acid indigestion.
• Pepcid AC prevents heartburn and acid indigestion brought on by consuming food and beverages.
It contains famotidine, a prescription-proven medicine.
The ingredient in PEPCID AC, famotidine, has been prescribed by doctors for years to treat millions of patients safely and effectively. The active ingredient in PEPCID AC has been taken safely with many frequently prescribed medications.

Action:

It is normal for the stomach to produce acid, especially after consuming food and beverages. However, acid in the wrong place (the esophagus), or too much acid, can cause burning pain and discomfort that interfere with everyday activities.

• **Heartburn—Caused by acid in the esophagus**

In clinical studies, PEPCID AC was significantly better than placebo pills in relieving and preventing heartburn.

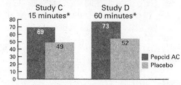

A valve-like muscle called the lower esophageal sphincter (LES) is relaxed in an open position — Burning pain/discomfort — Excess acid moves up into esophagus

Percent of heartburn episodes completely relieved

Study A: Pepcid AC 69, Placebo 41
Study B: Pepcid AC 67, Placebo 53

Percent of patients with prevention or reduction of heartburn symptoms

Study C 15 minutes*: Pepcid AC 69, Placebo 49
Study D 60 minutes*: Pepcid AC 73, Placebo 52

*Time taken before eating a meal that is expected to cause symptoms.

Uses:

• **For Relief** of heartburn, associated with acid indigestion, and sour stomach;
• **For Prevention** of heartburn associated with acid indigestion and sour stomach brought on by consuming food and beverages.

Tips for Managing Heartburn:
• Do not lie flat or bend over soon after eating.
• Do not eat late at night, or just before bedtime.
• Avoid food or drinks that are more likely to cause heartburn, such as rich, spicy, fatty, and fried foods, chocolate, caffeine, alcohol, and even some fruits and vegetables.
• Eat slowly and do not eat big meals.
• If you are overweight, lose weight.
• If you smoke, quit smoking.
• Raise the head of your bed.
• Wear loose fitting clothing around your stomach.

Warnings:
Allergy alert Do not use if you are allergic to famotidine or other acid reducers
Do not use:
• if you have trouble swallowing
• with other acid reducers
Stop use and ask a doctor if:
• stomach pain continues
• you need to take this product for more than 14 days
If pregnant or breast-feeding, ask a health professional before use.
Keep out of reach of children. In case of overdose, get medical help or contact a Poison Control Center right away.

Directions:
• Tablet: To relieve symptoms, swallow 1 tablet with a glass of water.
  Chewable Tablet: To relieve symptoms, chew one tablet thoroughly
  Gelcap: To relieve symptoms, swallow one gelcap with a glass of water.
• Tablet & Gelcap: To prevent symptoms, swallow one tablet or gelcap with a glass of water any time from 15 to 60 minutes before eating food or drinking beverages that cause heartburn.
• Chewable Tablet: To prevent symptoms, chew one chewable tablet before swallowing any time from 15 to 60 minutes before eating food or drinking beverages that cause heartburn.
• Can be used up to twice daily (up to 2 tablets or gelcaps in 24 hours).
• This product should not be given to children under 12 years old unless directed by a doctor.

Other Information:
• read the directions and warnings before use
• protect from moisture
• keep the carton and package insert, they contain important information
• store at 25°–33°C (77°–86°F)
in addition to the above the following also applies to the chewable tablet
• do not use if individual pouch is open or torn
• phenylketonurics: contains phenylalanine 1.4 mg per chewable tablet

How Supplied:

Pepcid AC Tablet is available as a rose-colored tablet identified as 'PEPCID AC'. NDC 16837-872
Pepcid AC Gelcap is available as a rose and white gelatin coated, capsule shaped tablet identified as 'PEPCID AC'. NDC 16837-856
Pepcid AC Chewable Tablet is available as a rose-colored chewable tablet identified as 'PEPCID AC'. NDC 16837-873

Shown in Product Identification Guide, page 508

Pepcid® Complete
Acid Reducer + Antacid with DUAL ACTION
Reduces and Neutralizes Acid

Description: Pepcid Complete combines an acid reducer (famotidine) with antacids (calcium carbonate and magnesium hydroxide) to relieve heartburn in two different ways: Acid reducers decrease the production of new stomach acid; antacids neutralize acid that is already in the stomach. The active ingredients in PEPCID COMPLETE have been used for years to treat acid-related problems in millions of people safely and effectively.

Uses: To relieve heartburn associated with acid indigestion and sour stomach.

Active Ingredients: (in each chewablet tablet)	Purpose:
Famotidine 10mg	Acid Reducer
Calcium Carbonate 800 mg	Antacid
Magnesium Hydroxide 165 mg	Antacid

Inactive Ingredients:
Cellulose acetate, corn starch, dextrates, flavors, hydroxypropyl cellulose, hydroxypropyl methylcellulose, lactose, magnesium stearate, pregelatinized starch, red iron oxide, sodium lauryl sulfate, sugar

In clinical studies, PEPCID COMPLETE was significantly better than placebo pills in relieving heartburn.

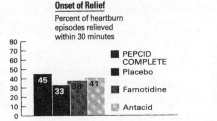

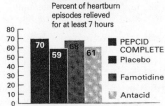

Sodium Content:
Each chewable tablet contains 0.5 mg of sodium.

Acid Neutralizing Capacity:
Each chewable tablet contains 21.7 mEq of acid neutralizing capacity.

Action:
It is normal for the stomach to produce acid, especially after consuming food and beverages. However, acid in the stomach may move up into the wrong place (the esophagus), causing burning pain and discomfort that interfere with everyday activities.

Heartburn—Caused by acid in the esophagus
- Burning pain/discomfort in esophagus
- A valve-like muscle called the lower esophageal sphincter (LES) is relaxed in an open position
- Acid moves up from stomach

PROVEN EFFECTIVE IN CLINICAL STUDIES
[See graphic above]

Directions:
- Adults and children 12 years and over:
  - **do not swallow tablet whole; chew completely.**
  - to relieve symptoms, chew 1 tablet before swallowing.
  - do not use more than 2 chewable tablets in 24 hours.
- Children under 12 years: ask a doctor.

Warnings:
- **Allergy alert:** Do not use if you are allergic to famotidine or other acid reducers.
- **Do not use:** if you have trouble swallowing.
- With other famotidine products or acid reducers.
- **Ask a doctor or pharmacist before use if you are** taking a prescription drug. Antacids may interact with certain prescription drugs.
- **Stop use and ask a doctor if** stomach pain continues
- You need to take this product for more than 14 days.
- **If pregnant or breast-feeding,** ask a health professional before use.
- **Keep out of reach of children.** In case of overdose, get medical help or contact a poison control center right away.

Tips For Managing Heartburn
- Do not lie flat or bend over soon after eating.

- Do not eat late at night, or just before bedtime.
- Certain foods or drinks are more likely to cause heartburn, such as rich, spicy, fatty, and fried foods, chocolate, caffeine, alcohol, and even some fruits and vegetables.
- Eat slowly and do not eat big meals.
- If you are overweight, lose weight.
- If you smoke, quit smoking.
- Raise the head of your bed.
- Wear loose fitting clothing around your stomach.

Other Information:
- read the directions and warnings before use.
- keep the carton and package insert. They contain important information.
- store at 25°–30°C (77°–86° F).
- protect from moisture.

How Supplied:
Pepcid Complete is available as a rose-colored chewable tablet identified by 'P'. NDC 16837-888

Shown in Product Identification Guide, page 508

Lederle Consumer Health

A Division of Whitehall-Robins Healthcare
FIVE GIRALDA FARMS
MADISON, NJ 07940

Direct Inquiries to:
Lederle Consumer Product Information
(800) 282-8805

FIBERCON®
[fĭ-bĕr-cŏn]
Calcium Polycarbophil
Bulk-Forming Laxative

Active ingredient
(in each caplet):
Calcium polycarbophil 625 mg (eqivalent to 500 mg polycarbophil)

Inactive ingredients: calcium carbonate, caramel, crospovidone, hydroxypropyl methylcellulose, magnesium stearate, microcrystalline cellulose, mineral oil, povidone, silica gel and sodium lauryl sulfate

Uses:
- relieves constipation to help restore and maintain regularity
- this product generally produces bowel movement in 12 to 72 hours

Directions:
- take this product (child or adult dose) with at least 8 ounces (a full glass) of water or other fluid. Taking this product without enough liquid may cause choking. See choking warning.
- FiberCon works naturally so continued use for one to three days is normally required to provide full benefit. Dosage may vary according to diet, exercise, previous laxative use or severity of constipation.

[See table below]

Warnings:
Choking: Taking this product without adequate fluid may cause it to swell and block your throat or esophagus and may cause choking. Do not take this product if you have difficulty in swallowing. If you experience chest pain, vomiting, or difficulty in swallowing or breathing after taking this product, seek immediate medical attention.

Ask a doctor before use if you have:
- abdominal pain, nausea, or vomiting
- a sudden change in bowel habits that persists over a period of 2 weeks

When using this product:
- do not use for more than 7 days unless directed by a doctor
- do not take caplets more than 4 times in a 24 hour period unless directed by a doctor

Stop use and ask a doctor if rectal bleeding occurs or if you fail to have a bowel movement after use of this or any other laxative. These could be signs of a serious condition

Drug Interaction precaution: Each caplet contains 122mg calcium. If you are taking any form of tetracycline antibiotic, FiberCon should be taken at least 1 hour before or 2 hours after you have taken the antibiotic

Keep out of reach of children. In case of overdose, get medical help or contact a Poison Control Center right away

Storage: Protect contents from moisture. Store at 20–25°C (68–77°F)

How Supplied: Film-coated scored caplets.

Package of 36 caplets, and

Bottles of 60, 90 and 150 caplets.

Age	Recommended dose	Daily maximum
adults & children over 12	2 caplets once a day	up to 4 times a day
children 6 to 12 years	1 caplet once a day	up to 4 times a day
children under 6 years	consult a physician	

3M

BUILDING 304-1-01
ST PAUL, MN 55144-1000

Direct Inquiries to:
Customer Service
(800) 537-2191

For Medical Emergencies Contact:
(651) 733-2882 (answered 24 hrs.)

3M™ TITRALAC™ ANTACID AND TITRALAC™ EXTRA STRENGTH ANTACID
[T ĭ ' tră lăc]

Active Ingredients: Calcium Carbonate: *Regular:* 420mg./tablet (168 mg. elemental calcium). *Extra Strength:* 750mg/tablet (300 mg. elemental calcium).

Inactive Ingredients: Glycine, Magnesium Stearate, Saccharin, Spearmint Oil, Starch.

Indications: A spearmint flavored non-chalky antacid tablet which quickly relieves heartburn, sour stomach, acid indigestion and upset stomach associated with these symptoms.

Dosage and Administration: *Regular:* Two tablets every two or three hours as symptoms occur or as directed by a physician. Tablets can be chewed, swallowed or allowed to melt in the mouth. *Extra Strength:* One or two tablets every two or three hours as symptoms occur or as directed by a physician. Tablets can be chewed, swallowed or allowed to melt in the mouth.

Warnings: *Regular:* Do not take more than 19 tablets in a 24-hour period or use maximum dosage for more than two weeks, except under the advice and supervision of a physician. *Extra Strength:* Do not take more than ten tablets in a 24-hour period or use maximum dosage for more than two weeks, except under the advice and supervision of a physician. **Keep this and all medication out of the reach of children**

Drug Interaction Precaution: Antacids may interact with certain prescription drugs. If you are presently taking a prescription drug, do not take this product without checking with your physician or other health professional.

Dietary Information: Titralac antacid tablets are sugar free. They have a very low sodium content (1.1 mg/tablet) and a low aluminum content (2.0 mg/tablet).

How Supplied: *Regular:* Available in bottles of 40, 100, 1000 tablets. *Extra Strength:* Available in bottles of 100 tablets.
Shown in Product Identification Guide, page 508

3M™ TITRALAC™ PLUS ANTACID
[T ĭ 'tră lăc]

Active Ingredients: Calcium Carbonate: 420 mg/tablet (168 mg elemental calcium), Simethicone: 21 mg/tablet.

Inactive Ingredients: Glycine, Magnesium Stearate, Saccharin, Spearmint Oil, Starch. May also contain Croscarmellose Sodium.

Indications: A spearmint flavored non-chalky antacid which quickly relieves heartburn, sour stomach, acid indigestion, and accompanying gas often associated with these symptoms.

Dosage and Administration: Two tablets every two or three hours as symptoms occur or as directed by a physician. Tablets can be chewed, swallowed or allowed to melt in the mouth.

Warnings: Do not take more than 19 tablets in a 24-hour period or use maximum dosage for more than two weeks, except under the advice and supervision of a physician. **Keep this and all medication out of the reach of children.**

Drug Interaction Precaution: Antacids may interact with certain prescription drugs. If you are presently taking a prescription drug, do not take this product without checking with your physician or other health professional.

Dietary Information: Tablets are sugar free. They have a very low sodium content (1.1 mg/tablet) and a low aluminum content (1.0 mg/tablet).

How Supplied: Available in bottles of 100 tablets.
Shown in Product Identification Guide, page 508

Matol Botanical International, Ltd.

1111, 46th AVENUE
LACHINE, QUEBEC
CANADA H8T 3C5

Direct Inquiries to:
Ph: (800) 363-3890
website: www.matol.com

BIOMUNE OSF™ EXPRESS
Homeopathic nasal and throat spray for the relief of the symptoms associated with the common cold, influenza, sinusitis, otitis media and similar conditions

Active Ingredients: Silicea Compound—Silicea (Quartz) 22X, Argentum Nitricum 21X, Atropa Belladonna ex-herba 15X.

Inactive Ingredients: Filtered water, proprietary extract of whey permeate, 2-deoxy-d-glucose, eucalyptus oil, disodium EDTA, thimerosal, benzalkonium chloride, sodium hydroxide.

Indications: For the relief of symptoms of the common cold, influenza, sinusitis, otitis media and similar conditions.

Directions: For children 3 years to adult. One to two sprays in each nostril every four to six hours during acute symptoms and two to three times per day with chronic symptoms. Shake well before using.

Warning: Do not use if the imprinted seal is broken or missing. If symptoms persist for more than five days or worsen, contact a licensed health professional. As with any drug, if you are pregnant or nursing a baby, seek the advice of a licensed health care professional before using the product. Keep this and all medication out of the reach of children. Store at room temperature.

How Supplied: Biomune OSF™ Express comes in .75 fluid ounce in metered spray bottle.

Clinical Study: *The Use of Matol Biomune OSF™ Express, a Homeopathic Medicine, in the Prevention and Treatment of Recurrent Otitis Media by Jesse A. Stoff, MD* Abstract: The study using matol Biomune OSF™ Express, a homeopathic medicine with the active ingredient Silicea Compound, as compared to pharmaceutical intervention, was carried out with twenty-six (26) children with a history of recurrent acute otitis media (RAOM).
Discussion: The use of the product was shown to be safe, rapid and effective and is indicated as a clear alternative to pharmaceutical intervention for the treatment of upper respiratory infection and recurrent otitis media in young children.
Shown in Product Identification Guide, page 508

McNeil Consumer Healthcare

Division of McNeil-PPC, Inc.
FORT WASHINGTON, PA 19034

Direct Inquiries to:
Consumer Relationship Center
Fort Washington, PA 19034
(215) 273-7000

Maximum Strength Gas Aid Softgels

Description: Each softgel of Maximum Strength GasAid contains simethicone 125 mg.

Actions: Simethicone acts in the stomach and intestines by altering the surface tension of gas bubbles enabling them to

coalesce, thereby freeing and eliminating the gas more easily by belching or passing flatus.

Uses: Relieves bloating, pressure, fullness or stuffed feeling commonly referred to as gas.

Directions: adults and children 12 years and older: take 1–2 softgels as needed after meals and at bedtime. Do not take more than 4 softgels in 24 hours unless directed by a doctor.

Warnings: Keep out of reach of children.

Other Information:
• do not use if carton or any blister unit is open or broken
• Store at room temperature. Avoid high humidity and excessive heat (40°C). Protect from light.

Inactive Ingredients: D&C yellow #10, FD&C blue #1, FD&C red #40, gelatin, glycerin, peppermint oil, titanium dioxide.

How Supplied: Softgels in 12s, 24s, and 48s blister packaging. Each Maximum Strength GasAid softgel is oval, green in color, and imprinted with "I-G" on one side.

Shown in Product Identification Guide, page 509

IMODIUM® A–D Liquid and Caplets
(loperamide hydrochloride)

Description: Each 5 mL (teaspoon) of *IMODIUM® A-D* liquid contains loperamide hydrochloride 1 mg. *IMODIUM® A-D* liquid is stable, cherry-mint flavored, and clear in color. Each caplet of *IMODIUM® A-D* contains 2 mg of loperamide and is scored and colored green.

Actions: *IMODIUM® A-D* contains a clinically proven antidiarrheal medication. Loperamide HCl acts by slowing intestinal motility and by affecting water and electrolyte movement through the bowel.

Indication: *IMODIUM® A-D* controls the symptoms of diarrhea, including Traveler's Diarrhea.

Directions: Use the enclosed cup to accurately measure Imodium® A-D Liquid. Drink plenty of clear fluids to help prevent dehydration, which may accompany diarrhea.

ADULTS AND CHILDREN 12 YEARS OF AGE AND OLDER: Take 4 teaspoonfuls (1 dosage cup) or 2 caplets after the first loose bowel movement and 2 teaspoonfuls or 1 caplet after each subsequent loose bowel movement but no more than 8 teaspoonfuls or 4 caplets a day for no more than 2 days.

CHILDREN 9–11 YEARS OLD (60–95 LBS): Take 2 teaspoonfuls (1/2 dosage cup) or 1 caplet after the first loose bowel movement and 1 teaspoonful or 1/2 caplet after each subsequent loose bowel

movement but no more than 6 teaspoonfuls or 3 caplets a day for no more than 2 days.

CHILDREN 6–8 YEARS OLD (48–59 LBS): Take 2 teaspoonfuls (1/2 dosage cup) or 1 caplet after the first loose bowel movement and 1 teaspoonful or 1/2 caplet after each subsequent loose bowel movement but no more than 4 teaspoonfuls or 2 caplets a day for no more than 2 days. Professional Dosage Schedule for children 2–5 years old (24–47 lbs): 1 teaspoonful after first loose bowel movement, followed by 1 after each subsequent loose bowel movement. Do not exceed 3 teaspoonfuls a day.

Warnings: KEEP THIS AND ALL DRUGS OUT OF THE REACH OF CHILDREN. Do not use for more than two days unless directed by a physician. DO NOT USE IF DIARRHEA IS ACCOMPANIED BY HIGH FEVER (GREATER THAN 101°F), OR IF BLOOD OR MUCUS IS PRESENT IN THE STOOL, OR IF YOU HAVE HAD A RASH OR OTHER ALLERGIC REACTION TO LOPERAMIDE HCl. If you are taking antibiotics or have a history of liver disease, consult a physician before using this product. As with any drug, if you are pregnant or nursing a baby, seek the advice of a health professional before using this product. In case of accidental overdose, seek professional assistance or contact a poison control center immediately.

Professional Information:
Overdosage Information Overdosage of loperamide HCl in man may result in constipation, CNS depression and nausea. A slurry of activated charcoal administered promptly after ingestion of loperamide hydrochloride can reduce the amount of drug which is absorbed. If vomiting occurs spontaneously upon ingestion, a slurry of 100 grams of activated charcoal should be administered orally as soon as fluids can be retained. If vomiting has not occurred, and CNS depression is evident, gastric lavage should be performed followed by administration of 100 gms of the activated charcoal slurry through the gastric tube. In the event of overdosage, patients should be monitored for signs of CNS depression for at least 24 hours. Children may be more sensitive to central nervous system effects than adults. If CNS depression is observed, naloxone may be administered. If responsive to naloxone, vital signs must be monitored carefully for recurrence of symptoms of drug overdose for at least 24 hours after the last dose of naloxone.

Inactive Ingredients:
Liquid: Benzoic acid, citric acid, flavors, glycerin, propylene glycol, purified water, sodium benzoate, sorbitol, sucrose, contains 0.5% alcohol.
Caplets: Dibasic calcium phosphate, magnesium stearate, microcrystalline cellulose, colloidal silicon dioxide, FD&C Blue #1 and D&C Yellow #10.

How Supplied:
Liquid: Cherry-mint flavored liquid (clear) 2 fl. oz., and 4 fl. oz. tamper evident bottles with child resistant safety caps and special dosage cups. Store between 20–25 °C (69–77 °F). Avoid excessive heat.
Caplets: Green scored caplets in 6s, 12s, 18s, 24s and 48s blister packaging which is tamper evident and child resistant. Store at 15–30°C (59–86°F)

Shown in Product Identification Guide, page 509

IMODIUM® ADVANCED
Chewable Tablets
(loperamide HCl/simethicone)

Description: Each mint-flavored chewable tablet of *Imodium® Advanced* contains loperamide HCl 2 mg/simethicone 125 mg.

Actions: *Imodium® Advanced* combines original prescription strength Imodium® to control the symptoms of diarrhea plus simethicone to relieve bloating, pressure and cramps commonly referred to as gas. Loperamide HCl acts by slowing intestinal motility and by affecting water and electrolyte movement through the bowel. Simethicone acts in the stomach and intestines by altering the surface tension of gas bubbles enabling them to coalesce, thereby freeing and eliminating the gas more easily by belching or passing flatus.

Uses: Controls the symptoms of diarrhea plus bloating, pressure, and cramps commonly referred to as gas.

Directions: Chew the first dose and take with water after the first loose stool. If needed, chew the next dose and take with water after the next loose stool. Drink plenty of clear liquids to prevent dehydration.

Adults aged 12 years and over: Chew 2 tablets and take with water after the first loose stool. If needed, chew 1 tablet and take with water after the next loose stool. Do not exceed 4 tablets a day.

Children 9-11 years (60-95 lbs): Chew 1 tablet and take with water after the first loose stool. If needed, chew 1/2 tablet and take with water after the next loose stool. Do not exceed 3 tablets a day.

Children 6-8 years (48-59 lbs): Chew 1 tablet and take with water after the first loose stool. If needed, chew 1/2 tablet and take with water after the next loose stool. Do not exceed 2 tablets a day.

Children under 6 years old (up to 47 lbs): Consult a physician. Not intended for use in children under 6 years old.

Warnings:
Do Not Use If:
• You have a high fever (over 101° F)
• Blood or mucus is in your stool
• You have had a rash or other allergic reaction to Loperamide HCl

Continued on next page

Imodium Advanced—Cont.

Do Not Use Without Asking A Doctor:
• For more than 2 days
• If you are taking antibiotics
• If you have a history of liver disease
As with any drug, If you are pregnant or nursing a baby, seek the advice of a health professional before using this product.
• **Keep this and all drugs out of the reach of children.**
• In case of accidental overdose, seek professional assistance or call a poison control center immediately.

Professional Information:
Overdosage Information Overdosage of loperamide HCl in man may result in constipation, CNS depression and nausea. A slurry of activated charcoal administered promptly after ingestion of loperamide hydrochloride can reduce the amount of drug which is absorbed. If vomiting occurs spontaneously upon ingestion, a slurry of 100 grams of activated charcoal should be administered orally as soon as fluids can be retained. If vomiting has not occurred, and CNS depression is evident, gastric lavage should be performed followed by administration of 100 gms of the activated charcoal slurry through the gastric tube. In the event of overdosage, patients should be monitored for signs of CNS depression for at least 24 hours. Children may be more sensitive to central nervous system effects than adults. If CNS depression is observed, naloxone may be administered. If responsive to naloxone, vital signs must be monitored carefully for recurrence of symptoms of drug overdose for at least 24 hours after the last dose of naloxone. No treatment is necessary for the simethicone ingestion in this circumstance.

Inactive Ingredients: Cellulose acetate, corn starch, D&C Yellow No. 10, dextrates, FD&C Blue No. 1, flavors, microcrystalline cellulose, polymethacrylates, saccharin sodium, sorbitol, stearic acid, sucrose, tribasic calcium phosphate.

How Supplied: Mint Chewable Tablets in 6's, 12's, 18's, 30's, and 42's blister packaging which is tamper evident and child resistant. Each Imodium® Advanced tablet is round, light green in color and has "IMODIUM" embossed on one side and "2/125" on the other side. Store at 15–30°C (59–86°F).

Shown in Product Identification Guide, page 509

MOTRIN® IB ibuprofen Pain Reliever/Fever Reducer Tablets, Caplets and Gelcaps

Description:
Each *MOTRIN® IB Tablet, Caplet and Gelcap* contains ibuprofen 200 mg.

Indications:
MOTRIN® IB Tablets, Caplets and Gelcaps: For the temporary relief of head-ache, muscular aches, the minor pain of arthritis, toothache, backache, minor aches and pains associated with the common cold, the pain of menstrual cramps, and for reduction of fever.

Directions:
Do not take more than directed. Adults: Take 1 tablet, caplet or gelcap every 4 to 6 hours while symptoms persist. If pain or fever does not respond to 1 tablet, caplet or gelcap, 2 tablets, caplets or gelcaps may be used, but do not exceed 6 tablets, caplets or gelcaps in 24 hours, unless directed by a doctor. The smallest effective dose should be used. Take with food or milk if occasional and mild heartburn, upset stomach or stomach pain occurs with use. Consult a doctor if these symptoms are more than mild or if they persist. **Children:** Do not give this product to children under 12 except under the advice and supervision of a doctor.

Warnings:
Do not take for pain for more than 10 days or for fever for more than 3 days unless directed by a doctor. If pain or fever persists or gets worse, if new symptoms occur, or if the painful area is red or swollen, consult a doctor. These could be signs of a serious illness. If you are under a doctor's care for any serious condition, consult a doctor before taking this product. As with aspirin and acetaminophen, if you have any condition which requires you to take prescription drugs, or if you have had any problems or serious side effects from taking any non-prescription pain reliever, do not take MOTRIN® IB without first discussing it with your doctor. If you experience any symptoms which are unusual or seem unrelated to the condition for which you took ibuprofen, consult a doctor before taking any more of it. Although ibuprofen is indicated for the same conditions as aspirin and acetaminophen, it should not be taken with them except under a doctor's direction. Do not combine this product with any other ibuprofen-containing product. Keep this and all drugs out of the reach of children. In case of accidental overdose, seek professional assistance or contact a poison control center immediately. As with any drug, if you are pregnant or nursing a baby, seek the advice of a health professional before using this product. IT IS ESPECIALLY IMPORTANT NOT TO USE IBUPROFEN DURING THE LAST 3 MONTHS OF PREGNANCY UNLESS SPECIFICALLY DIRECTED TO DO SO BY A DOCTOR BECAUSE IT MAY CAUSE PROBLEMS IN THE UNBORN CHILD OR COMPLICATIONS DURING DELIVERY.

Allergy Alert: ibuprofen may cause a severe allergic reaction which may include: hives, facial swelling, asthma (wheezing), shock.

Do not use if you have ever had an allergic reaction to any other pain reliever/fever reducer.

Stop use and ask a doctor if an allergic reaction occurs. Seek medical help right away.

Alcohol Warning: If you consume 3 or more alcoholic drinks every day, ask your doctor whether you should take ibuprofen or other pain relievers/fever reducers. Ibuprofen may cause stomach bleeding.

Professional Information:
Overdosage Information for Adult Motrin®
IBUPROFEN
The *toxicity of ibuprofen* overdose is dependent upon the amount of drug ingested and the time elapsed since ingestion, though individual response may vary, which makes it necessary to evaluate each case individually. Although uncommon, serious toxicity and death have been reported in the medical literature with ibuprofen overdosage. The most frequently reported symptoms of ibuprofen overdose include abdominal pain, nausea, vomiting, lethargy and drowsiness. Other central nervous system symptoms include headache, tinnitus, CNS depression and seizures. Metabolic acidosis, coma, acute renal failure and apnea (primarily in very young children) may rarely occur. Cardiovascular toxicity, including hypotension, bradycardia, tachycardia and atrial fibrillation, also have been reported. The *treatment of acute ibuprofen overdose* is primarily supportive. Management of hypotension, acidosis and gastrointestinal bleeding may be necessary. In cases of acute overdose, the stomach should be emptied through ipecac-induced emesis or lavage. Emesis is most effective if initiated within 30 minutes of ingestion. Orally administered activated charcoal may help in reducing the absorption and reabsorption of ibuprofen. In children, the estimated amount of ibuprofen ingested per body weight may be helpful to predict the potential for development of toxicity although each case must be evaluated. Ingestion of less than 100 mg/kg is unlikely to produce toxicity. Children ingesting 100 to 200 mg/kg may be managed with induced emesis and a minimal observation time of four hours. Children ingesting 200 to 400 mg/kg of ibuprofen should have immediate gastric emptying and at least four hours observation in a health care facility. Children ingesting greater than 400 mg/kg require immediate medical referral, careful observation and appropriate supportive therapy. Ipecac-induced emesis is not recommended in overdoses greater than 400 mg/kg because of the risk of convulsions and the potential for aspiration of gastric contents. In adult patients the history of the dose reportedly ingested does not appear to be predictive of toxicity. The need for referral and follow-up must be judged by the circumstances at the time of the overdose ingestion. Symptomatic adults should be admitted to a health care facility for observation.
Our Adult MOTRIN® combination products contain pseudoephedrine in addition to ibuprofen. For basic overdose information regarding pseudoephed-

rine, please see below. For additional emergency information, please contact your local poison control center.

PSEUDOEPHEDRINE

Symptoms from pseudoephedrine overdose consist most often of mild anxiety, tachycardia and/or mild hypertension. Symptoms usually appear within 4 to 8 hours and are transient, usually requiring no treatment.

Inactive Ingredients:

Tablets and Caplets: Carnauba wax, corn starch, FD&C Yellow #6, hydroxypropyl methylcellulose, iron oxide, polydextrose, polyethylene glycol, silicon dioxide, stearic acid, titanium dioxide.

Gelcaps: Benzyl alcohol, butylparaben, butyl alcohol, castor oil, colloidal silicon dioxide, cornstarch, edetate calcium disodium, FDC Yellow No. 6, gelatin, hydroxypropyl methylcellulose, iron oxide black, magnesium stearate, methylparaben, microcrystalline cellulose, povidone, pregelatinized starch, propylene glycol, propylparaben, SDA 3A alcohol, sodium lauryl sulfate, sodium propionate, sodium starch glycolate, and titanium dioxide.

How Supplied:

Tablets: (orange, printed "MOTRIN IB" in black) in tamper evident packaging of 24, 50, 100, 130, 135, and 165. Store between 20°–25° C (68°–77° F)

Caplets: (orange, printed "MOTRIN IB" in black) in tamper evident packaging of 24, 50, 60, 100, 130, 135, 165, 250 and 500. Store between 20°–25° C (68°–77° F)

Gelcaps: (colored orange and white, printed "MOTRIN IB" in black) in tamper evident packaging of 24 and 50. Store between 20°–25° C (68°–77° F)

Shown in Product Identification Guide, page 510

MOTRIN® Sinus/Headache Caplets

Description: Each MOTRIN® Sinus/Headache Caplet contains ibuprofen 200 mg and pseudoephedrine HCl 30 mg.

Indications: MOTRIN® Sinus/Headache Caplets are indicated for the temporary relief of symptoms associated with sinusitis, the common cold or flu including nasal congestion, headache, body aches, pains and fever.

Directions: Do not take more than directed. *Adults and children 12 years of age and older:* Take 1 caplet every 4 to 6 hours while symptoms persist. If symptoms do not respond to 1 caplet, 2 caplets may be used but do not exceed 6 caplets in 24 hours, unless directed by a doctor. The smallest effective dose should be used. Take with food or milk if occasional and mild heartburn, upset stomach, or stomach pain occurs with use. Consult a doctor if these symptoms are more than mild or if they persist. *Children:* Do not

give this product to children under 12 years of age except under the advice and supervision of a doctor.

Warnings: Do not take for more than 7 days. If symptoms do not improve, or are accompanied by fever that persists for more than 3 days, or if new symptoms occur, consult a doctor. These could be signs of a serious illness. As with aspirin and acetaminophen, if you have any condition which requires you to take prescription drugs or if you have had any problems or serious side effects from taking any non-prescription pain reliever, do not take this product without first discussing it with your doctor. IF YOU EXPERIENCE ANY SYMPTOMS WHICH ARE UNUSUAL OR SEEM UNRELATED TO THE CONDITION FOR WHICH YOU TOOK THIS PRODUCT CONSULT A DOCTOR BEFORE TAKING ANY MORE OF IT. If you are under a doctor's care for any serious condition, consult a doctor before taking this product. **Do not exceed recommended dosage.** If nervousness, dizziness, or sleeplessness occur, discontinue use and consult a doctor. Do not take this product if you have heart disease, high blood pressure, thyroid disease, diabetes, or difficulty in urination due to enlargement of the prostate gland, unless directed by a doctor. Do not combine this product with other non-prescription pain relievers. Do not combine this product with any other ibuprofen-containing product. Keep this and all drugs out of the reach of children. In case of accidental overdose, seek professional assistance or contact a poison control center immediately. As with any drug, if you are pregnant or nursing a baby, seek the advice of a health professional before using this product. IT IS ESPECIALLY IMPORTANT NOT TO USE THIS PRODUCT DURING THE LAST 3 MONTHS OF PREGNANCY UNLESS SPECIFICALLY DIRECTED TO DO SO BY A DOCTOR BECAUSE IT MAY CAUSE PROBLEMS IN THE UNBORN CHILD OR COMPLICATIONS DURING DELIVERY.

Allergy Alert: ibuprofen may cause a severe allergic reaction which may include: hives, facial swelling, asthma (wheezing), shock.

Do not use if you have ever had an allergic reaction to any other pain reliever/fever reducer.

Stop use and ask a doctor if an allergic reaction occurs. Seek medical help right away.

Alcohol Warning: If you consume 3 or more alcoholic drinks every day, ask your doctor whether you should take ibuprofen or other pain relievers/fever reducers. Ibuprofen may cause stomach bleeding.

Drug Interaction Precaution:

Do not use this product if you are now taking a prescription monoamine oxidase inhibitor (MAOI) (certain drugs for depression, psychiatric or emotional conditions, or Parkinson's disease), or for 2

weeks after stopping the MAOI drug. If you are uncertain whether your drug contains an MAOI, consult a health professional before taking this product.

Professional Information: Overdosage Information

For overdosage information, please refer to pgs. 642–643.

Inactive Ingredients: Caplets: Carnauba Wax, Cellulose, Corn Starch, FD&C Red #40, Hydroxypropyl Methylcellulose, Silicon Dioxide, Sodium Lauryl Sulfate, Sodium Starch Glycolate, Stearic Acid, Titanium Dioxide, Triacetin.

How Supplied: Caplets: (white, printed "Motrin Sinus/Headache" in red) in blister packs of 20 and 40.

Store between 20–25°C (68–77°F). Avoid excessive heat.

Shown in Product Identification Guide, page 510

Infants' MOTRIN® ibuprofen Concentrated Drops

Children's MOTRIN® ibuprofen Oral Suspension and Chewable Tablets

Junior Strength MOTRIN® ibuprofen Caplets and Chewable Tablets

Product information for all dosages of Children's MOTRIN have been combined under this heading

Description: *Infants' MOTRIN® Concentrated Drops* is an alcohol-free, berry-flavored suspension. Each 1.25 mL (dropperful) contains ibuprofen 50 mg. *Children's MOTRIN® Oral Suspension* is an alcohol-free, berry, bubblegum or grape-flavored suspension. Each 5 mL (teaspoon) of *Children's MOTRIN® Oral Suspension* contains ibuprofen 100 mg. Each *Children's MOTRIN® Chewable Tablet* contains 50 mg of ibuprofen and is available as orange or grape-flavored chewable tablets. *Junior Strength MOTRIN® Chewable Tablets* and *Junior Strength MOTRIN® Caplets* contain ibuprofen 100 mg. *Junior Strength MOTRIN® Chewable Tablets* are available in orange or grape flavors. *Junior Strength MOTRIN® Caplets* are available as easy-to-swallow caplets (capsule-shaped tablet).

Uses:

temporarily:

• reduces fever

• relieves minor aches and pains due to the common cold, flu, sore throat, headaches and toothaches

Directions: See Table 1: Children's Motrin Dosing Chart on pg. 645.

Warnings: *Infants' MOTRIN® Concentrated Drops, Children's MOTRIN® Chewable Tablets & Junior Strength MOTRIN® Caplets and Chewable Tablets.*

Continued on next page

Motrin Infants'—Cont.

Allergy alert: ibuprofen may cause a severe allergic reaction which may include:

- hives • facial swelling
- asthma (wheezing) • shock

Sore throat warning: severe or persistent sore throat or sore throat accompanied by high fever, headache, nausea, and vomiting may be serious. Consult doctor promptly. Do not use more than 2 days or administer to children under 3 years of age unless directed by a doctor.

Do not use if the children has ever had an allergic reaction to any pain reliever/fever reducer.

Ask a doctor before use if the child has:

- not been drinking fluids
- lost a lot of fluid due to continued vomiting or diarrhea
- stomach pain
- problems or serious side effects from taking fever reducers or pain relievers

Ask a doctor or pharmacist before use if child is:

- under a doctor's care for any serious condition
- taking any other drug
- taking any other product that contains ibuprofen, or any other pain reliever/fever reducer

Infants' MOTRIN® Concentrated Drops and Junior Strength MOTRIN® Caplets:

When using this product give with food or milk if stomach upset occurs

Children's MOTRIN® Chewable Tablets and Junior Strength MOTRIN® Chewable Tablets:

When using this product mouth or throat burning may occur; give with food or water

- if stomach upset occurs, give with food or milk

Stop use and ask a doctor if:

- an allergic reaction occurs. Seek medical help right away
- fever or pain gets worse or lasts more than 3 days
- the child does not get any relief within the first day (24 hours) of treatment
- stomach pain or upset gets worse or lasts
- redness or swelling is present in the painful area
- any new symptoms appear

Keep out of reach of children. In case of overdose, get medical help or contact a Poison Control Center right away.

Children's MOTRIN® Oral Suspension:

Allergy Alert: Ibuprofen may cause a severe allergic reaction which may include

- hives • facial swelling
- asthma (wheezing) • shock

Do not use if you have ever had an allergic reaction to any pain reliever/fever reducer

Stop use and ask a doctor if an allergic reaction occurs. Seek medical help right away.

Call Your Doctor If:

- Your child is under a doctor's care for any serious condition or is taking any other drug.

- Your child has problems or serious side effects from taking fever reducers or pain relievers.
- Your child does not get any relief within the first day (24 hours) of treatment, or pain or fever gets worse.
- Stomach upset gets worse or lasts.
- Redness or swelling is present in the painful area.
- Sore throat is severe, lasts for more than 2 days or occurs with fever, headache, rash, nausea or vomiting.
- Any new symptoms appear.

Do Not Use:

- With any other product that contains ibuprofen, or other pain reliever/fever reducer, unless directed by a doctor
- For more than **3 days** for fever or pain unless directed by a doctor.
- For stomach pain unless directed by a doctor.
- If your child is dehydrated (significant fluid loss) due to continued vomiting, diarrhea, or lack of fluid intake.
- **If plastic carton wrap or bottle wrap imprinted "Safety Seal®" is broken or missing.**

Keep this and all drugs out of the reach of children. In case of accidental overdose, seek professional assistance or contact a poison control center immediately.

Other Information:

Infants', Children's and Junior Strength MOTRIN® products:

- Store at 20–25°C (68–77°F)

Infants' MOTRIN® Concentrated Drops:

- **Do not use if plastic bottle wrap imprinted "Safety Seal®" and "Use With Enclosed Dropper Only" is broken or missing.**

Children's MOTRIN® Chewable Tablets:

- Phenylketonurics: Contains phenylalanine 1.4 mg per tablet
- do not use if neck wrap or foil inner seal imprinted "Safety Seal®" is broken or missing

Junior Strength MOTRIN® Caplets and Chewable Tablets:

- phenylketonurics: contains phenylalanine 2.8 mg per tablet (tablet only)
- **Do not use if neck wrap or foil inner seal imprinted "Safety Seal®" is broken or missing**

Professional Information:

Overdosage Information for all Infants', Children's & Junior Strength Motrin® Products

IBUPROFEN: The *toxicity of ibuprofen* overdose is dependent upon the amount of drug ingested and the time elapsed since ingestion, though individual response may vary, which makes it necessary to evaluate each case individually. Although uncommon, serious toxicity and death have been reported in the medical literature with ibuprofen overdosage. The most frequently reported symptoms of ibuprofen overdose include abdominal pain, nausea, vomiting, lethargy and drowsiness. Other central nervous system symptoms include headache, tinnitus, CNS depression and seizures. Metabolic acidosis, coma, acute renal failure and apnea (primarily in very young children) may rarely occur. Cardiovascular toxicity, including hypotension, bradycardia, tachycardia and

atrial fibrillation, also have been reported.

The *treatment of acute ibuprofen overdose* is primarily supportive. Management of hypotension, acidosis and gastrointestinal bleeding may be necessary. In cases of acute overdose, the stomach should be emptied through ipecac-induced emesis or lavage. Emesis is most effective if initiated within 30 minutes of ingestion. Orally administered activated charcoal may help in reducing the absorption and reabsorption of ibuprofen. In children, the estimated amount of ibuprofen ingested per body weight may be helpful to predict the potential for development of toxicity although each case must be evaluated. Ingestion of less than 100 mg/kg is unlikely to produce toxicity. Children ingesting 100 to 200 mg/kg may be managed with induced emesis and a minimal observation time of four hours. Children ingesting 200 to 400 mg/kg of ibuprofen should have immediate gastric emptying and at least four hours observation in a health care facility. Children ingesting greater than 400 mg/kg require immediate medical referral, careful observation and appropriate supportive therapy. Ipecac-induced emesis is not recommended in overdoses greater than 400 mg/kg because of the risk of convulsions and the potential for aspiration of gastric contents.

In adults patients the history of the dose reportedly ingested does not appear to be predictive of toxicity. The need for referral and follow-up must be judged by the circumstances at the time of the overdose ingestion. Symptomatic adults should be admitted to a health care facility for observation.

Our Children's MOTRIN® Cold products contain pseudoephedrine in addition to ibuprofen. The following is basic overdose information regarding pseudoephedrine.

PSEUDOEPHEDRINE: Symptoms from pseudoephedrine overdose consist most often of mild anxiety, tachycardia and/or mild hypertension. Symptoms usually appear within 4 to 8 hours of ingestion and are transient, usually requiring no treatment.

For additional emergency information, please contact your local poison control center.

Inactive Ingredients:

Infants' MOTRIN® Concentrated Drops: Artificial flavors, citric acid, corn starch, FD&C Red #40, glycerin polysorbate 80, purified water, sodium benzoate, sorbitol, sucrose, xanthan gum.

Children's MOTRIN® Oral Suspension: **Berry-Flavored:** Acesulfame potassium, citric acid, cornstarch, D&C Yellow #10, FD&C Red #40, glycerin, natural and artificial flavors, polysorbate 80, purified water, sodium benzoate, sucrose, xanthan gum. **Bubble Gum-Flavored:** Acesulfame potassium, citric acid, cornstarch, FD&C Red #40, natural and arti-

Table 1. Children's Motrin® Dosing Chart

PRODUCT FORM	INGREDIENTS	0-5 mos* (6-11 lbs)	6-11 mos (12-17 lbs)	12-23 mos (18-23 lbs)	2-3 yrs (24-35 lbs)	4-5 yrs (36-47 lbs)	6-8 yrs (48-59 lbs)	9-10 yrs (60-71 lbs)	11 yrs (72-95 lbs)	Maximum doses/24 hrs
AGE GROUP* / **WEIGHT** (if possible use weight to dose; otherwise use age)	**Dose to be administered based on weight or age†**									
Infants' Drops Per dropperful (1.25 mL)										
Infants' Motrin Concentrated Drops	Ibuprofen 50 mg	—	1 dropperful (1.25 mL)	1½ dropperful (1.875 mL)	—	—	—	—	—	4 times in 24 hrs
Children's Liquid Per 5 mL teaspoonful (TSP)										
Children's Motrin Suspension	Ibuprofen 100 mg	—	—	—	1 TSP	1½ TSP	2 TSP	2½ TSP	3 TSP	4 times in 24 hrs
Children's Motrin Cold Suspension Liquid†	Ibuprofen 100 mg Pseudoephedrine 15 mg	—	—	—	1 TSP	1 TSP	2 TSP	2 TSP	2 TSP	4 times in 24 hrs
Children's Tablets & Caplets Per tablet/caplet										
Children's Motrin Chewable Tablets	Ibuprofen 50 mg	—	—	—	—	3 tablets	4 tablets	5 tablets	6 tablets	4 times in 24 hrs
Junior Strength Motrin Chewable Tablets	Ibuprofen 100 mg	—	—	—	—	—	2 tablets	2½ tablets	3 tablets	4 times in 24 hrs
Junior Strength Motrin Caplets	Ibuprofen 100 mg	—	—	—	—	—	2 caplets	2½ caplets	3 caplets	4 times in 24 hrs

† Do not give, take or chew more than directed. If needed, repeat dose every 6-8 hours; except for Children's Motrin Cold which is every 6 hours.

* Under 6 mos, call a doctor.

- Infants' Motrin Drops are more concentrated than Children's Motrin Liquids. The Infants' Concentrated Drops have been specifically designed for use only with enclosed dropper. Do not use any other dosing device with this product.
- Children's Motrin Liquids are less concentrated than Infants' Motrin Drops. The Children's Motrin Liquids have been specifically designed for use with the enclosed measuring cup. Use only enclosed measuring cup to dose this product.
- Children's Motrin Chewable Tablets are not the same concentration as Junior Strength Motrin Chewable Tablets.
- Junior Strength Motrin Chewable Tablets contain twice as much medicine as Children's Motrin Chewable Tablets.

Motrin Infants'—Cont.

ficial flavors, glycerin, polysorbate 80, purified water, sodium benzoate, sucrose, xanthan gum. **Grape-Flavored:** Acesulfame potassium, citric acid, cornstarch, D&C Red #33, FD&C Blue #1, FD&C Red #40, natural and artificial flavors, glycerin, polysorbate 80, purified water, sodium benzoate, sucrose, xanthan gum.

Children's MOTRIN® Chewable Tablets: **Orange-Flavored:** acesulfame K, aspartame, cellulose, citric acid, FD&C Yellow #6, flavor, fumaric acid, hydroxyethyl cellulose, hydroxypropyl methylcellulose, magnesium stearate, mannitol, povidone, sodium lauryl sulfate, sodium starch glycolate. **Grape-Flavored:** acesulfame K, aspartame, cellulose, citric acid, D&C red #7, D&C red #30, FD&C blue #1, flavor, fumaric acid, hydroxyethyl cellulose, hydroxypropyl methylcellulose, magnesium stearate, mannitol, povidone, sodium lauryl sulfate, sodium starch glycolate.

Junior Strength MOTRIN® Chewable Tablets: **Orange-Flavored:** acesulfame K, aspartame, cellulose, citric acid, FD&C yellow #6, flavor, fumaric acid, hydroxyethyl cellulose, hydroxypropyl methylcellulose, magnesium stearate, mannitol, povidone, sodium lauryl sulfate, sodium starch glycolate. **Grape-Flavored:** acesulfame K, aspartame, cellulose, citric acid, D&C red #7, D&C red #30, FD&C blue #1, flavor, fumaric acid, hydroxyethyl cellulose, hydroxypropyl methylcellulose, magnesium stearate, mannitol, povidone, sodium lauryl sulfate, sodium starch glycolate. **Easy-To-Swallow Caplets:** carnauba wax, corn starch, D&C Yellow #10, FD&C Yellow #6, hydroxypropyl methylcellulose, microcrystalline cellulose, polydextrose, polyethylene glycol, propylene glycol, silicon dioxide, sodium starch glycolate, titanium dioxide, triacetin.

How Supplied: *Infants' MOTRIN® Concentrated Drops:* Berry-flavored, pink-colored liquid in ½ fl. oz. bottles.

Children's MOTRIN® Oral Suspension: Berry-flavored, orange-colored; Bubble Gum-flavored, pink-colored and Grape-flavored, purple-colored liquid in tamper evident bottles of 2 and 4 fl. oz.

Children's MOTRIN® Chewable Tablets: Orange-flavored, orange-colored and Grape-flavored, purple-colored chewable tablets in 24 count bottles.

Junior Strength MOTRIN® Chewable Tablets: Orange-flavored, orange-colored chewable tablets or Grape-flavored, purple-colored chewable tablets in 24 count bottles.

Junior Strength MOTRIN® Caplets: Easy-to-swallow caplets (capsule shaped tablets) in 24 count bottles.

Shown in Product Identification Guide, page 509

Children's MOTRIN® Cold ibuprofen/pseudoephedrine HCl Oral Suspension

Description: *Children's MOTRIN® Cold Oral Suspension* is an alcohol-free, berry or grape-flavored suspension. Each 5 mL (teaspoonful) contains the pain reliever/fever reducer ibuprofen 100 mg and the nasal decongestant pseudoephedrine 15 mg.

Uses: *Children's MOTRIN® Cold Oral Suspension:* temporarily relieves these cold, sinus and flu symptoms: •nasal and sinus congestion •stuffy nose •headache •sore throat •minor body aches and pains •fever

Directions: See Table 2: Children's Motrin Dosing Chart on pg. 645.

Warnings: Allergy alert: Ibuprofen may cause a severe allergic reaction which may include: •hives •facial swelling •asthma (wheezing) •shock

Sore throat warning: Severe or persistent sore throat or sore throat accompanied by high fever, headache, nausea, and vomiting may be serious. Consult a doctor promptly. Do not use more than 2 days or administer to children under 3 years of age unless directed by doctor.

Do not use:
- if the child has ever had an allergic reaction to any other pain reliever/fever reducer and/or nasal decongestant
- in a child who is taking a prescription monoamine oxidase inhibitor [MAOI] (certain drugs for depression, psychiatric or emotional conditions, or Parkinson's disease), or for 2 weeks after stopping the MAOI drug. If you do not know if your child's prescription drug contains an MAOI, ask a doctor or pharmacist before giving this product.

Ask a doctor before use if the child has:
- not been drinking fluids
- lost a lot of fluid due to continued vomiting or diarrhea
- problems or serious side effects from taking pain relievers, fever reducers or nasal decongestants
- stomach pain
- heart disease
- high blood pressure
- thyroid disease
- diabetes

Ask a doctor or pharmacist before use if the child is:
- under a doctor's care for any continuing medical condition
- taking any other drug
- taking any other product that contains ibuprofen or pseudoephedrine
- taking any other pain reliever/fever reducer and/or nasal decongestant

When using this product:
- do not exceed recommended dosage
- give with food or milk if stomach upset occurs

Stop use and ask a doctor if:
- an allergic reaction occurs. Seek medical help right away.
- the child does not get any relief within first day (24 hours) of treatment
- fever, pain or nasal congestion gets worse, or lasts for more than 3 days
- stomach pain or upset gets worse or lasts
- symptoms continue or get worse

- redness or swelling is present in the painful area
- the child gets nervous, dizzy, sleepless or sleepy
- any new symptoms appear

Keep out of reach of children. In case of overdose, get medical help or contact a Poison Control Center right away.

Other information:
- do not use if plastic carton wrap or bottle wrap imprinted "Safety Seal®" is broken or missing.
- Store at 20–25°C (68–77°F)

Professional Information:
Overdosage Information
For overdosage information, please refer to pg. 644.

Inactive Ingredients: *Children's MOTRIN® Cold Oral Suspension:* Berry Flavor: acesulfame potassium, citric acid, corn starch, D&C yellow #10, FD&C red #40, flavors, glycerin, polysorbate 80, purified water, sodium benzoate, sucrose, xanthan gum. *Children's MOTRIN® Cold Oral Suspension:* Grape Flavor: acesulfame potassium, citric acid, corn starch, D&C red #33, FD&C blue #1, FD&C red #40, flavors, glycerin, polysorbate 80, purified water, sodium benzoate, sucrose, xanthan gum.

How Supplied: Berry-flavored, orange-colored and grape-flavored, purple-colored liquid in tamper evident bottles of 4 fl. oz.

Shown in Product Identification Guide, page 509

Children's Motrin® Dosing Chart
[See table on previous page]

MOTRIN® MIGRAINE PAIN CAPLETS

Description: Each *Motrin® Migraine Pain Caplet* contains ibuprofen 200 mg.

Use: Treats pain of migraine headache

Directions:
Adults:
- take 1 or 2 caplets with a glass of water
- the smallest effective dose should be used
- if symptoms persist or worsen, ask your doctor
- do not take more than 2 caplets in 24 hours for pain of migraine unless directed by a doctor

Under 18 years of age:
- ask a doctor

Warnings: Allergy alert: ibuprofen may cause a severe allergic reaction which may include:
- hives • facial swelling
- asthma (wheezing) • shock

Alcohol warning: If you consume 3 or more alcoholic drinks every day, ask your doctor whether you should take ibuprofen or other pain relievers/fever reducers. Ibuprofen may cause stomach bleeding.

Do not use if you have ever had an allergic reaction to any other pain relievers/fever reducers

Ask a doctor before use if you have:

- never had migraines diagnosed by a health professional
- a headache that is different from your usual migraines
- the worst headache of your life
- fever and stiff neck
- headaches beginning after or caused by head injury, exertion, coughing or bending
- experienced your first headache after the age of 50
- daily headaches
- a migraine headaches so severe as to require bed rest
- problems or serious side effects from taking pain relievers or fever reducers
- stomach pain
- vomiting with your migraine headache

Ask a doctor or pharmacist before use if you are:

- under a doctor's care for any serious condition
- take any other drug
- taking any other product that contain ibuprofen, or any other pain reliever/fever reducer

Stop use and ask a doctor if:

- an allergic reaction occurs. Seek medical help right away.
- migraine headache pain is not relieved or gets worse after first dose
- stomach pain or upset gets worse or lasts
- new or unexpected symptoms occur

If pregnant or breast-feeding, ask a health professional before use. It is especially important not to use ibuprofen during the last 3 months of pregnancy unless definitely directed to do so by a doctor because it may cause problems in the unborn child or complications during delivery.

Keep out of reach of children. In case of overdose, get medical help or contact a Poison Control Center right away.

Other Information:

- do not use if neck wrap or foil inner seal imprinted **"Safety Seal"** is broken or missing
- store at 20–25°C (68–77°F)

Professional Information:
Overdosage Information

For overdosage information, please refer to pgs. 642–643.

Inactive Ingredients: carnauba wax, corn starch, hydroxypropyl methylcellulose, iron oxide black, pregelatinized starch, propylene glycol, silicon dioxide, stearic acid, titanium dioxide.

How Supplied: Caplets (white printed "Motrin M" in black) in tamper evident packaging of 24, 50, and 100

Shown in Product Identification Guide, page 510

NIZORAL® A-D
KETOCONAZOLE SHAMPOO 1%

Description: *Nizoral® A-D (Ketoconazole Shampoo 1%) Anti-Dandruff Shampoo* is a light-blue liquid for topical application, containing the broad spectrum synthetic antifungal agent Ketoconazole in a concentration of 1%.

Use: *Nizoral® A-D* controls the flaking, scaling, and itching associated with dandruff.

Directions: Adults and children over 12 years of age:

- wet hair thoroughly
- apply shampoo, generously lather, rinse thoroughly. Repeat.
- use every 3–4 days for up to 8 weeks if needed, or as directed by a doctor. Then use only as needed to control dandruff.

Children under 12 years of age: Ask a doctor.

Warnings:
Do Not Use:
- on scalp that is broken or inflamed
- if you are allergic to ingredients in this product

When Using This Product:
- do not get into eyes
- if product gets into eyes, rinse thoroughly with water

Stop Using This Product If:
- rash appears
- condition worsens or does not improve in 2–4 weeks

Ask a doctor. These may be signs of a serious condition.

For external use only.

As with any drug, if you are pregnant or nursing a baby, seek the advice of a health professional before using this product.

Keep this and all drugs out of the reach of children.

In case of accidental ingestion, seek professional assistance or contact a Poison Control Center immediately.

Storage: Store between 35° and 86°F (2° and 30°C). Protect from light. Protect from freezing.

Professional Information:
Overdosage Information *Nizoral® A-D (Ketoconazole) 1% Shampoo* is intended for external use only. In the event of accidental ingestion, supportive measures should be employed. Induced emesis and gastric lavage should usually be avoided.

Inactive Ingredients: Water, Sodium Laureth Sulfate, Cocamide MEA, Sodium Cocoyl Sarcosinate, Glycol Distearate, Acrylic Acid Polymer (Carbomer 1342), Fragrance, Sodium Chloride, Tetrasodium EDTA, Butylated Hydroxytoluene, Quaternium-15, Polyquaternium-7, Sodium Hydroxide and/or Hydrochloric Acid, FD&C Blue No. 1.

How Supplied: Available in 4 and 7 fl. oz. bottles and Travel size packets - 10 packets 0.2 fl oz (6 mL) each.

Shown in Product Identification Guide, page 510

SIMPLY SLEEP™
Nighttime Sleep Aid

Description: *SIMPLY SLEEP™* is a non habit-forming nighttime sleep aid. Each *SIMPLY SLEEP™* Caplet contains diphenhydramine HCl 25 mg.

Actions: *SIMPLY SLEEP™* contains an antihistamine (diphenhydramine HCl) which has sedative properties.

Uses: For relief of occasional sleeplessness.

Directions: Adults and Children 12 years of age and older: Take 2 Caplets at bedtime if needed or as directed by a doctor.
Children under 12 years of age: Do not give this product to children under 12 years of age.

Precautions: If a rare sensitivity reaction occurs, the drug should be discontinued.

Warnings: Do not give to children under 12 years of age. If sleeplessness persists continuously for more than 2 weeks, consult your doctor. Insomnia may be a symptom of serious underlying medical illness. Do not take this product, unless directed by a doctor, if you have a breathing problem such as emphysema or chronic bronchitis, or if you have glaucoma or difficulty in urination due to enlargement of the prostate gland. Avoid alcoholic beverages while taking this product. Do not take this product if you are taking sedatives or tranquilizers, without first consulting your doctor.

Keep this and all drugs out of the reach of children. In case of accidental overdose, contact a doctor or poison control center immediately. As with any drug, if you are pregnant or nursing a baby, seek the advice of a health care professional before using this product.

Do not use if carton is opened or blister unit is broken.

Inactive Ingredients: Cellulose, Croscarmellose Sodium, Dibasic Calcium Phosphate, Dihydrate, FD&C Blue #1, Hydroxypropyl Methylcellulose, Magnesium Stearate, Polyethylene Glycol, Polysorbate 80, Titanium Dioxide.

How Supplied: Light blue mini-caplets embossed with "SL" on one side in blister packs of 24 and 48. Store at room temperature.

Shown in Product Identification Guide, page 510

Regular Strength TYLENOL®
acetaminophen Tablets
Extra Strength TYLENOL®
acetaminophen Gelcaps, Geltabs, Caplets, Tablets
Extra Strength TYLENOL®
acetaminophen Adult Liquid Pain Reliever
TYLENOL® acetaminophen
Arthritis Pain Extended Relief Caplets

Product information for all dosage forms of Adult TYLENOL acetaminophen have been combined under this heading.

Description: *Each Regular Strength TYLENOL® Tablet* contains acetamino-

Continued on next page

Tylenol Reg. Strength—Cont.

phen 325 mg. *Each Extra Strength TYLENOL® Gelcap, Geltab, Caplet, or Tablet contains acetaminophen 500 mg. Each 15 mL (1/2 fl oz or one tablespoonful) of Extra Strength TYLENOL® Adult Liquid Pain Reliever contain 500 mg acetaminophen (alcohol 7%). Each TYLENOL® Arthritis Pain Extended Relief Caplet contains acetaminophen 650 mg.*

Actions: Acetaminophen is a clinically proven analgesic/antipyretic. Acetaminophen produces analgesia by elevation of the pain threshold and antipyresis through action on the hypothalamic heat-regulating center. Acetaminophen is equal to aspirin in analgesic and antipyretic effectiveness and it is unlikely to produce many of the side effects associated with aspirin and aspirin-containing products. *Tylenol Arthritis Pain Extended Relief* uses a unique, patented bilayer caplet. The first layer dissolves quickly to provide prompt relief while the second layer is time released to provide up to 8 hours of relief.

Uses: *Regular Strength TYLENOL® Tablets, Extra Strength TYLENOL® Gelcaps, Geltabs, Caplets, or Tablets. Extra Strength TYLENOL® Adult Liquid Pain Reliever:* For the temporary relief of minor aches and pains associated with headache, muscular aches, backache, minor arthritis pain, common cold, toothache, menstrual cramps and for the reduction of fever.
TYLENOL® Arthritis Pain Extended Relief Caplets: temporarily relieves minor aches and pains due to:
* arthritis
* the common cold
* headache
* toothache
* muscular aches
* backache
* menstrual cramps

Directions: *Regular Strength TYLENOL® Tablets:* **Adults and Children 12 years of Age and Older:** Take 2 tablets every 4 to 6 hours as needed. Do not take more than 12 tablets in 24 hours, or as directed by a doctor. **Children 6–11 years of age:** Take 1 tablet every 4 to 6 hours as needed. Do not take more than 5 tablets in 24 hours. **Children under 6 years of age:** Do not use this adult Regular Strength product in children under 6 years of age. This will provide more than the recommended dose (overdose) of TYLENOL® and could cause serious health problems.
Extra Strength TYLENOL® Gelcaps, Geltabs, Caplets, or Tablets: **Adults and Children 12 years of age and older:** Take 2 gelcaps, geltabs, caplets, or tablets every 4 to 6 hours as needed. Do not take more than 8 gelcaps, geltabs, caplets or tablets in 24 hours, or as directed by a doctor. **Children under 12 years:** Do not use this adult Extra Strength product in children under 12 years of age. This will provide more than the recommended dose (overdose) of

TYLENOL® and could cause serious health problems. *Extra Strength TYLENOL® Adult Liquid Pain Reliever:* **Adults and children 12 years of age and older:** Take 2 Tablespoons (tbsp.) in dose cup provided every 4 to 6 hours as needed. Do not take more than 8 Tablespoons in 24 hours, or as directed by a doctor. **Children under 12 years:** Do not use this adult Extra Strength product in children under 12 years of age. This will provide more than the recommended dose (overdose) of TYLENOL® and could cause health problems.
TYLENOL® Arthritis Pain Extended Relief Caplets:
* do not take more than directed adults:
* take 2 caplets every 8 hours with water
* swallow whole – do not crush, chew or dissolve
* do not take more than 6 caplets in 24 hours
* do not use for more than 10 days unless directed by a doctor
under 18 years of age:
* ask a doctor

Precautions:
If a rare sensitivity reaction occurs, the drug should be discontinued.

Warnings:
Regular Strength TYLENOL® Tablets, Extra Strength TYLENOL® Gelcaps, Geltabs, Caplets, or Tablets, Extra Strength TYLENOL® Adult Liquid Pain Reliever:
Alcohol Warning: If you consume 3 or more alcoholic drinks every day, ask your doctor whether you should take acetaminophen or other pain relievers/fever reducers. Acetaminophen may cause liver damage. **Do not use if carton is opened or red neck wrap or foil seal imprinted with "Safety Seal®" is broken.**
Do not Use:
* with any other product containing acetaminophen.
* for more than 10 days for pain unless directed by doctor.
* for more than 3 days for fever unless directed by a doctor.
Stop Using And Ask a Doctor If:
* symptoms do not improve
* new symptoms occur
* pain or fever persists or gets worse
* redness or swelling is present
Do not exceed recommended dose. Keep this and all drugs out of the reach of children. In case of accidental overdose, contact a poison control center immediately. Prompt medical attention is critical for adults as well as for children even if you do not notice any signs or symptoms. As with any drug, if you are pregnant or nursing a baby, seek the advise of a health professional before using this product.
TYLENOL® Arthritis Pain Extended Relief Caplets: **Alcohol Warning:** If you consume 3 or more alcoholic drinks every day, ask your doctor whether you should take acetaminophen or other pain relievers/fever reducers. Acetaminophen may cause liver damage.

Do not Use
* with any other product containing acetaminophen.
Stop use and ask a doctor if
* New symptoms occur
* Redness or swelling is present
* Pain gets worse or lasts for more than 10 days
If pregnant or breast-feeding, ask a health professional before use.
Keep out of the reach of children. In case of overdose, get medical help or contact a Poison Control Center right away. Quick medical attention is critical for adults as well as for children even if you do not notice signs or symptoms.
Other information
* **do not use if carton is opened or red neck wrap or foil inner seal with "Safety Seal®" is broken**
* store at 20–25°C (68–77°F)
* avoid excessive heat at 40°C (104°F)

Professional Information:
Overdosage Information for all Adult Tylenol products

ACETAMINOPHEN: Acetaminophen in massive overdosage may cause hepatic toxicity in some patients. In adults and adolescents ($\geq$ 12 years of age), hepatic toxicity may occur following ingestion of greater than 7.5 to 10 grams over a period of 8 hours or less. Fatalities are infrequent (less than 3–4% of untreated cases) and have rarely been reported with overdoses of less than 15 grams. In children (<12 years of age), an acute overdosage of less than 150 mg/kg has not been associated with hepatic toxicity. Early symptoms following a potentially hepatotoxic overdose may include: nausea, vomiting, diaphoresis and general malaise. Clinical and laboratory evidence of hepatic toxicity may not be apparent until 48 to 72 hours postingestion. In adults and adolescents, any individual presenting with an unknown amount of acetaminophen ingested or with a questionable or unreliable history about the time of ingestion should have a plasma acetaminophen level drawn and be treated with *N*-acetylcysteine. For full prescribing information, refer to the *N*-acetylcysteine package insert. Do not await results of assays for plasma acetaminophen levels before initiating treatment with *N*-acetylcysteine. The following additional procedures are recommended: Promptly initiate gastric decontamination of the stomach. A plasma acetaminophen assay should be obtained as early as possible, but no sooner than four hours following ingestion. If an acetaminophen *extended release* product is involved, it may be appropriate to obtain an additional plasma acetaminophen level 4–6 hours following the initial acetaminophen level. If either acetaminophen level plots above the treatment line on the acetaminophen overdose nomogram, *N*-acetylcysteine treatment should be continued for a full course of therapy. Liver function studies should be obtained initially and repeated at 24-hour intervals. Serious toxicity or fatalities have been extremely infrequent

following an acute acetaminophen overdose in young children, possibly because of differences in the way they metabolize acetaminophen. In children, the maximum potential amount ingested can be more easily estimated. If more than 150 mg/kg or an unknown amount was ingested, obtain a plasma acetaminophen level as soon as possible, but no sooner than 4 hours following ingestion. If an acetaminophen *extended release* product is involved, it may be appropriate to obtain an additional plasma acetaminophen level 4–6 hours following the initial acetaminophen level. If either acetaminophen level plots above the treatment line on the acetaminophen overdose nomogram, *N*-acetylcysteine treatment should be initiated and continued for a full course of therapy. If an assay cannot be obtained and the estimated acetaminophen ingestion exceeds 150 mg/kg, dosing with *N*-acetylcysteine should be initiated and continued for a full course of therapy. For additional emergency information, call your regional poison center or call the Rocky Mountain Poison Center toll-free, (1-800-525-6115).

Our adult Tylenol® combination products contain active ingredients in addition to acetaminophen. The following is basic overdose information regarding those ingredients.

CHLORPHENIRAMINE: Chlorpheniramine toxicity should be treated as you would an anthihistamine/anticholinergic overdose and is likely to be present within a few hours after acute ingestion.

DEXTROMETHORHPHAN: Acute dextromethorphan overdose usually does not result in serious signs and symptoms unless massive amounts have been ingested. Signs and symptoms of a substantial overdose may include nausea and vomiting, visual disturbances, CNS disturbances and urinary retention

DIPHENHYDRAMINE: Diphenhydramine toxicity should be treated as you would an antihistamine/anticholinergic overdose and is likely to be present within a few hours after acute ingestion.

DOXYLAMINE: Doxylamine toxicity should be treated as you would an antihistamine/anticholinergic overdose and is likely to be present within a few hours after acute ingestion.

GUAIFENESIN: Guaifenesin should be treated as a nontoxic ingestion.

PAMABROM: Acute overexposure of diuretics is primarily associated with fluid and electrolyte loss. Fluid loss should be treated with the appropriate intravenous and/or oral fluids.

PSEUDOEPHEDRINE: Symptoms from pseudoephedrine overdose consist most often of mild anxiety, tachycardia and/or mild hypertension. Symptoms usually appear within 4 to 8 hours of ingestion and are transient, usually requiring no treatment.

For additional emergency information, please contact your local poison control center.

Alcohol Information: Chronic heavy alcohol abusers may be at increased risk of liver toxicity from excessive acetaminophen use, although reports of this event are rare. Reports usually involve cases of severe chronic alcoholics and the dosages of acetaminophen most often exceed recommended doses and often involve substantial overdose. Healthcare professionals should alert their patients who regularly consume large amounts of alcohol not to exceed recommended doses of acetaminophen.

Inactive Ingredients: *Regular Strength TYLENOL®:* Tablets: Cellulose, Corn Starch, Magnesium Stearate, Sodium Starch Glycolate.

Extra Strength TYLENOL®: Tablets: Cellulose, Corn Starch, Magnesium Stearate, Sodium Starch Glycolate. Caplets: Cellulose, Corn Starch, FD&C Red No. 40, Hydroxypropyl Methylcellulose, Magnesium Stearate, Polyethylene Glycol, Sodium Starch Glycolate. Gelcaps: Benzyl Alcohol, Blue #1 and #2, Butylparaben, Castor Oil, Cellulose, Corn Starch, Edetate Calcium Disodium, Gelatin, Hydroxypropyl Methylcellulose, Magnesium Stearate, Methylparaben Propylparaben, Red #40, Sodium Lauryl Sulfate, Sodium Propionate, Sodium Starch Glycolate, Titanium Dioxide, and Yellow #10. Geltabs: Benzyl Alcohol, Blue #1 and 2, Butylparaben, Castor Oil, Cellulose, Corn Starch, Edetate Calcium Disodium, Gelatin, Hydroxypropyl Methylcellulose, Magnesium Stearate, Methylparaben Propylparaben, Red #40, Sodium Lauryl Sulfate, Sodium Propionate, Sodium Starch Glycolate, Titanium Dioxide, and Yellow #10.

Extra Strength TYLENOL® Adult Liquid Pain Reliever: Alcohol (7%), Citric Acid, D&C Yellow #10, FD&C Blue #1, FD&C Yellow #6, Flavor, Glycerin, Polyethylene Glycol, Purified Water, Sodium Benzoate, Sorbitol, Sucrose.

TYLENOL® Arthritis Pain Extended Relief Caplets: Corn Starch, Hydroxyethyl Cellulose, Hydroxypropyl Methylcellulose, Magnesium Stearate, Microcrystalline Cellulose, Povidone, Powdered Cellulose, Pregelatinized Starch, Sodium Starch Glycolate, Titanium Dioxide, Triacetin.

How Supplied: *Regular Strength TYLENOL®:* Tablets (colored white, scored, imprinted "TYLENOL" and "325")—tamper-evident bottles of 100. Store at room temperature.

Extra Strength TYLENOL®: Tablets (colored white, imprinted "TYLENOL" and "500")—tamper-evident bottles of 30, 60, 100, and 200. Store at room temperature. Caplets (colored white, imprinted "TYLENOL 500 mg")—vials of 10, 10 blister packs, and tamper-evident bottles of 24, 50, 100, 175, and 250. Store at room temperature. Gelcaps (colored yellow and red, imprinted "Tylenol 500") tamper-evident bottles of 24, 50, 100, and 225. Store at room temperature; avoid high humidity and excessive heat 40°C (104°F). Geltabs (colored yellow

and red, imprinted "Tylenol 500") tamper-evident bottles of 24, 50, and 100. Store at room temperature; avoid high humidity and excessive heat 40°C (104°F).

Extra Strength TYLENOL® Adult Liquid Pain Reliever: Mint-flavored liquid (colored green) 8 fl. oz. tamper-evident bottle with child resistant safety cap and special dosage cup. Store at room temperature.

TYLENOL® Arthritis Pain Extended Relief Caplets: (colored white, engraved "TYLENOL ER") tamper-evident bottles of 24, 50, and 100, 150 and 290's. Store at room temperature. Avoid excessive heat (40°C).

Shown in Product Identification Guide, page 511

TYLENOL® Severe Allergy Caplets

Maximum Strength
TYLENOL® Allergy Sinus NightTime Caplets

Maximum Strength
TYLENOL® Allergy Sinus Caplets, Gelcaps and Geltabs

Product information for all dosage forms of TYLENOL Allergy have been combined under this heading.

Description:
Each *TYLENOL® Severe Allergy Caplet* contains acetaminophen 500 mg and diphenhydramine HCl 12.5 mg. Each *Maximum Strength TYLENOL® Allergy Sinus NightTime Caplet* contains acetaminophen 500 mg, diphenhydramine HCl 25 mg, and pseudoephedrine HCl 30 mg. Each *Maximum Strength TYLENOL® Allergy Sinus Caplet Gelcap and Geltab* contains acetaminophen 500 mg, chlorpheniramine maleate 2 mg, and pseudoephedrine HCl 30 mg.

Actions:
TYLENOL® Severe Allergy Caplets contain a clinically proven analgesic-antipyretic and antihistamine. Acetaminophen produces analgesia by elevation of the pain threshold and antipyresis through action on the hypothalamic heat regulating center. Acetaminophen is equal to aspirin in analgesic and antipyretic effectiveness, and it is unlikely to produce many of the side effects associated with aspirin and aspirin-containing products. Diphenhydramine HCl is an antihistamine which helps provide temporary relief of itchy, watery eyes, runny nose, sneezing, itching of the nose or throat due to hay fever or other respiratory allergies.

Maximum Strength TYLENOL® Allergy Sinus NightTime Caplets contain, in addition to the above ingredients, a decongestant, pseudoephedrine HCl. Pseudoe-

Continued on next page

Tylenol Allergy—Cont.

phedrine is a sympathomimetic amine which provides temporary relief of nasal and sinus congestion.

Maximum Strength TYLENOL® Allergy Sinus Caplets, Gelcaps and Geltabs contain acetaminophen, pseudoephedrine HCl and the antihistamine, chlorpheniramine maleate. Chlorpheniramine is an antihistamine which helps provide temporary relief of runny nose, sneezing and watery and itchy eyes.

Uses:

TYLENOL® Severe Allergy: For the temporary relief of itchy, watery eyes, runny nose, sneezing, sore or scratchy throat and itching of the nose or throat due to hay fever or other upper respiratory allergies.

Maximum Strength TYLENOL® Allergy Sinus NightTime and TYLENOL® Allergy Sinus: For the temporary relief of nasal congestion, sinus congestion and pressure, sinus pain, headache, runny nose, sneezing, itching of the nose or throat and itchy watery eyes due to hay fever or other respiratory allergies.

Precautions:

TYLENOL® Severe Allergy, Maximum Strength TYLENOL® Allergy Sinus NightTime and *Maximum Strength TYLENOL® Allergy Sinus:* If a rare sensitivity reaction occurs, the drug should be discontinued.

Directions:

TYLENOL® Severe Allergy: **Adults and children 12 years of age and older:** Take 2 caplets every 4–6 hours. Do not take more than 8 caplets in 24 hours, or as directed by a doctor. **Children under 12 years:** Do not use this adult product in children under 12 years of age. This will provide more than the recommended dose (overdose) and could cause serious health problems.

Maximum Strength TYLENOL® Allergy Sinus NightTime: **Adults and children 12 years of age and older:** Take 2 caplets at bedtime. May repeat every 4–6 hours. Do not take more than 8 caplets in 24 hours, or as directed by a doctor. **Children under 12 years:** Do not use this adult product in children under 12 years of age. This will provide more than the recommended dose (overdose) and could cause serious health problems.

Maximum Strength TYLENOL® Allergy Sinus: **Adults and children 12 years of age and older:** Take two every 4–6 hours. Do not take more than 8 in 24 hours, or as directed by a doctor. **Children under 12 years:** Do not use this adult product in children under 12 years of age. This will provide more than the recommended dose (overdose) and could cause serious health problems.

Warnings:

Alcohol Warning: If you consume 3 or more alcoholic drinks every day, ask your doctor whether your should take acetaminophen or other pain relievers/fever reducers. Acetaminophen may cause liver damage.

TYLENOL® Severe Allergy: **Do not use if carton is opened or if blister unit is broken.** Do not take for pain for more than 7 days or for fever for more than 3 days unless directed by a doctor. If pain or fever persists, or gets worse, if new symptoms occur, or if redness or swelling is present, consult a doctor because these could be signs of a serious condition. If sore throat is severe, persists for more than 2 days, is accompanied or followed by fever, headache, rash, nausea or vomiting, consult a doctor promptly. May cause excitability especially in children. If nervousness, dizziness or sleeplessness occur, discontinue use and consult a doctor. May cause marked drowsiness; alcohol, sedatives and tranquilizers may increase the drowsiness effect. Avoid alcoholic beverages while taking this product. Do not take this product if you are taking sedatives or tranquilizers without first consulting your doctor. Use caution while driving a motor vehicle or operating machinery. Do not take this product, unless directed by a doctor, if you have a breathing problem such as emphysema or chronic bronchitis, or if you have glaucoma or difficulty in urination due to enlargement of the prostate gland.

Do not exceed recommended dosage. Keep this and all drugs out of the reach of children. In case of accidental overdose, contact a doctor or poison control center immediately. Prompt medical attention is critical for adults as well as for children even if you do not notice any signs or symptoms. As with any drug, if you are pregnant or nursing a baby, seek the advice of a health professional before using this product. Do not use with other products containing acetaminophen.

Maximum Strength TYLENOL® Allergy Sinus NightTime: **Do not use if carton is open or if a blister unit is broken.** Do not take for pain for more than 7 days or for fever for more than 3 days unless directed by a doctor. If pain or fever persists, or gets worse, if new symptoms occur, or if redness or swelling is present, consult a doctor because these could be signs of a serious condition. May cause excitability especially in children. If nervousness, dizziness or sleeplessness occur, discontinue use and consult a doctor. May cause marked drowsiness; alcohol, sedatives and tranquilizers may increase the drowsiness effect. Avoid alcoholic beverages while taking this product. Do not take this product if you are taking sedatives or tranquilizers without first consulting your doctor. Use caution when driving a motor vhicle or operating machinery. Do not take this product, unless directed by a doctor, if you have a breathing problem such as emphysema or chronic bronchitis, or if you have glaucoma, or difficulty in urination due to enlargement of the prostate gland. Do not take this product if you have heart disease, high blood pressure, thyroid disease or diabetes unless directed by a doctor.

Do not exceed recommended dosage. Keep this and all drugs out of the reach of children. In case of accidental overdose, contact a doctor or poison control center immediately. Prompt medical attention is critical for adults as well as for children even if you do not notice any signs or symptoms. As with any drug, if you are pregnant or nursing a baby, seek the advice of a health professional before using this product. Do not use with other products containing acetaminophen.

Maximum Strength TYLENOL® Allergy Sinus: **Do not use if carton is opened or if blister unit is broken.** Do not take for pain for more than 7 days or for fever for more than 3 days unless directed by a doctor. If pain or fever persists, or gets worse, if new symptoms occur, or if redness or swelling is present, consult a doctor because these could be signs of a serious condition. May cause excitability especially in children. If nervousness, dizziness or sleeplessness occur, discontinue use and consult a doctor. May cause drowsiness; alcohol, sedatives and tranquilizers may increase the drowsiness effect. Avoid alcoholic beverages while taking this product. Do not take this product if you are taking sedatives or tranquilizers, without first consulting your doctor. Use caution when driving a motor vehicle or operating machinery. Do not take this product, unless directed by a doctor, if you have a breathing problem such as emphysema or chronic bronchitis, or if you have glaucoma, or difficulty in urination due to enlargement of the prostate gland. Do not take this product if you have heart disease, high blood pressure, thyroid disease or diabetes unless directed by a doctor.

Do not exceed recommended dosage. Keep this and all drugs out of the reach of children. In case of accidental overdose, contact a doctor or poison. control center immediately. Prompt medical attention is critical for adults as well as for children even if you do not notice any signs or symptoms. As with any drug, if you are pregnant or nursing a baby, seek the advice of a health professional before using this product. Do not use with other products containing acetaminophen.

Drug Interaction Precaution

Maximum Strength TYLENOL® Allergy Sinus NightTime and *TYLENOL® Allergy Sinus:* Do not use this product if you are now taking a prescription monamine oxidase inhibitor (MAOI) (certain drugs for depression, psychiatric or emotional condition, or Parkinson's disease), or for 2 weeks after stopping the MAOI drug. If you are uncertain whether your prescription drug contains an MAOI, consult a health professional before taking this product.

Professional Information:
Overdosage Information

For overdosage information, please refer to pgs. 648–649.

Inactive Ingredients:

TYLENOL® Severe Allergy: **Caplets:** Carnauba Wax, Cellulose, Corn Starch, D&C Yellow #10, FD&C Yellow #6, Hydroxpropyl Cellulose, Hydroxypropyl Methylcellulose, Iron Oxide, Magnesium Stearate, Polyethylene Glycol, Sodium Citrate, Sodium Starch Glycolate, Titanium Dioxide.

Maximum Strength TYLENOL® Allergy Sinus NightTime: **Caplets:** Carnauba Wax, Cellulose, Corn Starch, D&C Yellow #10, FD&C Blue #1, Hydroxypropyl Methylcellulose, Iron Oxide, Magnesium Stearate, Polyethylene Glycol, Polysorbate 80, Sodium Citrate, Sodium Starch Glycolate, Titanium Dioxide.

Maximum Strength TYLENOL® Allergy Sinus: **Caplets:** Carnauba Wax, Cellulose, Corn Starch, D&C Yellow #10, FD&C Yellow #6, Hydroxypropyl Cellulose, Hydroxypropyl Methylcellulose, Magnesium Stearate, Polyethylene Glycol, Sodium Starch Glycolate, Titanium Dioxide. **Gelcaps and Geltabs:** Benzyl Alcohol, Butylparaben, Castor Oil, Cellulose, Corn Starch, D&C Yellow #10, Edetate Calcium Disodium, FD&C Blue #1, FD&C Blue #2, Gelatin, Hydroxypropyl Methylcellulose, Magnesium Stearate, Methylparaben, Propylparaben, Sodium Lauryl Sulfate, Sodium Propionate, Sodium Starch Glycolate, Titanium Dioxide.

How Supplied:

TYLENOL® Severe Allergy: **Caplets:** Yellow film-coated, imprinted with "TYLENOL Severe Allergy" on one side—blister packs of 24. Store at room temperature.

Maximum Strength TYLENOL® Allergy Sinus NightTime: **Caplets:** Light blue film-coated, imprinted with "TYLENOL A/S NightTime" on one side—blister packs of 24. Store at room temperature.

Maximum Strength TYLENOL® Allergy Sinus: **Caplets:** Yellow film-coated, imprinted with "TYLENOL Allergy Sinus" on one side—blister packs of 24. Store at room temperature.

Gelcaps and Geltabs: Green and yellow-colored, imprinted with "TYLENOL A/S"—blister packs of 24 and 48. Store at room temperature; avoid high humidity and excessive heat 40°C (104°F).

Shown in Product Identification Guide, page 511

**Multi-Symptom
TYLENOL® Cold Non-Drowsy
Caplets and Gelcaps**

**Multi-Symptom
TYLENOL® Cold Complete
Formula Caplets**

Product information for all dosage forms of TYLENOL Cold have been combined under this heading.

Description:

Each *Multi-Symptom TYLENOL® Cold Non-Drowsy Caplet and Gelcap* contains acetaminophen 325 mg, dextromethorphan HBr 15 mg, and pseudoephedrine HCl 30 mg.

Each *Multi-Symptom TYLENOL® Cold Complete Formula Caplet* contains acetaminophen 325 mg, chlorpheniramine maleate 2 mg, dextromethorphan HBr 15 mg, and pseudoephedrine HCl 30 mg.

Actions:

Multi-Symptom TYLENOL® Cold Non-Drowsy contains a clinically proven analgesic-antipyretic, a decongestant and a cough suppressant. Acetaminophen produces analgesia by elevation of the pain threshold and antipyresis through action on the hypothalamic heat regulating center. Acetaminophen is equal to aspirin in analgesic and antipyretic effectiveness and it is unlikely to produce many of the side effects associated with aspirin and aspirin-containing products. Pseudoephedrine is a sympathomimetic amine which provides temporary relief of nasal congestion. Dextromethorphan is a cough suppressant which provides temporary relief of coughs due to minor throat irritations that may occur with the common cold.

Multi-Symptom TYLENOL® Cold Complete Formula Caplets contain, in addition to the above ingredients, an antihistamine. Chlorpheniramine is an antihistamine which helps provide temporary relief of runny nose, sneezing and watery and itchy eyes.

Uses:

Multi-Symptom TYLENOL® Cold Non-Drowsy: For the temporary relief of these cold symptoms: minor aches and pains, headaches, sore throat, nasal congestion, coughs. For the reduction of fever.

Multi-Symptom TYLENOL® Cold Complete Formula: For the temporary relief of these cold symptoms: minor aches and pains, headaches, sore throat, nasal congestion, runny nose, coughs, sneezing, watery and itchy eyes. For the reduction of fever.

Directions:

Multi-Symptom TYLENOL® Cold Non Drowsy and Multi-Symptom TYLENOL® Cold Complete Formula: **Adults and children 12 years of age and older:** Take 2 every 6 hours. Do not take more than 8 in 24 hours, or as directed by a doctor. **Children 6–11 years of age:** Take 1 every 6 hours. Do not take more than 4 in 24 hours, or as directed by a doctor. **Children under 6 years of age:** Do not use this product in children under 6 years of age. This will provide more than the recommended dose (overdose) and could cause serious health problems.

Precautions:

If a rare sensitivity reaction occurs, the drug should be discontinued.

Warnings:

Alcohol Warning: If you consume 3 or more alcoholic drinks every day, ask your doctor whether you should take acetaminophen or other pain relievers/fever reducers. Acetaminophen may cause liver damage.

Multi-Symptom TYLENOL® Cold Non Drowsy: **Do not use if carton is opened or if blister unit is broken.** Do not take for pain for more than 7 days or for fever for more than 3 days unless directed by a doctor. If pain or fever persists, or gets worse, if new symptoms occur, or if redness or swelling is present, consult a doctor because these could be signs of a serious condition. If sore throat is severe, persists for more than 2 days, is accompanied or followed by fever, headache, rash, nausea or vomiting, consult a doctor promptly. A persistent cough may be a sign of a serious condition. If cough persists for more than 1 week, tends to recur or is accompanied by fever, rash or persistent headache, consult a doctor. Do not take this product for persistent or chronic cough such as occurs with smoking, asthma, emphysema or if cough is accompanied by excessive phlegm (mucus) unless directed by a doctor.

Do not exceed recommended dosage. If nervousness, dizziness or sleeplessness, occur, discontinue use and consult a doctor. Do not take this product if you have heart disease, high blood pressure, thyroid disease, diabetes or difficulty in urination due to enlargement of the prostate gland unless directed by a doctor.

Keep this and all drugs out of the reach of children. In case of accidental overdose, contact a doctor or poison control center immediately. Prompt medical attention is critical for adults as well as for children even if you do not notice any signs or symptoms. As with any drug, if you are pregnant or nursing a baby, seek the advice of a health professional before using this product. Do not use with other products containing acetaminophen.

Multi-Symptom TYLENOL® Cold Complete Formula: **Do not use if carton is opened or if blister unit is broken.** Do not take for pain for more than 7 days or for fever for more than 3 days unless directed by a doctor. If pain or fever persists, or gets worse, if new symptoms occur, or if redness or swelling is present, consult a doctor because these could be signs of a serious condition. If sore throat is severe, persists for more than 2 days, is accompanied or followed by fever, headache, rash, nausea or vomiting, consult a doctor promptly. A persistent cough may be a sign of a serious condition. If cough persists for more than 1 week, tends to recur or is accompanied by fever, rash or persistent headache, consult a doctor. Do not take this product for persistent or chronic cough such as occurs with smoking, asthma, emphysema or if cough is accompanied by excessive phlegm (mucus) unless directed by a doctor.

Do not exceed recommended dosage. If nervousness, dizziness or sleeplessness occur, discontinue use and consult a

Continued on next page

Tylenol Cold—Cont.

doctor. May cause excitability especially in children. Do not take this product unless directed by a doctor, if you have a breathing problem such as emphysema or chronic bronchitis, or if you have glaucoma or difficulty in urination due to enlargement of the prostate gland. Do not take this product if you have heart disease, high blood pressure, thyroid disease or diabetes unless directed by a doctor. May cause drowsiness; alcohol, sedatives and tranquilizers may increase the drowsiness effect. Avoid alcoholic beverages while taking this product. Do not take this product if you are taking sedatives or tranquilizers without first consulting your doctor. Use caution when driving a motor vehicle or operating machinery.

Keep this and all drugs out of the reach of children. In case of accidental overdose, contact a doctor or poison control center immediately. Prompt medical attention is critical for adults as well as for children even if you do not notice any signs or symptoms. As with any drug, if you are pregnant or nursing a baby, seek the advice of a health professional before using this product. Do not use with other products containing acetaminophen.

Drug Interaction Precaution

Do not use this product if you are now taking a prescription monoamine oxidase inhibitor (MAOI) (certain drugs for depression, psychiatric or emotional conditions, or Parkinson's disease), or for 2 weeks after stopping the MAOI drug. If you are uncertain whether your prescription drug contains an MAOI, consult a health professional before taking this product.

Professional Information:
Overdosage Information

For overdosage information, please refer to pgs. 648–649.

Inactive Ingredients:

Multi-Symptom TYLENOL® Cold Non Drowsy Formula: **Caplets:** Carnauba Wax, Cellulose, Corn Starch, D&C Yellow #10, FD&C Blue #1, Hydroxypropyl Methylcellulose, Iron Oxide, Magnesium Stearate, Sodium Starch Glycolate, Titanium Dioxide, Triacetin.

Gelcaps: Benzyl Alcohol, Butylparaben, Castor Oil, Cellulose, Corn Starch, D&C Yellow #10, Edetate Calcium Disodium, FD&C Red #40, Gelatin, Hydroxypropyl Methylcellulose, Iron Oxide, Magnesium Stearate, Methylparaben, Propylparaben, Sodium Lauryl Sulfate, Sodium Propionate, Sodium Starch Glycolate, Titanium Dioxide.

Multi-Symptom TYLENOL® Cold Complete Formula: **Caplets:** Carnauba Wax, Cellulose, Corn Starch, D&C Yellow #10, FD&C Blue #1, FD&C Yellow #6, Hydroxypropyl Methylcellulose, Iron Oxide, Magnesium Stearate, Sodium Starch Glycolate, Titanium Dioxide, Triacetin.

How Supplied:

Multi-Symptom TYLENOL® Cold Non Drowsy: **Caplets:** White-colored, imprinted with "TYLENOL Cold"—blister packs of 24. Store at room temperature. **Gelcaps:** Red- and tan-colored, imprinted with "TYLENOL COLD"—blister packs of 24. Store at room temperature. Avoid high humidity and excessive heat 40°C (104°F).

Multi-Symptom TYLENOL® Cold Complete Formula: **Caplets:** Yellow-colored, imprinted with "TYLENOL Cold"—blister packs of 24. Store at room temperature.

Shown in Product Identification Guide, page 512

Multi-Symptom
TYLENOL® Cold
Severe Congestion Non-Drowsy

Description:

Each *Multi-Symptom TYLENOL® Cold Severe Congestion Non-Drowsy Caplet* contains acetaminophen 325 mg, dextromethorphan HBr 15 mg, guaifenesin 200 mg and pseudoephedrine HCl 30 mg.

Actions:

Multi-Symptom TYLENOL® Cold Severe Congestion Non-Drowsy Caplets contains a clinically proven analgesic-antipyretic, decongestant, expectorant and cough suppressant. Acetaminophen produces analgesia by elevation of the pain threshold and antipyresis through action on the hypothalamic heat regulating center. Acetaminophen is equal to aspirin in analgesic and antipyretic effectiveness and is unlikely to produce many of the side effects associated with aspirin and aspirin-containing products. Pseudoephedrine is a sympathomimetic amine which provides temporary relief of nasal congestion. Guaifenesin is an expectorant which helps loosen phlegm (mucus) and thin bronchial secretions to make coughs more productive. Dextromethorphan is a cough suppressant which provides temporary relief of coughs due to minor throat irritations that may occur with the common cold.

Uses:

Multi-Symptom TYLENOL® Cold Severe Congestion Non-Drowsy Caplets: For the temporary relief of these cold symptoms: minor aches and pains, headaches, sore throat, nasal congestion, chest congestion, cough. For the reduction of fever.

Directions:

Adults and children 12 years of age and older: Take 2 caplets every 6–8 hours. Do not take more than 8 caplets in 24 hours, or as directed by a doctor. **Children 6–11 years of age:** Take 1 caplet every 6–8 hours. Do not take more than 4 caplets in 24 hours, or as directed by a doctor. **Children under 6 years of age:** Do not use this product in children under 6 years of age. This will pro-

vide more than the recommended dose (overdose) and could cause serious health problems.

Precautions:

If a rare sensitivity reaction occurs, the drug should be discontinued.

Warnings:

Alcohol Warning: If you consume 3 or more alcoholic drinks every day, ask your doctor whether you should take acetaminophen or other pain relievers/fever reducers. Acetaminophen may cause liver damage.

Do not use if carton is opened or if blister unit is broken. Do not take for pain for more than 7 days or for fever for more than 3 days unless directed by a doctor. If pain or fever persists, or gets worse, if new symptoms occur, or if redness or swelling is present, consult a doctor because these could be signs of a serious condition. If sore throat is severe, persists for more than 2 days, is accompanied or followed by fever, headache, rash, nausea or vomiting, consult a doctor promptly. A persistent cough may be a sign of a serious condition. If cough persists for more than 1 week, tends to recur or is accompanied by fever, rash or persistent headache, consult a doctor. Do not take this product for persistent or chronic cough such as occurs with smoking, asthma, emphysema or if cough is accompanied by excessive phlegm (mucus) unless directed by a doctor. **Do not exceed recommended dosage.** If nervousness, dizziness, or sleeplessness occur, discontinue use and consult a doctor. Do not take this product if you have heart disease, high blood pressure, thyroid disease, diabetes or difficulty in urination due to enlargement of the prostate gland unless directed by a doctor.

Keep this and all drugs out of the reach of children. In case of accidental overdose, contact a doctor or poison control center immediately. Prompt medical attention is critical for adults as well as for children even if you do not notice any signs or symptoms. As with any drug, if you are pregnant or nursing a baby, seek the advice of a health professional before using this product. Do not use with other products containing acetaminophen.

Drug Interaction Precaution:

Do not use this product if you are now taking a prescription monoamine oxidase inhibitor (MAOI) (certain drugs for depression, psychiatric or emotional conditions, or Parkinson's disease), or for 2 weeks after stoppping the MAOI drug. If you are uncertain whether your prescription drug contains an MAOI, consult a health professional before taking this product.

Professional Information:
Overdosage Information

For overdosage information, please refer to pgs. 648–649.

Inactive Ingredients:

Carnauba Wax, Cellulose, Corn Starch, D&C Yellow #10, FD&C Blue #1, FD&C

Yellow #6, Hydroxypropyl Methylcellulose, Iron Oxide, Povidone, Silicon Dioxide, Sodium Starch Glycolate, Stearic Acid, Titanium Dioxide, Triacetin.

How Supplied:

Caplets: Buttery-tan-colored, imprinted with *"TYLENOL COLD SC"* in green ink—blister packs of 24. Store at room temperature. Avoid high humidity and excessive heat (40°C).

Shown in Product Identification Guide, page 512

Maximum Strength TYLENOL® Flu Non-Drowsy Gelcaps

Maximum Strength TYLENOL® Flu NightTime Gelcaps

Maximum Strength TYLENOL® Flu NightTime Liquid

Product information for all dosage forms of TYLENOL Flu have been combined under this heading.

Description: Each *Maximum Strength TYLENOL® Flu Non-Drowsy Gelcap* contains acetaminophen 500 mg, dextromethorphan HBr 15 mg and pseudoephedrine HCl 30 mg. Each *Maximum Strength TYLENOL® Flu NightTime Gelcap* contains acetaminophen 500 mg, diphenhydramine HCl 25 mg and pseudoephedrine HCl 30 mg. *Maximum Strength TYLENOL® Flu NightTime Liquid:* Each 30 mL (2 tablespoonsful) contains acetaminophen 1000 mg, dextromethorphan HBr 30 mg, doxylamine succinate 12.5 mg, and pseudoephedrine HCl 60 mg.

Actions: *Maximum Strength TYLENOL® Flu Non-Drowsy Gelcaps* contain a clinically proven analgesic-antipyretic, a decongestant and a cough suppressant. Acetaminophen produces analgesia by elevation of the pain threshold and antipyresis through action on the hypothalamic heat regulating center. Acetaminophen is equal to aspirin in analgesic and antipyretic effectiveness and it is unlikely to produce many of the side effects associated with aspirin and aspirin-containing products. Pseudoephedrine hydrochloride is a sympathomimetic amine which provides temporary relief of nasal congestion. Dextromethorphan is a cough suppressant which provides temporary relief of coughs due to minor throat irritations that may occur with the common cold. *Maximum Strength TYLENOL® Flu NightTime Gelcaps* contains the same clinically proven analgesic-antipyretic and decongestant as *Maximum Strength TYLENOL® Flu Non-Drowsy Gelcaps* along with an antihistamine. Diphenhydramine is an antihistamine which helps provide temporary relief of runny nose and sneezing. *Maximum Strength TYLENOL® Flu NightTime Liquid* contains the same clinically proven analgesic-antipyretic, decongestant and cough suppressant as *Maximum Strength TYLENOL Flu Non-Drowsy Gelcaps* along with an antihistamine. Doxylamine succinate is an antihistamine which helps provide temporary relief of runny nose and sneezing.

Uses: *Maximum Strength TYLENOL® Flu Non-Drowsy Gelcaps:* For the temporary relief of these cold and flu symptoms: minor aches and pains, headaches, sore throat, nasal congestion, coughs. For the reduction of fever.
Maximum Strength TYLENOL® Flu NightTime Gelcaps: For the temporary relief of these cold and flu symptoms: minor aches and pains, headaches, sore throat, nasal congestion, runny nose, sneezing. For the reduction of fever.
Maximum Strength TYLENOL® Flu NightTime Liquid: For the temporary relief of: body aches and headache, coughing, nasal congestion, sore throat, runny nose/sneezing. For the reduction of fever.

Directions: *Maximum Strength TYLENOL® Flu Non-Drowsy Gelcaps:*
Adults and children 12 years of age and older: Take 2 gelcaps every 6 hours. Do not take more than 8 gelcaps in 24 hours, or as directed by a doctor. **Children under 12 years:** Do not use this adult product in children under 12 years of age. This will provide more than the recommended dose (overdose) and could cause serious health problems.
Maximum Strength TYLENOL® Flu NightTime Gelcaps: **Adults and children 12 years of age and older:** Take 2 gelcaps at bedtime. May repeat every 6 hours. Do not take more than 8 gelcaps in 24 hours, or as directed by a doctor. **Children under 12 years:** Do not use this adult product in children under 12 years of age. This will provide more than the recommended dose (overdose) and could cause serious health problems.
Maximum Strength TYLENOL® Flu NightTime Liquid: **Adults and children 12 years of age and older:** Take 2 Tablespoons (tbsp). May repeat every 6 hours. Do not use more than 4 times in 24 hours, or as directed by a doctor. **Children under 12 years:** Do not use this adult product in children under 12 years of age. This will provide more than the recommended dose (overdose) and could cause serious health problems.

Precautions: If a rare sensitivity reaction occurs, the drug should be discontinued.

Warnings: Alcohol Warning: If you consume 3 or more alcoholic drinks every day, ask your doctor whether you should take acetaminophen or other pain relievers/fever reducers. Acetaminophen may cause liver damage.
Maximum Strength TYLENOL® Flu Non-Drowsy Gelcaps: **Do not use if carton is opened or if blister unit is broken.** Do not take for pain for more than 7 days or for fever for more than 3 days unless directed by a doctor. If pain or fever persists, or gets worse, if new symptoms occur, or if redness or swelling is present, consult a doctor because these could be signs of a serious condition. If sore throat is severe, persists for more than 2 days, is accompanied or followed by fever, headache, rash, nausea or vomiting, consult a doctor promptly. A persistent cough may be a sign of a serious condition. If cough persists for more than 1 week, tends to recur or is accompanied by fever, rash or persistent headache, consult a doctor. Do not take this product for persistent or chronic cough such as occurs with smoking, asthma, emphysema or if cough is accompanied by excessive phlegm (mucus) unless directed by a doctor.

Do not exceed recommended dosage. If nervousness, dizziness or sleeplessness occur, discontinue use and consult a doctor. Do not take this product if you have heart disease, high blood pressure, thyroid disease, diabetes, or difficulty in urination due to enlargement of the prostate gland unless directed by a doctor.

Keep this and all drugs out of the reach of children. In case of accidental overdose, contact a doctor or poison control center immediately. Prompt medical attention is critical for adults as well as for children even if you do not notice any signs or symptoms. As with any drug, if you are pregnant or nursing a baby, seek the advice of a health professional before using this product. Do not use with other products containing acetaminophen.

Maximum Strength TYLENOL® Flu NightTime Gelcaps: **Do not use if carton is opened or if blister unit is broken.** Do not take for pain for more than 7 days or for fever for more than 3 days unless directed by a doctor. If pain or fever persists, or gets worse, if new symptoms occur, or if redness or swelling is present, consult a doctor because these could be signs of a serious condition. If sore throat is severe, persists for more than 2 days, is accompanied by fever, headache, rash, nausea or vomiting, consult a doctor promptly.

Do not exceed recommended dosage. If nervousness, dizziness, or sleeplessness occur, discontinue use and consult a doctor. May cause excitability, especially in children. Do not take this product, unless directed by a doctor, if you have a breathing problem such as emphysema or chronic bronchitis, or if you have glaucoma or difficulty in urination due to enlargement of the prostate gland. Do not take this product if you have heart disease, high blood pressure, thyroid disease, or diabetes unless directed by a doctor. May cause marked drowsiness; alcohol, sedatives and tranquilizers may increase the drowsiness effect. Avoid alcoholic beverages while taking this product. Do not take this product if you are taking sedatives or tranquilizers without first consulting your doctor. Use caution when driving a motor vehicle or operating machinery.

Continued on next page

Tylenol Flu—Cont.

Keep this and all drugs out of the reach of children. In case of accidental overdose, contact a doctor or poison control center immediately. Prompt medical attention is critical for adults as well as for children even if you do not notice any signs or symptoms. As with any drug, if you are pregnant or nursing a baby, seek the advice of a health professional before using this product. Do not use with other products containing acetaminophen.

Maximum Strength TYLENOL® Flu NightTime Liquid: **Do not use if carton is opened or if bottle wrap or foil inner seal imprinted "Safety Seal®" is broken or missing.** Do not take for pain for more than 7 days or for fever for more than 3 days unless directed by a doctor. If pain or fever persists, or gets worse, if new symptoms occur, or if redness or swelling is present, consult a doctor because these could be signs of a serious condition. If sore throat is severe, persists for more than 2 days, is accompanied or followed by fever, headache, rash, nausea, or vomiting, consult a doctor promptly. A persistent cough may be a sign of a serious condition. If cough persists for more than 1 week, tends to recur or is accompanied by fever, rash or persistent headache, consult a doctor. Do not take this product for persistent or chronic cough such as occurs with smoking, asthma, or emphysema or if cough is accompanied by excessive phlegm (mucus) unless directed by a doctor. **Do not exceed recommended dosage.** If nervousness, dizziness or sleeplessness occur, discontinue use and consult a doctor. May cause excitability especially in children. Do not take this product, unless directed by a doctor, if you have a breathing problem such as emphysema or chronic bronchitis, or if you have glaucoma or difficulty in urination due to enlargement of the prostate gland. Do not take this product if you have heart disease, high blood pressure, thyroid disease or diabetes unless directed by a doctor.

May cause marked drowsiness; alcohol, sedatives and tranquilizers may increase the drowsiness effect. Avoid alcoholic beverages while taking this product. Do not take this product if you are taking sedatives or tranquilizers, without first consulting your doctor. Use caution when driving a motor vehicle or operating machinery.

Keep this and all drugs out of the reach of children. In case of accidental overdose, contact a doctor or poison control center immediately. Prompt medical attention is critical for adults as well as for children even if you do not notice any signs or symptoms. As with any drug, if you are pregnant or nursing a baby, seek the advice of a health professional before using this product. Do not use with other products containing acetaminophen.

Drug Interaction Precaution: Do not use this product if you are now taking a prescription monoamine oxidase inhibitor (MAOI) (certain drugs for depression, psychiatric or emotional conditions, or Parkinson's disease), or for 2 weeks after stopping the MAOI drug. If you are uncertain whether your prescription drug contains an MAOI, consult a health professional before taking this product.

Professional Information:
Overdosage Information
For overdosage information, please refer to pgs. 648–649.

Inactive Ingredients: *Maximum Strength TYLENOL® Flu Non-Drowsy Gelcaps:* Benzyl Alcohol, Butylparaben, Castor Oil, Cellulose, Corn Starch, Edetate Calcium Disodium, FD&C Blue #1, FD&C Red #40, Gelatin, Hydroxypropyl Methylcellulose, Iron Oxide, Magnesium Stearate, Methylparaben, Propylparaben, Sodium Lauryl Sulfate, Sodium Propionate, Sodium Starch Glycolate, Titanium Dioxide.

Maximum Strength TYLENOL® Flu NightTime Gelcaps: Benzyl Alcohol, Butylparaben, Castor Oil, Cellulose, Corn Starch, D&C Red #28, Edetate Calcium Disodium, FD&C Blue #1, Gelatin, Hydroxypropyl Methylcellulose, Iron Oxide, Magnesium Stearate, Methylparaben, Propylparaben, Sodium Citrate, Sodium Lauryl Sulfate, Sodium Propionate, Sodium Starch Glycolate, Titanium Dioxide.

Maximum Strength TYLENOL® Flu NightTime Liquid: Citric Acid, Corn Syrup, D&C Red #33, FD&C Red #40, Flavors, Polyethylene Glycol, Propylene Glycol, Purified Water, Saccharin Sodium, Sodium Benzoate, Sorbitol.

How Supplied: *Maximum Strength TYLENOL® Flu Non-Drowsy:* **Gelcaps:** Burgundy- and white-colored gelcap, imprinted with "TYLENOL FLU" in gray ink—blister packs of 24. Store at room temperature. Avoid high humidity and excessive heat 40°C (104°F).

Maximum Strength TYLENOL® Flu NightTime: **Gelcaps:** Blue and white-colored gelcap, imprinted with "TYLENOL FLU NT" gray ink—blister packs of 12 and 24. Store at room temperature. Avoid high humidity and excessive heat 40°C (104°F). **Liquid:** Red-colored—bottles of 8 fl. oz with child resistant safety cap and tamper evident packaging. Store at room temperature.

Shown in Product Identification Guide, page 512

Extra Strength
TYLENOL® PM
Pain Reliever/Sleep Aid Caplets, Geltabs and Gelcaps

Description: Each *Extra Strength TYLENOL® PM Caplet, Geltab* or *Gelcap* contains acetaminophen 500 mg and diphenhydramine HCl 25 mg.

Actions: *Extra Strength TYLENOL® PM Caplets, Geltabs* and *Gelcaps* contain a clinically proven analgesic-antipyretic and an antihistamine. Maximum allowable non-prescription levels of acetaminophen and diphenhydramine provide temporary relief of occasional headaches and minor aches and pains accompanying sleeplessness. Acetaminophen is equal to aspirin in analgesic and antipyretic effectiveness and it is unlikely to produce many of the side effects associated with aspirin containing products. Acetaminophen produces analgesia by elevation of the pain threshold. Diphenhydramine HCl is an antihistamine with sedative properties.

Uses: *Extra Strength TYLENOL® PM Caplets, Geltabs* and *Gelcaps:* For the temporary relief of occasional headaches and minor aches and pains with accompanying sleeplessness.

Directions: Adults and children 12 years of age and older: Take 2 caplets, geltabs or gelcaps at bedtime or as directed by a doctor. **Children under 12 years of age:** Do not use this adult product in children under 12 years of age. This will provide more than the recommended dose (overdose) and could cause serious health problems.

Precautions: If a rare sensitivity reaction occurs, the drug should be discontinued.

Warnings: Alcohol Warning: If you consume 3 or more alcoholic drinks every day, ask your doctor whether you should take acetaminophen or other pain relievers/fever reducers. Acetaminophen may cause liver damage.

Do not use if carton is opened or neck wrap or foil inner seal imprinted with "Safety Seal®" is broken. If sleeplessness persists continuously for more than 2 weeks, consult your doctor. Insomnia may be a symptom of serious underlying medical illness. Do not take for pain for more than 10 days or for fever for more than 3 days unless directed by a doctor. If pain or fever persists, or gets worse, if new symptoms occur, or if redness or swelling is present, consult a doctor because these could be signs of a serious condition. Do not take this product, unless directed by a doctor, if you have a breathing problem such as emphysema or chronic bronchitis, or if you have glaucoma or difficulty in urination due to enlargement of the prostate gland. Avoid alcoholic beverages while taking this product. Do not take this product if your are taking sedatives or tranquilizers without first consulting your doctor. **Do not exceed recommended dose.** Keep this and all drugs out of the reach of children. In case of accidental overdose, contact a physician or poison control center immediately. Prompt medical attention is critical for adults as well as for children even if you do not notice any signs or symptoms. As with any drug, if you are pregnant or nursing a baby, seek the advice of a health professional before using this product. Do not use with other products containing acetaminophen.

CAUTION: This product will cause drowsiness. Do not drive a motor vehicle or operate machinery after use.

Professional Information:
Overdosage Information
For overdosage information, please refer to pgs. 648–649.

Inactive Ingredients: Caplets: Cellulose, Cornstarch, FD&C Blue #1, FD&C Blue #2, Hydroxypropyl Methylcellulose, Magnesium Stearate, Polyethylene Glycol, Polysorbate 80, Sodium Citrate, Sodium Starch Glycolate, Titanium Dioxide.
Geltabs/Gelcaps: Benzyl Alcohol, Butylparaben, Castor Oil, Cellulose, Corn Starch, D&C Red #28, Edetate Calcium Disodium, FD&C Blue #1, Gelatin, Hydroxypropyl Methylcellulose, Magnesium Stearate, Methylparaben, Propylparaben, Sodium Citrate, Sodium Lauryl Sulfate, Sodium Propionate, Sodium Starch Glycolate, Titanium Dioxide.

How Supplied: Caplets (colored light blue imprinted "Tylenol PM") tamper-evident bottles of 24, 50, 100, and 150. Store at room temperature.
Gelcaps (colored blue and white imprinted "TYLENOL PM") tamper-evident bottles of 24 and 50. Store at room temperature; avoid high humidity and excessive heat 40°C (104°F).
Geltabs (colored blue and white imprinted "TYLENOL PM") tamper-evident bottles of 24, 50, and 100. Store at room temperature; avoid high humidity and excessive heat 40°C (104°F).

Shown in Product Identification Guide, page 512

**Maximum Strength
TYLENOL® Sinus Non-Drowsy**
Geltabs, Gelcaps, Caplets and Tablets

**Maximum Strength
TYLENOL® Sinus
NightTime Caplets**

Product information for all dosage forms of TYLENOL Sinus have been combined under this heading.

Description: Each *Maximum Strength TYLENOL® Sinus Non-Drowsy Geltab, Gelcap, or Caplet* contains acetaminophen 500 mg and pseudoephedrine HCl 30 mg. Each *Maximum Strength TYLENOL® Sinus NightTime Caplet* contains acetaminophen 500 mg, doxylamine succinate 6.25 mg and pseudoephedrine HCl 30 mg.

Actions: *Maximum Strength TYLENOL® Sinus Non-Drowsy* contains a clinically proven analgesic-antipyretic and a decongestant. Maximum allowable non-prescription levels of acetaminophen and pseudoephedrine provide temporary relief of sinus pain and headache and congestion. Acetaminophen is equal to aspirin in analgesic and antipyretic effectiveness and it is unlikely to produce many of the side effects associated with aspirin and aspirin-containing products. Acetaminophen produces analgesia by elevation of the pain threshold and antipyresis through action on the hypothalamic heat regulating center. Pseudoephedrine hydrochloride is a sympathomimetic amine which promotes sinus cavity drainage by reducing nasopharyngeal mucosal congestion.
Maximum Strength TYLENOL® Sinus NightTime Caplets contain, in addition to the above ingredients, an antihistamine which provides temporary relief of runny nose and itching of the nose or throat.

Uses: *Maximum Strength TYLENOL® Sinus Non-Drowsy:* For the temporary relief of sinus pain and headaches and nasal and sinus congestion.
Maximum Strength TYLENOL® Sinus NightTime: For the temporary relief of nasal congestion, sinus congestion and pressure, sinus pain, headache, runny nose, and itching of the nose or throat.

Precautions: If a rare sensitivity reaction occurs, the drug should be discontinued.

Directions: *Maximum Strength TYLENOL® Sinus Non-Drowsy:* **Adults and children 12 years of age and older:** Take 2 every 4–6 hours. Do not take more than 8 in 24 hours, or as directed by a doctor.
Children under 12 years: Do not use this adult product in children under 12 years of age. This will provide more than the recommended dose (overdose) and could cause serious health problems.
Maximum Strength TYLENOL® Sinus NightTime: **Adults and children 12 years of age and older:** Take 2 caplets at bedtime. May repeat every 4 to 6 hours. Do not take more than 8 caplets in 24 hours, or as directed by a doctor.
Children under 12 years: Do not use this adult product in children under 12 years of age. This will provide more than the recommended dose (overdose) and could cause serious health problems.

Warnings: Alcohol Warning: If you consume 3 or more alcoholic drinks every day, ask your doctor whether you should take acetaminophen or other pain relievers/fever reducers. Acetaminophen may cause liver damage.
Maximum Strength TYLENOL® Sinus Non-Drowsy: **Do not use if carton is opened or if blister unit is broken.** Do not take for pain for more than 7 days or for fever for more than 3 days unless directed by a doctor. If pain or fever persists, or gets worse, if new symptoms occur, or if redness or swelling is present, consult a doctor because these could be signs of a serious condition. If nervousness, dizziness or sleeplessness occur, discontinue use and consult a doctor. Do not take this product if you have heart disease, high blood pressure, thyroid disease, diabetes, or difficulty in urination due to enlargement of the prostate gland unless directed by a doctor.

Do not exceed recommended dosage. Keep this and all drugs out of the reach of children. In case of accidental overdose, contact a doctor or poison control center immediately. Prompt medical attention is critical for adults as well as for children even if you do not notice any signs or symptoms. As with any drug, if you are pregnant or nursing a baby, seek the advice of a health professional before using this product. Do not use with other products containing acetaminophen.
Maximum Strength TYLENOL® Sinus NightTime Caplets: **Do not use if carton is opened or if blister unit is broken.** Do not take for pain for more than 7 days or for fever for more than 3 days unless directed by a doctor. If pain or fever persists, or gets worse, if new symptoms occur, or if redness or swelling is present, consult a doctor because these could be signs of a serious condition. May cause excitability especially in children. If nervousness, dizziness or sleeplessness occur, discontinue use and consult a doctor. May cause marked drowsiness; alcohol, sedatives and tranquilizers may increase the drowsiness effect. Avoid alcoholic beverages while taking this product. Do not take this product if you are taking sedatives or tranquilizers, without first consulting your doctor. Use caution when driving a motor vehicle or operating machinery. Do not take this product, unless directed by a doctor, if you have a breathing problem such as emphysema or chronic bronchitis, or if you have glaucoma, or difficulty in urination due to enlargement of the prostate gland. Do not take this product if you have heart disease, high blood pressure, thyroid disease or diabetes unless directed by a doctor.
Do not exceed recommended dosage. Keep this and all drugs out of the reach of children. In case of accidental overdose, contact a doctor or poison control center immediately. Prompt medical attention is critical for adults as well as for children even if you do not notice any signs or symptoms. As with any drug. If you are pregnant or nursing a baby, seek the advice of a health professional before using this product. Do not use with other products containing acetaminophen.

Drug Interaction Precaution: Do not use this product if you are now taking a prescription monoamine oxidase inhibitor (MAOI) (certain drugs for depression, psychiatric or emotional conditions, or Parkinson's disease), or for 2 weeks after stopping the MAOI drug. If you are uncertain whether your prescription drug contains an MAOI, consult a health professional before taking this product.

Professional Information:
Overdosage Information
For overdosage information, please refer to pgs. 648–649.

Inactive Ingredients: *Maximum Strength TYLENOL® Sinus Non-Drowsy Formula:* **Caplets:** Carnauba

Continued on next page

Tylenol Sinus—Cont.

Wax, Cellulose, Corn Starch, D&C Yellow #10, FD&C Blue #1, FD&C Red #40, Hydroxypropyl Methylcellulose, Iron Oxide, Magnesium Stearate, Polyethylene Glycol, Polysorbate 80, Sodium Starch Glycolate, Titanium Dioxide.

Gelcaps and Geltabs: Benzyl Alcohol, Butylparaben, Castor Oil, Cellulose, Corn Starch, D&C Yellow #10, Edetate Calcium Disodium, FD&C Blue #1, Gelatin, Hydroxypropyl Methylcellulose, Iron Oxide, Magnesium Stearate, Methylparaben, Propylparaben, Sodium Lauryl Sulfate, Sodium Propionate, Sodium Starch Glycolate, Titanium Dioxide.

Maximum Strength TYLENOL® Sinus NightTime Caplets: Cellulose, Corn Starch, FD&C Blue #1, FD&C Blue #2, Hydroxypropyl Methylcellulose, Iron Oxide, Silicon Dioxide, Sodium Starch Glycolate, Stearic Acid, Titanium Dioxide, Triacetin.

How Supplied: *Maximum Strength TYLENOL® Sinus Non-Drowsy Formula:*

Caplets: Light green-colored, imprinted with "TYLENOL Sinus" in green ink—blister packs of 24 and 48. Store at room temperature.

Gelcaps: Green- and white-colored, imprinted with "TYLENOL Sinus" in dark green ink—blister packs of 24 and 48. Store at room temperature; avoid high humidity and excessive heat 40°C (104°F).

Geltabs: Green-colored on one side and white-colored on opposite side, imprinted with "TYLENOL Sinus" in gray ink—blister packs of 24 and 48. Store at room temperature; avoid high humidity and excessive heat 40°C (104°F).

Maximum Strength TYLENOL® Sinus NightTime Caplets: Green-colored, imprinted with "Tylenol Sinus NT"—blister packs of 24. Store at room temperature.

Shown in Product Identification Guide, page 512

Maximum Strength TYLENOL® Sore Throat Adult Liquid

Description:
Maximum Strength TYLENOL® Sore Throat Liquid is available in Honey Lemon Flavor or Cherry Flavor and contains acetaminophen 1000 mg in each 30 mL (2 Tablespoonsful).

Actions:
Acetaminophen is a clinically proven analgesic/antipyretic. Acetaminophen produces analgesia by elevation of the pain threshold and antipyresis through action on the hypothalamic heat regulating center. Acetaminophen is equal to aspirin in analgesic and antipyretic effectiveness and it is unlikely to produce many of the side effects associated with aspirin and aspirin-containing products.

Uses:
For the temporary relief of minor aches and pains associated with sore throat, headache, muscular aches, common cold. For the reduction of fever.

Directions:
Adults and children 12 years of age and older: Take 2 Tablespoons (tbsp.) every 4 to 6 hours as needed. Do not use more than 4 times in 24 hours, or as directed by a doctor.
Children under 12 years: Do not use this adult product in children under 12 years of age. This will provide more than the recommended dose (overdose) of TYLENOL® and could cause serious health problems.

Precautions:
If a rare sensitivity reaction occurs, the drug should be discontinued.

Warnings:
Alcohol Warning: If you consume 3 or more alcoholic drinks every day, ask your doctor whether you should take acetaminophen or other pain relievers/fever reducers. Acetaminophen may cause liver damage.
Do Not Use:
• with any other product containing acetaminophen
• for more than 10 days for pain unless directed by a doctor
• for more than 3 days for fever unless directed by a doctor
Stop Using and Ask a Doctor if:
• symptoms do not improve
• new symptoms occur
• pain or fever persists or gets worse
• redness or swelling is present
• sore throat is severe, persists for more than 2 days, is accompanied or followed by fever, headache, rash, nausea or vomiting
Do not exceed recommended dose. Keep this and all drugs out of the reach of children. In case of accidental overdose, contact a physician or poison control center immediately. Prompt medical attention is critical for adults as well as for children even if you do not notice any signs or symptoms. As with any drug, if you are pregnant or nursing a baby, seek the advice of a health professional before using this product. **Do not use if carton is opened or if bottle wrap or foil inner seal imprinted "Safety Seal®" is broken or missing.**

Professional Information:
Overdosage Information
For overdosage information, please refer to pgs. 648–649.

Inactive Ingredients:
Maximum Strength TYLENOL® Sore Throat Honey-Lemon-Flavored Adult Liquid: Carmel color, Citric Acid, Flavor, High Fructose Corn Syrup, Polyethylene Glycol, Propylene Glycol, Purified Water, Saccharin Sodium, Sodium Benzoate, Sorbitol
Maximum Strength TYLENOL® Sore Throat Cherry-Flavored Adult Liquid: Citric Acid, D&C Red No. 33, FD&C Red No. 40, Flavor, High Fructose Corn Syrup, Polyethylene Glycol, Propylene Glycol, Purified Water, Saccharin Sodium, Sodium Benzoate, Sorbitol

How Supplied:
Honey lemon-flavored or cherry-flavored liquid in child-resistant tamper-evident bottles of 8 fl. oz. Store at room temperature.

Shown in Product Identification Guide, page 512

Women's TYLENOL® Multi-Symptom Menstrual Relief Pain Reliever/Diuretic Caplets

Description: Each *Women's Tylenol Multi-Symptom Menstrual Relief Caplet* contains acetaminophen 500 mg and pamabrom 25 mg.

Actions: *Women's TYLENOL® Multi-Symptom Menstrual Relief Caplets* contain a clinically proven analgesic-antipyretic and a diuretic. Maximum allowable non-prescription levels of acetaminophen and pamabrom provide temporary relief of minor aches and pains due to cramps, headache, and backache and water retention, weight gain, bloating, swelling and full feeling associated with the premenstrual and menstrual periods. Acetaminophen is equal to aspirin in analgesic and antipyretic effectiveness and it is unlikely to produce many of the side effects associated with aspirin containing products. Acetaminophen produces analgesia by elevation of the pain threshold. Pamabrom is a diuretic which relieves water retention.

Uses: *Women's TYLENOL® Multi-Symptom Menstrual Relief Caplets:* For the temporary relief of minor aches and pains due to cramps, headache, backache. Temporarily relieves water weight gain, bloating, swelling and full feeling associated with the premenstrual and menstrual periods.

Directions: **Do not take more than directed**
adults and children 12 years and over: Take 2 caplets every 4 to 6 hours, do not take more than 8 caplets in 24 hours, or as directed by a doctor.
children under 12 years: Do not use this adult product in children under 12 years of age; this will provide more than the recommended dose (overdose) and could cause serious health problems.

Precautions: If a rare sensitivity reaction occurs, the drug should be discontinued.

Warnings: Alcohol Warning: If you consume 3 or more alcoholic drinks every day, ask your doctor whether you should take acetaminophen or other pain relievers/fever reducers. Acetaminophen may cause liver damage.
Do not use:
• with any other product containing acetaminophen
Stop use and ask a doctor if:
• new symptoms occur
• redness or swelling is present
• pain gets worse or lasts for more than 10 days
If pregnant or breast-feeding, ask a health professional before use

Keep out of reach of children.
In case of overdose, immediately get medical help or contact a Poison Control Center right away. Prompt medical attention is critical for adults as well as for children even if you do not notice any signs or symptoms.

Other information:
• **do not use if carton is opened, or if neck wrap or foil inner seal imprinted "Safety Seal®" is broken or missing**
• store at room temperature, avoid excessive heat 104°F (40°C)

Professional Information:
Overdosage Information
For overdosage information, please refer to pgs. 648–649.

Inactive Ingredients: cellulose, corn starch, hydroxypropyl methylcellulose, magnesium stearate, polydextrose, polyethylene glycol, sodium starch glycolate, titanium dioxide, triacetin.

How Supplied: Caplets—white capsule shaped caplets with TYME printed on one side in tamper-evident bottles of 24 and 40.

Shown in Product Identification Guide, page 512

**Infants' TYLENOL®
acetaminophen Concentrated
Drops**

**Children's TYLENOL®
acetaminophen Suspension Liquid
and Soft Chews Chewable Tablets**

**Junior Strength TYLENOL®
acetaminophen Soft Chews
Chewable Tablets**

Product information for all dosages of Children's TYLENOL have been combined under this heading

Description: *Infants' TYLENOL® Concentrated Drops* are stable, alcohol-free, grape-flavored and purple in color or cherry-flavored and red in color. Each 1.6 mL (2 dropperfuls) contains 160 mg acetaminophen. *Infants' TYLENOL® Concentrated Drops* features the SAFE-TY-LOCK™ Bottle. The SAFE-TY-LOCK™ Bottle has a unique safety barrier inside the bottle which helps make administration easier. The integrated dropper promotes proper administration. The innovative design eliminates excess product on dropper. The star-shaped barrier inside the bottle minimizes spills and discourages pouring into a spoon. *Children's TYLENOL® Suspension Liquid* is stable, alcohol-free, cherry-flavored and red in color, or bubble gum-flavored and pink in color, or grape-flavored and purple in color. Each 5 mL (one teaspoonful) contains 160 mg acetaminophen. Each *Children's TYLENOL® Soft Chews Chewable Tablet* contains 80 mg acetaminophen in a grape, bubble gum, or fruit flavor. *Each Junior Strength TYLENOL® Soft Chews Chewable Tablet* contain 160 mg acetaminophen in a grape or fruit-flavored chewable tablet.

Actions: Acetaminophen is a clinically proven analgesic/antipyretic. Acetaminophen produces analgesia by elevation of the pain threshold and antipyresis through action on the hypothalamic heat-regulating center. Acetaminophen is equal to aspirin in analgesic and antipyretic effectiveness and it is unlikely to produce many of the side effects associated with aspirin and aspirin-containing products.

Uses: *Infants' TYLENOL® Concentrated Drops and Children's TYLENOL® Suspension Liquid, Soft Chews Chewable Tablets:* For the reduction of fever. For the temporary relief of minor aches and pains associated with a cold, flu, headache, sore throat, immunizations, toothache. *Junior Strength TYLENOL® Soft Chews Chewable Tablets:* For the temporary relief of minor aches and pains associated with: a cold, flu, headache, muscle aches, sprains, overexertion. For the reduction of fever.

Directions: See Table 2: Children's Tylenol Dosing Chart on pgs. 660-662.

Precautions: If a rare sensitivity reaction occurs, the drug should be discontinued.

Warnings: Do Not Use:
• with any other products containing acetaminophen
• for more than 3 days for fever unless directed by a doctor.
• for more than 5 days for pain unless directed by a doctor.
Stop Using This Product and Ask a Doctor If:
• symptoms do not improve.
• new symptoms occur.
• pain or fever persists or gets worse.
• redness or swelling is present.
• sore throat is severe, lasts for more than 2 days or occurs with fever, headache, rash, nausea or vomiting (this statement applies only to Infants' & Children's Tylenol)
Do not exceed recommended dose.
Taking more than the recommended dose (overdose) may not provide more relief and could cause serious health problems. Keep this and all drugs out of the reach of children. In case of accidental overdose, contact a physician or poison control center immediately. Prompt medical attention is critical even if you do not notice any signs or symptoms.
Infants' TYLENOL® Concentrated Drops: **Do not use if plastic carton wrap or bottle wrap imprinted "Safety Seal®" is broken or missing.**
Children's TYLENOL® Suspension Liquid: **Do not use if plastic carton wrap, bottle wrap, or foil inner seal imprinted "Safety Seal®" is broken or missing.** *Children's TYLENOL® Soft Chews Chewable Tablets:* **Do not use if carton is opened or if neck wrap or foil inner seal imprinted "Safety Seal®" is broken or missing.** Phenylketonurics: grape contains phenylalanine 5 mg per tablet, bubble gum contains 6 mg per tablet, fruit contains 6 mg per tablet. *Junior Strength*

TYLENOL® Soft Chews Chewable Tablets: Phenylketonurics: grape soft chew contains phenylalanine 10 mg per tablet, fruit soft chew contains phenylalanine 12 mg per tablet. **Do not use if carton is opened or if blister unit is broken.**

Professional Information:
Overdosage Information for all Infants', Children's & Junior Strength Tylenol® Products

ACETAMINOPHEN: Acetaminophen in massive overdosage may cause hepatic toxicity in some patients. In adults and adolescents ($\geq$ 12 years of age), hepatic toxicity may occur following ingestion of greater than 7.5 to 10 grams over a period of 8 hours or less. Fatalities are infrequent (less than 3–4% of untreated cases) and have rarely been reported with overdoses of less than 15 grams. In children (<12 years of age), an acute overdosage of less than 150 mg/kg has not been associated with hepatic toxicity. Early symptoms following a potentially hepatotoxic overdose may include: nausea, vomiting, diaphoresis and general malaise. Clinical and laboratory evidence of hepatic toxicity may not be apparent until 48 to 72 hours postingestion. In adults and adolescents, any individual presenting with an unknown amount of acetaminophen ingested or with a questionable or unreliable history about the time of ingestion should have a plasma acetaminophen level drawn and be treated with N-acetylcysteine. For full prescribing information, refer to the N-acetylcysteine package insert. Do not await results of assays for plasma acetaminophen levels before initiating treatment with N-acetylcysteine. The following additional procedures are recommended: Promptly initiate gastric decontamination of the stomach. A plasma acetaminophen assay should be obtained as early as possible, but no sooner than four hours following ingestion. If an acetaminophen *extended release* product is involved, it may be appropriate to obtain an additional plasma acetaminophen level 4–6 hours following the initial acetaminophen level. If either acetaminophen level plots above the treatment line on the acetaminophen overdose nomogram, N-acetylcysteine treatment should be continued for a full course of therapy. Liver function studies should be obtained initially and repeated at 24-hour intervals. Serious toxicity or fatalities have been extremely infrequent following an acute acetaminophen overdose in young children, possibly because of differences in the way they metabolize acetaminophen. In children, the maximum potential amount ingested can be more easily estimated. If more than 150 mg/kg or an unknown amount was ingested, obtain a plasma acetaminophen level as soon as possible, but no sooner than 4 hours following ingestion. If an acetaminophen *extended release* product is involved, it may be appropri-

Continued on next page

Tylenol Infants—Cont.

ate to obtain an additional plasma acetaminophen level 4–6 hours following the initial acetaminophen level. If either acetaminophen level plots above the treatment line on the acetaminophen overdose nomogram, *N*-acetylcysteine treatment should be initiated and continued for a full course of therapy. If an assay cannot be obtained and the estimated acetaminophen ingestion exceeds 150 mg/kg, dosing with *N*-acetylcysteine should be initiated and continued for a full course of therapy. For additional emergency information, call your regional poison center or call the Rocky Mountain Poison Center toll-free, (1-800-525-6115).

Our pediatric Tylenol® combination products contain active ingredients in addition to acetaminophen. The following is basic overdose information regarding those ingredients.
CHLORPHENIRAMINE: Chlorpheniramine toxicity should be treated as you would an anthihistamine/anticholinergic overdose and is likely to be present within a few hours after acute ingestion.
DEXTROMETHORPHAN: Acute dextromethorphan overdose usually does not result in serious signs and symptoms unless massive amounts have been ingested. Signs and symptoms of a substantial overdose may include nausea and vomiting, visual disturbances, CNS disturbances and urinary retention.
DIPHENHYDRAMINE: Diphenhydramine toxicity should be treated as you would an antihistamine/anticholinergic overdose and is likely to be present within a few hours after acute ingestion.
PSEUDOEPHEDRINE: Symptoms from pseudoephedrine overdose consist most often of mild anxiety, tachycardia and/or mild hypertension. Symptoms usually appear within 4 to 8 hours of ingestion and are transient, usually requiring no treatment.
For additional emergency information, please contact your local poison control center.

Inactive Ingredients: *Infants' TYLENOL® Concentrated Drops:* **Cherry-Flavored:** Butylparaben, Cellulose, Citric Acid, Corn Syrup, FD&C Red #40, Flavors, Glycerin, Propylene Glycol, Purified Water, Sodium Benzoate, Sorbitol, Xanthan Gum. **Grape-Flavored:** Butylparaben, Cellulose, Citric Acid, Corn Syrup, D&C Red #33, FD&C Blue #1, Flavors, Glycerin, Propylene Glycol, Purified Water, Sodium Benzoate, Sorbitol, Xanthan Gum.
Children's TYLENOL® Suspension Liquid: Butylparaben, Cellulose, Citric Acid, Corn Syrup, Flavors, Glycerin, Propylene Glycol, Purified Water, Sodium Benzoate, Sorbitol, Xanthan Gum. In addition to the above ingredients cherry-flavored suspension contains FD&C Red #40, bubble gum-flavored suspension contains D&C Red #33 and FD&C Red #40, and grape-flavored suspension contains D&C Red #33 and FD&C Blue #1.
Junior Strength TYLENOL® Soft Chews Chewable Tablets: **Fruit-Flavored:** Aspartame, Cellulose, Citric Acid, D&C Red #7, Flavors, Magnesium Stearate, Mannitol. May contain Ethylcellulose or Cellulose Acetate and Povidone. **Grape-Flavored:** Aspartame, Cellulose, Citric Acid, D&C Red #7, D&C Red #30, FD&C Blue #1, Flavors, Magnesium Stearate, Mannitol. May contain Ethylcellulose or Cellulose Acetate and Povidone.
Children's TYLENOL® Soft Chews Chewable Tablets: **Fruit-Flavored:** Aspartame, Cellulose, Citric Acid, D&C Red #7, Flavors, Magnesium Stearate, Mannitol. May contain Ethylcellulose or Cellulose Acetate and Povidone. **Grape-Flavored:** Aspartame, Cellulose, Citric Acid, D&C Red #7, D&C Red #30, FD&C Blue #1, Flavors, Magnesium Stearate, Mannitol. May contain Ethylcellulose or Cellulose Acetate and Povidone. **Bubble Gum-Flavored:** Asparatame, Cellulose, D&C Red #7, Flavors, Magnesium Stearate, Mannitol. May contain Ethylcellulose or Cellulose Actate and Povidone.

How Supplied: *Infants' TYLENOL® Concentrated Drops:* (purple-colored grape): bottles of ½ oz (15 mL) and 1 oz (30 mL); (red-colored cherry): bottles of ½ oz and 1 oz, each with calibrated plastic dropper. Store at room temperature.
Children's TYLENOL® Suspension Liquid: (red-colored cherry): bottles of 2 and 4 fl oz. (pink-colored bubble gum and purple-colored grape): bottles of 4 fl. oz. Store at room temperature.
Children's TYLENOL® Soft Chews Chewable Tablets: (pink-colored fruit, purple-colored grape, pink-colored bubble gum, scored, imprinted "TY80"). Bottles of 30 and also blister packaged 60's and 96's (fruit). Bubble gum and fruit: Store at room temperature; Grape: Store at room temperature and keep product away from direct light.
Junior Strength TYLENOL® Soft Chews Chewable Tablets: (purple-colored grape or pink-colored fruit, imprinted "TYLENOL 160") Package of 24. Fruit: Store at room temperature. Avoid excessive heat: 40°C (104°F); Grape: Store at room temperature. Avoid excessive heat: 40°C (104°F). Keep product away from direct light. All packages listed above are safety sealed and use child-resistant safety caps or blisters.
Shown in Product Identification Guide, page 510, 511

Children's TYLENOL® Allergy-D Liquid

Description: *Children's TYLENOL® Allergy-D Liquid* is Bubble Gum Blast-flavored and contains no alcohol or aspirin. Each teaspoonful (5 mL) contains acetaminophen 160 mg, diphenhydramine HCl 12.5 mg and pseudoephedrine HCl 15 mg.

Actions: *Children's TYLENOL® Allergy-D Liquid* combines the analgesic-antipyretic acetaminophen with the antihistamine diphenhydramine hydrochloride and the decongestant pseudoephedrine hydrochloride to provide fast, effective, temporary relief of all your child's symptoms associated with hay fever and other respiratory allergies including sneezing, sore throat, itchy throat, itchy/watery eyes, runny nose, stuffy nose and nasal congestion. Acetaminophen is equal to aspirin in analgesic and antipyretic effectiveness and it is unlikely to produce the side effects often associated with aspirin or aspirin-containing products.

Uses: For the reduction of fever. For the temporary relief of these hay fever and other upper respiratory allergy symptoms: sneezing, sore throat, nasal congestion, itchy/watery eyes, runny nose, stuffy nose, nasal congestion.

Directions: See Table 2: Children's Tylenol Dosing Chart on pgs. 660-662.

Precautions: If a rare sensitivity reaction occurs, the drug should be discontinued.

Warnings: Do not take for pain for more than 5 days or for fever for more than 3 days unless directed by a doctor. If pain or fever persists, or gets worse, if new symptoms occur, or if redness or swelling is present, consult a doctor because these could be signs of a serious condition. If sore throat is severe, persists for more than 2 days, is accompanied or followed by fever, headache, rash, nausea or vomiting, consult a doctor promptly. If nervousness, dizziness or sleeplessness occur, discontinue use and consult a doctor. May cause excitability especially in children. Do not give this product to children who have a breathing problem such as chronic bronchitis, or who have glaucoma, heart disease, high blood pressure, thyroid disease, or diabetes without first consulting the child's doctor. May cause marked drowsiness; sedatives and tranquilizers may increase the drowsiness effect. Do not give this product to children who are taking sedatives or tranquilizers without first consulting the child's doctor. **Do not exceed recommended dosage.** Taking more than the recommended dose (overdose) may not provide more relief and could cause serious health problems. Keep this and all drugs out of the reach of children. In case of accidental overdose, contact a doctor or poison control center immediately. Prompt medical attention is critical for adults as well as for children even if you do not notice any signs or symptoms. Do not use with other products containing acetaminophen.

Drug Interaction Precaution: Do not give this product to a child who is taking a prescription monoamine oxidase inhibitor (MAOI) (certain drugs for depression, psychiatric or emotional conditions, or Parkinson's disease), or for 2 weeks after stopping the MAOI drug. If you are uncertain whether your child's

prescription drug contains an MAOI, consult a health professional before giving this product.

Professional Information: Overdosage Information

For overdosage information, please refer to pgs. 657–658.

Inactive Ingredients: Benzoic Acid, Citric Acid, Corn Syrup, D&C Red #33, FD&C Red #40, Flavors, Polyethylene Glycol, Propylene Glycol, Purified Water, Sodium Benzoate, Sorbitol.

How Supplied: Pink-colored–child-resistant bottles of 4 fl. oz. Store at room temperature. Avoid excessive heat, 104°F (40°C).

Shown in Product Identification Guide, page 510

Infants' TYLENOL® Cold Decongestant & Fever Reducer Concentrated Drops

Infants' TYLENOL® Cold Decongestant & Fever Reducer Concentrated Drops Plus Cough

Children's TYLENOL® Cold Suspension Liquid and Chewable Tablets

Children's TYLENOL® Cold Plus Cough Suspension Liquid and Chewable Tablets

Description: *Infants' TYLENOL® Cold Decongestant & Fever Reducer Concentrated Drops* are alcohol-free, aspirin-free, BubbleGum Blast-flavored and red in color. Each 1.6 mL (2 dropperfuls) contains acetaminophen 160 mg and pseudoephedrine HCl 15 mg. *Infants' TYLENOL® Cold Decongestant & Fever Reducer Concentrated Drops Plus Cough* are alcohol-free, aspirin-free, Wild-Cherry-flavored and red in color. Each 1.6 mL (2 dropperfuls) contains acetaminophen 160 mg, dextromethorphan HBr 5 mg, and pseudoephedrine HCl 15 mg. *Children's TYLENOL® Cold Suspension Liquid* is Great Grape-flavored and contains no alcohol or aspirin. Each teaspoonful (5 mL) contains acetaminophen 160 mg, chlorpheniramine maleate 1 mg and pseudoephedrine HCl 15 mg. *Children's TYLENOL® Cold Chewable Tablets* are Great Grape-flavored and each tablet contains acetaminophen 80 mg, chlorpheniramine maleate 0.5 mg and pseudoephedrine HCl 7.5 mg. *Children's TYLENOL® Cold Plus Cough Suspension Liquid* is Wild-Cherry-flavored and contains no alcohol or aspirin. Each teaspoonful (5 mL) contains acetaminophen 160 mg, chlorpheniramine maleate 1 mg, dextromethorphan HBr 5 mg and pseudoephedrine HCl 15 mg. *Children's TYLENOL® Cold Plus Cough Chewable Tablets* are Wild-Cherry-flavored and each tablet contains acetaminophen 80 mg, chlorpheniramine maleate 0.5 mg, dextromethorphan HBr 2.5 mg, and pseudoephedrine HCl 7.5 mg.

Actions: Acetaminophen is a clinically proven analgesic/antipyretic. Acetaminophen produces analgesia by elevation of the pain threshold and antipyresis through action on the hypothalamic heat-regulating center. Acetaminophen is equal to aspirin in analgesic and antipyretic effectiveness and it is unlikely to produce many of the side effects associated with aspirin and aspirin-containing products.

Pseudoephedrine hydrochloride is a sympathomimetic amine which provides temporary relief of nasal congestion. Chlorpheniramine maleate is an antihistamine that provides temporary relief of runny nose, sneezing and watery and itchy eyes.

Dextromethorphan hydrobromide is a cough suppressant which helps relieve coughs.

Uses: *Infants' TYLENOL® Cold Decongestant & Fever Reducer Concentrated Drops:* For the reduction of fever. For the temporary relief of these cold symptoms: minor aches and pains, nasal congestion, headaches. *Infants' TYLENOL® Cold Decongestant & Fever Reducer Concentrated Drops Plus Cough:* For the reduction of fever. For the temporary relief of these cold symptoms: coughs, nasal congestion, minor aches and pains, sore throat, headaches. *Children's TYLENOL® Cold Suspension Liquid* and *Chewable Tablets:* For the temporary relief of these cold symptoms: nasal congestion, runny nose, sore throat, sneezing, minor aches and pains, headaches and fever. *Children's TYLENOL® Cold Plus Cough Suspension Liquid* and *Chewable Tablets:* For the temporary relief of these cold symptoms: minor aches and pains, sore throat, coughs, nasal congestion, headaches, fever, sneezing, runny nose.

Directions: See Table 2: Children's Tylenol Dosing Chart on pgs. 660-662.

Precautions: If a rare sensitivity reaction occurs, the drug should be discontinued.

Warnings: Do not take for pain for more than 5 days or for fever for more than 3 days unless directed by a doctor. If pain or fever persists, or gets worse, if new symptoms occur, or if redness or swelling is present, consult a doctor because these could be signs of a serious condition. If nervousness, dizziness, or sleeplessness occur, discontinue use and consult a doctor. **Do not exceed recommended dosage.** Taking more than the recommended dose (overdose) may not provide more relief and could cause serious health problems. Keep this and all drugs out of the reach of children. In case of accidental overdose, contact a doctor or poison control center immediately. Prompt medical attention is critical even if you do not notice any signs or symptoms. Do not use with other products containing acetaminophen.

Drug Interaction Precaution: Do not give this product to a child who is taking

a prescription monamine oxidase inhibitor (MAOI) (certain drugs for depression, psychiatric or emotional conditions or Parkinson's disease), or for 2 weeks after stopping the MAOI drug. If you are uncertain whether your child's prescription drug contains an MAOI, consult a health professional before giving this product.

Infants' TYLENOL® Cold Decongestant & Fever Reducer Concentrated Drops: Do not give this product to children who have heart disease, high blood pressure, thyroid disease, or diabetes without first consulting the child's doctor. **Do not use if plastic carton wrap or bottle wrap imprinted "Safety Seal®" is broken or missing.**

Infants' TYLENOL® Cold Decongestant & Fever Reducer Concentrated Drops Plus Cough: If sore throat is severe, persists for more than 2 days, is accompanied or followed by fever, headache, rash, nausea, or vomiting, consult a doctor promptly. Do not give this product to children who have heart disease, high blood pressure, thyroid disease, or diabetes without first consulting the child's doctor. A persistent cough may be a sign of a serious condition. If cough persists for more than 1 week, tends to recur or is accompanied by fever, rash or persistent headache, consult a doctor. Do not give this product for persistent or chronic cough such as occurs with asthma or if cough is accompanied by excessive phlegm (mucus) unless directed by a doctor. **Do not use if plastic carton wrap or bottle wrap imprinted "Safety Seal®" is broken or missing.**

Children's TYLENOL® Cold Suspension Liquid and *Chewable Tablets:* If sore throat is severe, persists for more than 2 days, is accompanied or followed by fever, headache, rash, nausea, or vomiting, consult a doctor promptly. May cause excitability especially in children. Do not give this product to children who have a breathing problem such as chronic bronchitis, or who have glaucoma, heart disease, high blood pressure, thyroid disease, or diabetes without first consulting the child's doctor. May cause drowsiness. Sedatives and tranquilizers may increase the drowsiness effect. Do not give this product to children who are taking sedatives or tranquilizers, without first consulting the child's doctor. **Suspension Liquid: Do not use if plastic carton wrap, bottle wrap, or foil inner seal imprinted "Safety Seal®" is broken or missing. Chewable Tablets: Do not use if carton is opened or if blister unit is broken.** Phenylketonurics: contains phenylalanine 6 mg per tablet.

Children's TYLENOL ® Cold Plus Cough Suspension Liquid and *Chewable Tablets:* If sore throat is severe, persists for more than 2 days, is accompanied or followed by fever, headache, rash, nausea, or vomiting, consult a doctor promptly. May cause excitability especially in children. Do not give this product to children who have a breathing

Continued on next page

TABLE 2
Children's Tylenol® Dosing Chart

PRODUCT FORM / INGREDIENTS	AGE GROUP: 0-3 mos	4-11 mos	12-23 mos	2-3 yrs	4-5 yrs	6-8 yrs	9-10 yrs	11 yrs	12 yrs	Maximum doses/24 hrs
WEIGHT (if possible use weight to dose; otherwise use age)	6-11 lbs	12-17 lbs	18-23 lbs	24-35 lbs	36-47 lbs	48-59 lbs	60-71 lbs	72-95 lbs	Over 96 lbs	
Dose	to be	administered	based	on	weight	or	age†			
Infants' Drops — Per dropperful (0.8 mL)										
Infants' Tylenol Concentrated Drops — Acetaminophen 80 mg	½ dropperful (0.4 mL)*	1 dropperful (0.8 mL)*	1½ dropperfuls (0.8 + 0.4 mL)*	2 dropperfuls (0.8 + 0.8 mL)	—	—	—	—	—	5 times in 24 hrs
Infants' Tylenol Cold Decongestant & Fever Reducer Concentrated Drops — Acetaminophen 80 mg Pseudoephedrine HCl 7.5 mg	½ dropperful (0.4 mL)*	1 dropperful (0.8 mL)*	1½ dropperfuls (0.8 + 0.4 mL)*	2 dropperfuls (0.8 + 0.8 mL)	—	—	—	—	—	4 times in 24 hrs
Infants' Tylenol Cold Decongestant & Fever Reducer Concentrated Drops Plus Cough — Acetaminophen 80 mg Dextromethorphan HBr 2.5 mg Pseudoephedrine HCl 7.5 mg	½ dropperful (0.4 mL)*	1 dropperful (0.8 mL)*	1½ dropperfuls (0.8 + 0.4 mL)*	2 dropperfuls (0.8 + 0.8 mL)	—	—	—	—	—	4 times in 24 hrs
Children's Liquids — Per 5 mL teaspoonful (TSP)										
Children's Tylenol Suspension Liquid — Acetaminophen 160 mg	—	½ TSP*	¾ TSP*	1 TSP	1½ TSP	2 TSP	2½ TSP	3 TSP	—	5 times in 24 hrs
Children's Tylenol Cold Suspension Liquid — Acetaminophen 160 mg Chlorpheniramine Maleate 1 mg Pseudoephedrine HCl 15 mg	—	½ TSP**	¾ TSP**	1 TSP**	1½ TSP**	2 TSP	2½ TSP	3 TSP	—	4 times in 24 hrs

Product	Ingredients		½ TSP	¾ TSP	1 TSP	1½ TSP	2 TSP	2½ TSP	3 TSP		Frequency
Children's Tylenol Cold Plus Cough Suspension Liquid	Acetaminophen 160 mg, Chlorpheniramine Maleate 1 mg, Dextromethorphan HBr 5 mg, Pseudoephedrine HCl 15 mg	—	½ TSP**	¾ TSP**	1 TSP**	1½ TSP**	2 TSP	2½ TSP	3 TSP	—	4 times in 24 hrs
Children's Tylenol Flu Suspension Liquid†	Acetaminophen 160 mg, Chlorpheniramine Maleate 1 mg, Dextromethorphan HBr 7.5 mg, Pseudoephedrine HCl 15 mg	—	½ TSP**	¾ TSP**	1 TSP**	1½ TSP**	2 TSP	2½ TSP	3 TSP	—	4 times in 24 hrs
Children's Tylenol Sinus Suspension Liquid	Acetaminophen 160 mg, Pseudoephedrine HCl 15 mg	—	½ TSP*	¾ TSP*	1 TSP	1½ TSP	2 TSP	2½ TSP	3 TSP	—	4 times in 24 hrs
Children's Tylenol Allergy-D Liquid	Acetaminophen 160 mg, Diphenhydramine HCl 12.5 mg, Pseudoephedrine HCl 15 mg	—	½ TSP**	¾ TSP**	1 TSP**	1½ TSP**	2 TSP	2½ TSP	3 TSP	—	4 times in 24 hrs

†All products may be dosed every 4 hours, if needed; except for Children's Tylenol Flu which is dosed every 6–8 hrs, if needed.
*Under 2 years (under 24 lbs), consult a doctor.   **Under 6 years (under 48 lbs), consult a doctor.
•Infants' Tylenol Drops are more concentrated than Children's Tylenol Liquids. The Infants' Concentrated Drops have been specifically designed for use only with enclosed dropper. Do not use any other dosing device with this product.
•Children's Tylenol Liquids are less concentrated than Infants' Tylenol Concentrated Drops. The Children's Tylenol Liquids have been specifically designed for use with the enclosed measuring cup. Use only enclosed measuring cup to dose this product.
•Children's Tylenol Soft Chews Chewable Tablets are not the same concentration as Junior Strength Tylenol Soft Chews Chewable Tablets.
•Junior Strength Tylenol Soft Chews Chewable Tablets contain twice as much medicine as Children's Tylenol Soft Chews Chewable Tablets.

Table continued on next page

TABLE 2
Children's Tylenol® Dosing Chart (continued)

AGE GROUP	0–3 mos	4–11 mos	12–23 mos	2–3 yrs	4–5 yrs	6–8 yrs	9–10 yrs	11 yrs	12 yrs	Maximum doses/24 hrs
WEIGHT (if possible use weight to dose; otherwise use age)	6–11 lbs	12–17 lbs	18–23 lbs	24–35 lbs	36–47 lbs	48–59 lbs	60–71 lbs	72–95 lbs	Over 96 lbs	
PRODUCT FORM / **INGREDIENTS** Per tablet	Dose	to be	administered	based	on	weight	or	age†		
Children's Tablets										
Children's Tylenol Soft Chews Chewable Tablets — Acetaminophen 80 mg	—	—	—	2 tablets	3 tablets	4 tablets	5 tablets	6 tablets	—	5 times in 24 hrs
Children's Tylenol Cold Chewable Tablets — Acetaminophen 80 mg, Chlorpheniramine Maleate 0.5 mg, Pseudoephedrine HCl 7.5 mg	—	—	—	2 tablets**	3 tablets**	4 tablets	5 tablets	6 tablets	—	4 times in 24 hrs
Children's Tylenol Cold Plus Cough Chewable Tablets — Acetaminophen 80 mg, Chlorpheniramine Maleate 0.5 mg, Dextromethorphan HBr 2.5 mg, Pseudoephedrine HCl 7.5 mg	—	—	—	2 tablets**	3 tablets**	4 tablets	5 tablets	6 tablets	—	4 times in 24 hrs
Junior Strength Tylenol Soft Chews Chewable Tablets — Acetaminophen 160 mg	—	—	—	—	—	2 tablets	2½ tablets	3 tablets	4 tablets	5 times in 24 hrs

†All products may be dosed every 4 hours, if needed; except for Children's Tylenol Flu which is dosed every 6–8 hrs, if needed.
*Under 2 years (under 24 lbs), consult a doctor.　　**Under 6 years (under 48 lbs), consult a doctor.
•Infants' Tylenol Drops are more concentrated than Children's Tylenol Liquids. The Infants' Concentrated Drops have been specifically designed for use only with enclosed dropper. Do not use any other dosing device with this product.
•Children's Tylenol Liquids are less concentrated than Infants' Tylenol Concentrated Drops. The Children's Tylenol Liquids have been specifically designed for use with the enclosed measuring cup. Use only enclosed measuring cup to dose this product.
•Children's Tylenol Soft Chews Chewable Tablets are not the same concentration as Junior Strength Tylenol Soft Chews Chewable Tablets.
•Junior Strength Tylenol Soft Chews Chewable Tablets contain twice as much medicine as Children's Tylenol Soft Chews Chewable Tablets.

problem such as chronic bronchitis, or who have glaucoma, heart disease, high blood pressure, thyroid disease, or diabetes without first consulting the child's doctor. May cause drowsiness. Sedatives and tranquilizers may increase the drowsiness effect. Do not give this product to children who are taking sedatives or tranquilizers, without first consulting the child's doctor. A persistent cough may be a sign of a serious condition. If cough persists for more than 1 week, tends to recur or is accompanied by fever, rash or persistent headache, consult a doctor. Do not give this product for persistent or chronic cough such as occurs with asthma or if cough is accompanied by excessive phlegm (mucus) unless directed by a doctor. **Liquid: Do not use if plastic carton wrap, bottle wrap, or foil inner seal imprinted "Safety Seal®" is broken or missing. Tablets: Do not use if carton is opened or if blister unit is broken.** Phenylketonurics: contains phenylalanine 4 mg per tablet.

Professional Information:
Overdosage Information
For overdosage information, please refer to pgs. 657–658.

Inactive Ingredients:
Infants' TYLENOL® Cold Decongestant & Fever Reducer Concentrated Drops: Citric Acid, Corn Syrup, FD&C Red #40, Flavors, Polyethylene Glycol, Propylene Glycol, Saccharin, Sodium Benzoate.
Infants' TYLENOL® Cold Decongestant & Fever Reducer Concentrated Drops Plus Cough: Acesulfame Potassium, Citric Acid, Corn Syrup, FD&C Red #40, Flavors, Polyethylene Glycol, Propylene Glycol, Sodium Benzoate.
Children's TYLENOL® Cold: **Suspension Liquid:** acesulfame potassium, butylparaben, cellulose, citric acid, corn syrup, D&C Red #33, FD&C Blue #1, FD&C Red #40, flavors, glycerin, propylene glycol, purified water, sodium benzoate, sodium carboxymethylcellulose, sorbitol, xanthan gum. **Chewable Tablets:** Aspartame, Basic Polymethacrylate, Cellulose, Cellulose Acetate, Citric Acid, D&C Red #7, FD&C Blue #1, Flavors, Hydroxypropyl Methylcellulose, Magnesium Stearate, Mannitol.
Children's TYLENOL® Cold Plus Cough: **Suspension Liquid:** Acesulfame K, Butylparaben, Cellulose, Citric Acid, Corn Syrup, D&C Red #33, FD&C Red #40, Flavors, Glycerin, Propylene Glycol, Purified Water, Sodium Benzoate, Sodium Carboxymethylcellulose, Sorbitol, Xanthan Gum: **Chewable Tablets:** Aspartame, Basic Polymethacrylate, Cellulose, Cellulose Acetate, D&C Red #7, Flavors, Hydroxypropyl Methylcellulose, Magnesium Stearate, Mannitol.

How Supplied:
Infants' TYLENOL® Cold Decongestant & Fever Reducer Concentrated Drops, Infants' TYLENOL® Cold Decongestant & Fever Reducer Concentrated Drops Plus Cough: Red-colored drops in bottles of $^1/_2$ fl. oz. Store at room temperature.

Children's TYLENOL® Cold: **Suspension Liquid:** Purple-colored-bottles of 4 fl. oz. Store at room temperature.
Chewable Tablets: Purple-colored, imprinted "TYLENOL COLD" on one side and "TC" on opposite side- blisters of 24. Store at room temperature.
Children's TYLENOL® Cold Plus Cough: **Suspension Liquid:** Red-colored suspension-bottles of 4 fl. oz. Store at room temperature.
Chewable Tablets: Red-colored, imprinted TYLENOL C/C" on one side and "TC/C" on the opposite side- blisters of 24. Store at room temperature.
Shown in Product Identification Guide, page 510

Children's TYLENOL® Flu Suspension Liquid

Description: *Children's TYLENOL® Flu Suspension Liquid* is Bubble Gum Blast-flavored and contains no alcohol or aspirin. Each teaspoonful (5 mL) contains acetaminophen 160 mg, chlorpheniramine maleate 1 mg, dextromethorphan HBr 7.5 mg and pseudoephedrine HCl 15 mg.

Actions: *Children's TYLENOL® Flu Suspension Liquid* combines the analgesic-antipyretic acetaminophen with the decongestant pseudoephedrine hydrochloride, the cough suppressant dextromethorphan hydrobromide and the antihistamine chlorpheniramine maleate to provide fast, effective, temporary relief of all your child's symptoms associated with flu including fever, body aches, headache, stuffy nose, runny nose, sore throat and coughs. Acetaminophen is equal to aspirin in analgesic and antipyretic effectiveness and it is unlikely to produce the side effects often associated with aspirin or aspirin-containing products.

Uses: For the temporary relief of these cold and flu symptoms: minor aches and pains, sore throat, coughs, nasal congestion, headaches, fever, and runny nose.

Directions: See Table 2: Children's Tylenol Dosing Chart on pgs. 660-662.

Precautions: If a rare sensitivity reaction occurs, the drug should be discontinued.

Warnings: **Do not use if plastic carton wrap, bottle wrap, or foil inner seal imprinted "Safety Seal"® is broken or missing.** Do not take for pain for more than 5 days or for fever for more than 3 days unless directed by a doctor. If pain or fever persists, or gets worse, if new symptoms occur, or if redness or swelling is present, consult a doctor because these could be signs of a serious condition. If sore throat is severe, persists for more than 2 days, is accompanied or followed by fever, headache, rash, nausea or vomiting, consult a doctor promptly. If nervousness, dizziness or sleeplessness occur, discontinue use and

consult a doctor. May cause excitability especially in children. Do not give this product to children who have a breathing problem such as chronic bronchitis, or who have glaucoma, heart disease, high blood pressure, thyroid disease or diabetes without first consulting the child's doctor. May cause drowsiness. Sedatives and tranquilizers may increase the drowsiness effect. Do not give this product to children who are taking sedatives or tranquilizers without first consulting the child's doctor. A persistent cough may be a sign of a serious condition. If cough persists for more than 1 week, tends to recur, or is accompanied by fever, rash, or persistent headache, consult a doctor. Do not give this product for persistent or chronic cough such as occurs with asthma or if cough is accompanied by excessive phlegm (mucus) unless directed by a doctor. **Do not exceed recommended dosage.** Taking more than the recommended dose (overdose) may not provide more relief and could cause serious health problems. Keep this and all drugs out of the reach of children. In case of accidental overdose, contact a doctor or poison control center immediately. Prompt medical attention is critical even if you do not notice any signs or symptoms. Do not use with other products containing acetaminophen.

Drug Interaction Precaution: Do not give this product to a child who is taking a prescription monoamine oxidase inhibitor (MAOI) (certain drugs for depression, psychiatric or emotional conditions, or Parkinson's disease) or for 2 weeks after stopping the MAOI drug. If you are uncertain whether your child's prescription drug contains an MAOI, consult a health professional before giving this product.

Professional Information:
Overdosage Information
For overdosage information, please refer to pgs. 657–658.

Inactive Ingredients: Acesulfame K, Butylparaben, Cellulose, Citric Acid, Corn Syrup, D&C Red #33, FD&C Red #40, Flavors, Glycerin, Propylene Glycol, Purified Water, Sodium Benzoate, Sodium Carboxymethylcellulose, Sorbitol, Xanthan Gum.

How Supplied: Pinkish-red-colored suspension liquid in bottles of 4 fl. oz. Store at room temperature.
Shown in Product Identification Guide, page 511

Children's TYLENOL® Sinus Suspension Liquid

Description: *Children's TYLENOL® Sinus Suspension Liquid* is Fruit Burst-flavored and contains no alcohol or aspirin. Each teaspoonful (5 mL) contains acetaminophen 160 mg and pseudoephedrine HCl 15 mg.

Continued on next page

Tylenol Children's—Cont.

Actions: *Children's TYLENOL® Sinus Suspension Liquid* combines the analgesic-antipyretic acetaminophen with the decongestant pseudoephedrine hydrochloride to provide fast, effective, temporary relief of all your child's sinus symptoms including stuffy nose, sinus headache, sinus pressure, sinus pain, and nasal congestion. Acetaminophen is equal to aspirin in analgesic and antipyretic effectiveness and is unlikely to produce the side effects often associated with aspirin or aspirin-containing products.

Uses: For the reduction of fever. For the temporary relief of minor aches, pains and headaches, sinus congestion, stuffy nose and sinus pressure.

Directions: See Table 2: Children's Tylenol Dosing Chart on pgs. 660-662.

Precautions: If a rare sensitivity reaction occurs, the drug should be discontinued.

Warnings: Do not take for pain for more than 5 days or for fever for more than 3 days unless directed by a doctor. If pain or fever persists, or gets worse, if new symptoms occur, or if redness or swelling is present, consult a doctor because these could be signs of a serious condition. If nervousness, dizziness or sleeplessness occur, discontinue use and consult a doctor. Do not give this product to children who have heart disease, high blood pressure, thyroid disease, or diabetes without first consulting the child's doctor. **Do not exceed recommended dosage.** Taking more than the recommended dose (overdose) may not provide more relief and could cause serious health problems. Keep this and all drugs out of the reach of children. In case of accidental overdose, contact a doctor or poison control center immediately. Prompt medical attention is critical even if you do not notice any signs or symptoms. Do not use with other products containing acetaminophen. **Do not use if plastic carton wrap, bottle wrap, or foil inner seal imprinted "Safety Seal®" is broken or missing.**

Drug Interaction Precaution: Do not give this product to a child who is taking a prescription monoamine oxidase inhibitor (MAOI) (certain drugs for depression, psychiatric or emotional conditions, or Parkinson's disease), or for 2 weeks after stopping the MAOI drug. If you are uncertain whether your child's prescription drug contains an MAOI, consult a health professional before giving this product.

Professional Information:
Overdosage Information
For overdosage information, please refer to pgs. 657-658.

Inactive Ingredients: acesulfame potassium, butylparaben, cellulose, citric acid, corn syrup, D&C Red #33, FD&C Red #40, flavors, glycerin, propylene glycol, purified water, sodium benzoate, sodium carboxymethylcellulose, sorbitol, xanthan gum.

How Supplied: Red-colored–child resistant bottles of 4 fl. oz. Store at room temperature. Avoid excessive heat, 104°F (40°C).

Shown in Product Identification Guide, page 511

Children's Tylenol® Dosing Chart

[See table on pages 660, 661 and 662]

Medeva Pharmaceuticals, Inc.

PO BOX 31710
ROCHESTER, NY 14603

Direct Inquiries to:
Customer Service Department
P.O. Box 31766
Rochester, NY 14603
(716) 274-5300
(888) 9–MEDEVA

DELSYM® Cough Formula
[*del 'sĭm*]
(dextromethorphan polistirex)
Extended-Release Suspension
12-Hour Cough Relief

Active Ingredient: Each teaspoonful (5 mL) contains dextromethorphan polistirex equivalent to 30 mg dextromethorphan hydrobromide.

Inactive Ingredients: Alcohol 0.26%, citric acid, ethylcellulose, FD&C Yellow No. 6, flavor, high fructose corn syrup, methylparaben, polyethylene glycol 3350, polysorbate 80, propylene glycol, propylparaben, purified water, sucrose, tragacanth, vegetable oil, xanthan gum.

Indications: Temporarily relieves cough due to minor throat and bronchial irritation as may occur with the common cold or inhaled irritants.

Warnings: Do not take this product for persistent or chronic cough such as occurs with smoking, asthma, or emphysema, or if cough is accompanied by excessive phlegm (mucus) unless directed by a physician. A persistent cough may be a sign of a serious condition. If cough persists for more than 1 week, tends to recur, or is accompanied by fever, rash, or persistent headache, consult a physician. As with any drug, if you are pregnant or nursing a baby, seek the advice of a health professional before using this product. **Keep this and all drugs out of the reach of children.** In case of accidental overdose, seek professional assistance or contact a Poison Control Center immediately.

Drug Interaction Precaution: Do not use this product if you are now taking a prescription monoamine oxidase inhibitor (MAOI) (certain drugs for depression, psychiatric or emotional conditions, or Parkinson's disease), or for 2 weeks after stopping the MAOI drug. If you are uncertain whether your prescription drug contains an MAOI, consult a health professional before taking this product.

Directions: **Shake Bottle Well Before Using.** Dose as follows or as directed by a physician.
Adults and Children 12 years of age and over: 2 teaspoonfuls every 12 hours, not to exceed 4 teaspoonfuls in 24 hours.
Children 6 to under 12 years of age: 1 teaspoonful every 12 hours, not to exceed 2 teaspoonfuls in 24 hours.
Children 2 to under 6 years of age: $1/2$ teaspoonful every 12 hours, not to exceed 1 teaspoonful in 24 hours.
Children under 2 years of age: Consult a physician.

How Supplied: 89 mL (3 fl oz) bottles NDC 53014-842-61
Store at 15°–30°C (59°–86°F).
®Fisons Investment Inc.
Medeva Pharmaceuticals, Inc.
Rochester, NY 14623 USA

Medtech

488 MAIN AVENUE
NORWALK, CT 06851

Address Questions and Comments to:
(800) 443-4908

Other Medtech Products:
APF Arthritis Pain Formula
Freezone Corn & Callus Liquid
Heet Pain Relieving Liniment
Oxipor Psoriasis Lotion
Zincon Medicated Dandruff Shampoo

COMPOUND W® One Step Wart Remover Pads
COMPOUND W® One Step Plantar Pads
COMPOUND W® One Step Pads For Kids
Salicylic Acid

Indications: Compound W® One Step and One Step Pads for Kids: For the removal of common warts. The common wart is easily recognized by the rough "cauliflower-like" appearance of the surface.

Active Ingredient: **Purpose:**
40% Salicylic Acid in a
plaster vehicle ... Plantar/Wart Remover

Indications: Compound W® One Step Plantar Pads: For the removal of plantar warts on the bottom of the foot. The plan-

tar wart is recognized by its location only on the bottom of the foot, its tenderness, and the interruption of the footprint pattern.

Warnings:
Do Not Use If:
• you are diabetic • you have poor blood circulation.
Do Not Use On:
• irritated skin • any area that is infected or reddened • moles • birthmarks • warts with hair growing from them • genital warts • warts on the face • warts on mucous membranes, such as inside mouth, nose, anus, genitals, lips
Stop Using This Product and See Your Doctor If:
• discomfort persists.
For external use only. Keep this and all drugs out of the reach of children. In case of accidental ingestion, seek professional assistance or contact a poison control center immediately.

Directions: Wash affected area. May soak wart in warm water for 5 minutes. Dry area thoroughly. Remove medicated pad from backing paper by pulling from center of pad. Then apply. Repeat procedure every 48 hours as needed (until wart is removed) for up to 12 weeks.
Adult Supervision of Compound W Pads For Kids recommended.

Inactive Ingredients: Lanolin, Polybutene, Rosin Ester, Rubber.
Store at room temperature. Avoid excessive heat (37°C, 99°F).

How Supplied: Compound W One Step Pads: 14 Medicated One Step Pads **Compound W One Step Plantar Warts:** 20 Medicated One Step Pads **Compound W One Step Pads for Kids:** 12 Medicated Pads
Mfg. for Medtech, Jackson WY 83001 USA, Made in Japan, Questions? 1-800-443-4908

©Medtech R 2/99

COMPOUND W® Wart Remover
LIQUID & GEL
Maximum Strength
Salicylic Acid

Active Ingredient   Purpose
Salicylic Acid 17% w/w....Wart Remover

Indications: For the removal of common warts. The common wart is easily recognized by the rough "cauliflower-like" appearance of the surface.

Warnings: LIQUID
Do Not Use If:
• you are diabetic • you have poor blood circulation.
Do Not Use On:
• irritated skin • any area that is infected or reddened • moles • birthmarks
• warts with hair growing from them • genital warts • warts on the face
• warts on mucous membranes, such as inside mouth, nose, anus, genitals, lips.

When Using This Product:
• avoid contact with eyes. If product gets into eyes, flush with water for 15 minutes.
Stop Using This Product and See Your Doctor If:
• discomfort persists.
Extremely flammable. Keep away from fire or flame. Cap bottle tightly and store at room temperature away from heat. Avoid inhaling vapors. **For external use only.** Keep this and all drugs out of the reach of children. In case of accidental ingestion, seek professional assistance or contact a poison control center immediately.

Warnings: GEL
Do Not Use If:
• you are diabetic • you have poor blood circulation.
Do Not Use On:
• irritated skin • any area that is infected or reddened • moles • birthmarks
• warts with hair growing from them • genital warts • warts on the face • warts on mucous membranes, such as inside mouth, nose, anus, genitals, lips.
When Using This Product:
• avoid contact with eyes. If product gets into eyes, flush with water for 15 minutes.
Stop Using This Product and See Your Doctor If:
• discomfort persists.
Extremely flammable. Keep away from fire or flame. Cap tube tightly and store at room temperature away from heat. Avoid inhaling vapors. **For external use only.** Keep this and all drugs out of the reach of children. In case of accidental ingestion, seek professional assistance or contact a poison control center immediately.

Directions:
LIQUID: Wash affected area. May soak wart in warm water for 5 minutes. Dry area thoroughly. Using the applicator apply Compound W Liquid to each wart. Let dry. Repeat procedure once or twice daily as needed (until wart is removed) for up to 12 weeks.
GEL: Wash affected area. May soak wart in warm water for 5 minutes. Dry area thoroughly. By squeezing the tube gently, apply one drop at a time to sufficiently cover each wart. Let dry. Repeat procedure once or twice daily as needed (until wart is removed) for up to 12 weeks.

Inactive Ingredients:
LIQUID: Alcohol 21.2%, Camphor, Castor Oil, Collodion, Ether 63.6%, Ethylcellulose, Hypophosphorous Acid, Menthol, Polysorbate 80
GEL: Alcohol 67.5% by vol., Camphor, Castor Oil, Collodion, Colloidal Silicon Dioxide, Hydroxypropyl Cellulose, Hypophosphorous Acid, Polysorbate 80

How Supplied:
LIQUID: .31 FL OZ
GEL: Net Wt .25 oz (7g)

Mfg. for Medtech, Jackson WY 83001 USA

Question? 1-800-443-4908
LIQUID: © Medtech, R5/99
GEL: © Medtech, R6/99

PERCOGESIC®
EXTRA STRENGTH
• **PAIN RELIEVER**
• **FEVER REDUCER**
• **ANTIHISTAMINE**
Aspirin Free

Active Ingredient Per Coated Caplet: Purpose:
Acetaminophen
  500 mg .... Pain Reliever, Fever Reducer
Diphenhydramine HCl 12.5 mg .... Antihistamine

Indications: For the temporary relief of minor aches and pains associated with headaches, muscular aches, backaches, premenstrual and menstrual discomfort, colds, the flu, toothaches, minor pain from arthritis, to reduce fever, as well as temporary relief of runny nose, sneezing, itching of the nose or throat, and itchy, watery eyes due to hayfever.

Directions: Adults (12 years and over): 2 caplets every 6 hours while symptoms persist. Maximum daily dose 8 caplets. Children under 12 years of age: consult a doctor.
Store at room temperature. Avoid excessive heat.

Inactive Ingredients: Corn Starch, FD&C Yellow #6 Aluminum Lake, Hydroxypropylmethylcellulose, Magnesium Stearate, Microcrystalline Cellulose, Polydextrose, Polyethylene Glycol, Povidone, Silicon Dioxide, Stearic Acid, Titanium Dioxide, Triacetin.

Warnings: May cause marked drowsiness; alcohol, sedatives, and tranquilizers may increase the drowsiness effect. Avoid alcoholic beverages while taking this product. Use caution when driving a motor vehicle or operating machinery. May cause excitability, especially in children. Do not give to children for arthritis pain, unless directed by a doctor. **Do Not Use (unless directed by a doctor): If you are:** • taking sedatives or tranquilizers **If you have:** • a breathing problem such as emphysema or chronic bronchitis • glaucoma • difficulty in urination due to enlargement of the prostate gland **Stop Using This Product and Consult a Doctor If:** pain persists for more than 10 days (adults) or 5 days (children) • fever persists more than 3 days (unless directed by a doctor) • condition worsens or new symptoms occur • redness or swelling is present. **These may be signs of a serious condition.** As with any drug, if you are pregnant or nursing a baby, seek the advice of a health professional before using this product. **Keep**

Continued on next page

Percogesic—Cont.

this and all drugs out of the reach of children. In case of accidental overdose, contact a physician or poison control center immediately. Prompt medical attention is critical for adults as well as for children even if you do not notice any signs or symptoms.

Alcohol Warning: If you consume 3 or more alcoholic drinks every day, ask your doctor whether you should take acetaminophen or other pain relievers/fever reducers. Acetaminophen may cause liver damage.

How Supplied 40 Coated caplets
Mfg. for Medtech, Jackson, WY 83001 USA
Questions? 800-443-4908 © Medtech, R10/98

DERMOPLAST®
Hospital Strength
Pain Relieving Spray

Active Ingredients:	**Purpose:**
Benzocaine USP 20%	Topical Anesthetic
Menthol 0.5%	Antipruritic

Indications: For temporary relief of pain and itching associated with •sunburn •insect bites •minor cuts •scrapes •minor burns •minor skin irritations

Warnings:
When Using This Product: •use only as directed •avoid contact with eyes Stop Using This Product If: •condition worsens •symptoms persist for more than 7 days •symptoms clear up and recur within a few days. **Consult a physician.** For external use only. Contents under pressure. Do not puncture or incinerate. Do not expose to heat or temperature above 120° F. Do not use near open flame. **Keep this and all drugs out of reach of children.** If accidentally ingested, seek professional assistance or contact a poison control center immediately. Intentional misuse by deliberately concentrating and inhaling the contents can be harmful or fatal.

Directions: Children under 2 years of age: do not use. Consult physician. Adults and children 2 years and older: clean and apply to affected area not more than 3 to 4 times daily. Hold can 6 to 12 inches away from affected area. Point spray nozzle and press button. To apply to face, spray in palm of hand.

Other information: Store at room temperature (approximately 25° C, 77° F).

Inactive Ingredients: Acetylated Lanolin Alcohol, Aloe Vera Oil, Butane, Cetyl Acetate, Hydrofluorocarbon, Methylparaben, PEG-8 Laurate, Polysorbate 85.

How Supplied: NET WT. 2¾ FL OZ (81 ml)

Manufactured for
Medtech, Jackson WY 83001 USA
Questions? 1-800-443-4908

DERMOPLAST® Antibacterial Spray
Hospital Strength
Antiseptic * Anesthetic

Active Ingredients:	**Purpose:**
Benzethonium Chloride USP 0.2%	Antibacterial.
Benzocaine USP 20%	Topical Anesthetic

Indications: First aid to help prevent infection and provide temporary relief of pain and itching associated with •sunburn •insect bites •minor cuts •scrapes •minor burns •minor skin irritations

Warnings:
Do Not Use: •in eyes •on deep or puncture wounds, animal bites or serious burns. Consult a doctor
When Using This Product: •use only as directed •do not apply over large areas of the body •do not use longer than 1 week, unless directed by a doctor
Stop Using This Product And Consult A Doctor If: •condition worsens •symptoms persist for more than 7 days •symptoms clear up and recur within a few days.
For external use only. Contents under pressure. Do not puncture or incinerate. Do not expose to heat or temperature above 120 F. Do not use near open flame. **Keep this and all drugs out of reach of children.** If accidentally ingested, seek professional assistance or contact a poison control center immediately. Intentional misuse by deliberately concentrating and inhaling the contents can be harmful or fatal.

Directions: Children under 2 years of age: do not use. Consult a doctor. Adults and children 2 years and older: clean and apply to affected area not more than 3 times daily. Hold can 6 to 12 inches away from affected area. Point spray nozzle and press button. May be covered with a sterile bandage. If bandaged, let dry first

Other information: Store at room temperature (approximately 25° C, 77° F).

Inactive Ingredients: Acetulan, Aloe Vera Oil, Menthol, Methylparaben USP, N-Butane/P152a (65:35), PEG 400, Monolaurate, Polysorbate 85.

How Supplied: 2¾ FL OZ (81 ml)
Manufactured for
Medtech, Jackson WY 83001 USA
Questions? 1-800-443-4908

MOMENTUM® Bachache Relief
Magnesium Salicylate
Extra Strength Analgesic

Active Ingredient Per Caplet: Magnesium Salicylate Tetrahydrate 580mg (Equivalent to 467mg of Magnesium Salicylate Anhydrous).

Purpose: Analgesic

Uses: For temporary relief of minor aches and pains associated with:
• Backache and muscular aches
• Back pain due to muscle strain or spasm
• Muscle stiffness
Provides maximum dosage of Magnesium Salicylate back pain medicine available without a prescription

Warnings:
• Do not take this product if you are taking a prescription drug for anticoagulation (thinning of the blood), diabetes, gout, or arthritis unless directed by a doctor.
• Do not take for pain for more than 10 days unless directed by a doctor.
• Children or teenagers should not use this product for chicken pox or flu symptoms before a doctor is consulted about Reye Syndrome, a rare but serious illness.

Alcohol Warning: If you consume 3 or more alcoholic drinks every day, ask your doctor whether you should take magnesium salicylate or other pain relievers/fever reducers. Magnesium salicylate may cause stomach bleeding.

Ask a Doctor Before Use:
If you are:
• Allergic to salicylates (including aspirin)
If you have:
• Recurring stomach problems such as heartburn, nausea, pain
• Ulcers or bleeding problems
Consult a Doctor After Use If:
• Pain persists or gets worse
• Redness or swelling is present
• New or unexpected symptoms occur
• You experience ringing in the ears or a loss of hearing
These could be signs of a serious condition.
As with any drug, if you are pregnant or nursing a baby, seek the advice of a health professional before using this product.
Keep this and all drugs out of reach of children. In case of accidental overdose, seek professional assistance or contact a poison control center immediately.

Directions:

Adults:	Take with a full glass of water. Take 2 caplets every 6 hours while symptoms persist. Do not take more than 8 caplets in 24 hours.
Children under 12 yrs:	Consult a doctor.

How Supplied: 48 Coated Caplets
Do not use if imprinted foil seal under cap is broken or missing.
Store at room temperature between 15°–30°C (59°–86°F).

Inactive Ingredients: Hydrogenated Vegetable Oil, Hydroxypropyl Methylcel-

lulose Microcrystalline Cellulose, Polyethylene Glycol, Polysorbate 80, Titanium Dioxide
Manufactured for Medtech, Jackson, WY 83001 USA
Questions? 800-443-4908

NEW SKIN® Liquid Bandage
Antiseptic For Minor Cuts & Scrapes

Description: New-Skin dries rapidly to form a tough protective cover that is antiseptic, flexible, waterproof and lets skin breathe. Completely covers the entire wound to keep out dirt and germs. New-Skin Liquid is suited for smaller areas. Try New-Skin Spray for large areas on legs and arms.

Uses: • **Protects cuts and scrapes** • **Prevents and protects blisters** • **Helps prevent the formation of calluses** • **Covers painful hangnails** • **Particularly useful for bowlers, golfers, tennis players, fisherman and musicans**

Caution: For use on minor cuts and abrasions only. Do not apply to infected areas or wounds that are draining. Consult physician for: deep cuts, serious bleeding, puncture wounds, or application over sutures; if diabetic or have poor circulation; if redness, swelling or pain persists or increases; if infection occurs. Intentional misuse by deliberately concentrating and inhaling contents can be harmful or fatal. For topical external use only. Keep away from eyes and other mucous membranes.

Directions: Thoroughly clean affected area with soap and water. Dry. Apply a coating of New-Skin. Let dry. A second coating may be applied for extra protection. New-Skin may be applied as necessary. A standard coating will last 24–48 hours. Do not apply in conjunction with other first aid products, lotions, drugs, or creams. May temporarily sting upon application.
TO REMOVE: Apply more New-Skin and quickly wipe off. Finger nail polish remover may dissolve New-Skin.

Warning: FLAMMABLE: Do not use or store near heat or open flame • **Keep this and all drugs out of the reach of children** • **In case of accidental ingestion, seek medical assistance or contact your poison control center immediately** • **Do not allow to come in contact with floors, countertops or other finished surfaces - will stain.**

Contains: Pyroxylin Solution, Alcohol 6.7%, Oil of Cloves, 8-hydroxyquinoline

How Supplied: .3 FL. OZ. also available in 1 FL OZ and 1 FL OZ SPRAY
Mfg. for Medtech, Jackson WY 83001 USA Questions? 800-443-4908
© Medtech, R5/99

PERCOGESIC®
Aspirin-Free Pain Reliever

Active Ingredient per caplet:

	Purpose:
Acetaminophen 325 mg, Phenyltoloxamine Citrate 30 mg	Analgesic

Indications: For the temporary relief of minor aches and pains associated with headaches, muscular aches, backaches, premenstrual and menstrual periods, colds, the flu, toothaches, as well as for minor pain from arthritis, and to reduce fever.

Directions: Adults (12 years and over) – 1 or 2 tablets every 4 hours. Maximum daily dose – 8 tablets. Children (6 to under 12 years) – 1 tablet every 4 hours. Maximum daily dose – 4 tablets. Children under 6 years of age: Consult a doctor.

Warnings: Do not take this product for pain for more than 10 days (adults) or 5 days (children), and do not take for fever for more than 3 days unless directed by a doctor. If pain or fever persists or worsens, new symptoms occur or redness or swelling is present, consult a doctor, as these could be signs of a serious condition. Do not give to children for arthritis pain unless directed by a doctor. May cause excitability, especially in children. Do not take this product, unless directed by a doctor, if you have a breathing problem such as emphysema or chronic bronchitis, or if you have glaucoma or difficulty in urination due to enlargement of the prostate gland. May cause marked drowsiness; alcohol, sedatives, and tranquilizers may increase the drowsiness effect. Avoid alcoholic beverages while taking this product. Do not take this product if you are taking sedatives or tranquilizers without first consulting your doctor. Use caution when driving a motor vehicle or operating machinery.

Alcohol Warning: If you consume 3 or more alcoholic drinks every day, ask your doctor whether you should take acetaminophen or other pain relievers/fever reducers. Acetaminophen may cause liver damage.

KEEP THIS AND ALL DRUGS OUT OF THE REACH OF CHILDREN. In case of accidental overdose, seek professional assistance or contact a poison control center immediately. Prompt medical attention is critical for adults as well as for children even if you do not notice any signs or symptoms. As with any drug, if you are pregnant or nursing a baby, seek the advice of a health professional before using this product.

How Supplied: 24 Coated Tablets; 50 coated tablets*; 90 coated tablets

---

STORE AT ROOM TEMPERATURE. AVOID EXCESSIVE HEAT.

---

*Percogesic Aspirin Free Analgesic 50 tablets package is for Households without young children.

Active Ingredients: Each tablet contains Acetaminophen 325 mg, Phenyltoloxamine Citrate 30 mg.

Inactive Ingredients: Cellulose, FD&C Yellow No. 6, Flavor, Hydroxypropyl Methylcellulose, Magnesium Stearate, Polyethylene Glycol, Povidone, Silica Gel, Starch, Stearic Acid, Sucrose. Mfg. for Medtech Jackson, WY 83001 U.S.A.

Mission Pharmacal Company
**10999 IH 10 WEST
SUITE 1000
SAN ANTONIO, TX 78230-1355**

Direct Inquiries to:
PO Box 786099
San Antonio, TX 78278-6099
TOLL FREE: (800) 292-7364
(210) 696-8400
FAX: (210) 696-6010
For Medical Information Contact:
In Emergencies:
George Alexandrides
(830) 249-9822
FAX: (830) 816-2545

THERA-GESIC®
[thĕr'ə-jē-zik]
**(Methyl Salicylate 15%, Menthol 1%)
Topical Therapeutic Analgesic Creme**

Description: THERA-GESIC® contains methyl salicylate and menthol in a rapidly absorbed greaseless base containing carbomer 934, dimethicone, glycerine, methylparaben, propylparaben, sodium lauryl sulfate, trolamine, and water.

Indications: For the temporary relief of minor aches and pains of muscles and joints associated with arthritis, simple backache, strains, sprains and sports injuries.

Warnings: FOR EXTERNAL USE ONLY. Use only as directed. Keep away from children to avoid accidental poisoning. Keep away from eyes, mucous membranes, broken or irritated skin. Do not use THERA-GESIC® if you have skin sensitive to oil of wintergreen (methyl salicylate). If skin irritation develops, if pain lasts 7 days or more, or if redness is present, discontinue use and consult a physician immediately. **DO NOT SWALLOW.** If swallowed induce vomiting, call a phy-

Continued on next page

Thera-Gesic—Cont.

sician. Contact a physician before applying this medicine to children, including teenagers, with chicken pox or flu.

Directions: ADULTS AND CHILDREN 12 OR MORE YEARS OF AGE: An application of THERA-GESIC® is the gentle massaging of several thin layers of creme into and around the sore or painful area. The number of thin layers controls the intensity of the action. One thin layer provides a mild effect, two thin layers provide a strong effect and three thin layers provide a very strong effect. Do not apply more than 3 to 4 times daily. Once THERA-GESIC® has penetrated the skin, the area may be washed, leaving it dry, clean and fragrance-free without decreasing the effectiveness of the product. IF YOU INTEND TO WRAP, BANDAGE OR COVER THE AREA WHERE YOU HAVE APPLIED THERA-GESIC®, IT MUST BE WASHED THOROUGHLY TO AVOID EXCESSIVE IRRITATION. DO NOT USE A HEATING PAD AFTER APPLICATION OF THERA-GESIC®.

How Supplied:
NDC 0178-0320-03   3 oz. tube
NDC 0178-0320-05   5 oz. tube
Store at room temperature.

Novartis Consumer Health, Inc.
**560 MORRIS AVE.
SUMMIT, NJ 07901-1312**

Direct Product Inquiries to:
Consumer & Professional Affairs
(800) 452-0051
Fax: (800) 635-2801
Or write to above address.

DESENEX® ANTIFUNGALS
[dess 'i-nex]

All products are Prescription Strength
Shake Powder
Liquid Spray
Spray Powder
Jock Itch Spray Powder

Indications: Cures athlete's foot (tinea pedis), jock itch (tinea cruris) and ringworm (tinea corporis). For effective relief of the itching, burning, cracking and scaling which can accompany these conditions. Desenex powders also help keep feet dry.

Active Ingredient: *Shake Powder*, *Liquid Spray*, *Spray Powder*, and *Jock Itch Spray Powder*—Miconazole nitrate 2%.

Inactive Ingredients:
SHAKE POWDER—Corn starch, corn starch/acrylamide/sodium acrylate polymer, fragrance, talc.

LIQUID SPRAY—Polyethylene glycol 300, polysorbate 20, SD alcohol 40-B (15% w/w).
Propellant: Dimethyl ether.
SPRAY POWDER—Aloe vera gel, aluminum starch octenyl succinate, isopropyl myristate, propylene carbonate, SD alcohol 40-B (10% w/w), sorbitan monooleate, stearalkonium hectorite.
Propellant: Isobutane/propane.
JOCK ITCH SPRAY POWDER—Aloe vera gel, aluminum starch octenyl succinate, isopropyl myristate, propylene carbonate, SD alcohol 40-B (10% w/w), sorbitan monooleate, stearalkonium hectorite.
Propellant: Isobutane/propane.

Warnings: Do not use on children under 2 years of age unless directed by a doctor. For external use only. Avoid contact with the eyes. If irritation occurs, or if there is no improvement within 4 weeks (for athlete's foot or ringworm) or within 2 weeks for jock itch, discontinue use and consult a doctor. **Keep this and all drugs out of the reach of children.** In case of accidental ingestion, seek professional assistance or contact a poison control center immediately. Use only as directed. *For Spray Powders and Liquid Spray*—Avoid inhaling. Avoid contact with the eyes or other mucous membranes. Contents under pressure. Do not puncture or incinerate. Flammable mixture, do not use near fire or flame. Do not expose to heat or temperatures above 49°C (120°F). Use only as directed. Intentional misuse by deliberately concentrating and inhaling the contents can be harmful or fatal.

Directions: Clean the affected area and dry thoroughly. Apply a thin layer of the product over affected area twice daily (morning and night) or as directed by a doctor. (For Sprays: **Shake Spray can well,** and hold 4″ to 6″ from skin when applying.) For athlete's foot, pay special attention to the spaces between the toes. Wear well-fitting, ventilated shoes and change shoes and socks at least once daily. For athlete's foot or ringworm, use daily for 4 weeks. For jock itch, use daily for 2 weeks. If condition persists longer, consult a doctor. Supervise children in the use of this product. This product is not effective on the scalp or nails.

How Supplied:
Shake Powder—1.5 oz, 3 oz, 4 oz. plastic bottles.
Spray Powder—3 oz, 4 oz. cans.
Liquid Spray—3.5 oz, 4.6 oz. cans.
Store **powders/spray powders** and **liquid sprays** at room temperature, 15°–30°C (59°–86°F). See container bottom for lot number and expiration date. Spray powders: Tamper-resistant aerosol can for your protection. If clogging occurs, remove button and clean nozzle with pin.

DesenexMax Cream®
Active Ingredient: Terbinafine hydrohloride 1%

Inactive Ingredients: benzyl alcohol, cetyl alcohol, cetyl palmitate, isopropyl myristate, polysorbate 60, purified water, sodium hydroxide, sorbitan monostearate, stearyl alcohol.

Warnings: For external use only.
Do not use:
• On nails or scalp
• In or near the mouth or the eyes
• For vaginal yeast infections
When using this produt do not get into the eyes. If eye contact occurs, rinse thoroughly with water. Stop use and ask a doctor if too much irritaiton occurs or gets worse. Keep out of reach of children. Of swallowed, get medical help or contact a poison control center right away.

Directions: Adults and children 12 years and over:
• Use the tip of the cap to break the seal and open the tube
• Wash the affected skin with soap and water and dry completely before applying
• For athlete's foot wear well-fitting, ventilated shoes. Change shoes and socks at least once daily.
• **Between the toes only:** apply twice a day (morning and night) for 1 week or as directed by a doctor.

1 week between the toes

• **on the bottom or sides of the foot:** apply twice a day (morning and night) for 2 weeks or as directed by a doctor.

2 weeks on the bottom or sides of the foot

• **for jock itch and ringworm:** apply once a day (morning or night) for 1 week or as directed by a doctor.
• wash hands after each use
• children under 12 years: ask a doctor

How Supplied: 0.42 oz. (12 gram) and 0.85 oz. (24 gram) tubes
Do not use if seal on tube is broken or is not visible. Store between 5° and 30° C (41° and 86° F).
Questions: Call 1-800-452-0051 24 hours a day, 7 days a week
Novartis Consumer Health Inc.
Summit NJ 07901-1312
©2001
Shown in Product Identification Guide, page 512

DULCOLAX®
[dul 'co-lax]
**brand of bisacodyl USP
Tablets of 5 mg
Suppositories of 10 mg
Laxative**

Indications: For the relief of occasional constipation and irregularity. Tablets:

Expect results in 8–12 hours if taken at bedtime or within 6 hours if taken before breakfast.

Suppositories: This product generally provides a bowel movement in 15 minutes to 1 hour.

Active Ingredients: Dulcolax Tablets-Bisacodyl USP 5 mg.
Dulcolax Suppositories-Bisacodyl USP 10 mg.

Inactive Ingredients: Dulcolax Tablets-acacia, acetylated monoglyceride, carnauba wax, cellulose acetate phthalate, corn starch, D&C Red No. 30 aluminum lake, D&C Yellow No. 10 aluminum lake, dibutyl phthalate, docusate sodium, gelatin, glycerin, iron oxides, kaolin, lactose, magnesium stearate, methylparaben, pharmaceutical glaze, polyethylene glycol, povidone, propylparaben, sodium benzoate, sorbitan monooleate, sucrose, talc, titanium dioxide, white wax. **Dulcolax Suppositories**-Hydrogenated vegetable oil.

Sodium Content: Tablets and suppositories contain less than 0.2 mg per dosage unit and are thus dietetically sodium free.

Directions:
Tablets
Adults and children 12 years of age and over: Take 2 or 3 tablets (usually 2) in a single dose once daily.
Children 6 to under 12 years of age: Take 1 tablet once daily.
Children under 6 years of age: Consult a physician.
Suppositories
Adults and children 12 years of age and over: 1 suppository once daily. Remove foil wrapper. Lie on your side and, with pointed end first, push suppository high into the rectum so it will not slip out. Retain it for 15 to 20 minutes. If you feel the suppository must come out immediately, it was not inserted high enough and should be pushed higher.
Children 6 to under 12 years of age: $^{1}/_{2}$ suppository once daily.
Children under 6 years of age: Consult a physician.
If the suppository seems soft, hold in foil wrapper under cold water for one or two minutes before use. In the presence of anal fissures or hemorrhoids, suppository may be coated at the tip with petroleum jelly before insertion.

Warnings: Do not use laxative products when abdominal pain, nausea, or vomiting are present unless directed by a physician. If you have noticed a sudden change in bowel habits that persists over a period of 2 weeks, consult a physician before using a laxative. Restoration of normal bowel function by using this product may cause abdominal discomfort including cramps. Laxative products should not be used for a period longer than 1 week unless directed by a physician. Rectal bleeding or failure to have a bowel movement after use of a laxative may indicate a serious condition. If this occurs, discontinue use and consult your physician. As with any drug, if you are pregnant or nursing a baby, seek the advice of a health care professional before using this product. **Keep this and all drugs out of the reach of children.** In case of accidental overdose or ingestion, seek professional assistance or contact a poison control center immediately. For tablets: Do not chew or crush. Do not give to children under 6 years of age unless directed by a physician. Do not take this product within 1 hour after taking an antacid or milk.

How Supplied: Dulcolax, brand of bisacodyl: Yellow, enteric-coated tablets of 5 mg in boxes of 10, 25, 50 and 100; suppositories of 10 mg in boxes of 4, 8, 16 and 50.

Store Dulcolax suppositories and tablets at temperatures below 77°F (25°C). Avoid excessive humidity.

Also Available: Dulcolax® Bowel Prep Kit. Each kit contains:
  1 Dulcolax suppository of 10 mg bisacodyl;
  4 Dulcolax tablets of 5 mg bisacodyl;
  Complete patient instructions.

Professional Labeling

Description and Clinical Pharmacology: Dulcolax is a contact stimulant laxative, administered either orally or rectally, which acts directly on the colonic mucosa to produce normal peristalsis throughout the large intestine. The active ingredient in Dulcolax, bisacodyl, is a colorless, tasteless compound that is practically insoluble in water or alkaline solution. Its chemical name is: bis(p-acetoxyphenyl)-2-pyridylmethane. Bisacodyl is very poorly absorbed, if at all, in the small intestine following oral administration, nor in the large intestine following rectal administration. On contact with the mucosa or submucosal plexi of the large intestine, bisacodyl stimulates sensory nerve endings to produce parasympathetic reflexes resulting in increased peristaltic contractions of the colon. It has also been shown to promote fluid and ion accumulation in the colon, which increases the laxative effect. A bowel movement is usually produced approximately 6 hours after oral administration (8–12 hours if taken at bedtime), and approximately 15 minutes to 1 hour after rectal administration, providing satisfactory cleansing of the bowel which may, under certain circumstances, obviate the need for colonic irrigation.

Indications and Usage: For use as part of a bowel cleansing regimen in preparing the patient for surgery or for preparing the colon for x-ray endoscopic examination. Dulcolax will not replace the colonic irrigations usually given patients before intracolonic surgery, but is useful in the preliminary emptying of the colon prior to these procedures.
Also for use as a laxative in postoperative care (i.e., restoration of normal bowel hygiene), antepartum care, postpartum care, and in preparation for delivery.

Contraindications: Stimulant laxatives, such as Dulcolax, are contraindicated for patients with acute surgical abdomen, appendicitis, rectal bleeding, gastroenteritis, or intestinal obstruction.

Precautions: Long-term administration of Dulcolax is not recommended in the treatment of chronic constipation.

Dosage and Administration: Preparation for x-ray endoscopy: For barium enemas, no food should be given following oral administration to prevent reaccumulation of material in the cecum, and a suppository should be administered one to two hours prior to examination. Children under 6 years of age: Oral administration is not recommended due to the requirement to swallow tablets whole. For rectal administration, the suppository dosage is 5 mg ($^{1}/_{2}$ of 10 mg suppository) in a single daily dose.

Shown in Product Identification Guide, page 513

EX–LAX® Chocolated Laxative Pieces

Active Ingredient: Sennosides, USP, 15mg

Use: For Relief of
• OCCASIONAL CONSTIPATION (IRREGULARITY). This product generally produces bowel movement in 6 to 12 hours.

Directions: Adults and children 12 years of age and over: chew 2 chocolated pieces once or twice daily. Children 6 to under 12 years of age: chew 1 chocolated piece once or twice daily. Children under 6 years of age: consult a doctor.

Warnings:
• as with any drug, if you are pregnant or nursing a baby, seek the advice of a health professional before using the product.
Unless directed by a doctor, do not use
• laxative products when abdominal pain, nausea, or vomiting is present.
• laxative products for a period longer than 1 week.
Consult a doctor before using a laxative if
• you have noticed a sudden change in bowel habits that persists over a period of 2 weeks.
Consult a doctor and stop using a laxative if
• rectal bleeding occurs or you fail to have a bowel movement after use because this may indicate a serious condition.
Keep this and all drugs out of the reach of children
In case of accidental overdose, seek professional assistance or contact a poison control center immediately.

Continued on next page

Information on Novartis Consumer Health, Inc., products appearing on these pages is effective as of November 2000.

Ex-Lax Chocolated—Cont.

Inactive Ingredients: cocoa, confectioners sugar, hydrogenated palm kernel oil, lecithin, non-fat dry milk, vanillin. Store at controlled room temperature 20–25°C (68–77°F)

How Supplied: Available in boxes of 6, 18, 48, chewable chocolated pieces.
Shown in Product Identification Guide, page 513

EX-LAX® Gentle Strength Laxative Plus Stool Softener

Active Ingredients: Docusate sodium, 65 mg and Sennosides, USP, 10 mg, per caplet

Use: For Relief of
• OCCASIONAL CONSTIPATION (IRREGULARITY). This product generally produces bowel movement in 6 to 12 hours.

Directions: Adults and children 12 years of age and over: Take 2 caplets once or twice daily with a glass of water. Children 6 to under 12 years of age: take 1 caplet once or twice daily with a glass of water. Children under 6 years of age: consult a doctor.

Warnings:
• as with any drug, if you are pregnant or nursing a baby, seek the advice of a health professional before using this product.
Unless directed by a doctor, do not use a laxative:
• when abdominal pain, nausea or vomiting is present.
• for a period longer than 1 week.
Consult a doctor before using a laxative if:
• you are presently taking mineral oil.
• you have noticed a sudden change in bowel habits that persists over a period of 2 weeks.
Consult a doctor and stop using a laxative if:
• rectal bleeding occurs or you fail to have a bowel movement after use because this may indicate a serious condition.
Keep this and all drugs out of the reach of children.
In case of accidental overdose, seek professional assistance or contact a poison control center immediately.

Inactive Ingredients: croscarmellose sodium, D&C Red No. 27 lake, FD&C Blue No. 1 lake, FD&C Yellow No. 6 lake, hydroxypropyl methylcellulose, lactose, methylparaben, polydextrose, polyethylene glycol, pregelatinized starch, silicon dioxide, sodium benzoate, stearic acid, titanium dioxide, traicetin

Sodium content: 5 mg per caplet.

How Supplied: Available in boxes of 24 caplets.

Store at room temperature

©1998 Novartis Consumer Health, Inc. Summit, NJ 07901-1312

4323-22
Shown in Product Identification Guide, page 513

EX–LAX® Laxative Pills
Regular Strength Ex-Lax® Laxative Pills
Maximum Strength Ex-Lax® Laxative Pills

Active Ingredients: *Regular Strength Ex-Lax Laxative Pills:* Sennosides, USP, 15 mg. *Maximum Relief Formula Ex-Lax Laxative Pills:* Sennosides, USP, 25 mg.

Use: For Relief of
• OCCASIONAL CONSTIPATION (IRREGULARITY). This product generally produces bowel movement in 6 to 12 hours.

Warnings:
• as with any drug, if you are pregnant or nursing a baby, seek the advice of a health professional before using this product.
Unless directed by a doctor, do not use:
• laxative products when abdominal pain, nausea, or vomiting is present.
• laxative products for a period longer than 1 week.
Consult a doctor before using a laxative if:
• you have noticed a sudden change in bowel habits that persists over a period of 2 weeks.
Consult a doctor and stop using a laxative if:
• rectal bleeding occurs or you fail to have a bowel movement after use because this may indicate a serious condition.
Keep this and all drugs out of the reach of children. In case of accidental overdose, seek professional assistance or contact a poison control center immediately.

Dosage and Administration: *Regular Strength Ex-Lax Laxative Pills, and Maximum Strength Ex-Lax Laxative Pills*—Adults and children 12 years of age and over: take 2 pills once or twice daily with a glass of water. Children 6 to under 12 years of age: take 1 pill once or twice daily with a glass of water. Children under 6 years of age: consult a doctor.

Inactive Ingredients: *Regular Strength Ex-Lax Laxative Pills*—acacia, alginic acid, carnauba wax, colloidal silicon dioxide, dibasic calcium phosphate, iron oxides, magnesium stearate, microcrystalline cellulose, sodium benzoate, sodium lauryl sulfate, starch, stearic acid, sucrose, talc, titanium dioxide. Sodium-free. *Maximum Strength Ex-Lax Laxative Pills:* acacia, alginic acid, FD&C Blue No. 1 aluminum lake, carnauba wax, colloidal silicon dioxide, dibasic calcium phosphate, magnesium stearate, microcrystalline cellulose, povidone, sodium benzoate, sodium lauryl sulfate, starch, stearic acid, sucrose, talc, titanium dioxide. Very low sodium.

Store at controlled room temperature 20–25°C (68–77°F)

How Supplied: *Regular Strength Ex-Lax Laxative Pills*—Available in boxes of 8, 30, and 60 pills. *Maximum Strength Ex-Lax Laxative Pills*—Available in boxes of 24, 48, and 90 pills.
Shown in Product Identification Guide, page 513

Ex-Lax® Milk of Magnesia STIMULANT FREE Liquid: Laxative/Antacid, Chocolate Creme, Mint, Raspberry Creme

Indications: As a Laxative: To relieve occasional constipation (irregularity). This saline laxative product generally produces bowel movement in ½ to 6 hours.
As an Antacid: To relieve acid indigestion, sour stomach and heartburn.

Active Ingredient: Magnesium hydroxide – 400 mg per teaspoon (5 ml)

Inactive Ingredients:
Chocolate Creme: Carboxymethylcellulose sodium, flavors, glycerin, hydroxypropyl methylcellulose, microcrystalline cellulose, purified water, saccharin sodium, simethicone, sorbitol.
Mint: Carboxymethylcellulose sodium, flavor, glycerin, hydroxypropyl methylcellulose, microcrystalline cellulose, purified water, saccharin sodium, simethicone, sorbitol.
Raspberry Creme: Carboxymethylcellulose sodium, flavor, glycerin, hydroxypropyl methylcellulose, microcrystalline cellulose, purified water, saccharin sodium, simethicone, sorbitol.

Directions: Shake well before using.
Keep tightly closed and avoid freezing.
For Laxative Use: Adults/Children – 12 years and older: 2–4 tablespoonsful (TBSP) at bedtime or upon arising, followed by a full glass (8 oz.) of liquid.
Children: DO NOT USE DOSAGE CUP – 6–11 years: 1–2 tablespoonsful (TBSP), followed by a full glass (8 oz.) of liquid.
2–5 years: 1–3 teaspoonsful, followed by a full glass (8 oz.) of liquid.
Under 2 years: Consult a doctor.
FOR ANTACID USE: DO NOT USE DOSAGE CUP – Adults/Children - 12 years and older: 1–3 teaspoonsful with a little water, up to four times a day or as directed by a doctor.

Drug Interaction Precaution: Antacids may interact with certain prescription drugs. If you are presently taking a prescription drug, do not take this product without checking with your doctor or other health professional.

Laxative Warnings: Do not take any laxative if abdominal pain, nausea, vomiting or kidney disease are present unless directed by a doctor. If you have noticed a sudden change in bowel habits persisting for over 2 weeks, consult a doctor before using a laxative. Laxative products should not be used for a period

longer than 1 week, unless directed by a doctor. Rectal bleeding or failure to have a bowel movement after use of a laxative may indicate a serious condition. Discontinue use and consult your doctor.

Antacid Warnings: Do not take more than the maximum recommended daily dosage in a 24 hour period (See Directions), or use the maximum dosage of this product for more than two weeks, or use this product if you have kidney disease, except under the advice and supervision of a doctor. May have laxative effect.

As with any drug, if you are pregnant or nursing a baby, seek the advice of a health professional before using this product. Keep this and all drugs out of the reach of children. In case of accidental overdose, seek professional assistance or contact a poison control central immediately.

How Supplied: EX-LAX MILK OF MAGNESIA is available in Chocolate Creme, Mint, and Raspberry Creme and comes in 12 oz (355 ml) and 26 oz (769 ml) bottles.
Store at controlled room temperature 20–25°C (68–77°F).
Distributed by:
NOVARTIS
Novarits Consumer Health, Inc.
Summit, NJ 07901-1312
Shown in Product Identification Guide, page 513

EX-LAX® STOOL SOFTENER CAPLETS
docusate sodium 100mg
stimulant-free
mild, natural-feeling relief
for sensitive systems

Active Ingredient: Docusate Sodium, 100 mg per caplet.

Use: For the relief of occasional constipation (irregularity), especially for sensitive systems. Useful in constipation due to hard stools and conditions where ease of passage is desirable. This gentle, stimulant-free formula generally works within 12–72 hours after the first dose.

Directions: Take Ex-Lax stool softener caplets with a glass of water at any time. Adults and children 12 years of age and over: 1 to 3 caplets daily as needed. Children 2 to under 12 years of age: 1 caplet daily. This dose may be taken as a single daily dose or in divided doses. Children under 2 years of age: consult a doctor.

Warnings:
• as with any drug, if you are pregnant or nursing a baby, seek the advice of a health professional before using this product.
Unless directed by a doctor, do not use
• laxative products when abdominal pain, nausea, or vomiting is present.
• laxative products for a period longer than 1 week.

Consult a doctor before using a laxative if
• you have noticed a sudden change in bowel habits that persists over a period of 2 weeks.
Consult a doctor and stop using a laxative if
• rectal bleeding occurs or you fail to have a bowel movement after use because this may indicate a serious condition.
Keep this and all drugs out of the reach of children. In case of accidental overdose, seek professional assistance or contact a poison control center immediately.

Inactive Ingredients: Alginic Acid, Blue 1, Colloidal Silicon Dioxide, Croscarmellose Sodium, Dibasic Calcium Phosphate, Hydroxypropyl Methylcellulose, Magnesium Stearate, Methylparaben, Microcrystalline Cellulose, Polydextrose, Polyethylene Glycol, Silicon Dioxide, Sodium Benzoate, Stearic Acid, Talc, Titanium Dioxide, Triacetin, Yellow 10. Sodium content: 8 mg per caplet.

Drug Interaction Precaution: Do not take this product if you are presently taking mineral oil, unless directed by a doctor.
Store at controlled room temperature 15°–30°C (59°–86°F). Protect from moisture.

How Supplied: Available in boxes of 40 caplets.
Shown in Product Identification Guide, page 513

GAS–X®
EXTRA STRENGTH GAS-X®
MAXIMUM STRENGTH GAS-X®
Antiflatulent, Anti-Gas Chewable Tablets
Extra Strength Softgels
Extra Strength Liquids
Maximum Strength Softgels

Active Ingredients: GAS-X®—Each chewable tablet contains simethicone 80 mg.
EXTRA STRENGTH GAS-X®—Each chewable tablet contains simethicone, 125 mg, each swallowable softgel contains simethicone, USP, 125 mg and each teaspoon of liquid contains simethicone, 50 mg; USP
MAXIMUM STRENGTH GAS-X®— Each Swallowable softgel contains sinethicone, USP, 166 mg.

Inactive Ingredients:
EXTRA STRENGTH PEPPERMINT CREME: calcium phosphate tribasic, colloidal silicon dioxide, D&C Yellow 10 aluminum lake, dextrose, flavors, maltodextrin.
EXTRA STRENGTH CHERRY CREME: calcium phosphate tribasic, colloidal silicon dioxide, D&C Red 30 aluminum lake, dextrose, flavors, maltodextrin.
GAS-X PEPPERMINT CREME: calcium carbonate, dextrose, flavors, maltodextrin.

GAS-X CHERRY CREME: calcium carbonate, D&C Red 30, dextrose, flavors, maltodextrin.
EXTRA STRENGTH SOFTGELS: D&C Yellow 10, FD&C Blue 1, FD&C Red 40, gelatin, glycerin, peppermint oil, purified water, sorbitol, titanium dioxide.
MAXIMUM STRENGTH SOFTGELS: D&C Red 33, FD&C Blue 1, FD&C Red 40, gelatin, glycerin, peppermint oil, purified water, sorbitol.
Liquids: benzoic acid, carboxymethylcellulose sodium, flavors, hydrochloric acid, microcrystalline cellulose, propylene glycol, propylparaben, purified water, sucrose, titanium dioxide, (cherry creme contains FD&C Red 40).

Indications: Relieves the symptoms referred to as gas.

Actions: GAS-X relieves the bloating, pressure and fullness commonly referred to as gas.

Warning: Keep out of reach of children.

Drug Interaction Precautions: No known drug interaction.

Dosage and Administration: For Chewable Tablets: Adults: Chew thoroughly and swallow one or two tablets as needed after meals or at bedtime. Do not exceed six GAS-X chewable tablets or four EXTRA STRENGTH GAS-X chewable tablets in 24 hours. Do not increase dosage unless recommended by your physician.
For EXTRA STRENGTH GAS-X SOFTGELS: Adults: Swallow with water 1 or 2 softgels as needed after meals or at bedtime. Do not exceed 4 softgels in 24 hours unless recommended by your physician.
For MAXIMUM STRENGTH SOFTGELS: Adults: Swallow with water one or two softgels as needed after meals or at bedtime. Do not exceed 3 softgels in 24 hours except under the advice and supervision of a physician.
For EXTRA STRENGTH GAS-X LIQUIDS: Adults: 2–4 teaspoons as needed after meals or at bedtime. Do not exceed 10 teaspoons in a 24 hour period. Children (2–12 years): 1 teaspoon as needed after meals or at bedtime. Do not exceed 4 teaspoons in 24 hours. Consult a physician before increasing dosage.

Professional Labeling: GAS-X may be used in the alleviation of postoperative bloating/pressure, and for use in endoscopic examination.

How Supplied: GAS-X Chewable tablets are available in peppermint creme and cherry creme flavored, chewable, scored tablets in boxes of 12 tablets and 36 tablets.

Continued on next page

Information on Novartis Consumer Health, Inc., products appearing on these pages is effective as of November 2000.

Gas-X—Cont.

EXTRA STRENGTH GAS-X Chewable tablets are available in peppermint creme and cherry creme flavored, chewable, scored tablets in boxes of 18 tablets and 48 tablets.

Easy-to-swallow, tasteless/EXTRA STRENGTH GAS-X SOFTGELS are available in boxes of 10 pills, 30 pills, 50 pills and 60 pills.

Easy-to-swallow, tasteless/MAXIMUM STRENGTH GAS-X SOFTGELS are available in box of 50 pills.

EXTRA STRENGTH GAS-X LIQUIDS are available in peppermint creme and cherry creme in 10 oz. bottles.

Shown in Product Identification Guide, page 513

LAMISIL® AT™ ANTIFUNGAL
TERBINAFINE HYDROCHLORIDE CREAM 1%
CURES ATHLETE'S FOOT
CURES JOCK ITCH
CURES RINGWORM

Description: For effective relief of itching and burning. Full prescription strength. Dries fast. Not greasy.

Active ingredient:
Terbinafine hydrochloride 1%
Purpose: Antifungal

Inactive ingredients: benzyl alcohol, cetyl alcohol, cetyl palmitate, isopropyl myristate, polysorbate 60, purified water, sodium hydroxide, sorbitan monostearate, stearyl alcohol.

Uses:
For Athlete's Foot:
•cures athlete's foot (tinea pedis) •cures jock itch (tinea cruris) and ringworm (tinea corporis) •relieves itching, burning, cracking and scaling which accompany these conditions
For Jock Itch and Ringworm
•cures jock itch (tinea cruris) •relieves itching, burning, cracking and scaling which accompany this condition

Warnings:
For external use only
Do not use on nails or scalp, in or near the mouth or the eyes, for vaginal yeast infections.
When using this product do not get into the eyes. If eye contact occurs, rinse thoroughly with water.
Stop use and ask a doctor if too much irritation occurs or gets worse.
Keep out of reach of children. If swallowed, get medical help or contact a poison control center right away.

Directions:
• adults and children 12 years and over:
 • use the tip of the cap to break the seal and open the tube
 • wash the affected skin with soap and water and dry completely before applying
 • **for athlete's foot** wear well-fitting, ventilated shoes. Change shoes and socks at least once daily.

• **between the toes only:** apply twice a day (morning and night) for **1 week** or as directed by a doctor.

1 week between the toes

• **on the bottom or sides of the foot:** apply twice a day (morning and night) for **2 weeks** or as directed by a doctor.

2 weeks on the bottom or sides of the foot

 • wash hands after each use
• children under 12 years: ask a doctor
For Jock Itch and Ringworm
• adults and children 12 years and over
 • use the tip of the cap to break the seal and open the tube
 • wash the affected skin with soap and water and dry completely before applying
 • apply once a day (morning **or** night) for **1 week** or as directed by a doctor.
 • wash hands after each use
• children under 12 years: ask a doctor

How Supplied: Athlete's Foot — Net wt. 12g (.42 oz) tube and 24g (.85 oz.) tube, Jock Itch — Net wt. 12g (.42 oz.) tube.

Other information: •do not use if seal on tube is broken or is not visible
•store between 5° and 30° C (41° and 86° F)

Questions?
Call 1-800-452-0051
24 hours a day, 7 days a week.
Novartis Consumer Health, Inc.,
Summit, NJ 07901-1312 ©2001
Shown in Product Identification Guide, page 513

LAMISIL® AT™ ANTIFUNGAL
TERBINAFINE HYDROCHLORIDE SOLUTION 1%
CURE'S ATHLETE'S FOOT
CURES JOCK ITCH
CURES RING WORM

Description: For effective relief of itching and burning. Full prescription strength. Dries fast. Not greasy.

Active Ingredient: Terbinafine Hydrochloride 1%.
Purpose: Antifungal

Inactive Ingredients: Cetomacrogol, Ethanol, Propylene Glycol, Purified Water USP

Uses:
Lamisil® AT™ Solution Dropper and Lamisil® AT™ Spray Pump – For Athlete's Foot and Jock Itch:

• Cures athlete's foot (tinea pedis) between the toes. Effectiveness on the bottom or sides of foot is unknown.
• Cures jock itch (tinea cruris), and ringworm (tinea corporis)
• Relieves itching, burning, cracking, and scaling which accompany these conditions

Warnings:
For external use only:
Do not use:
• on nails or scalp
• in or near the mouth or the eyes
• for vaginal yeast infections
When using this product do not get into eyes. If contact occurs, rinse eyes thoroughly with water.
Stop use and ask a doctor if too much irritation occurs or gets worse.
Keep out of reach of children. If swallowed, get medical help or contact a poison control center right away.

Directions:
Lamisil® AT™ Solution Dropper For Athlete's Foot
• adults and children 12 years and older
 • wash the affected skin with soap and water and dry completely before applying
 • **for athlete's foot between the toes** apply twice a day (morning and night) for 1 week or as directed by a doctor. Wear well-fitting, ventilated shoes. Change shoes and socks at least once daily.
 • **for jock itch and ringworm** apply to affected area once a day (morning or night) for 1 week or as directed by a doctor

1 week between the toes

• wash hands after each use
• children under 12 years: ask a doctor
Lamisil® AT™ Spray Pump For Athlete's Foot
• adults and children 12 years and older
 • wash the affected skin with soap and water and dry completely before applying
 • **for athlete's foot between the toes** apply twice a day (morning and night) for 1 week or as directed by a doctor. Wear well-fitting, ventilated shoes. Change shoes and socks at least once daily.
 • **for jock itch and ringworm** apply to affected area once a day (morning or night) for 1 week or as directed by a doctor

1 week between the toes

• wash hands after each use
• children under 12 years: ask a doctor
Lamisil® AT™ Spray Pump For Jock Itch:
• adults and children 12 years and older
 • wash the affected skin with soap and water and dry completely before applying
 • spray affected area once a day (morning **or** night) for 1 week or as directed by a doctor.
 • wash hands after each use
 • children under 12 years: ask a doctor

How Supplied: Bottle of 30 ml (1 fl. oz.). Spray Pump or Solution Dropper

Other Information: Store at 8°–25°C (46°–77°F).

Questions?

Call 1-800-452-0051 24 hours a day, 7 days a week.

Novartis Consumer Health, Inc., Summit, NJ 07901-1312 ©2001

Shown in Product Identification Guide, page 513

MAALOX® MAX MAXIMUM STRENGTH ANTACID/ANTI-GAS Liquid
Oral Suspension Antacid/Anti-Gas

Liquids
☐ Lemon
☐ Cherry
☐ Mint
☐ Vanilla Crème
☐ Peaches n' Crème
☐ Wild Berry

Description: MAALOX® Max Maximum Strength Antacid/Anti-Gas, a balanced combination of magnesium and aluminum hydroxides plus simethicone, is an antacid/anti-gas product to provide symptomatic relief of acid indigestion, heartburn, sour stomach, upset stomach associated with these symptoms and relief of pressure and bloating commonly referred to as gas.

Composition: To provide symptomatic relief of hyperacidity plus alleviation of gas symptoms, each teaspoonful contains:

Active Ingredients	Maximum Strength Maalox® Max Antacid/Anti-Gas Per Tsp. (5 mL)
Magnesium Hydroxide	400 mg
Aluminum Hydroxide (equivalent to dried gel, USP)	400 mg
Simethicone	40 mg

Inactive Ingredients: Butylparaben, Carboxymethylcellulose Sodium, D&C Yellow #10 (Lemon Flavor only), Flavor, Hydroxypropyl Methylcyllulose, Microcrystalline Cellulose, Potassium Citrate, Polyparaben, Purified Water, Saccharin Sodium, Sorbitol.

Directions for Use: 2 to 4 teaspoonfuls, 4 times per day, or as directed by a physician.

Patient Warnings: Do not take more than 12 teaspoonfuls in a 24-hour period or use the maximum dosage for more than 2 weeks or use if you have kidney disease except under the advise and supervision of a physician. **Keep this and all drugs out of the reach of children.**

Drug Interaction Precaution: Antacids may interact with certain prescription drugs. If you are presently taking a prescription drug, do not take this product without checking with your physician or other health professional.

To aid in establishing proper dosage schedules, the following information is provided:

MAALOX® Max Maximum Strength Antacid/Anti-Gas

	Per 2 Tsp. (10 mL) (Minimum Recommended Dosage)
Acid neutralizing capacity	38.8 mEq

Professional Labeling

Indications: As an antacid for symptomatic relief of hyperacidity associated with the diagnosis of peptic ulcer, gastritis, peptic esophagitis, gastric hyperacidity, heartburn, or hiatal hernia. As an antiflatulent to alleviate the symptoms of gas, including postoperative gas pain.

Warnings: Prolonged use of aluminum-containing antacids in patients with renal failure may result in or worsen dialysis osteomalacia. Elevated tissue aluminum levels contribute to the development of the dialysis encephalopathy and osteomalacia syndromes. Small amounts of aluminum are absorbed from the gastrointestinal tract and renal excretion of aluminum is impaired in renal failure. Aluminum is not well removed by dialysis because it is bound to albumin and transferrin, which do not cross dialysis membranes. As a result, aluminum is deposited in bone, and dialysis osteomalacia may develop when large amounts of aluminum are ingested orally by patients with impaired renal function. Aluminum forms insoluble complexes with phosphate in the gastrointestinal tract, thus decreasing phosphate absorption. Prolonged use of aluminum-containing antacids by normophosphatemic patients may result in hypophosphatemia if phosphate intake is not adequate. In its more severe forms, hypophosphatemia can lead to anorexia, malaise, muscle weakness, and osteomalacia.

Advantages: In addition to the fast acting antacid ingredients, Aluminum Hydroxide and Magnesium Hydroxide, MAALOX® Max Maximum Strength Antacid/Antigas contains the powerful antigas ingredient, simethicone, to provide concurrent fast relief from discomfort associated with entrapped gas.

How Supplied:
MAALOX® MAX MAXIMUM STRENGTH

ANTACID/ANTI-GAS Liquid
Oral Suspension Antacid/Anti-Gas

Lemon is available in plastic bottles of 5 fl. oz. (148 mL), 12 fl. oz. (355 mL), and 26 fl. oz. (769 mL).

Cherry is available in plastic bottles of 12 fl. oz. (355 mL) and 26 fl. oz. (769 mL).

Mint is available in plastic bottles of 12 fl. oz. (355 mL) and 26 fl. oz. (769 mL).

Peaches n' Crème is available in Plastic Bottles of 12 fl. Oz. (355 mL).

Vanilla Crème is available in Plastic Bottles of 12 fl. Oz. (355 mL).

Wild Berry is available in Plastic Bottles of 12 fl. Oz. (355 mL).

Shown in Product Identification Guide, page 514

MAALOX®
Oral Suspension
Antacid/Anti-Gas

Liquids
Cooling Mint
Smooth Cherry
Refreshing Lemon

Description: Maalox® Antacid/Anti-Gas, a balanced combination of magnesium and aluminum hydroxides plus simethicone, is an Antacid/Anti-Gas product to provide relief of acid indigestion, heartburn, sour stomach, upset stomach associated with these symptoms, and relief of pressure and bloating commonly referred to as gas.

Active Ingredients	Maalox Suspension 5 mL teaspoon
Magnesium Hydroxide	200 mg
Aluminum Hydroxide (equivalent to dried gel, USP)	200 mg
Simethicone	20 mg

Inactive Ingredients: Butylparaben, Carboxymethylcellulose Sodium, D&C Yellow #10, (Lemon Flavors only), Flavor, Hydroxypropyl Methylcellulose, Microcrystalline Cellulose, Propylparaben, Purified Water, Saccharin Sodium, Sorbitol.

Maalox Suspension Per 2 Tsp. (10 mL) (Minimum Recommended Dosage)	
Acid neutralizing capacity	19.4 mEq

Continued on next page

Information on Novartis Consumer Health, Inc., products appearing on these pages is effective as of November 2000.

Maalox Antacid Liquid—Cont.

Directions for Use: Two to four teaspoonfuls, four times a day or as directed by a physician.

Patient Warnings: Do not take more than 16 teaspoonfuls in a 24-hour period or use the maximum dosage for more than 2 weeks or use if you have kidney disease except under the advice and supervision of a physician. **Keep this and all drugs out of the reach of children.**

Drug Interaction Precaution: Antacids may interact with certain prescription drugs. If you are presently taking a prescription drug, do not take this product without checking with your physician or other health professional.

Professional Labeling
Indications: As an antacid for symptomatic relief of hyperacidity associated with the diagnosis of peptic ulcer, gastritis, peptic esophagitis, gastric hyperacidity, heartburn, or hiatal hernia. As an antiflatulent to alleviate the symptoms of gas, including postoperative gas pain.

Warnings: Prolonged use of aluminum-containing antacids in patients with renal failure may result in or worsen dialysis osteomalacia. Elevated tissue aluminum levels contribute to the development of the dialysis encephalopathy and osteomalacia syndromes. Small amounts of aluminum are absorbed from the gastrointestinal tract and renal excretion of aluminum is impaired in renal failure. Aluminum is not well removed by dialysis because it is bound to albumin and transferrin, which do not cross dialysis membranes. As a result, aluminum is deposited in bone, and dialysis osteomalacia may develop when large amounts of aluminum are ingested orally by patients with impaired renal function. Aluminum forms insoluble complexes with phosphate in the gastrointestinal tract, thus decreasing phosphate absorption. Prolonged use of aluminum-containing antacids by normophosphatemic patients may result in hypophosphatemia if phosphate intake is not adequate. In its more severe forms, hypophosphatemia can lead to anorexia, malaise, muscle weakness, and osteomalacia.

Advantages: In addition to the fast acting antacid ingredients, Aluminum Hydroxide and Magnesium Hydroxide, MAALOX® Antacid/Antigas contains the powerful antigas ingredient, simethicone, to provide concurrent fast relief from discomfort associated with entrapped gas.

How Supplied:
Maalox® Cooling Mint Suspension is available in plastic bottles of 5 oz. (148 mL), 12 oz. (355 mL) and 26 oz. (769 mL)
Maalox® Smooth Cherry Suspension is available in plastic bottles of 12 oz. (355 mL) and 26 oz. (769 mL)

Maalox® Refreshing Lemon Suspension is available in plastic bottles of 12 oz. (355 mL) and 26 oz. (769 mL)
Shown in Product Identification Guide, page 514

**Quick Dissolve
MAALOX® Regular Strength
Antacid and MAALOX® Max
Maximum Strength Antacid/
Antigas.
Calcium Carbonate (and
Simethicone in Maximum
Strength) Chewable Tablets
Assorted, Lemon, Wildberry and
Wintergreen Flavors. Fast Dissolving
Tablets**

Description: Quick Dissolve Maalox® Antacid Calcium Carbonate Chewable Tablets have a unique form that dissolves quickly to relieve heartburn, acid indigestion, and sour stomach fast.
Maximum Strength Quick Dissolve MAALOX® Max provides the additional benefit of relief of pressure and bloating commonly referred to as gas.

Active Ingredients:
Regular Strength—600 mg Calcium Carbonate
Maximum Strength—1000 mg Calcium Carbonate and 60 mg Simethicone
The acid neutralizing capacity (per two tablets) for Regular Strength is 21.6 mEq; for Maximum Strength is 84 mEq.

Inactive Ingredients: Regular Strength–Aspartame, colloidal silicon dioxide, croscarmellose sodium, dextrose, flavors, magnesium stearate, maltodextrin, mannitol, pregelatinized starch. Depending on the flavor, may also contain FD&C Blue 1 aluminum lake, D&C Red 30 aluminum lake, D&C yellow 10 aluminum lake.
Sodium Content: 1 mg per tablet for Regular Strength; 2 mg per tablet for Maximum Strength.
Maximum Strength—Dextrose, mannitol, croscarmellose sodium, maltodextrin, flavors, magnesium stearate, pregelantinized starch, colloidal silicon dioxide, acesulfame K, depending on the flavor, may also contain FD&C Red no. 40 lake, FD&C Yellow no. 5 lake, FD&C Yellow no. 6 lake.

Directions for Use: Regular Strength—Chew 2 to 4 tablets as symptoms occur or as directed by a physician.
Maximum Strength—Chew 1 to 2 tablets as symptoms occur or as directed by a physician.

Patient Warnings: Do not take more than 12 (8 for Maximum Strength) tablets in a 24-hour period or use the maximum dosage for more than 2 weeks except under the advice and supervision of a physician.
Keep out of reach of children.
Phenylketonurics: Regular Strength contains Phenylalanine .5 mg per tablet.

Maximum Strength does not contain Phenylalanine but does contain FD&C Yellow no. 5 lake (tartrazine) as a color additive.

Drug Interaction Precaution: Ask a doctor before use if you are presently taking a prescription drug. Antacids may interact with certain prescription drugs.

Advantages: Quick Dissolve Maalox® Calcium Carbonate Antacid Tablets have a unique form that dissolves quickly to relieve heartburn fast.
Maximum Strength Quick Dissolve MAALOX® Max also contains simethicone to alleviate discomfort associated with entrapped gas.

How Supplied: Regular Strength Quick Dissolve MAALOX®
Lemon — Plastic Bottles of 45 and 85 Tablets.
Wildberry — Plastic Bottles of 85 Tablets.
Wintergreen — Plastic Bottles of 45 Tablets.
Assorted — Plastic Bottles of 45, 85, and 145 Tablets.
Maximum Strength Quick Dissolve MAALOX® Max
Lemon — Plastic Bottles of 35 and 65 Tablets.
Wildberry — Plastic Bottles of 35 and 65 Tablets.
Assorted — Plastic Bottles of 35, 65, and 90 Tablets.
Shown in Product Identification Guide, page 514

**Overnight Relief
PERDIEM®**
[pĕr "dē 'ŭm]
Natural Bulk Fiber Plus Vegetable Laxative

Use: Provides overnight relief of constipation within 6 to 12 hours.

Description: Overnight Relief Perdiem® is a 100% Natural Fiber *plus* Vegetable Laxative. Perdiem's unique combination of natural laxative ingredients provides gentle, predictable overnight relief of constipation without chemical additives. Perdiem's unique form is easy to swallow and requires no mixing.

Active Ingredients:
(in each 6 gram teaspoonful): Purpose:
Psyllium 3.25 g .... Bulk fiber laxative
Senna 0.74 g .... Stimulant laxative

Warnings: Allery alert: do not use if you have a history of psyllium allergy.
CHOKING: TAKING THIS PRODUCT WITHOUT ADEQUATE FLUID MAY CAUSE IT TO SWELL AND BLOCK YOUR THROAT OR ESOPHAGUS AND MAY CAUSE CHOKING. DO NOT TAKE THIS PRODUCT IF YOU HAVE DIFFICULTY IN SWALLOWING. IF YOU EXPERIENCE CHEST PAIN, VOMITING, OR DIFFICULTY IN SWALLOWING OR

BREATHING AFTER TAKING THIS PRODUCT, SEEK IMMEDIATE MEDICAL ATTENTION.

Do not use:
- if you experience abdominal pain, nausea, or vomiting
- if you have difficulty in swallowing
- if you have esophageal narrowing

Ask a doctor or pharmacist before use if you have noticed a sudden change in bowel habits that persists over a period of 2 weeks

When using this product:
- do not use this product for a period longer than 1 week

Stop use and ask a doctor if:
- rectal bleeding or failure to have a bowel movement occur after use of a laxative. These may be signs of a serious condition.

If pregnant or breast-feeding, ask a health care professional before use.

Keep out of reach of children. In case of overdose, get medical help or contact a Poison Control Center right away.

Directions:
- **TAKE THIS PRODUCT (CHILD OR ADULT DOSE) WITH AT LEAST 8 OUNCES (A FULL GLASS) OF COOL WATER OR OTHER FLUID. TAKING THIS PRODUCT WITHOUT ENOUGH LIQUID MAY CAUSE CHOKING. SEE CHOKING WARNING.**
- Perdiem should not be chewed.
  1. Moisten your mouth with a drink of water or any cool beverage.
  2. Place a teaspoonful of granules on your tongue. If you prefer, take only a partial teaspoonful at a time.
  3. Without chewing, wash granules down with water or any cool beverage.
  4. Repeat last three steps until the recommended dose has been swallowed. Be sure to drink at least 8 ounces of cool liquid.
- Adults and Children 12 years and older: In the evening and/or before breakfast, 1 to 2 rounded teaspoonfuls 1 to 2 times daily should be placed in the mouth and swallowed with at least 8 ounces of cool liquid.
- Children 7 to 11 years: 1 rounded teaspoonful 1 to 2 times daily with at least 8 ounces of cool liquid.

Four easy steps for using Perdiem

1. Moisten your mouth with a drink of water or any cool beverage.

2. Place a teaspoonful of granules on your tongue. If you prefer take only a partial teaspoonful at a time.

3. Without chewing, wash granules down with water or any cool beverage.

4. Repeat steps 1–3 until the recommended dose has

been swallowed. Be sure to drink at least 8 ounces of cool liquid.

Other information:
- Store at controlled room temperature 15°–30°C (59°–86°F).
- Protect from moisture.

Inactive Ingredients: acacia, iron oxides, natural flavors, paraffin, sucrose, talc

How Supplied: Granules: 250-gram (8.8 oz) canisters, 400-gram (14 oz) canisters, and 600-gram (21 oz) canisters.

Shown in Product Identification Guide, page 514

FIBER THERAPY PERDIEM®
[pĕr "dē 'ŭm]
Bulk Fiber Laxative

Use: For relief of occasional constipation (irregularity)-generally in 12–72 hrs.

Description: Fiber Therapy Perdiem® is a 100% Natural Bulk-Forming Fiber that helps maintain regularity and prevent constipation (irregularity) without chemical stimulants. Perdiem's unique form is easy to swallow and requires no mixing.

Active Ingredients
Each rounded (6 gram) teaspoonful contains:
4.03 grams psyllium, 36.1 mg potassium, 1.80 mg sodium. only **4 calories**

Warnings: Allergy alert:
- do not use if you have a history of psyllium allergy.

CHOKING: TAKING THIS PRODUCT WITHOUT ADEQUATE FLUID MAY CAUSE IT TO SWELL AND BLOCK YOUR THROAT OR ESOPHAGUS AND MAY CAUSE CHOKING. DO NOT TAKE THIS PRODUCT IF YOU HAVE DIFFICULTY IN SWALLOWING. IF YOU EXPERIENCE CHEST PAIN, VOMITING, OR DIFFICULTY IN SWALLOWING OR BREATHING AFTER TAKING THIS PRODUCT, SEEK IMMEDIATE MEDICAL ATTENTION.

Do not use:
- if you experience abdominal pain, nausea, or vomiting
- if you have difficulty in swallowing
- if you have esophageal narrowing

Ask a doctor or pharmacist before use if you have noticed a sudden change in bowel habits that persists over a period of 2 weeks

When using this product • do not use this product for a period longer than 1 week

Stop use and ask a doctor if • rectal bleeding or failure to have a bowel movement occur after use of a laxative. These may be signs of a serious condition.

If pregnant or breast-feeding, ask a health care professional before use.

Keep out of reach of children. In case of overdose, get medical help or contact a Poison Control Center right away.

Directions:
- **TAKE THIS PRODUCT (CHILD OR ADULT DOSE) WITH AT LEAST 8 OUNCES (A FULL GLASS) OF COOL WATER OR OTHER FLUID. TAKING THIS PRODUCT WITHOUT ENOUGH LIQUID MAY CAUSE CHOKING. SEE CHOKING WARNING.**
- Perdiem should not be chewed.
  1. Moisten your mouth with a drink of water or any cool beverage.
  2. Place a teaspoonful of granules on your tongue. If you prefer, take only a partial teaspoonful at a time.
  3. Without chewing, wash granules down with water or any cool beverage.
  4. Repeat last three steps until the recommended dose has been swallowed. Be sure to drink at least 8 ounces of cool liquid.
- Adults and Children 12 years and older: In the evening and/or before breakfast, 1 to 2 rounded teaspoonfuls 1 to 2 times daily should be placed in the mouth and swallowed with at least 8 ounces of cool liquid.
- Children 7 to 11 years: 1 rounded teaspoonful 1 to 2 times daily with at least 8 ounces of cool liquid

Four easy steps for using Perdiem

1. Moisten your mouth with a drink of water or any cool beverage.

2. Place a teaspoonful of granules on your tongue. If you prefer, take only a partial teaspoonful at a time.

3. Without chewing, wash granules down with water or any cool beverage.

4. Repeat steps 1–3 until the recommended dose has been swallowed. Be sure to drink at least 8 ounces of cool liquid.

Other information
- Store at controlled room temperature 15°–30°C (59°–86°F).
- Protect from moisture.

Inactive Ingredients: acacia, iron oxides, natural flavors, paraffin, sucrose, talc, titanium dioxide

How Supplied: Granules: 250-gram (8.8 oz) canisters.

Shown in Product Identification Guide, page 514

Continued on next page

Information on Novartis Consumer Health, Inc., products appearing on these pages is effective as of November 2000.

TAVIST® Allergy
Antihistamine Tablets
Nonprescription Drug
Clemastine Fumarate

Active ingredient:
(in each tablet)
Clemastine fumarate, USP 1.34 mg
(equivalent to 1 mg
clemastine) .... Antihistamine

Uses: Temporarily reduces these symptoms of the common cold, hay fever, and other respiratory allergies:
• runny nose
• itchy, watery eyes
• sneezing
• itching of the nose or throat

Warnings:
Ask a doctor before use if you have:
• a breathing problem such as emphysema or chronic bronchitis
• glaucoma
• trouble urinating due to an enlargement of the prostate gland
Ask a doctor or pharmacist before use if you are taking sedatives or tranquilizers
When using this product
• avoid alcoholic drinks
• drowsiness may occur
• alcohol, sedatives, and tranquilizers may increase drowsiness
• be careful when driving a motor vehicle or operating machinery
• excitability may occur, especially in children
If pregnant or breast-feeding, ask a health professional before use.
Keep out of reach of children. In case of overdose, get medical help or contact a poison control center right away.

Directions:
• adults and children 12 years of age and older: take 1 tablet every 12 hours, not more than 2 tablets in 24 hours unless directed by a doctor
• children under 12 years of age: consult a doctor

Other information:
• sodium free
• store at controlled room temperature 20–25°C (68–77°F)

Inactive Ingredients lactose, povidone, starch, stearic acid, talc.

How Supplied: Packets of 8 and 16 Tablets
Novartis Consumer Health, Inc.
Summit, NJ 07901-1312
Shown in Product Identification Guide, page 514

TAVIST•D® TABLETS and CAPLETS

Information on replacement products that do not contain Phenylpropanolamine as part of the formulation will be forthcoming in 2001.

TAVIST® SINUS
Non-Drowsy Coated Caplets
Pain Reliever/Nasal Decongestant

Drug Facts:

Active ingredients:
(in each caplet): **Purpose:**
Acetaminophen
500 mg .... Pain reliever

Pseudoephedrine HCl
30 mg .... Nasal decongestant

Uses: Temporarily relieves:
• nasal and sinus congestion and pressure
• sinus pain
• minor aches and pains associated with the common cold
• headache

Warnings
Alcohol Warning if you consume 3 or more alcoholic drinks every day, ask your doctor whether you should take acetaminophen or other pain relievers/fever reducers. Acetaminophen may cause liver damage.
Do not use if you are now taking
• a prescription monoamine oxidase inhibitor (MAOI) (certain drugs for depression, psychiatric or emotional conditions, or Parkinson's disease), or for 2 weeks after stopping the MAOI drug. If you do not know if your prescription drug contains an MAOI, ask a doctor or pharmacist before taking this product.
• together with another product containing acetaminophen.
Ask a doctor before use if you have:
• heart disease
• high blood pressure
• thyroid disease
• diabetes
• difficulty urinating due to an enlarged prostate gland
When using this product
• do not use more than directed
Stop use and ask a doctor if:
• nervousness, dizziness, or sleeplessness occurs
• symptoms do not improve for 7 days or occur with a fever
• symptoms do not improve for 10 days (pain) or for 3 days (fever). These could be signs of a serious condition.
If pregnant or breast-feeding, ask a health professional before use.
Keep out of reach of children. In case of overdose, get medical help or contact a poison control center right away. Prompt medical attention is critical for adults as well as for children even if you do not notice any signs or symptoms.

Directions:
• adults and children 12 years of age and over: take 2 caplets every 6 hours, not to exceed 8 caplets in 24 hours or as directed by a doctor
• children under 12 years of age: consult a doctor

Other information:
• each caplet contains: sodium 3 mg
• store at controlled room temperature 20–25°C (68–77°F)

Inactive Ingredients colloidal silicon dioxide, croscarmellose sodium, hydroxypropyl cellulose, hydroxypropyl methylcellulose, lactose monohydrate, magnesium stearate, methylparaben, polydextrose powder, polyethylene glycol, pregelatinized starch, purified water, titanium dioxide, triacetin.

Question? call 1-800-452-0051 24 hours a day, 7 days a week.

How Supplied: Packets of 24 Coated and 48 Caplets.
Novartis Consumer Health, Inc.
Summit, NJ 07901-1312 ©2001
Shown in Product Identification Guide, page 514

THERAFLU® REGULAR STRENGTH
Cold & Sore Throat Night Time Medicine
Cold & Cough Night Time Medicine

Description: Each packet of TheraFlu Regular Strength **Cold & Sore Throat Night Time Medicine** contains: acetaminophen 650 mg, pseudoephedrine hydrochloride 60 mg, and chlorpheniramine maleate 4 mg. Each packet of TheraFlu Regular Strength **Cold & Cough Night Time Medicine** also contains dextromethorphan hydrobromide 20 mg.

Inactive ingredients: ascorbic acid, citric acid, D&C Yellow 10, natural lemon flavors, pregelatinized starch, silicon dioxide, sodium citrate, sucrose, titanium dioxide and tribasic calcium phosphate.

Each packet contains: sodium 25 mg

Indications: Temporarily relieves these symptoms: headache, minor aches and pains, fever, minor sore throat pain, nasal and sinus congestion, runny nose, itchy nose or throat, itchy, watery eyes and sneezing. TheraFlu Regular Strength **Cold & Cough Night Time Medicine** also suppresses coughs due to minor throat and bronchial irritation.

Warnings: Keep this and all drugs out of the reach of children. In case of accidental overdose, seek professional assistance or contact a poison control center immediately. Prompt medical attention is critical for adults as well as children even if you do not notice any signs or symptoms.
Do not exceed recommended dosage. If nervousness, dizziness, or sleeplessness occur, discontinue use and consult a doctor. If symptoms do not improve within 7 days or are accompanied by fever, consult a doctor. May cause excitability especially in children. Do not take this product if you have heart disease, high blood pressure, thyroid disease, diabetes, glaucoma, a breathing problem such as emphysema or chronic bronchitis, or difficulty in urination due to enlargement of the prostate gland, unless directed by a doctor.
Do not take this product for pain for more than 10 days or for fever for more than 3 days unless directed by a doctor. If pain or fever persists or gets worse, if new symptoms occur, or if redness or swelling is present, consult a doctor because these could be signs of a serious condition. If sore throat is severe, persists for more than 2 days, is accompanied or followed by fever, headache, rash, nausea, or vomiting, consult a doctor promptly.

May cause marked drowsiness; alcohol, sedatives, and tranquilizers may increase the drowsiness effect. Avoid alcoholic beverages while taking this product. Do not take this product if you are taking sedatives or tranquilizers, without first consulting your doctor. Use caution when driving a motor vehicle or operating machinery.

A persistent cough may be a sign of a serious condition. If cough persists for more than 1 week, tends to recur, or is accompanied by a fever, rash, or persistent headache, consult a doctor. Do not take this product for persistent or chronic cough such as occurs with smoking, asthma, or emphysema, or if cough is accompanied by excessive phlegm (mucus) unless directed by a doctor.

As with any drug, if you are pregnant or nursing a baby, seek the advice of a health professional before using this product.

Alcohol Warning: If you consume 3 or more alcoholic drinks every day, ask your doctor whether you should use acetaminophen or other pain relievers/fever reducers. Acetaminophen may cause liver damage.

Drug Interaction Precaution: Do not use this product if you are now taking a prescription monoamine oxidase inhibitor [MAOI] (certain drugs for depression, psychiatric or emotional conditions, or Parkinson's disease), or for 2 weeks after stopping the MAOI drug. If you are uncertain whether your prescription drug contains an MAOI, consult a health professional before taking this product.

Directions: Adults and children 12 years of age and over: dissolve contents of one packet in 6 oz. hot water; sip while hot. One packet every 4 to 6 hours; not to exceed 4 packets in 24 hours, or as directed by a doctor. Children under 12 years of age: consult a doctor. **Microwave heating instructions:** Add contents of packet and 6 oz. of cool water to a microwave-safe cup and stir briskly. Microwave on high 1¹/₂ minutes or until hot. Do not boil water or overheat, and remember to stir liquid between reheatings. Sweeten to taste if desired.

How Supplied: TheraFlu Regular Strength **Cold & Sore Throat Night Time Medicine** powder in foil packets, 6 packets per carton. TheraFlu Regular Strength **Cold & Cough Night Time Medicine** powder in foil packets, 6 or 12 packets per carton.

Shown in Product Identification Guide, page 515

THERAFLU® MAXIMUM STRENGTH
Flu & Sore Throat Night Time Hot Liquid Medicine

Each packet of Theraflu Maximum Strength **Flu & Sore Throat Night Time Hot Liquid Medicine** contains: aceta-minophen 1000 mg, pseudoephedrine HCl 60 mg, chlorpheniramine maleate 4 mg.

Inactive Ingredients: Acesulfame K, ascorbic acid, aspartame, citric acid, D&C Yellow 10, FD&C Blue 1, FD&C Red 40, maltodextrin, natural apple and cinnamon flavors, silicon dioxide, sodium citrate, sucrose and tribasic calcium phosphate.

Each packet contains: sodium 30 mg Phenylketonurics: contains phenylalanine 25 mg per adult dose

Indications: Temporarily relieves these symptoms: headache, minor aches and pains, itchy nose and throat, itchy watery eyes, fever, minor sore throat pain, nasal and sinus congestion, runny nose and sneezing.

Warnings: Keep this and all drugs out of the reach of children. In case of accidental overdose, seek professional assistance or contact a poison control center immediately. Prompt medical attention is critical for adults as well as children even if you do not notice any signs or symptoms.

Do not exceed recommended dosage. If nervousness, dizziness, or sleeplessness occur, discontinue use and consult a doctor. If symptoms do not improve within 7 days or are accompanied by fever, consult a doctor. May cause excitability, especially in children. Do not take this product if you have heart disease, high blood pressure, thyroid disease, diabetes, glaucoma, a breathing problem such as emphysema or chronic bronchitis, or difficulty in urination due to enlargement of the prostate gland, unless directed by a doctor.

Do not take this product for pain for more than 10 days or for fever for more than 3 days unless directed by a doctor. If pain or fever persists or gets worse, if new symptoms occur, or if redness or swelling is present, consult a doctor because these could be signs of a serious condition. If sore throat is severe, persists for more than 2 days, is accompanied or followed by fever, headache, rash, nausea, or vomiting, consult a doctor promptly.

May cause drowsiness; alcohol, sedatives and tranquilizers may increase the drowsiness effect. Avoid alcoholic beverages while taking this product. Do not take this product if you are taking sedatives or tranquilizers without first consulting your doctor. Use caution when driving a motor vehicle or operating machinery.

As with any drug, if you are pregnant or nursing a baby, seek the advice of a health professional before using this product.

Alcohol Warning: If you consume 3 or more alcoholic drinks every day ask your doctor whether you should take acetaminophen or other pain relievers/fever reducers. Acetaminophen may cause liver damage.

Drug Interaction Precaution: Do not use this product if you are now taking a prescription monoamine oxidase inhibitor [MAOI] (certain drugs for depression, psychiatric or emotional conditions, or Parkinson's Disease), or for 2 weeks after stopping the MAOI drug. If you are uncertain whether your prescription drug contains an MAOI, consult a health professional before taking this product.

Directions: Adults and children 12 years of age and over: dissolve one packet in 6 oz. of hot water; sip while hot. One packet every 6 hours, not to exceed 4 packets in 24 hours, or as directed by a doctor. Children under 12 years of age: consult a doctor. **Microwave Heating Instructions:** Add contents of packet and 6 oz. of cool water to a microwave-safe cup and stir briskly. Microwave on high 1 ¹/₂ minutes or until hot. Do not boil water or overheat, and remember to stir liquid between reheatings. Sweeten to taste if desired.

How Supplied: Theraflu Maximum Strength **Flu & Sore Throat Night Time Hot Liquid Medicine** powder in foil packets, 6 packets per carton.

Shown in Product Identification Guide, page 515

THERAFLU® MAXIMUM STRENGTH
Flu & Congestion Non-Drowsy Hot Liquid Medicine

Description: Each packet of TheraFlu Maximum Strength **Flu & Congestion Non-Drowsy Hot Liquid Medicine** contains: acetaminophen 1000 mg, guaifenesin 400 mg, pseudoephedrine HCl 60 mg, dextromethorphan HBr 30 mg.

Inactive Ingredients: acesulfame K, aspartame, D&C yellow 10, maltodextrin, flavors, silicon dioxide, sucrose.

Each packet contains: sodium 1 mg Phenylketonurics: contains phenylalanine 25 mg per adult dose

Indications: Temporarily relieves these symptoms: headache, minor aches and pains, chest congestion, fever, minor sore throat pain, nasal and sinus congestion. TheraFlu Maximum Strength **Flu & Congestion Non-Drowsy Hot Liquid Medicine** also suppresses coughs due to minor throat and bronchial irritation.

Warnings: Keep this and all drugs out of the reach of children. In case of overdose, get medical help or contact a Poison Control Center immediately. Prompt medical attention is critical for adults as well as for children even if you do not notice any signs or symptoms. As

Continued on next page

Information on Novartis Consumer Health, Inc., products appearing on these pages is effective as of November 2000.

Theraflu Flu/Cong.—Cont.

with any drug, if you are pregnant or nursing a baby, seek the advice of a health professional before using this product.

Do not exceed recommended dosage. If nervousness, dizziness, or sleeplessness occur, discontinue use and consult a doctor. Do not take this product if you have heart disease, high blood pressure, thyroid disease, diabetes, or difficulty in urination due to enlargement of the prostate gland.

If symptoms do not improve within 7 days or are accompanied by fever, consult a doctor. Do not take this product for pain for more than 10 days. A persistent cough may be a sign of a serious condition. If cough persists for more than 7 days, tends to recur, or is accompanied by fever, rash or persistent headache, fever that lasts for more than 3 days, or if new symptoms occur consult a doctor. Do not take this product: 1) cough is accompanied by excessive phlegm (mucus), 2) for persistent or chronic cough such as occurs with smoking, asthma, emphysema or chronic bronchitis, 3) if sore throat persists for more than 2 days, is accompanied or followed by fever, headache, rash, nausea, or vomiting, unless directed by a doctor.

Alcohol Warning: If you consume 3 or more alcoholic drinks every day, ask your doctor whether you should take acetaminophen or other pain relievers/fever reducers. Acetaminophen may cause liver damage.

Drug Interaction Precaution: Do not use this product if you are now taking a prescription monoamine oxidase inhibitor (MAOI) (certain drugs for depression, psychiatric or emotional conditions, or Parkinson's disease), or for 2 weeks after stopping the MAOI drug. If you are uncertain whether your prescription drug contains an MAOI, consult a health professional before taking this product.

Directions: Adults and children 12 years of age and over: dissolve contents of one packet in 6 oz. hot water; sip while hot. One packet every 6 hours, not to exceed 4 packets in 24 hours, or as directed by a doctor. Children under 12 years of age: consult a doctor.

Microwave heating instructions: Add contents of one packet and 6 oz. of cool water to a microwave-safe cup and stir briskly. Microwave on high 1 1/2 minutes or until hot. Do not boil water or overheat, and remember to stir liquid between reheatings.

Sweeten to taste if desired.

How Supplied: TheraFlu Maximum Strength **Flu & Congestion Non-Drowsy Hot Liquid Medicine** is available in 6 foil packets per carton.

Shown in Product Identification Guide, page 515

THERAFLU® MAXIMUM STRENGTH
Flu & Cough Night Time Hot Liquid Medicine

Active Ingredients: Each packet of TheraFlu Maximum Strength **Flu & Cough Night Time Hot Liquid Medicine** contains: acetaminophen 1,000 mg, pseudoephedrine HCl 60 mg, dextromethrophan HBr 30 mg, chlorpheniramine maleate 4 mg.

Inactive Ingredients: acesulfame K, ascorbic acid, aspartame, cherry flavor, citric acid, FD&C Blue 1, FD&C Red 40, maltodextrin, silicon dioxide, sodium citrate, sucrose, tribasic calcium phosphate.

Each packet contains: sodium 26 mg
Phenylketonurics: contains phenylalanine 26 mg per adult dose

Indications: Temporarily relieves these symptoms: headache, minor aches and pains, itchy nose and throat, itchy, watery eyes, fever, minor sore throat pain, nasal and sinus congestion, runny nose and sneezing. TheraFlu Maximum Strength **Flu & Cough Night Time Hot Liquid Medicine** also suppresses coughs due to minor throat and bronchial irritation.

Warnings: Keep this and all drugs out of the reach of children. In case of accidental overdose, seek professional assistance or contact a Poison Control Center immediately. Prompt medical attention is critical for adults as well as for children even if you do not notice any signs or symptoms.

Do not exceed recommended dosage. If nervousness, dizziness, or sleeplessness occur, discontinue use and consult a doctor. If symptoms do not improve within 7 days or are accompanied by fever, consult a doctor. May cause excitability, especially in children. Do not take this product if you have heart disease, high blood pressure, thyroid disease, diabetes, glaucoma, a breathing problem such as emphysema or chronic bronchitis, or difficulty in urination due to enlargement of the prostate gland, unless directed by a doctor.

A persistent cough may be a sign of a serious condition. If cough persists for more than 1 week, tends to recur, or is accompanied by fever, rash, or persistent headache, consult a doctor. Do not take this product for persistent or chronic cough such as occurs with smoking, asthma, emphysema, or if cough is accompanied by excessive phlegm (mucus) unless directed by a doctor.

Do not take this product for pain for more than 10 days or for fever for more than 3 days unless directed by a doctor. If pain or fever persists or gets worse, if new symptoms occur, or if redness or swelling is present, consult a doctor because these could be signs of a serious condition. If sore throat is severe, persists for more than 2 days, is accompa-

nied or followed by fever, headache, rash, nausea, or vomiting, consult a doctor promptly.

May cause marked drowsiness; alcohol, sedatives, and tranquilizers may increase the drowsiness effect. Avoid alcoholic beverages while taking this product. Do not take this product if you are taking sedatives or tranquilizers, without first consulting your doctor. Use caution when driving a motor vehicle or operating machinery.

As with any drug, if you are pregnant or nursing a baby, seek the advice of a health professional before using this product.

Alcohol Warning: If you consume 3 or more alcoholic drinks every day, ask your doctor whether you should take acetaminophen or other pain relievers/fever reducers. Acetaminophen may cause liver damage.

Drug interaction Precaution: Do not use this product if you are now taking a prescription monoamine oxide inhibitor [MAOI] (certain drugs for depression, psychiatric or emotional conditions, or Parkinson's disease), or for 2 weeks after stopping the MAOI drug. If you are uncertain whether your prescription drug contains an MAOI, consult a health professional before taking this product.

Directions: Adults and children 12 years of age and over: dissolve contents of one packet in 6 oz. hot water; sip while hot. One packet every 6 hours, not to exceed 4 packets in 24 hours, or as directed by a doctor. Children under 12 years of age: consult a doctor.

Microwave heating instructions: Add contents of one packet and 6 oz. of cool water to a microwave-safe cup and stir briskly. Microwave on high 1½ minutes or until hot. Do not boil water or overheat, and remember to stir liquid between reheatings.

Sweeten to taste if desired.

How Supplied: TheraFlu Maximum Strength **Flu & Cough Night Time Hot Liquid Medicine** is available in 6 foil packets per carton.

Shown in Product Identification Guide, page 515

THERAFLU® MAXIMUM STRENGTH
Severe Cold & Congestion Night Time Hot Liquid Medicine and Caplets

Description: Each packet of TheraFlu Maximum Strength **Severe Cold & Congestion Night Time Hot Liquid Medicine** contains: acetaminophen 1000 mg, dextromethorphan HBr 30 mg, pseudoephedrine HCl 60 mg, and chlorpheniramine maleate 4 mg.

Inactive Ingredients: ascorbic acid, citric acid, D&C Yellow 10, maltol, natural lemon flavors, pregelatinized starch, silicon dioxide, sodium citrate, sucrose,

titanium dioxide and tribasic calcium phosphate.

Each packet contains: Sodium 25 mg

TheraFlu **Maximum Strength Severe Cold & Congestion Night Time Caplets:** each caplet contains acetaminophen 500 mg, pseudoephedrine HCl 30 mg, dextromethorphan HBr 15 mg, and chlorpheniramine maleate 2 mg.

Inactive Ingredients: colloidal silicon dioxide, croscarmellose sodium, D&C Yellow 10, FD&C Blue 1, FD&C Yellow 6, gelatin, hydroxypropyl cellulose, hydroxypropyl methylcellulose, lactose, magnesium stearate, methylparaben, polydextrose, polyethylene glycol, pregelatinized starch, titanium dioxide and triacetin.

Sodium content: 6 mg per caplet.

Indications: TheraFlu Hot Liquid and Caplets provide temporary relief of these symptoms: headache, minor aches and pains, itchy nose and throat, itchy watery eyes, fever, minor sore throat pain, nasal and sinus congestion, runny nose, sneezing, and coughs due to minor throat and bronchial irritation.

Warnings: Keep this and all drugs out of the reach of children. In case of accidental overdose, seek professional assistance or contact a poison control center immediately. Prompt medical attention is critical for adults as well as children even if you do not notice any signs or symptoms.
Do not exceed recommended dosage. If nervousness, dizziness, or sleeplessness occur, discontinue use and consult a doctor. If symptoms do not improve within 7 days or are accompanied by fever, consult a doctor. May cause excitability, especially in children. Do not take this product if you have heart disease, high blood pressure, thyroid disease, diabetes, glaucoma, a breathing problem such as emphysema or chronic bronchitis, or difficulty in urination due to enlargement of the prostate gland, unless directed by a doctor. A persistent cough may be a sign of a serious condition. If cough persists for more than 1 week, tends to recur, or is accompanied by a fever, rash, or persistent headache, consult a doctor. Do not take this product for persistent or chronic cough such as occurs with smoking, asthma, or emphysema, or if cough is accompanied by excessive phlegm (mucus) unless directed by a doctor.
Do not take this product for pain for more than 10 days or for fever for more than 3 days unless directed by a doctor. If pain or fever persists or gets worse, if new symptoms occur, or if redness or swelling is present, consult a doctor because these could be signs of a serious condition. If sore throat is severe, persists for more than 2 days, is accompanied or followed by fever, headache, rash, nausea, or vomiting, consult a doctor promptly.
May cause marked drowsiness; alcohol, sedatives, and tranquilizers may in-

crease the drowsiness effect. Avoid alcoholic beverages while taking this product. Do not take this product if you are taking sedatives or tranquilizers, without first consulting your doctor. Use caution when driving a motor vehicle or operating machinery.
As with any drug, if you are pregnant or nursing a baby, seek the advice of a health professional before using this product.

Alcohol Warning: If you consume 3 or more alcoholic drinks every day ask your doctor whether you should take acetaminophen or other pain relievers/fever reducers. Acetaminophen may cause liver damage.

Drug Interaction Precaution: Do not use this product if you are now taking a prescription monoamine oxidase inhibitor [MAOI] (certain drugs for depression, psychiatric or emotional conditions, or Parkinson's disease), or for 2 weeks after stopping the MAOI drug. If you are uncertain whether your prescription drug contains an MAOI, consult a health professional before taking this product.

Directions: TheraFlu® Maximum Strength Severe Cold & Congestion Night Time Hot Liquid Medicine: Adults and children 12 years of age and over: dissolve contents of one packet in 6 oz. cup of hot water; sip while hot. Take every 6 hours, not to exceed 4 packets in 24 hours, or as directed by a doctor. Children under 12 years of age: consult a doctor. **Microwave Heating Instructions:** Add contents of one packet and 6 oz. of cool water to a microwave-safe cup and stir briskly. Microwave on high $1^{1}/_{2}$ minutes or until hot. Do not boil water or overheat, and remember to stir liquid between reheatings. Sweeten to taste if desired.

TheraFlu Maximum Strength Severe Cold & Congestion Night Time Caplets: Adults and children 12 years of age and over: two caplets every 6 hours, not to exceed 8 caplets in 24 hours or as directed by a doctor. Children under 12 years of age: consult a doctor.

How Supplied: TheraFlu Maximum Strength **Severe Cold & Congestion Night Time Hot Liquid Medicine** powder in foil packets, 6, or 12, packets per carton. TheraFlu Maximum Strength **Severe Cold & Congestion Night Time** Caplets in blister packs of 12's and 24's.

Shown in Product Identification Guide, page 515

THERAFLU® MAXIMUM STRENGTH
Severe Cold & Congestion Non-Drowsy Hot Liquid Medicine and Caplets

Description: Each packet of TheraFlu Maximum Strength **Severe Cold & Congestion Non-Drowsy Hot Liquid Medicine** contains: acetaminophen 1000

mg, pseudoephedrine HCl 60 mg, dextromethorphan HBr 30 mg. **Inactive Ingredients:** Ascorbic acid, citric acid, D&C Yellow 10, maltol, natural lemon flavors, pregelatinized starch, silicon dioxide, sodium citrate, sucrose, titanium dioxide and tribasic calcium phosphate.

Each packet contains: sodium 25 mg

Each TheraFlu Maximum Strength **Severe Cold & Congestion Non-Drowsy Caplet** contains: Acetaminophen 500 mg, pseudoephedrine HCl 30 mg, dextromethorphan HBr 15 mg.

Inactive ingredients: colloidal silicon dioxide, croscarmellose sodium, D&C Yellow 10, FD&C Red 40, FD&C Yellow 6, gelatin, hydroxypropyl cellulose, hydroxypropyl methylcellulose, lactose, magnesium stearate, methylparaben, polydextrose, polyethylene glycol, pregelatinized starch, titanium dioxide and triacetin.

Sodium content: 6 mg per caplet.

Indications: Temporarily relieves these symptoms: headache, minor aches and pains, fever, minor sore throat pain, nasal and sinus congestion. TheraFlu Maximum Strength **Severe Cold & Congestion Non-Drowsy Medicine** also suppresses cough due to minor throat and bronchial irritation.

Warnings: Keep this and all drugs out of the reach of children. In case of accidental overdose, seek professional assistance or contact a poison control center immediately. Prompt medical attention is critical for adults as well as children even if you do not notice any signs or symptoms.
Do not exceed recommended dosage. If nervousness, dizziness, or sleeplessness occur, discontinue use and consult a doctor. If symptoms do not improve within 7 days or are accompanied by fever, consult a doctor. Do not take this product if you have heart disease, high blood pressure, thyroid disease, diabetes, or difficulty in urination due to enlargement of the prostate gland unless directed by a physician.
A persistent cough may be a sign of a serious condition. If cough persists for more than 1 week, tends to recur, or is accompanied by a fever, rash, or persistent headache, consult a doctor. Do not take this product for persistent or chronic cough such as occurs with smoking, asthma, or emphysema, or if cough is accompanied by excessive phlegm (mucus) unless directed by a doctor.
Do not take this product for pain for more than 10 days or for fever for more than 3 days unless directed by a doctor. If pain or fever persists or gets worse, if

Continued on next page

Information on Novartis Consumer Health, Inc., products appearing on these pages is effective as of November 2000.

Theraflu Cold/Cong.—Cont.

new symptoms occur, or if redness or swelling is present, consult a doctor, because these could be signs of a serious condition. If sore throat is severe, persists for more than 2 days, is accompanied or followed by fever, headache, rash, nausea, or vomiting, consult a doctor promptly.

As with any drug, if you are pregnant or nursing a baby, seek the advice of a health professional before using this product.

Alcohol Warning: If you consume 3 or more alcoholic drinks every day ask your doctor whether you should take acetaminophen or other pain relievers/fever reducers. Acetaminophen may cause liver damage.

Drug Interaction Precaution: Do not take this product if you are now taking a prescription monoamine oxidase inhibitor [MAOI] (certain drugs for depression, psychiatric or emotional conditions, or Parkinson's disease), or for 2 weeks after stopping the MAOI drug. If you are uncertain whether your prescription drug contains an MAOI, consult a health professional before taking this product.

Directions: TheraFlu® Maximum Strength Severe Cold & Congestion Non-Drowsy Hot Liquid Medicine: Adults and children 12 years of age and over: dissolve one packet in 6 oz. cup of hot water; sip while hot. Take every 6 hours, not to exceed 4 packets in 24 hours, or as directed by a doctor. Children under 12 years of age: consult a doctor. Microwave Heating Instructions: Add contents of one packet and 6 oz. of cool water to a microwave-safe cup and stir briskly. Microwave on high 1 1/2 minutes or until hot. Do not boil or overheat, and remember to stir liquid between reheatings. Sweeten to taste if desired.

TheraFlu Maximum Strength Severe Cold & Congestion Non-Drowsy Caplet: Adults and Children 12 years of age and over: two caplets every 6 hours, not to exceed eight caplets in 24 hours or as directed by a doctor. Children under 12 years of age: Consult a doctor.

How Supplied: TheraFlu Maximum Strength **Severe Cold & Congestion Non-Drowsy Hot Liquid Medicine** powder in foil packets, 6 packets per carton. TheraFlu Maximum Strength **Severe Cold & Congestion Non-Drowsy gelatin coated caplets** in blister packs of 12 and 24.

Shown in Product Identification Guide, page 515

TRIAMINIC® Allergy Congestion
Nasal Decongestant-Orange Flavor

Drug Facts

Active ingredient
(in each 5 mL, 1 teaspoon)

Pseudoephedrine HCl, USP,
15 mg .... Nasal decongestant

Uses temporarily relieves these symptoms:
• hay fever or other upper respiratory allergies • nasal and sinus congestion

Warnings
Do not use in a child who is taking a prescription monoamine oxidase inhibitor (MAOI) (certain drugs for depression, psychiatric or emotional conditions, or Parkinson's disease), or for 2 weeks after stopping the MAOI drug. If you do not know if the child's prescription drug contains an MAOI, ask a doctor or pharmacist before giving this product.

Ask a doctor before use if the child has
• heart disease • high blood pressure
• thyroid disease • diabetes

When using this product
• do not use more than directed

Stop use and ask a doctor if
• nervousness, dizziness, or sleeplessness occurs • symptoms do not improve within 7 days or occur with a fever. These could be signs of a serious condition.

Keep out of reach of children. In case of overdose, get medical help or contact a poison control center right away.

Dosage and Administration • take every 4 to 6 hours; not more than 4 doses in 24 hours or as directed by a doctor

Age	Weight	Dose
4 months to under 1 year[1]	12 to 17 lb	¼ tsp (1.25 mL)
1 to under 2 years[1]	18 to 23 lb	½ tsp (2.5 mL)
2 to under 6 years	24 to 47 lb	1 tsp (5 mL)
6 to under 12 years	48 to 95 lb	2 tsp (10 mL)
12 years to adult	96+ lb	4 tsp (20 mL)

[1]The dosage for children under 2 years should be determined by the physician on the basis of the patient's weight, physical condition or other appropriate considerations. Dosages are provided as guidelines.

Other Information
• each teaspoon contains: **sodium 1 mg**
• contains no aspirin • store at controlled room temperature 20–25°C (68–77°F).

Inactive Ingredients benzoic acid, edetate disodium, flavors, purified water, sodium hydroxide, sorbitol, sucrose

How Supplied Bottle of 4 fl. oz. (118 mL)

Questions: call **1-800-452-0051**
**For more information about Triaminic®
visit our website at www.triaminic.com**
NOVARTIS
Novartis Consumer Health, Inc.

Summit, NJ 07901-1312 ©2001
Shown in Product Identification Guide, page 515

TRIAMINIC® Chest Congestion
Expectorant, Nasal Decongestant
Citrus Flavor

Drug Facts
Active ingredients
(in each 5 mL, 1 teaspoon)
Guaifenesin,
USP, 50 mg .... Expectorant
Pseudoephedrine HCl,
USP, 15 mg .... Nasal decongestant

Uses temporarily relieves these symptoms:
• chest congestion by loosening phlegm (mucus) to help clear bronchial passageways • nasal and sinus congestion

Warnings
Do not use in a child who is taking a prescription monoamine oxidase inhibitor (MAOI) (certain drugs for depression, psychiatric or emotional conditions, or Parkinson's disease), or for 2 weeks after stopping the MAOI drug. If you do not know if the child's prescription drug contains an MAOI, ask a doctor or pharmacist before giving this product.

Ask a doctor before use if the child has
• heart disease • high blood pressure
• thyroid disease • diabetes • glaucoma
• cough that occurs with too much phlegm (mucus) • chronic cough that lasts or a breathing problem such as asthma or chronic bronchitis

Ask a doctor or pharmacist before use if the child is taking sedatives or tranquilizers.

When using this product
• do not use more than directed

Stop use and ask a doctor if
• nervousness, dizziness, or sleeplessness occur • symptoms do not improve within 7 days or occur with a fever
• cough persists for more than 7 days, comes back, or occurs with a fever, rash, or persistent headache. These could be signs of a serious condition.

Keep out of reach of children. In case of overdose, get medical help or contact a poison control center right away.

Dosage and Administration
take every 4 to 6 hours; not more than 4 doses in 24 hours or as directed by a doctor

Age	Weight	Dose
4 months to under 1 year[1]	12 to 17 lb	¼ tsp (1.25 mL)
1 to under 2 years[1]	18 to 23 lb	½ tsp (2.5 mL)
2 to under 6 years	24 to 47 lb	1 tsp (5 mL)
6 to under 12 years	48 to 95 lb	2 tsp (10 mL)
12 years to adult	96+ lb	4 tsp (20 mL)

[1] The dosage for children under 2 years should be determined by the physician on the basis of the patient's weight, physical condition or other appropriate considerations. Dosages are provided as guidelines.

Other Information
- each teaspoon contains: **sodium 2 mg**
- contains no aspirin • store at controlled room temperature 20–25°C (68–77°F)

Inactive Ingredients benzoic acid, D&C Yellow 10, edetate disodium, FD&C Yellow 6, flavors, glycerin, hydrochloric acid, polyethylene glycol, propylene glycol, purified water, sorbitol, sucrose

How Supplied: Bottles of 4 fl. oz. (118 mL) and 8 fl. oz. (236 mL)
Questions: call **1-800-452-0051**
For more information about Triaminic® visit our website at www.triaminic.com
NOVARTIS
Novartis Consumer Health, Inc.
Summit, NJ 07901-1312 ©2001
Shown in Product Identification Guide, page 515

TRIAMINIC® Cold & Allergy
Nasal Decongestant, Antihistamine
Orange Flavor
TRIAMINIC® Cold & Cough
Nasal Decongestant, Cough Suppressant
Antihistamine-Cherry Flavor
TRIAMINIC® Cold, Cough & Fever
Fever Reducer-Pain Reliever,
Nasal Decongestant, Cough Suppressant
Antihistamine-Bubble Gum Flavor
TRIAMINIC® Cold & Night Time Cough
Nasal Decongestant, Cough Suppressant
Antihistamine-Grape Flavor

Drug Facts
Active ingredients
(in each 5 mL, 1 teaspoon)
TRIAMINIC® Cold & Allergy
Orange Flavor
Pseudoephedrine HCl,
USP, 15 mg .... Nasal decongestant
Chlorpheniramine maleate,
USP, 1 mg .... Antihistamine
TRIAMINIC® Cold & Cough
Cherry Flavor
Pseudoephedrine HCl,
USP, 15 mg .... Nasal decongestant
Dextromethorphan HBr,
USP, 5 mg .... Cough suppressant
Chlorpheniramine maleate,
USP, 1 mg .... Antihistamine
TRIAMINIC® Cold, Cough & Fever
Bubble Gum Flavor
Acetaminophen,
USP, 160 mg ..... Fever reducer, Pain reliever
Pseudoephedrine HCl,
USP, 15 mg .... Nasal decongestant
Dextromethorphan HBr,
USP, 7.5 mg .... Cough suppressant

Chlorpheniramine maleate,
USP, 1 mg .... Antihistamine
TRIAMINIC® Cold & Night Time Cough
Grape Flavor
Pseudoephedrine HCl,
USP, 15 mg .... Nasal decongestant
Dextromethorphan HBr,
USP, 7.5 mg .... Cough suppressant
Chlorpheniramine maleate,
USP, 1 mg .... Antihistamine

Uses temporarily relieves these symptoms:
TRIAMINIC® Cold & Allergy
Nasal Decongestant, Antihistamine
Orange Flavor
- itchy, watery eyes • runny nose • itchy nose or throat • sneezing • nasal and sinus congestion
TRIAMINIC® Cold & Cough
Nasal Decongestant, Cough Suppressant
Antihistamine-Cherry Flavor
- cough due to minor throat and bronchial irritation • runny nose • nasal and sinus congestion • sneezing • itchy nose or throat • itchy, watery eyes
TRIAMINIC® Cold, Cough & Fever
Fever Reducer-Pain Reliever,
Nasal Decongestant, Cough Suppressant
Antihistamine-Bubble Gum Flavor
- fever • minor aches and pains • headache and sore throat • cough due to minor throat and bronchial irritation • nasal and sinus congestion • sneezing • itchy nose or throat • itchy, watery eyes
TRIAMINIC® Cold & Night Time Cough
Nasal Decongestant, Cough Suppressant
Antihistamine-Grape Flavor
- cough due to minor throat and bronchial irritation • runny nose • nasal and sinus congestion • sneezing • itchy nose or throat • itchy, watery eyes

Warnings
Do not use in a child who is taking a prescription monoamine oxidase inhibitor (MAOI) (certain drugs for depression, psychiatric or emotional conditions, or Parkinson's disease), or for 2 weeks after stopping the MAOI drug. If you do not know if the child's prescription drug contains an MAOI, ask a doctor or pharmacist before giving this product.
Specific to Cold, Cough & Fever: other products containing acetaminophen
Specific to Cold & Night Time Cough: if a child is on a sodium-restricted diet unless directed by a doctor
Ask a doctor before use if the child has
- heart disease • high blood pressure
- thyroid disease • diabetes • glaucoma
- cough that occurs with too much phlegm (mucus) (does not apply to Cold & Allergy) • breathing problems such as asthma or chronic bronchitis • chronic cough that lasts (does not apply to Cold & Allergy)
Ask a doctor or pharmacist before use if the child is taking sedatives or tranquilizers.
When using this product
- do not use more than directed • excitability may occur, especially in children

- marked drowsiness may occur • sedatives and tranquilizers may increase drowsiness
Stop use and ask a doctor if
- nervousness, dizziness, or sleeplessness occur
- symptoms do not improve within 7 days or occur with a fever
- sore throat persists for more than 2 days or occurs with headache, fever, rash, nausea or vomiting
- cough persists for more than 7 days, comes back, or occurs with fever, rash, or persistent headache (does not apply to Cold & Allergy)
Specific to Cold, Cough & Fever:
- symptoms do not improve within 5 days (pain) or 3 days (fever).
These could be signs of a serious condition.
Keep out of reach of children. In case of overdose, get medical help or contact a poison control center right away. Prompt medical attention is critical even if you do not notice any signs or symptoms.

Dosage and Administration[1]
TRIAMINIC® Cold & Allergy
Nasal Decongestant, Antihistamine
Orange Flavor
TRIAMINIC® Cold & Cough
Nasal Decongestant, Cough Suppressant
Antihistamine-Cherry Flavor
Take every 4 to 6 hours; not more than 4 doses in 24 hours or as directed by a doctor.
TRIAMINIC® Cold, Cough & Fever
Fever-Reducer-Pain Reliever,
Nasal Decongestant, Cough Suppressant
Antihistamine-Bubble Gum Flavor
TRIAMINIC® Cold & Night Time Cough
Nasal Decongestant, Cough Suppressant
Antihistamine-Grape Flavor
Take every 6 hours; not more than 4 doses in 24 hours or as directed by a doctor.

Age	Weight	Dose
4 months to under 1 year[2]	12–17 lb	¼ tsp (1.25 mL)
1 to under 2 years[2]	18–23 lb	½ tsp (2.5 mL)
2 to under 6 years[1]	24–47 lb	1 tsp (5 mL)
6 to under 12 years	48–95 lb	2 tsp (10 mL)
12 years to adult	96+ lb	4 tsp (20 mL)

[1] As with any antihistamine-containing product, use of Triaminic® Formulas containing antihistamines in children under 6 years of age should be only un-

Continued on next page

Information on Novartis Consumer Health, Inc., products appearing on these pages is effective as of November 2000.

Triaminic Cold—Cont.

der the advice and supervision of a physician.
[2] The dosage for children under 2 years should be determined by the physician on the basis of patients weight, physical condition or other appropriate considerations. Dosages are provided as guidelines. Antihistamines should not be given to neonates and are contraindicated in newborns.

Other Information

TRIAMINIC® Cold & Allergy
Nasal Decongestant, Antihistamine
Orange Flavor
- each teaspoon contains: **sodium 2 mg**
- contains no aspirin
- store at controlled room temperature 20–25°C (68–77°F).

TRIAMINIC® Cold & Cough
Nasal Decongestant, Cough Suppressant
Antihistamine-Cherry Flavor
- each teaspoon contains: **sodium 10 mg**
- contains no aspirin
- store at controlled room temperature 20–25°C (68–77°F).

TRIAMINIC® Cold, Cough & Fever
Fever Reducer-Pain Reliever,
Nasal Decongestant, Cough Suppressant
Antihistamine-Bubble Gum Flavor
- each teaspoon contains: **sodium 3 mg**
- contains no aspirin
- protect from light
- store at controlled room temperature 20–25°C (68–77°F).

TRIAMINIC® Cold & Night Time Cough
Nasal Decongestant, Cough Suppressant
Antihistamine-Grape Flavor
- each teaspoon contains: **sodium 22 mg**
- contains no aspirin
- store at controlled room temperature 20–25°C (68–77°F).

Inactive Ingredients

TRIAMINIC® Cold & Allergy
Nasal Decongestant, Antihistamine
Orange Flavor
benzoic acid, edetate disodium, FD&C Yellow 6, flavors, purified water, sorbitol, sucrose

TRIAMINIC® Cold & Cough
Nasal Decongestant, Cough Suppressant
Antihistamine-Cherry Flavor
benzoic acid, FD&C Red 40, flavors, propylene glycol, purified water, sodium chloride, sorbitol, sucrose

TRIAMINIC® Cold, Cough & Fever
Fever Reducer-Pain Reliever,
Nasal Decongestant, Cough Suppressant
Antihistamine-Bubble Gum Flavor
acesulfame K, benzoic acid, citric acid, D&C Red 33, dibasic potassium phosphate, disodium edetate, FD&C Red 40, flavors, glycerin, polyethylene glycol, potassium chloride, propylene glycol, purified water, sucrose, other ingredients

TRIAMINIC® Cold & Night Time Cough
Nasal Decongestant, Cough Suppressant
Antihistamine-Grape Flavor
benzoic acid, citric acid, D&C Red 33, dibasic sodium phosphate, FD&C Blue 1, flavors, propylene glycol, purified water, sorbitol, sucrose

How Supplied

TRIAMINIC® Cold & Allergy
TRIAMINIC® Cold & Cough
TRIAMINIC® Cold & Night Time Cough
Bottles of 4 fl. oz. (118 mL) and 8 fl.oz. (236 mL)
TRIAMINIC® Cold, Cough & Fever
Bottle of 4 fl. oz. (118 mL)
Questions: call **1-800-452-0051**
For more information about Triaminic® visit our website at www.triaminic.com
NOVARTIS
Novartis Consumer Health, Inc.
Summit, NJ 07901-1312 ©2001
Shown in Product Identification Guide, page 515

TRIAMINIC® Cough
Nasal Decongestant, Cough Suppressant
Berry Flavor

TRIAMINIC® Cough & Congestion
Nasal Decongestant, Cough Suppressant
Orange Strawberry Flavor

TRIAMINIC Cough & Sore Throat
Pain Reliever-Fever Reducer, Nasal Decongestant, Cough Suppressant
Grape Flavor

Drug Facts
Active ingredients
(in each 5 mL, 1 teaspoon)
TRIAMINIC® Cough
Berry Flavor
Pseudoephedrine, HCl,
USP, 15 mg .... Nasal decongestant
Dextromethorphan HBr,
USP 5 mg .... Cough suppressant
TRIAMINIC® Cough & Congestion
Orange Strawberry Flavor
Pseudoephedrine, HCl,
USP, 15 mg .... Nasal decongestant
Dextromethorphan HBr,
USP, 7.5 mg .... Cough suppressant
TRIAMINIC® Cough & Sore Throat
Grape Flavor
Acetaminophen,
USP, 160 mg ..... Fever reducer, Pain reliever
Pseudoephedrine HCl,
USP, 15 mg .... Nasal decongestant
Dextromethorphan HBr,
USP, 7.5 mg .... Cough suppressant

Uses temporarily relieves these symptoms:
TRIAMINIC® Cough
Nasal Decongestant, Cough Suppressant
Berry Flavor
TRIAMINIC® Cough & Congestion
Nasal Decongestant, Cough Suppressant
Orange Strawberry Flavor
- cough due to minor throat and bronchial irritation • nasal and sinus congestion
TRIAMINIC® Cough & Sore Throat
Pain Reliever-Fever Reducer, Nasal Decongestant, Cough Suppressant
Grape Flavor
- sore throat pain • minor aches and pains • cough due to minor throat and bronchial irritations • nasal and sinus congestion

Warnings
Do not use in a child who is taking a prescription monoamine oxidase inhibitor

(MAOI) (certain drugs for depression, psychiatric or emotional conditions, or Parkinson's disease), or for 2 weeks after stopping the MAOI drug. If you do not know if the child's prescription drug contains an MAOI, ask a doctor or pharmacist before giving this product.
Specific to Cough & Sore Throat: other products containing acetaminophen
Specific to Cough: if child is on a sodium-restricted diet unless directed by a doctor
Ask a doctor before use if the child has
- heart disease • high blood pressure
- thyroid disease • diabetes • glaucoma
- cough that occurs with too much phlegm (mucus) • chronic cough that lasts or a breathing problem such as asthma or chronic bronchitis
Ask a doctor or pharmacist before use if the child is taking sedatives or tranquilizers.
When using this product
- do not use more than directed
Stop use and ask a doctor if
- nervousness, dizziness, or sleeplessness occurs • cough persists for more than 7 days, comes back, or occurs with fever, rash, or persistent headache
Specific to Cough & Sore Throat:
- sore throat persists for more than 2 days, or occurs with headache, fever, rash, nausea, or vomiting. These could be signs of a serious condition. • symptoms do not improve for 5 days (pain) or 3 days (fever)
Keep out of reach of children. In case of overdose, get medical help or contact a poison control center right away. Prompt medical attention is critical even if you do not notice any signs or symptoms.

Dosage and Administration
Triaminic® Cough
Nasal Decongestant, Cough Suppressant
Berry Flavor
Take every 4 to 6 hours; not more than 4 doses in 24 hours or as directed by a doctor.
Triaminic® Cough & Congestion
Nasal Decongestant, Cough Suppressant
Orange Strawberry Flavor
Triaminic® Cough & Sore Throat
Pain Reliever-Fever Reducer, Nasal Decongestant, Cough Suppressant
Grape Flavor
Take every 6 hours; not more than 4 doses in 24 hours or as directed by a doctor.

Age	Weight	Dose
4 mos. to under 1 yr[1]	12–17 lb	¼ tsp (1.25 mL)
1 to under 2 years[1]	18–23 lb	½ tsp (2.5 mL)
2 to under 6 years	24–47 lb	1 tsp (5 mL)
6 to under 12 years	48–95 lb	2 tsp (10 mL)
12 years to adult	96 + lb	4 tsp (20 mL)

¹The dosage for children under 2 years should be determined by the physician on the basis of patients weight, physical condition or other appropriate considerations. Dosages are provided as guidelines.

Other Information
TRIAMINIC® Cough
Nasal Decongestant, Cough Suppressant
Berry Flavor
• each teaspoon contains: **sodium 20 mg**
• contains no aspirin • store at controlled room temperature 20–25°C (68–77°F)

TRIAMINIC® Cough & Congestion
Nasal Decongestant, Cough Suppressant
Orange Strawberry Flavor
• each teaspoon contains: **sodium 7 mg**
• contains no aspirin • store at controlled room temperature 20–25°C (68–77°F)

TRIAMINIC® Cough & Sore Throat
Pain Reliever-Fever Reducer, Nasal Decongestant, Cough Suppressant
Grape Flavor
• each teaspoon contains: **sodium 11 mg**
• contains no aspirin • store at controlled room temperature 20–25°C (68–77°F)

Inactive Ingredients
TRIAMINIC® Cough
Nasal Decongestant, Cough Suppressant
Berry Flavor
benzoic acid, FD&C Blue 1, FD&C Red 40, flavors, propylene glycol, purified water, sodium chloride, sorbitol, sucrose

TRIAMINIC® Cough & Congestion
Nasal Decongestant, Cough Suppressant
Orange Strawberry Flavor
benzoic acid, citric acid, dibasic sodium phosphate, edetate disodium, flavors, propylene glycol, purified water, sorbitol, sucrose

TRIAMINIC® Cough & Sore Throat
Pain Reliever-Fever Reducer, Nasal Decongestant, Cough Suppressant
Grape Flavor
benzoic acid, D&C Red 33, dibasic sodium phosphate, edetate disodium, FD&C Blue 1, FD&C Red 40, flavors, glycerin, polyethylene glycol, propylene glycol, purified water, sucrose, tartaric acid

How Supplied
Triaminic® Cough
Triaminic® Cough & Congestion
Bottles of 4 fl. oz. (118 mL)

Triaminic® Cough & Sore Throat
Bottles of 4 fl. oz. (118 mL) and 8 fl. oz (236 mL)

Questions: call **1-800-452-0051**
For more information about Triaminic® visit our website at www.triaminic.com
NOVARTIS
Novartis Consumer Health, Inc.
Summit, NJ 07901-1312 ©2001
Shown in Product Identification Guide, page 515

TRIAMINIC® Softchews®
Cold & Allergy
Nasal Decongestant,
Antihistamine-Orange Flavor
TRIAMINIC® Softchews®
Cold & Cough
Nasal Decongestant, Cough Suppressant, Antihistamine-Cherry Flavor

Drug Facts
Active ingredients (in each tablet)
TRIAMINIC® Softchews® Cold & Allergy-Orange Flavor
Pseudoephedrine, HCl, USP,
15 mg .... Nasal decongestant
Chlorpheniramine maleate, USP,
1 mg .... Antihistamine
TRIAMINIC® Softchews® Cold & Cough-Cherry Flavor
Pseudoephedrine HCl, USP,
15 mg .... Nasal decongestant
Dextromethorphan HBr, USP,
5 mg .... Cough suppressant
Chlorpheniramine maleate, USP,
1 mg .... Antihistamine

Uses Temporarily relieves these symptoms:
TRIAMINIC® Softchews® Cold & Allergy
Nasal Decongestant, Antihistamine
Orange Flavor
• nasal and sinus congestion • runny nose • sneezing • itchy nose or throat • itchy, watery eyes
TRIAMINIC® Softchews® Cold & Cough
Nasal Decongestant, Cough Suppressant
Antihistamine-Cherry Flavor
• cough due to minor throat and bronchial irritation • runny nose • nasal and sinus congestion • sneezing • itchy nose or throat • itchy, watery eyes

Warnings
Do not use in a child who is taking a prescription monoamine oxidase inhibitor (MAOI) (certain drugs for depression, psychiatric or emotional conditions, or Parkinson's disease), or for 2 weeks after stopping the MAOI drug. If you do not know if the child's prescription drug contains an MAOI, ask a doctor or pharmacist before giving this product.
Ask a doctor before use if the child has
• heart disease • high blood pressure • thyroid disease • diabetes • glaucoma • a breathing problem such as chronic bronchitis or asthma
Specific to Cold & Cough: cough that occurs with too much phlegm (mucus) or chronic cough that lasts.
Ask a doctor or pharmacist before use if the child is taking sedatives or tranquilizers.
When using this product
• do not use more than directed • drowsiness may occur • sedatives and tranquilizers may increase drowsiness • excitability may occur, especially in children
Stop use and ask a doctor if
• nervousness, dizziness, or sleeplessness occurs • cough persists for more than 7 days • symptoms do not improve

within 7 days, or occur with fever, rash, or persistent headache. These could be signs of a serious condition.
Keep out of reach of children. In case of overdose, get medical help or contact a poison control center right away.

Dosage and Administration¹
• Let Softchews® tablet dissolve in mouth or chew Softchews® tablet before swallowing, whichever is preferred
• take every 4 to 6 hours; not more than 4 doses in 24 hours or as directed by a doctor

Age	Weight	Dose
2 to under 6 years¹	24 to 47 lb	1 tablet
6 to under 12 years	48 to 95 lb	2 tablets
12 years to adult	96 + lb	4 tablets

¹ As with any antihistamine-containing product, use of Triaminic® Formulas containing antihistamines in children under 6 years of age should be only under the advice and supervision of a physician.

Other Information
• each Softchews® tablet contains:
sodium 5 mg • contains no aspirin
• store at controlled room temperature 20–25°C (68–77°F)
Triaminic® Softchews® Cold & Allergy
Nasal Decongestant, Antihistamine
Orange Flavor • **Phenylketonurics:** Contains: **Phenylalanine, 17.5 mg** per Softchews® tablet
Triaminic® Softchews® Cold & Cough
Nasal Decongestant, Cough Suppressant
Antihistamine-Cherry Flavor • **Phenylketonurics:** Contains: **Phenylalanine, 17.7 mg** per Softchews® tablet

Inactive Ingredients
TRIAMINIC® Softchews® Cold & Allergy
Nasal Decongestant, Antihistamine-Orange Flavor
aspartame, carnauba wax, citric acid, crospovidone, D&C Red 27 aluminum lake, D&C Yellow 10 aluminum lake, ethylcellulose, flavors, glycerides, hydroxypropyl methylcellulose, magnesium stearate, mannitol, mono- and diglycosides, silicon dioxide, sodium bicarbonate, sucrose
TRIAMINIC® Softchews® Cold & Cough
Nasal Decongestant, Cough Suppressant
Antihistamine-Cherry Flavor
aspartame, carnauba wax, citric acid, crospovidone, D&C Red 27, aluminum

Continued on next page

Information on Novartis Consumer Health, Inc., products appearing on these pages is effective as of November 2000.

Triaminic Softchews Cold—Cont.

lake, D&C Red 30 aluminum lake, ethylcellulose, FD&C Blue 2 aluminum lake, flavors, hydroxypropyl methylcellulose, magnesium stearate, mannitol, microcrystalline cellulose, mono- and diglycerides, povidone, silicone dioxide, sodium bicarbonate, sucrose

How Supplied: 18 Softchews® Tablets.

Questions: call **1-800-452-0051**
For more information about Triaminic®
visit our website at www.triaminic.com
NOVARTIS
Novartis Consumer Health, Inc.
Summit, NJ 07901-1312 ©2001
Shown in Product Identification Guide, page 515

TRIAMINIC® Softchews® Cough
Cough Suppressant-Strawberry Flavor
TRIAMINIC® Softchews® Cough & Sore Throat
Pain Reliever-Fever Reducer, Nasal Decongestant, Cough Suppressant-Grape Flavor

Drug Facts
Active Ingredient (in each tablet)
TRIAMINIC® Softchews® Cough
Strawberry Flavor
Dextromethorphan HBr, USP,
7.5 mg .... Cough suppressant
TRIAMINIC® Softchews® Cough & Sore Throat
Grape Flavor
Acetaminophen, USP,
160 mg ...... Fever reducer, Pain reliever
Pseudoephedrine HCl, USP,
15 mg .... Nasal decongestant
Dextromethorphan HBr, USP,
5 mg .... Cough suppressant

Uses Temporarily relieves these symptoms:
TRIAMINIC® Softchews® Cough
Cough Suppressant-Strawberry Flavor
• cough due to minor throat and bronchial irritation associated with the common cold
TRIAMINIC® Softchews® Cough & Sore Throat
Pain Reliever-Fever Reducer, Nasal Decongestant, Cough Suppressant Grape Flavor
• fever • minor aches and pains • headache and sore throat • cough due to minor throat and bronchial irritation • nasal and sinus congestion

Warnings
Do not use in a child who is taking a prescription monoamine oxidase inhibitor (MAOI) (certain drugs for depression, psychiatric or emotional conditions, or Parkinson's disease), or for 2 weeks after stopping the MAOI drug. If you do not know if the child's prescription drug contains an MAOI, ask a doctor or pharmacist before giving this product.
Specific to Cough & Sore Throat: other products containing acetaminophen
Ask a doctor before use if the child has

• a breathing problem such as chronic bronchitis or asthma • heart disease • high blood pressure • thyroid disease • diabetes • glaucoma
Specific to Cough & Sore Throat: cough that occurs with too much phlegm or chronic cough that lasts
Ask a doctor or pharmacist before use if the child is taking sedatives or tranquilizers
When using this product
• do not use more than directed
Stop use and ask a doctor if
• nervousness, dizziness, or sleeplessness occurs • symptoms do not improve within 7 days, or occur with fever, rash, or persistent headache. These could be signs of a serious condition.
Specific to Cough & Sore Throat:
• symptoms do not improve for 5 days (pain) or 3 days (fever) • sore throat persists for more than 2 days or occurs with persistant headache, fever, rash, nausea or vomiting. These could be signs of a serious condition.
Keep out of reach of children In case of overdose, get medical help or contact a poison control center right away.

Dosage and Administration
Let *Softchews®* tablet dissolve in mouth or chew *Softchews®* tablet before swallowing, whichever is preferred.
TRIAMINIC® Softchews® Cough
Strawberry Flavor • take every 6 to 8 hours • not more than 4 doses in 24 hours
TRIAMINIC® Softchews® Cough & Sore Throat-Grape Flavor • take every 4 to 6 hours • not more than 4 doses in 24 hours.

Age	Weight	Dose
2 to under 6 years	24 to 47 lb	1 tablet
6 to under 12 years	48–97 lb	2 tablets
12 years to adult	96+ lb	4 tablets

Other Information
• contains no aspirin • store at controlled room temperature 20°–25°C (68°–77°F)
TRIAMINIC® Softchews® Cough
Cough Suppressant-Strawberry Flavor
• each Softchews® tablet contains:
sodium 5 mg • Phenylketonurics: Contains **Phenylalanine 22.5 mg** per tablet
TRIAMINIC® Softchews® Cough & Sore Throat
Pain Reliever-Fever Reducer, Nasal Decongestant, Cough Suppressant Grape Flavor
• each Softchews® tablet contains **sodium 8 mg**
• Phenylketonurics: Contains **Phenylalanine, 28.1 mg** per tablet

Inactive Ingredients
TRIAMINIC® Softchews® Cough
Cough Suppressant-Strawberry Flavor

aspartame, citric acid, crospovidone, ethylcellulose, FD&C Red 40 aluminum lake, flavors, magnesium stearate, mannitol, microcrystalline cellulose, povidone, silicon dioxide (colloidal), sodium bicarbonate
TRIAMINIC® Softchews® Cough & Sore Throat
Pain Reliever-Fever Reducer, Nasal Decongestant, Cough Suppressant Grape Flavor
aspartame, citric acid, crospovidone, D&C Red 27 aluminum lake, ethylcellulose, FD&C Blue 1 aluminum lake, flavors, magnesium stearate, mannitol, microcrystalline cellulose, povidone, silicon dioxide, sodium bicarbonate

How Supplied: 18 Softchews® Tablets
Questions: call **1-800-452-0051**
For more information about Triaminic®
visit our website at www.triaminic.com
NOVARTIS
Novartis Consumer Health, Inc.
Summit, NJ 07901-1312 ©2001
Shown in Product Identification Guide, page 515

TRIAMINIC® Vapor Patch -Mentholated Cherry Scent Cough Suppressant
TRIAMINIC® Vapor Patch -Menthol Scent Cough Suppressant

Drug Facts
Active ingredients (in each patch)
Camphor 4.7% .... Cough suppressant
Menthol 2.6% .... Cough suppressant

Uses temporarily relieves these symptoms:
• cough due to a cold • cough due to minor throat and bronchial irritation • cough to help you sleep

Warnings
For external use only
Flammable: Keep away from fire or flame
Do not use
• near an open flame • by adding to hot water • in a microwave oven • in a container in which water is being heated
Ask a doctor before use if the child has
• cough that occurs with too much phlegm (mucus) • a persistent or chronic cough such as occurs with asthma
When using this product
• do not use more than directed • do not take by mouth or place in nostrils • do not apply to eyes, wounds, or damaged skin
Stop use and ask a doctor if
• a cough persists for more than 7 days, comes back, or occurs with fever, rash, or persistent headache. These could be signs of a serious condition • too much skin irritation occurs or gets worse
Keep out of reach of children. If swallowed, get medical help or contact a poison control center right away.

Dosage and Administration

Children 2 to under 12 years of age:
• Remove plastic backing • Apply to the throat or chest • Clothing should be left loose about the throat and chest to help the vapors rise to reach the nose and mouth • More than one patch may be used • Applications may be repeated up to three times daily or as directed by a doctor • May use with other cough suppressant products

Children under 2 years of age: Ask a doctor

Other Information:
• store at controlled room temperature 20–25°C (68–77°F) • protect from excessive heat

Inactive Ingredients
TRIAMINIC® Vapor Patch
-Mentholated Cherry Scent Cough Suppressant

acrylic ester copolymer, aloe vera gel, eucalyptus oil, glycerin, karaya, propylene glycol, purified water, wild cherry fragrance

TRIAMINIC® Vapor Patch
-Menthol Scent Cough Suppressant
acrylic ester, copolymer, aloe vera gel, eucalyptus oil, glycerin, karaya, purified water, spirits of turpentine

How Supplied: Packet of 6 patches, ointment on a breathable cloth patch.
Questions: call **1-800-452-0051**
For more information about Triaminic® visit our website at www.triaminic.com
NOVARTIS
Novartis Consumer Health, Inc.,
Summit, NJ 07901-1312   ©2001
Shown in Product Identification Guide, page 515

The Parthenon Co., Inc.
3311 W. 2400 SOUTH
SALT LAKE CITY, UTAH 84119

Direct Inquiries to:
(801) 972-5184
FAX: (801) 972-4734

For Medical Emergency Contact:
Nick G. Mihalopoulos
(801) 972-5184

DEVROM® CHEWABLE TABLETS

Description: DEVROM® is a safe and effective internal (oral) deodorant. Each tablet contains 200 mg of Bismuth Subgallate powder.

Indications: DEVROM® is indicated for the control of odors from ileostomies, colostomies and fecal incontinence.

Dosage: Take one or two tablets of DEVROM® three times a day with meals or as directed by physician. Chew or swallow whole if desired.

Note: The beneficial ingredient in **DEVROM®** may coat the tongue which may also darken in color. This condition is harmless and temporary. Darkening of the stool is also possible and equally harmless.

Warning: This product cannot be expected to be effective in the reduction of odor due to faulty personal hygiene.
KEEP THIS BOTTLE AND ALL MEDICATION OUT OF THE REACH OF CHILDREN.

Inactive Ingredients: Xylitol USP, MCC, Starch Pregelatinized, Natural Banana Flavor USP, Talc, Magnesium Stearate.
NO PHYSICIAN'S PRESCRIPTION IS NECESSARY

How Supplied: DEVROM® is supplied in bottles of 100 chewable tablets and capsules.
　DO NOT USE IF PRINTED OUTER SAFETY SEAL OR PRINTED INNER
　SAFETY SEAL IS BROKEN.
THE PARTHENON CO., INC.
3311 W. 2400 So.
Salt Lake City, Utah 84119

Pfizer Inc,
Warner-Lambert
Consumer Group
201 TABOR ROAD
MORRIS PLAINS, NJ 07950

Direct Inquiries to:
1-(800) 223-0182

For Consumer Product Information Call:
1-(800) 524-2854 – Celestial Seasonings Soothers (only)
1-(800) 223-0182

CELESTIAL SEASONINGS® SOOTHERS™ Herbal Throat Drops

Active Ingredients: Menthol and Pectin.

Inactive Ingredients: *HARVEST CHERRY*—Ascorbic Acid (Vitamin C); Cherry and Elderberry Juices; Citric Acid; Corn Syrup; Natural Flavoring; Oils of Angelica Root, Anise Star, Ginger, Lemon Grass, Sage and White Thyme; Sodium Ascorbate and Sucrose. *HONEY-LEMON CHAMOMILE*—Ascorbic Acid (Vitamin C); Chamomile Flower Extract; Citric Acid; Corn Syrup; Honey; Lemon Juice; Natural Flavoring; Oils of Angelica Root, Anise Star, Ginger, Lemon Grass, Sage and White Thyme; Sodium Ascorbate; Sucrose and Tea Extract. *SUNSHINE CITRUS*—Ascorbic Acid (Vitamin C); Beta Carotene; Citric Acid; Corn Syrup; Natural Flavoring; Oils of Angelica Root, Anise Star, Ginger, Lemon Grass, Sage and White Thyme; Orange Juice; Sodium Ascorbate, and Sucrose.

Indications: For temporary relief of occasional minor irritation, pain, sore mouth and sore throat. Provides temporary protection of irritated areas in sore mouth and sore throat.

Warnings: If sore throat is severe, persists for more than 2 days, is accompanied or followed by fever, headache, rash, nausea, or vomiting, consult a doctor promptly. If sore mouth symptoms do not improve in 7 days, see your dentist or doctor promptly. KEEP THIS AND ALL DRUGS OUT OF THE REACH OF CHILDREN.

Dosage and Administration: Adults and children 5 years and over: Dissolve 2 drops (one at a time) slowly in the mouth. May be repeated every 2 hours as needed or as directed by a dentist or doctor. Children under 5 years: Consult a dentist or doctor.

How Supplied: Celestial Seasonings Soothers Throat Drops are available in bags of 24 drops. They are available in four flavors: Harvest Cherry, Honey-Lemon Chamomile, Sunshine Citrus.
Shown in Product Identification Guide, page 515

CERTS® Cool Mint Drops® with a Retsyn® Center
[*Surts cul mint drops*]

Ingredients: *PEPPERMINT:* Sugar, Modified Food Starch, Glucose Syrup, Artificial and Natural Flavoring*, Maltodextrin, Gum Arabic, Rice Starch, Magnesium Stearate, Blue 2 Lake, Partially Hydrogenated Cottonseed Oil*, and Copper Gluconate*.
FRESHMINT: Sugar, Modified Food Starch, Glucose Syrup, Artificial and Natural Flavoring*, Maltodextrin, Gum Arabic, Rice Starch, Magnesium Stearate, Blue 2 Lake, Yellow 5 Lake, Partially Hydrogenated Cottonseed Oil* and Copper Gluconate*.
CINNAMINT: Sugar, Modified Food Starch, Glucose Syrup, Artificial and Natural Flavoring*, Maltodextrin, Gum Arabic, Rice Starch, Magnesium Stearate, Red 40 Lake, Partially Hydrogenated Cottonseed Oil* and Copper Gluconate*.

Description: Oval breath drop.

Directions: Take 1 mint as desired.

How Supplied: Certs® Cool Mint Drops® with a Retsyn® Center are available in Peppermint, Freshmint and Cin-

Continued on next page

Certs Cool Mint—Cont.

namint Flavors in slide-top cartons of about 27 pressed mints each.
Shown in Product Identification Guide, page 515

CERTS® Powerful Mints with Retsyn® Crystals
[*Surts pau wur ful mints*]

Ingredients: *PEPPERMINT:* Sorbitol, Maltodextrin, Natural Flavoring*, Aspartame, Magnesium Stearate, Partially Hydrogenated Cottonseed Oil*, Copper Gluconate* and Blue 1 *Retsyn®. PHENYLKETONURICS: CONTAINS PHENYLALANINE.
SPEARMINT: Sorbitol, Artificial and Natural Flavoring*, Maltodextrin, Aspartame, Magnesium Stearate, Partially Hydrogenated Cottonseed Oil*, Copper Gluconate*, Yellow 5 and Blue 1. Retsyn® PHENYLKETONURICS: CONTAINS PHENYLALANINE*.

*RETSYN®: A combination of Partially Hydrogenated Cottonseed Oil, Copper Gluconate and Flavoring.

Description: Breath Freshening Mint.

Directions: Take 1 tablet as desired.

How Supplied: Certs® Powerful Mints with Retsyn® Crystals are available in Peppermint and Spearmint flavors in a credit card size vial of 50 tablets each.
Shown in Product Identification Guide, page 516

HALLS® MENTHO–LYPTUS®
Cough Suppressant Drops
[*Hols*]

Active Ingredient: *MENTHO-LYPTUS®:* Menthol 7 mg per drop. *CHERRY:* Menthol 7.6 mg per drop. *HONEY-LEMON:* Menthol 8.6 mg per drop. *ICE BLUE PEPPERMINT:* Menthol 12 mg per drop. *SPEARMINT:* Menthol 6 mg per drop. *STRAWBERRY:* Menthol 3.5 mg per drop.

Inactive Ingredients: *MENTHO-LYPTUS®:* Eucalyptus Oil, Flavoring, Glucose Syrup and Sucrose. *CHERRY:* Blue 2, Eucalyptus Oil, Flavoring, Glucose Syrup, Red 40 and Sucrose. *HONEY-LEMON:* Beta Carotene, Eucalyptus Oil, Flavoring, Glucose Syrup and Sucrose. *ICE BLUE PEPPERMINT:* Blue 1, Eucalyptus Oil, Flavoring, Glucose Syrup and Sucrose. *SPEARMINT:* Beta Carotene, Blue 1, Eucalyptus Oil, Flavoring, Glucose Syrup and Sucrose. *STRAWBERRY:* Eucalyptus Oil, Flavoring Glucose Syrup, Red 40 and Sucrose.

Indications: For temporary relief of minor throat irritation and coughs due to colds or inhaled irritants.

Warnings: A persistent cough may be a sign of a serious condition. If cough persists for more than 1 week, tends to recur, or is accompanied by fever, rash or persistent headache, consult a doctor. Do not take this product for persistent or chronic cough such as occurs with smoking, asthma, or emphysema, or if cough is accompanied by excessive phlegm (mucus) unless directed by a doctor. If sore throat is severe, persists for more than 2 days, is accompanied or followed by fever, headache, rash, swelling, nausea, or vomiting, consult a doctor promptly. KEEP THIS AND ALL DRUGS OUT OF THE REACH OF CHILDREN.

Dosage and Administration: *MENTHO-LYPTUS®, CHERRY, HONEY LEMON, ICE BLUE PEPPERMINT* and *SPEARMINT:* Adults and children 5 years and over: dissolve 1 drop slowly in mouth. Repeat every hour as needed or as directed by a doctor. Children under 5 years: consult a doctor.
STRAWBERRY: Adults and children 5 years and over: for sore throat dissolve at 2 drops (one at a time) slowly in the mouth. Repeat every hour as needed or as directed by a doctor. Children under 5 years: consult a doctor.

How Supplied: Halls® *Mentho-Lyptus®* Cough Suppressant Drops are available in single sticks of 9 drops each and in bags of 30. They are available in six flavors: *Regular Mentho-Lyptus®, Cherry, Honey-Lemon, Ice Blue Peppermint, Spearmint* and *Strawberry*. Regular Mentho-Lyptus®, Cherry and Honey-Lemon flavors are also available in bags of 80 drops. *Mentho-Lyptus®* and *Cherry* are also available in bags of 200 drops.
Shown in Product Identification Guide, page 516

HALLS® PLUS
Cough Suppressant/Throat Drops
[*Hols*]

Active Ingredients: Each drop contains Menthol 10 mg and Pectin.

Inactive Ingredients: MENTHO-LYPTUS®: Carrageenan, Eucalyptus Oil, Flavoring, Glucose Syrup, Glycerin and Sucrose. CHERRY: Blue 2, Carrageenan, Eucalyptus Oil, Flavoring, Glucose Syrup, Glycerin, Red 40 and Sucrose. HONEY-LEMON: Beta Carotene, Carrageenan, Eucalyptus Oil, Flavoring, Glucose Syrup, Glycerin, Honey and Sucrose.

Indications: For temporary relief of minor throat irritation and coughs due to colds or inhaled irritants. Provides temporary protection of irritated areas in sore throat.

Warnings: A persistent cough may be a sign of a serious condition. If cough persists for more than 1 week, tends to recur, or is accompanied by fever, rash, or persistent headache, consult a doctor. Do not take this product for persistent or chronic cough such as occurs with smoking, asthma, or emphysema, or if cough is accompanied by excessive phlegm (mucous) unless directed by a doctor. If sore throat is severe, persists for more than 2 days, is accompanied or followed by fever, headache, rash, swelling, nausea, or vomiting, consult a doctor promptly. KEEP THIS AND ALL DRUGS OUT OF THE REACH OF CHILDREN.

Dosage and Administration: Adults and children 5 years and over: dissolve 1 drop slowly in the mouth. Repeat every hour as needed or as directed by a doctor. Children under 5 years: consult a doctor.

How Supplied: Halls® Plus Cough Suppressant / Throat Drops are available in single sticks of 10 drops each and in bags of 25 drops. They are available in three flavors: Regular Mentho-Lyptus®, Cherry and Honey-Lemon.
Shown in Product Identification Guide, page 516

HALLS® SUGAR FREE
HALLS® SUGAR FREE SQUARES
MENTHO-LYPTUS®
Cough Suppressant Drops
[*Hols*]

Active Ingredient: Halls® Sugar Free: BLACK CHERRY and CITRUS BLEND: Menthol 5 mg per drop. MOUNTAIN MENTHOL: Menthol 5.8 mg per drop.
Halls® Sugar Free Squares: BLACK CHERRY: Menthol 5.8 mg per drop. MOUNTAIN MENTHOL: Menthol 6.8 mg per drop.

Inactive Ingredients: BLACK CHERRY: Acesulfame Potassium, Aspartame, Blue 1, Citric Acid, Eucalyptus Oil, Flavoring, Isomalt and Red 40. **Phenylketonurics: Contains 2 mg Phenylalanine Per Drop.** CITRUS BLEND: Acesulfame Potassium, Aspartame, Citric Acid, Eucalyptus Oil, Flavoring, Isomalt and Yellow 5 (Tartrazine). **Phenylketonurics: Contains 2 mg Phenylalanine Per Drop.** MOUNTAIN MENTHOL: Acesulfame Potassium, Aspartame, Eucalyptus Oil, Flavoring and Isomalt. **Phenylketonurics: Contains 2 mg Phenylalanine Per Drop.**

Indications: For temporary relief of minor throat irritation and coughs due to colds or inhaled irritants.

Warnings: A persistent cough may be a sign of a serious condition. If cough persists for more than 1 week, tends to recur, or is accompanied by fever, rash, or persistent headache, consult a doctor. Do not take this product for persistent or chronic cough such as occurs with smoking, asthma, or emphysema, or if cough is accompanied by excessive phlegm (mucus) unless directed by a doctor. If sore throat is severe, persists for more than 2 days, is accompanied or followed by fever,

headache, rash, swelling, nausea, or vomiting, consult a doctor promptly. KEEP THIS AND ALL DRUGS OUT OF THE REACH OF CHILDREN.

Dosage and Administration: Adults and children 5 years and over: dissolve 1 drop slowly in mouth. Repeat every hour as needed or as directed by a doctor. Children under 5 years: consult a doctor.

Additional Information:
Halls® Sugar Free:
Exchange Information*:
1 Drop = Free Exchange
10 Drops = 1 Fruit
*The dietary exchanges are based on the *Exchange Lists for Meal Planning,* Copyright ©1989 by the American Diabetes Association, Inc. and the American Dietetic Association.
Excess consumption may have a laxative effect.

How Supplied: Halls® Sugar Free: Halls® Sugar Free Mentho-Lyptus® Cough Suppressant Drops are available in bags of 25 drops. They are available in three flavors: Black Cherry, Citrus Blend and Mountain Menthol. Halls® Sugar Free Squares: Halls® Sugar Free Squares Mentho-Lyptus® Cough Suppressant Drops are available in single sticks of 9 drops each. They are available in two flavors: Black Cherry and Mountain Menthol.
Shown in Product Identification Guide, page 516

HALLS DEFENSE™ Vitamin C Supplement Drops
[Hols]

Ingredients: *ASSORTED CITRUS FLAVORS:* Sugar, Glucose Syrup, Sodium Ascorbate, Citric Acid, Natural Flavoring, Ascorbic Acid, Color Added and Red 40. *STRAWBERRY:* Sugar, Glucose Syrup, Sodium Ascorbate, Citric Acid, Ascorbic Acid, Natural and Artificial Flavoring, Color Added. *HARVEST CHERRY MULTIBLEND:* (vitamin C, Echinacea, Zinc); Sugar, Glucose Syrup, Sodium Ascorbate, Citric Acid, Cotton Seed Oil, Natural Flavoring, Ascorbic Acid, Zinc Sulfate, Red 40, Blue 1, Oils of Angelica Root, Anise Star, Ginger, Lemon Grass, Sage and White Thyme.

Description: Halls Defense™ Vitamin C Supplement Drops are a delicious way to get 100% of the Daily Value of Vitamin C. Each drop provides 60 mg of Vitamin C (100% of the Daily Value).

Indications: Dietary Supplement.

How Supplied: Halls Defense™ Vitamin C Supplement Drops are available in all-natural citrus Assortment (lemon, sweet grapefruit, orange) and Strawberry in sticks of 9 drops each and in bags of 30 drops. Also available in Harvest Cherry Multiblend (Vitamin C, Echinacea, and Zinc) in bags of 25 drops.
Shown in Product Identification Guide, page 516

TRIDENT ADVANTAGE® MINTS
Sugarless Mints with Recaldan™
(Tri-dent Ad-van-tage Mints)

Ingredients: *PEPPERMINT:* Sorbitol, Calcium Casein Peptone-Calcium Phosphate (Lactose-Free Milk Derivative)**, Magnesium Stearate, Artificial and Natural Flavoring, Aspartame and Acesulfame Potassium. **Contains a Milk-Based Ingredient.** PHENYLKETONURICS: CONTAINS PHENYLALANINE.
WINTERGREEN: Sorbitol, Calcium Casein Peptone-Calcium Phosphate (Lactose-Free Milk Derivative)**, Artificial and Natural Flavoring, Magnesium Stearate, Aspartame and Acesulfame Potassium. **Contains a Milk-Based Ingredient.** PHENYLKETONURICS: CONTAINS PHENYLALANINE.
RECALDENT™**: A patented ingredient derived from casein, a bovine phosphoprotein found in milk. RECALDANT™ is a trademark of Bonlac Foods Limited.

Description: Trident Advantage® Mints offer remineralization (teeth strengthening) and breath freshening in a great tasting, sugarless mint.

Directions: Allowing Trident Advantage® Mints to dissolve in the mouth promotes salivary flow, which supports the mouth's natural ability to strengthen teeth.

How Supplied: Sugarless Trident Advantage® Mints with Recaldent™ are available in Peppermint and Wintergreen Flavors in a 12-mint plastic vial.
Shown in Product Identification Guide, page 516

TRIDENT ADVANTAGE®
Sugarless Gum with Recaldent™
[Tri-dent Ad-van-tage]

Ingredients: *PEPPERMINT:* Gum Base, Xylitol, Maltitol, Mannitol, Sorbitol, Sodium Bicarbonate (Baking Soda), Artificial and Natural Flavoring, Acacia, Calcium Casein Peptone-Calcium Phosphate (Lactose-Free Milk Derivative)**, Titanium Dioxide (Color), Aspartame, Acesulfame Potassium and Candelilla Wax. **Contains a Milk-Based Ingredient.** PHENYLKETONURICS: CONTAINS PHENYLALANINE.
COOLMINT®: Gum Base, Xylitol, Maltitol, Sorbitol, Sodium Bicarbonate (Baking Soda), Artificial and Natural Flavoring, Acacia, Calcium Casein Peptone-Calcium Phosphate (Lactose-Free Milk Derivative)**, Titanium Dioxide (Color), Aspartame, Acesulfame Potassium and Candelilla Wax. **Contains a Milk-Based Ingredient.** PHENYLKETONURICS: CONTAINS PHENYLALANINE.
RECALDENT™**: A patented ingredient derived from casein, a bovine phosphoprotein found in milk. RECALDENT™ is a trademark of Bonlac Foods Limited.

Description: Trident Advantage® is a dental care gum that comes in pellet form offering remineralization (teeth strengthening), unsightly plaque reduction and teeth whitening benefits.

Directions: Each time you chew two pieces of Trident Advantage® it promotes salivary flow, which supports the mouth's natural ability to strengthen teeth. With regular use, chewing two pieces after eating has been shown to reduce unsightly plaque.

How Supplied: Trident Advantage® with Recaldent™ is available in Peppermint and Coolmint® Flavors in a 12 pellet blister foil.
Shown in Product Identification Guide, page 516

TRIDENT FOR KIDS™
Sugarless Gum with Recaldent™
[Tri-dent for kids]

Ingredients: *BERRY BUBBLE GUM:* Sorbitol, Gum Base, Mannitol, Glycerin, Artificial and Natural Flavoring, Xylitol, Calcium Casein Peptone-Calcium Phosphate (Lactose-Free Milk Derivative)**, Soy Lecithin, Acetylated Monoglycerides, Sucralose, Red 40 Lake and Blue 2 Lake. **Contains a Milk-Based Ingredient.**

RECALDENT™**: A patented ingredient derived from casein, a bovine phosphoprotein found in milk. RECALDENT™ is a trademark of Bonlac Foods Limited.

Description: Trident For Kids™ is a dental care gum that remineralizes tooth enamel by safely delivering calcium directly to teeth. In addition to strengthening teeth, chewing Trident for Kids™ may reduce the risk of tooth decay.

Directions: Trident For Kids™ chewed after meals provides an ideal way to deliver the benefits of Recaldent™, to help remove food particles that may adhere to teeth, and to help minimize plaque acids.

How Supplied: Trident For Kids™ with Recaldent™ is available in Berry Bubble Gum Flavor in an 8-stick pack.
Shown in Product Identification Guide, page 516

UNKNOWN DRUG?
Consult the
Product Identification Guide
(Gray Pages)
for full-color photos of
leading over-the-counter
medications

Continued on next page

Pfizer Inc,
Warner-Lambert
Consumer Healthcare
201 TABOR ROAD
MORRIS PLAINS, NJ 07950

Address Questions & Comments to:
Consumer Affairs, Pfizer CHC
182 Tabor Road
Morris Plains, NJ 07950
For Medical Emergencies/Information Contact:
1-(800)-223-0182
1-(800)-732-7529 (BenGay, Bonine, Cortizone, Desitin Unisom, Visine, and Wart-Off products)
1-(800)-378-1783 (e.p.t.)
1-(800)-337-7266 (e.p.t.-Spanish)

ACTIFED® Cold & Allergy Tablets
[ăk 'tuh-fĕd]

Active Ingredients: Each tablet contains Pseudoephedrine Hydrochloride 60 mg and Triprolidine Hydrochloride 2.5 mg.

Inactive Ingredients: Corn Starch, Flavor, Hydroxypropyl Methylcellulose, Lactose, Magnesium Stearate, Polyethylene Glycol, Potato Starch, Povidone, Sucrose, and Titanium Dioxide.

Indications: Temporarily relieves nasal congestion due to the common cold. Temporarily dries runny nose and alleviates sneezing, itching of the nose or throat, and itchy, watery eyes due to hay fever or other upper respiratory allergies.

Directions: Adults and children 12 years of age and over: 1 tablet. Children 6 to under 12 years of age: $^1/_2$ tablet. Dosage may be repeated every 4 to 6 hours, not to exceed 4 doses in 24 hours, or as directed by a doctor. Children under 6 years of age: consult a doctor.

Warnings: Do not exceed recommended dosage. If nervousness, dizziness, or sleeplessness occur, discontinue use and consult a doctor. If symptoms do not improve within 7 days or are accompanied by fever, consult a doctor. Do not take this product, unless directed by a doctor, if you have heart disease, high blood pressure, thyroid disease, diabetes, a breathing problem such as emphysema or chronic bronchitis, or if you have glaucoma or difficulty in urination due to enlargement of the prostate gland. May cause excitability especially in children. May cause drowsiness; alcohol, sedatives, and tranquilizers may increase the drowsiness effect. Avoid alcoholic beverages while taking this product. Do not take this product if you are taking sedatives or tranquilizers, without first consulting your doctor. Use caution when driving a motor vehicle or operating machinery. As with any drug, if you are

pregnant or nursing a baby, seek the advice of a health professional before using this product. **KEEP THIS AND ALL DRUGS OUT OF THE REACH OF CHILDREN.** In case of accidental overdose, seek professional assistance or contact a Poison Control Center immediately.

Drug Interaction Precaution: Do not use this product if you are now taking a prescription monoamine oxidase inhibitor (MAOI) (certain drugs for depression, psychiatric or emotional conditions, or Parkinson's disease), or for 2 weeks after stopping the MAOI drug. If you are uncertain whether your prescription drug contains an MAOI, consult a health professional before taking this product.

How Supplied: Boxes of 12 and 24 tablets.
Store at 15° to 25°C (59° to 77°F) in a dry place and protect from light.
Shown in Product Identification Guide, page 516

ACTIFED® Cold & Sinus Caplets and Tablets
Maximum Strength
[ak 'tuh-fed]

Active Ingredients: Each coated caplet and tablet contains Acetaminophen 500 mg, Pseudoephedrine Hydrochloride 30 mg and Chlorpheniramine Maleate 2 mg.

Inactive Ingredients: Calcium Stearate, Candelilla Wax, Croscarmellose Sodium, Crospovidone, D&C Yellow No. 10 Aluminum Lake, FD&C Yellow No. 6 Aluminum Lake, Hydroxypropyl Methylcellulose, Microcrystalline Cellulose, Polyethylene Glycol, Polysorbate 80, Povidone, Pregelatinized Starch, Stearic Acid, and Titanium Dioxide.

Indications: Temporarily relieves nasal congestion due to the common cold or associated with sinusitis. Helps decongest sinus openings and passages; temporarily relieves sinus congestion and pressure. For the temporary relief of minor aches, pains, headache, and fever associated with a cold, and runny nose and sneezing, itching of the nose or throat, and itchy, watery eyes due to hay fever.

Directions: Adults and children 12 years of age and over: 2 caplets. Dosage may be repeated every 6 hours while symptoms persist, not to exceed 8 caplets in 24 hours, or as directed by a doctor. Children under 12 years of age: consult a doctor.

Warnings: Do not exceed recommended dosage. If nervousness, dizziness, or sleeplessness occur, discontinue use and consult a doctor. Do not take this product for more than 10 days. If symptoms do not improve or are accompanied by fever that lasts for more than 3 days, or if new symptoms occur, consult a doctor. Do not take this product, unless di-

rected by a doctor, if you have heart disease, high blood pressure, thyroid disease, diabetes, a breathing problem such as emphysema or chronic bronchitis, or if you have glaucoma or difficulty in urination due to enlargement of the prostate gland. May cause excitability especially in children. May cause drowsiness; alcohol, sedatives, and tranquilizers may increase the drowsiness effect. Avoid alcoholic beverages while taking this product. Do not take this product if you are taking sedatives or tranquilizers, without first consulting your doctor. Use caution when driving a motor vehicle or operating machinery. As with any drug, if you are pregnant or nursing a baby, seek the advice of a health professional before using this product. **KEEP THIS AND ALL DRUGS OUT OF THE REACH OF CHILDREN.** In case of accidental overdose, seek professional assistance or contact a Poison Control Center immediately. Prompt medical attention is critical for adults as well as for children even if you do not notice any signs or symptoms.

Alcohol Warning: If you consume 3 or more alcoholic drinks every day, ask your doctor whether you should take acetaminophen or other pain relievers/fever reducers. Acetaminophen may cause liver damage.

Drug Interaction Precaution: Do not use this product if you are now taking a prescription monoamine oxidase inhibitor (MAOI) (certain drugs for depression, psychiatric or emotional conditions, or Parkinson's disease), or for 2 weeks after stopping the MAOI drug. If you are uncertain whether your prescription drug contains an MAOI, consult a health professional before taking this product.

How Supplied: Boxes of 20.
Store at 59° to 77°F in a dry place.
Shown in Product Identification Guide, page 516

ANUSOL®
Hemorrhoidal Ointment
[ă'nū-sōl"]

Active Ingredient: Pramoxine HCl 1%, Zinc Oxide 12.5%, and Mineral Oil. Also contains: Benzyl Benzoate, Calcium Phosphate Dibasic, Cocoa Butter, Glyceryl Monooleate, Glyceryl Monostearate, Kaolin, Peruvian Balsam and Polyethylene Wax.

Actions: Anusol Ointment helps to relieve burning, itching and discomfort arising from irritated anorectal tissues. Pramoxine Hydrochloride in Anusol Ointment is a rapidly acting local anesthetic for the skin and mucous membranes in the lower portion of the anal canal. Pramoxine HCl is also chemically distinct from procaine, cocaine, and dibucaine and can often be used in the patient previously sensitized to other surface anesthetics. Surface analgesia lasts for several hours.

Indications: Temporarily relieves the pain, soreness, burning and itching associated with hemorrhoids and anorectal disorders while temporarily forming a protective coating over inflamed tissues to help prevent the drying of tissues. Anusol Ointment is to be applied externally or in the lower portion of the anal canal (The enclosed dispensing cap is designed to control dispersion of the ointment to the affected area in the lower portion of the anal canal only.)

Warnings: If condition worsens or does not improve within 7 days, consult a physician. Certain persons can develop allergic reactions to ingredients in this product. If the symptom being treated does not subside or if redness, irritation, swelling, pain or other symptoms develop or increase, discontinue use and consult a physician promptly. Do not exceed the recommended daily dosage unless directed by a physician. Do not put this product into the rectum by using fingers or any mechanical device or applicator. KEEP THIS AND ALL DRUGS OUT OF THE REACH OF CHILDREN. In case of accidental ingestion seek professional assistance or contact a Poison Control Center immediately.

Directions: Adults: When practical, cleanse the affected area with mild soap and warm water and rinse thoroughly. Gently dry by patting or blotting with toilet tissue or a soft cloth before application of this product. Apply externally to the affected area up to 5 times daily. To use dispensing cap, attach it to tube, lubricate well, then gently insert part way into the anal canal. Squeeze tube to deliver medication. Thoroughly cleanse dispensing cap after use. Children under 12 years of age: Consult a physician.

How Supplied:—1-oz (28.3g) tubes with plastic applicator. Store at room temperature (59° to 77°F).

Shown in Product Identification Guide, page 516

ANUSOL®
Hemorrhoidal Suppositories
[ă′nū-sŏl″]

Active Ingredient: Topical Starch 51%. Also contains: Benzyl Alcohol, Hydrogenated Vegetable Oil, Tocopheryl Acetate.

Actions: Anusol Suppositories helps to relieve burning, itching and discomfort arising from irritated anorectal tissues. They have a soothing, lubricant action on the intrarectal mucous membrane.

Indications: Gives temporary relief from the itching, burning and discomfort associated with hemorrhoids and other anorectal disorders and provides a coating to protect irritated tissue.

Warnings: Do not exceed the recommended daily dosage unless directed by a physician. If condition worsens or does

not improve within 7 days, consult a physician. In case of bleeding consult a physician promptly.
KEEP THIS AND ALL DRUGS OUT OF THE REACH OF CHILDREN. In case of accidental ingestion seek professional assistance or contact a Poison Control Center immediately. As with any drug, if you are pregnant or nursing a baby, seek the advice of a health professional before using this product.

Directions: Adults—when practical, cleanse the affected area with mild soap and warm water and rinse thoroughly. Gently dry by patting or blotting with toilet tissue or a soft cloth before application of this product.
1. Detach (1) one suppository from the strip of suppositories.
2. Remove wrapper before inserting into the rectum as follows: Hold suppository upright (with words "pull apart" at top) and carefully separate foil by inserting tip of fingernail at foil split.

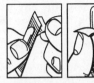

3. Peel foil slowly and evenly down both sides, exposing suppository.
4. Avoid excessive handling of suppository which is designed to melt at body temperature. If suppository seems soft, hold in foil wrapper under cold water for 2 or 3 minutes.
5. Insert one (1) suppository rectally up to six times daily or after each bowel movement.
Children under 12 years of age: consult a physician.

How Supplied: In boxes of 12 or 24 in silver foil strips. Store at 59–77°F to avoid melting.

Shown in Product Identification Guide, page 516

ANUSOL HC-1 Hydrocortisone Anti-Itch
[ă′nū-sŏl″]

Active Ingredient: Hydrocortisone Acetate (equivalent to 1% Hydrocortisone). Also contains: Diazolidinyl Urea, Methylparaben, Microcrystalline Wax, Mineral Oil, Propylene Gylcol, Propylparaben, Sorbitan Sesquioleate and White Petrolatum.

Indications: For temporary relief of itching associated with minor skin irritations, rashes and for external anal itching. Other uses of this product should be only under the advice and supervision of a physician.

Warnings: For external use only. Avoid contact with the eyes. If condition worsens or if symptoms persist for more than 7 days or clear up and occur again within a few days, stop use of this product and do not begin use of any other hydrocorti-

sone product unless you have consulted a physician. Do not exceed the recommended daily dosage unless directed by a physician. In case of bleeding, consult a physician promptly. Do not put this product into the rectum by using fingers or any mechanical device or applicator. Do not use for treatment of diaper rash. Consult a physician. KEEP THIS AND ALL DRUGS OUT OF THE REACH OF CHILDREN. In case of accidental ingestion, seek professional assistance or contact a Poison Control Center immediately.

Directions: Adults: When practical, cleanse the affected area with mild soap and warm water and rinse thoroughly. Gently dry by patting or blotting with toilet tissue or soft cloth before application of this product. Apply to affected area not more than 3 to 4 times daily. Children under 12 years: consult a physician.

How Supplied: 0.7oz (19.8g) tube. Store at 59° to 77°F.

Shown in Product Identification Guide, page 516

BENADRYL® ALLERGY CHEWABLES
[bĕ ′nă-drĭl]

Active Ingredients: Each chewable tablet contains: Diphenhydramine Hydrochloride 12.5 mg.

Inactive Ingredients: Aspartame, Dextrates, D&C Red No. 27 Aluminum Lake, FD&C Blue No. 1 Aluminum Lake, Flavors, Magnesium Stearate, Magnesium Trisilicate, and Tartaric Acid.

Indications: Temporarily relieves runny nose and sneezing, itching of the nose or throat, and itchy, watery eyes due to hay fever or other upper respiratory allergies, and runny nose and sneezing associated with the common cold.

Directions: Follow dosage recommendations, or use as directed by your doctor. Chew tablets thoroughly before swallowing. Adults and children 12 years of age and over: 2 to 4 tablets (25 to 50 mg) every 4 to 6 hours. Not to exceed 24 tablets in 24 hours. Children 6 to under 12 years of age: 1 to 2 tablets (12.5 to 25 mg) every 4 to 6 hours. Not to exceed 12 tablets in 24 hours. Children under 6 years of age: consult a doctor.

Continued on next page

This product information was prepared in November 2000. On these and other Pfizer Consumer Healthcare Products, detailed information may be obtained by addressing Pfizer, Inc. Warner-Lambert Consumer Healthcare Products, Morris Plains, NJ 07950

Benadryl Allergy—Cont.

Warnings: May cause excitability especially in children. Do not take this product, unless directed by a doctor, if you have a breathing problem such as emphysema or chronic bronchitis, or if you have glaucoma or difficulty in urination due to enlargement of the prostate gland. May cause marked drowsiness; alcohol, sedatives, and tranquilizers may increase the drowsiness effect. Avoid alcoholic beverages while taking this product. Do not take this product if you are taking sedatives or tranquilizers, without first consulting your doctor. Use caution when driving a motor vehicle or operating machinery. **Do not use any other products containing diphenhydramine while using this product.** As with any drug, if you are pregnant or nursing a baby, seek the advice of a health professional before using this product. KEEP THIS AND ALL DRUGS OUT OF THE REACH OF CHILDREN. In case of accidental overdose, seek professional assistance or contact a Poison Control Center immediately. **Phenylketonurics: Contains Phenylalanine 4.2 mg. Per Tablet.**

How Supplied: Benadryl® Allergy Chewables are supplied in boxes of 24 tablets. Store at 59° to 77°F in a dry place.

Shown in Product Identification Guide, page 517

BENADRYL® Allergy Liquid Medication
[bĕ 'nă-drĭl]

Active Ingredient: Each teaspoonful (5 mL) contains Diphenhydramine Hydrochloride 12.5 mg.

Inactive Ingredients: Citric Acid, D&C Red No. 33, FD&C Red No. 40, Flavors, Glycerin, Poloxamer 407, Purified Water, Sodium Benzoate, Sodium Chloride, Sodium Citrate, and Sugar.

Indications: Temporarily relieves runny nose and sneezing, itching of the nose or throat, and itchy, watery eyes due to hay fever or other upper respiratory allergies, and runny nose and sneezing associated with the common cold.

Directions: Follow dosage recommendations below, or use as directed by your doctor.

Benadryl® Allergy
Liquid Medication

AGE	DOSAGE
Children under 6 years of age	Consult a doctor.
Children 6 to under 12 years of age	**1 to 2 teaspoonfuls (12.5 to 25 mg)** every 4 to 6 hours. Not to exceed 12 teaspoonfuls in 24 hours.
Adults and children 12 years of age and over	**2 to 4 teaspoonfuls (25 to 50 mg)** every 4 to 6 hours. Not to exceed 24 teaspoonfuls in 24 hours.

Warnings: May cause excitability especially in children. Do not take this product, unless directed by a doctor, if you have a breathing problem such as emphysema, or chronic bronchitis, or if you have glaucoma or difficulty in urination due to enlargment of the prostate gland. May cause marked drowsiness; alcohol, sedatives, and tranquilizers may increase the drowsiness effect. Avoid alcoholic beverages while taking this product. Do not take this product if you are taking sedatives or tranquilizers, without first consulting your doctor. Use caution when driving a motor vehicle or operating machinery. **Do not use any other products containing diphenhydramine while using this product.** As with any drug, if you are pregnant or nursing a baby, seek the advice of a health professional before using this product. KEEP THIS AND ALL DRUGS OUT OF THE REACH OF CHILDREN. In case of accidental overdose, seek professional assistance or contact a Poison Control Center immediately.

How Supplied: Benadryl Allergy Liquid Medication is supplied in 4 and 8 fluid ounce bottles.

Store at 59° to 77°F.

Shown in Product Identification Guide, page 517

BENADRYL® Dye-Free Allergy Liquid Medication
[bĕ 'nă-drĭl]

Bubble Gum Flavor

Active Ingredients: Each teaspoonful (5 mL.) contains Diphenhydramine Hydrochloride 12.5 mg.

Inactive Ingredients: Carboxymethylcellulose Sodium, Citric Acid, Flavor, Glycerin, Purified Water, Saccharin Sodium, Sodium Benzoate, Sodium Citrate, and Sorbitol Solution.

Indications: Temporarily relieves runny nose and sneezing, itching of the nose or throat, and itchy, watery eyes due to hay fever or other upper respiratory allergies, and runny nose and sneezing associated with the common cold.

Directions: Follow dosage recommendations below, or use as directed by your doctor.

Benadryl® Dye-Free Allergy
Liquid Medication

AGE	DOSAGE
Children under 6 years of age	Consult a doctor.
Children 6 to under 12 years of age	**1–2 teaspoonfuls (12.5 to 25 mg)** every 4 to 6 hours. Not to exceed 12 teaspoonfuls in 24 hours.
Adults and children 12 years of age and over	**2–4 teaspoonfuls (25 to 50 mg)** every 4 to 6 hours. Not to exceed 24 teaspoonfuls in 24 hours.

Warnings: May cause excitability especially in children. Do not take this product, unless directed by a doctor, if you have a breathing problem such as emphysema or chronic bronchitis, or if you have glaucoma or difficulty in urination due to enlargement of the prostate gland. May cause marked drowsiness; alcohol, sedatives, and tranquilizers may increase the drowsiness effect. Avoid alcoholic beverages while taking this product. Do not take this product if you are taking sedatives or tranquilizers, without first consulting your doctor. Use caution when driving a motor vehicle or operating machinery. **Do not use any other products containing diphenhydramine while using this product.** As with any drug, if you are pregnant or nursing a baby, seek the advice of a health professional before using this product. KEEP THIS AND ALL DRUGS OUT OF THE REACH OF CHILDREN. In case of accidental overdose, seek professional assistance or contact a Poison Control Center immediately.

How Supplied: Benadryl Dye-Free Allergy Liquid Medication is supplied in 4 fl. oz. bottles.

Store at 59°–77°F.
Protect from freezing.
Shown in Product Identification Guide, page 517

BENADRYL® Dye-Free Allergy Liqui-Gels® Softgel
[bĕ 'nă-drĭl]

Active Ingredients: Each softgel contains: Diphenhydramine Hydrochloride 25 mg.

Inactive Ingredients: Gelatin, Glycerin, Polyethylene Glycol 400 and Sorbitol.

Indications: Temporarily relieves runny nose and sneezing, itching of the nose or throat, and itchy, watery eyes due

to hay fever or other upper respiratory allergies, and runny nose and sneezing associated with the common cold.

Directions: Follow dosage recommendations below, or use as directed by your doctor.

Benadryl® Dye-Free Allergy
Liqui-Gels® Softgel

AGE	DOSAGE
Adults and children 12 years of age and over	25 to 50 mg (1 to 2 softgels) every 4 to 6 hours. Not to exceed 12 softgels in 24 hours.
Children 6 to under 12 years of age See ** symbol below	12.5** to 25 mg (1 softgel) every 4 to 6 hours. Not to exceed 6 softgels in 24 hours.
Children under 6 years of age	Consult a doctor.

**12.5 mg dosage strength is not available in this package. Do not attempt to break softgels. This dosage is available in bubble gum flavored Benadryl® Dye-Free Allergy Liquid Medication.

Warnings: May cause excitability especially in children. Do not take this product, unless directed by a doctor, if you have a breathing problem such as emphysema or chronic bronchitis, or if you have glaucoma or difficulty in urination due to enlargement of the prostate gland. May cause marked drowsiness; alcohol, sedatives, and tranquilizers may increase the drowsiness effect. Avoid alcoholic beverages while taking this product. Do not take this product if you are taking sedatives or tranquilizers, without first consulting your doctor. Use caution when driving a motor vehicle or operating machinery. **Do not use any other products containing diphenhydramine while using this product.** As with any drug, if you are pregnant or nursing a baby, seek the advice of a health professional before using this product. KEEP THIS AND ALL DRUGS OUT OF THE REACH OF CHILDREN. In case of accidental overdose, seek professional assistance or contact a Poison Control Center immediately.

How Supplied: Benadryl® Dye-Free Allergy Liqui-Gels® Softgels are supplied in boxes of 24.

Store at 59° to 77°F in a dry place.

Liqui-Gels is a registered trademark of R.P. Scherer Corporation.

Shown in Product Identification Guide, page 517

BENADRYL® Allergy Ultratab™ Tablets and Kapseal® Capsules
[bĕ 'nă-drĭl]

Active Ingredients: Each Tablet/Capsule contains: Diphenhydramine Hydrochloride 25 mg.

Inactive Ingredients: Each Tablet contains: Candelilla Wax, Crospovidone, Dibasic Calcium Phosphate Dihydrate, D&C Red No. 27 Aluminum Lake, Hydroxypropyl Methylcellulose, Magnesium Stearate, Microcrystalline Cellulose, Polyethylene Glycol, Polysorbate 80, Pregelatinized Starch, Stearic Acid, and Titanium Dioxide.
Each Capsule contains: Lactose and Magnesium Stearate. The Banded Kapseals capsule shell contains: D&C Red No. 28, FD&C Red No. 3, FD&C Red No. 40, FD&C Blue No. 1, Gelatin, Glyceryl Monooleate, and Titanium Dioxide.

Indications: Temporarily relieves runny nose and sneezing, itching of the nose or throat, and itchy, watery eyes due to hay fever or other upper respiratory allergies, and runny nose and sneezing associated with the common cold.

Directions: Follow dosage directions or use as directed by your doctor. Adults and children 12 years of age and over: 25 to 50 mg (1 to 2 tablets/capsules) every 4 to 6 hours. Not to exceed 12 tablets/capsules in 24 hours. Children 6 to under 12 years of age: 12.5 mg** to 25 mg (1 tablet/capsule) every 4 to 6 hours, not to exceed 6 tablets/capsules in 24 hours. Children under 6 years of age: consult your doctor.

** This dosage is not available in this package. Do not attempt to break tablet/capsule. This dosage is available in pleasant tasting Benadryl Allergy Liquid Medication.

Warnings: May cause excitability especially in children. Do not take this product, unless directed by a doctor, if you have a breathing problem such as emphysema or chronic bronchitis, or if you have glaucoma or difficulty in urination due to enlargement of the prostate gland. May cause marked drowsiness; alcohol, sedatives, and tranquilizers may increase the drowsiness effect. Avoid alcoholic beverages while taking this product. Do not take this product if you are taking sedatives or tranquilizers, without first consulting your doctor. Use caution when driving a motor vehicle or operating machinery. **Do not use any other products containing diphenhydramine while using this product.** As with any drug, if you are pregnant or nursing a baby, seek the advice of a health professional before using this product. KEEP THIS AND ALL DRUGS OUT OF THE REACH OF CHILDREN. In case of accidental overdose, seek professional assistance or contact a Poison Control Center immediately.

How Supplied: Benadryl tablets are supplied in boxes of 24 and 48, bottle of 100; capsules are supplied in boxes of 24 and 48.
Store at 59° to 77°F in a dry place.
Shown in Product Identification Guide, page 516

BENADRYL® ALLERGY/COLD TABLETS
[bĕ 'nă-drĭl]

Active Ingredients: Each tablet contains: Diphenhydramine Hydrochloride 12.5 mg, Pseudoephedrine Hydrochloride 30 mg and Acetaminophen 500 mg.

Inactive Ingredients: Candelilla Wax, Croscarmellose Sodium, Hydroxypropyl Cellulose, Hydroxypropyl Methylcellulose, Magnesium Stearate, Microcrystalline Cellulose, Polyethylene Glycol, Pregelatinized Starch, Propylene Glycol, Sodium Starch Glycolate, Starch, Stearic Acid, Titanium Dioxide, and Zinc Stearate. Printed with edible blue ink.

Indications: For the temporary relief of minor aches, pains, headache, muscular aches, sore throat, fever, runny nose and sneezing, itching of the nose or throat, and itchy, watery eyes due to hay fever, and nasal congestion due to the common cold.

Directions: Follow dosage recommendations, or use as directed by your doctor. Adults and children 12 years of age and over: two (2) tablets every 6 hours while symptoms persist. Not to exceed 8 tablets in 24 hours. Children under 12 years of age: consult a doctor.

Warnings: Do not exceed recommended dosage. If nervousness, dizziness, or sleeplessness occur, discontinue use and consult a doctor. Do not take this product for more than 10 days. If symptoms do not improve or are accompanied by fever that lasts for more than 3 days, or if new symptoms occur, consult a doctor. If sore throat is severe, persists for more than 2 days, is accompanied or followed by fever, headache, rash, nausea, or vomiting, consult a doctor promptly. Do not take this product, unless directed by a doctor, if you have a breathing problem such as emphysema or chronic bronchitis, heart disease, high blood pressure, thyroid disease, diabetes, or if you have glaucoma or difficulty in urination due to enlargement of the prostate gland. May

Continued on next page

This product information was prepared in November 2000. On these and other Pfizer Consumer Healthcare Products, detailed information may be obtained by addressing Pfizer, Inc. Warner-Lambert Consumer Healthcare Products, Morris Plains, NJ 07950

Benadryl Allergy/Cold—Cont.

cause excitability especially in children. May cause marked drowsiness; alcohol, sedatives, and tranquilizers may increase the drowsiness effect. Avoid alcoholic beverages while taking this product. Do not take this product if you are taking sedatives or tranquilizers, without first consulting your doctor. Use caution when driving a motor vehicle or operating machinery. Do not use any other products containing diphenhydramine while using this product. As with any drug, if you are pregnant or nursing a baby, seek the advice of a health professional before using this product. KEEP THIS AND ALL DRUGS OUT OF THE REACH OF CHILDREN. In case of accidental overdose, seek professional assistance or contact a Poison Control Center immediately. Prompt medical attention is critical for adults as well as for children even if you do not notice any signs or symptoms.

Alcohol Warning: If you consume 3 or more alcoholic drinks every day, ask your doctor whether you should take acetaminophen or other pain relievers/fever reducers. Acetaminophen may cause liver damage.

Drug Interaction Precaution: Do not use this product if you are now taking a prescription monoamine oxidase inhibitor (MAOI) (certain drugs for depression, psychiatric or emotional conditions, or Parkinson's disease), or for 2 weeks after stopping the MAOI drug. If you are uncertain whether your prescription drug contains an MAOI, consult a health professional before taking this product.

How Supplied: Benadryl® Allergy/Cold tablets are supplied in boxes of 24 tablets. Store at 59° to 77°F in a dry place.

Shown in Product Identification Guide, page 517

BENADRYL® CHILDREN'S ALLERGY/COLD FASTMELT
[bĕ 'nă-drĭl]
Antihistamine/Cough Suppressant/ Nasal Decongestant

Indications: For the temporary relief of runny nose, sneezing, itching of the nose or throat, itchy, watery eyes and nasal congestion due to hay fever, and runny nose, sneezing and nasal congestion due to the common cold. Temporarily relieves cough due to minor throat and bronchial irritation occurring with the common cold or inhaled irritants.

Directions: Adults and children 12 years of age and over: two (2) tablets every 4 hours. Not to exceed 8 tablets in 24 hours, or as directed by your doctor. Children 6 to under 12 years of age: one (1) tablet every 4 hours. Not to exceed 4 tablets in 24 hours, or as directed by your doctor.

Warnings: Do not exceed recommended dosage. If nervousness, dizziness, or sleeplessness occur, discontinue use and consult a doctor. If symptoms do not improve within 7 days or are accompanied by fever, consult a doctor. A persistent cough may be a sign of a serious condition. If cough persists for more than 1 week, tends to recur, or is accompanied by fever, rash, or persistent headache, consult a doctor. Do not take this product for persistent or chronic cough such as occurs with smoking, asthma, or emphysema, or if cough is accompanied by excessive phlegm (mucus) unless directed by a doctor. Do not take this product, unless directed by a doctor, if you have a breathing problem such as emphysema or chronic bronchitis, heart disease, high blood pressure, thyroid disease, diabetes, or if you have glaucoma or difficulty in urination due to enlargement of the prostate gland. May cause excitability especially in children. May cause marked drowsiness; alcohol, sedatives, and tranquilizers may increase the drowsiness effect. Avoid alcoholic beverages while taking this product. Do not take this product if you are taking sedatives or tranquilizers, without first consulting your doctor. Use caution when driving a motor vehicle or operating machinery. **Do not use any other products containing diphenhydramine while using this product.** As with any drug, if you are pregnant or nursing a baby, seek the advice of a health professional before using this product. KEEP THIS AND ALL DRUGS OUT OF THE REACH OF CHILDREN. In case of accidental overdose, seek professional assistance or contact a Poison Control Center immediately. **Phenylketonurics: Contains Phenylalanine 1.2 mg Per Tablet**

Drug Interaction Precaution: Do not use this product if you are now taking a prescription monoamine oxidase inhibitor (MAOI) (certain drugs for depression, psychiatric or emotional conditions, or Parkinson's disease), or for 2 weeks after stopping the MAOI drug. If you are uncertain whether your prescription drug contains an MAOI, consult a health professional before taking this product.

Active Ingredients: Each tablet contains: Diphenhydramine Citrate 19 mg and Pseudoephedrine Hydrochloride 30 mg. Also contains: Aspartame, Citric Acid, Ethylcellulose, D&C Red No. 7 Calcium Lake, Flavor, Lactitol, Magnesium Stearate, Mannitol, and Stearic Acid. Store at 59° to 77°F in a dry place.

How Supplied: Cherry Flavor: Available in 20 dissolving tablets.
Shown in Product Identification Guide, page 517

BENADRYL®
Allergy/Congestion Tablets
[bĕ 'nă-drĭl]

Active Ingredients: Each tablet contains: Diphenhydramine Hydrochloride 25 mg and Pseudoephedrine Hydrochloride 60 mg.

Inactive Ingredients: Each tablet contains: Croscarmellose Sodium, Dibasic Calcium Phosphate Dihydrate, FD&C Blue No. 1 Aluminum Lake, Hydroxypropyl Methylcellulose, Microcrystalline Cellulose, Polyethylene Glycol, Polysorbate 80, Pregelatinized Starch, Stearic Acid, Titanium Dioxide and Zinc Stearate.

Indications: Temporarily relieves nasal congestion, runny nose and sneezing, itching of the nose or throat, and itchy, watery eyes due to hay fever or other upper respiratory allergies, and runny nose, sneezing, and nasal congestion associated with the common cold.

Directions: Follow dosage recommendation, or use as directed by your doctor. Adults and children 12 years of age and over: one (1) tablet every 4 to 6 hours, not to exceed 4 tablets in 24 hours. Children under 12 years of age: consult a doctor.

Warning: Do not exceed recommended dosage. If nervousness, dizziness, or sleeplessness occur, discontinue use and consult a doctor. If symptoms do not improve within 7 days or are accompanied by fever, consult a doctor. Do not take this product, unless directed by a doctor, if you have a breathing problem such as emphysema or chronic bronchitis, heart disease, high blood pressure, thyroid disease, diabetes, or if you have glaucoma or difficulty in urination due to enlargement of the prostate gland. May cause excitability especially in children. May cause marked drowsiness; alcohol, sedatives, and tranquilizers may increase the drowsiness effect. Avoid alcoholic beverages while taking this product. Do not take this product if you are taking sedatives or tranquilizers, without first consulting your doctor. Use caution when driving a motor vehicle or operating machinery. Do not use any other products containing diphenhydramine while using this product. As with any drug, if you are pregnant or nursing a baby, seek the advice of a health professional before using this product. KEEP THIS AND ALL DRUGS OUT OF THE REACH OF CHILDREN. In case of accidental overdose, seek professional assistance or contact a Poison Control Center immediately.

Drug Interaction Precaution: Do not use this product if you are now taking a prescription monoamine oxidase inhibitor (MAOI) (certain drugs for depression, psychiatric or emotional conditions, or Parkinson's disease), or for 2 weeks after stopping the MAOI drug. If you are uncertain whether your prescription drug contains an MAOI, consult a health professional before taking this product.

How Supplied: Benadryl Allergy/Congestion Tablets are supplied in boxes of 24.

Store at 59° to 77°F in a dry place.
Shown in Product Identification Guide, page 517

BENADRYL®
[bĕ'nădrĭl]
Antihistamine/Nasal Decongestant
For Allergy Plus Sinus Pressure Relief

[See table above right]

Inactive Ingredients: Aspartame, citric acid, ethylcellulose, D&C red no. 7 calcium lake, flavor, lactitol, magnesium stearate, mannitol, and stearic acid

Uses:
- temporarily relieves these symptoms of hay fever or the common cold:
- runny nose
- sneezing
- nasal congestion
- temporarily relieves these additional symptoms of hay fever:
- itching of the nose or throat
- itchy, watery eyes

Warnings:
Do not use:
- if you are now taking a prescription monoamine oxidase inhibitor (MAOI) (certain drugs for depression, psychiatric or emotional conditions, or Parkinson's disease), or for 2 weeks after stopping the MAOI drug. If you do not know if your prescription drug contains an MAOI, ask a doctor or pharmacist before taking this product.
- with any other product containing diphenhydramine, including one applied topically.

Ask a doctor before use if you have:
- heart disease
- high blood pressure
- thyroid disease
- trouble urinating due to an enlarged prostate gland
- diabetes
- glaucoma
- a breathing problem such as emphysema or chronic bronchitis

Ask a doctor or pharmacist before use if you are taking sedatives or tranquilizers
When using this product:
- **do not use more than directed**
- marked drowsiness may occur
- avoid alcoholic drinks
- excitability may occur, especially in children
- alcohol, sedatives, and tranquilizers may increase drowsiness
- be careful when driving a motor vehicle or operating machinery

Stop use and ask a doctor if:
- you get nervous, dizzy or sleepless
- symptoms do not improve within 7 days or are accompanied by fever
If pregnant or breast-feeding, ask a health professional before use.
Keep out of reach of children. In case of overdose, get medical help or contact a Poison Control Center right away.

Directions:
- adults and children 12 years of age and over: 2 tablets
- place in mouth and allow to dissolve
- take every 4 to 6 hours
- do not take more than 8 tablets in 24 hours, or as directed by a doctor
Other information:
- **Phenylketonurics:** Contains Phenylalanine 1.2 mg Per Tablet
- Store at 59° to 77°F in a dry place
How Supplied: Available in 20 count dissolving tablets.

Shown in Product Identification Guide, page 517

Active Ingredients (in each tablet):	Purposes:
Diphenhydramine citrate 19 mg*	Antihistamine
Pseudoephedrine HCl 30 mg	Nasal decongestant

*equivalent to 12.5 mg of diphenhydramine HCl

BENADRYL®
Allergy & Sinus
Liquid Medication
[bĕ 'nă-drĭl]

Active Ingredients: Each teaspoonful (5 mL) contains: Diphenhydramine Hydrochloride 12.5 mg and Pseudoephedrine Hydrochloride 30 mg.

Inactive Ingredients: Citric Acid, FD&C Blue No. 1, FD&C Red No. 40, Flavors, Glycerin, Poloxamer 407, Polysorbate 20, Purified Water, Saccharin Sodium, Sodium Benzoate, Sodium Chloride, Sodium Citrate and Sorbitol Solution.

Indications: Temporarily relieves nasal congestion, runny nose and sneezing, itching of the nose or throat, and itchy, watery eyes due to hay fever or other upper respiratory allergies, and runny nose, sneezing, and nasal congestion associated with the common cold.

Directions: Follow dosage recommendations below, or use as directed by your doctor.

Benadryl® Allergy & Sinus
Liquid Medication

AGE	DOSAGE
Children under 6 years of age	Consult a doctor.
Children 6 to under 12 years of age	One (1) teaspoonful every 4 to 6 hours. Not to exceed 4 teaspoonfuls in 24 hours.
Adults and children 12 years of age and over	Two (2) teaspoonfuls every 4 to 6 hours. Not to exceed 8 teaspoonfuls in 24 hours.

Warnings: Do not exceed recommended dosage. If nervousness, dizziness, or sleeplessness occur, discontinue use and consult a doctor. If symptoms do not improve within 7 days or are accompanied by fever, consult a doctor. Do not take this product, unless directed by a doctor, if you have a breathing problem such as emphysema or chronic bronchitis, heart disease, high blood pressure, thyroid disease, diabetes, or if you have glaucoma or difficulty in urination due to enlargement of the prostate gland. May cause excitability especially in children. May cause marked drowsiness; alcohol, sedatives, and tranquilizers may increase the drowsiness effect. Avoid alcoholic beverages while taking this product. Do not take this product if you are taking sedatives or tranquilizers, without first consulting your doctor. Use cau-

---

tion when driving a motor vehicle or operating machinery. **Do not use any other products containing diphenhydramine while using this product.** As with any drug, if you are pregnant or nursing a baby, seek the advice of a health professional before using this product. KEEP THIS AND ALL DRUGS OUT OF THE REACH OF CHILDREN. In case of accidental overdose, seek professional assistance or contact a Poison Control Center immediately.

Drug Interaction Precaution: Do not use this product if you are now taking a prescription monoamine oxidase inhibitor (MAOI) (certain drugs for depression, psychiatric or emotional conditions, or Parkinson's disease), or for 2 weeks after stopping the MAOI drug. If you are uncertain whether your prescription drug contains an MAOI, consult a health professional before taking this product.

How Supplied: Benadryl Allergy & Sinus Liquid Medication is supplied in 4 fl. oz. bottles.
Store at room temperature (59°–86°F). Protect from freezing.
Shown in Product Identification Guide, page 517

BENADRYL® Allergy Sinus
Headache Caplets & Gelcaps
[bĕ 'nă-drĭl]

Action: BENADRYL ALLERGY/SINUS HEADACHE is specially formulated to provide effective relief of your upper respiratory allergy symptoms complicated by sinus and headache problems. It combines the strength of BENADRYL to relieve your runny nose, sneezing, itchy, water eyes, itchy nose or throat, with a maximum strength NASAL DECONGESTANT to relieve nasal and sinus congestion, and a maximum strength non-aspirin PAIN RELIEVER to relieve sinus pain and headache.

Active Ingredients: Each caplet and gelcap contains Diphenhydramine Hydrochloride 12.5 mg, Pseudoephedrine Hydrochloride 30 mg and Acetaminophen 500 mg.

Inactive Ingredients: For Caplet: Candelilla Wax, Croscarmellose Sodium,

Continued on next page

This product information was prepared in November 2000. On these and other Pfizer Consumer Healthcare Products, detailed information may be obtained by addressing Pfizer, Inc. Warner-Lambert Consumer Healthcare Products, Morris Plains, NJ 07950

Benadryl All./Sinus—Cont.

D&C Yellow No. 10 Aluminum Lake, FD&C Blue No. 1 Aluminum Lake, FD&C Yellow No. 6 Aluminum Lake, Hydroxypropyl Cellulose, Hydroxypropyl Methylcellulose, Microcrystalline Cellulose, Polyethylene Glycol, Polysorbate 80, Pregelatinized Starch, Sodium Starch Glycolate, Starch, Stearic Acid, Titanium Dioxide, and Zinc Stearate.

For Gelcaps: Colloidal Silicon Dioxide, Croscarmellose Sodium, D&C Yellow No. 10 Aluminum Lake, FD&C Green No. 3 Aluminum Lake, Gelatin, Hydroxypropyl Methylcellulose, Polysorbate 80, Sodium Lauryl Sulfate, Stearic Acid, and Titanium Dioxide.

Indications: For the temporary relief of minor aches, pains, and headache, runny nose and sneezing, itching of the nose or throat, and itchy, watery eyes due to hay fever, and nasal congestion due to the common cold, hay fever, or other upper respiratory allergies. Helps decongest sinus openings and passages; temporarily relieves sinus congestion and pressure.

Directions: Adults and children 12 years of age and over: two (2) caplets or gelcaps every 6 hours while symptoms persist. Not to exceed 8 caplets or gelcaps in 24 hours. Children under 12 years of age: consult a doctor.

Warnings: Do not exceed recommended dosage. If nervousness, dizziness, or sleeplessness occur, discontinue use and consult a doctor. Do not take this product for more than 10 days. If symptoms do not improve or are accompanied by fever that lasts for more than 3 days, or if new symptoms occur, consult a doctor. Do not take this product, unless directed by a doctor, if you have a breathing problem such as emphysema or chronic bronchitis, heart disease, high blood pressure, thyroid disease, diabetes, or if you have glaucoma or difficulty in urination due to enlargement of the prostate gland. May cause excitability especially in children. May cause marked drowsiness; alcohol, sedatives, and tranquilizers may increase the drowsiness effect. Avoid alcoholic beverages while taking this product. Do not take this product if you are taking sedatives or tranquilizers, without first consulting your doctor. Use caution when driving a motor vehicle or operating machinery. Do not use any other products containing diphenhydramine while using this product. As with any drug, if you are pregnant or nursing a baby, seek the advice of a health professional before using this product. KEEP THIS AND ALL DRUGS OUT OF THE REACH OF CHILDREN. In case of accidental overdose, seek professional assistance or contact a Poison Control Center immediately. Prompt medical attention is critical for adults as well as for children even if you do not notice any signs or symptoms.

Alcohol Warning: If you consume 3 or more alcoholic drinks every day, ask your doctor whether you should take acetaminophen or other pain relievers/fever reducers. Acetaminophen may cause liver damage.

Drug Interaction Precaution: Do not use this product if you are now taking a prescription monoamine oxidase inhibitor (MAOI) (certain drugs for depression, psychiatric or emotional conditions, or Parkinson's disease), or for 2 weeks after stopping the MAOI drug. If you are uncertain whether your prescription drug contains an MAOI, consult a health professional before taking this product.

How Supplied: Benadryl Allergy Sinus Headache is available in boxes of 24 and 48 caplets, and box of 24 gelcaps. Store at 59°–77° in a dry place. Protect from moisture.

Shown in Product Identification Guide, page 517

BENADRYL® SEVERE ALLERGY & SINUS HEADACHE† MAXIMUM STRENGTH
[bĕ′nă drĭl]
Antihistamine/Nasal Decongestant/ Pain Reliever
†Upper Respiratory Allergies Only

Benadryl Severe Allergy & Sinus Headache is specially formulated to provide effective relief of your upper respiratory allergy symptoms complicated by sinus and headache problems. It combines the maximum strength of BENADRYL to relieve your runny nose, sneezing, itchy, watery eyes, itchy nose or throat, with a maximum strength NASAL DECONGESTANT to relieve nasal and sinus congestion, and a maximum strength non-aspirin PAIN RELIEVER to relieve sinus pain and headache.

Indications: For the temporary relief of minor aches, pains, and headache, runny nose and sneezing, itching of the nose or throat, and itchy, watery eyes due to hay fever, and nasal congestion due to the common cold, hay fever, or other respiratory allergies. Helps decongest sinus openings and passages; temporarily relieves sinus congestion and pressure.

Directions: Follow dosage recommendations below, or use as directed by a doctor.
[See table below]

Warnings: Do not exceed recommended dosage. If nervousness, dizziness, or sleeplessness occur, discontinue use and consult a doctor. Do not take this product for more than 10 days. If symptoms do not improve or are accompanied by fever that lasts for more than 3 days, or if new symptoms occur, consult a doctor. Do not take this product, unless directed by a doctor, if you have a breathing problem such as emphysema or chronic bronchitis, heart disease, high blood pressure, thyroid disease, diabetes, or if you have glaucoma or difficulty in urination due to enlargement of the prostate gland. May cause excitability especially in children. May cause marked drowsiness; alcohol, sedatives, and tranquilizers may increase the drowsiness effect. Avoid alcoholic beverages while taking this product. Do not take this product if you are taking sedatives or tranquilizers, without first consulting your doctor. Use caution when driving a motor vehicle or operating machinery. Do not use any other products containing diphenhydramine while using this product. As with any drug, if you are pregnant or nursing a baby, seek the advice of a health professional before using this product. KEEP THIS AND ALL DRUGS OUT OF THE REACH OF CHILDREN. In case of accidental overdose, seek professional assistance or contact a Poison Control Center immediately. Prompt medical attention is critical for adults as well as for children even if you do not notice any signs or symptoms.

Alcohol Warning: If you consumer 3 or more alcoholic drinks every day, ask your doctor whether you should take acetaminophen or other pain relievers/fever reducers. Acetaminophen may cause liver damage.

Drug Interaction Precaution: Do not use this product if you are now taking a prescription monoamine oxidase inhibitor (MAOI) (certain drugs for depression, psychiatric or emotional conditions, or Parkinson's disease), or for 2 weeks after stopping the MAOI drug. If you are uncertain whether your prescription drug contains an MAOI, consult a health professional before taking this product.

Active Ingredients: Each caplet contains: Diphenhydramine Hydrochloride 25 mg, Pseudoephedrine Hydrochloride 30 mg, and Acetaminophen 500 mg. Also contains: Carnauba Wax, Crospovidone, FD&C Blue No. 1 Aluminum Lake, Hydroxypropyl Methylcellulose, Magnesium Stearate, Microcrystalline Cellulose, Polyethylene Glycol, Polysorbate 80, Povidone, Pregelatinized Starch, Sodium Starch Glycolate, Stearic Acid, and Titanium Dioxide

Store at 59° to 77°F in a dry place and protect from light.

AGE	DOSAGE
Adults and children 12 years of age and over	Two (2) caplets every 6 hours while symptoms persist. Not to exceed 8 caplets in 24 hours.
Children under 12 years of age	Consult a doctor.

How Supplied: Available in 20 Caplets (capsule-shaped tablets).

Shown in Product Identification Guide, page 517

BENADRYL® Itch Relief Stick Extra Strength
Topical Analgesic/Skin Protectant
[bě 'nă-drĭl]

Active Ingredients: Diphenhydramine Hydrochloride 2%, Zinc Acetate 0.1%.

Inactive Ingredients: Alcohol 73.5% v/v, Glycerin, Povidone, Purified Water and Tromethamine.

Indications: For the temporary relief of itching and pain associated with insect bites, minor skin irritations and rashes due to poison ivy, poison oak, or poison sumac. Dries the oozing and weeping of poison ivy, poison oak and poison sumac.

Warnings: FOR EXTERNAL USE ONLY. Do not use on chicken pox, measles, blisters, or on extensive areas of skin, except as directed by a physician. Avoid contact with the eyes. If condition worsens, or does not improve within 7 days or if symptoms persist for more than 7 days or clear up and occur again within a few days, discontinue use of this product and consult a physician. Do not use on children under 6 years of age without consulting a physician. **Do not use any other drugs containing diphenhydramine while using this product.** KEEP THIS AND ALL DRUGS OUT OF THE REACH OF CHILDREN. In case of accidental ingestion, seek professional assistance or contact a Poison Control Center immediately. Flammable. Keep away from fire or flame.

Directions: Adults and children 6 years of age and older: Apply to the affected area not more than 3 to 4 times daily. Children under 6 years of age: Consult a physician.

How Supplied: Benadryl® Itch Relief Stick is available in a .47 fl. oz (14 mL) dauber.

Shown in Product Identification Guide, page 517

BENADRYL® Itch Stopping Cream
Original Strength & Extra Strength
[bě 'nă-drĭl]

Active Ingredients:
Original Strength: Diphenhydramine Hydrochloride 1% and Zinc Acetate 0.1%.
Extra Strength: Diphenhydramine Hydrochloride 2% and Zinc Acetate 0.1%.

Inactive Ingredients: Cetyl Alcohol, Diazolidinyl Urea, Methylparaben, Polyethylene Glycol Monostearate 1000, Propylene Glycol, Propylparaben and Purified Water.

Indications: For the temporary relief of itching and pain associated with insect bites, minor skin irritations and rashes due to poison ivy, poison oak or poison sumac. Dries the oozing and weeping of poison ivy, poison oak and poison sumac.

Actions: Benadryl Itch Stopping Cream:
• Stops your itch at the source by blocking the histamine that causes itch.
• Provides local anesthetic itch and pain relief in a greaseless vanishing cream.
• Blocks the histamine hydrocortisone can't.
Original Strength:
• Contains 1% diphenhydramine hydrochloride - for itch relief that is appropriate for the whole family to use (ages 2 and up).
Extra Strength:
• Contains the maximum amount of diphenhydramine hydrochloride - for times when you need extra strength itch relief.

Warnings: FOR EXTERNAL USE ONLY.
Original Strength: Do not use on chicken pox, measles, blisters or on extensive areas of skin, except as directed by a physician. Avoid contact with the eyes. If condition worsens, or does not improve within 7 days or if symptoms persist for more than 7 days or clear up and occur again within a few days, discontinue use of this product and consult a physician. Do not use on children under 2 years of age without consulting a physician. **Do not use any other drugs containing diphenhydramine while using this product.** KEEP THIS AND ALL DRUGS OUT OF THE REACH OF CHILDREN. In case of accidental ingestion, seek professional assistance or contact a Poison Control Center immediately.

Extra Strength: Do not use on chicken pox, measles, blisters or on extensive areas of skin, except as directed by a physician. Avoid contact with the eyes. If condition worsens, or does not improve within 7 days or if symptoms persist for more than 7 days or clear up and occur again within a few days, discontinue use of this product and consult a physician. Do not use on children under 12 years of age without consulting a physician. **Do not use any other drugs containing diphenhydramine while using this product.** KEEP THIS AND ALL DRUGS OUT OF THE REACH OF CHILDREN. In case of accidental ingestion, seek professional assistance or contact a Poison Control Center immediately.

Directions: Original Strength: Adults and children 2 years of age and older: Apply to affected area not more than 3 to 4 times daily. Children under 2 years of age: Consult a physician. Extra Strength: Adults and children 12 years of age and older: Apply to affected area not more than 3 to 4 times daily. Children under 12 years of age: Consult a physician.

How Supplied: Benadryl Itch Stopping Cream is available in 1 oz (28.3 g) Original Strength and 1 oz (28.3 g) Extra Strength tubes.

Shown in Product Identification Guide, page 517

BENADRYL® Itch Stopping Gel
Original Strength & Extra Strength
[bě 'nă-drĭl]

Active Ingredients:
Original Strength: Diphenhydramine Hydrochloride 1%.
Extra Strength: Diphenhydramine Hydrochloride 2%.

Inactive Ingredients: SD Alcohol 38B, Camphor, Citric Acid, Diazolidinyl Urea, Glycerin, Hydroxypropyl Methylcellulose, Methylparaben, Propylene Glycol, Propylparaben, Purified Water, and Sodium Citrate.

Indications: For the temporary relief of itching and pain associated with insect bites, minor skin irritations and rashes due to poison ivy, poison oak or poison sumac.

Actions: Original Strength: Benadryl Original Strength Gel stops your itch at the source by blocking the histamine that causes itch. It contains 1% diphenhydramine hydrochloride for itch relief appropriate for the whole family to use (ages 6 and up). It provides local anesthetic itch and pain relief. Benadryl Itch Stopping Gel blocks the histamine hydrocortisone can't!
Extra Strength: Benadryl Extra Strength Gel stops your itch at the source by blocking the histamine that causes itch. It contains the maximum amount of diphenhydramine hydrochloride for times when you need extra stength itch relief. It provides local anesthetic itch and pain relief. Benadryl Itch Stopping Gel blocks the histamine hydrocortisione can't!

Warnings: FOR EXTERNAL USE ONLY.
Do not use on chicken pox, measles, blisters or on extensive areas of skin, except as directed by a physician. Avoid contact with the eyes. If condition worsens, or if symptoms persist for more than 7 days

Continued on next page

This product information was prepared in November 2000. On these and other Pfizer Consumer Healthcare Products, detailed information may be obtained by addressing Pfizer, Inc. Warner-Lambert Consumer Healthcare Products, Morris Plains, NJ 07950

Benadryl Itch Gel—Cont.

or clear up and occur again within a few days, discontinue use of this product and consult a physician. **Do not use any other drugs containing diphenhydramine while using this product.** KEEP THIS AND ALL DRUGS OUT OF THE REACH OF CHILDREN. In case of accidental ingestion, seek professional assistance or contact a Poison Control Center immediately.

Directions: Original Strength: Shake well. Adults and children 6 years of age and older: Apply to affected area not more than 3 to 4 times daily. Children under 6 years of age: Consult a physician.
Extra Strength: Shake well. Adults and children 12 years of age and older: Apply to affected area not more than 3 to 4 times daily. Children under 12 years of age: Consult a physician.

How Supplied: Benadryl Itch Stopping Gel is supplied in 4 fl. oz. (118mL) bottles in both Original and Extra.

Shown in Product Identification Guide, page 517

BENADRYL® Itch Stopping Spray Original Strength & Extra Strength
[bĕ ʹnă-drĭl]

Active Ingredients:
Original Strength: Diphenhydramine Hydrochloride 1% and Zinc Acetate 0.1%.
Extra Strength: Diphenhydramine Hydrochloride 2% and Zinc Acetate 0.1%.

Inactive Ingredients: Alcohol up to 73.6% v/v, Glycerin, Povidone, Purified Water and Tromethamine.

Indications: For the temporary relief of itching and pain associated with insect bites, minor skin irritations and rashes due to poison ivy, poison oak or poison sumac. Dries the oozing and weeping of poison ivy, poison oak and poison sumac.

Warnings: FOR EXTERNAL USE ONLY.
Original Strength: Do not use on chicken pox, measles, blisters or on extensive areas of skin, except as directed by a physician. Avoid contact with the eyes. If condition worsens or does not improve within 7 days, or if symptoms persist for more than 7 days or clear up and occur again within a few days, discontinue use of this product and consult a physician. Do not use on children under 2 years of age without consulting a physician. **Do not use any other drugs containing diphenhydramine while using this product.** KEEP THIS AND ALL DRUGS OUT OF THE REACH OF CHILDREN. In case of accidental ingestion, seek professional assistance or contact a Poison Control Center immediately. Flammable. Keep away from fire or flame.

Extra Strength: Do not use on chicken pox, measles, blisters or on extensive areas of skin, except as directed by a physician. Avoid contact with the eyes. If condition worsens or does not improve within 7 days, or if symptoms persist for more than 7 days or clear up and occur again within a few days, discontinue use of this product and consult a physician. Do not use on children under 12 years of age without consulting a physician. **Do not use any other drugs containing diphenhydramine while using this product.** KEEP THIS AND ALL DRUGS OUT OF THE REACH OF CHILDREN. In case of accidental ingestion, seek professional assistance or contact a Poison Control Center immediately. Flammable. Keep away from fire or flame.

Directions: Original Strength: Adults and children 2 years of age and older: Apply to affected area not more than 3 to 4 times daily. Children under 2 years of age: Consult a physician. Extra Strength: Adults and children 12 years of age and older: Apply to affected area not more than 3 to 4 times daily. Children under 12 years of age: Consult a physician.

How Supplied: Benadryl Itch Stopping Spray Original and Extra Strength is available in a 2 fl. oz. (59mL) pump spray bottle.

Shown in Product Identification Guide, page 517

BENGAY® External Analgesic Products

Description: BENGAY products contain menthol in an alcohol base gel, combinations of methyl salicylate and menthol in cream and ointment bases, as well as a combination of methyl salicylate, menthol and camphor in a non-greasy cream base; all suitable for topical application.
In addition to the Original Formula Pain Relieving Ointment (methyl salicylate, 18.3%; menthol, 16%), BENGAY is offered as BENGAY Greaseless Pain Relieving Cream (methyl salicylate, 15%; menthol, 10%), an Arthritis Formula NonGreasy Pain Relieving Cream (methyl salicylate, 30%; menthol, 8%), an Ultra Strength NonGreasy Pain Relieving Cream (methyl salicylate 30%; menthol 10%; camphor 4%), Vanishing Scent NonGreasy Pain Relieving Gel (2.5% menthol), and S.P.A. (Site Penetrating Action) Pain Relieving Cream (10% menthol) with a fresh scent.

Action and Uses: Methyl salicylate, menthol and camphor are external analgesics which stimulate sensory receptors of warmth and/or cold. This produces a counter-irritant response which provides temporary relief of minor aches and pains of muscles and joints associated with simple backache, arthritis, strains and sprains.

Several double-blind clinical studies of BENGAY products containing menthol-methyl salicylate have shown the effectiveness of this combination in counteracting minor pain of skeletal muscle stress and arthritis.
Three studies involving a total of 102 normal subjects in which muscle soreness was experimentally induced showed statistically significant beneficial results from use of the active product vs. placebo for lowered Muscle Action Potential (spasms), greater rise in threshold of muscular pain and greater reduction in perceived muscular pain.
Six clinical studies of a total of 207 subjects suffering from minor pain due to osteoarthritis and rheumatoid arthritis showed the active product to give statistically significant beneficial results vs. placebo for greater relief of perceived pain, increased range of motion of the affected joints and increased digital dexterity. In two studies designed to measure the effect of topically applied BENGAY vs. placebo on muscular endurance, discomfort, onset of exercise pain and fatigue, 30 subjects performed a submaximal three-hour run and another 30 subjects performed a maximal treadmill run. BENGAY was found to significantly decrease the discomfort during the submaximal and maximal runs, and increase the time before onset of fatigue during the maximal run.
Applied before workouts, BENGAY relaxes tight muscles and increases circulation to make exercising more comfortable, longer.
To help reduce muscle ache and soreness after exercise, BENGAY can be applied and allowed to work before taking a shower.

Directions: Apply generously and gently massage into painful area until BENGAY disappears. Repeat 3 to 4 times daily.

Warnings: For external use only. Do not use with a heating pad. Keep away from children to avoid accidental poisoning. Do not bandage tightly. Do not swallow. If swallowed, induce vomiting and call a physician. Keep away from eyes, mucous membranes, broken or irritated skin. If skin redness or irritation develops, pain lasts for more than 10 days, or with arthritis—like conditions in children under 12, do not use and call a physician.
Shown in Product Identification Guide, page 518

BENYLIN® Adult Formula Cough Suppressant
[bĕ ʹ-nă-lĭn]

Active Ingredient: Each teaspoonful (5 mL) contains: Dextromethorphan Hydrobromide 15 mg.

Inactive Ingredients: Caramel, Citric Acid, D&C Red No. 33, FD&C Red No. 40, Flavors, Glycerin, Poloxamer 407,

Polysorbate 20, Purified Water, Saccharin Sodium, Sodium Benzoate, Sodium Carboxymethyl Cellulose, Sodium Citrate, and Sorbitol Solution.

Indication: Temporarily relieves cough due to minor throat and bronchial irritation occurring with the common cold.

Directions: Follow dosage recommendations below, or as directed by a doctor. Dosage may be repeated every 6 to 8 hours, not to exceed 4 doses in 24 hours.

Benylin® Adult Formula

AGE	DOSAGE
Adults and children 12 years of age and over	Two (2) teaspoonfuls
Children 6 to under 12 years of age	One (1) teaspoonful
Children 2 to under 6 years of age	One-half (¹/₂) teaspoonful
Children under 2 years of age	Consult a doctor

Warnings: A persistent cough may be a sign of a serious condition. If cough persists for more than 1 week, tends to recur, or is accompanied by fever, rash or persistent headache, consult a doctor. Do not take this product for persistent or chronic cough such as occurs with smoking, asthma, emphysema, or if cough is accompanied by excessive phlegm (mucus) unless directed by a doctor. As with any drug, if you are pregnant or nursing a baby, seek the advice of a health professional before using this product. **KEEP THIS AND ALL DRUGS OUT OF THE REACH OF CHILDREN.** In case of accidental overdose, seek professional assistance or contact a Poison Control Center immediately.

Drug Interaction Precaution: Do not use this product if you are now taking a prescription monoamine oxidase inhibitor (MAOI) (certain drugs for depression, psychiatric or emotional conditions, or Parkinson's disease), or for 2 weeks after stopping the MAOI drug. If you are uncertain whether your prescription drug contains an MAOI, consult a health professional before taking this product.

Store at room temperature (59–86°F).

How Supplied: Benylin Adult Formula is supplied in 4 fl. oz. (118 mL) bottles.

Shown in Product Identification Guide, page 518

BENYLIN® Expectorant
Cough Suppressant/Expectorant
[bĕ '-nă-lĭn]

Active Ingredients: Each teaspoonful (5 mL) contains Guaifenesin 100 mg and Dextromethorphan Hydrobromide 5 mg.

Inactive Ingredients: Caramel, Citric Acid, D&C Red No. 33, Disodium Edetate, FD&C Red No. 40, Flavors, Poloxamer 407, Polyethylene Glycol, Propyl Gallate, Propylene Glycol, Purified Water, Saccharin Sodium, Sodium Benzoate, Sodium Chloride, Sodium Citrate, and Sorbitol Solution.

Indications: Temporarily relieves cough due to minor throat and bronchial irritation occurring with the common cold. Helps loosen phlegm (mucus) and thin bronchial secretions to drain bronchial tubes and make coughs more productive.

Directions: Follow dosage recommendations below, or as directed by a doctor. Dosage may be repeated every 4 hours, not to exceed 6 doses in 24 hours.

Benylin® Expectorant

AGE	DOSAGE
Adults and children 12 years of age and over	Four (4) teaspoonfuls
Children 6 to under 12 years of age	Two (2) teaspoonfuls
Children 2 to under 6 years of age	One (1) teaspoonful
Children under 2 years of age	Consult a doctor

Warning: A persistent cough may be a sign of a serious condition. If cough persists for more than 1 week, tends to recur, or is accompanied by fever, rash, or persistent headache, consult a doctor. Do not take this product for persistent or chronic cough such as occurs with smoking, asthma, chronic bronchitis, or emphysema, or where cough is accompanied by excessive phlegm (mucus) unless directed by a doctor. As with any drug, if you are pregnant or nursing a baby, seek the advice of a health professional before using this product. **KEEP THIS AND ALL DRUGS OUT OF THE REACH OF CHILDREN.** In case of accidental overdose, seek professional assistance or contact a Poison Control Center immediately.

Drug Interaction Precaution: Do not use this product if you are now taking a prescription monoamine oxidase inhibitor (MAOI) (certain drugs for depression, psychiatric or emotional conditions, or Parkinson's disease), or for 2 weeks after stopping the MAOI drug. If you are uncertain whether your prescription drug contains an MAOI, consult a health professional before taking this product. Store at room temperature (59°–86°F).

How Supplied: Benylin Expectorant is available in 4 fl. oz. (118 mL) bottles.

Shown in Product Identification Guide, page 518

BENYLIN® Multi-Symptom Cough
Suppressant/Expectorant/Nasal
Decongestant
[bĕ '-nă-lĭn]

Active Ingredients: Each teaspoonful (5 mL) contains Guaifenesin 100 mg, Pseudoephedrine Hydrochloride 15 mg, and Dextromethorphan Hydrobromide 5 mg.

Inactive Ingredients: Caramel, Citric Acid, D&C Red No. 33, Edetate Disodium, FD&C Red No. 40, Flavors, Poloxamer 407, Polyethylene Glycol 1450, Propyl Gallate, Propylene Glycol, Purified Water, Saccharin Sodium, Sodium Benzoate, Sodium Chloride, Sodium Citrate, and Sorbitol Solution.

Indications: Temporarily relieves cough due to minor throat and bronchial irritation and nasal congestion occurring with the common cold. Helps loosen phlegm (mucus) and thin bronchial secretions to drain bronchial tubes and make coughs more productive.

Directions: Follow dosage recommendations below, or use as directed by a doctor. Dosage may be repeated every 4 hours, not to exceed 4 doses in 24 hours.

Benylin® Multisymptom

AGE	DOSAGE
Adults and children 12 years and over	Four (4) teaspoonfuls
Children 6 to under 12 years of age	Two (2) teaspoonfuls
Children 2 to under 6 years of age	One (1) teaspoonful
Children under 2 years of age	Consult a doctor

Continued on next page

This product information was prepared in November 2000. On these and other Pfizer Consumer Healthcare Products, detailed information may be obtained by addressing Pfizer, Inc. Warner-Lambert Consumer Healthcare Products, Morris Plains, NJ 07950

Benylin Multisymptom—Cont.

Warnings: Do not exceed recommended dosage. If nervousness, dizziness, or sleeplessness occur, discontinue use and consult a doctor. If symptoms do not improve within 7 days or are accompanied by fever, consult a doctor. Do not take this product if you have heart disease, high blood pressure, thyroid disease, diabetes, or difficulty in urination due to enlargement of the prostate gland unless directed by a doctor. A persistent cough may be a sign of a serious condition. If cough persists for more than 1 week, tends to recur, or is accompanied by a fever, rash or persistent headache, consult a doctor. Do not take this product for persistent or chronic cough such as occurs with smoking, asthma, chronic bronchitis, or emphysema, or where cough is accompanied by excessive phlegm (mucus) unless directed by a doctor. As with any drug, if you are pregnant or nursing a baby, seek the advice of a health professional before using this product. **KEEP THIS AND ALL DRUGS OUT OF THE REACH OF CHILDREN.** In case of accidental overdose, seek professional assistance or contact a Poison Control Center immediately.

Drug Interaction Precaution: Do not use this product if you are now taking a prescription monoamine oxidase inhibitor (MAOI) (certain drugs for depression, psychiatric or emotional conditions, or Parkinson's disease), or for 2 weeks after stopping the MAOI drug. If you are uncertain whether your prescription drug contains an MAOI, consult a health professional before taking this product. Store at room temperature (59°–86°F).

How Supplied: Benylin Multisymptom is available in 4 fl. oz. (118 mL) bottles.

Shown in Product Identification Guide, page 518

BENYLIN® Pediatric
Cough Suppressant
[bĕ '-nă-lĭn]

Active Ingredient: Each teaspoonful (5 mL) contains: Dextromethorphan Hydrobromide 7.5 mg.

Inactive Ingredients: Citric Acid, FD&C Blue No. 1, FD&C Red No. 40, Flavors, Glycerin, Poloxamer 407, Polysorbate 20, Purified Water, Saccharin Sodium, Sodium Benzoate, Sodium Carboxymethyl Cellulose, Sodium Citrate, and Sorbitol Solution.

Indications: Temporarily relieves cough due to minor throat and bronchial irritation occurring with the common cold.

Directions: Follow dosage recommendations below, or as directed by a doctor. Dosage may be repeated every 6 to 8 hours, not to exceed 4 doses in 24 hours.

Benylin® Pediatric	
AGE	**DOSAGE**
Children under 2 years of age	Consult a doctor
Children 2 to under 6 years of age	One (1) teaspoonful
Children 6 to under 12 years of age	Two (2) teaspoonfuls
Adults and children 12 years of age and over	Four (4) teaspoonfuls

Warnings: A persistent cough may be a sign of a serious condition. If cough persists for more than 1 week, tends to recur, or is accompanied by fever, rash, or persistent headache, consult a doctor. Do not take this product for persistent or chronic cough such as occurs with smoking, asthma or emphysema, or if cough is accompanied by excessive phlegm (mucus) unless directed by a doctor. As with any drug, if you are pregnant or nursing a baby, seek the advice of a health professional before using this product. **KEEP THIS AND ALL DRUGS OUT OF THE REACH OF CHILDREN**. In case of accidental overdose, seek professional assistance or contact a Poison Control Center immediately.

Drug Interaction Precaution: Do not use this product if you are now taking a prescription monoamine oxidase inhibitor (MAOI) (certain drugs for depression, psychiatric or emotional conditions, or Parkinson's disease), or for 2 weeks after stopping the MAOI drug. If you are uncertain whether your prescription drug contains an MAOI, consult a health professional before taking this product. Store at room temperature (59°–86°F).

How Supplied: Benylin Pediatric is supplied in 4 fl. oz. (118 mL) bottles.
Shown in Product Identification Guide, page 518

BONINE®
(Meclizine hydrochloride)
Chewable Tablets

Action: BONINE (meclizine HCl) is an H₁ histamine receptor blocker of the piperazine side chain group. It exhibits its action by an effect on the Central Nervous System (CNS), possibly by its ability to block muscarinic receptors in the brain.

Indications: BONINE is effective in the management of nausea, vomiting and dizziness associated with motion sickness.

Contraindications: Do not take this product, unless directed by a doctor, if you have a breathing problem such as emphysema or chronic bronchitis, or if you have glaucoma or difficulty in urination due to enlargement of the prostate gland.

Warnings: May cause drowsiness; alcohol, sedatives and tranquilizers may increase the drowsiness effect. Avoid alcoholic beverages while taking this product. Do not take this product if you are taking sedatives or tranquilizers without first consulting your doctor. Do not drive or operate dangerous machinery while taking this medication.

Usage in Children: Clinical studies establishing safety and effectiveness in children have not been done; therefore, usage is not recommended in children under 12 years of age.

Usage in Pregnancy: As with any drug, if you are pregnant or nursing a baby, seek advice of a health care professional before taking this product.

Adverse Reactions: Drowsiness, dry mouth, and on rare occasions, blurred vision have been reported.

Dosage and Administration: For motion sickness, take one or two tablets of Bonine once daily, one hour before travel starts, for up to 24 hours of protection against motion sickness. The tablet can be chewed with or without water or swallowed whole with water. Thereafter, the dose may be repeated every 24 hours for the duration of the travel.

How Supplied: BONINE (meclizine HCl) is available in convenient packets of 8 and 16 chewable tablets of 25 mg. meclizine HCl.

Inactive Ingredients: FD&C Red #40, Lactose, Magnesium Stearate, Purified Siliceous Earth, Raspberry Flavor, Saccharin Sodium, Starch, Talc.
Shown in Product Identification Guide, page 518

CALADRYL® Lotion
CALADRYL® Clear™ Lotion
[că 'lă drĭl "]

Active Ingredients: Caladryl Lotion: Calamine 8%, and Pramoxine Hydrochloride 1%.
Caladryl Clear Lotion: Pramoxine Hydrochloride 1% and Zinc Acetate 0.1%.

Inactive Ingredients: Caladryl Lotion: Alcohol USP, Camphor, Diazolidinyl Urea, Fragrance, Hydroxypropyl Methylcellulose, Methylparaben, Oil of Lavender, Oil of Rosemary, Polysorbate 80, Propylene Glycol, Propylparaben, Purified Water and Xanthan Gum.
Caladryl Clear Lotion: Alcohol USP, Camphor, Citric Acid, Diazolidinyl Urea, Fragrance, Glycerin, Hydroxypropyl Methylcellulose, Methylparaben, Oil of Lavender, Oil of Rosemary, Polysorbate 40, Propylene Glycol, Propylparaben, Purified Water and Sodium Citrate.

Indications: For the temporary relief of itching and pain associated with rashes due to poison ivy, poison oak or poison sumac, insect bites and minor skin irritations. Dries the oozing and weeping of poison ivy, poison oak and poison sumac.

Warnings: FOR EXTERNAL USE ONLY. Avoid contact with the eyes. If condition worsens or does not improve within 7 days, or if symptoms persist for more than 7 days or clear up and occur again within a few days, discontinue use of this product and consult a physician. KEEP THIS AND ALL DRUGS OUT OF THE REACH OF CHILDREN. In case of accidental ingestion, seek professional assistance or contact a Poison Control Center immediately.
Caladryl Clear Lotion: Do not use on children under 2 years of age without consulting a physician.

Directions: SHAKE WELL Before application, wash affected area of skin. Adults and children 2 years of age and older: Apply to affected area not more than 3 to 4 times daily. Children under 2 years of age: Consult a physician.

How Supplied: Caladryl Clear Lotion—6 fl. oz. (177 mL) bottles
Caladryl Lotion—6 fl. oz. (177 mL) bottles
Shown in Product Identification Guide, page 518

CORTIZONE•5®
Creme and Ointment
CORTIZONE FOR KIDS™
Creme Anti-itch
(0.5% hydrocortisone)

Description: CORTIZONE•5® creme (with aloe) and ointment are topical anti-itch preparations.

Active Ingredient: Hydrocortisone 0.5%.

Inactive Ingredients: Creme: Aloe Barbadensis Gel, Aluminum Sulfate, Calcium Acetate, Cetearyl Alcohol, Glycerin, Light Mineral Oil, Maltodextrin, Methylparaben, Potato Dextrin, Propylparaben, Purified Water, Sodium Cetearyl Sulfate, Sodium Lauryl Sulfate, White Petrolatum, White Wax.
Ointment: Aloe Barbadensis Extract, White Petrolatum.

Indications: CORTIZONE•5® is recommended for the temporary relief of itching associated with minor skin irritations, inflammation and rashes due to: eczema, insect bites, poison ivy, oak, sumac, soaps, detergents, cosmetics, jewelry, seborrheic dermatitis, psoriasis, external anal and genital itching. Other uses of this product should be only under the advice and supervision of a doctor.

Warnings: For external use only. Avoid contact with the eyes. If condition worsens, or if symptoms persist for more than 7 days or clear up and occur again within

a few days, stop use of this product and do not begin use of any other hydrocortisone product unless you have consulted a doctor. Do not use in genital area if you have a vaginal discharge, consult a doctor. Do not use for the treatment of diaper rash or for the treatment of chicken pox, consult a doctor.
Warnings For External Anal Itching Users: Do not exceed the recommended daily dosage unless directed by a doctor. In case of bleeding, consult a doctor promptly. Do not put this product into the rectum by using fingers or any mechanical device or applicator.
Keep this and all drugs out of the reach of children. In case of accidental ingestion, seek professional assistance or contact a poison control center immediately.

Dosage and Administration: Adults and children 2 years of age and older: Apply to affected area not more than 3 to 4 times daily. Children under 2 years of age: Do not use, consult a doctor.

Directions For External Anal Itching Users: Adults: When practical, cleanse the affected area with mild soap and warm water and rinse thoroughly. Gently dry by patting or blotting with toilet tissue or a soft cloth before application of this product. Children under 12 years of age: Consult a doctor.

How to Store: Store at controlled room temperature 15°–30°C (59°–86°F).

How Supplied: CORTIZONE•5® creme: 1 oz. and 2 oz. tubes. CORTIZONE•5® ointment: 1 oz. tube. CORTIZONE for KIDS™ creme: $1/2$ oz. and 1 oz. tubes.
Shown in Product Identification Guide, page 518

CORTIZONE•10®
Creme and Ointment
CORTIZONE•10®
Quick Shot Spray

Description: CORTIZONE•10® creme (with aloe), ointment and Quick Shot Spray are topical anti-itch preparations and are the maximum strength available without a prescription.

Active Ingredient: Hydrocortisone 1%.

Inactive Ingredients: Creme: Aloe Barbadensis Gel, Aluminum Sulfate, Calcium Acetate, Cetearyl Alcohol, Glycerin, Light Mineral Oil, Maltodextrin, Methylparaben, Potato Dextrin, Propylparaben, Purified Water, Sodium Cetearyl Sulfate, Sodium Lauryl Sulfate, White Petrolatum, White Wax.
Ointment: White Petrolatum.
Quick Shot Spray: Benzyl Alcohol, Propylene Glycol, Purified Water, SD Alcohol 40-2 (60% v/v).

Indications: Cortizone•10® is recommended for the temporary relief of itching associated with minor skin irritations, inflammation and rashes due to: eczema, insect bites, poison ivy, oak, su-

mac, soaps, detergents, cosmetics, jewelry, seborrheic dermatitis, psoriasis, external anal and genital itching. Other uses of this product should be only under the advice and supervision of a doctor.

Warnings: For external use only. Avoid contact with the eyes. If condition worsens, or if symptoms persist for more than 7 days or clear up and occur again within a few days, stop use of this product and do not begin use of any other hydrocortisone product unless you have consulted a doctor. Do not use in genital area if you have a vaginal discharge, consult a doctor. Do not use for the treatment of diaper rash, consult a doctor.
CORTIZONE•10® Creme and Ointment only: **Warnings For External Anal Itching Users:** Do not exceed the recommended daily dosage unless directed by a doctor. In case of bleeding, consult a doctor promptly. Do not put this product into the rectum by using fingers or any mechanical device or applicator.
Keep this and all drugs out of the reach of children. In case of accidental ingestion, seek professional assistance or contact a poison control center immediately.

Dosage and Administration: Adults and children 2 years of age and older: Apply to affected area not more than 3 to 4 times daily. Children under 2 years of age: Do not use, consult a doctor.
CORTIZONE•10® Creme and Ointment Only:

Directions For External Anal Itching Users: Adults: When practical, cleanse the affected area with mild soap and warm water. Rinse thoroughly. Gently dry by patting or blotting with toilet tissue or a soft cloth before application of this product. Children under 12 years of age: Consult a doctor.

How to Store: Store at controlled room temperature 15°–30°C (59°–86°F).
Quick Shot Spray only:
Flammable—Keep away from fire or flame.

How Supplied: CORTIZONE•10® creme: .5 oz, 1 oz. and 2 oz. tubes. CORTIZONE•10® ointment: 1 oz. and 2 oz. tubes.
CORTIZONE•10® Quick Shot Spray: 1.5 oz. pump bottle.
Shown in Product Identification Guide, page 518

Continued on next page

This product information was prepared in November 2000. On these and other Pfizer Consumer Healthcare Products, detailed information may be obtained by addressing Pfizer, Inc. Warner-Lambert Consumer Healthcare Products, Morris Plains, NJ 07950

CORTIZONE•10® Plus
Creme

Description: CORTIZONE•10® Plus creme is a topical anti-itch preparation containing 10 moisturizers.

Active Ingredient: Hydrocortisone 1%.

Inactive Ingredients: Aloe Barbadensis Gel, Aluminum Sulfate, Calcium Acetate, Cetearyl Alcohol, Cetyl Alcohol, Corn Oil, Glycerin, Isopropyl Palmitate, Light Mineral Oil, Maltodextrin, Methylparaben, Potato Dextrin, Propylene Glycol, Propylparaben, Purified Water, Sodium Cetearyl Sulfate, Sodium Lauryl Sulfate, Vitamin A Palmitate, Vitamin D, Vitamin E, White Petrolatum, White Wax.

Indications: CORTIZONE•10® Plus is recommended for the temporary relief of itching associated with minor skin irritations, inflammation and rashes due to: eczema, insect bites, poison ivy, oak, sumac, soaps, detergents, cosmetics, jewelry, seborrheic dermatitis, psoriasis, external anal and genital itching. Other uses of this product should be only under the advice and supervision of a doctor.

Warnings: For external use only. Avoid contact with the eyes. If condition worsens, or if symptoms persist for more than 7 days or clear up and occur again within a few days, stop use of this product and do not begin use of any other hydrocortisone product unless you have consulted a doctor. Do not use in genital area if you have a vaginal discharge, consult a doctor. Do not use for the treatment of diaper rash consult a doctor.

Warnings For External Anal Itching Users: Do not exceed the recommended daily dosage unless directed by a doctor. In case of bleeding, consult a doctor promptly. Do not put this product into the rectum by using fingers or any mechanical device or applicator.

Keep this and all drugs out of the reach of children. In case of accidental ingestion, seek professional assistance or contact a poison control center immediately.

Dosage and Administration: Adults and children 2 years of age and older: Apply to affected area not more than 3 to 4 times daily. Children under 2 years of age: Do not use, consult a doctor.

Directions For External Anal Itching Users: Adults: When practical, cleanse the affected area with mild soap and warm water and rinse thoroughly. Gently dry by patting or blotting with toilet tissue or a soft cloth before application of this product. Children under 12 years of age: Consult a doctor.

How to Store: Store at controlled room temperature 15°–30°C (59°–86°F).

How Supplied: CORTIZONE•10® Plus creme: 1 oz and 2 oz. tubes.

Shown in Product Identification Guide, page 518

DESITIN® CORNSTARCH BABY POWDER
(with Zinc Oxide)

Description: Desitin Cornstarch Baby Powder combines zinc oxide (10%) with topical starch (cornstarch) for topical application. Also contains: fragrance and tribasic calcium phosphate.

Actions and Uses: Desitin Cornstarch Baby Powder with zinc oxide and topical starch (cornstarch) is designed to protect from wetness, help prevent and treat diaper rash, and other minor skin irritations. It offers all the benefits of a talc-free, absorbent cornstarch powder, but with the addition of zinc oxide, the same protective ingredient found in Desitin Ointment. Cornstarch also prevents friction. Zinc oxide provides an additional physical barrier by forming a protective coating over the skin or mucous membranes which serves to reduce further effects of irritants on affected areas.

Directions: Change wet and soiled diapers promptly, cleanse the diaper area, and allow to dry.
Apply powder close to the body away from child's face. Carefully shake the powder into the diaper or into the hand and apply to diaper area. Apply liberally as often as necessary with each diaper change, especially at bedtime, or anytime when exposure to wet diapers may be prolonged. Use liberally in all body creases, and whenever chafing, prickly heat or other minor skin irritations occur.

Warning: For external use only. Do not use on broken skin. Avoid contact with eyes. Keep powder away from child's face to avoid inhalation. If diaper rash worsens or does not improve within 7 days, consult a doctor.

How Supplied: Desitin Cornstarch Baby Powder with Zinc Oxide is available in 14 ounce (397g) containers with sifter-top caps.

Shown in Product Identification Guide, page 518

DESITIN® CREAMY WITH ALOE and VITAMIN E
Diaper Rash Ointment
(10% Zinc Oxide)

Description: Desitin Creamy with Aloe and Vitamin E contains Zinc Oxide (10%) in a white petrolatum base suitable for topical application. Also contains: aloe barbadensis gel, cyclomethicone, dimethicone, fragrance, methylparaben, microcrystalline wax, mineral oil, propylparaben, purified water, sodium borate, sorbitan sesquioleate, Vitamin E, white petrolatum and white wax.

Actions and Uses: Desitin Creamy treats diaper rash and soothes irritated skin. It also prevents diaper rash by forming a protective barrier that helps seal out wetness and irritants that can cause diaper rash. Desitin Creamy has a pleasant hypoallergenic formula that is easy to apply, easy to clean off, and has a fresh scent.

Directions: 1) Change wet and soiled diapers promptly. 2) Cleanse the diaper area. 3) Allow to dry. 4) Apply ointment liberally as often as necessary, with each diaper change, especially at bedtime or anytime when exposure to wet diapers may be prolonged.

Warnings: For external use only. Avoid contact with eyes. If condition worsens or does not improve within 7 days, consult your doctor. Keep this and all drugs out of the reach of children. In case of accidental ingestion, seek professional assistance or contact a poison control center immediately. Store between 15° and 30°C (59° and 86°F).

How Supplied: Desitin Creamy with Aloe and Vitamin E is available in 2 oz. (57g) and 4 oz. (113g) tubes.

Shown in Product Identification Guide, page 518

DESITIN® OINTMENT

Description: Desitin Ointment combines Zinc Oxide (40%) with Cod Liver Oil in a petrolatum-lanolin base suitable for topical application. Also contains: BHA, fragrance, methylparaben, talc and water.

Actions and Uses: Desitin Ointment helps treat and prevent diaper rash. Desitin also protects chafed skin due to diaper rash and helps seal out wetness. In addition to healing diaper rash, Desitin is excellent first aid to treat and protect minor burns, cuts, scrapes, sunburn, and skin irritations. Use for superficial non-infected wounds and burns only.
Relief and protection is afforded by Zinc Oxide in a unique hypoallergenic formula. This ingredient together with cod liver oil and the petrolatum-lanolin base provide a physical barrier by forming a protective coating over skin or mucous membranes which serves to reduce further effects of irritants on the affected area and relieves burning, pain or itch produced by them.
Several studies have shown the effectiveness of Desitin Ointment in the relief and prevention of diaper rash.
Two clinical studies involving 90 infants demonstrated the effectiveness of Desitin Ointment in curing diaper rash. The diaper rash area was treated with Desitin Ointment at each diaper change for a period of 24 hours, while the untreated site served as controls. A significant reduction was noted in the severity and area of diaper dermatitis on the treated area.
Ninety-seven (97) babies participated in a 12-week study to show that Desitin Ointment helps prevent diaper rash. Approximately half of the infants (49) were treated with Desitin Ointment on a reg-

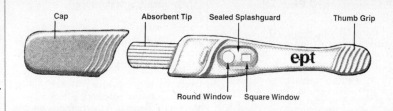

ular daily basis. The other half (48) received the ointment as necessary to treat any diaper rash which occurred. The incidence as well as the severity of diaper rash was significantly less among the babies using the ointment on a regular daily basis.

In a comparative study of the efficacy of Desitin Ointment vs. a baby powder, forty-five (45) babies were observed for a total of eight (8) weeks. Results support the conclusion that Desitin Ointment is a better prophylactic against diaper rash than the baby powder.

In another study, Desitin was found to be dramatically more effective in reducing the severity of medically diagnosed diaper rash than a commercially available diaper rash product in which only anhydrous lanolin and petrolatum were listed as ingredients. Fifty (50) infants participated in the study, half of whom were treated with Desitin and half with the other product. In the group (25) treated with Desitin, seventeen (17) infants showed significant improvement within 10 hours which increased to twenty-three improved infants within 24 hours. Of the group (25) treated with the other product, only three showed improvement at ten hours with a total of four improved within twenty-four hours. These results are statistically valid to conclude that Desitin Ointment reduces severity of diaper rash within ten hours.

Several other studies show that Desitin Ointment helps relieve other skin disorders, such as contact dermatitis.

Directions: To treat and prevent diaper rash, change wet and soiled diapers promptly, cleanse the diaper area and allow to dry. Apply Desitin Ointment liberally as often as necessary, with each diaper change, especially at bedtime or anytime when exposure to wet diapers may be prolonged.

Treatment: If diaper rash is present, or at the first sign of redness, minor skin irritation or chafing, simply apply Desitin Ointment three or four times daily as needed. In superficial noninfected surface wounds and minor burns, apply a thin layer of Desitin Ointment, using a gauze dressing, if necessary. For external use only.

Warnings: For external use only. Avoid contact with eyes. If condition worsens or does not improve within 7 days, consult your doctor. Keep this and all drugs out of the reach of children. In case of accidental ingestion, seek professional assistance or contact a poison control center immediately. Store between 15° and 30°C (59° and 86°F).

How Supplied: Desitin Ointment is available in 1 ounce (28g), 2 ounce (57g),and 4 ounce (114g) tubes, and 9 ounce (255g) and 1 lb. (454g) jars.

Shown in Product Identification Guide, page 518

e.p.t® PREGNANCY TEST
Over 99% Accurate in Laboratory Tests

PLEASE READ INSTRUCTIONS CAREFULLY:
[See graphic above]
How to use: Remove the **e.p.t.** test stick from its foil packet just prior to use. Remove the purple cap to expose the absorbent tip. Hold the test stick by its thumb grip. Point the absorbent tip downward. Place the absorbent tip in the urine flow for just 5 seconds, or dip the absorbent tip into a clean container of urine for just 5 seconds.

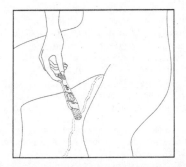

Place the test stick of a flat surface with the windows facing up for at least 3 minutes. (If you wish, replace the cap to cover the absorbent tip.) You may notice a light pink color moving across the windows.
Important: To avoid affecting the test result, wait at least 3 minutes before lifting the stick.

How to Read the Results:
Wait 3 minutes to read the result. A line will appear in the square window showing the test is complete. Be sure to read the result before 20 minutes have passed.

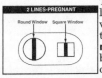

Two distinct parallel lines, one in each window, indicate that you are **pregnant**. The lines can be different shades of pink. Please see your doctor to discuss your pregnancy and the next steps. Early prenatal care is important to ensure the health of you and your baby.

One line in the square window but none in the round window indicates that you are **not pregnant**. If your period does not

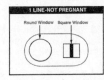

start within a week, repeat the test. If you still get a negative result and your period has not started, please see your doctor.

Important: If no line appears in the square window, the test result is invalid. Do not read the result. Call toll-free number 1-800-378-1783 (1-800-EPT-1STEP).

Questions? Call toll-free 1-800-378-1783 Registered nurses available 8:30 am - 5:00 pm EST weekdays, consumer specialists available until 8:00 pm, and recorded help available 24 hours, (including weekends).

Questions and Answers about e.p.t.®
When can I use e.p.t?
e.p.t can be used any time of day as soon as you miss your period and any day thereafter.

How does e.p.t work?
e.p.t detects hCG (human Chorionic Gonadotropin), a hormone present in urine only during pregnancy. **e.p.t** can detect hCG in your urine as early as the first day your period is late.

What if the lines in the round and square windows are different shades of pink? As long as 2 parallel lines appear, one in each window, the result is positive, even if the two lines are different shades of pink.

What if I think the test result is incorrect? Following the instructions carefully should yield an accurate reading. If you think the result is incorrect, or if it is difficult to detect a line in the round window, repeat test after 2–3 days with a new **e.p.t** stick.

Are there any factors that can affect the test result? Yes. Certain drugs which contain hCG or are used in combination with hCG (such as Humegon™, Pregnyl, Profasi, Pergonal, APL) and rare medical

Continued on next page

This product information was prepared in November 2000. On these and other Pfizer Consumer Healthcare Products, detailed information may be obtained by addressing Pfizer, Inc. Warner-Lambert Consumer Healthcare Products, Morris Plains, NJ 07950

E.P.T. Pregnancy Test—Cont.

conditions. If you repeat the test and continue to get an unexpected result, contact your doctor.

Using **e.p.t** within 8 weeks of giving birth or having a miscarriage may cause a false positive result. The test may detect hCG still in your system from a previous pregnancy. You should ask your doctor for help in interpreting the result of your **e.p.t** test if you have recently been pregnant.

Factors which should <u>not</u> affect the test result include alcohol, analgesics (pain killers), antibiotics, birth control pills or hormone therapies containing clomiphene citrate (Clomid or Serophen). Store at room temperature 15°–30°C (59°–86°F). FOR IN-VITRO DIAGNOSTIC USE. (NOT FOR INTERNAL USE.) KEEP OUT OF THE REACH OF CHILDREN.

Please call our toll-free number 1-800-378-1783 with any questions about using e.p.t.

Shown in Product Identification Guide, page 518

LISTERINE® Antiseptic
[lĭs 'tərēn]

Active Ingredients: Thymol 0.064%, Eucalyptol 0.092%, Methyl Salicylate 0.060% and Menthol 0.042%.

Inactive Ingredients: Water, Alcohol 26.9%, Benzoic Acid, Poloxamer 407, Sodium Benzoate and Caramel.

Indications: To help prevent and reduce plaque and gingivitis/For bad breath.

Actions: Listerine® Antiseptic has been shown to help prevent and reduce supragingival plaque accumulation and gingivitis when used in a conscientiously applied program of oral hygiene and regular professional care. Its effect on periodontitis has not been determined. Listerine is the only leading nonprescription mouthrinse that has received the American Dental Association's Council on Scientific Affairs Seal of Acceptance for helping to prevent and reduce plaque above the gumline and gingivitis.

Directions: Rinse full strength for 30 seconds with 20 ml ($^2/_3$ fl. ounce or 4 teaspoonfuls) morning and night. If bad breath persists, see your dentist.

Warnings: Do not administer to children under twelve years of age. Keep this and all drugs out of the reach of children. Do not swallow. In case of accidental overdose, seek professional assistance or contact a poison control center immediately.

How Supplied: Listerine® Antiseptic is supplied in 250 ml, 500 ml, 1.0 liter and 1.5 liter bottles, as well as 3 fl. oz. bottles. It is also available to professionals in 3 fl. oz. bottles and in gallons.

Shown in Product Identification Guide, page 518

COOL MINT LISTERINE®
[lĭs 'tərēn]

Active Ingredients: Thymol 0.064%, Eucalyptol 0.092%, Methyl Salicylate 0.060% and Menthol 0.042%.

Inactive Ingredients: Water, Alcohol 21.6%, Sorbitol Solution, Flavor, Poloxamer 407, Benzoic Acid, Sodium Saccharin, Sodium Benzoate and FD&C Green No. 3.

Indications: To help prevent and reduce plaque and gingivitis/For bad breath.

Actions: Cool Mint Listerine® Antiseptic has been shown to help prevent and reduce supragingival plaque accumulation and gingivitis when used in a conscientiously applied program of oral hygiene and regular professional care. Its effect on periodontitis has not been determined. Listerine is the only leading nonprescription mouthrinse that has received the American Dental Association's Council on Scientific Affairs Seal of Acceptance for helping to prevent and reduce plaque above the gumline and gingivitis.

Directions: Rinse full strength for 30 seconds with 20 ml ($^2/_3$ fl. ounce or 4 teaspoonfuls) morning and night. If bad breath persists, see your dentist.

Warnings: Do not administer to children under twelve years of age. Keep this and all drugs out of the reach of children. Do not swallow. In case of accidental overdose, seek professional assistance or contact a poison control center immediately.

How Supplied: Cool Mint Listerine® Antiseptic is supplied in 250 ml, 500 ml, 1.0 liter and 1.5 liter bottles, as well as 3 and 58 fl. oz. bottles. It is also available to professionals in gallon bottles.

Shown in Product Identification Guide, page 518

FRESHBURST LISTERINE®
[lĭs 'tərēn]

Active Ingredients: Thymol 0.064%, Eucalyptol 0.092%, Methyl Salicylate 0.060% and Menthol 0.042%.

Inactive Ingredients: Water, Alcohol 21.6%, Sorbitol Solution, Flavor, Poloxamer 407, Benzoic Acid, Sodium Saccharin, Sodium Benzoate, D&C Yellow No. 10 and FD&C Green No. 3.

Indications: To help prevent and reduce plaque and gingivitis/For bad breath.

Actions: FreshBurst Listerine® Antiseptic has been shown to help prevent and reduce supragingival plaque accumulation and gingivitis when used in a conscientiously applied program of oral hygiene and regular professional care. Its effect on periodontitis has not been

determined. Listerine is the only leading nonprescription mouthrinse that has received the American Dental Association's Council on Scientific Affairs Seal of Acceptance for helping to prevent and reduce plaque above the gumline and gingivitis.

Directions: Rinse full strength for 30 seconds with 20 ml ($^2/_3$ fl. ounce or 4 teaspoonfuls) morning and night. If bad breath persists, see your dentist.

Warnings: Do not administer to children under twelve years of age. Keep this and all drugs out of the reach of children. Do not swallow. In case of accidental overdose, seek professional assistance or contact a poison control center immediately.

How Supplied: FreshBurst Listerine® antiseptic is supplied in 250 ml, 500 ml, 1.0 liter and 1.5 liter bottles, as well as 3 fl. oz. bottles. It is also available to professionals in gallon bottles.

Shown in Product Identification Guide, page 519

TARTAR CONTROL LISTERINE® Antiseptic
[lys'tərĕn]

Active Ingredients: Thymol 0.064%, Eucalyptol 0.092%, Methyl Salicylate 0.060%, and Menthol 0.042.%.

Inactive Ingredients: Water, Alcohol (21.6%), Sorbitol Solution, Flavoring, Poloxamer 407, Sodium Saccharin, Benzoic Acid, Zinc Chloride, Sodium Benzoate, and FD&C Blue # 1.

Actions: To help prevent and reduce plaque and gingivitis, prevent tartar buildup, and fight bad breath. Use Tartar Control Listerine Antiseptic twice daily to help:
• Prevent & Fight Tartar
• Prevent & Reduce Plaque
• Prevent & Reduce Gingivitis
• Fight Bad Breath
• Kill Germs Between Teeth

Tartar Control Listerine® Antiseptic has been shown to help prevent and reduce supragingival plaque accumulation and gingivitis when used in a conscientiously applied program of oral hygiene and regular professional care. Its effect on periodontitis has not been determined. Listerine is the only leading nonprescription mouthrinse that has received the American Dental Association's Council on Scientific Affairs Seal of Acceptance for helping to prevent and reduce plaque above the gumline and gingivitis.

Directions: Rinse full strength for 30 seconds with 20ml (2/3 fluid ounce or 4 teaspoonfuls) morning and night. If bad breath persists, see your dentist. [See graphic at top of next page]

Warnings: Do not administer to children under twelve years of age. **KEEP THIS AND ALL DRUGS OUT OF THE REACH OF CHILDREN.** Do not swallow. In case of accidental ingestion, seek pro-

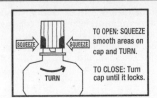

SQUEEZE ← → SQUEEZE

TO OPEN: SQUEEZE smooth areas on cap and TURN.

TURN

TO CLOSE: Turn cap until it locks.

fessional assistance or contact a Poison Control Center immediately. **Cold weather may cloud Tartar Control Listerine. Its antiseptic properties are not affected.** Store at 59° to 77°F.

How Supplied: Tartar Control Listerine® Antiseptic is suppled in 250 ml, 500 ml, 1.0 litter and 1.5 litter bottles, as well as 3 fl. oz. bottles.

Shown in Product Identification Guide, page 519

LISTERMINT®
Alcohol-Free Mouthrinse
[lĭs 'tər mĭnt]

Ingredient: Water, Glycerin, Poloxamer 335, PEG 600, Flavors, Sodium Lauryl Sulfate, Sodium Benzoate, Sodium Saccharin, Benzoic Acid, Zinc Chloride, D&C Yellow No. 10, FD&C Green No. 3.

Indications: Freshens breath; contains no fluoride.

Directions: Rinse with 30 ml (1 fl. oz.) for 30 seconds to freshen breath in the morning and after meals as needed.

Warnings: Do not swallow. Keep out of reach of children.

How Supplied: Listermint® is supplied to consumers in a 32 fl. oz. bottle and is available to professionals in 3 fl. oz. bottles and in gallons.

Shown in Product Identification Guide, page 519

LUBRIDERM®
Skin Therapy Moisturizing Lotion
[lū brĭ dĕrm]

Ingredients: Scented—Water, Mineral Oil, Petrolatum, Sorbitol Solution, Stearic Acid, Lanolin, Lanolin Alcohol, Cetyl Alcohol, Glyceryl Stearate/PEG-100 Stearate, Triethanolamine, Dimethicone, Propylene Glycol, Microcrystalline Wax, Tri(PPG-3 Myristyl Ether) Citrate, Disodium EDTA, Methylparaben, Ethylparaben, Propylparaben, Fragrance, Xanthan Gum, Butylparaben, Methyldibromo Glutaronitrile.
Fragrance Free—Contains Water, Mineral Oil, Petrolatum, Sorbitol Solution, Stearic Acid, Lanolin, Lanolin Alcohol, Cetyl Alcohol, Glyceryl Stearate/PEG-100 Stearate, Triethanolamine, Dimethicone, Propylene Glycol, Microcrystalline Wax, Tri(PPG-3 Myristyl Ether) Citrate, Disodium EDTA, Methylparaben, Eth-

ylparaben, Propylparaben, Xanthan Gum, Butylparaben, Methyldibromo Glutaronitrile.

Uses: Lubriderm provides the essential moisturizing elements that contribute to healthy skin. Its unique combination of emollients penetrate dry skin to effectively moisturize without leaving a greasy feel. Lubriderm helps heal and protect skin from dryness, absorbs rapidly for a clean, natural feel and is non-comedogenic so it won't clog pores.

Directions: Smooth on hands and body every day. Particularly effective when used after showering or bathing. For external use only.

How Supplied:
Scented: Available in 6, 10, 16 and 32 fl. oz. plastic bottles, and a 2.5 fl. oz. tube.
Fragrance Free: Available in 6, 10 and 16 fl. oz. plastic bottles, and a 2.5 fl. oz. and 3.3 fl. oz. tube.

Shown in Product Identification Guide, page 519

LUBRIDERM®
Seriously Sensitive® Lotion
[lū brĭ dĕrm]

Ingredients: Water, Butylene Glycol, Mineral Oil, Petrolatum, Glycerin, Cetyl Alcohol, Propylene Glycol Dicaprylate/Dicaprate, PEG-40 Stearate, C11-13 Isoparaffin, Glyceryl Stearate, Tri (PPG-3 Myristyl Ether) Citrate, Emulsifying Wax, Dimethicone, DMDM Hydantoin, Methylparaben, Carbomer 940, Ethylparaben, Propylparaben, Titanium Dioxide, Disodium EDTA, Sodium Hydroxide, Butylparaben, Xanthan Gum.

Uses: Lubriderm Seriously Sensitive Lotion's unique combination of emollients provides sensitive dry skin with the moisture it needs while helping to create a protective layer. It is non-comedogenic, 100% lanolin free, fragrance free, and dye free so its appropriate for skin that is sensitive to these ingredients. It is nongreasy feeling and absorbs quickly.

Directions: Smooth on hands and body everyday. Particularly effective when used after showering or bathing. For external use only.

How Supplied: Available in 1, 6, 10, and 16 fl. oz. plastic bottles and 3.3 fl. oz. tube.

Shown in Product Identification Guide, page 519

LUBRIDERM® Advanced Therapy
Creamy Lotion
[lū brĭ dĕrm]

Ingredients: Water, Cetyl Alcohol, Glycerin, Mineral Oil, Cyclomethicone, Propylene Glycol Dicaprylate/Dicaprate, PEG-40 Stearate, Isopropyl Isostearate, Emulsifying Wax, Lecithin, Carbomer

940, Diazolidinyl Urea, Titanium Dioxide, Sodium Benzoate, BHT, Tri(PPG-3 Myristyl Ether) Citrate, Disodium EDTA, Retinyl Palmitate, Tocopheryl Acetate, Sodium Pyruvate, Iodopropynyl Butylcarbamate, Fragrance, Sodium Hydroxide, Xanthan Gum.

Uses: Lubriderm Advanced Therapy's nourishing, rich and creamy formula helps heal extra-dry skin. Its unique combination of nutrient-enriched moisturizers penetrate dry skin leaving you with soft, smooth and comfortable skin. This non-greasy feeling lotion absorbs quickly and is non-comedogenic.

Directions: Smooth Lubriderm on hands and body every day. For external use only.

How Supplied: Available in 6, 10, 16 fl. oz plastic bottles and a 3.3 fl. oz. tube.

Shown in Product Identification Guide, page 519

LUBRIDERM® Daily UV Lotion
w/Sunscreen
[lū brĭ dĕrm]

Active Ingredients: Octyl Methoxycinnamate 7.5%, Octyl Salicylate 4%, Oxybenzone 3%. **Inactive Ingredients:** Purified Water, C12-15 Alkyl Benzoate, Cetearyl Alcohol (and) Ceteareth-20, Cetyl Alcohol, Glyceryl Monostearate, Propylene Glycol, Petrolatum, Diazolidinyl Urea, Triethanolamine, Disodium EDTA, Xanthan Gum, Acrylates/C10-30 Alkyl Acrylate Crosspolymer, Tocopheryl Acetate, Iodopropynyl Butylcarbamate, Fragrance, Carbomer.

Actions and Uses: Lubriderm Daily UV Lotion's unique formula combines light, daily moisturization with dermatologist-recommended SPF 15 sun protection. This non-greasy feeling lotion moisturizes dry skin and helps protect against the damaging rays of the sun.

Directions: Apply liberally as often as necessary. Children under 6 months of age: consult a doctor.

Warnings: For external use only. Avoid contact with the eyes. If contact occurs, rinse eyes thoroughly with water. Discontinue use if signs of irritation or rash appear. If irritation or rash persists, consult a doctor. Keep out of reach of children. In case of accidental ingestion, seek professional assistance or contact a Poison Control Center immediately.

Continued on next page

This product information was prepared in November 2000. On these and other Pfizer Consumer Healthcare Products, detailed information may be obtained by addressing Pfizer, Inc. Warner-Lambert Consumer Healthcare Products, Morris Plains, NJ 07950

Lubriderm Daily UV—Cont.

Store between 59°–77°F.

How Supplied: Available in 6, 10, 16 fl. oz plastic bottles and a 3.3 fl. oz. tube.
Shown in Product Identification Guide, page 519

NEOSPORIN® Ointment
[nē ´uh-spō ´rŭn]

Each Gram Contains: Polymyxin B Sulfate 5,000 units, Bacitracin Zinc 400 units and Neomycin 3.5 mg. Also contains a base of Cocoa Butter*, Cottonseed Oil*, Olive Oil*, Sodium Pyruvate*, Tocopheryl Acetate* and White Petrolatum. *U.S. Patent # 5,652,274

Indications: First aid to help prevent infection in minor cuts, scrapes, and burns.

Directions: Clean the affected area. Apply a small amount of this product (an amount equal to the surface area of the tip of a finger) on the area 1 to 3 times daily. May be covered with a sterile bandage.

Warnings: For external use only. Do not use in the eyes or apply over large areas of the body. In case of deep or puncture wounds, animal bites, or serious burns, consult a physician. Stop use and consult a physician if the condition persists or gets worse, or if a rash or other allergic reaction develops. Do not use if you are allergic to any of the ingredients. Do not use longer than 1 week unless directed by a physician. KEEP THIS AND ALL DRUGS OUT OF THE REACH OF CHILDREN. In case of accidental ingestion, seek professional assistance or contact a Poison Control Center immediately.

How Supplied: Tubes, $1/2$ oz (14.2 g) (with applicator tip), 1 oz (28.3 g), $1/32$ oz (0.9 g) foil packets packed 10 per box (Neo To Go™) or 144 per box. Store at 59° to 77°F.
Shown in Product Identification Guide, page 519

NEOSPORIN® + PAIN RELIEF MAXIMUM STRENGTH Cream
[nē ´uh-spō ´rŭn]

Each Gram Contains: Polymyxin B Sulfate 10,000 units, Neomycin 3.5 mg, and Pramoxine Hydrochloride 10 mg. Also contains: Emulsifying Wax, Methylparaben 0.25% (added as a preservative), Mineral Oil, Poloxamer 188, Propylene Glycol, Purified Water, and White Petrolatum.

Indications: First aid to help prevent infection and provide temporary relief of pain or discomfort in minor cuts, scrapes, and burns.

Directions: Adults and children 2 years of age and older: Clean the affected area. Apply a small amount of this product (an amount equal to the surface area of the tip of a finger) on the area 1 to 3 times daily. May be covered with a sterile bandage. Children under 2 years of age: Consult a physician.

Warnings: For external use only. Do not use in the eyes or apply over large areas of the body. In case of deep or puncture wounds, animal bites, or serious burns, consult a physician. Stop use and consult a physician if the condition persists or gets worse, or if symptoms persist for more than 1 week or clear up and occur again within a few days, or if a rash or other allergic reaction develops. Do not use if you are allergic to any of the ingredients. Do not use longer than 1 week unless directed by a physician. KEEP THIS AND ALL DRUGS OUT OF THE REACH OF CHILDREN. In case of accidental ingestion, seek professional assistance or contact a Poison Control Center immediately.

How Supplied: $1/2$ oz (14.2 g) (with applicator tip) tubes. Store at 59° to 77°F.
Shown in Product Identification Guide, page 519

NEOSPORIN® + PAIN RELIEF MAXIMUM STRENGTH Ointment
[nē ´uh-spō ´rŭn]

Each Gram Contains: Polymyxin B Sulfate 10,000 units, Bacitracin Zinc 500 units, Neomycin 3.5 mg, and Pramoxine Hydrochloride 10 mg, in a custom blend of White Petrolatum.

Indications: First aid to help prevent infection and provide temporary relief of pain or discomfort in minor cuts, scrapes, and burns.

Directions: Adults and children 2 years of age and older: Clean the affected area. Apply a small amount of this product (an amount equal to the surface area of the tip of a finger) on the area 1 to 3 times daily. May be covered with a sterile bandage. Children under 2 years of age: Consult a physician.

Warnings: For external use only. Do not use in the eyes or apply over large areas of the body. In case of deep or puncture wounds, animal bites, or serious burns, consult a physician. Stop use and consult a physician if the condition persists or gets worse, or if symptoms persist for more than 1 week or clear up and occur again within a few days, or if a rash or other allergic reaction develops. Do not use if you are allergic to any of the ingredients. Do not use longer than 1 week unless directed by a physician. KEEP THIS AND ALL DRUGS OUT OF THE REACH OF CHILDREN. In case of accidental ingestion, seek professional assistance or contact a Poison Control Center immediately.

How Supplied: $1/2$ oz (14.2 g) (with applicator tip) and 1 oz (28.3 g) tubes. Store at 59° to 77°F.
Shown in Product Identification Guide, page 519

NIX® Creme Rinse
Permethrin
Lice Treatment
[nĭks]

Each Fluid Ounce Contains: Active Ingredient: permethrin 280 mg (1%). Also contains: balsam canada, cetyl alcohol, citric acid, FD&C Yellow No. 6, fragrance, hydrolyzed animal protein, hydroxyethylcellulose, polyoxyethylene 10 cetyl ether, propylene glycol, stearalkonium chloride, water, isopropyl alcohol 5.6 g (20%), methylparaben 56 mg (0.2%), and propylparaben 22 mg (0.08%).

Product Benefits: Nix Creme Rinse kills lice and their unhatched eggs with usually only one application. Nix protects against head lice reinfestation for 14 days. The creme rinse formula leaves hair manageable and easy to comb.

Indications: For the treatment of head lice.

Directions for Use: Nix Creme Rinse should be used after hair has been washed with your regular shampoo, rinsed with water and towel dried. A sufficient amount should be applied to saturate hair and scalp (especially behind the ears and on the nape of the neck). Leave on hair for 10 minutes but no longer. Rinse with water. A single application is usually sufficient. If live lice are observed seven days or more after the first application of this product, a second treatment should be given. For proper head lice management, remove nits with the nit comb provided.

Head lice live on the scalp and lay small white eggs (nits) on the hair shaft close to the scalp. The nits are most easily found on the nape of the neck or behind the ears. All personal headgear, scarfs, coats, and bed linen should be disinfected by machine washing in hot water and drying, using the hot cycle of a dryer for at least 20 minutes. Personal articles of clothing or bedding that cannot be washed may be dry-cleaned, sealed in a plastic bag for a period of about 2 weeks, or sprayed with a product specifically designed for this purpose. Personal combs and brushes may be disinfected by soaking in hot water (above 130°F) for 5 to 10 minutes. Thorough vacuuming of rooms inhabited by infected patients is recommended.

Shake well before using.

Warnings: For external use only. Keep out of eyes when rinsing hair. Adults and children: Close eyes and do not open eyes until product is rinsed out. If product gets into the eyes, immediately flush

with water. Do not use near the eyes or permit contact with mucous membranes, such as inside the nose, mouth, or vagina, as irritation may occur. Children: Also protect children's eyes with a washcloth, towel, or other suitable material or method. This product should not be used on children less than 2 months of age. Itching, redness, or swelling of the scalp may occur. If skin irritation persists or infection is present or develops, discontinue use and consult a doctor. Consult a doctor if infestation of eyebrows or eyelashes occurs. This product may cause breathing difficulty or an asthmatic episode in susceptible persons. As with any drug, if you are pregnant or nursing a baby, seek the advice of a health professional before using this product. Keep this and all drugs out of the reach of children. In case of accidental ingestion, seek professional assistance or contact a Poison Control Center immediately.

Professional Labeling:
Indications: For the treatment of head lice. For prophylactic use during head lice epidemics.

Warnings: For external use only. Keep out of eyes when rinsing hair. Adults and children: Close eyes and do not open eyes until product is rinsed out. If product gets into the eyes, immediately flush with water. Do not use near the eyes or permit contact with mucous membranes, such as inside the nose, mouth, or vagina, as irritation may occur. Children: Also protect children's eyes with a washcloth, towel, or other suitable material or method. This product should not be used on pediatric patients less than 2 months of age. Itching, redness, or swelling of the scalp may occur. If skin irritation persists or infection is present or develops, discontinue use and consult a doctor. Consult a doctor if infestation of eyebrows or eyelashes occurs. This product may cause breathing difficulty or an asthmatic episode in susceptible persons. As with any drug, if you are pregnant or nursing a baby, seek the advice of a health professional before using this product. Keep this and all drugs out of the reach of children. In case of accidental ingestion, seek professional assistance or contact a Poison Control Center immediately.

Dosage and Administration
Treatment
Nix Creme Rinse should be used after hair has been washed with patient's regular shampoo, rinsed with water and towel dried. A sufficient amount should be applied to saturate hair and scalp (especially behind the ears and on the nape of the neck). Leave on hair for 10 minutes but no longer. Rinse with water. A single application is usually sufficient. If live lice are observed seven days or more after the first application of this product, a second treatment should be given. For proper head lice management, remove nits with the nit comb provided.

Head lice live on the scalp and lay small white eggs (nits) on the hair shaft close to the scalp. The nits are most easily found on the nape of the neck or behind the ears. All personal headgear, scarfs, coats, and bed linen should be disinfected by machine washing in hot water and drying, using the hot cycle of a dryer for a least 20 minutes. Personal articles of clothing or bedding that cannot be washed may be dry-cleaned, sealed in a plastic bag for a period of about 2 weeks, or sprayed with a product specifically designed for this purpose. Personal combs and brushes may be disinfected by soaking in hot water (above 130°F) for 5 to 10 minutes. Thorough vacuuming of rooms inhabited by infected patients is recommended.

Prophylaxis
Prophylactic use of Nix Creme Rinse is only recommended for individuals exposed to head lice epidemics in which at least 20% of the population at an institution are infested and for immediate household members of infested individuals. Casual use is strongly discouraged. The method of application of Nix Creme Rinse for prophylaxis is identical to that described above for treatment of a lice infestation except nit removal is not required.

Directions for Use
One application of Nix Creme Rinse has been shown to protect greater than 95% of patients against reinfestation for at least two weeks. In epidemic settings, a second prophylactic application is recommended two weeks after the first because the life cycle of a head louse is approximately four weeks.

How Supplied: Bottles of 2 fl. oz. (59 mL) with nit removal comb and Family Pack of 2 bottles, 2 fl. oz. (59 mL) each, with two nit removal combs. Store at 15° to 25°C (59° to 77°F).
Shown in Product Identification Guide, page 519

NIX® LICE CONTROL SPRAY
For Bedding and Furniture

NOT FOR USE IN HUMANS

Directions for Use: It is a violation of Federal law to use this product in a manner inconsistent with its labeling.

FOR USE IN NON-FOOD AREA OF HOMES
Indoor Application: Surface Spraying: To kill lice, spray in an inconspicuous area to test for possible staining or discoloration. Inspect again after drying, then proceed to spray entire area to be treated. Spray from a distance of 8 to 10 inches. Treat only those garments and parts of bedding, including mattresses and furniture that cannot be either laundered or dry cleaned. Allow all treated articles to dry thoroughly before use.
Do not use in food/feed areas of food/feed handling establishments, restaurants or other areas where food/feed is commercially prepared or processed. Do not use in serving areas while food is exposed or facility is in operation. Serving areas or areas where prepared foods are served such as dinning rooms, but excluding areas where foods may be prepared or held.

In the home, cover all food handling surfaces, cover or remove all food and cooking utensils or wash thoroughly after treatment.

Do not apply to classrooms while in use.

Not for use in Federally Inspected Meat and Poultry Plants.

Storage and Disposal: Do not contaminate water, food or feed by storing or disposal.

Pesticide Storage and Spill Procedures: Keep from freezing. Store upright at room temperature. Avoid exposure to extreme temperatures. In case of spill or leakage, soak up with an absorbent material such as sand, sawdust, earth, fuller's earth, etc. Dispose of with chemical waste.

Pesticide Disposal: Pesticide or rinse water that cannot be used according to label instructions must be disposed of at or by an approved waste disposal facility.

Container Disposal: Do not reuse empty container. Wrap container and put in trash collection.

READ ENTIRE LABEL BEFORE EACH USE.

> Observe all precautionary statements and follow directions for use carefully.

Environmental Hazards: This product is extremely toxic to fish and aquatic organisms. Do not apply directly to any body of water. Do not contaminate water when disposing of equipment washwater. This pesticide is toxic to honey bees and other beneficial pollinators exposed to an application. Do not apply when bees are actively visiting blooming plants (vegetables, flowers, fruit/ornamental trees) Do not allow this product to come in direct contact with bee hives at any time.

QUESTIONS OR COMMENTS:
Call Toll Free 1-888-542-3546
Shown in Product Identification Guide, page 519

Continued on next page

This product information was prepared in November 2000. On these and other Pfizer Consumer Healthcare Products, detailed information may be obtained by addressing Pfizer, Inc. Warner-Lambert Consumer Healthcare Products, Morris Plains, NJ 07950

POLYSPORIN® Ointment
[pŏl 'ē-spō 'rŭn]

Each Gram Contains: Polymyxin B Sulfate 10,000 units and Bacitracin Zinc 500 units in a special White Petrolatum Base.

Indications: First aid to help prevent infection in minor cuts, scrapes, and burns.

Directions: Clean the affected area. Apply a small amount of this product (an amount equal to the surface area of the tip of a finger) on the area 1 to 3 times daily. May be covered with a sterile bandage.

Warnings: For external use only. Do not use in the eyes or apply over large areas of the body. In case of deep or puncture wounds, animal bites, or serious burns, consult a physician. Stop use and consult a physician if the condition persists or gets worse, or if a rash or other allergic reaction develops. Do not use if you are allergic to any of the ingredients. Do not use longer than 1 week unless directed by a physician. KEEP THIS AND ALL DRUGS OUT OF THE REACH OF CHILDREN. In case of accidental ingestion, seek professional assistance or contact a Poison Control Center immediately.

How Supplied: Tubes, $1/2$ oz (14.2 g) with applicator tip, 1 oz (28.3 g); $1/32$ oz (0.9 g) foil packets packed in cartons of 144.
Store at 59° to 77°F.
Shown in Product Identification Guide, page 519

POLYSPORIN® Powder
[pŏl 'ē-spō 'rŭn]

Each Gram Contains: Polymyxin B Sulfate 10,000 units and Bacitracin Zinc 500 units in a Lactose Base.

Indications: First aid to help prevent infection in minor cuts, scrapes, and burns.

Directions: Clean the affected area. Apply a light dusting of the powder on the area 1 to 3 times daily. May be covered with a sterile bandage.

Warnings: For external use only. Do not use in the eyes or apply over large areas of the body. In case of deep or puncture wounds, animal bites, or serious burns, consult a physician. Stop use and consult a physician if the condition persists or gets worse, or if a rash or other allergic reaction develops. Do not use if you are allergic to any of the ingredients. Do not use longer than 1 week unless directed by a physician. KEEP THIS AND ALL DRUGS OUT OF THE REACH OF CHILDREN. In case of accidental ingestion, seek professional assistance or contact a Poison Control Center immediately.

How Supplied: 0.35 oz (10 g) shaker-vial.
Store at 15° to 25°C (59° to 77°F). Do not store under refrigeration.

ROLAIDS® Antacid Tablets
Original Peppermint, Spearmint, and Cherry

Active Ingredients: Calcium Carbonate 550 mg and Magnesium Hydroxide 110 mg per tablet.

Inactive Ingredients: *Peppermint and Spearmint Flavors:* Dextrose, Flavoring, Magnesium Stearate, Polyethylene Glycol, Pregelatinized Starch and Sucrose.
Cherry Flavor: Dextrose, Flavoring, Magnesium Stearate, Polyethylene Glycol, Pregelatinized Starch, Sucrose and D&C Red No. 27 Aluminum Lake.

Indications: For the relief of heartburn, sour stomach or acid indigestion and upset stomach associated with these symptoms.

Actions: Rolaids® provides rapid neutralization of stomach acid. Each tablet has an acid-neutralizing capacity of 14.7 mEq and the ability to maintain the pH of stomach contents at 3.5 or greater for a significant period of time.

Warnings: Do not take more than 12 tablets in a 24 hour period or use the maximum dosage of this product for more than 2 weeks except under the advice and supervision of a physician. KEEP THIS AND ALL DRUGS OUT OF THE REACH OF CHILDREN.

Drug Interaction Precaution: Antacids may interact with certain prescription drugs. If you are presently taking a prescription drug, do not take this product without checking with your physician or other health professional.

Dosage and Administration: Chew 2 to 4 tablets as symptoms occur. Repeat hourly if symptoms return, or as directed by a physician.

How Supplied: Rolaids® is available in 12-tablet rolls, 3-packs containing three 12-tablet rolls and in bottles containing 150 or 300 tablets.
Shown in Product Identification Guide, page 519

EXTRA STRENGTH ROLAIDS®
Antacid Tablets
Freshmint and Fruit Flavors

Active Ingredients: Calcium Carbonate 675 mg and Magnesium Hydroxide 135 mg per tablet.
Inactive Ingredients: *Freshmint Flavor:* Dextrose, Flavoring, Magnesium Stearate, Polyethylene Glycol, Pregelatinized Starch and Sucrose.
Fruit Flavor: Dextrose, Flavoring, Magnesium Stearate, Polyethylene Glycol,

Pregelatinized Starch, Sucrose and FD & C Yellow No. 5 Aluminum Lake (tartrazine).

Indications: For the relief of heartburn, sour stomach or acid indigestion and upset stomach due to these symptoms.

Actions: Extra Strength Rolaids® provides rapid neutralization of stomach acid. Each tablet has an acid-neutralizing capacity of 18.2 mEq and the ability to maintain the pH of stomach contents at 3.5 or greater for a significant period of time.

Warnings: Do not take more than 10 tablets in a 24 hour period or use the maximum dosage of this product for more than 2 weeks except under the advice of and supervision of a physician. KEEP THIS AND ALL DRUGS OUT OF THE REACH OF CHILDREN.

Drug Interaction Precaution: Antacids may interact with certain prescription drugs. If you are presently taking a prescription drug, do not take this product without checking with your physician or other health professional.

Dosage and Administration: Chew 2 to 4 tablets as symptoms occur. Repeat hourly if symptoms return, or as directed by a physician.

How Supplied: Extra Strength Rolaids® is available in 10-tablet rolls, 3-packs containing three 10-tablet rolls and in bottle containing 100 and 250 tablets.
Shown in Product Identification Guide, page 519

SINUTAB® Non-Drying
Liquid Caps
[sĭn 'ū tăb]

Active Ingredients: Each liquid cap contains: Pseudoephedrine Hydrochloride 30 mg., Guaifenesin 200 mg.

Inactive Ingredients: FD&C Blue No. 1, Gelatin, Glycerin, Polyethylene Glycol 400, Povidone, Propylene Glycol, and Sorbitol. Printed with edible white ink.

Indications: Temporarily relieves nasal congestion associated with sinusitis. Helps loosen phlegm (mucus) and thin bronchial secretions to drain bronchial tubes.

Dosage and Administration: Adults and children 12 years of age and over: swallow 2 liquid caps every 4 hours, not to exceed 8 liquid caps in 24 hours, or as directed by a doctor. Children under 12 years of age: consult a doctor.

Warnings: Do not exceed recommended dosage. If nervousness, dizziness, or sleeplessness occur, discontinue use and consult a doctor. If symptoms do not improve within 7 days or are accompanied by fever, consult a doctor. Do not

take this product if you have heart disease, high blood pressure, thyroid disease, diabetes, or difficulty in urination due to enlargement of the prostate gland unless directed by a doctor. A persistent cough may be a sign of a serious condition. If cough persists for more than 1 week, tends to recur, or is accompanied by a fever, rash, or persistent headache, consult a doctor. Do not take this product for persistent or chronic cough such as occurs with smoking, asthma, chronic bronchitis, or emphysema, or where cough is accompanied by excessive phlegm (mucus) unless directed by a doctor. As with any drug, if you are pregnant or nursing a baby, seek the advice of a health professional before using this product. **KEEP THIS AND ALL DRUGS OUT OF THE REACH OF CHILDREN.** In case of accidental overdose, seek professional assistance or contact a Poison Control Center immediately.

Drug Interaction Precaution: Do not use this product if you are now taking a prescription monoamine oxidase inhibitor (MAOI) (certain drugs for depression, psychiatric or emotional conditions, or Parkinson's disease), or for 2 weeks after stopping the MAOI drug. If you are uncertain whether your prescription drug contains an MAOI, consult a health professional before taking this product.

How Supplied: Sinutab® Non-Drying supplied in a box of 24 liquid caps. Store at 59°–77°F. Protect from heat and humidity.

Shown in Product Identification Guide, page 520

**SINUTAB® Sinus Allergy Medication, Maximum Strength Formula,
Tablets and Caplets**
[sîn 'ū tăb]

Active Ingredients: Each tablet/caplet contains: Acetaminophen 500 mg., Chlorpheniramine Maleate 2 mg., Pseudoephedrine Hydrochloride 30 mg.

Inactive Ingredients: Croscarmellose Sodium, Crospovidone, D&C Yellow No. 10 Aluminum Lake, FD&C Yellow No. 6 Aluminum Lake, Microcrystalline Cellulose, Povidone, Pregelatinized Starch and Stearic Acid. May also contain Calcium Stearate, Candelilla Wax, Carnauba Wax, Hydroxypropyl Cellulose, Hydroxypropyl Methylcellulose, Polyethylene Glycol, Polysorbate 80, Titanium Dioxide and Zinc Stearate. See package for complete listing.

Indications: For the temporary relief of minor aches, pains and headache and nasal congestion associated with sinusitis. Temporarily relieves runny nose, sneezing itching of the nose or throat, and itchy, watery eyes due to hay fever or other upper respiratory allergies.

Dosage: Adults and children 12 years of age and over: 2 tablets or caplets every 6 hours while symptoms persist, not to exceed 8 tablets or caplets in 24 hours, or as directed by a doctor. Children under 12 years of age: consult a doctor.

Warnings: Do not exceed recommended dosage. If nervousness, dizziness, or sleeplessness occur, discontinue use and consult a doctor. Do not take this product for more than 10 days. If symptoms do not improve or are accompanied by fever that lasts for more than 3 days, or if new symptoms occur, consult a doctor. Do not take this product, unless directed by a doctor, if you have heart disease, high blood pressure, thyroid disease, diabetes, a breathing problem such as emphysema or chronic bronchitis, or if you have glaucoma or difficulty in urination due to enlargement of the prostate gland. May cause excitability especially in children. May cause drowsiness; alcohol, sedatives, and tranquilizers may increase the drowsiness effect. Avoid alcoholic beverages while taking this product. Do not take this product if you are taking sedatives or tranquilizers, without first consulting your doctor. Use caution when driving a motor vehicle or operating machinery. As with any drug, if you are pregnant or nursing a baby, seek the advice of a health professional before using this product. **KEEP THIS AND ALL DRUGS OUT OF THE REACH OF CHILDREN.** In case of accidental overdose, seek professional assistance or contact a Poison Control Center immediately. Prompt medical attention is critical for adults as well as for children even if you do not notice any signs or symptoms.

Alcohol Warning: If you consume 3 or more alcoholic drinks every day, ask your doctor whether you should take acetaminophen or other pain relievers/fever reducers. Acetaminophen may cause liver damage.

Drug Interaction Precaution: Do not use this product if you are now taking a prescription monoamine oxidase inhibitor (MAOI) (certain drugs for depression, psychiatric or emotional conditions, or Parkinson's disease), or for 2 weeks after stopping the MAOI drug. If you are uncertain whether your prescription drug contains an MAOI, consult a health professional before taking this product.

How Supplied: Sinutab® Sinus Allergy Medication, Maximum Strength Formula, Caplets and Tablets are supplied in child-resistant blister packs in boxes of 24 tablets or caplets.

Store at 59° to 77°F in a dry place.
Shown in Product Identification Guide, page 520

SINUTAB® Sinus Medication, Maximum Strength Without Drowsiness Formula, Tablets and Caplets
[sîn 'ū tăb]

Active Ingredients: Each tablet/caplet contains: Acetaminophen 500 mg., Pseudoephedrine Hydrochloride 30 mg.

Inactive Ingredients: Croscarmellose Sodium, Crospovidone, FD&C Yellow No. 6 Aluminum Lake, Microcrystalline Cellulose, Povidone, Pregelatinized Starch and Stearic Acid. May also contain: Calcium Stearate, Candelilla Wax, Carnauba Wax, D&C Yellow No. 10 Aluminum Lake, Hydroxypropyl Cellulose, Hydroxypropyl Methylcellulose, Polyethylene Glycol, Polysorbate 80, Titanium Dioxide, and Zinc Stearate. See package for complete listing.

Indications: For the temporary relief of minor aches, pains, and headache and nasal congestion associated with sinusitis.

Dosage: Adults and children 12 years of age and over: 2 tablets or caplets every 6 hours while symptoms persist, not to exceed 8 tablets or caplets in 24 hours, or as directed by a doctor. Children under 12 years of age: consult a doctor.

Warnings: Do not exceed recommended dosage. If nervousness, dizziness, or sleeplessness occur, discontinue use and consult a doctor. Do not take this product for more than 10 days. If symptoms do not improve or are accompanied by fever that lasts for more than 3 days, or if new symptoms occur, consult a doctor. Do not take this product if you have heart disease, high blood pressure, thyroid disease, diabetes, or difficulty in urination due to enlargement of the prostate gland unless directed by a doctor. As with any drug, if you are pregnant or nursing a baby, seek the advice of a health professional before using this product. **KEEP THIS AND ALL DRUGS OUT OF THE REACH OF CHILDREN.** In case of accidental overdose, seek professional assistance or contact a Poison Control Center immediately. Prompt medical attention is critical for adults as well as for children even if you do not notice any signs or symptoms.

Alcohol Warning: If you consume 3 or more alcoholic drinks every day, ask your doctor whether you should take acetaminophen or other pain relievers/fever re-

Continued on next page

This product information was prepared in November 2000. On these and other Pfizer Consumer Healthcare Products, detailed information may be obtained by addressing Pfizer, Inc. Warner-Lambert Consumer Healthcare Products, Morris Plains, NJ 07950

Sinutab Sinus—Cont.

ducers. Acetaminophen may cause liver damage.

Drug Interaction Precaution: Do not use this product if you are now taking a prescription monoamine oxidase inhibitor (MAOI) (certain drugs for depression, psychiatric or emotional conditions, or Parkinson's disease), or for 2 weeks after stopping the MAOI drug. If you are uncertain whether your prescription drug contains an MAOI, consult a health professional before taking this product.

How Supplied: Sinutab® Sinus Medication, Maximum Strength Without Drowsiness Formula, Caplets and Tablets are supplied in child-resistant blister packs in boxes of 24 tablets or caplets. Store at 59° to 77°F in a dry place.
Shown in Product Identification Guide, page 520

SUDAFED® 12 Hour Caplets*
[sū 'duh-fĕd]
*Capsule-shaped Tablets

Description: Sudafed 12 Hour is a long-acting nasal decongestant providing temporary relief of nasal and sinus congestion due to a cold, allergy, or sinusitis for up to 12 hours. Sudafed 12 Hour helps clear nasal congestion and release sinus pressure to restore freer breathing without drowsiness.

Active Ingredient: Each coated extended-release tablet contains Pseudoephedrine Hydrochloride 120 mg.

Inactive Ingredients: Hydroxypropyl Methylcellulose, Magnesium Stearate, Microcrystalline Cellulose, Polyethylene Glycol, Povidone, and Titanium Dioxide. Printed with edible blue ink. May also contain Carnauba Wax or Candelilla Wax.

Indications: For the temporary relief of nasal congestion due to the common cold, hay fever, or other upper respiratory allergies, and nasal congestion associated with sinusitis. Promotes nasal and/or sinus drainage; temporarily relieves sinus congestion and pressure. Temporarily restores freer breathing through the nose.

Directions: Adults and children 12 years and over—One tablet every 12 hours, not to exceed two tablets in 24 hours. Sudafed 12 Hour is not recommended for children under 12 years of age.

Warnings: Do not exceed recommended dosage. If nervousness, dizziness, or sleeplessness occur, discontinue use and consult a doctor. If symptoms do not improve within 7 days or are accompanied by fever, consult a doctor. Do not take this product if you have heart disease, high blood pressure, thyroid disease, diabetes, or difficulty in urination

due to enlargement of the prostate gland unless directed by a doctor. As with any drug, if you are pregnant or nursing a baby, seek the advice of a health professional before using this product. **KEEP THIS AND ALL DRUGS OUT OF THE REACH OF CHILDREN.** In case of accidental overdose, seek professional assistance or contact a Poison Control Center immediately.

Drug Interaction Precaution: Do not use this product if you are now taking a prescription monoamine oxidase inhibitor (MAOI) (certain drugs for depression, psychiatric or emotional conditions, or Parkinson's disease), or for 2 weeks after stopping the MAOI drug. If you are uncertain whether your prescription drug contains an MAOI, consult a health professional before taking this product.

How Supplied: Boxes of 10 and 20. Store at 15° to 25°C (59° to 77°F) in a dry place and protect from light.
Shown in Product Identification Guide, page 520

SUDAFED® 24 Hour Tablets Non-Drowsy
[sū 'duh-fĕd]

Description: Sudafed 24 Hour is specially formulated to provide relief for 24 hours with a one tablet, once daily dosage. Each Sudafed 24 Hour tablet releases an outer coating of medication immediately and then continues to work by releasing medication at a precisely controlled rate for 24 hours of relief. Sudafed 24 Hour contains a nasal decongestant that provides relief without drowsiness.

Active Ingredient: Each Sudafed 24 Hour tablet contains a total of 240 mg pseudoephedrine hydrochloride, 60 mg immediate release and 180 mg controlled release.

Inactive Ingredients: Cellulose, cellulose acetate, hydroxypropyl cellulose, hydroxypropyl methylcellulose, magnesium stearate, polyethylene glycol, polysorbate 80, povidone, sodium chloride, and titanium dioxide.

Indications: Provides temporary relief of nasal congestion due to the common cold, hay fever, or other upper respiratory allergies, and nasal congestion associated with sinusitis; reduces swelling of nasal passages; shrinks swollen membranes; relieves sinus pressure, and temporarily restores freer breathing through the nose.

Directions: Adults and children 12 years of age and over: Take just one tablet with fluid every 24 hours. **DO NOT EXCEED ONE TABLET IN 24 HOURS.** SWALLOW EACH TABLET WHOLE; DO NOT DIVIDE, CRUSH, CHEW OR DISSOLVE THE TABLET. The tablet does not completely dissolve and may be seen in the stool (this is normal). Not for use in children under 12 years of age.

Warnings: DO NOT EXCEED RECOMMENDED DOSAGE. If nervousness, dizziness, or sleeplessness occur, discontinue use and consult a physician. Do not take this product for more than 7 days. If symptoms do not improve or are accompanied by fever, consult a physician. Do not take this product if you have heart disease, high blood pressure, thyroid disease, diabetes, or difficulty in urination due to enlargement of the prostate gland, unless directed by a physician.
Rarely, tablets of this kind may cause bowel obstruction (blockage), usually in people with severe narrowing of the bowel (esophagus, stomach or intestine). If you have had obstruction or narrowing of the bowel, do not take this product without consulting your physician. Contact your physician if you experience persistent abdominal pain or vomiting. As with any drug, if you are pregnant or nursing a baby, seek the advice of a health professional before using this product. **KEEP THIS AND ALL DRUGS OUT OF THE REACH OF CHILDREN.** In case of accidental overdose, seek professional assistance or contact a Poison Control Center immediately.

Drug Interaction Precaution: Do not use this product if you are now taking a prescription monoamine oxidase inhibitor (MAOI) (certain drugs for depression, psychiatric or emotional conditions, or Parkinson's disease), or for 2 weeks after stopping the MAOI drug. If you are uncertain whether your prescription drug contains an MAOI, consult a health professional before taking this product.

How Supplied: Box of 5 tablets and 10 tablets. Store in a dry place between 4° and 30°C (39° and 86°F). **BLISTER PACKAGED FOR YOUR PROTECTION. DO NOT USE IF INDIVIDUAL SEALS ARE BROKEN.**
Shown in Product Identification Guide, page 520

SUDAFED® Cold & Allergy Tablets
[sū 'duh-fĕd]

Description: Sudafed Cold & Allergy provides temporary, maximum strength relief of nasal congestion and allergy symptoms. Sudafed Cold & Allergy helps dry a runny nose and relieve sneezing, and itchy, watery eyes due to allergies.

Active Ingredients: Each tablet contains: Chlorpheniramine Maleate 4 mg. and Pseudoephedrine Hydrochloride 60 mg.

Inactive Ingredients: May also contain: Candelilla Wax, Crospovidone, Hydroxypropyl Methylcellulose, Microcrystalline Cellulose, Poloxamer 407, Polyethylene Glycol, Polyethylene Oxide, Potato Starch, Povidone, Pregelatinized Starch, Silicon Dioxide, Sodium Lauryl Sulfate, Stearic Acid, Titanium Dioxide. See package for complete listing.

Indications: For the temporary relief of runny nose, sneezing and nasal congestion due to the common cold. For the temporary relief of runny nose, sneezing, itching of the nose or throat, itchy, watery eyes, and nasal congestion due to hay fever (allergic rhinitis).

Directions: To be given every 4 to 6 hours. Do not exceed 4 doses in 24 hours, or as directed by a doctor. Adults and children 12 years of age and over: 1 tablet. Children 6 to under 12 years of age: $1/2$ tablet. Children under 6 years of age: consult a doctor.

Warnings: Do not exceed recommended dosage. If nervousness, dizziness, or sleeplessness occur, discontinue use and consult a doctor. If symptoms do not improve within 7 days or are accompanied by fever, consult a doctor. Do not take this product, unless directed by a doctor, if you have a breathing problem such as emphysema or chronic bronchitis, heart disease, high blood pressure, thyroid disease, diabetes, or if you have glaucoma or difficulty in urination due to enlargement of the prostate gland. May cause excitability especially in children. May cause drowsiness; alcohol, sedatives, and tranquilizers may increase the drowsiness effect. Avoid alcoholic beverages while taking this product. Do not take this product if you are taking sedatives or tranquilizers, without first consulting your doctor. Use caution when driving a motor vehicle or operating machinery. As with any drug, if you are pregnant or nursing a baby, seek the advice of a health professional before using this product. **KEEP THIS AND ALL DRUGS OUT OF THE REACH OF CHILDREN.** In case of accidental overdose, seek professional assistance or contact a Poison Control Center immediately.

Drug Interaction Precaution: Do not use this product if you are now taking a prescription monoamine oxidase inhibitor (MAOI) (certain drugs for depression, psychiatric or emotional conditions, or Parkinson's disease), or for 2 weeks after stopping the MAOI drug. If you are uncertain whether your prescription drug contains an MAOI, consult a health professional before taking this product.

How Supplied: Boxes of 24 tablets. Store at 59° to 77°F in a dry place and protect from light.
Shown in Product Identification Guide, page 520

SUDAFED® Cold & Cough Liquid Caps
[sū 'duh-fĕd]

Description: Sudafed Cold & Cough Liquid Caps provide temporary relief of colds and coughs. Sudafed Cold & Cough helps clear nasal and chest congestion and relieve sinus pressure while reliev-ing headaches, fever, body aches, coughs and sore throats due to colds without drowsy or overdrying side effects.

Active Ingredients: Each liquid cap contains: Acetaminophen 250 mg, Guaifenesin 100 mg, Pseudoephedrine Hydrochloride 30 mg, and Dextromethorphan Hydrobromide 10 mg.

Inactive Ingredients: D&C Yellow No. 10, FD&C Red No. 40, Gelatin, Glycerin, Polyethylene Glycol 400, Povidone, Propylene Glycol, Purified Water, and Sorbitol. Printed with edible white ink.

Indications: For the temporary relief of nasal congestion, minor aches, pains, headache, muscular aches, sore throat, and fever associated with the common cold. Temporarily relieves cough occurring with a cold. Helps loosen phlegm (mucus) and thin bronchial secretions to drain bronchial tubes and make coughs more productive.

Directions: Adults and children 12 years of age and over: 2 liquid caps every 4 hours, while symptoms persist, not to exceed 8 liquid caps in 24 hours, or as directed by a doctor. Children under 12 years of age: consult a doctor.

Warnings: Do not exceed recommended dosage. If nervousness, dizziness, or sleeplessness occur, discontinue use and consult a doctor. Do not take this product for more than 10 days. A persistent cough may be a sign of a serious condition. If symptoms do not improve of if cough persists for more than 7 days, tends to recur, or is accompanied by rash, persistent headache, fever that lasts for more than 3 days, or if new symptoms occur, consult a doctor. Do not take this product for persistent or chronic cough such as occurs with smoking, asthma, chronic bronchitis, or emphysema, or where cough is accompanied by excessive phlegm (mucus) unless directed by a doctor. If sore throat is severe, persists for more than 2 days, is accompanied or followed by fever, headache, rash, nausea, or vomiting, consult a doctor promptly. Do not take this product if you have heart disease, high blood pressure, thyroid disease, diabetes, or difficulty in urination due to enlargement of the prostate gland unless directed by a doctor. As with any drug, if you are pregnant or nursing a baby, seek the advice of a health professional before using this product. **KEEP THIS AND ALL DRUGS OUT OF THE REACH OF CHILDREN.** In case of accidental overdose, seek professional assistance or contact a Poison Control Center immediately. Prompt medical attention is critical for adults as well as for children even if you do not notice any signs or symptoms.

Alcohol Warning: If you consume 3 or more alcoholic drinks every day, ask your doctor whether you should take acetaminophen or other pain relievers/fever reducers. Acetaminophen may cause liver damage.

Drug Interaction Precaution: Do not use this product if you are now taking a prescription monoamine oxidase inhibitor (MAOI) (certain drugs for depression, psychiatric or emotional conditions, or Parkinson's disease), or for 2 weeks after stopping the MAOI drug. If you are uncertain whether your prescription drug contains an MAOI, consult a health professional before taking this product.

How Supplied: Boxes of 10 and 20. Store at 59° to 77°F in a dry place and protect from light.
Shown in Product Identification Guide, page 520

CHILDREN'S SUDAFED®
Cold & Cough Liquid
[sū 'duh-fĕd]

Description: Children's Sudafed Cold and Cough Liquid provides temporary relief for a child's stuffy nose and coughing due to the common cold. It also comes in a great tasting cherry-berry flavor that makes it easy to give to children.

Active Ingredients: Each teaspoonful (5 mL) contains Pseudoephedrine Hydrochloride 15 mg and Dextromethorphan Hydrobromide 5 mg.

Inactive Ingredients: Carboxymethylcellulose Sodium, Citric Acid, D&C Red No. 33, FD&C Red No. 40, Flavors, Glycerin, Poloxamer 407, Polyethylene Glycol 1450, Purified Water, Saccharin Sodium, Sodium Benzoate, Sodium Chloride, Sodium Citrate and Sorbitol Solution.

Indications: For the temporary relief of nasal congestion due to the common cold; temporarily quiets cough due to minor throat and bronchial irritation occurring with a cold or inhaled irritants. Suppresses cough impulses without narcotics.

Directions: Follow dosage recommendations below, or as directed by a doctor. Dosage may be repeated every 4 hours, not to exceed 4 doses in 24 hours.

Children's Sudafed®
Cold & Cough Liquid

AGE	DOSAGE
Children under 2 years of age	Consult a doctor
Children 2 to under 6 years of age	One (1) teaspoonful

Continued on next page

This product information was prepared in November 2000. On these and other Pfizer Consumer Healthcare Products, detailed information may be obtained by addressing Pfizer, Inc. Warner-Lambert Consumer Healthcare Products, Morris Plains, NJ 07950

Sudafed Children's C & C—Cont

| Children 6 to under 12 years of age | Two (2) teaspoonfuls |
| Adults and children 12 years of age and over | Four (4) teaspoonfuls |

Warnings: Do not exceed recommended dosage. If nervousness, dizziness, or sleeplessness occur, discontinue use and consult a doctor. If symptoms do not improve within 7 days or are accompanied by fever, consult a doctor. Do not take this product if you have heart disease, high blood pressure, thyroid disease, diabetes, or difficulty in urination due to enlargement of the prostate gland unless directed by a doctor. A persistent cough may be a sign of a serious condition. If cough persists for more than 1 week, tends to recur, or is accompanied by fever, rash, or persistent headache, consult a doctor. Do not take this product for persistent or chronic cough such as occurs with smoking, asthma or emphysema, or if cough is accompanied by excessive phlegm (mucus) unless directed by a doctor. As with any drug, if you are pregnant or nursing a baby, seek the advice of a health professional before using this product. **KEEP THIS AND ALL DRUGS OUT OF THE REACH OF CHILDREN.** In case of accidental overdose, seek professional assistance or contact a Poison Control Center immediately.

Drug Interaction Precaution: Do not use this product if you are now taking a prescription monoamine oxidase inhibitor (MAOI) (certain drugs for depression, psychiatric or emotional conditions, or Parkinson's disease), or for 2 weeks after stopping the MAOI drug. If you are uncertain whether your prescription drug contains an MAOI, consult a health professional before taking this product.

How Supplied: Sudafed Children's Cold and Cough Liquid is supplied in 4 fl. oz. bottles.
Store at 59° to 77°F.
Shown in Product Identification Guide, page 520

SUDAFED® COLD & SINUS
Liquid Caps
[sū 'duh-fĕd]

Description: Sudafed Cold & Sinus temporarily relieves cold symptoms and sinus pain. Sudafed Cold & Sinus contains Sudafed's maximum strength nasal decongestant to help clear nasal congestion and relieve sinus pressure, plus a pain reliever to alleviate the headache, fever, sore throat, and body aches for relief without drowsy or overdrying side effects.

Active Ingredients: Each liquid cap contains: Acetaminophen 325 mg and

Pseudoephedrine Hydrochloride 30 mg.

Inactive Ingredients: FD&C Blue No. 1, FD&C Red No. 40, Gelatin, Glycerin, Pharmaceutical Glaze, Polyethylene Glycol, Povidone, Purified Water, Sodium Acetate, Sorbitol Special, and Titanium Dioxide.

Indications: For the temporary relief of nasal congestion, minor aches, pains, headache, muscular aches, sore throat, and fever due to the common cold. Temporarily relieves nasal congestion associated with sinusitis. Reduces swelling of nasal passages; shrinks swollen membranes. Promotes nasal and/or sinus drainage; temporarily relieves sinus congestion and pressure. Temporarily restores freer breathing through the nose.

Directions: Adults and children 12 years of age and over: 2 liquid caps every 4 to 6 hours, while symptoms persist, not to exceed 8 liquid caps in 24 hours, or as directed by a doctor. Children under 12 years of age: consult a doctor.

Warnings: Do not exceed recommended dosage. If nervousness, dizziness, or sleeplessness occur, discontinue use and consult a doctor. Do not take this product for more than 10 days. If symptoms do not improve or are accompanied by fever that lasts for more than 3 days, or if new symptoms occur, consult a doctor. If sore throat is severe, persists for more than 2 days, is accompanied or followed by fever, headache, rash, nausea, or vomiting, consult a doctor promptly. Do not take this product if you have heart disease, high blood pressure, thyroid disease, diabetes, or difficulty in urination due to enlargement of the prostate gland unless directed by a doctor. As with any drug, if you are pregnant or nursing a baby, seek the advice of a health professional before using this product. **KEEP THIS AND ALL DRUGS OUT OF THE REACH OF CHILDREN.** In case of accidental overdose, seek professional assistance or contact a Poison Control Center immediately. Prompt medical attention is critical for adults as well as for children even if you do not notice any signs or symptoms.

Alcohol Warning: If you consume 3 or more alcoholic drinks every day, ask your doctor whether you should take acetaminophen or other pain relievers/fever reducers. Acetaminophen may cause liver damage.

Drug Interaction Precaution: Do not use this product if you are now taking a prescription monoamine oxidase inhibitor (MAOI) (certain drugs for depression, psychiatric or emotional conditions, or Parkinson's disease), or for 2 weeks after stopping the MAOI drug. If you are uncertain whether your prescription drug contains an MAOI, consult a health professional before taking this product.

How Supplied: Boxes of 10 and 20 liquid caps. Store at 15° to 25°C (59° to 77°F) in a dry place and protect from light.
Shown in Product Identification Guide, page 520

SUDAFED® Nasal Decongestant Tablets 30 mg.
[sū 'duh-fĕd]

Description: Sudafed Nasal Decongestant tablets provide temporary, maximum strength relief of nasal and sinus congestion due to a cold, allergy, or sinusitis. Sudafed Nasal Decongestant helps clear nasal congestion and relieve sinus pressure to restore freer breathing without drowsy or overdrying side effects.

Active Ingredient: Each tablet contains Pseudoephedrine Hydrochloride 30 mg.

Inactive Ingredients: Acacia, Corn Starch, FD&C Red No. 40 Aluminum Lake, FD&C Yellow No. 6 Aluminum Lake, Magnesium Stearate, Pharmaceutical Glaze, Polysorbate 60, Povidone, Sodium Benzoate, Stearic Acid, Sucrose, and Titanium Dioxide. May also contain: Candelilla Wax, Carnauba Wax, Dibasic Calcium Phosphate, Hydroxypropyl Methylcellulose, Lactose Monohydrate, Poloxamer 407, Polyethylene Glycol, Polyethylene Oxide, Potato Starch, Propylene Glycol, Silicon Dioxide, Sodium Lauryl Sulfate and Talc. See package for complete listing. Printed with edible black ink.

Indications: For the temporary relief of nasal congestion due to the common cold, hay fever or other upper respiratory allergies, and nasal congestion associated with sinusitis. Helps decongest sinus openings and passages; temporarily relieves sinus congestion and pressure. Temporarily restores freer breathing through the nose.

Directions: To be given every 4 to 6 hours. Do not exceed 4 doses in 24 hours. Adults and children 12 years of age and over: 2 tablets. Children 6 to under 12 years of age: 1 tablet. Children 2 to under 6 years of age: use Children's Sudafed Liquid. Children under 2 years of age: consult a doctor.

Warnings: Do not exceed recommended dosage. If nervousness, dizziness or sleeplessness occur, discontinue use and consult a doctor. If symptoms do not improve within 7 days or are accompanied by fever, consult a doctor. Do not take this product if you have heart disease, high blood pressure, thyroid disease, diabetes, or difficulty in urination due to enlargement of the prostate gland unless directed by a doctor. As with any drug, if you are pregnant or nursing a baby, seek the advice of a health professional before using this product. **KEEP THIS AND ALL DRUGS OUT OF THE REACH OF CHILDREN.** In case of accidental overdose, seek professional assistance or contact a Poison Control Center immediately.

Drug Interaction Precaution: Do not use this product if you are now taking a prescription monoamine oxidase inhibitor (MAOI) (certain drugs for depres-

sion, psychiatric or emotional conditions, or Parkinson's disease), or for 2 weeks after stopping the MAOI drug. If you are uncertain whether your prescription drug contains an MAOI, consult a health professional before taking this product.

How Supplied: Boxes of 24, 48 and 96. Store at 59° to 77°F in a dry place.

Shown in Product Identification Guide, page 520

CHILDREN'S SUDAFED®
Nasal Decongestant Chewables
[sū ' duh-fĕd]

Description: Children's Sudafed Nasal Decongestant Chewables provides temporary relief for a child's stuffy nose and head due to a cold, allergy, or sinusitis. It also comes in a wonderful orange flavor chewable tablet that makes it easy to give to children.

Active Ingredient: Each chewable tablet contains Pseudoephedrine Hydrochloride 15 mg.

Inactive Ingredients: Ascorbic Acid, Aspartame, Carnauba Wax, Citric Acid, Crospovidone, FD&C Yellow No. 6 Aluminum Lake, Flavors, Hydroxypropyl Methylcellulose, Magnesium Stearate, Mannitol, Microcrystalline Cellulose, Sodium Chloride, Tartaric Acid.

Indications: For the temporary relief of nasal congestion due to the common cold, hay fever or other upper respiratory allergies, and nasal congestion associated with sinusitis. Promotes nasal and/or sinus drainage; temporarily relieves sinus congestion and pressure.

Directions: Do not exceed 4 doses in a 24-hour period. Children 6 to under 12 years of age: 2 chewable tablets every 4 to 6 hours. Children 2 to under 6 years of age: 1 chewable tablet every 4 to 6 hours. Children under 2 years of age: consult a doctor.

Warnings: Do not exceed recommended dosage. If nervousness, dizziness, or sleeplessness occur, discontinue use and consult a doctor. If symptoms do not improve within 7 days or are accompanied by fever, consult a doctor. Do not give this product to a child who has heart disease, high blood pressure, thyroid disease, or diabetes unless directed by a doctor. **KEEP THIS AND ALL DRUGS OUT OF THE REACH OF CHILDREN.** In case of accidental overdose, seek professional assistance or contact a Poison Control Center immediately. **Phenylketonurics: Contains Phenylalanine 0.78 mg Per Tablet.**

Drug Interaction Precaution: Do not give this product to a child who is taking a prescription monoamine oxidase inhibitor (MAOI) (certain drugs for depression, psychiatric or emotional conditions), or for 2 weeks after stopping the MAOI drug. If you are uncertain whether your child's prescription drug contains an MAOI, consult a health professional before giving this product.

How Supplied: Box of 24 chewable tablets. Store at 59° to 77°F in a dry place and protect from light.

Shown in Product Identification Guide, page 520

SUDAFED®
CHILDREN'S NASAL DECONGESTANT LIQUID MEDICATION
[sū 'duh-fĕd]

Description: Children's Sudafed Nasal Decongestant Liquid provides temporary relief for a child's stuffy nose and head due to a cold or allergy. It also comes in a wonderful grape flavor that makes it easy to give to children.

Active Ingredient: Each teaspoonful (5 mL) contains Pseudoephedrine Hydrochloride 15 mg.

Inactive Ingredients: Citric Acid, Edetate Disodium, FD&C Red No. 40, FD&C Blue No. 1, Flavors, Glycerin, Poloxamer 407, Polyethylene Glycol 1450, Povidone K-90, Purified Water, Saccharin Sodium, Sodium Benzoate, Sodium Citrate and Sorbitol Solution.

Indications: For the temporary relief of nasal congestion due to the common cold, hay fever or other upper respiratory allergies, and nasal congestion associated with sinusitis. Promotes nasal and/or sinus drainage; temporarily relieves sinus congestion and pressure.

Directions: Follow dosage recommendations below. Dosage may be repeated every 4 to 6 hours, not to exceed 4 doses in 24 hours.

Sudafed® Children's Nasal Decongestant Liquid Medication

Age	Dosage
Children under 2 years of age	Consult a doctor
Children 2 to under 6 years of age	One (1) teaspoonful
Children 6 to under 12 years of age	Two (2) teaspoonfuls
Adults and children 12 years of age and over	Four (4) teaspoonfuls

Warnings: Do not exceed recommended dosage. If nervousness, dizziness, or sleeplessness occur, discontinue use and consult a doctor. If symptoms do not improve within 7 days or are accompanied by fever, consult a doctor. Do not take this product if you have heart disease, high blood pressure, thyroid disease, diabetes, or difficulty in urination due to enlargement of the prostate gland unless directed by a doctor. As with any drug, if you are pregnant or nursing a baby, seek the advice of a health professional before using this product. **KEEP THIS AND ALL DRUGS OUT OF THE REACH OF CHILDREN.** In case of accidental overdose, seek professional assistance or contact a Poison Control Center immediately.

Drug Interaction Precaution: Do not use this product if you are now taking a prescription monoamine oxidase inhibitor (MAOI) (certain drugs for depression, psychiatric or emotional conditions, or Parkinson's disease), or for 2 weeks after stopping the MAOI drug. If you are uncertain whether your prescription drug contains an MAOI, consult a health professional before taking this product.

How Supplied: Sudafed Children's Nasal Decongestant is supplied in 4 fl. oz. bottles
Store at 59° to 77°F.

Shown in Product Identification Guide, page 521

SUDAFED® Severe Cold Formula
Caplets and Tablets
[sū 'duh-fĕd]

Description: Sudafed Severe Cold Formula contains maximum strength ingredients to temporarily relieve the worst cold symptoms. Sudafed Severe Cold Formula helps clear nasal congestion and relieve sinus pressure while relieving headaches, fever, body aches, coughs and sore throats due to colds without drowsy or overdrying side effects.

Active Ingredients: Each coated caplet/tablet contains: Acetaminophen 500 mg, Pseudoephedrine Hydrochloride 30 mg, and Dextromethorphan Hydrobromide 15 mg.

Inactive Ingredients: Crospovidone, Hydroxypropyl Methylcellulose, Magnesium Stearate, Microcrystalline Cellulose, Polyethylene Glycol, Povidone, Pregelatinized Corn Starch, Stearic Acid and Titanium Dioxide. May also contain: Candelilla Wax, Carnauba Wax, Poloxamer 407, Polyethylene Oxide, Silicon Dioxide or Sodium Lauryl Sulfate. See package for complete listing.

Indications: For the temporary relief of nasal congestion, minor aches, pains,

Continued on next page

This product information was prepared in November 2000. On these and other Pfizer Consumer Healthcare Products, detailed information may be obtained by addressing Pfizer, Inc. Warner-Lambert Consumer Healthcare Products, Morris Plains, NJ 07950

Sudafed Severe Cold—Cont.

headache, muscular aches, sore throat, and fever associated with the common cold. Temporarily relieves cough occurring with a cold.

Directions: Adults and children 12 years of age and over: 2 caplets or tablets every 6 hours, while symptoms persist, not to exceed 8 caplets or tablets in 24 hours, or as directed by a doctor. Children under 12 years of age: consult a doctor.

Warnings: Do not exceed recommended dosage. If nervousness, dizziness, or sleeplessness occur, discontinue use and consult a doctor. Do not take this product for more than 10 days. A persistent cough may be a sign of a serious condition. If symptoms do not improve or if cough persists for more than 7 days, tends to recur, or is accompanied by rash, persistent headache, fever that lasts for more than 3 days, or if new symptoms occur, consult a doctor. Do not take this product for persistent or chronic cough such as occurs with smoking, asthma or emphysema, or if cough is accompanied by excessive phlegm (mucus) unless directed by a doctor. If sore throat is severe, persists for more than 2 days, is accompanied or followed by fever, headache, rash, nausea, or vomiting, consult a doctor promptly. Do not take this product if you have heart disease, high blood pressure, thyroid disease, diabetes, or difficulty in urination due to enlargement of the prostate gland unless directed by a doctor. As with any drug, if you are pregnant or nursing a baby, seek the advice of a health professional before using this product. **KEEP THIS AND ALL DRUGS OUT OF THE REACH OF CHILDREN.** In case of accidental overdose, seek professional assistance or contact a Poison Control Center immediately. Prompt medical attention is critical for adults as well as for children even if you do not notice any signs or symptoms.

Alcohol Warning: If you consume 3 or more alcoholic drinks every day, ask your doctor whether you should take acetaminophen or other pain relievers/fever reducers. Acetaminophen may cause liver damage.

Drug Interaction Precaution: Do not use this product if you are now taking a prescription monoamine oxidase inhibitor (MAOI) (certain drugs for depression, psychiatric or emotional conditions, or Parkinson's disease), or for 2 weeks after stopping the MAOI drug. If you are uncertain whether your prescription drug contains an MAOI, consult a health professional before taking this product.

How Supplied: Boxes of 12 and 24 caplets; boxes of 12 tablets.
Store at 59° to 77°F in a dry place.

Shown in Product Identification Guide, page 520

SUDAFED® NON-DRYING SINUS LIQUID CAPS
[sū 'duh-fěd]

Description: Sudafed Non-Drying Sinus provides temporary, maximum strength relief of nasal congestion and sinus pressure due to sinusitis, colds, or allergies. Sudafed Non-Drying Sinus contains ingredients that help clear nasal congestion, relieve sinus pressure without overdrying sensitive nasal tissue or causing drowsiness and temporarily relieves chest congestion.

Active Ingredients: Each liquid cap contains Guaifenesin 200 mg. and Pseudoephedrine Hydrochloride 30 mg.

Inactive Ingredients: FD&C Blue No. 1, Gelatin, Glycerin, Polyethylene Glycol 400, Povidone, Propylene Glycol and Sorbitol. Printed with edible white ink.

Indications: For the temporary relief of nasal congestion associated with sinusitis. Promotes nasal and/or sinus drainage; temporarily relieves sinus congestion and pressure. Helps loosen phlegm (mucus) and thin bronchial secretions to rid the bronchial passageways of bothersome mucus and make coughs more productive.

Directions: Adults and children 12 years of age and over: swallow 2 liquid caps every 4 hours, not to exceed 8 liquid caps in 24 hours, or as directed by a doctor. Children under 12 years of age: consult a doctor.

Warnings: Do not exceed recommended dosage. If nervousness, dizziness, or sleeplessness occur, discontinue use and consult a doctor. If symptoms do not improve within 7 days or are accompanied by fever, consult a doctor. Do not take this product if you have heart disease, high blood pressure, thyroid disease, diabetes, or difficulty in urination due to enlargement of the prostate gland unless directed by a doctor. A persistent cough may be a sign of a serious condition. If cough persists for more than 1 week, tends to recur, or is accompanied by a fever, rash, or persistent headache, consult a doctor. Do not take this product for persistent or chronic cough such as occurs with smoking, asthma, chronic bronchitis, or emphysema, or where cough is accompanied by excessive phlegm (mucus) unless directed by a doctor. As with any drug, if you are pregnant or nursing a baby, seek the advice of a health professional before using this product. **KEEP THIS AND ALL DRUGS OUT OF THE REACH OF CHILDREN.** In case of accidental overdose, seek professional assistance or contact a Poison Control Center immediately.

Drug Interaction Precaution: Do not use this product if you are now taking a prescription monoamine oxidase inhibitor (MAOI) (certain drugs for depression, psychiatric or emotional conditions, or Parkinson's disease), or for 2 weeks af-

ter stopping the MAOI drug. If you are uncertain whether your prescription drug contains an MAOI, consult a health professional before taking this product.

How Supplied: Sudafed Non-Drying Sinus is supplied in boxes of 24 liquid caps.
Store at 15° to 25°C (59° to 77°F) in a dry place and protect from light.

Shown in Product Identification Guide, page 520

SUDAFED® Sinus Headache Caplets and Tablets
[sū 'duh-fěd]

Description: Sudafed Sinus Headache Caplets contains Sudafed's maximum strength decongestant and a maximum strength pain reliever to temporarily relieve sinus symptoms. Sudafed Sinus Headache helps clear nasal congestion and relieve sinus pressure while relieving sinus headaches due to sinusitis, allergies or colds without drowsy or overdrying side effects.

Active Ingredients: Each coated caplet/tablet contains: Acetaminophen 500 mg and Pseudoephedrine Hydrochloride 30 mg.

Inactive Ingredients: Caplets and Tablets contain Crospovidone, FD&C Yellow No. 6 Aluminum Lake, Hydroxypropyl Methylcellulose, Microcrystalline Cellulose, Polyethylene Glycol, Polysorbate 80, Povidone, Pregelatinized Starch, Stearic Acid and Titanium Dioxide.
May also contain: Carnauba Wax or Candelilla Wax, Calcium Stearate, Magnesium Stearate and Croscarmellose Sodium. See package for complete listing.

Indications: For the temporary relief of nasal congestion associated with sinusitis. Helps decongest sinus openings and passages; temporarily relieves sinus congestion and pressure. Temporarily relieves headache, minor aches, and pains. Temporarily restores freer breathing through the nose.

Directions: Adults and children 12 years and over: 2 caplets or tablets every 6 hours, while symptoms persist, not to exceed 8 caplets or tablets in 24 hours, or as directed by a doctor. Children under 12 years of age: consult a doctor.

Warnings: Do not exceed recommended dosage. If nervousness, dizziness, or sleeplessness occur, discontinue use and consult a doctor. Do not take this product for more than 10 days. If symptoms do not improve or are accompanied by fever that lasts for more than 3 days, or if new symptoms occur, consult a doctor. Do not take this product if you have heart disease, high blood pressure, thyroid disease, diabetes, or difficulty in urination due to enlargement of the prostate gland unless directed by a doctor. As with any drug, if you are pregnant or nursing a baby, seek the advice of a

health professional before using this product. **KEEP THIS AND ALL DRUGS OUT OF THE REACH OF CHILDREN.** In case of accidental overdose, seek professional assistance or contact a Poison Control Center immediately. Prompt medical attention is critical for adults as well as for children even if you do not notice any signs or symptoms.

Alcohol Warning: If you consume 3 or more alcoholic drinks every day, ask your doctor whether you should take acetaminophen or other pain relievers/fever reducers. Acetaminophen may cause liver damage.

Drug Interaction Precaution: Do not use this product if you are now taking a prescription monoamine oxidase inhibitor (MAOI) (certain drugs for depression, psychiatric or emotional conditions, or Parkinson's disease), or for 2 weeks after stopping the MAOI drug. If you are uncertain whether your prescription drug contains an MAOI, consult a health professional before taking this product.

How Supplied: Boxes of 24 and 48 caplets; boxes of 24 tablets. Store at 59° to 77°F in a dry place.
Shown in Product Identification Guide, page 520

TUCKS®
Pre-moistened Hemorrhoidal/Vaginal Pads
[tŭks]

Active Ingredients: Soft pads are pre-moistened with a solution containing Witch Hazel 50%.

Inactive Ingredients: Water, Glycerin, Alcohol, Propylene Glycol, Sodium Citrate, Diazolidinyl Urea, Citric Acid, Methylparaben, Propylparaben.

Indications: For the temporary relief of external itching, burning and irritation associated with hemorrhoids.

Other Uses:
Hygienic Wipe: TUCKS Pads are effective for everyday personal hygienic use on outer rectal and vaginal areas. Used in place of toilet tissue, TUCKS Pads gently and thoroughly remove irritation-causing matter. They are especially handy during menstrual periods.
Vaginal Care: Gentle, soft TUCKS Pads can be used daily to freshen and cleanse.
Moist Compress: For additional relief, TUCKS Pads can be folded and used as a compress on inflamed tissue. TUCKS Pads are particularly helpful in relieving discomfort following childbirth, rectal or vaginal surgery.
Baby Care: TUCKS Pads are recommended as a final cleansing step at diaper changing time.

Directions: For external use only. *As a hemorrhoidal treatment* —Adults: When practical, cleanse the affected area with mild soap and warm water and rinse

thoroughly. Gently dry by patting or blotting with toilet tissue or soft cloth before application of this product. Gently apply to affected area by patting and then discard. Can be used up to six times daily or after each bowel movement. Children under 12 years of age: consult a physician. *As a hygienic wipe* —Use as a wipe instead of toilet tissue.
As a moist compress —For soothing relief, fold pad and place in contact with irritated tissue. Leave in place for 5 to 15 minutes. Repeat as needed.

Warnings: If condition worsens or does not improve within 7 days, consult a physician. Do not exceed recommended daily dosage unless directed by a physician. In case of bleeding, consult a physician promptly. Do not put this product into the rectum by using fingers or any mechanical device or applicator. **KEEP THIS AND ALL DRUGS OUT OF THE REACH OF CHILDREN.** In case of accidental ingestion, seek professional assistance or contact a Poison Control Center immediately.
Store at 59° to 77°F.

How Supplied: Jars of 40 and 100 pads. Also available TUCKS® individual foil-wrapped towelettes.
Shown in Product Identification Guide, page 521

MAXIMUM STRENGTH UNISOM SLEEPGELS®
Nighttime Sleep Aid

Description: Maximum Strength Unisom SleepGels are liquid-filled, blue soft gelatin capsules.
Active Ingredient: Diphenhydramine Hydrochloride 50 mg.
Inactive Ingredients: FD&C Blue No. 1, Gelatin, Glycerin, Pharmaceutical Glaze, Polyethylene Glycol, Propylene Glycol, Purified Water, Sorbitol, Titanium Dioxide.

Indications: Helps to reduce difficulty falling asleep.

Action: Diphenhydramine Hydrochloride is an ethanolamine antihistamine with anticholinergic and sedative effects.

Administration and Dosage: Adults and children 12 years of age and over: Oral dosage is one softgel (50 mg) at bedtime if needed, or as directed by a doctor.

Warnings: Do not take this product, unless directed by a doctor, if you have a breathing problem such as emphysema or chronic bronchitis, or if you have glaucoma or difficulty in urination due to enlargement of the prostate gland. Do not take this product if pregnant or nursing a baby.
- Do not give to children under 12 years of age.
- If sleeplessness persists continuously for more than two weeks, consult your doctor. Insomnia may be a symptom of serious underlying medical illness.
- Avoid alcoholic beverages while taking this product. Do not take this product

if you are taking sedatives or tranquilizers, without first consulting your doctor.
- **Do Not Use:** with any other product containing diphenhydramine, including one applied topically.
- Keep this and all drugs out of the reach of children.
- In case of accidental overdose, seek professional assistance or contact a poison control center immediately.

Drug Interaction: Monoamine oxidase (MAO) inhibitors prolong and intensify the anticholinergic effects of antihistamines. The CNS depressant effect is heightened by alcohol and other CNS depressant drugs.

Symptoms of Oral Overdosage: Antihistamine overdosage reactions may vary from central nervous system depression to stimulation.
Stimulation is particularly likely in children. Atropine-like signs and symptoms, such as dry mouth, fixed and dilated pupils, flushing, and gastrointestinal symptoms, may also occur.

Attention: Use only if softgel blister seals are unbroken.

How Supplied: Boxes of 16 liquid filled softgels in child resistant blisters and boxes of 8 with non-child resistant packaging. Also in a 32 count easy to open child resistant bottle.
Store between 15° and 30°C (59° and 86°F)

UNISOM® SleepTabs™
[yu 'na-som]
Nighttime Sleep Aid
(doxylamine succinate)

PRODUCT OVERVIEW

Key Facts: Unisom is an ethanolamine antihistamine (doxylamine) which characteristically shows a high incidence of sedation. It produces a reduced latency to end of wakefulness and early onset of sleep.

Major Uses: Unisom has been shown to be clinically effective as a sleep aid when 1 tablet is given 30 minutes before retiring.

Safety Information: Unisom is contraindicated in pregnancy and nursing mothers. It is also contraindicated in patients with asthma, glaucoma, and enlargement of the prostate. Caution

Continued on next page

This product information was prepared in November 2000. On these and other Pfizer Consumer Healthcare Products, detailed information may be obtained by addressing Pfizer, Inc. Warner-Lambert Consumer Healthcare Products, Morris Plains, NJ 07950

Unisom—Cont.

should be used if taken when alcohol is being consumed. Caution is also indicated when taken concurrently with other medications due to the anticholinergic properties of antihistamines.

Description: Pale blue oval scored tablets containing 25 mg. of doxylamine succinate, 2-[α-(2-dimethylaminoethoxy)α-methylbenzyl]pyridine succinate.

Inactive Ingredients: Dibasic Calcium Phosphate, FD&C Blue #1 Aluminum Lake, Magnesium Stearate, Microcrystalline Cellulose, Sodium Starch Glycolate.

Administration and Dosage: One tablet 30 minutes before going to bed. Take once daily or as directed by a doctor. Not for children under 12 years of age.

Warnings: Do not take this product, unless directed by a doctor, if you have a breathing problem such as emphysema or chronic bronchitis, or if you have glaucoma or difficulty in urination due to enlargement of the prostate gland. Do not take this product if pregnant or nursing a baby.
- If sleeplessness persists continuously for more than two weeks, consult your doctor. Insomnia may be a symptom of a serious underlying medical illness.
- Do not take this product if presently taking any other drug, without consulting your doctor or pharmacist.
- Take this product with caution if alcohol is being consumed.
- For adults only. Do not give to children under 12 years of age.
- Keep this and all medications out of the reach of children. This product contains an antihistamine and will cause drowsiness. It should be used only at bedtime.

Side Effects: Occasional anticholinergic effects may be seen.

Attention: Use only if tablet blister seals are unbroken.

How Supplied: Boxes of 8, 32 and 48 tablets in child resistant packaging. Boxes of 16 tablets in non-child resistant packaging.

Shown in Product Identification Guide, page 521

ADVANCED RELIEF VISINE®
Lubricant/Redness Reliever Eye Drops

Description: Advanced Relief Visine is a sterile, isotonic, buffered ophthalmic solution containing polyethylene glycol 400 1%, povidone 1%, dextran 70 0.1%, tetrahydrozoline hydrochloride 0.05%. Advanced Relief Visine is an ophthalmic solution combining the effects of the decongestant, tetrahydrozoline hydrochloride, with the demulcent effects of polyethylene glycol, povidone and dextran 70. It provides symptomatic relief of con-

junctival edema and hyperemia secondary to minor irritations. Tetrahydrozoline hydrochloride is a sympathomimetic agent, which brings about decongestion by vasoconstriction. Reddened eyes are rapidly whitened by this effective vasoconstrictor, which limits the local vascular response by constricting the small blood vessels. The onset of vasoconstriction becomes apparent within minutes. Additional effects include amelioration of burning, irritation and excessive lacrimation. Relief is afforded by three moisturizers: polyethylene glycol 400, povidone and dextran 70.

Polyethylene glycol 400, povidone and dextran 70 are ophthalmic demulcents which have been shown to be effective for the temporary relief of discomfort of minor irritations of the eye due to exposure to wind or sun. They are effective as protectants and lubricants against further irritation or to relieve dryness of the eye. The effectiveness of tetrahydrozoline hydrochloride in relieving conjunctival hyperemia and associated symptoms has been demonstrated by numerous clinicals, including several double-blind studies, involving more than 2,000 subjects suffering from acute or chronic hyperemia induced by a variety of conditions. Advanced Relief Visine is a unique eye drop formulation that combines the redness-relieving effects of a vasoconstrictor and the soothing, moisturizing and protective effects of three demulcents.

Indications: Relieves redness of the eye due to minor eye irritations. For use as a protectant against further irritation or to relieve dryness.

Directions: Instill 1 to 2 drops in the affected eye(s) up to 4 times daily.

Active Ingredients: Polyethylene glycol 400 1%; povidone 1%; dextran 70 0.1%; tetrahydrozoline hydrochloride 0.05%.

Inactive Ingredients: Benzalkonium chloride; boric acid; edetate disodium; purified water; sodium borate; sodium chloride.

Warnings: If you experience eye pain, changes in vision, continued redness or irritation of the eye, or if the condition worsens or persists for more than 72 hours, discontinue use and consult a physician. If you have glaucoma, do not use this product except under the advice and supervision of a physician. As with any drug, if you are pregnant or nursing a baby, seek the advice of a health professional before using this product. Overuse of this product may produce increased redness of the eye. If solution changes color or becomes cloudy, do not use. To avoid contamination, do not touch tip of container to any surface. Replace cap after using. Remove contact lenses before using this product.

Parents Note: Before using with children under 6 years of age, consult your physician. Keep this and all drugs out of the reach of children. In case of ac-

cidental ingestion, seek professional assistance or contact a Poison Control Center immediately.

Caution: Should not be used if Visine-imprinted neckband on bottle is broken or missing.

Storage: Store between 15° and 30°C (59° and 86°F).

How Supplied: In 0.5 fl. oz. and 1.0 fl. oz. plastic dispenser bottle.

Shown in Product Identification Guide, page 521

VISINE®-A™
Eye Allergy Relief
Itching & Redness Reliever
Eye Drops
ANTIHISTAMINE & REDNESS RELIEVER

Visine-A is an antihistamine and redness reliever eye drop, clinically proven to temporarily relieve itching and redness of the eye.

Indications: For the temporary relief of itching and redness of the eye due to pollen, ragweed, grass, animal hair and dander.

Directions: Adults and children 6 years of age or older: Place 1 or 2 drops in the affected eye(s) up to four times a day. Some users may experience a brief tingling sensation.

Active Ingredients: pheniramine maleate 0.3%, naphazoline hydrochloride 0.025%.

Inactive Ingredients: boric acid and sodium borate buffer system preserved with benzalkonium chloride (0.01%) and edetate disodium (0.1%), sodium hydroxide and/or hydrochloric acid (to adjust pH) and purified water. The solution has a pH of 5.5–6.5 and a tonicity of 245—305 mOsm/Kg.

Warnings: If you experience eye pain, changes in vision, continued redness or irritation of the eye, or if the condition worsens or persists for more than 72 hours, discontinue use and consult a physician.

Do not use this product if you have heart disease, high blood pressure, difficulty in urination due to enlargement of the prostate gland or narrow angle glaucoma unless directed by a physician.

To avoid contamination of this product, do not touch tip of container to any surface. Replace cap after using. Do not use if solution changes color or becomes cloudy.

Remove contact lenses before using.

Overuse of this product may produce increased redness of the eye. When using this product pupils may become enlarged temporarily.

Use before the expiration date marked on the carton or bottle.

Keep this and all drugs out of the reach of children. If swallowed, get medical help or contact a Poison Control Center

right away. Accidental swallowing by infants and children may lead to coma and marked reduction in body temperature. Store between 15° and 25°C (59° and 77°F).

Parents Note: Before using with children under 6 years of age, consult your physician. Keep this and all drugs out of the reach of children. In case of accidental ingestion, seek professional assistance or contact a Poison Control Center immediately.

Caution: Do not use if Pfizer imprinted neckband on bottle is broken or missing.

Distributed By:
CONSUMER HEALTH CARE GROUP, PFIZER INC, NEW YORK, NEW YORK 10017

Shown in Product Identification Guide, page 521

VISINE® L.R.™ Long Lasting
Oxymetazoline Hydrochloride/
Redness Reliever Eye Drops

Description: Visine L.R. is a sterile, isotonic, buffered ophthalmic solution containing the vasoconstrictor, oxymetazoline hydrochloride. Visine L.R. is specially formulated to relieve redness of the eye in minutes with effective relief that lasts up to 6 hours.

Indications: Visine L.R. is a decongestant ophthalmic solution designed for the relief of redness of the eye due to minor eye irritations.

Directions: Adults and children 6 years of age or older: Place 1 or 2 drops in the affected eye(s). This may be repeated as needed every 6 hours or as directed by a physician.

Active Ingredients: Oxymetazoline hydrochloride 0.025%.

Inactive Ingredients: Sodium chloride; boric acid; sodium borate; with benzalkonium chloride 0.01% and edetate disodium 0.1% added as preservatives; purified water.

Warnings: If you experience eye pain, changes in vision, continued redness or irritation of the eye, or if the condition worsens or persists for more than 72 hours, discontinue use and consult a physician. If you have glaucoma, do not use this product except under the advice and supervision of a physician. As with any drug, if you are pregnant or nursing a baby, seek the advice of a health professional before using this product. Overuse of this product may produce increased redness of the eye. If solution changes color or becomes cloudy, do not use. To avoid contamination, do not touch tip of container to any surface. Replace cap after using. Remove contact lenses before using this product.

Parents: Before using with children under 6 years of age, consult your physician. Keep this and all drugs out of the

reach of children. In case of accidental ingestion, seek professional assistance or contact a Poison Control Center immediately.

Caution: Should not be used if Visine-imprinted neckband on bottle is broken or missing.

Storage: Store between 15° and 30°C (59° and 86°F).

How Supplied: In 0.5 fl. oz. and 1 fl. oz. plastic dispenser bottle.

Shown in Product Identification Guide, page 521

VISINE A.C.®
Seasonal Relief From Pollen & Dust
Astringent/Redness Reliever Eye Drops

Description: Visine A.C. is a sterile, isotonic, buffered ophthalmic solution containing tetrahydrozoline hydrochloride 0.05% and zinc sulfate 0.25%. Visine A.C. is a fast-acting, dual-action ophthalmic solution combining the effects of the vasoconstrictor, tetrahydrozoline hydrochloride, with the astringent effects of zinc sulfate. The vasoconstrictor provides temporary relief of conjunctival edema, hyperemia and discomfort, while zinc sulfate helps to relieve itching and burning discomfort due to airborne irritants such as pollen, dust and ragweed.

Tetrahydrozoline hydrochloride is a sympathomimetic agent, which brings about decongestion by vasoconstriction. Reddened eyes are rapidly whitened by this effective vasoconstrictor which limits the local vascular response by constricting the small blood vessels. The onset of vasoconstriction becomes apparent within minutes. Zinc sulfate is an ocular astringent which, by precipitating protein, helps to clear mucus from the outer surface of the eye. The effectiveness of Visine A.C. in temporarily relieving conjunctival hyperemia and eye discomfort due to pollen, dust and ragweed has been clinically demonstrated. In one double-blind study of subjects who experienced acute episodes of minor eye irritation, Visine A.C. produced statistically significant beneficial results versus a placebo of normal saline solution in relieving irritation of bulbar conjunctivae, irritation of palpebral conjunctivae and mucus buildup. Treatment with Visine A.C. also significantly relieved eye discomfort.

Indications: For temporary relief of discomfort and redness due to minor eye irritations.

Directions: Instill 1 to 2 drops in the affected eye(s) up to 4 times daily.

Note: As drops go to work, some users may notice a brief tingling sensation which will quickly pass.

Active Ingredients: Zinc sulfate 0.25%; tetrahydrozoline hydrochloride 0.05%.

Inactive Ingredients: Benzalkonium chloride; boric acid; edetate disodium; purified water; sodium chloride; sodium citrate.

Warnings: If you experience eye pain, changes in vision, continued redness or irritation of the eye, or if the condition worsens or persists for more than 72 hours, discontinue use and consult a physician. If you have glaucoma, do not use this product except under the advice and supervision of a physician. As with any drug, if you are pregnant or nursing a baby, seek the advice of a health professional before using this product. Overuse of this product may produce increased redness of the eye. If solution changes color or becomes cloudy, do not use. To avoid contamination, do not touch tip of container to any surface. Replace cap after using. Remove contact lenses before using this product.

Parents Note: Before using with children under 6 years of age, consult your physician. Keep this and all drugs out of the reach of children. In case of accidental ingestion, seek professional assistance or contact a Poison Control Center immediately.

Caution: Should not be used if Visine-imprinted neckband on bottle is broken or missing.

Storage: Store between 15° and 30°C (59° and 86°F).

How Supplied: In 0.5 fl. oz. and 1.0 fl. oz. plastic dispenser bottle.

Shown in Product Identification Guide, page 521

VISINE® ORIGINAL
Tetrahydrozoline Hydrochloride/
Redness Reliever Eye Drops

Description: Visine is a sterile, isotonic, buffered ophthalmic solution containing tetrahydrozoline hydrochloride 0.05%. Visine is a decongestant ophthalmic solution designed to provide symptomatic relief of conjunctival edema and hyperemia secondary to minor irritations, due to conditions such as smoke, dust, other airborne pollutants and swimming. Relief is afforded by tetrahydrozoline hydrochloride, a sympathomimetic agent, which brings about decongestion by vasoconstriction. Reddened eyes are rapidly whitened by this effective vasoconstrictor, which limits the lo-

Continued on next page

This product information was prepared in November 2000. On these and other Pfizer Consumer Healthcare Products, detailed information may be obtained by addressing Pfizer, Inc. Warner-Lambert Consumer Healthcare Products, Morris Plains, NJ 07950

Visine Original—Cont.

cal vascular response by constricting the small blood vessels. The onset of vasoconstriction becomes apparent within minutes.

The effectiveness of Visine in relieving conjunctival hyperemia has been demonstrated by numerous clinicals, including several double-blind studies, involving more than 2,000 subjects suffering from acute or chronic hyperemia induced by a variety of conditions. Visine was found to be efficacious in providing relief from conjunctival hyperemia.

Indications: Relieves redness of the eye due to minor eye irritations.

Directions: Instill 1 to 2 drops in the affected eye(s) up to four times daily.

Active Ingredient: Tetrahydrozoline hydrochloride 0.05%.

Inactive Ingredients: Benzalkonium chloride; boric acid; edetate disodium; purified water; sodium borate; sodium chloride.

Warnings: If you experience eye pain, changes in vision, continued redness or irritation of the eye, or if the condition worsens or persists for more than 72 hours, discontinue use and consult a physician. If you have glaucoma, do not use this product except under the advice and supervision of a physician. As with any drug, if you are pregnant or nursing a baby, seek the advice of a health professional before using this product. Overuse of this product may produce increased redness of the eye. If solution changes color or becomes cloudy, do not use. To avoid contamination, do not touch tip of container to any surface. Replace cap after using. Remove contact lenses before using this product.

Parents Note: Before using with children under 6 years of age, consult your physician. Keep this and all drugs out of the reach of children. In case of accidental ingestion, seek professional assistance or contact a Poison Control Center immediately.

Caution: Should not be used if Visine-imprinted neckband on bottle is broken or missing.

Storage: Store between 15° and 30°C (59° and 86°F).

How Supplied: In 0.5 fl. oz. and 1.0 fl. oz. plastic dispenser bottle and 0.5 fl. oz. plastic bottle with dropper.
Shown in Product Identification Guide, page 521

VISINE® TEARS™
Lubricant Eye Drops

Description:
Visine® Tears™
Visine® Tears™ Lubricant Eye Drops cools and comforts your dry, scratchy, irritated eyes, and helps them feel their best. It relieves the dryness caused by

computer use, reading, wind, heat and air conditioning, while it protects your eyes from further irritation. Visine Tears is safe to use as often as needed.

Indications: For the temporary relief of burning and irritation due to dryness of the eye and for use as a protectant against further irritation.

Directions: Instill 1 to 2 drops in the affected eye(s) as needed.

Active Ingredients: Polyethylene glycol 400 1%; glycerin 0.2%; hydroxypropyl methylcellulose 0.2%.

Inactive Ingredients: Ascorbic acid; benzalkonium chloride; boric acid; dextrose; disodium phosphate; glycine; magnesium chloride; potassium chloride; purified water; sodium borate; sodium chloride; sodium citrate; sodium lactate.

Warnings: If you experience eye pain, changes in vision, continued redness or irritation of the eye, or if the condition worsens or persists for more than 72 hours, discontinue use and consult a physician. As with any drug, if you are pregnant or nursing a baby, seek the advice of a health professional before using this product. If solution changes color or becomes cloudy, do not use. To avoid contamination, do not touch tip of container to any surface. Replace cap after using. Remove contact lenses before using this product.

Parents note: Before using with children under 6 years of age, consult your physician. Keep this and all drugs out of the reach of children. In case of accidental ingestion, seek professional assistance or contact a Poison Control Center immediately.

Caution: Should not be used if Visine-imprinted neckband on bottle is broken or missing.

Storage: Store between 15° and 30°C (59° and 86°F).

How Supplied: In 0.5 fl. oz. and 1 fl. oz. plastic dispenser bottle.
Shown in Product Identification Guide, page 521

VISINE® TEARS™
Preservative Free, Single-Use Containers
Lubricant Eye Drops

Description:
Visine® Tears™ Preservative Free Lubricant Eye Drops
Visine Tears Preservative Free cools and comforts your dry, scratchy, irritated eyes, and helps them feel their best. It relieves the dryness caused by computer use, reading, wind, heat and air conditioning, while it actually protects your eyes from further irritation. Visine Tears Preservative Free is specially formu-

lated for people whose eyes are sensitive to preservatives and is safe to use as often as needed. It is also sealed in convenient single-use containers.

Indications: For the temporary relief of burning and irritation due to dryness of the eye and for use as a protectant against further irritation.

Directions: Instill 1 to 2 drops in the affected eye(s) as needed.
How to use:
1. To open, completely twist off tab.
2. Instill 1 to 2 drops in the affected eye(s) as needed.
3. Once opened, discard.

Active Ingredients: Polyethylene glycol 400 1%; glycerin 0.2%; hydroxypropyl methylcellulose 0.2%.

Inactive Ingredients: Ascorbic acid; dextrose; disodium phosphate; glycine; magnesium chloride; potassium chloride; purified water; sodium chloride; sodium citrate; sodium lactate; sodium phosphate.

Warnings: If you experience eye pain, changes in vision, continued redness or irritation of the eye, or if the condition worsens or persists for more than 72 hours, discontinue use and consult a physician. As with any drug, if you are pregnant or nursing a baby, seek the advice of a health professional before using this product. If solution changes color or becomes cloudy, do not use. To avoid contamination, do not touch tip of container to any surface. Do not reuse. Once opened, discard. Remove contact lenses before using this product.

Parents note:
Before using with children under 6 years of age, consult your physician. Keep this and all drugs out of the reach of children. In case of accidental ingestion, seek professional assistance or contact a Poison Control Center immediately.

Caution: Use only if unit dose container is intact.
Storage: Store between 15° and 30° C (59° and 86° F).

How Supplied: 1 box contains 28 single-use containers, 0.01 fl. oz. (0.4 mL) each
Shown in Product Identification Guide, page 521

WART–OFF®
Liquid

Active Ingredient: Salicylic Acid 17% w/w.

Inactive Ingredients: Alcohol, 26.3% w/w, *t*-Butyl Alcohol, Denatonium Benzoate, Flexible Collodion, Propylene Glycol Dipelargonate.

Indications: For the removal of common warts and plantar warts on the bot-

tom of the foot. The common wart is easily recognized by the rough "cauliflower-like" appearance of the surface. The plantar wart is recognized by its location only on the bottom of the foot, its tenderness, and the interruption of the footprint pattern.

Warnings: For external use only. Keep this and all medications out of the reach of children to avoid accidental poisoning. In case of accidental ingestion, contact a physician or a Poison Control Center immediately. Do not use this product on irritated skin, on any area that is infected or reddened, if you are a diabetic, or if you have poor blood circulation. Do not use on moles, birthmarks, warts with hair growing from them, genital warts, or warts on the face or mucous membranes. If product gets into the eye, flush with water for 15 minutes. Avoid inhaling vapors. If discomfort persists, see your doctor.

Extremely Flammable—Keep away from fire or flame. Cap bottle tightly and store at room temperature (59°–86°F) (15°–30°C) and keep away from heat.

Directions: Read warnings. Wash affected area. Dry area thoroughly. Apply one drop at a time to sufficiently cover each wart. Apply Wart-Off to warts only—not to surrounding skin. Let dry. Repeat this procedure once or twice daily as needed (until wart is removed) for up to 12 weeks. Replace cap tightly to prevent evaporation.

How Supplied: 0.45 fluid ounce (13.3mL) bottle.

ZANTAC® 75
Ranitidine Tablets 75 mg
Acid Reducer
[zan ' tak]

Active Ingredient: Each tablet contains: 84 mg ranitidine hydrochloride (equivalent to 75 mg ranitidine).

Inactive Ingredients: Hydroxypropyl methylcellulose, magnesium stearate, microcrystalline cellulose, synthetic red iron oxide, titanium dioxide and triacetin. Zantac 75 tablets are sodium and sugar free.

Uses:
- For **relief** of heartburn associated with acid indigestion and sour stomach.
- For **prevention** of heartburn associated with acid indigestion and sour stomach brought on by certain foods and beverages.

Directions:
- For **relief** of symptoms, swallow 1 tablet with a glass of water.
- To **prevent** symptoms, swallow 1 tablet with a glass of water **30 to 60 minutes before** eating food or drinking beverages that cause heartburn.
- Can be used up to twice daily (up to 2 tablets in 24 hours).
- This product should not be given to children under 12 years old unless directed by a doctor.

Warnings:
- **Allergy Warning:** Do not use if you are allergic to Zantac (ranitidine hydrochloride) or other acid reducers.
- Do not use with other acid reducers.
- Do not take the maximum daily dose for more than 14 consecutive days, unless directed by your doctor.
- If you have trouble swallowing or persistent abdominal pain, see your doctor promptly. You may have a serious condition that may need different treatment.
- As with any drug, if you are pregnant or nursing a baby, seek the advice of a health professional before using this product.
- Keep this and all drugs out of the reach of children.
- In case of accidental overdose, seek professional assistance or contact a poison control center immediately.

Read the Label: Read the directions, consumer information leaflet and warnings before use. Keep the carton. It contains important information.

How Supplied: Zantac 75 is available in convenient blister packs in boxes of 4, 10, 20 and 30 tablets, and in bottles of 60, 80 and 90 count. Store between 20°–25°C (68°–77°F). Avoid excessive heat or humidity.

Zantac is a registered trademark of the Glaxo Wellcome group of companies.

Questions or Comments? Call us Toll-Free at 1-800-223-0182 weekdays between 9:00 am and 5:00 pm EST.

Shown in Product Identification Guide, page 521

Pharmacia Consumer Healthcare
PEAPACK, NJ 07977

For Medical and Pharmaceutical Information, Including Emergencies:
(616) 833-8244
(800) 253-8600 ext. 3-8244

CORTAID®
Maximum Strength, Sensitive Skin and Intensive Therapy
Cream and Ointment
(hydrocortisone 1% and $^1/_2$%)
Anti-itch products

Indications: Use CORTAID for the temporary relief of itching associated with minor skin irritations, inflammation, and rashes due to eczema, psoriasis, seborrheic dermatitis, poison ivy, poison oak, or poison sumac, insect bites, soaps, detergents, cosmetics, jewelry, and for external feminine and anal itching. Other uses of this product should be only under the advice and supervision of a physician.

Description: CORTAID provides safe, effective relief of many different types of itches and rashes and no brand is recom-

mended by more physicians and pharmacists. CORTAID Maximum Strength 1% hydrocortisone is the same strength and form of hydrocortisone relief formerly available only with a prescription. CORTAID Sensitive Skin has been specially formulated with aloe and $^1/_2$% hydrocortisone. CORTAID Intensive Therapy's special formula of 1% hydrocortisone is specific for eczema and psoriasis sufferers. CORTAID is available in 1) a greaseless, odorless vanishing cream that leaves no residue; 2) a soothing, lubricating ointment.

Active Ingredients: CORTAID Maximum Strength Cream: Hydrocortisone 1%

CORTAID Maximum Strength Ointment: Hydrocortisone acetate 1%

CORTAID Intensive Therapy Cream: Hydrocortisone 1%

CORTAID Sensitive Skin Cream: Hydrocortisone acetate $^1/_2$%

Other Ingredients:

Maximum Strength Products: *Maximum Strength Cream:* Aloe vera, benzyl alcohol, ceteareth-20, cetearyl alcohol, cetyl palmitate, glycerin, isopropyl myristate, isostearyl neopentanoate, methylparaben, and purified water.

Maximum Strength Ointment: butylparaben, cholesterol, methylparaben, microcrystalline wax, mineral oil, and white petrolatum.

Sensitive Skin Products:

Sensitive Skin Cream: aloe vera, butylparaben, cetyl palmitate, glyceryl stearate, methylparaben, polyethylene glycol, stearamidoethyl diethylamine, and purified water.

Intensive Therapy Products:

Intensive Therapy Cream: cetyl alcohol, citric acid, glyceryl stearate, isopropyl myristate, methylparaben, polyoxyl 40 stearate, polysorbate 60, propylene glycol, propylparaben, purified water, sodium citrate, sorbic acid, sorbitan monostearate, stearyl alcohol and white wax.

Uses: The vanishing action of CORTAID Cream makes it cosmetically acceptable when the skin itch or rash treated is on exposed parts of the body such as the hands or arms. CORTAID Ointment is best used where protection, lubrication, and soothing of dry and scaly lesions are required. The ointment is also recommended for treating itchy genital and anal areas.

Warnings: For external use only. Avoid contact with the eyes. If condition wors-

Continued on next page

Cortaid—Cont.

ens, or if symptoms persist for more than 7 days or clear up and occur again within a few days, stop use of this product and do not begin use of any other hydrocortisone product unless you have consulted a physician. Do not use for the treatment of diaper rash. Consult a physician. For external feminine itching, do not use if you have a vaginal discharge. Consult a physician. For external anal itching, do not exceed the recommended daily dosage unless directed by a physician. In case of bleeding, consult a physician promptly. Do not put this product into the rectum by using fingers or any mechanical device or applicator. **Keep this and all drugs out of the reach of children. In case of accidental ingestion, seek professional assistance or contact a Poison Control Center immediately.**

Dosage and Administration: *Adults and children 2 years of age and older:* Apply to affected area not more than 3 to 4 times daily. *Children under 2 years of age:* Do not use, consult a physician. *Adults:* For external anal itching, when practical, cleanse the affected area with mild soap and warm water and rinse thoroughly by patting or blotting with an appropriate cleansing pad. Gently dry by patting or blotting with toilet tissue or a soft cloth before application of this product. *Children under 12 years of age:* For external anal itching, consult a physician.

How Supplied: Maximum Strength Cream: $^{1}/_{2}$ oz., 1 oz., and 2 oz. tubes Maximum Strength Ointment: $^{1}/_{2}$ oz. and 1 oz. tubes
Sensitive Skin Cream: $^{1}/_{2}$ oz. tube
Intensive Therapy Cream: 2 oz. tube

DRAMAMINE® Original Formula Tablets
(dimenhydrinate USP)
DRAMAMINE® Chewable Formula Tablets
(dimenhydrinate USP)

Indications: For the prevention and treatment of the nausea, vomiting, or dizziness associated with motion sickness.

Description: Dimenhydrinate is the chlorotheophylline salt of the antihistaminic agent diphenhydramine. Dimenhydrinate contains not less than 53% and not more than 56% of diphenhydramine, and not less than 44% and not more than 47% of 8-chlorotheophylline, calculated on the dried basis.

Active Ingredients: DRAMAMINE Tablets and Chewable Tablets: Dimenhydrinate 50 mg.

Inactive Ingredients: DRAMAMINE Original Formula Tablets: Colloidal Silicon Dioxide, Croscarmellose Sodium, Lactose, Magnesium Stearate, Microcrystalline Cellulose.
DRAMAMINE Chewable Formula Tablets: Aspartame, Citric Acid, FD&C Yellow No. 5 (Tartrazine) and FD&C Yellow No. 6 as color additives, Flavor, Magnesium Stearate, Methacrylic Acid Copolymer, Sorbitol.
Phenylketonurics: Contains Phenylalanine 1.5 mg per tablet.

Actions: While the precise mode of action of dimenhydrinate is not known, it is thought to have a depressant action on hyperstimulated labyrinthine function.

Directions:
DRAMAMINE Original Formula Tablets and Chewable Formula Tablets: To prevent motion sickness, the first dose should be taken one half to one hour before starting activity. **Adults:** 1 to 2 tablets every 4 to 6 hours, not to exceed 8 tablets in 24 hours or as directed by a doctor.
Children 6 to under 12 years: $^{1}/_{2}$ to 1 tablet every 6 to 8 hours, not to exceed 3 tablets in 24 hours or as directed by a doctor.
Children 2 to under 6 years: $^{1}/_{4}$ to $^{1}/_{2}$ tablet every 6 to 8 hours not to exceed $1^{1}/_{2}$ tablets in 24 hours or as directed by a doctor.

Warnings: Do not take this product, unless directed by a doctor, if you have a breathing problem such as emphysema or chronic bronchitis, or if you have glaucoma or difficulty in urination due to enlargement of the prostate gland. Do not give to children under 2 years of age unless directed by a doctor. May cause marked drowsiness; alcohol, sedatives, and tranquilizers may increase the drowsiness effect. Avoid alcoholic beverages while taking this product. Do not take this product if you are taking sedatives or tranquilizers, without first consulting your doctor. Use caution when driving a motor vehicle or operating machinery. Not for frequent or prolonged use except on advice of a doctor. Do not exceed recommended dosage. Keep this and all drugs out of the reach of children. **In case of accidental overdose, seek professional assistance or Contact a Poison Control Center immediately. As with any drug, if you are pregnant or nursing a baby, seek the advice of a health professional before using this product.**

How Supplied: *Tablets*—scored, white tablets available in 12 ct. vials, 36 ct. and 100 ct. packages; *Chewables*—scored, orange tablets available in packages of 8 ct. and 24 ct.

DRAMAMINE® Less Drowsy Formula
(Meclizine hydrochloride)

Indications: For the prevention and treatment of the nausea, vomiting, or dizziness associated with motion sickness.

Description: Meclizine hydrochloride is an antihistamine of the piperazine class with antiemetic action.

Actions: While the precise mode of action of meclizine hydrochloride is not known, it is thought to have a depressant action on hyperstimulated labyrinthine function.

Active Ingredients: Each tablet contains 25 mg of meclizine hydrochloride.

Inactive Ingredients: Colloidal silicon dioxide, Corn starch, D&C Yellow No. 10 (Aluminum Lake), Lactose, Magnesium Stearate, Microcrystalline Cellulose.

Directions: To prevent motion sickness, the first dose should be taken one hour before starting your activity. **Adults (12 years and older):** Take 1 to 2 tablets daily or as directed by a doctor. Do not exceed 2 tablets in 24 hours.

Warnings: Do not take this product, unless directed by a doctor, if you have a breathing problem such as emphysema or chronic bronchitis, or if you have glaucoma or difficulty in urination due to enlargement of the prostate gland. Do not give to children under 12 years of age unless directed by a doctor. May cause drowsiness; alcohol, sedatives, and tranquilizers may increase the drowsiness effect. Avoid alcoholic beverages while taking this product. Do not take this product if you are taking sedatives or tranquilizers, without first consulting your doctor. Use caution when driving a motor vehicle or operating machinery. Not for frequent or prolonged use except on the advice of a doctor. Do not exceed recommended dosage. **Keep this and all drugs out of reach of children. In case of accidental overdose, seek professional assistance or contact a Poison Control Center immediately.** As with any drug, if you are pregnant or nursing a baby, seek the advice of a health professional before using this product.

How Supplied: DRAMAMINE Less Drowsy Formula is supplied as a yellow tablet in 8 ct. vials.

EMETROL®
(Phosphorated Carbohydrate Solution)
For the relief of nausea associated with upset stomach

Description: EMETROL is an oral solution containing balanced amounts of dextrose (glucose) and levulose (fructose) and phosphoric acid with controlled hydrogen ion concentration. Available in original lemon-mint or cherry flavor.

Active Ingredients: Each 5 mL teaspoonful contains dextrose (glucose), 1.87 g; levulose (fructose), 1.87 g; and phosphoric acid, 21.5 mg.

Inactive Ingredients: glycerin, methylparaben, purified water; D&C

Yellow No. 10 and natural lemon-mint flavor in lemon-mint EMETROL; FD&C Red No. 40 and artificial cherry flavor in cherry EMETROL.

Action: EMETROL quickly relieves nausea by local action on the wall of the hyperactive G.I. tract.

Indications: For the relief of nausea due to upset stomach from intestinal flu and food or drink indiscretions. For other conditions, take only as directed by your physician.

Usual Adult Dose: One or two tablespoonfuls (1 tbsp equals 3 tsps). Repeat every 15 minutes until distress subsides.

Usual Children's Dose (2 to 12 years): One or two teaspoonfuls. Repeat dose every 15 minutes until distress subsides.

Important: For maximum effectiveness never dilute EMETROL or drink fluids of any kind immediately before or after taking a dose.

Caution: Not to be taken for more than one hour (5 doses) without consulting a physician. If upset stomach continues or recurs frequently, consult a physician promptly as it may be a sign of a serious condition.

Warning: This product contains fructose and should not be taken by persons with hereditary fructose intolerance (HFI).
As with any drug, if you are pregnant or nursing a baby, seek the advice of a health professional before using this product.
This product contains sugar and should not be taken by diabetics except under the advice and supervision of a physician.
KEEP THIS AND ALL MEDICATIONS OUT OF THE REACH OF CHILDREN.
In case of accidental overdose, contact a Poison Control Center, emergency medical facility, or physician immediately for advice.

How Supplied: Yellow, Lemon-Mint: Bottles of 4 & 8 fluid ounces.
Red, Cherry:
Bottles of 4 & 8 fluid ounces.

NASALCROM™ Nasal Spray
Nasal Allergy Symptom Controller

Description: NASALCROM Nasal Spray contains a liquid formulation of cromolyn sodium that stabilizes mast cells that release histamine. By using NASALCROM Nasal Spray prior to exposure to nasal allergens, degranulation and the release of histamine from mast cells is reduced. NASALCROM Nasal Spray works only in the nose and is not known to cause side effects such as drowsiness, nervousness, or rebound congestion. NASALCROM NS has no known drug interactions and is safe to use with other medications including other allergy medications. NASALCROM does not contain corticosteroids, antihistamines or decongestants.

Indications: NASALCROM Nasal Spray is indicated for the prevention and treatment of the symptoms of seasonal and perennial allergic rhinitis such as runny/itchy nose, sneezing, and allergic stuffy nose.

Ingredients: Each   mL   of NASALCROM Nasal Spray contains 40 mg of cromolyn sodium in purified water with 0.01% benzalkonium chloride to preserve and 0.01% EDTA (edetate disodium) to stabilize the solution. Each metered spray releases the same amount of medicine, 5.2 mg cromolyn sodium.

Directions:
Adults and children 6 years of age and older:
- Spray once into each nostril. Repeat 3–4 times a day (every 4–6 hours). If needed, may be used up to 6 times a day. Directions on how to use pump spray are detailed on carton and package insert.
- Use every day while in contact with the cause of the allergies (pollens, molds, pets, and dust).
- To **prevent** nasal allergy symptoms, use before contact with the cause of the allergies. For best results, start using up to one week before contact.
- If desired, NASALCROM Nasal Spray can be used with other allergy medications.

Children under 6 years of age: Do not use unless directed by a doctor.

Warnings:
Ask a doctor before use if you have:
- Fever
- Discolored nasal discharge
- Sinus pain
- Wheezing

When using this product:
- It may take several days of use to notice an effect. The best effect may not be seen for 1 to 2 weeks.
- Brief stinging or sneezing may occur right after use.
- Do not use this product to treat sinus infection, asthma, or cold symptoms.
- Do not share this bottle with anyone else as this may spread germs.

Stop using this product if:
- Symptoms worsen.
- New symptoms occur.
- Symptoms do not begin to improve within two weeks.

See your doctor because these could be signs of a serious illness.
As with any drug, if you are pregnant or nursing a baby, seek the advice of a healthcare professional before using this product. Keep this and all drugs out of the reach of children. In case of accidental ingestion/overdose, seek professional assistance or contact a Poison Control Center immediately.

Do not use if printed plastic bottle wrap imprinted with "Safety Seal®" is broken or missing.

How Supplied: NASALCROM Nasal Spray is available in 13mL (100 metered sprays) and 26mL (200 metered sprays) sizes.

PEDIACARE® Cough-Cold Liquid
PEDIACARE® NightRest
Cough-Cold Liquid
PEDIACARE® Infants' Drops
Decongestant
PEDIACARE® Infants' Drops
Decongestant Plus Cough

Description: Each 5 mL of **PEDIACARE® Cough-Cold Liquid** contains pseudoephedrine hydrochloride 15 mg, chlorpheniramine maleate 1 mg and dextromethorphan hydrobromide 5 mg. Each 0.8 mL oral dropper of **PEDIACARE® Infants' Drops Decongestant** contains pseudoephedrine hydrochloride 7.5 mg. Each 0.8 mL of **PEDIACARE® Infants' Drops Decongestant Plus Cough** contains pseudoephedrine hydrochloride 7.5 mg and dextromethorphan hydrobromide 2.5 mg. Each 5 mL of **PEDIACARE® NightRest Cough-Cold Liquid** contains pseudoephedrine hydrochloride 15 mg, chlorpheniramine maleate 1 mg and dextromethorphan hydrobromide 7.5 mg. **PEDIACARE® Cough-Cold Liquid** and **NightRest Cough-Cold Liquid** are stable, cherry flavored and red in color. **PEDIACARE® Infants' Drops** is fruit flavored alcohol free and red in color. **PEDIACARE® Infants' Drops Decongestant Plus Cough** is cherry flavored, alcohol free and clear, non-staining in color.

Actions: **PEDIACARE** products are available in four different formulas, allowing you to select the ideal product to temporarily relieve your patient's symptoms. **PEDIACARE® Cough-Cold Liquid** contains an antihistamine, chlorpheniramine maleate, a nasal decongestant, pseudoephedrine HCl, and a cough suppressant, dextromethorphan hydrobromide, to provide temporary relief of nasal congestion, runny nose, sneezing and coughing due to the common cold, hay fever or other upper respiratory allergies. **PEDIACARE® NightRest Cough-Cold Liquid** contains a decongestant, pseudoephedrine hydrochloride, an antihistamine, chlorpheniramine maleate, and a cough suppressant, dextromethorphan hydrobromide, to provide temporary relief of coughs, nasal congestion, runny nose and sneezing due to the common cold hayfever or other upper respiratory allergies. **PEDIACARE® NightRest Cough-Cold Liquid** may be used day or night to relieve cough and cold symptoms. **PEDIACARE® Infants' Drops Decongestant** contains a decongestant, pseudoephedrine hydrochloride, to provide temporary relief of nasal congestion due to the common cold, hay fever or other upper respiratory allergies. **PEDIACARE® Infants' Drops Decongestant Plus Cough** contains a decongestant, pseudoephedrine hydrochloride, and a cough suppressant, dextromethorphan hydrobromide to provide temporary relief of nasal congestion and coughing due to common cold, hay fever or other upper respiratory allergies.

Continued on next page

PediaCare—Cont.

Professional Dosage: A calibrated dosage cup is provided for accurate dosing of the **PEDIACARE** Liquid formulas. A calibrated oral dropper is provided for accurate dosing of **PEDIACARE® Infants' Drops**. All doses of **PEDIACARE® Cough-Cold Liquid**, as well as **PEDIACARE® Infants' Drops** may be repeated every 4–6 hours, not to exceed 4 doses in 24 hours. **PEDIACARE® NightRest Liquid** may be repeated every 6–8 hrs, not to exceed 4 doses in 24 hours.
[See table below]

Warnings: DO NOT USE IF CARTON IS OPENED, OR IF PRINTED PLASTIC BOTTLE WRAP OR FOIL INNER SEAL IS BROKEN. KEEP THIS AND ALL MEDICATION OUT OF THE REACH OF CHILDREN. IN CASE OF ACCIDENTAL OVERDOSAGE, CONTACT A PHYSICIAN OR POISON CONTROL CENTER IMMEDIATELY.
The following information appears on the appropriate package labels:
PEDIACARE® Cough-Cold Liquid and Night Rest Cough-Cold Liquid: Do not exceed recommended dosage. If nervousness, dizziness or sleeplessness occur, discontinue use and consult a doctor. If symptoms do not improve within 7 days or are accompanied by fever, consult a doctor. A persistent cough may be a sign of a serious condition. If cough persists for more than one week, tends to recur or is accompanied by fever, rash, or persistent headache, consult a doctor. Do not give this product for persistent or chronic cough such as occurs with asthma or if cough is accompanied by excessive phlegm (mucus) unless directed by a doctor. May cause excitability especially in children. May cause drowsiness. Sedatives and tranquilizers may increase the drowsiness effect. Do not give this product to children who are taking sedatives or tranquilizers without first consulting the child's doctor. Do not give this product to children who have a breathing problem such as chronic bronchitis, or who have glaucoma, heart disease, high blood pressure, thyroid disease or diabetes, without first consulting the child's doctor.

PEDIACARE® Infants' Drops Decongestant: Do not exceed the recommended dosage. If nervousness, dizziness or sleeplessness occur discontinue use and consult a doctor. If symptoms do not improve within 7 days or are accompanied by fever, consult a physician. Do not give this product to a child who has heart disease, high blood pressure, thyroid disease or diabetes unless directed by a doctor. Take by mouth only. Not for nasal use.

PEDIACARE® Infants' Drops Decongestant Plus Cough: Do not exceed recommended dosage. If nervousness, dizziness, or sleeplessness occur, discontinue use and consult a doctor. If symptoms do not improve within 7 days or are accompanied by fever, consult a doctor. A persistent cough may be a sign of a serious condition. If cough persists for more than one week, tends to recur or is accompanied by fever, rash, or persistent headache, consult a doctor. Do not give this product for persistent or chronic cough such as occurs with asthma or if cough is accompanied by excessive phlegm (mucus) unless directed by a doctor. Do not give this product to a child who has heart disease, high blood pressure, thyroid disease or diabetes unless directed by a doctor. Take by mouth only. Not for nasal use.

Drug Interaction Precaution: Do not give this product to a child who is taking a prescription monoamine oxidase inhibitor (MAOI) (certain drugs for depression, psychiatric or emotional conditions), or for 2 weeks after stopping the MAOI drug. If you are uncertain whether your child's prescription drug contains an MAOI, consult a health professional before giving this product.

Inactive Ingredients: PEDIACARE® Cough-Cold Liquid: Citric acid, corn syrup, flavors, glycerin, propylene glycol, sodium benzoate, sodium carboxymethylcellulose, sorbitol, purified water and Red #40.

PEDIACARE® NightRest Cough-Cold Liquid: Citric acid, corn syrup, flavors, glycerin, propylene glycol, sodium benzoate, sodium carboxymethylcellulose, sorbitol, purified water and Red #40.

PEDIACARE® Infants' Drops Decongestant: Benzoic acid, citric acid, flavors, glycerin, polyethylene glycol, propylene glycol, purified water, sodium benzoate, sorbitol, sucrose and Red #40.

PEDIACARE® Infants' Drops Decongestant Plus Cough: Citric acid, flavors, glycerin, purified water, sodium benzoate, and sorbitol.

Overdosage: Acute dextromethorphan overdose usually does not result in serious signs and symptoms unless massive amounts have been ingested. Signs and symptoms of a substantial overdose may include nausea and vomiting, visual disturbances, CNS disturbances, and urinary retention. Symptoms from pseudoephedrine overdose consist most often of mild anxiety, tachycardia and/or mild hypertension. Symptoms usually appear within 4 to 8 hours of ingestion and are transient, usually requiring no treatment. Chlorpheniramine toxicity should be treated as you would an antihistamine/anticholinergic overdose and is likely to be present within a few hours after acute ingestion.

How Supplied: PEDIACARE® Cough-Cold Liquid and NightRest Cough-Cold Liquid (colored red)—bottles of 4 fl. oz. (120 mL) with child-resistant safety cap and calibrated dosage cup. **PEDIACARE® Infants' Drops Decongestant** (colored red) and **PEDIACARE® Infants' Drops Decongestant Plus Cough** (clear)—bottles of $^{1}/_{2}$ fl. oz. (15 mL) with calibrated dropper.

Age Group	0–3 mos	4–11 mos	12–23 mos	2–3 yrs	4–5 yrs	6–8 yrs	9–10 yrs	11 yrs	Dosage
Weight (lbs)	6–11 lbs	12–17 lbs	18–23 lbs	24–35 lbs	36–47 lbs	48–59 lbs	60–71 lbs	72–95 lbs	
PEDIACARE® Infants' Drops Decongestant*	$^{1}/_{2}$ dropper (0.4 mL)	1 dropper (0.8 mL)	$1^{1}/_{2}$ droppers (1.2 mL)	2 droppers (1.6 mL)					q4–6h
PEDIACARE® Infants' Drops Decongestant Plus Cough*	$^{1}/_{2}$ dropper (0.4 mL)	1 dropper (0.8 mL)	$1^{1}/_{2}$ droppers (1.2 mL)	2 droppers (1.6 mL)					q4–6h
PEDIACARE® Cough-Cold Liquid**				1 tsp	$1^{1}/_{2}$ tsp	2 tsp	$2^{1}/_{2}$ tsp	3 tsp	q4–6h
PEDIACARE® NightRest Liquid**				1 tsp	$1^{1}/_{2}$ tsp	2 tsp	$2^{1}/_{2}$ tsp	3 tsp	q6–8h

*Administer to children under 2 years only on the advice of a physician.
**Administer to children under 6 years only on the advice of a physician.

ROGAINE® EXTRA STRENGTH FOR MEN
Hair Regrowth Treatment
(5% Minoxidil Topical Solution)

Description: ROGAINE Extra Strength For Men is a colorless solution for use only on the scalp to help regrow hair in men.

Active Ingredient: Minoxidil 5% w/v

Inactive Ingredients: Alcohol, 30% v/v, propylene glycol, 50% v/v, and purified water.

Indication: To regrow hair on the scalp.

Directions: FOR EXTERNAL USE ONLY. Apply 1 mL (twice a day, every day, directly onto the scalp) in the hair loss area. Using more or using more often will not improve results. Do not apply to other parts of the body.

Warnings:
Not for use by women: May grow facial hair. May be harmful if used during pregnancy or breast-feeding.
Do not use ROGAINE Extra Strength if you are:
• a woman
• not sure of the reason for your hair loss
• under 18 years of age. Not for babies and children.
• using other medicines on the scalp
Do not use if you have:
• no family history of hair loss
• sudden and/or patchy hair loss
• a red, inflamed, infected, irritated or painful scalp
Stop use and see a doctor if you get:
• chest pain, a rapid heartbeat faintness, or dizziness
• sudden unexplained weight gain
• swollen hands or feet
• scalp irritation that continues or worsens
For external use only.
Avoid contact with eyes. In case of accidental contact, rinse with large amounts of cool tap water. As with any drug, if you are pregnant or nursing a baby, seek the advice of a healthcare professional before using this product.
Keep this and all drugs out of the reach of children. Do not use on babies and children. In case of accidental ingestion, seek professional assistance or contact a Poison Control Center immediately.

Additional Information:
ROGAINE Extra Strength For Men will not prevent or improve hair loss which may occur with the use of some prescription and non-prescription medications, certain severe nutritional problems (very low body iron; too much vitamin A intake), low thyroid states (hypothyroidism), chemotherapy, or diseases and conditions which cause scarring of the scalp.

How Supplied: ROGAINE Extra Strength For Men is available in packs of one, three, or four 60 mL bottles. (One 60 mL bottle is a one-month supply.)

How Stored:
Store at controlled room temperature 20° to 25°C (68° to 77°F)

ROGAINE® For Women
Hair Regrowth Treatment
2% Minoxidil Topical Solution

Description: ROGAINE is a colorless liquid medication use on the scalp to help regrow hair.

Active Ingredient: Minoxidil 2% w/v

Inactive Ingredients: Alcohol, 60% v/v, propylene glycol, and purified water.

Indication: To regrow hair on the scalp.

Directions: FOR EXTERNAL USE ONLY. Apply 1 mL (2 times a day, every day, directly onto the scalp) in the hair loss area. Using more or using more often will not improve results.

Warnings:
Do not use ROGAINE and see your doctor if you:
• Have no family history of hair loss
• Have sudden hair loss
• Have patchy hair loss
• Do not know the reason for your hair loss
Do not use ROGAINE if you:
• Are less than 18 years old. Do not use on babies and children
• Have ever had an allergic reaction to ROGAINE
Do not apply ROGAINE on scalp if the skin is:
• Red or inflamed
• Infected
• Irritated
• Painful to touch (such as severe sunburn)
Stop using ROGAINE and see your doctor if you get:
• Unwanted facial hair growth
• Chest pain
• Rapid heartbeat
• Faintness and/or dizziness
• Sudden, unexplained weight gain
• Swollen hands or feet
• Redness or irritation on treated areas of your scalp
For external use only.
AVOID CONTACT WITH EYES. IN CASE OF ACCIDENTAL CONTACT, RINSE WITH LARGE AMOUNTS OF COOL TAP WATER. As with any drug, if you are pregnant or nursing a baby, seek the advice of a healthcare professional before using this product. Do not use if your hair loss is associated with childbirth.
Keep this and all drugs out of the reach of children. In case of accidental ingestion, seek professional assistance or contact a Poison Control Center immediately.

Side Effects:
The most common side effects are itching and other skin irritations of the treated area of the scalp. If scalp irritation continues, stop use and see a doctor.
Although unwanted facial hair growth has been reported on the face and on other parts of the body, such reports have been infrequent. The unwanted hair growth may be caused by the transfer of ROGAINE to areas other than the scalp, or by absorption into the circulatory system of low levels of the active ingredient, or by a medical condition not related to the use of ROGAINE. If you experience unwanted hair growth, discontinue using ROGAINE and see your doctor for recommendations about appropriate treatment. After stopping use of ROGAINE, the unwanted hair, if caused by the use of ROGAINE, should go away over time.

How Supplied: ROGAINE For Women is available in packs of one, two, or three 60 mL bottles. (One 60 mL bottle is a one-month supply.)
Store at Controlled Room Temperature 20° to 25°C (68° to 77°F).

SURFAK® LIQUI-GELS®
Stool Softener Laxative

Indications: SURFAK®, a stool softener, is indicated for the relief of occasional constipation. SURFAK is a convenient, once a day therapy, which provides gentle prevention and superior relief from the discomfort associated with passing stools related to trauma, lifestyle, or aging. It works gently by drawing water into the stool, making it softer and easier to pass. Regularity can be expected to return in 12 to 72 hours.

Active Ingredients: Each soft gelatin Liqui-Gel contains 240 mg docusate calcium.

Inactive Ingredients: Also contains corn oil, FD&C Blue #1 and Red #40, gelatin, glycerin, parabens, sorbitol, and other ingredients.

Dosage and Administration: Adults and children 12 years of age and over: one capsule by mouth daily for several days or until bowel movements are normal. For use in children under 12, consult a physician.

Warnings: Do not use laxative products when abdominal pain, nausea, or vomiting are present unless directed by a doctor. If you have noticed a sudden change in bowel habits that persists over a period of 2 weeks, consult a doctor before using a laxative. Laxative products should not be used for a period longer than 1 week unless directed by a doctor. Rectal bleeding or failure to have a bowel movement after use of a laxative may indicate a serious condition. Discontinue use and consult your doctor. Keep this and all drugs out of the reach of children. In case of accidental overdose, seek professional assistance or contact a Poison Control Center immediately. As with any drug, if you are pregnant or nursing a baby, seek the advice of a health professional before using this product.

Drug Interaction Precaution: Do not take this product if you are presently taking mineral oil, unless directed by a doctor.

How Supplied: Red soft gelatin capsules in packages of 10, 30 and 100 and Unit Dose 100s (10 × 10 strips).

Continued on next page

Surfak—Cont.

LIQUI-GELS® is a registered trademark of RP Scherer Corp.

Procter & Gamble

P. O. BOX 5516
CINCINNATI, OH 45201

Direct Inquiries to:
Charles Lambert
(800) 358-8707

For Medical Emergencies:
Call Collect: (513) 636-5107

METAMUCIL® Fiber Laxative
[met uh-mū sil]
(psyllium husk)
Also see Metamucil Dietary Fiber Supplement in Dietary Supplement Section

Description: Metamucil contains psyllium husk (from the plant *Plantago ovata*), a bulk forming, natural therapeutic fiber for restoring and maintaining regularity when recommended by a physician. Metamucil contains no chemical stimulants and does not disrupt normal bowel function. Each dose contains approximately 3.4 grams of psyllium husk (or 2.4 grams of soluble fiber). Inactive ingredients, sodium, calcium, potassium, calories, carbohydrate, dietary fiber, and phenylalanine content are shown in the following table for all versions and flavors. Metamucil Smooth Texture Sugar-Free Regular Flavor contains no sugar and no artificial sweeteners; Metamucil Smooth Texture Sugar-Free Orange Flavor contains aspartame (phenylalanine content per dose is 25 mg). Metamucil powdered products are gluten-free. Metamucil Fiber Wafers contain gluten: Apple Crisp contains 0.7g/dose, Cinnamon Spice contains 0.5g/dose. Each two-wafer dose contains 5 grams of fat.

Actions: The active ingredient in Metamucil is psyllium husk, a natural fiber which promotes elimination due to its bulking effect in the colon. This bulking effect is due to both the water-holding capacity of undigested fiber and the increased bacterial mass following partial fiber digestion. These actions result in enlargement of the lumen of the colon, and softer stool, thereby decreasing intraluminal pressure and straining, and speeding colonic transit in constipated patients.

Indications: Metamucil is indicated for the treatment of occasional constipation, and when recommended by a physician, for chronic constipation and constipation associated with irritable bowel syndrome, diverticulosis, hemorrhoids, convalescence, senility and pregnancy. Pregnancy: Category B. If considering use of Metamucil as part of a cholesterol-lowering program, see **Metamucil Dietary Fiber Supplement** in Dietary Supplement Section.

Contraindications: Intestinal obstruction, fecal impaction, allergy to any component.

Warnings: Patients are advised they should consult a doctor before using this product if they have abdominal pain, nausea, vomiting or rectal bleeding, if they have noticed a sudden change in

Metamucil Fiber Laxative/Dietary Fiber Supplement

Versions/Flavors	Ingredients (alphabetical order)	Sodium mg/dose	Calcium mg/dose	Potassium mg/dose	Calories kcal/dose	Total Carbohydrate g/dose	Dietary Fiber/(Soluble) g/dose	Dosage (Weight in gms)	How Supplied
Smooth Texture Orange Flavor Metamucil Powder	Citric Acid, FD&C Yellow #6, Natural and Artificial Flavor, Psyllium Husk, Sucrose	5	7	30	45	12	3 (2.4)	1 rounded tablespoon ~12g	Canisters: Doses: 48, 72, 114; Cartons: 30 single-dose packets.
Smooth Texture Sugar-Free Orange Flavor Metamucil Powder	Aspartame, Citric Acid, FD&C Yellow #6, Maltodextrin, Natural and Artificial Flavor, Psyllium Husk	5	7	30	20	5	3 (2.4)	1 rounded teaspoon ~5.8g	Canisters: Doses: 48, 72 114, 180; Cartons: 30 single-dose packets.
Smooth Texture Sugar-Free Regular Flavor Metamucil Powder	Citric Acid, Maltodextrin, Psyllium Husk	4	7	30	20	5	3 (2.4)	1 rounded teaspoon ~5.4g	Canisters: Doses: 48, 72 114.
Original Texture Regular Flavor Metamucil Powder	Psyllium Husk, Sucrose	3	6	30	25	6	3 (2.4)	1 rounded teaspoon ~7g	Canisters: Doses: 48, 72 114.
Original Texture Orange Flavor Metamucil Powder	Citric Acid, FD&C Yellow #6, Natural and Artificial Flavor, Psyllium Husk, Sucrose	5	6	30	40	10	3 (2.4)	1 rounded tablespoon ~11g	Canisters: Doses: 48,72 114.
Fiber Laxative									
Wafers									
Apple Crisp Metamucil Wafers	(1)	20	14	60	120	17	6	2 wafers 25 g	Cartons: 12 doses
Cinnamon Spice Metamucil Wafers	(2)	20	14	60	120	17	6	2 wafers 25 g	Cartons: 12 doses

(1) Ascorbic Acid, Brown Sugar, Cinnamon, Corn Oil, Flavoring, Fructose, Lecithin, Modified Food Starch, Molasses, Oat Hull Fiber, Sodium Bicarbonate, Sucrose, Water, Wheat Flour
(2) Ascorbic Acid, Cinnamon, Corn Oil, Flavoring, Fructose, Lecithin, Modified Food Starch, Molasses, Nutmeg, Oat Hull Fiber, Oats, Sodium Bicarbonate, Sucrose, Water, Wheat Flour

bowel habits that persists over a period of two weeks, or if they are considering use of this product as part of a cholesterol-lowering program. Patients are advised to consult a physician if constipation persists for longer than one week, as this may be a sign of a serious medical condition. **Patients are cautioned that taking this product without adequate fluid may cause it to swell and block the throat or esophagus and may cause choking. They should not take the product if they have difficulty in swallowing. If they experience chest pain, vomiting, or difficulty in swallowing or breathing after taking this product, they are advised to seek immediate medical attention.** Psyllium products may cause allergic reaction in people sensitive to inhaled or ingested psyllium. Keep out of the reach of children. In case of accidental overdose, seek professional assistance or contact a poison control center immediately.

Precaution: Notice to Health Care Professionals: To minimize the potential for allergic reaction, health care professionals who frequently dispense powdered psyllium products should avoid inhaling airborne dust while dispensing these products. Handling and Dispensing: To minimize generating airborne dust, spoon product from the canister into a glass according to label directions.

Dosage and Administration: The usual adult dosage is one rounded teaspoon, or tablespoon, depending on the product version. Some versions are available in single-dose packets. For children (6 to 12 years old) use ½ the adult dose; for children under 6, consult a doctor. The appropriate dose should be mixed with 8 oz. of liquid (e.g., cool water, fruit juice, milk) following the label instructions. Metamucil Fiber Wafers should be consumed with 8 oz. of liquid. **The product (child or adult dose) should be taken with at least 8 oz. (a full glass) of water or other fluid. Taking this product without enough liquid may cause choking (see warnings).** Metamucil can be taken one to three times per day, depending on the need and response. It may require continued use for 2 to 3 days to provide optimal benefit. Generally produces effect in 12–72 hours.

Laxatives, including bulk fibers, may affect how well other medicines work. If you are taking a prescription medicine by mouth, take this product at least 2 hours before or 2 hours after the prescribed medicine. As your body adjusts to increased fiber intake, you may experience changes in bowel habits or minor bloating.

How Supplied: Powder: canisters and cartons of single-dose packets. Wafers: cartons of single dose packets. (See Table 1)

[See table at bottom of previous page]

Shown in Product Identification Guide, page 521

PEPTO-BISMOL® ORIGINAL LIQUID, ORIGINAL AND CHERRY TABLETS AND EASY-TO-SWALLOW CAPLETS
For upset stomach, indigestion, diarrhea, heartburn and nausea.

Multi-symptom Pepto-Bismol contains bismuth subsalicylate and is the only leading OTC stomach remedy clinically proven effective for both upper and lower GI symptoms. It has been clinically proven in double-blind placebo-controlled trials for relief of upset stomach symptoms and diarrhea.

Description: Each tablespoon (15 ml) of Pepto-Bismol Liquid contains 262 mg bismuth subsalicylate. Each tablespoonful of liquid contains a total of 130 mg non-aspirin salicylate. Pepto-Bismol Liquid contains no sugar. Inactive ingredients: benzoic acid, D&C Red No. 22, D&C Red No. 28, flavor, magnesium aluminum silicate, methylcellulose, saccharin sodium, salicylic acid, sodium salicylate, sorbic acid and water.

Each Pepto-Bismol Tablet contains 262 mg bismuth subsalicylate. Each tablet contains a total of 102 mg non-aspirin salicylate (99 mg non-aspirin salicylate for Cherry). Pepto-Bismol Tablets contain no sugar. Inactive ingredients include: adipic acid (in Cherry only), calcium carbonate, D&C Red No. 27 aluminum lake, FD&C Red No. 40 aluminum lake (in Cherry only), flavor, magnesium stearate, mannitol, povidone, saccharin sodium and talc.

Each Pepto-Bismol Caplet contains 262 mg bismuth subsalicylate. Each caplet contains a total of 99 mg non-aspirin salicylate. Caplets contain no sugar. Inactive ingredients include: calcium carbonate, D&C Red No. 27 aluminum lake, magnesium stearate, mannitol, microcrystalline cellulose, povidone, polysorbate 80, silicon dioxide, and sodium starch glycolate.

Indications: Pepto-Bismol controls diarrhea within 24 hours, relieving associated abdominal cramps; soothes heartburn and indigestion without constipating; and relieves nausea and upset stomach.

Actions: For upset stomach symptoms (i.e., indigestion, heartburn, nausea and fullness caused by over-indulgence), the active ingredient is believed to work via a topical effect on the stomach mucosa. For diarrhea, it is believed to work by several mechanisms in the gastrointestinal tract, including: 1) normalizing fluid movement via an antisecretory mechanism, 2) binding bacterial toxins and 3) antimicrobial activity.

Warnings: Children and teenagers who have or are recovering from chicken pox or flu should not use this medicine to treat nausea or vomiting. If nausea or vomiting is present, patients are advised to consult a doctor because this could be an early sign of Reye syndrome, a rare but serious illness.

This product contains non-aspirin salicylates. If taken with aspirin and ringing in the ears occurs, discontinue use. This product does not contain aspirin, but should not be administered to those patients who have a known allergy to aspirin or other non-aspirin salicylates as an adverse reaction may occur. Caution is advised in the administration to patients taking medication for anticoagulation, diabetes and gout.

If diarrhea is accompanied by a high fever or continues more than 2 days, patients are advised to consult a physician. As with any drug, caution is advised in the administration to pregnant or nursing women.

Keep all medicines out of the reach of children.

Note: This medication may cause a temporary and harmless darkening of the tongue and/or stool. Stool darkening should not be confused with melena.

Overdosage: In case of overdose, patients are advised to contact a physician or Poison Control Center. Emesis induced by ipecac syrup is indicated in large ingestions provided ipecac can be administered within one hour of ingestion. Activated charcoal should be administered after gastric emptying. Patients should be evaluated for signs and symptoms of salicylate toxicity.

Dosage and Administration: Liquid: Shake well before using.

Adults—2 tablespoonsful
(1 dose cup, 30 ml)

Children (according to age)—

9–12 yrs. 1 tablespoonful
(½ dose cup, 15 ml)

6–9 yrs. 2 teaspoonsful
(⅓ dose cup, 10 ml)

3–6 yrs. 1 teaspoonful
(⅙ dose cup, 5 ml)

Repeat dosage every ½ to 1 hour, if needed, to a maximum of 8 doses in a 24-hour period. Drink plenty of clear fluids to help prevent dehydration which may accompany diarrhea.

For children under 3 years of age, consult a physician.

Tablets:

Adults—Two tablets

Children (according to age)—

9–12 yrs. 1 tablet

6–9 yrs. ⅔ tablet

3–6 yrs. ⅓ tablet

Chew or dissolve in mouth. Repeat every ½ to 1 hour as needed, to a maximum of 8 doses in a 24-hour period. Drink plenty of clear fluids to help pre-

Continued on next page

Pepto-Bismol Original—Cont.

vent dehydration, which may accompany diarrhea. For children under 3 years of age, consult a physician.

Caplets:
Adults—Two caplets
Children (according to age)—
9–12 yrs. 1 caplet
6–9 yrs. $^2/_3$ caplet
3–6 yrs. $^1/_3$ caplet

Swallow caplet(s) with water, do not chew. Repeat every $^1/_2$ to 1 hour as needed, to a maximum of 8 doses in a 24-hour period. Drink plenty of clear fluids to help prevent dehydration, which may accompany diarrhea. For children under 3 years of age, consult a physician.

How Supplied: Pepto-Bismol Liquid is available in: 4, 8, 12, and 16 FL OZ bottles. Pepto-Bismol Tablets are pink, round, chewable tablets imprinted with a debossed triangle and "Pepto-Bismol" on one side. Tablets are available in: boxes of 30 and 48. Caplets are available in bottles of 24 and 40. Caplets are imprinted with "Pepto-Bismol" on one side.

Shown in Product Identification Guide, page 521

PEPTO-BISMOL®
MAXIMUM STRENGTH LIQUID
For upset stomach, indigestion, diarrhea, heartburn and nausea.

Multi-symptom Pepto-Bismol contains bismuth subsalicylate and is the only leading OTC stomach remedy clinically proven effective for both upper and lower GI symptoms. It has been clinically-proven in double-blind placebo-controlled trials for relief of upset stomach symptoms and diarrhea.

Description: Each tablespoonful (15 ml) of Maximum Strength Pepto-Bismol Liquid contains 525 mg bismuth subsalicylate (236 mg non-aspirin salicylate). Maximum Strength Pepto-Bismol Liquid contains no sugar. Inactive ingredients include: benzoic acid, D&C Red No. 22, D&C Red No. 28, flavor, magnesium aluminum silicate, methylcellulose, saccharin sodium, salicylic acid, sodium salicylate, sorbic acid and water.

Indications: Maximum Strength Pepto-Bismol soothes upset stomach and indigestion without constipating; controls diarrhea within 24 hours, relieving associated abdominal cramps; and relieves heartburn and nausea.

Actions: For upset stomach symptoms (i.e. indigestion, heartburn, nausea and fullness caused by over-indulgence), the active ingredient is believed to work via a topical effect on the stomach mucosa. For diarrhea, it is believed to work by several mechanisms in the gastrointestinal tract, including: 1) normalizing fluid movement via an antisecretory mechanism, 2) binding bacterial toxins, and 3) antimicrobial activity.

Warnings: Children and teenagers who have or are recovering from chicken pox or flu should not use this medicine to treat nausea or vomiting. If nausea or vomiting is present, patients are advised to consult a doctor because this could be an early sign of Reye syndrome, a rare but serious illness.

This product contains non-aspirin salicylates. If taken with aspirin and ringing in the ears occurs, discontinue use. This product does not contain aspirin, but should not be administered to those patients who have a known allergy to aspirin or other non-aspirin salicylates as an adverse reaction may occur. Caution is advised in the administration to patients taking medication for anticoagulation, diabetes and gout.

If diarrhea is accompanied by a high fever or continues more than 2 days, patients are advised to consult a physician. As with any drug, caution is advised in the administration to pregnant or nursing women.

Keep all medicines out of the reach of children.

Note: This medication may cause a temporary and harmless darkening of the tongue and/or stool. Stool darkening should not be confused with melena.

Overdosage: In case of overdose, patients are advised to contact a physician or Poison Control Center. Emesis induced by ipecac syrup is indicated in large ingestions provided ipecac can be administered within one hour of ingestion. Activated charcoal should be administered after gastric emptying. Patients should be evaluated for signs and symptoms of salicylate toxicity.

Dosage and Administration: Shake well before using.

Adults— 2 tablespoonsful
(1 dose cup, 30 ml)
Children (according to age)—
9–12 yrs. 1 tablespoonful
($^1/_2$ dose cup, 15 ml)
6–9 yrs. 2 teaspoonsful
($^1/_3$ dose cup, 10 ml)
3–6 yrs. 1 teaspoonful
($^1/_6$ dose cup, 5 ml)

Repeat dosage every hour, if needed, to a maximum of 4 doses in a 24-hour period. Drink plenty of clear fluids to help prevent dehydration, which may accompany diarrhea.

How Supplied: Maximum Strength Pepto-Bismol is available in: 4, 8, and 12 FL OZ bottles.

VICKS® 44® COUGH
RELIEF
Dextromethorphan HBr/
Cough Suppressant
Alcohol 5%

Active Ingredient
per 3 tsp. (15 ml):
Dextromethorphan Hydrobromide 30 mg

Inactive Ingredients: Alcohol, Blue 1, Carboxymethylcellulose Sodium, Citric Acid, Flavor, High Fructose Corn Syrup, Polyethylene Oxide, Polyoxyl 40 Stearate, Propylene Glycol, Purified Water, Red 40, Saccharin Sodium, Sodium Benzoate, Sodium Citrate.

SODIUM CONTENT: 31 mg per 15 mL dose.

Use: Temporarily relieves cough due to minor throat and bronchial irritation associated with a cold.

Directions: **Use teaspoon (tsp) or dose cup.**

Under 6 yrs.: Ask a doctor.

6–11 yrs.	1$^1/_2$ tsp or 7$^1/_2$ ml
12 yrs. & older	3 tsp or 15 ml

Repeat every 6–8 hours, not to exceed 4 doses per day or use as directed by a doctor.

Warnings: A persistent cough may be a sign of a serious condition. If cough persists for more than 1 week, tends to recur, or is accompanied by fever, rash, or persistent headache, ask a doctor. Do not take this product for persistent or chronic cough such as occurs with smoking, asthma, emphysema, or if cough is accompanied by excessive phlegm (mucus) unless directed by a doctor. **Keep this and all drugs out of the reach of children.** In case of accidental overdose, seek professional advice or contact a poison control center immediately. As with any drug, if you are pregnant or nursing a baby, seek the advice of a health professional before using this product.

Drug Interaction Precaution: Do not use this product without first asking a doctor if you take a prescription monoamine oxidase inhibitor (MAOI) (certain drugs for depression, psychiatric or emotional conditions, or Parkinson's disease), or for 2 weeks after stopping the MAOI drug or if you are uncertain whether your prescription drug contains an MAOI.

How Supplied: Available in 4 FL OZ (118 ml) plastic bottle. A calibrated dose cup accompanies each bottle.

VICKS® 44D®
COUGH & HEAD CONGESTION
RELIEF
Cough Suppressant/
Nasal Decongestant
Alcohol 5%

Active Ingredients per 3 tsp. (15 ml): Dextromethorphan Hydrobromide 30 mg, Pseudoephedrine Hydrochloride 60 mg.

Inactive Ingredients: Alcohol, Blue 1, Carboxymethylcellulose Sodium, Cit-

ric Acid, Flavor, High Fructose Corn Syrup, Polyethylene Oxide, Polyoxyl 40 Stearate, Propylene Glycol, Purified Water, Red 40, Saccharin Sodium, Sodium Benzoate, Sodium Citrate.

Sodium Content: 31 mg per 15 mL dose.

Uses: Temporarily relieves cough and nasal congestion due to a common cold.

Directions: Use teaspoon (tsp) or dose cup.

Under 6 yrs.: Ask a doctor.

6–11 yrs.	1½ tsp or 7½ ml
12 yrs. & older	3 tsp or 15 ml

Repeat every 6 hours, not to exceed 4 doses per day or use as directed by a doctor.

Warnings: Do not exceed recommended dosage.

If nervousness, dizziness, or sleeplessness occur, discontinue use and ask a doctor.

Do not take unless directed by a doctor if you have:
• heart disease
• asthma
• emphysema
• thyroid disease
• diabetes
• high blood pressure
• excessive phlegm (mucus)
• persistent or chronic cough
• cough associated with smoking
• difficulty in urination due to enlarged prostate gland

Keep this and all drugs out of the reach of children. In the case of accidental overdose, seek professional advice or contact a poison control center immediately. As with any drug, if you are pregnant or nursing a baby, seek the advice of a health professional before using this product.

Drug Interaction Precaution: Do not use this product without first asking a doctor if you take a prescription monoamine oxidase inhibitor (MAOI) (certain drugs for depression, psychiatric or emotional conditions, or Parkinson's disease), or for 2 weeks after stopping the MAOI drug or if you are uncertain whether your prescription drug contains an MAOI.

Dosing Duration and When to Ask a Doctor:
• If symptoms do not improve within 7 days or are accompanied by fever.
• If a cough persists for more than 7 days, recurs, or is accompanied by fever, rash or persistent headache. A persistent cough may be the sign of a serious condition.

How Supplied: Available in 4 FL OZ (118 ml) and 8 FL OZ (236 ml) plastic bottles. A calibrated dose cup accompanies each bottle.

VICKS® 44E®
Cough & Chest Congestion Relief
Cough Suppressant/Expectorant
Alcohol 5%

Active Ingredients: per 3 teaspoons (15 ml): Dextromethorphan Hydrobromide 20 mg, Guaifenesin 200 mg

Inactive Ingredients: Alcohol, Blue 1, Carboxymethylcellulose Sodium, Citric Acid, Flavor, High Frutose Corn Syrup, Polyethylene Oxide, Polyoxyl 40 Stearate, Propylene Glycol, Purified Water, Red 40, Saccharin Sodium, Sodium Benzoate, Sodium Citrate.

Sodium Content: 31 mg per 15 mL dose.

Uses: Temporarily relieves cough due to a common cold. Helps loosen phlegm to rid the bronchial passageways of bothersome mucus.

Directions: Use teaspoon (tsp) or dose cup.

Under 6 yrs.: Ask a doctor.

6–11 yrs.	1½ tsp or 7½ ml
12 yrs. & older	3 tsp or 15 ml

Repeat every 4 hours, not to exceed 6 doses per day or use as directed by a doctor.

Warnings: *Do not take unless directed by a doctor if you have:*
• asthma
• emphysema
• excessive phlegm (mucus)
• persistent or chronic cough
• chronic bronchitis
• cough associated with smoking

Keep this and all drugs out of the reach of children.

In the case of accidental overdose, seek professional advice or contact a poison control center immediately. As with any drug, if you are pregnant or nursing a baby, seek the advice of a health professional before using this product. Do not use this product if you are on a sodium-restricted diet unless directed by a doctor.

Drug Interaction Precaution: Do not use this product without first asking a doctor if you take a prescription monoamine oxidase inhibitor (MAOI) (certain drugs for depression, psychiatric or emotional conditions, or Parkinson's disease), or for 2 weeks after stopping the MAOI drug or if you are uncertain whether your prescription drug contains an MAOI.

Dosing Duration & When to Ask a Doctor:
• If a cough persists for more than 7 days, recurs, or is accompanied by fever, rash or persistent headache. A persistent cough may be the sign of a serious condition.

How Supplied: Available in 4 FL OZ (118 ml) and 8 FL OZ (236 ml) plastic bottles. A calibrated dose cup accompanies each bottle.

VICKS® 44M®
COUGH, COLD & FLU RELIEF
Cough Suppressant/Nasal Decongestant/Antihistamine/
Pain Reliever–Fever Reducer
Alcohol 10%

Active Ingredients: per 4 tsp. (20 ml): Dextromethorphan Hydrobromide 30 mg, Pseudoephedrine Hydrochloride 60 mg, Chlorpheniramine Maleate 4 mg, Acetaminophen 650 mg

Inactive Ingredients: Alcohol, Blue 1, Carboxymethylcellulose Sodium, Citric Acid, Flavor, High Fructose Corn Syrup, Polyethylene Glycol, Polyethylene Oxide, Propylene Glycol, Purified Water, Red 40, Saccharin Sodium, Sodium Citrate.

Sodium Content: 32 mg per 20 mL dose.

Uses: Temporarily relieves cough/cold/flu symptoms:
• cough
• nasal congestion
• runny nose
• sneezing
• headache
• fever
• muscular aches
• sore throat pain

Directions: Use teaspoon (tsp) or dose cup.

12 yrs. & older	4 tsp or 20 ml

Under 12 yrs.: Ask a doctor.
Repeat every 6 hours, not to exceed 4 doses per day, or use as directed by a doctor.
Failure to follow these warnings could result in serious consequences.

Warnings: Do not exceed recommended dosage. Do not use with other products containing Acetaminophen.

If nervousness, dizziness, or sleeplessness occur, discontinue use and ask a doctor. May cause drowsiness. May cause excitability especially in children.
Do not take unless directed by a doctor if you have:
• heart disease
• asthma
• emphysema
• thyroid disease
• diabetes
• glaucoma
• high blood pressure
• excessive phlegm (mucus)
• breathing problems
• chronic bronchitis
• difficulty in breathing
• persistent or chronic cough
• cough associated with smoking
• difficulty in urination due to enlarged prostate gland

Alcohol Warning: If you generally consume 3 or more alcoholic drinks per day, ask your doctor whether you should take acetaminophen or other pain relievers/fever reducers. Acetaminophen may cause liver damage.

Keep this and all drugs out of the reach of children. In the case of accidental

Continued on next page

Vicks 44M—Cont.

overdose, seek professional advice or contact a poison control center immediately. Prompt medical attention is critical for adults as well as for children even if you do not notice any signs or symptoms. As with any drug, if you are pregnant or nursing a baby, seek the advice of a health professional before using this product.

Alcohol, sedatives, and tranquilizers may increase the drowsiness effect. Avoid alcoholic beverages while taking this product. Use caution when driving a motor vehicle or operating machinery.

Drug Interaction Precaution: Do not use this product without first asking a doctor if you take:
- sedatives
- tranquilizers
- a prescription monoamine oxidase inhibitor (MAOI) (certain drugs for depression, psychiatric or emotional conditions, or Parkinson's disease), or for 2 weeks after stopping the MAOI drug or if you are uncertain whether your prescription drug contains an MAOI.

Dosing Duration: Do not use over 7 days. *Ask a Doctor:*
- If sore throat is severe, persists for more than 2 days, is accompanied or followed by fever, headache, rash, nausea, or vomiting.
- If symptoms do not improve or are accompanied by a fever that lasts more than 3 days, or if new symptoms occur.
- If a cough presists for more than 7 days, recurs, or is accompanied by a rash or persistent headache. A persistent cough may be the sign of a serious condition.

How Supplied: Available in 4 FL OZ (118 ml) and 8 FL OZ (236 ml) plastic bottles. A calibrated dose cup accompanies each bottle.

CHILDREN'S VICKS® NYQUIL® COLD/COUGH RELIEF
Antihistamine/Nasal Decongestant/Cough Suppressant

Children's NyQuil was specially formulated with three effective ingredients to relieve nighttime cough, nasal congestion, and runny nose so children can rest. Children's NyQuil® is alcohol free and analgesic free and has a pleasant cherry flavor.

Uses: Temporarily relieves cold symptoms:
- cough
- sneezing
- runny nose
- nasal congestion
[See table below]

Inactive Ingredients: Citric Acid, Flavor, Potassium Sorbate, Propylene Glycol, Purified Water, Red 40, Sodium Citrate, Sucrose. **Sodium Content:** 160 mg per 30 ml dose.

Directions: [See table below]

Warnings:
Do not use
- if you are on a sodium-restricted diet
- if you are now taking a prescription monoamine oxidase inhibitor (MAOI) (certain drugs for depression, psychiatric or emotional conditions, or Parkinson's disease), or for 2 weeks after stopping the MAOI drug. If you do not know if your prescription drug contains an MAOI, ask a doctor or pharmacist before taking this product.

Ask a doctor before use if you have:
- heart disease
- asthma
- emphysema
- thyroid disease
- diabetes
- glaucoma
- high blood pressure
- excessive phlegm (mucus)
- breathing problems
- chronic bronchitis
- persistent or chronic cough
- cough associated with smoking
- trouble urinating due to an enlarged prostate gland

Ask a doctor or pharmacist before use if you are taking sedatives or tranquilizers.

When using this product:
- do not use more than directed
- excitability may occur, especially in children
- drowsiness may occur
- avoid alcoholic drinks
- be careful when driving a motor vehicle or operating machinery
- alcohol, sedatives, and tranquilizers may increase drowsiness

Stop use and ask a doctor if:
- you get nervous, dizzy or sleepless
- new symptoms occur
- you need to use more than 7 days
- symptoms do not get better within 7 days or accompanied by a fever
- cough lasts more than 7 days, comes back, or occurs with fever, rash, or headache that lasts.

These could be the signs of a serious condition.

If pregnant or breast-feeding, ask a health professional before use.

Keep out of reach of children. In case of overdose, get medical help or contact a Poison Control Center right away. Quick medical attention is critical for adults as well as for children even if you do not notice any signs or symptoms.

Other Information:
- store at room temperature
- **each tablespoon contains** sodium 70.5 mg

How Supplied: Available in 4 FL OZ (115 ml) plastic bottles with child-resistant, tamper-evident cap and a calibrated medicine cup.

VICKS® Cough Drops
Menthol Cough Suppressant/Oral Anesthetic
Menthol and Cherry Flavors

Uses: temporarily relieves:
- sore throat
- coughs due to colds or inhaled irritants
[See table at top of next page]

Inactive Ingredients:
[Cherry]
Ascorbic Acid, Blue 1, Citric Acid, Corn Syrup, Eucalyptus Oil, Flavor, Red 40, Sucrose
[Menthol]
Ascorbic Acid, Caramel, Corn Syrup, Eucalyptus Oil, Sucrose

Directions:
- under 5 yrs.: ask a doctor
- adults & children 5 yrs. & older:
[menthol]
allow 2 drops to dissolve slowly in mouth
[cherry]
allow 3 drops to dissolve slowly in mouth
Cough: may be repeated every hour. Sore Throat: may be repeated every 2 hours.

Other Information:
Store at room temperature

Warnings:
Ask a doctor before use if you have:
- cough associated with excessive phlegm (mucus)
- persistent or chronic cough such as those caused by asthma, emphysema, or smoking
- a severe sore throat accompanied by difficulty in breathing or that lasts more than 2 days
- a sore throat accompanied or followed by fever, headache, rash, swelling, nausea or vomiting

Stop use and ask a doctor if:
- you need to use more than 7 days
- cough lasts more than 7 days, comes back, or occurs with fever, rash, or headache that lasts.

A persistent cough could be the sign of a serious condition.

If pregnant or breast-feeding, ask a health professional before use.

Keep out of reach of children.

How Supplied: Vicks® Cough Drops are available in boxes of 20 triangular drops. Each red or green drop is debossed with "V."

Questions? 1-800-358-8707

Active ingredients (per tablespoon):	Purpose:
Chlorpheniramine maleate 2 mg	Antihistamine
Dextromethorphan HBr 15 mg	Cough suppressant
Pseudoephedrine HCl 30 mg	Nasal decongestant

- use tablespoon (TBSP) or dose cup
  - under 6 yrs .... ask a doctor
  - 6–11 yrs .... 1 TBSP (15 ml)
  - 12 yrs. & older .... 2 TBSP (30 ml)
- Repeat every 6 hours, not to exceed 4 doses per day.

Active Ingredients (per drop): **Purpose:**
[CHERRY]
Menthol 1.7 mg .... Cough suppressant/oral anesthetic
[MENTHOL]
Menthol 3.3 mg .... Cough suppressant/oral anesthetic

VICKS® DAYQUIL® LIQUID
VICKS® DAYQUIL® LIQUICAPS®
Multi-Symptom Cold/Flu Relief
Nasal Decongestant/
Pain Reliever/Cough
Suppressant/Fever Reducer

Uses:
Temporarily relieves common cold/flu symptoms:
• minor aches
• pains
• headache
• muscular aches
• sore throat pain
• fever
• nasal congestion
• cough

Active Ingredients
(per tablespoon): **Purpose:**
Acetaminophen
325 mg .... Pain reliever/fever reducer
Dextromethorphan HBr
10 mg .... Cough suppressant
Pseudoephedrine HCl
30 mg .... Nasal decongestant

Active Ingredients
(per softgel): **Purpose:**
Acetaminophen
250 mg .... Pain reliever/fever reducer
Dextromethorphan HBr
10 mg .... Cough suppressant
Pseudoephedrine HCl
30 mg .... Nasal decongestant

Inactive Ingredients: *VICKS®*
DAYQUIL® LIQUID: Citric Acid, Flavor, Glycerin, Polyethylene Glycol, Propylene Glycol, Purified Water, Saccharin Sodium, Sodium Citrate, Sucrose, Yellow 6.
VICKS® DAYQUIL® LIQUICAPS: Gelatin, Glycerin, Polyethylene Glycol, Povidone, Propylene Glycol, Purified Water, Red 40, Sorbitol Special, Yellow 6.

Directions:
[6 & 10 oz bottle]
• use teaspoon (tsp), tablespoon (TBSP) or dose cup
  under 6 yrs .... ask a doctor
  6–11 yrs ...... 1 TBSP or 3 tsp or 15 ml
  12 yrs. & older ...... 2 TBSP or 6 tsp or 30 ml
• Repeat every 4 hours, not to exceed 4 doses per day or use as directed by a doctor. If taking NyQuil® and DayQuil, limit total to 4 doses per day.
[LIQUICAPS]
  under 6 yrs .... ask a doctor
  6–11 yrs .... 1 softgel with water
  12 yrs. & older .. 2 softgels with water
• Repeat every 4 hours, not to exceed 4 doses per day or use as directed by a doctor. If taking NyQuil® and DayQuil, limit total to 4 doses per day.

Other Information:
• store at room temperature
Warnings:
Alcohol warning If you consume 3 or more alcoholic drinks every day, ask your doctor whether you should take acetaminophen or other pain relievers/fever reducers. Acetaminophen may cause liver damage.
Sore throat warning Severe or persistent sore throat or sore throat that occurs with high fever, headache, nausea, and vomiting may be serious. Ask a doctor right away. Do not use more than 2 days or give to children under 6 years of age unless directed by a doctor.
Do not use
• if you are on a sodium-restricted diet
• if you are now taking a prescription monoamine oxidase inhibitor (MAOI) (certain drugs for depression, psychiatric or emotional conditions, or Parkinson's disease), or for 2 weeks after stopping the MAOI drug. If you do not know if your prescription drug contains an MAOI, ask a doctor or pharmacist before taking this product.
Ask a doctor before use if you have:
• heart disease
• asthma
• emphysema
• thyroid disease
• diabetes
• cough associated with smoking
• high blood pressure
• excessive phlegm (mucus)
• breathing problems
• persistent or chronic cough
• trouble urinating due to enlarged prostate gland
When using this product
• do not use more than directed
• avoid alcoholic drinks
• do not use with other products containing acetaminophen
Stop use and ask a doctor if:
• you get nervous, dizzy or sleepless
• fever gets worse or lasts more than 3 days
• new sysmptoms occur
• symptoms do not get better within 7 days
• you need to use more than 7 days (adults) or 5 days (children)
• cough lasts more than 7 days (adults) or 5 days (chidren), comes back, or occurs with fever, rash, or headache that lasts. These could be the signs of a serious condition.
If pregnant or breast-feeding, ask a health professional before use.
Keep out of the reach of children. In case of overdose, get medical help or contact a Poison Control Center right away. Quick medical attention is critical for adults as well as for children even if you do not notice any signs or symptoms.

How Supplied: Available in: **LIQUID** 6 FL OZ (175 ml) and 10 FL OZ (295 ml) plastic bottles with child-resistant, tamper-evident cap and a calibrated medicine cup.
LIQUICAP: in 12-count child-resistant packages and 20- and 36-count nonchild-resistant packages. Each softgel is imprinted: "DayQuil."
Questions? 1-800-251-3374

VICKS® NYQUIL® LIQUICAPS®
VICKS® NYQUIL® LIQUID
(Original and Cherry)
Multi-Symptom Cold/Flu Relief
Antihistamine/Cough
Suppressant/Pain Reliever/
Nasal Decongestant/
Fever Reducer

Uses: Temporarily relieves common cold/flu symptoms:
• minor aches
• pains
• headache
• muscular aches
• sore throat pain
• fever
• runny nose and sneezing
• nasal congestion
• cough due to minor throat and bronchial irritation

Active Ingredients:
[See tables at bottom of next page]

Inactive Ingredients:
VICKS® NYQUIL® LIQUICAPS®: Blue 1, Gelatin, Glycerin, Polyethylene, Glycol, Povidone, Propylene Glycol, Purified Water, Sodium Carbonate, Sorbitol Special, Yellow 10.
VICKS® NYQUIL® LIQUID: [ORIGINAL] Alcohol, Citric Acid, Flavor, Green 3, High Fructose Corn Syrup, Polyethylene Glycol, Propylene Glycol, Purified Water, Saccharin Sodium, Sodium Citrate, Yellow 6, Yellow 10.
[CHERRY] Alcohol, Blue 1, Citric Acid, Flavor, Fructose Corn Syrup, Polyethylene Glycol, Propylene Glycol, Purified Water, Red 40, Saccharin Sodium, Sodium Citrate.

Directions:
VICKS® NYQUIL® LIQUICAPS®:
• do not use in children under 12 yrs.
• 12 yrs. & older: swallow 2 softgels with water, repeat every 6 hours; no more than 4 doses daily. If taking NyQuil and DayQuil®. limit total to 4 doses daily.
VICKS® NYQUIL® LIQUID®:
[6 & 10 oz bottle]

Directions:
• do not use in children under 12 yrs.
• 12 yrs. & older: take 2 tablespoons (TBSP) or 30 ml (dose cup), repeat every 6 hours; no more than 4 doses daily. If taking NyQuil® and DayQuil®, limit total to 4 doses daily.
[1 oz bottle]

Directions:
• do not use in children under 12 yrs.
• 12 yrs. & older: take 2 tablespoons (TBSP), repeat every 6 hours; no more than 4 doses daily. If taking NyQuil and DayQuil®, limit total to 4 doses daily. [1 oz cherry pouch]

Directions:
• do not use in children under 12 yrs.
• 12 yrs. & older: cut corner of pouch with scissors to open. Take 1 fluid ounce (contents of pouch), repeat every 6 hrs; no more than 4 doses dialy. If taking NyQuil® and DayQuil®, limit total to 4 doses daily.

Other Information:
• Store at room temperature
• **each softgel contains** sodium 2 mg

Continued on next page

Vicks Nyquil—Cont.

Warnings:

Alcohol warning If you consume 3 or more alcoholic drinks every day, ask your doctor whether you should take acetaminophen or other pain relievers/fever reducers. Acetaminophen may cause liver damage.

Sore throat warning Severe or persistent sore throat or sore throat that occurs with high fever, headache, nausea, and vomiting may be serious. Ask a doctor right away. Do not use more than 2 days or give to children under 12 years of age unless directed by a doctor.

Do not use if you are now taking a prescription monoamine oxidase inhibitor (MAOI) (certain drugs for depression, psychiatric, or emotional conditions, or Parkinson's disease), or for 2 weeks after stopping the MAOI drug. If you do not know if your prescription drug contains an MAOI, ask a doctor or pharmacist before taking this product.

Ask a doctor before use if you have:
- heart disease
- asthma
- emphysema
- thyroid disease
- diabetes
- glaucoma
- high blood pressure
- excessive phlegm (mucus)
- breathing problems
- chronic bronchitis
- persistent or chronic cough
- cough associated with smoking
- trouble urinating due to an enlarged prostate gland

Ask a doctor or pharmacist before use if you are taking sedatives or tranquilizers.

When using this product:
- do not use more than directed
- excitability may occur, especially in children
- marked drowsiness may occur
- avoid alcoholic drinks
- be careful when driving a motor vehicle or operating machinery
- do not use with other products containing acetaminophen
- alcohol, sedatives, and tranquilizers may increase drowsiness

Stop use and ask a doctor if:
- you get nervous, dizzy or sleepless
- new symptoms occur
- symptoms do not get better
- fever gets worse or lasts more than 3 days
- you need to use more than 7 days
- cough lasts more than 7 days, comes back, or occurs with fever, rash, or headache that lasts.

These could be signs of a serious condition.

If pregnant or breast-feeding, ask a health professional before use.

Keep out of reach of children. In case of overdose, get medical help or contact a Poison Control Center right away. Quick medical attention is critical for adults as well as for children even if you do not notice any signs or symptoms.

How Supplied: **(LiquiCaps®)** Available in 12- and 36-count child-resistant blister packages and 20-count non-child resistant blister packages. Each softgel is imprinted "NyQuil".
(Liquid) Available in 6 and 10 FL OZ (175 and 295 ml, respectively) plastic bottles with child-resistant, tamper-evident cap and calibrated medicine cup.
Questions? 1-800-362-1683

PEDIATRIC VICKS® 44e®
Cough & Chest Congestion Relief

Active Ingredients:
per 1 tablespoon (TBSP.) (15 ml): Dextromethorphan Hydrobromide 10 mg, Guaifenesin 100 mg.

CONTAINS NO ALCOHOL

Inactive Ingredients: Carboxymethylcellulose Sodium, Citric Acid, Flavor, High Fructose Corn Syrup, Polyethylene Oxide, Polyoxyl 40 Stearate, Propylene Glycol, Purified Water, Red 40, Saccharin Sodium, Sodium Benzoate, Sodium Citrate.
Sodium Content: 60 mg per 30 mL dose.

Uses: Temporarily relieves cough due to a common cold. Helps loosen phlegm to rid the bronchial passageways of bothersome mucus.

Directions: Use Tablespoon (TBSP) or dose cup.

Under 2 yrs.	Ask a doctor.
2–5 yrs.	$1/_2$ TBSP or $7^1/_2$ ml
6–11 yrs.	1 TBSP or 15 ml
12 yrs. & older	2 TBSP or 30 ml

Repeat every 4 hours. Not to exceed 6 doses per day or use as directed by a doctor.

Active Ingredients (per softgel): Purpose:
Acetaminophen 325 mg .... Pain reliever/fever reducer
Dextromethorphan HBr 15 mg .... Cough suppressant
Doxylamine succinate 6.25 mg .... Antihistamine
Pseudoephedrine HCl 30 mg .... Nasal decongestant

---

Active Ingredients (per tablespoon): Purpose:
Acetaminophen 500 mg .... Pain reliever/fever reducer
Dextromethorphan HBr 15 mg .... Cough suppressant
Doxylamine succinate 6.25 mg .... Antihistamine
Pseudoephedrine HCl 30 mg .... Nasal decongestant

---

*Professional Dosage:

Physicians: Suggested doses for children under 2 years of age.

Age	Dose
* 6–11 mo.	1 teaspoon (tsp.) (5 ml)
*12–23 mo.	$1^1/_4$ teaspoon (tsp.) (6.25 ml)

Repeat every 4 hours. Not to exceed 6 doses per day or use as directed by doctor.

*Based on extrapolation from studies on the safety and efficacy of active ingredients conducted among older children and adults. Use caution in treating children under 2 years who were born prematurely.

Warnings:
Do not take unless directed by a doctor if you have:
- asthma
- emphysema
- excessive phlegm (mucus)
- persistent or chronic cough
- chronic bronchitis
- cough associated with smoking

Keep this and all drugs out of the reach of children.
In the case of accidental overdose, seek professional advice or contact a poison control center immediately. As with any drug, if you are pregnant or nursing a baby, seek the advice of a health professional before using this product. Do not use this product if you are on a sodium-restricted diet unless directed by a doctor.
Drug Interaction Precaution: Do not use this product without first asking a doctor if you are take a prescription monoamine oxidase inhibitor (MAOI) (certain drugs for depression, psychiatric or emotional conditions, or Parkinson's disease), or for 2 weeks after stopping the MAOI drug or if you are uncertain whether your prescription drug contains an MAOI.
Dosing Duration & When to Ask a Doctor:
- If a cough persists for more than 7 days, recurs, or is accompanied by fever, rash or persistent headache. A persistent cough may be the sign of a serious condition.

How Supplied: 4 FL OZ (118 ml) plastic bottles. A calibrated dose cup accompanies each bottle.

PEDIATRIC VICKS® 44m®
Cough & Cold Relief
Cough Suppressant/Nasal Decongestant/Antihistamine

Active Ingredients: Per 1 tablespoon (TBSP) (15 ml): Dextromethorphan Hydrobromide 15 mg, Pseudoephedrine Hydrochloride 30 mg, Chlorpheniramine Maleate 2 mg.

CONTAINS NO ALCOHOL

Inactive Ingredients: Carboxymethylcellulose Sodium, Citric Acid, Flavor, High Fructose Corn Syrup, Polyethylene Oxide, Polyoxyl 40 Stearate, Propylene Glycol, Purified Water, Red 40, Saccharin Sodium, Sodium Benzoate, Sodium Citrate.
Sodium Content: 60 mg per 30 mL dose.

Uses: Temporarily relieves cough/cold symptoms:
• cough
• nasal congestion
• runny nose
• sneezing

Directions: Use Tablespoon (TBSP) or dose cup.

Under 6 yrs.	Ask a doctor.
6–11 yrs.	1 TBSP or 15 ml
12 yrs. & older	2 TBSP or 30 ml

Repeat every 6 hours, not to exceed 4 doses per day or use as directed by a doctor.

Professional Dosage:

*Physicians: Suggested doses for children under 6 years of age.

Age	Dose
* 6–11 mo.	1 teaspoon (tsp.) (5 ml)
*12–23 mo.	1$^{1}/_{4}$ teaspoon (tsp.) (6.25 ml)
2–5 yrs.	$^{1}/_{2}$ TABLESPOON (TBSP.) (7.5 ml)

Repeat every 6 hours, no more than 4 doses in 24 hours, or as directed by doctor.

*Based on extrapolation from studies on the safety and efficacy of active ingredients conducted among older children and adults. Use caution in treating children under 2 years of age who were born prematurely.

Warnings: Do not exceed recommended dosage.
If nervousness, dizziness, or sleeplessness occur, discontinue use and ask a doctor. May cause drowsiness. May cause excitability especially in children. *Do not take unless directed by a doctor if you have:*
• heart disease
• asthma
• emphysema
• thyroid disease
• diabetes
• glaucoma
• high blood pressure
• excessive phlegm (mucus)
• breathing problems
• chronic bronchitis
• difficulty in breathing
• persistent or chronic cough
• cough associated with smoking
• difficulty in urination due to enlarged prostate gland
Keep this and all drugs out of the reach of children. In case of accidental overdose, seek professional advice or contact a poison control center immediately. As with any drug, if you are pregnant or nursing a baby, seek the advice of a health professional before using this product.
Alcohol, sedatives, and tranquilizers may increase the drowsiness effect. Avoid alcoholic beverages while taking this product. Use caution when driving a motor vehicle or operating machinery. Do not use this product if you are on a sodium-restricted diet unless directed by a doctor.
Drug Interaction Precaution: Do not take this product without first asking a doctor if you take:
• sedatives
• tranquilizers
• a prescription monoamine oxidase inhibitor (MAOI) (certain drugs for depression, psychiatric or emotional conditions, or Parkinson's disease), or for 2 weeks after stopping the MAOI drug or if you are uncertain whether your prescription drug contains an MAOI.
Dosing Duration: Do not use over 7 days. *Ask a Doctor:*
• If symptoms do not improve within 7 days or are accompanied by a fever.
• If a cough persists for more than 7 days, recurs, or is accompanied by fever, rash or persistent headache. A persistent cough may be a sign of a serious condition.

How Supplied: 4 fl oz (118 ml) plastic bottles. A calibrated dose cup accompanies each bottle.

VICKS® SINEX® NASAL SPRAY
[sī 'nĕx]
[Ultra Fine Mist] for Sinus Relief
Phenylephrine HCl Nasal Decongestant

Uses: temporarily relieves sinus/nasal congestion due to
• colds
• hay fever
• upper respiratory allergies
• sinusitis
[See table above]

Inactive Ingredients: Benzalkonium Chloride, Camphor, Chlorhexidine Gluconate, Citric Acid, Disodium EDTA, Eucalyptol, Menthol, Purified Water, Tyloxapol.

Directions:
[NASAL SPRAY]
• under 12 yrs. ask a doctor
• adults & children 12 yrs. & older: 2 or 3 sprays in each nostril without tilting your head, not more often than every 4 hours.
[ULTRA FINE MIST] Remove protective cap. Before using for the first time, prime the pump by firmly depressing its rim several times. Hold container with thumb at base and nozzle between first and second fingers. Without tilting your head, insert nozzle into nostril. Fully depress rim with a firm, even stroke and inhale deeply.

Active Ingredients: **Purpose:**
Phenylephrine hydrochloride [HCl] 0.5% .... Nasal decongestant

• under 12 yrs. ask a doctor
• adults and children 12 yrs. & older: 2 or 3 sprays in each nostril, not more often than every 4 hours.

Warnings:
Do not use
• this container by more than one person, it may spread infection
• for more than 3 days
Ask a doctor before use if you have
• heart disease
• thyroid disease
• diabetes
• high blood pressure
• trouble urinating due to an enlarged prostate gland
When using this product:
• do not exceed recommended dosage
• temporary burning, stinging, sneezing, or increased nasal discharge may occur
• frequent or prolonged use may cause nasal congestion to recur or worsen
Stop use and ask a doctor if:
• symptoms persist for more than 3 days
If pregnant or breast-feeding, ask a health professional before use.
Keep out of reach of children. In case of accidental ingestion, get medical help or contact a poison control center right away.

Other Information:
• store at room temperature

How Supplied: Available in $^{1}/_{2}$ fl oz (15 ml) plastic squeeze bottle and $^{1}/_{2}$ fl oz (15 ml) measured dose Ultra Fine mist pump.
Questions? 1 800 358-8707

VICKS® SINEX®
[sī 'nĕx]
12-HOUR [Nasal Spray]
[Ultra Fine Mist] for Sinus Relief
Oxymetazoline HCl
Nasal Decongestant

Uses:
Temporary relieves sinus/nasal congestion due to
• colds
• hay fever
• upper respiratory allergies
• sinusitis
[See table at top of next page]

Inactive Ingredients: Benzalkonium Chloride, Camphor, Chlorhexidine Gluconate, Disodium EDTA, Eucalyptol, Menthol, Potassium Phosphate, Purified Water, Sodium Chloride, Sodium Phosphate, Tyloxapol.

Directions:
[NASAL SPRAY]
• under 6 yrs. ask a doctor
• adults & children 6 yrs. & older (with adult supervision): 2 or 3 sprays in each nostril without tilting your head, not more often than every 10 to 12 hours. Do not exceed 2 applications in any 24-hour period.
[ULTRA FINE MIST] Remove protective cap. Before using for the first time,

Continued on next page

Vicks Sinex 12-Hour—Cont.

prime the pump by firmly depressing its rim several times. Hold container with thumb at base and nozzle between first and second fingers. Without tilting your head, insert nozzle into nostril. Fully depress rim with a firm, even stroke and inhale deeply.
- under 6 yrs. ask a doctor
- adults & children 6 yrs. & older (with adult supervision): 2 or 3 sprays in each nostril, not more often than every 10 to 12 hours. Do not exceed 2 applications in any 24-hour period.

Warnings:
Do not use:
This container by more than one person; it may spread infection
- for more than 3 days
Ask a doctor before use if you have
- heart disease
- thyroid disease
- diabetes
- high blood pressure
- trouble urinating due to an enlarged prostate gland
When using this product:
- do not exceed recommended dosage
- temporary burning, stinging, sneezing, or increased nasal discharge may occur
- frequent or prolonged use may cause nasal congestion to recur or worsen
Stop use and ask a doctor if:
- symptoms persist for more than 3 days
If pregnant or breast-feeding, ask a health professional before use.
Keep out of reach of children. In case of accidental ingestion, get medical help or contact a poison control center right away.

Other Information:
Store at room temperature

How Supplied: Available in $1/2$ FL OZ (15 ml) plastic squeeze bottle and $1/2$ FL OZ (15 ml) measured-dose Ultra Fine mist pump.
Questions? 1 800 358-8707

VICKS® VAPOR INHALER
Levmetamfetamine/Nasal Decongestant

Uses:
Temporarily relieves nasal congestion due to:
- colds
- hay fever
- upper respiratory allergies
- sinusitis
[See table below]

Inactive Ingredients: Bornyl Acetate, Camphor, Lavender Oil, Menthol

Directions:
- under 6 yrs. ask a doctor
- 6–11 yrs.: with adult supervision, 1 inhalation in each nostril not more often than every 2 hours.
- 12 yrs. & older: 2 inhalations in each nostril, not more often than every 2 hours.

Active Ingredients: **Purpose:**
Levmetamfetamine 50 mg .... Nasal decongestant

---

Active Ingredients: **Purpose:**
Oxymetazoline hydrochloride [HCl] 0.05% .... Nasal decongestant

Warnings:
Do not use
- this container by more than one person; it may spread infection
- for more than 3 days
Ask a doctor before use if you have
- heart disease
- high blood pressure
- thyroid disease
- diabetes
- trouble urinating due to an enlarged prostate gland
When using this product:
- do not exceed recommended dosage
- temporary burning, stinging, sneezing, or increased nasal discharge may occur
- frequent or prolonged use may cause nasal congestion to recur or worsen
Stop use and ask a doctor if:
- symptoms persist for more than 3 days
If pregnant or breast-feeding, ask a health professional before use.
Keep out of reach of children. In case of overdose, get medical help or contact a poison control center right away.

Other Information: Store at room temperature

How Supplied: Available as a cylindrical plastic nasal inhaler.
Net weight: 0.007 OZ (200 mg).
Questions? 1 800 358-8707

VICKS® VAPORUB®
VICKS® VAPORUB® CREAM
(greaseless)
[vā 'pō-rub]
Nasal Decongestant/Cough Suppressant/Topical Analgesic

Uses:
On chest & throat temporarily relieves:
- cough
- nasal congestion [due to the common cold]
On aching muscles temporarily relieves:
- minor aches & pains
[See table at top of next page]

Inactive Ingredients: Carbomer 954, Cedarleaf Oil, Cetyl Alcohol, Cetyl Palmitate, Cyclomethicone Copolyol, Dimethicone Copolyol, Dimethicone, EDTA, Glycerin, Imidazolidinyl Urea, Isopropyl Palmitate, Methylparaben, Nutmeg Oil, Peg-100 Stearate, Propylparaben, Purified Water, Sodium Hydroxide, Stearic Acid, Stearyl Alcohol, Thymol, Titanium Dioxide, Turpentine Oil.

Directions:
see important warnings under "When using this product"
- under 2 yrs. ask a doctor
- adults and children 2 yrs. & older: Rub a thick layer on chest & throat or rub on sore aching muscles. If desired, cover with a soft cloth but keep clothing loose. Repeat up to three times daily.

Warnings:
For external use only; avoid contact with eyes.
Do not use:
- by mouth
- with tight bandages
- in nostrils
- on wounds or damaged skin
Ask a doctor before use if you have:
- excessive phlegm (mucus)
- asthma
- emphysema
- persistent or chronic cough
- cough associated with smoking
When using this product do not:
- heat
- microwave
- use near an open flame
- add to hot water or any container where heating water. May cause splattering and result in burns.
Stop use and ask a doctor if:
- muscle aches/pains persist more than 7 days or come back
- cough lasts more than 7 days, comes back, or occurs with fever, rash, or headache that lasts.
These could be signs of a serious condition.
If pregnant or breast-feeding, ask a health professional before use.
Keep out of reach of children. In case of accidental ingestion, get medical help or contact a Poison Control Center right away.

Other Information:
Store at room temperature

How Supplied: **(ointment)** Available in 1.5 OZ (40 g), 3.0 OZ (90 g) and 6.0 OZ (170 g) plastic jars. **(cream)** 2.0 OZ (56 g) tube.
Questions? 1 800 358-8707

VICKS® VAPOSTEAM®
[vā 'pō "stēm]
Liquid Medication for Hot Steam Vaporizers.
Camphor/Cough Suppressant

Uses:
Temporarily relieves cough associated with a cold.
[See table at bottom of next page]

Inactive Ingredients:
Alcohol 78%, Cedarleaf Oil, Eucalyptus Oil, Laureth-7, Menthol, Nutmeg Oil, Poloxamer 124, Silicone

Directions:
See important warnings under "When using this product"
- under 2 yrs.: ask a doctor
- adults & children 2 yrs. & older: use 1 tablespoon of solution for each quart of water or 1 $1/2$ teaspoonful of solution for each pint of water
  - add solution directly to cold water only in a hot steam vaporizer
  - follow manufacturer's directions for using vaporizer. Breathe in medicated vapors. May be repeated up to 3 times a day.

Active Ingredients: | **Purpose:**

Camphor 5.2% .... Cough suppressant, nasal decongestant & topical analgesic
Eucalyptus oil 1.2% .... Cough suppressant & nasal decongestant
Menthol 2.8% .... Cough suppressant, nasal decongestant & topical analgesic

Warnings:

For external use only

Flammable Keep away from fire or flame. Cap container tightly and store at room temperature away from heat.

Ask a doctor before use if you have:
- a persistent or chronic cough
- cough associated with smoking
- emphysema
- excessive phlegm (mucus)
- asthma

When using this product do not:
- **heat**
- **microwave**
- **use near an open flame**
- **take by mouth**
- **direct steam from the vaporizer too close to the face**
- **add to hot water or any container where heating water except when adding to cold water only in a hot steam vaporizer. May cause splattering and result in burns.**

Stop use and ask a doctor if:
- cough lasts more than 7 days, comes back, or occurs with fever, rash, or headache that lasts. These could be the signs of a serious condition.

Keep out of reach of children. In case of eye exposure (flush eyes with water); or in case of accidental ingestion: seek medical help or contact a Poison Control Center right away.

How Supplied: Available in 4 FL OZ (118 mL) and 8 FL OZ (235 mL) bottles.

Questions? 1 800 358-8707

EDUCATIONAL MATERIAL

Procter & Gamble offers to health care professionals a variety of journal reprints and patient education materials on:
- fiber therapy and related bowel disorders (Metamucil),
- H. pylori research and healthy traveling advice (Pepto-Bismol),
- caffeine reduction (Folgers), and
- pharmacy practice issues (Pharmacy Digest newsletter).

Additionally, selected professional samples of Procter & Gamble Health Care and Skin Care products are available to targeted health care specialists.

For these materials, please call 1-800/358-8707, or write:

Charles Lambert
Manager, Scientific Communications
The Procter & Gamble Company
Two Procter & Gamble Plaza
Cincinnati, OH 45201

Active Ingredients: | **Purpose:**
Camphor 6.2% .... Cough suppressant

Products on Demand

1621 EAST FLAMINGO RD.
SUITE 15A
LAS VEGAS, NV 89119
www.vitara.com
(702) 765-5001

Direct Inquiries to:
Shaina M. Toppo
702-765-5001
www.vitara.com

Vitara™
Female Sexual Aid/Enhancer

Active Ingredients: N-methylnicotinate, (FDA Monograph) Wild Yam Plant Extract (Discoreae), DHEA

Inactive Ingredients: Water, Propylene Glycol, Glycerin, Polyquaternium-37/Propylene Glycol Dicaprylate Dicaprate & PPG1 Trideceth-6, Sorbic Acid, Methyl & Propyl Paraben, Fragrance

Description: Several studies have shown that in excess of 40% of females suffer from some type of sexual dysfunction. Sexual dysfunction has been divided into four subclasses. Three of these four subclasses can be attributed to a decrease in blood flow to the female genitalia. In particular, the lack of blood flow to the clitoris makes reaching orgasm very difficult or impossible to attain. Vitara™ causes increased blood flow instantaneously to the genitalia, which, with manual stimulation has shown to allow women to experience an orgasm. Also, the natural occurring estrogens and hormonal precursors found in the yams and DHEA increase vaginal moisture.

Actions: Used as directed, Vitara™ Female Sexual Enhancer causes immediate profound vasodialation to the female genitalia and with appropriate manipulation allows for female orgasm. Even in women who are diabetic, menopausal, or who take medication for high blood pressure, depression or anxiety. Also, women who have orgasms report greater intensity and frequency or orgasms. Vaginal mucosa also becomes more lubricated and women experience a very warm, "tingling" sensation wherever Vitara™ is applied.

Warnings: Vitara™ will cause vasodialation/dermal flush to any tissue.

How Supplied: Available in 1 Fl. oz Bottle.

Shown in Product Identification Guide, page 522

The Purdue Frederick Company

ONE STAMFORD FORUM
STAMFORD, CT 06901-3431

For Medical Information Contact:
Medical Department
(888) 726–7535

BETADINE® BRAND
First Aid Antibiotics
+ Moisturizer Ointment

Actions: Topical broad-spectrum antibiotics polymyxin B sulfate and bacitracin zinc in a cholesterolized ointment* (moisturizer) base to help prevent infection. Formulated with a special blend of waxes and oils to help retain vital moisture needed to aid in healing.

Indications: First aid to help prevent infection in minor cuts, scrapes and burns.

Administration: Clean affected area. Apply small amount of this product (an amount equal to the surface area of the tip of the finger) on the area 1 to 3 times daily. May be covered with a sterile bandage.

Warnings: For External Use Only. Do not use in the eyes or apply over large areas of the body. In case of deep or puncture wounds, animal bites, or serious burns, consult a physician. Stop use and consult a physician if the condition persists or gets worse, or if a rash or other allergic reaction develops. Do not use this product if you are allergic to any of the ingredients. Do not use longer than 1 week unless directed by a physician. Keep this and all medications out of the reach of children. In case of accidental ingestion, seek professional assistance or contact a Poison Control Center immediately.

Active Ingredients: Per gram: Polymyxin B Sulfate (10,000 IU) and Bacitracin Zinc (500 IU).

How Supplied: 1/2 oz. plastic tube with applicator tip. Store at room temperature.

* Formulated with Aquaphor®—a registered trademark of Beiersdorf AG.

Copyright 1998, 2001, The Purdue Frederick Company

Shown in Product Identification Guide, page 522

BETADINE® BRAND PLUS
First Aid Antibiotics + Pain Reliever
Ointment
[bā 'tăh-dīn"]

Actions: Topical broad-spectrum antibiotics polymyxin B sulfate and bacitra-

Continued on next page

Betadine Plus—Cont.

cin zinc plus topical anesthetic in a cholesterolized ointment* (moisturizer) base to help prevent infection and relieve pain.

Indications: First aid to help prevent infection and provide temporary pain relief in minor cuts, scrapes and burns.

Administration: Clean affected area. Apply small amount of this product (an amount equal to the surface area of the tip of the finger) on the area 1 to 3 times daily. May be covered with a sterile bandage. Children under 2 years of age: Consult a physician.

Warnings: For External Use Only. Do not use in the eyes or apply over large areas of the body. In case of deep or puncture wounds, animal bites, or serious burns, consult a physician. Stop use and consult a physician if the condition persists or gets worse, or if a rash or other allergic reaction develops. Do not use this product if you are allergic to any of the ingredients. Do not use longer than 1 week unless directed by a physician. Keep this and all medications out of the reach of children. In case of accidental ingestion, seek professional assistance or contact a Poison Control Center immediately.

Active Ingredients: Per gram: Polymyxin B Sulfate (10,000 IU), Bacitracin Zinc (500 IU), and Pramoxine HCl 10 mg.

How Supplied: 1/2 oz. plastic tube with an applicator tip. Store at room temperature.
*Formulated with Aquaphor® — a registered trademark of Beiersdorf AG.
Copyright 1998, 2001, The Purdue Frederick Company.
Shown in Product Identification Guide, page 521

BETADINE® OINTMENT
(povidone-iodine, 10%)
BETADINE® SOLUTION
(povidone-iodine, 10%)
BETADINE ® SKIN CLEANSER
(povidone-iodine, 7.5%)
Topical Antiseptic
Bactericide/Virucide

Action: Topical microbicides active against organisms commonly encountered in minor skin wounds and burns.

Indications: **Ointment**—For the prevention of infection in minor burns, cuts and abrasions. Kills microorganisms promptly. **Solution**—Kills microorganisms in minor burns, cuts and scrapes. First aid to help prevent infection in cuts, scrapes and minor burns. **Skin Cleanser**—Helps prevent infection in cuts, scrapes and minor burns. Use routinely for general hygiene.

Administration: **Ointment**—For the prevention of infection in minor burns, cuts and abrasions, apply directly to af-

fected areas as needed. Nonocclusive: allows air to reach the wound. May be bandaged. **Solution**—For minor cuts, scrapes and burns, apply directly to affected area as needed. May be covered with gauze or adhesive bandage. **Skin Cleanser**—Wet skin and apply a sufficient amount to work up a rich, golden lather. Allow lather to remain about 3 minutes and rinse off. Repeat 2–3 times a day or as directed by physician.

Warnings: For External Use Only. In case of deep or puncture wounds or serious burns, consult physician. If redness, irritation, swelling or pain persists or increases, or if infection occurs, discontinue use and consult physician. Keep out of reach of children.

How Supplied:
Ointment: 1/32 oz. and 1/8 oz. packettes and 1 oz. tubes
Solution: 1/2 oz., 4 oz., 8 oz., 16 oz. (1 pt.), 32 oz. (1 qt.), and 1 gal. plastic bottles.
Skin Cleanser: 4 fl. oz. plastic bottles
Avoid storing at excessive heat.
Copyright 1991, 2001, The Purdue Frederick Company
Shown in Product Identification Guide, page 522

BETADINE® PREPSTICK® APPLICATOR
[bā′ tăh-dīn′′]
[povidone-iodine, 10%]
Topical Antiseptic Bactericide/Virucide

Individually wrapped applicators are packaged dry with approximately 2.6 grams of microbicidal Betadine® Solution stored in the handle of the applicator. Antiseptic solution is released into the 1³⁄₈-inch-long, soft foam swab head by gently squeezing the 4-inch-long plastic handle.

Actions: Reduces bacterial load and the risk of infection.

Indications: For degerming skin and mucous membranes. Provides sufficient antiseptic solution for most kinds of site prepping—including prior to IM injections, venous punctures, and minor surgical procedures.

Administration: Tear wrapper on dotted line and discard top part of wrapper. With the tip still in the wrapper, gently squeeze plastic handle to break the seal. Release antiseptic solution into foam swab head by lightly squeezing handle. Apply to prep site with the moistened foam tip, working in a circular motion from inside to the outside. Apply as often as needed.

Warnings: For External Use Only. Do not use in the eyes. Discontinue use if irritation and redness develop. **Do not heat prior to application.**

How Supplied: 150 individually packaged applicators per dispensing unit. Each applicator contains approximately 2.6 grams of solution.

Avoid storing at excessive heat.
Copyright 1999, 2001, The Purdue Frederick Company
Shown in Product Identification Guide, page 522

SENOKOT® Tablets/Granules
SenokotXTRA® Tablets
(standardized senna concentrate)
SENOKOT® Syrup
SENOKOT® Children's Syrup
(extract of senna concentrate)
SENOKOT-S® Tablets
(standardized senna concentrate and docusate sodium)

Natural Vegetable Laxative

Actions: Senna provides a colon-specific action which is gentle, effective, and predictable, generally producing bowel movement in 6 to 12 hours. Senokot-S tablets also contain a stool softener for smoother, easier evacuation.

Indications: For the relief of occasional constipation. Senokot products generally produce bowel movement in 6 to 12 hours.

Dosage and Administration: Take according to product-package instructions or as directed by a doctor. Take preferably at bedtime. For use of Senokot Laxatives in children under 2 years of age, consult a doctor.

Warnings: Do not use a laxative product when abdominal pain, nausea or vomiting are present unless directed by a doctor. If you have noticed a sudden change in bowel movements that persists over a period of 2 weeks, consult a doctor before using a laxative. Do not use laxative products for longer than 1 week unless directed by a doctor. Rectal bleeding or failure to have a bowel movement after the use of a laxative may indicate a serious condition. Discontinue use and consult your doctor. As with any drug, if you are pregnant or nursing a baby, seek the advice of a health professional before using this product. In case of accidental overdose, seek professional assistance or contact a Poison Control Center immediately. Keep out of children's reach.

How Supplied: Senokot Tablets: Boxes of 20; bottles of 50, 100, and 1000; Unit Strip Packs in boxes of 100 individually sealed tablets. Each Senokot Tablet contains 8.6 mg sennosides.
SenokotXTRA Tablets: Boxes of 12 and 36. Each SenokotXTRA Tablet contains 17.2 mg sennosides.
Senokot-S Tablets: Packages of 10; bottles of 30, 60 and 1000; Unit Strip boxes of 100. Each Senokot-S Tablet contains 8.6 mg sennosides and 50 mg docusate sodium.
Senokot Granules: 2, 6, and 12 oz. plastic containers. Each teaspoon of Senokot Granules contains 15 mg sennosides.
Senokot Syrup: 2 and 8 fl. oz. bottles.
Senokot Children's Syrup: Chocolate-flavored, alcohol-free syrup in 2.5 fl. oz.

plastic bottle packaged with measuring cup. Each teaspoon of Senokot Syrup or Senokot Children's Syrup contains 8.8 mg sennosides.

Copyright 1991, 2001, The Purdue Frederick Company.

Shown in Product Identification Guide, page 522

EDUCATIONAL MATERIAL

Samples Available:
1) Senokot-S® Tablets Samples– 1 display of 12 (4 tablets per packette)
2) Betadine® Brand First Aid Antibiotics + Moisturizer Ointment Samples– 1 display of 48 packettes
3) Betadine® Brand Plus First Aid Antibiotics + Pain Reliever– 1 display of 48 packettes
4) **Up-to-date Information:** www.senokot.com provides dosing information for the Senokot® products family of laxatives, as well as patient education about constipation and its causes. A special section on toilet training, written by a pediatrician, describes the popular child-centered approach.

Richardson-Vicks Inc.
(See Procter & Gamble.)

Schering-Plough HealthCare Products
3 OAK WAY
BERKELEY HEIGHTS, NJ 07922

Direct Product Requests to:
Schering-Plough HealthCare Products
Attn: Managed Care Department
3 Oak Way
Berkeley Heights, NJ 07922

For Medical Emergencies Contact:
Consumer Relations Department
(901) 320-2998 (Business Hours)
(901) 320-2364 (After Hours)

A + D® Ointment with Zinc Oxide

Active Ingredients: Dimethicone 1%, Zinc Oxide 10%.

Inactive Ingredients: Aloe Extract, Benzyl Alcohol, Cod Liver Oil (contains Vitamin A and Vitamin D), Fragrance, Glyceryl Oleate, Light Mineral Oil, Ozokerite, Paraffin, Propylene Glycol, Sorbitol, Synthetic Beeswax, Water.

Indications: Helps treat and prevent diaper rash. Protects chafed skin or minor skin irritation associated with diaper rash and helps seal out wetness.

Directions: Change wet and soiled diapers promptly, cleanse the diaper area and allow to dry. Apply ointment liberally as often as necessary with each diaper change especially at bedtime or anytime when exposure to wet diapers may be prolonged.

Warning: For external use only. Avoid contact with eyes. If condition worsens or does not improve within 7 days, consult a doctor. Not to be applied over deep or puncture wounds, infections, or lacerations. Consult a doctor. Keep this and all drugs out of the reach of children. In case of accidental ingestion, seek professional assistance or contact a Poison Control Center immediately.

How Supplied: A and D® Ointment with Zinc Oxide is available in 1 $1/2$-ounce (42.5g) 3 ounce (81g) and 4-ounce (113g) tubes.
Store between 15° and 30°C (59° and 86°F).

Shown in Product Identification Guide, page 522

A + D ® Original Ointment

Active Ingredients: Petrolatum 53.4%, Lanolin 15.5%.

Inactive Ingredients: Cod Liver Oil (Contains Vitamin A and Vitamin D), Fragrance, Light Mineral Oil, Microcrystalline Wax, Paraffin.

A+D Original Ointment for Diaper Rash:

Indications: Helps treat and prevent diaper rash. Protects chafed skin or minor skin irritation associated with diaper rash and helps seal out wetness.

Directions: Change wet and soiled diapers promptly, cleanse the diaper area, and allow to dry. Apply **A+D Original Ointment** liberally as often as necessary with each diaper change especially at bedtime or anytime when exposure to wet diapers may be prolonged.

A+D Original Ointment for Skin Irritations:

Indications: Helps prevent and temporarily protects chafed, chapped, cracked or windburn skin and lips. Provides temporary protection of minor cuts, scrapes, burns and sunburn.

Directions: Apply **A+D Original Ointment** liberally as often as necessary.

Warnings: For external use only. Avoid contact with eyes. If condition worsens or does not improve within 7 days, consult a doctor. Not to be applied over deep or puncture wounds, infections or lacerations. Consult a doctor. Keep this and all drugs out of the reach of children. In case of acidental ingestion, seek professional assistance or contact a Poison Control Center immediately.

How Supplied: A and D Ointment is available in $1^1/_2$-ounce (42.5g) 3 ounce (81g) and 4-ounce (113g) tubes and 1-pound (454g) jars.
Store between 15° and 30°C (59° and 86°F)

Shown in Product Identification Guide, page 522

AFRIN® 12 Hour
[*á frin*]
Original Nasal Spray
Original Pump Mist
Sinus Nasal Spray
Severe Congestion Nasal Spray
Extra Moisturizing Nasal Spray

Description: AFRIN 12 Hour products contain oxymetazoline hydrochloride, the longest acting OTC topical nasal decongestant available.

Each mL of **AFRIN Original Nasal Spray and Pump Mist** contains Oxymetazoline Hydrochloride, 0.05%. **Also contains:** Benzalkonium Chloride, Edetate Disodium, Polyethylene Glycol, Povidone, Propylene Glycol, Sodium Phosphate Dibasic, Sodium Phosphate Monobasic, Water.

Each mL of **AFRIN Sinus Nasal Spray** contains Oxymetazoline Hydrochloride 0.05%. **Also contains:** benzalkonium chloride, benzyl alcohol, camphor, edetate disodium, eucalyptol, menthol, polysorbate 80, propylene glycol, sodium phosphate dibasic, sodium phosphate monobasic, water

Each mL of **AFRIN Extra Moisturizing Nasal Spray** contains Oxymetazoline Hydrochloride, 0.05%. **Also contains:** benzalkonium chloride, edetate disodium, glycerin, polyethylene glycol, povidone, propylene glycol, sodium phosphate dibasic, sodium phosphate monobasic, water

Each mL of **AFRIN Severe Congestion Nasal Spray** contains Oxymetazoline Hydrochloride 0.05%. **Also contains:** Benzalkonium Chloride, Benzyl Alcohol, Camphor, Edetate Disodium, Eucalyptol, Menthol, Polysorbate 80, Propylene Glycol, Sodium Phosphate Dibasic, Sodium Phosphate Monobasic, Water.

Indications: For the temporary relief of nasal congestion due to a cold, due to hay fever or other upper respiratory allergies, or associated with sinusitis. Shrinks swollen nasal membranes so you can breathe more freely.

Actions: The sympathomimetic action of AFRIN products constricts the smaller arterioles of the nasal passages, producing a prolonged, gentle and predictable

Continued on next page

Information on Schering-Plough HealthCare Products appearing on these pages is effective as of November 2000.

Afrin 12 Hour—Cont.

decongesting effect. In just a few seconds a single dose, as directed, provides immediate, temporary relief of nasal congestion that lasts 12 hours.

Warnings: Do not exceed recommended dosage. This product may cause temporary discomfort such as burning, stinging, sneezing, or an increase in nasal discharge. Do not use this product for more than 3 days. Use only as directed. Frequent or prolonged use may cause nasal congestion to recur or worsen. If symptoms persist, consult a doctor. The use of this container by more than one person may spread infection. Do not use this product if you have heart disease, high blood pressure, thyroid disease, diabetes, or difficulty in urination due to enlargement of the prostate gland unless directed by a doctor. As with any drug, if you are pregnant or nursing a baby, seek the advice of a health professional before using this product. Keep this and all drugs out of the reach of children. In case of accidental ingestion, seek professional assistance or contact a Poison Control Center immediately.

Directions for Afrin Original Nasal Spray, Sinus Nasal Spray, Severe Congestion Nasal Spray and Extra Moisturizing Nasal Spray: Adults and children 6 to under 12 years of age (with adult supervision): 2 or 3 sprays in each nostril not more often than every 10 to 12 hours. Do not exceed 2 doses in any 24-hour period. **Children under 6 years of age:** consult a doctor. To spray, squeeze bottle quickly and firmly. Do not tilt head backward while spraying. Wipe nozzle clean after use.

Directions for Afrin Original Pump Mist:

Adults and children 6 to under 12 years of age (with adult supervision): 2 or 3 sprays in each nostril not more often than every 10 to 12 hours. Do not exceed 2 doses in any 24-hour period. **Children under 6 years of age: consult a doctor.** To spray, remove protective cap. Hold bottle with thumb at base and nozzle between first and second fingers. Without tilting head, insert nozzle into nostril. Fully depress rim with a firm, even stroke and sniff deeply. Wipe nozzle clean after use. Before using the first time, remove the protective cap from the tip and prime metered pump by depressing pump firmly several times.

How Supplied: AFRIN Nasal Spray 0.05%-15 ml and 30 ml plastic squeeze bottles.
AFRIN Pump Mist 0.05% (1:2000)-15 ml pump bottle.
AFRIN Sinus Nasal Spray 0.05%-15 ml plastic squeeze bottles.
AFRIN Extra Moisturizing Nasal Spray 0.05%-15 ml plastic squeeze bottles.
AFRIN Severe Congestion Nasal Spray 0.05% (1:2000)-15 ml plastic squeeze bottle.

Store all nasal sprays between 2° and 30°C (36° and 86°F)
Shown in Product Identification Guide, page 522

AFRIN® Saline Aromatic Mist
[á frin]

Ingredients: Water, PEG-32, Propylene Glycol, Sodium Chloride, PVP, Disodium Phosphate, Sodium Phosphate, Benzyl Alcohol, Polysorbate 80, Benzalkonium Chloride, Menthol, Camphor, Eucalyptol, Disodium EDTA.

Indications: Provides gentle, soothing moisture to irritated, dry nasal passages due to colds, allergies, air pollution, smoke, dry air (low humidity) and air travel. Moisturizes to help make nasal passages feel clear and more comfortable. And since it is non-medicated, AFRIN Saline Mist is safe to use with cold, allergy and sinus medications; it is also safe enough for infants.

Directions: For infants, children and adults, 2 to 6 sprays/drops in each nostril as often as needed or as directed by a doctor. With head in a normal, upright position, put spray tip into nostril. Squeeze bottle with firm, quick pressure while inhaling. For a fine mist, keep bottle upright; for nose drops, keep bottle upside down; for a stream, keep bottle horizontal. Wipe nozzle clean after use. Keep out of the reach of children. The use of this dispenser by more than one person may spread infection.

How Supplied: Afrin Saline Aromatic Mist—45 mL plastic squeeze bottle.

AFRIN® Extra Moisturizing Saline Mist
[á frin]

Ingredients: Water, PEG-32, Sodium Chloride, PVP, Disodium Phosphate, Sodium Phosphate, Benzalkonium Chloride, Disodium EDTA.

CONTAINS NO ALCOHOL

Indications: Provides gentle soothing moisture to dry, irritated nasal passages caused by colds, allergies, air pollution, smoke, dry air (low humidity) and air travel. Contains special moisturizing ingredients to moisturize and help make nasal passages feel clear and more comfortable. Afrin Moisturizing Saline Mist can be used as often as needed, and is safe to use with cold, allergy, and sinus medications. It is also safe enough for infants.

Directions: For infants, children and adults, 2 to 6 sprays/drops in each nostril as often as needed or as directed by a doctor. With head in a normal, upright position, put spray tip into nostril. Squeeze bottle with firm, quick pressure while in-

haling. For a fine mist, keep bottle upright; for nose drops, keep bottle upside down; for a stream, keep bottle horizontal. Wipe nozzle clean after use.

Keep out of the reach of children.
The use of this dispenser by more than one person may spread infection.

How Supplied: Afrin Moisturizing Saline Mist—45 mL plastic squeeze bottle.
Shown in Product Identification Guide, page 522

AFRIN® NASAL DECONGESTANT CHILDREN'S Pump Mist
Phenylephrine Hydrochloride

- Safe for kids 6–12 years old
- #1 Pediatrician recommended ingredient
- Clears stuffy noses fast
- Specially formulated to be mild and moisturizing
- Easy action pump delivers a precise, measured dose each time

Active Ingredient: Phenylephrine Hydrochloride 0.25%.

Inactive Ingredients: Benzalkonium Chloride, Edetate Disodium, Glycerin, Polyethylene Glycol 1450, Propylene Glycol, Sodium Phosphate Dibasic, Sodium Phosphate Monobasic, Water.

Indications: For temporary relief of nasal congestion due to colds, hay fever or other upper respiratory allergies, or associated with sinusitis. Shrinks swollen nasal membranes so you can breathe more freely.

Warnings: Do not exceed recommended dosage. This product may cause temporary discomfort such as burning, stinging, sneezing, or an increase in nasal discharge. Do not use this product for more than 3 days. Use only as directed. Frequent or prolonged use may cause nasal congestion to recur or worsen. If symptoms persist, consult a doctor. The use of this container by more than one person may spread infection. Do not use this product if you have heart disease, high blood pressure, thyroid disease, diabetes, or difficulty in urination due to enlargement of the prostate gland unless directed by a doctor. As with any drug, if you are pregnant or nursing a baby, seek the advice of a health professional before using this product. Keep this and all drugs out of the reach of children. In case of accidental ingestion, seek professional assistance or contact a Poison Control Center immediately.

Important: RETAIN CARTON FOR FUTURE REFERENCE ON FULL LABELING AND WARNINGS.

Directions: Adults and children 6 to under 12 years of age (with adult supervision): 2 or 3 sprays in each nostril not more often than every 4 hours. Do not give to children under 6 years of age unless directed by a doctor.
To spray, remove protective cap. Hold bottle with thumb at base and nozzle be-

tween first and second fingers. Without tilting head, insert nozzle into nostril. Fully depress rim with a firm, even stroke and sniff deeply. Wipe nozzle clean after use. Before using the first time, remove the protective cap from the tip and prime metered pump by depressing pump firmly several times.

How Supplied: Afrin Nasal Decongestant
Children's Pump Mist—$1/2$ FL OZ (15 mL)
Store between 2° and 30°C (36° and 86°F).
21029700/05591-00
©1994, 1999 Distributed by Schering-Plough HealthCare Products, Inc., Memphis, TN 38151 USA. All rights reserved. Patent Pending. Made in USA.

Afrin® No Drip Nasal
Decongestant 12 Hour Pump Mist
 No Drip Original
 No Drip Extra Moisturizing
 No Drip Sinus
 No Drip Severe Congestion
Nonprescription Drugs
Oxymetazoline Hydrochloride

Description: Afrin No Drip contains oxymetazoline hydrochloride, the longest acting OTC topical nasal decongestant available.
Afrin® brand—Number One in Doctor and Pharmacist Recommendations
Afrin® No Drip is a breakthrough in nasal spray. It stays where you spray it without messy dripping from your nose or down your throat.

Uses: For temporary relief of nasal congestion due to a cold, hay fever or other upper respiratory allergies, or associated with sinusitis. Shrinks swollen nasal membranes so you can breathe more freely.
Afrin® No Drip Original
Active Ingredient: Oxymetazoline Hydrochloride, 0.05%
Inactive Ingredients: benzalkonium chloride, benzyl alcohol, carboxymethyl-cellulose sodium, edetate disodium, flavor, microcrystalline cellulose, polyethylene glycol, povidone, sodium phosphate dibasic, sodium phosphate monobasic, water
Afrin® No Drip Extra Moisturizing contains a special blend of ingredients that soothes and moisturizes dry irritated nasal passages. It starts to work in seconds, providing 12 hours of comfortable nasal congestion relief with no drowsiness—and no dripping.
Active Ingredient: Oxymetazoline Hydrochloride, 0.05%
Inactive Ingredients: benzalkonium chloride, benzyl alcohol, carboxymethyl-cellulose sodium, edetate disodium, flavor, glycerin, microcrystalline cellulose, polyethylene glycol, povidone, sodium phosphate dibasic, sodium phosphate monobasic, water

Afrin® No Drip Sinus contains a special blend of ingredients which works instantly to cool and soothe your sinuses. Afrin® No Drip Sinus' special formula also moisturizes dry, irritated nasal passages. It starts to work in seconds providing 12 hours of comfortable nasal congestion relief without drowsiness—and no dripping.
Active Ingredient: Oxymetazoline Hydrochloride, 0.05%
Inactive Ingredients: benzalkonium chloride, benzyl alcohol, camphor, carboxymethylcellulose sodium, edetate disodium, eucalyptol, menthol, microcrystalline cellulose, polyethylene glycol, povidone, sodium phosphate dibasic, sodium phosphate monobasic, water
Afrin® No Drip Severe Congestion is a maximum strength formula with the aromatic power of menthol. It starts to work in seconds providing 12 hours of nasal congestion relief without drowsiness—and no dripping.
Active Ingredient: Oxymetazoline Hydrochloride, 0.05%
Inactive Ingredients: benzalkonium chloride, benzyl alcohol, camphor, carboxymethylcellulose sodium, edetate disodium, eucalyptol, menthol, microcrystalline cellulose, polyethylene glycol, povidone, propylene glycol, sodium phosphate dibasic, sodium phosphate monobasic, water

Directions: Adults and children 6 to under 12 years of age (with adult supervision): 2 or 3 sprays in each nostril not more often than every 10 to 12 hours. Do not exceed 2 doses in any 24-hour period. **Children under 6 years of age:** consult a doctor.
Shake well before use.
Before using the first time, remove the protective cap from the tip and prime metered pump by depressing pump firmly several times.
To spray, remove protective cap. Hold bottle with thumb at base and nozzle between first and second fingers. Without tilting head, insert nozzle into nostril. Fully depress rim with a firm, even stroke and sniff deeply. Wipe nozzle clean after use.

Warnings: Do not exceed recommended dosage. This product may cause temporary discomfort such as burning, stinging, sneezing, or an increase in nasal discharge. Do not use this product for more than 3 days. Use only as directed. Frequent or prolonged use may cause nasal congestion to recur or worsen. If symptoms persist, consult a doctor. The use of this container by more than one person may spread infection. Do not use this product if you have heart disease, high blood pressure, thyroid disease, diabetes, or difficulty in urination due to enlargement of the prostate gland unless directed by a doctor. As with any drug, if you are pregnant or nursing a baby, seek the advice of a health professional before using this product. Keep this and all drugs out of the reach of chil-

dren. In case of accidental ingestion, seek professional assistance or contact a Poison Control Center immediately.
Important: RETAIN CARTON FOR FUTURE REFERENCE ON FULL LABELING AND WARNINGS.
Store between 15° and 25°C (59° and 77°F).

How Supplied: Afrin® No Drip Pump Mist—15 mL (0.5 fl. Oz.) pump bottle.
Shown in Product Identification Guide, page 522

CHLOR–TRIMETON®
[klor-tri 'mĕ-ton]
4 Hour Allergy Tablets
8 Hour Allergy Tablets
12 Hour Allergy Tablets

Active Ingredients: Each 4 Hour Allergy Tablet contains: 4 mg chlorpheniramine maleate, also contains: Corn Starch, D&C Yellow No. 10 Aluminum Lake, Lactose, Magnesium Stearate. **Each 8 Hour Allergy Tablet contains:** 8 mg chlorpheniramine maleate; also contains: Acacia, Butylparaben, Calcium Phosphate, Calcium Sulfate, Carnauba Wax, Corn Starch, D&C Yellow No. 10 Aluminum Lake, FD&C Yellow No. 6 Aluminum Lake, FD&C Yellow No. 6, Lactose, Magnesium Stearate, Neutral Soap, Oleic Acid, Potato Starch, Rosin, Sugar, Talc, White Wax, Zein.
Each 12 Hour Allergy Tablet contains: 12 mg chlorpheniramine maleate; also contains: Acacia, Butylparaben, Calcium Phosphate, Calcium Sulfate, Carnauba Wax, Corn Starch, D&C Yellow No. 10 Aluminum Lake, FD&C Blue No. 2 Aluminum Lake, FD&C Yellow No. 6, FD&C Yellow No. 6 Aluminum Lake, Lactose, Magnesium Stearate, Neutral Soap, Oleic Acid, Potato Starch, Rosin, Sugar, Talc, White Wax, Zein.

Indications: For effective temporary relief of sneezing, itchy, watery eyes, itchy nose or throat, and runny nose due to hay fever or other upper respiratory allergies.

Warnings: May cause excitability especially in children. Do not give the 8 Hour or 12 Hour Allergy Tablets to children under 12 years, or 4 Hour Allergy Tablets to children under 6 years except under the advice and supervision of a doctor. Do not take this product, unless directed by a doctor, if you have a breathing problem such as emphysema or chronic bronchitis, or if you have glaucoma, difficulty in urination due to enlargement of the prostate gland. May cause drowsiness; alco-

Continued on next page

Information on Schering-Plough HealthCare Products appearing on these pages is effective as of November 2000.

Chlor-Trimeton Allergy—Cont.

hol, sedatives and tranquilizers may increase the drowsiness effect. Avoid alcoholic beverages while taking this product. Do not take this product if you are taking sedatives or tranquilizers, without first consulting your doctor. Use caution when driving a motor vehicle or operating machinery. As with any drug, if you are pregnant or nursing a baby, seek the advice of a health professional before using this product. Keep this and all drugs out of the reach of children. In case of accidental overdose, seek professional assistance or contact a Poison Control Center immediately.

Dosage and Administration: 4 Hour Allergy Tablets—Adults and Children 12 years of age and over: Oral dosage is one tablet (4 mg) every 4 to 6 hours, not to exceed 6 tablets (24 mg) in 24 hours or as directed by a doctor. Children 6 to under 12 years of age: Oral dosage is one half the adult dose (2 mg) (break tablet in half) every 4 to 6 hours, not to exceed 3 whole tablets (12 mg) in 24 hours, or as directed by a doctor. Children under 6 years of age: consult a doctor.
8 Hour Allergy Tablets—Adults and Children 12 years and over—One tablet every 8 to 12 hours. Do not take more than one tablet every 8 hours or 3 tablets in 24 hours. Children under 12 years of age: Consult a doctor.
12 Hour Allergy Tablets—Adults and children 12 years and over—One tablet every 12 hours. Do not exceed 2 tablets in 24 hours. Children under 12 years of age: Consult a doctor.

How Supplied: CHLOR-TRIMETON 4 Hour Allergy Tablets, box of 24, bottles of 100.
CHLOR-TRIMETON 8 Hour Allergy Tablets, boxes of 15, bottles of 100.
CHLOR-TRIMETON 12 Hour Allergy Tablets, boxes of 10 and 24, bottles of 100.
Store between 2° and 30°C (36° and 86°F). Protect from excessive moisture.
Shown in Product Identification Guide, page 522

CHLOR–TRIMETON®

[*klortri ′mĕ-ton*]
4 Hour Allergy/Decongestant Tablets
12 Hour Allergy/Decongestant Tablets

Active Ingredients: Each 4 Hour Allergy/Decongestant Tablet contains: 4 mg chlorpheniramine maleate, and 60 mg pseudoephedrine sulfate; also contains: Corn Starch, FD&C Blue No. 1, Lactose, Magnesium Stearate, Povidone.
Each 12 Hour Allergy/Decongestant Tablet contains: 8 mg chlorpheniramine maleate and 120 mg pseudoephedrine sulfate; also contains: Acacia, Butylparaben, Calcium Sulfate, Carnauba Wax, Corn Starch, D&C Yellow No. 10 Aluminum Lake, FD&C Blue No. 1 Alu-

minum Lake, FD&C Yellow No. 6 Aluminum Lake, Gelatin, Lactose, Magnesium Stearate, Neutral Soap, Oleic Acid, Povidone, Rosin, Sugar, Talc, White Wax, Zein.
Indications: For the temporary relief of sneezing, itching of the nose or throat, itchy, watery eyes and runny nose due to hay fever or other upper respiratory allergies. Helps decongest sinus openings and passages. Reduces swelling of nasal passages, shrinks swollen membranes, and temporarily restores freer breathing through the nose.

Warnings: CHLOR-TRIMETON 4 HOUR ALLERGY/DECONGESTANT: Do not exceed recommended dosage. If nervousness, dizziness, or sleeplessness occur, discontinue use and consult a doctor. If symptoms do not improve within 7 days or are accompanied by fever, consult a doctor. Do not take this product unless directed by a doctor, if you have a breathing problem such as emphysema, chronic bronchitis, or if you have glaucoma, heart disease, high blood pressure, thyroid disease, diabetes, or difficulty in urination due to enlargement of the prostate gland. May cause excitability, especially in children. May cause drowsiness; alcohol, sedatives, and tranquilizers may increase the drowsiness effect. Avoid alcoholic beverages while taking this product. Do not take this product if you are taking sedatives or tranquilizers, without first consulting your doctor. Use caution when driving a motor vehicle or operating machinery. As with any drug, if you are pregnant or nursing a baby, seek the advice of a health professional before using this product. Keep this and all drugs out of the reach of children. In case of accidental overdose, seek professional assistance or contact a Poison Control Center immediately.

Drug Interaction Precaution: Do not use this product if you are now taking a prescription monoamine oxidase inhibitor (MAOI) (certain drugs for depression, psychiatric or emotional conditions, or Parkinson's disease), or for 2 weeks after stopping the MAOI drug. If you are uncertain whether your prescription drug contains an MAOI, consult a health professional before taking this product.
CHLOR-TRIMETON 12 HOUR ALLERGY/DECONGESTANT: Do not exceed recommended dosage. If nervousness, dizziness, or sleeplessness occur, discontinue use and consult a doctor. If symptoms do not improve within 7 days or are accompanied by fever, consult a doctor. Do not take this product unless directed by a doctor if you have a breathing problem such as emphysema, or chronic bronchitis, or if you have glaucoma, heart disease, high blood pressure, thyroid disease, diabetes, or difficulty in urination due to enlargement of the prostate gland, or give this product children under 12 years of age. May cause excitability especially in children. May cause

drowsiness; alcohol, sedatives, and tranquilizers may increase the drowsiness effect. Avoid alcoholic beverages while taking this product. Do not take this product if you are taking sedatives or tranquilizers without first consulting a doctor. Use caution when driving a motor vehicle or operating machinery. As with any drug, if you are pregnant or nursing a baby, seek the advice of a health professional before using this product. Keep this and all drugs out of the reach of children. In case of accidental overdose, seek professional assistance or contact a Poison Control Center immediately.
Drug Interaction Precaution: Do not use this product if you are now taking a prescription monoamine oxidase inhibitor (MAOI) (certain drugs for depression, psychiatric or emotional conditions, or Parkinson's disease), or for 2 weeks after stopping the MAOI drug. If you are uncertain whether your prescription drug contains an MAOI, consult a health professional before taking this product.

Dosage and Administration: 4 Hour Allergy/Decongestant Tablets—ADULTS AND CHILDREN 12 YEARS OF AGE AND OVER: Oral dosage is one tablet every 4 to 6 hours, not to exceed 4 tablets in 24 hours, or as directed by a doctor. CHILDREN 6 TO UNDER 12 YEARS OF AGE: Oral dosage is one half the adult dose (break tablet in half) every 4 to 6 hours, not to exceed 2 whole tablets in 24 hours, or as directed by a doctor. CHILDREN UNDER 6 YEARS OF AGE: Consult a doctor. **12 Hour Allergy/Decongestant Tablets—**ADULTS AND CHILDREN 12 YEARS AND OVER: one tablet every 12 hours. Do not exceed 2 tablets in 24 hours. CHILDREN UNDER 12 YEARS OF AGE: Consult a doctor.

How Supplied: CHLOR-TRIMETON 4 Hour Allergy/Decongestant Tablets—boxes of 24. CHLOR-TRIMETON 12 Hour Allergy/Decongestant Tablets boxes of 10 and 24.
Store these CHLOR-TRIMETON Products between 2° and 30°C (36°and 86°F); and protect from excessive moisture.
Shown in Product Identification Guide, page 522

Clear Away®
LIQUID WART REMOVER SYSTEM
Clear Away®
GEL with Aloe Wart Remover System

Uses:
For the removal of common and plantar warts. Common warts can be easily recognized by the rough cauliflower-like appearance of the surface. Plantar warts can be recognized by its location only on the bottom of the foot, its tenderness, and the interruption of the footprint pattern.

Active Ingredient:
Salicylic Acid 17% W/W.

Inactive Ingredients:
Clear Away® Liquid Wart Remover System: Acetone, Balsam Oregon (natural or synthetic), Flexible Collodion, Alcohol 17% (from SD alcohol 32), Ether 52%.
Clear Away® Gel with Aloe Wart Remover System: Alcohol 57.6% (w/w), Aloe Extract, Ether 16.4% (w/w), Ethyl Lactate, Flexible Collodion, Hydroxypropyl Cellulose, Polybutene

Directions:
Clear Away® Liquid Wart Remover System: Wash and dry affected area thoroughly. Apply one drop of liquid at a time to sufficiently cover each wart. Let dry. Self-adhesive cover-up discs may be used to conceal wart. Repeat procedure once or twice daily as needed [until wart is removed] for up to 12 weeks.
Clear Away® Gel with Aloe Wart Remover System: Wash and dry affected area thoroughly. Apply thin layer of gel to sufficiently cover each wart. Let dry. Self-adhesive cover-up discs may be used to conceal wart. Repeat procedure once or twice daily as needed [until wart is removed] for up to 12 weeks.

Warnings: For external use only. Do not use this product on irritated skin, on any area that is infected or reddened, if you are a diabetic, or if you have poor blood circulation. If discomfort persists, see your doctor. Do not use on moles, birthmarks, warts with hair growing from them, genital warts, or warts on the face or mucous membranes. If product gets into the eye, flush with water for 15 minutes. Avoid inhaling vapors. Extremely flammable. Keep away from fire or flame. Cap bottle/tube tightly and store at room temperature away from heat. Keep this and all drugs out of the reach of children. In case of accidental ingestion, seek professional help or contact a Poison Control Center immediately.

How Supplied:
Clear Away® Liquid Wart Remover System: Available in a 1/3 fluid ounce liquid with dropper. Cover up bandages help to hide wart while it is removed.
Clear Away® Gel with Aloe Wart Remover System: Available in a ½ ounce tube. Cover up bandages help to hide wart while it is removed.

CLEAR AWAY®
ONE STEP WART REMOVER
CLEAR AWAY®
ONE STEP WART REMOVER FOR KIDS
CLEAR AWAY®
ONE STEP PLANTAR WART REMOVER
CLEAR AWAY® WART REMOVER SYSTEM
CLEAR AWAY® CLEAR WART REMOVER

Active Ingredient: Salicylic Acid 40% in a synthetic rubber-based vehicle.

Uses: For removal of common and plantar warts. Common warts are easily recognized by the rough cauliflower-like appearance of the surface. Plantar warts are recognized by its location only on the bottom of the foot, its tenderness, and the interruption of the footprint pattern.

Warnings: For external use only. Do not use this product on irritated skin, on any area that is infected or reddened, if you are a diabetic, or if you have poor blood circulation. If discomfort persists, see your doctor. Do not use on moles, birthmarks, warts with hair growing from them, genital warts or warts on the face or mucous membranes. Keep this and all drugs out of the reach of children. In case of accidental ingestion, seek professional assistance or contact a Poison Control Center immediately.
Not recommended for children under the age of 2 except at the advice of a doctor.

Directions: Wash and dry affected area thoroughly.
Apply medicated disc, strip, or pad positioning medicated disc directly over wart. Wart Remover system and Clear Wart Remover contain cover-up pads which can be used to cover the medicated disc. Repeat procedure every 48 hours as needed (until wart is removed) for up to 12 weeks.

How Supplied: Clear Away One Step Wart Remover and Clear Away One Step Wart Remover for Kids contain 14 all-in-one medicated strips, Clear Away One Step Plantar Wart Remover contains 16 all-in-one medicated cushioning pads, Clear Away Wart Remover System contains 18 medicated discs and 20 cover-up pads, Clear Away Clear contains 18 medicated discs and 18 cover-up pads that protect and conceal while treatment is ongoing. Conceals as it Heals™.
Store between 15°C and 30°C (59° and 86°F).

Shown in Product Identification Guide, page 522

Coricidin D®
Cold, Flu & Sinus Tablets
[*kor-a-see'din*]

Active ingredients
(in each tablet): **Purpose:**
Acetaminophen
325 mg .... Pain reliever/fever reducer
Chlorpheniramine maleate
2 mg .... Antihistamine
Pseudoephedrine sulfate
30 mg .... Nasal decongestant

Inactive Ingredients: Carnauba Wax, Hydroxypropyl Methylcellulose, Iron Oxide, Lactose, Magnesium Stearate, Microcrystalline Cellulose, Polyethylene Glycol, Polysorbate 80, Povidone, Pregelatinized Starch, Propylene Glycol, Shellac, Stearic Acid, Titanium Dioxide

Uses: Temporarily relieves these cold and flu symptoms: • runny nose • sneezing • nasal congestion • minor aches and pains • stuffy nose • headache • helps decongest sinus openings and passages to temporarily relieve sinus congestion and pressure • temporarily reduces fever

Warnings: Alcohol warning: If you consume 3 or more alcoholic drinks every day, ask your doctor whether you should take acetaminophen or other pain relievers/fever reducers. Acetaminophen may cause liver damage.
Do not use if you are now taking a prescription monoamine oxidase inhibitor (MAOI) (certain drugs for depression, psychiatric or emotional conditions, or Parkinson's disease), or for 2 weeks after stopping the MAOI drug. If you do not know if your prescription drug contains an MAOI, ask a doctor or pharmacist before taking this product.
Ask a doctor before use if you have:
• a breathing problem such as emphysema or chronic bronchitis • glaucoma • heart disease • high blood pressure • thyroid disease • diabetes • trouble urinating due to an enlarged prostate gland
Ask a doctor or pharmacist before use if you are taking sedatives or tranquilizers
When using this product
• **do not use more than directed**
• drowsiness may occur
• excitability may occur, especially in children
• avoid alcoholic beverages
• alcohol, sedatives and tranquilizers may increase drowsiness
• use caution when driving a motor vehicle or operating machinery
Stop use and ask a doctor if
• symptoms last more than 7 days (for adults) or 5 days (for children 6 to under 12 years)
• nervousness, dizziness or sleeplessness occur
• symptoms do not improve
• new symptoms occur
• redness or swelling is present
• you also have a fever that lasts for more than 3 days
If pregnant or breast-feeding, ask a health professional before use.
Keep out of reach of children. In case of overdose, get medical help or contact a Poison Control Center right away. Prompt medical attention is critical for adults as well as children even if you do not notice any signs or symptoms.

Directions:

Adults and children 12 years and over	2 tablets every 4 to 6 hours, not more than 8 tablets in 24 hours
Children 6 to under 12 years	1 tablet every 4 hours, not more than 4 tablets in 24 hours

Continued on next page

Information on Schering-Plough HealthCare Products appearing on these pages is effective as of November 2000.

Coricidin D—Cont.

Children under | ask a doctor
6 years

CORICIDIN D® Decongestant Tablets—blisters of 24.

Store between 15° and 25°C (59° and 77°F).

PROTECT FROM EXCESSIVE MOISTURE.

Shown in Product Identification Guide, page 522

CORICIDIN HBP®
[kor-a-see'din]
Cold & Flu Tablets
Cough & Cold Tablets
Night-Time Cold & Flu Tablets
Maximum Strength Flu Tablets

Active Ingredients: CORICIDIN HBP® Cold & Flu Tablets—325 mg Acetaminophen, 2 mg Chlorpheniramine Maleate.
CORICIDIN HBP® Cough & Cold Tablets—4 mg Chlorpheniramine Maleate, 30 mg Dextromethorphan Hydrobromide.
CORICIDIN HBP® Night-Time Cold & Flu—Acetaminophen 325 mg, Diphenhydramine Hydrochloride 25 mg.
CORICIDIN HBP Maximum Strength Flu Tablets—(per tablet): Acetaminophen 500 mg, Chlorpheniramine Maleate 2 mg, Dextromethorphan Hydrobromide 15 mg.

Inactive Ingredients: CORICIDIN HBP® Cold & Flu Tablets—Acacia, Butylparaben, Calcium Sulfate, Carnauba Wax, Cellulose, Corn Starch, FD&C Red No. 40 Aluminum Lake, FD&C Yellow No. 6 Aluminum Lake, Lactose, Magnesium Stearate, Povidone, Sugar, Talc, Titanium Dioxide, White Wax.
CORICIDIN HBP® Cough & Cold Tablets—Acacia, Calcium Sulfate, Carnauba Wax, Croscarmellose Sodium, D&C Red No. 27 Aluminum Lake, FD&C Yellow No. 6 Aluminum Lake, Lactose, Magnesium Stearate, Microcrystalline Cellulose, Povidone, Sodium Benzoate, Sugar, Talc, Titanium Dioxide, White Wax.
CORICIDIN HBP® Night-Time Cold & Flu—Acacia, Butylparaben, Calcium Sulfate, Carnauba Wax, Hydroxypropyl Methylcellulose, Magnesium Stearate, Microcrystalline Cellulose, Silicon Dioxide, Sodium Starch, Glycolate, Sucrose, Talc, Titanium Dioxide, White Wax.
CORICIDIN HBP Maximum Strength Flu Tablets—Carnauba Wax, FD&C Red No. 40 Aluminum Lake, Hydroxypropyl Methylcellulose, Lactose, Magnesium Stearate, Microcrystalline Cellulose, Polyethylene Glycol, Povidone, Pregelatinized Starch, Stearic Acid.

Indications: CORICIDIN HBP® Cold & Flu Tablets temporarily relieve runny nose, sneezing and itchy watery eyes due to the common cold, hay fever, and other upper respiratory allergies; temporarily relieve minor aches, pains and headache, and reduce the fever associated with a cold or flu. **Unlike most cold remedies, CORICIDIN HBP® Cold & Flu Tablets do not contain a decongestant and therefore are suitable for hypertensive patients.**
CORICIDIN HBP® Cough & Cold Tablets temporarily relieve coughs due to minor throat irritations as may occur with a cold; temporarily relieve sneezing, runny nose and itchy, watery eyes due to the common cold, hay fever or other respiratory allergies. **Unlike most cold remedies, CORICIDIN HBP® Cough & Cold Tablets do not contain a decongestant and are suitable for hypertensive patients.**
CORICIDIN HBP® Night-Time Tablets temporarily relieve runny nose, sneezing, and itchy watery eyes due to the common cold, hay fever or other upper respiratory allergies; temporarily relieve minor aches, pains, sore throat and headache, and reduce the fever associated with a cold or flu. **Unlike most cold remedies, CORICIDIN HBP® Night-Time Tablets do not contain a decongestant and therefore are suitable for hypertensive patients.**
CORICIDIN HBP® Maximum Strength Flu Tablets—Temporarily relieves cough, runny nose and sneezing associated with the common cold. For the temporary relief of minor aches, pains, headache, muscular aches, and fever associated with cold and flu. **Unlike most cold remedies, CORICIDIN HBP® Maximum Strength Flu Tablets do not contain a decongestant and therefore are suitable for hypertensive patients.**

Warnings: CORICIDIN HBP® Cold & Flu Tablets—Do not take this product for pain for more than 10 days (adults) or 5 days (children 6 to under 12 years of age) and do not take for fever for more than 3 days unless directed by a doctor. If pain or fever persists or gets worse, if new symptoms occur, or if redness or swelling is present, consult a doctor because these could be signs of a serious condition. May cause excitability especially in children. Do not take this product, unless directed by a doctor, if you have a breathing problem such as emphysema or chronic bronchitis, or if you have glaucoma or difficulty in urination due to enlargement of the prostate gland. May cause drowsiness; alcohol, sedatives, and tranquilizers may increase the drowsiness effect. Avoid alcoholic beverages while taking this product. Do not take this product if you are taking sedatives or tranquilizers without first consulting your doctor. Use caution when driving a motor vehicle or operating machinery. As with any drug if you are pregnant or nursing a baby, seek the advice of a health professional before using this product. Keep this and all drugs out of the reach of children. In case of accidental overdose, seek professional assistance or contact a Poison Control Center immediately. Prompt medical attention is critical for adults as well as for children even if you do not notice any signs or symptoms.

Alcohol Warning: If you consume 3 or more alcoholic drinks every day, ask your doctor whether you should take acetaminophen or other pain relievers/fever reducers. Acetaminophen may cause liver damage.

CORICIDIN HBP® Cough & Cold Tablets—A persistent cough may be a sign of a serious condition. If cough persists for more than 1 week, tends to recur, or is accompanied by fever, rash or persistent headache, consult a doctor. Do not take this product for persistent or chronic cough such as occurs with smoking, asthma, emphysema, or if cough is accompanied by excessive phlegm (mucus) unless directed by a doctor. May cause excitability, especially in children. Do not take this product, unless directed by a doctor, if you have a breathing problem such as emphysema or chronic bronchitis, or if you have glaucoma or difficulty in urination due to enlargement of the prostate gland. May cause marked drowsiness; alcohol, sedatives, and tranquilizers may increase the drowsiness effect. Avoid alcoholic beverages while taking this product. Do not take this product if you are taking sedatives or tranquilizers, without first consulting your doctor. Use caution when driving a motor vehicle or operating machinery. As with any drug, if you are pregnant or nursing a baby, seek the advice of a health professional before using this product. Keep this and all drugs out of the reach of children. In case of accidental overdose, seek professional assistance or contact a Poison Control Center immediately.

DRUG INTERACTION PRECAUTION: Do not use this product if you are now taking a prescription monoamine oxidase inhibitor (MAOI) (certain drugs for depression, psychiatric or emotional conditions, or Parkinson's disease), or for 2 weeks after stopping the MAOI drug. If you are uncertain whether your prescription drug contains an MAOI, consult a health professional before taking this product.

CORICIDIN HBP® Night-Time Tablets—Do not take this product for pain for more than 10 days or for fever for more than 3 days unless directed by a doctor. If pain or fever persists or gets worse, if new symptoms occur, or if redness or swelling is present, consult a doctor because these could be signs of a serious condition. If sore throat is severe, persists for more than 2 days, is accompanied or followed by fever, headache, rash, nausea, or vomiting consult a doctor promptly. May cause excitability especially in children. Do not take this product, unless directed by a doctor, if you have a breathing problem such as emphysema or chronic bronchitis, or if you have glaucoma or difficulty in urination due to enlargement of the prostate gland. May cause marked drowsiness;

alcohol, sedatives and tranquilizers may increase the drowsiness effect. Avoid alcoholic beverages while taking this product. Do not take this product if you are taking sedatives or tranquilizers, without first consulting your doctor. Use caution when driving a motor vehicle or operating machinery. As with any drug, if you are pregnant or nursing a baby, seek the advice of a health professional before using this product. Keep this and all drugs out of the reach of children. In case of accidental overdose, seek professional assistance or contact a Poison Control Center immediately. Prompt medical attention is critical for adults as well as for children even if you do not notice any signs or symptoms.

Do not use with any other product containing diphenhydramine, includine one applied topically.

Alcohol Warning: If you consume 3 or more alcoholic drinks every day, ask your doctor whether you should take Acetaminophen or other pain relievers/fever reducers. Acetaminophen may cause liver damage.

CORICIDIN HBP® Maximum Strength Flu Tablets—May cause excitability especially in children. Do not take this product, unless directed by a doctor, if you have a breathing problem such as emphysema or chronic bronchitis, or if you have glaucoma or difficulty in urination due to enlargement of the prostate gland. May cause marked drowsiness; alcohol, sedatives, and tranquilizers may increase the drowsiness effect. Avoid alcoholic beverages while taking this product. Do not take this product if you are taking sedatives or tranquilizers, without first consulting your doctor. Use caution when driving a motor vehicle or operating machinery. A persistent cough may be a sign of a serious condition. If cough persists for more than 1 week, tends to recur, or is accompanied by fever, rash, or persistent headache, consult a doctor. Do not take this product for persistent or chronic cough such as occurs with smoking, asthma or emphysema, or if cough is accompanied by excessive phlegm (mucus) unless direct by a doctor.

Do not take this product for pain for more than 10 days or for fever for more than 3 days unless directed by a doctor. If pain or fever persists or gets worse, if new symptoms occur, or if redness or swelling is present, consult a doctor because these could be signs of a serious condition. As with any drug, if you are pregnant or nursing a baby, seek the advice of a health professional before using this product. Keep this and all drugs out of the reach of children. In case of accidental overdose, seek professional assistance or contact a Poison Control Center immediately. Prompt medical attention is critical for adults as well as for children even if you do not notice any signs or symptoms.

Drug Interaction Precaution: Do not use this product if you are now tak-

ing a prescription monoamine oxidase inhibitor (MAOI) (certain drugs for depression, psychiatric or emotional conditions, or Parkinson's disease), or for 2 weeks after stopping the MAOI drug. If you are uncertain whether your prescription drug contains an MAOI, consult a health professional before taking this product.

Alcohol Warning: If you consume 3 or more alcoholic drinks every day, ask your doctor whether you should take acetaminophen or other pain relievers/fever reducers. Acetaminophen may cause liver damage.

Dosage and Administration: CORICIDIN HBP® Cold & Flu Tablets—Adults and children 12 years of age and over: oral dosage is 2 tablets every 4 to 6 hours, not to exceed 12 tablets in 24 hours, or as directed by a doctor. **Children 6 to under 12 years of age:** oral dosage is 1 tablet every 4 to 6 hours, not to exceed 5 tablets in 24 hours, or as directed by a doctor. **Children under 6 years of age:** consult a doctor. **CORICIDIN HBP® Cough & Cold Tablets—Adults and Children 12 years of age and over:** one tablet every 6 hours, not to exceed 4 tablets in 24 hours. This product is not for children under 12 years of age.

CORICIDIN HBP® Night-Time Tablets—Adults and children 12 years of age and over: oral dosage is one to two tablets every 4 to 6 hours, not to exceed 12 tablets in 24 hours, or as directed by a doctor. **Children under 12 years of age:** consult a doctor.

CORICIDIN HBP® Maximum Strength Flu Tablets—Adults and children 12 years of age and over: 2 tablets every 6 hours, while symptoms persist, not to exceed 8 tablets in 24 hours, or as directed by a doctor. **Children under 12 years of age:** consult a doctor.

How Supplied: CORICIDIN HBP® Cold & Flu Tablets— Bottles of 48, and 100 tablets, blisters of 12 and 24. Store between 2° and 30°C (36° and 86°F). PROTECT FROM EXCESSIVE MOISTURE.

CORICIDIN HBP® Cough & Cold Tablets— blisters of 16. Store between 2° and 30°C (36° and 86°F). PROTECT FROM EXCESSIVE MOISTURE.

CORICIDIN HBP® Night-Time Tablets—24 Tablets. Store between 15° and 25°C (59° and 77°F). PROTECT FROM EXCESSIVE MOISTURE.

CORICIDIN HBP® Maximum Strength Flu Tablets—blisters of 20. Store between 15° and 25°C (59° and 77°F). PROTECT FROM EXCESSIVE MOISTURE.

Shown in Product Identification Guide, page 522

CORRECTOL®
Laxative Tablets and Caplets

Active Ingredient: Bisacodyl, 5 mg.

Inactive Ingredients: Acetylated monoglycerides, calcium sulfate, carnauba wax, D&C Red no. 7 calcium lake, gelatin, hydroxypropyl methylcellulose phthalate, lactose, magnesium stearate, sugar, talc, titanium dioxide, white wax.

Indications: For gentle, overnight relief of occasional constipation and irregularity. Correctol Laxative generally produces a bowel movement in 6 to 12 hours.

Warnings: Do not chew tablets or caplets. Do not give to children under 6 years of age, or to persons who cannot swallow without chewing, unless directed by a doctor. Do not take this product within 1 hour after taking an antacid or milk. Do not use laxative products when abdominal pain, nausea, or vomiting are present unless directed by a doctor. If you have noticed a sudden change in bowel habits that persists over a period of 2 weeks, consult a doctor before using a laxative. Laxative products should not be used for a period longer than 1 week unless directed by a doctor. Rectal bleeding or failure to have a bowel movement after use of a laxative may indicate a serious condition. Discontinue use and consult your doctor. All stimulant laxatives may cause abdominal discomfort, faintness, and cramps. As with any drug, if you are pregnant or nursing a baby, seek the advice of a health professional before using this product. Keep this and all drugs out of the reach of children. In case of accidental overdose, seek professional assistance or contact a Poison Control Center immediately. Store at temperatures not above 86°F (30°C). Protect from excessive moisture.

Directions: Adults and children 12 years of age and older: Take 1 to 3 tablets or caplets in a single dose once daily. **Children 6 to under 12 years of age:** Take 1 tablet or caplet once daily. **Children under 6 years of age:** consult a doctor. **Do not chew or crush tablets or caplets.**

Each laxative works differently. Adults and children over 12 may need fewer tablets or caplets of Correctol to get the same effect as more tablets or caplets of another brand. **We recommend you start with one Correctol tablet or caplet and take with water.** If one tablet or caplet does not produce desired results, then try two or three Correctol tablets or caplets daily. Do not take more than 3 tablets or caplets of Correctol daily.

How Supplied: Tablets: Individual foil-backed safety sealed blister packaging in boxes of 10, 30, 60, & 90 tablets. Caplets: Individual foil-backed safety sealed blister packaging in boxes of 30 caplets.

Shown in Product Identification Guide, page 523

Continued on next page

Information on Schering-Plough HealthCare Products appearing on these pages is effective as of November 2000.

DRIXORAL® COLD & ALLERGY
[dricks-or 'al]
Sustained-Action Tablets

Description: EACH DRIXORAL® COLD & ALLERGY SUSTAINED-ACTION TABLET CONTAINS: 120 mg of Pseudoephedrine Sulfate and 6 mg of Dexbrompheniramine Maleate. Half of the medication is released after the tablet is swallowed and the remaining amount of medication is released hours later providing continuous long-lasting relief for 12 hours.

Inactive Ingredients: Acacia, Butylparaben, Calcium Sulfate, Carnauba Wax, Corn Starch, D&C Yellow No. 10 Aluminum Lake, FD&C Blue No. 1 Aluminum Lake, FD&C Yellow No. 6 Aluminum Lake, Gelatin, Lactose, Magnesium Stearate, Neutral Soap, Oleic Acid, Povidone, Rosin, Sugar, Talc, White Wax, Zein.

Indications: The decongestant (pseudoephedrine sulfate) temporarily relieves nasal congestion due to the common cold, hay fever or other upper respiratory allergies, and associated with sinusitis. Helps decongest sinus openings and sinus passages. Reduces swelling of nasal passages; shrinks swollen membranes; and temporarily restores freer breathing through the nose. The antihistamine (dexbrompheniramine maleate) alleviates runny nose, sneezing, itching of the nose or throat and itchy and watery eyes as may occur in allergic rhinitis (such as hay fever).

Warnings: Do not exceed recommended dosage. If nervousness, dizziness, or sleeplessness occur, discontinue use and consult a doctor. If symptoms do not improve within 7 days, or are accompanied by fever, consult a doctor. May cause excitability especially in children. Do not take this product if you have a breathing problem such as emphysema or chronic bronchitis, or if you have glaucoma, heart disease, high blood pressure, thyroid disease, diabetes, or difficulty in urination due to enlargement of the prostate gland, or give this product to children under 12 years of age, unless directed by a doctor. May cause drowsiness; alcohol, sedatives, and tranquilizers may increase the drowsiness effect. Avoid alcoholic beverages while taking this product. Do not take this product if you are taking sedatives or tranquilizers without first consulting your doctor. Use caution when driving a motor vehicle or operating machinery. As with any drug, if you are pregnant or nursing a baby, seek the advice of a health professional before using this product. Keep this and all drugs out of the reach of children. In case of accidental overdose, seek professional assistance or contact a Poison Control Center immediately.

Drug Interaction Precaution: Do not use this product if you are now taking a prescription monoamine oxidase inhibitor (MAOI) (certain drugs for depression, psychiatric or emotional conditions, or Parkinson's disease),or for 2 weeks after stopping the MAOI drug. If you are uncertain whether your prescription drug contains an MAOI, consult a health professional before taking this product.

Dosage and Administration: ADULTS AND CHILDREN 12 YEARS AND OVER—one tablet every 12 hours. Do not exceed two tablets in 24 hours. Children under 12 years of age: Consult a doctor.

How Supplied: DRIXORAL® Cold & Allergy Sustained-Action Tablets, green, sugar-coated tablets branded in black with the product name, boxes of 10, 20, and 30.
Store between 2° and 25°C (36° and 77°F).
Protect from excessive moisture.
Shown in Product Identification Guide, page 523

DRIXORAL® Nasal Decongestant
[dricks-or 'al]

DRIXORAL® Nasal Decongestant Tablets contain 120 mg Pseudoephedrine Sulfate, a nasal decongestant, in an extended-release tablet providing up to 12 hours of continuous relief ...without drowsiness.

Inactive Ingredients: Acacia, Butylparaben, Calcium Sulfate, Carnauba Wax, Corn Starch, FD&C Blue No. 1 Aluminum Lake, Gelatin, Lactose, Magnesium Stearate, Neutral Soap, Oleic Acid, Povidone, Rosin, Sugar, Talc, White Wax, Zein.

Indications: For temporary relief of nasal congestion due to the common cold, hay fever or other upper respiratory allergies, and associated with sinusitis. Helps decongest sinus openings and sinus passages.

Directions: Adults and Children 12 Years and Over—One tablet every 12 hours. Do not exceed two tablets in 24 hours. **Children under 12 years of age:** Consult a doctor.

Warnings: Do not exceed recommended dosage. If nervousness, dizziness, or sleeplessness occur, discontinue use and consult a doctor. If symptoms do not improve within 7 days or are accompanied by fever, consult a doctor. Do not take this product if you have heart disease, high blood pressure, thyroid disease, diabetes, or difficulty in urination due to enlargement of the prostate gland, or give this product to children under 12 years of age, unless directed by a doctor. As with any drug, if you are pregnant or nursing a baby, seek the advice of a health professional before using this product. Keep this and all drugs out of the reach of children. In case of accidental overdose, seek professional assistance or contact a Poison Control Center immediately.

Drug Interaction Precaution: Do not use this product if you are now taking a prescription monoamine oxidase inhibitor (MAOI) (certain drugs for depression, psychiatric or emotional conditions, or Parkinson's disease), or for 2 weeks after stopping the MAOI drug. If you are uncertain whether your prescription drug contains an MAOI, consult a health professional before taking this product.

How Supplied: DRIXORAL® Nasal Decongestant Long-Acting Non-Drowsy Tablets are available in boxes of 10's and 20's.
Store between 2° and 25°C (36° and 77°F).
Protect from excessive moisture.
Shown in Product Identification Guide, page 523

DRIXORAL® COLD & FLU
[dricks-or 'al]
Tablets

Active Ingredients: 500 mg Acetaminophen, 3 mg Dexbrompheniramine Maleate, 60 mg Pseudoephedrine Sulfate.

Inactive Ingredients: Calcium Phosphate, Carnauba Wax, D&C Yellow No. 10 Aluminum Lake, FD&C Blue No. 1 Aluminum Lake, FD&C Yellow No. 6 Aluminum Lake, Hydroxypropyl Methylcellulose, Magnesium Stearate, Methylparaben, PEG, Propylparaben, Stearic Acid.
DRIXORAL® COLD & FLU Extended-Release Tablets combine a nasal decongestant and an antihistamine with a pain reliever-fever reducer in a special 12-hour continuous-acting timed-release tablet.

Indications: The *decongestant* temporarily relieves nasal congestion due to the common cold, hay fever or other upper respiratory allergies, and associated with sinusitis. Reduces swelling of nasal passages; shrinks swollen membranes; and temporarily restores freer breathing through the nose. Also helps decongest sinus openings, sinus passages. The pain reliever-fever reducer temporarily relieves minor aches, pains, and headache and reduces fever due to the common cold. The *antihistamine* temporarily relieves runny nose and sneezing associated with the common cold.

Directions: ADULTS AND CHILDREN 12 YEARS AND OVER—two tablets every 12 hours. Do not exceed four tablets in 24 hours. **CHILDREN UNDER 12 YEARS OF AGE:** Consult a doctor.

Warnings: Do not exceed recommended dosage. If nervousness, dizziness, or sleeplessness occur, discontinue use and consult a doctor. If symptoms do not improve within 7 days , or are accompanied by fever that lasts for more than 3 days or recurs, consult a doctor before continuing use. If pain or fever persists

or gets worse, if new symptoms occur, or if redness or swelling is present, consult a doctor because these could be signs of a serious condition. May cause excitability especially in children. Do not take this product if you have a breathing problem such as emphysema or chronic bronchitis, or if you have glaucoma, heart disease, high blood pressure, thyroid disease, diabetes, or difficulty in urination due to enlargement of the prostate gland, or give this product to children under 12 years of age, unless directed by a doctor. May cause drowsiness; alcohol, sedatives, and tranquilizers may increase the drowsiness effect. Avoid alcoholic beverages while taking this product. Do not take this product if you are taking sedatives or tranquilizers without first consulting your doctor. Use caution when driving a motor vehicle or operating machinery. As with any drug, if you are pregnant or nursing a baby, seek the advice of a health professional before using this product. Keep this and all drugs out of the reach of children. In case of accidental overdose, seek professional assistance or contact a Poison Control Center immediately. Prompt medical attention is critical for adults as well as for children even if you do not notice any signs or symptoms.

Alcohol Warning: If you consume 3 or more alcoholic drinks every day, ask your doctor whether you should take acetaminophen or other pain relievers/fever reducers. Acetaminophen may cause liver damage.

Drug Interaction Precaution: Do not use this product if you are now taking a prescription monoamine oxidase inhibitor (MAOI) (certain drugs for depression, psychiatric or emotional conditions, or Parkinson's disease), or for 2 weeks after stopping the MAOI drug. If you are uncertain whether your prescription drug contains an MAOI, consult a health professional before taking this product.

How Supplied: DRIXORAL® COLD & FLU Extended-Release Tablets are available in boxes of 12's.

Store between 2° and 25°C (36° and 77°F).

Protect from excessive moisture.

Shown in Product Identification Guide, page 523

DRIXORAL® ALLERGY/SINUS

[dricks-or 'al]

Nasal decongestant/Pain reliever/ Antihistamine

DRIXORAL® ALLERGY/SINUS Extended-Release Tablets combine a nasal decongestant, a non-aspirin pain-reliever, and an antihistamine in a 12-hour timed-release tablet.

Indications: The *decongestant* temporarily relieves nasal congestion due to sinusitis, the common cold, and hay fever or other upper respiratory allergies. Helps decongest sinus openings and si-

nus passages; relieves sinus pressure. Reduces swelling of nasal passages; shrinks swollen membranes; and temporarily restores freer breathing through the nose. The *pain reliever* temporarily relieves headaches, and minor aches and pains. The *antihistamine* alleviates runny nose, sneezing, itching of the nose or throat, and itchy and watery eyes as may occur in allergic rhinitis (such as hay fever).

Each DRIXORAL® ALLERGY/SINUS Extended-Release Tablet Contains: 60 mg of Pseudoephedrine Sulfate, 3 mg of Dexbrompheniramine Maleate, and 500 mg of Acetaminophen. These ingredients are released continuously, providing long-lasting relief for 12 hours.

Inactive Ingredients: Calcium Phosphate, Carnauba Wax, D&C Yellow No. 10 Aluminum Lake, FD&C Yellow No. 6 Aluminum Lake, Hydroxypropyl Methylcellulose, Magnesium Stearate, Methylparaben, PEG, Propylparaben, Stearic Acid.

Directions: ADULTS AND CHILDREN 12 YEARS AND OVER—two tablets every 12 hours. Do not exceed four tablets in 24 hours. **CHILDREN UNDER 12 YEARS OF AGE:** consult a physician. **Store between 2° and 25°C (36° and 77°F).** Protect from excessive moisture.

Warnings: Do not exceed recommended dosage. If nervousness, dizziness, or sleeplessness occur, discontinue use and consult a doctor. If symptoms do not improve within 7 days, or are accompanied by fever that lasts for more than 3 days or recurs, consult a doctor before continuing use. If pain or fever persists or gets worse, if new symptoms occur, or if redness or swelling is present, consult a doctor because these could be signs of a serious condition. May cause excitability especially in children. Do not take this product if you have a breathing problem such as emphysema or chronic bronchitis, or if you have glaucoma, heart disease, high blood pressure, thyroid disease, diabetes, or difficulty in urination due to enlargement of the prostate gland, or give this product to children under 12 years of age, unless directed by a doctor. May cause drowsiness; alcohol, sedatives, and tranquilizers may increase the drowsiness effect. Avoid alcoholic beverages while taking this product. Do not take this product if you are taking sedatives or tranquilizers without first consulting your doctor. Use caution when driving a motor vehicle or operating machinery. As with any drug, if you are pregnant or nursing a baby, seek the advice of a health professional before using this product. Keep this and all drugs out of the reach of children. In case of accidental overdose, seek professional assistance or contact a Poison Control Center immediately. Prompt medical attention is critical for adults as well as for children even if you do not notice any signs or symptoms.

Alcohol Warning: If you consume 3 or more alcoholic drinks every day, ask your doctor whether you should take acetaminophen or other pain relievers/fever reducers. Acetaminophen may cause liver damage.

Drug Interaction Precaution: Do not use this product if you are now taking a prescription monoamine oxidase inhibitor (MAOI) (certain drugs for depression, psychiatric or emotional conditions, or Parkinson's disease), or for 2 weeks after stopping the MAOI drug. If you are uncertain whether your prescription drug contains an MAOI, consult a health professional before taking this product.

How Supplied: DRIXORAL® ALLERGY/SINUS Extended-Release Tablets are available in boxes of 12's.

Shown in Product Identification Guide, page 523

GYNE-LOTRIMIN 3®

3-Day Treatment

Clotrimazole Vaginal Cream (2%)

Vaginal Antifungal

3 Disposable Applicators

Vaginal Cream

GYNE-LOTRIMIN 3® Vaginal Cream is a 3-day treatment that cures most vaginal yeast infections. **If this is the first time you have had vaginal itching and discomfort, talk to your doctor.** If you have had a doctor diagnose a vaginal yeast infection before and have the same symptoms now, use this cream as directed for 3 days in a row.

Active Ingredient: Clotrimazole 2% (100 mg per applicator).

Use:
- For the treatment of vaginal yeast infections *(candidiasis)*.

Warnings:
- **For vaginal use only. Do not use in eyes or take by mouth.**
- Do not use GYNE-LOTRIMIN 3 Vaginal Cream if you have any of the following symptoms:
  - fever (higher than 100°F).
  - pain in the lower abdomen, back, or either shoulder.
  - a foul-smelling vaginal discharge.
- While using GYNE-LOTRIMIN 3 Vaginal Cream, if you get a fever, abdominal pain, or a foul-smelling discharge, **stop using the product** and contact your doctor right away. You may have a more serious illness.
- If your symptoms do not improve in 3 days, or you still have symptoms after 7 days, you should call your doctor.
- If your symptoms return within 2 months, you should talk to your doctor. You could be pregnant or there could be a serious underlying medical cause for your symptoms, including diabetes

Continued on next page

Information on Schering-Plough HealthCare Products appearing on these pages is effective as of November 2000.

Gyne-Lotrimin 3—Cont.

or a weaken immune system (which may be due to HIV-the virus that causes AIDS).

- Contact your doctor if you get hives or a skin rash while using this product.
- Do not use tampons, douches, or spermicides while using this product.
- Do not rely on condoms or diaphragms to prevent sexually transmitted diseases or pregnancy. This product may damage condoms and diaphragms and cause them to fail.
- If pregnant or breast-feeding, ask a health professional before use.
- Do not use in girls less than 12 years of age.
- **Keep this and all drugs out of the reach of children.** If swallowed, get medical help or contact a Poison Control Center right away.

Directions: Applicator and instructions are enclosed.

- Before using, read the enclosed brochure for complete instructions.
- To open: use cap to break seal.
- Insert one applicatorful of cream into the vagina at bedtime for 3 days in a row.

Inactive Ingredients: Benzyl alcohol, cetearyl alcohol, cetyl esters wax, octyldodecanol, polysorbate 60, purified water, sorbitan monostearate.

Store at room temperature 15°–30°C (59°–86°F). Avoid heat over 30°C or 86°F. See end flap of carton and end of tube for lot number and expiration data.

Important: The tube opening should be sealed. If seal has been broken or the embossed *SP* design is not visible, do not use the product. Return the product to the store where you bought it.

Medical questions should be answered by your doctor. If you have any other questions, or need more information on this product, call our **TOLL-FREE Number, at 1-877-496-3568**, between 8:00 a.m. and 5:00 p.m. Eastern Standard Time, Monday through Friday.

Shown in Product Identification Guide, page 523

LOTRIMIN® AF ANTIFUNGAL
[lo-tre-min]
Clotrimazole
Cream 1%
Solution 1%
Lotion 1%
Jock Itch Cream 1%

Description: Lotrimin® AF Cream 1% is a white fully vanishing homogeneous cream containing 1% clotrimazole. The cream contains no sensitizing parabens and is totally grease free and nonstaining.

Lotrimin® AF Solution is a nonaqueous liquid, containing 1% clotrimazole. Also contains polyethylene glycol.

Lotrimin® AF Lotion is a light penetrating buffered emulsion containing 1% clotrimazole. Does not contain common sensitizing agents. Also is greaseless and nonstaining.

Indications: Lotrimin AF Cream, Solution and Lotion cure athlete's foot (tinea pedis), jock itch (tinea cruris) and ringworm (tinea corporis). For effective relief of the itching, cracking, burning, scaling and discomfort which can accompany these conditions.

Directions: Cleanse skin with soap and water and dry thoroughly. Apply a thin layer over affected area morning and evening or as directed by a doctor. For athlete's foot, pay special attention to the spaces between the toes. It is also helpful to wear well-fitting, ventilated shoes and to change shoes and socks at least once daily. Best results in athlete's foot and ringworm are usually obtained with 4 weeks use of this product, and in jock itch with 2 weeks use. If satisfactory results have not occurred within these times, consult a doctor or pharmacist. Children under 12 years of age should be supervised in the use of this product. This product is not effective on the scalp or nails.

Warnings: For external use only. Avoid contact with the eyes. Do not use on children under 2 years of age except under the advice and supervision of a doctor. If irritation occurs or if there is no improvement within 4 weeks (for athlete's foot or ringworm) or within 2 weeks (for jock itch), discontinue use and consult a doctor or pharmacist. Keep this and all drugs out of the reach of children. In case of accidental ingestion, seek professional assistance or contact a Poison Control Center immediately.

How Supplied: Lotrimin® AF Antifungal Cream is available in a 0.42 oz. tube (12 grams) and a 0.84 oz. tube (24 grams). Lotrimin® AF Jock Itch Cream is available in a 0.42 oz tube (12 grams).

Inactive Ingredients: Cetearyl alcohol, cetyl esters wax, octyldecanol, polysorbate, sorbitan monostearate and water and as a preservative, benzyl alcohol (1%).

Lotrimin® AF Antifungal Solution is available in a 0.33 fl. oz. (10 milliliters) bottle. Inactive ingredient is PEG.

Lotrimin® AF Antifungal Lotion is available in a 0.66 fl. oz. (20 milliliters) bottle. Inactive ingredients include cetearyl alcohol, cetyl esters wax, octyldodecanol, polysorbate, sodium biphosphate, sodium phosphate dibasic, sorbitan monostearate and water and as a preservative, benzyl alcohol (1%).

Storage: Keep Lotrimin® AF Cream and Solution products between 2° and 30°C (36° and 86°F), and Lotrimin® AF Lotion product between 2° and 25°C (36° and 77°F).

Shown in Product Identification Guide, page 523

LOTRIMIN® AF ANTIFUNGAL
Miconazole Nitrate 2%
Athlete's Foot Spray Liquid
Athlete's Foot Spray Powder
Athlete's Foot Spray Deodorant Powder
Athlete's Foot Powder
Jock Itch Spray Powder

Active Ingredients: SPRAY LIQUID contains Miconazole Nitrate 2%. Also contains: Alcohol SD-40 (17% w/w), Cocamide DEA, Isobutane, Propylene Glycol, Tocopherol (vitamin E).

SPRAY POWDER (Athlete's Foot) contains Miconazole Nitrate 2%. Also contains: Alcohol SD-40 (10% w/w), Isobutane, Starch/Acrylates/Acrylamide Copolymer, Stearalkonium Hectorite, Talc.

SPRAY POWDER (Jock Itch) contains Miconazole Nitrate 2%. Also contains Alcohol SD-40 (10% w/w), Isobutane, Stearalkonium Hectorite, Talc.

SPRAY DEODORANT POWDER contains Miconazole Nitrate 2%. Also contains: Isobutane, Alcohol SD-40 (10% w/w), Talc, Starch/Acrylates/Acrylamide Copolymer, Stearalkonium Hectorite, Fragrance.

POWDER contains Miconazole Nitrate 2%. Also contains: Benzethonium Chloride, Corn Starch, Kaolin, Sodium Bicarbonate, Starch/Acrylates/Acrylamide Copolymer, Zinc Oxide.

Indications: LOTRIMIN® AF Athlete's Foot Spray Liquid, Spray Powder, Spray Deodorant Powder and Powder are proven clinically effective in the treatment of athlete's foot (tinea pedis), jock itch (tinea cruris) and ringworm (tinea corporis). For effective relief of the itching, cracking, burning, scaling and discomfort that can accompany these conditions.

LOTRIMIN AF Powder also aids in the drying of naturally moist areas.

LOTRIMIN® AF Jock Itch Spray Powder cures jock itch (tinea cruris). For effective relief of the itching, burning, scaling and discomfort associated with jock itch.

Warnings: For Athlete's Foot Spray Powder, Spray Liquid, Spray Deodorant Powder and Jock Itch Spray Powder: Do not use on children under 2 years of age unless directed by a doctor. For external use only. Avoid contact with the eyes. If irritation occurs or if there is no improvement within 4 weeks (for athlete's foot and ringworm) or 2 weeks (for jock itch), discontinue use and consult a doctor. Flammable. Do not use while smoking or near heat or flame. Avoid spraying in eyes. Contents under pressure. Do not puncture or incinerate. Do not store at temperature above 120°F. Use only as directed. Intentional misuse by deliberately concentrating and inhaling contents can be harmful or fatal. Keep this and all drugs out of the reach of children. In case of accidental ingestion, seek professional assistance or contact a Poison Control Center immediately.

Lotrimin® AF Powder: Do not use on children under 2 years of age unless directed by a doctor. For external use only. Avoid contact with the eyes. If irritation occurs, or if there is no improvement within 4 weeks (for athlete's foot or ringworm) or within 2 weeks (for jock itch), discontinue use and consult a doctor. Keep this and all drugs out of the reach of children. In case of accidental ingestion, seek professional assistance or contact a Poison Control Center immediately.

Directions: For Athlete's Foot Spray Liquid, Spray Powder, Spray Deodorant Powder and Jock Itch Spray Powder: Wash affected area and dry thoroughly. Shake can well. Spray a thin layer of product over affected area twice daily (morning and night) or as directed by a doctor. Supervise children in the use of this product. For athlete's foot, pay special attention to the spaces between the toes; wear well-fitting, ventilated shoes and change shoes and socks at least once daily. For athlete's foot and ringworm use daily for 4 weeks; for jock itch use daily for 2 weeks. If condition persists longer, consult a doctor. This product is not effective on the scalp or nails.

Powder: Wash affected area and dry thoroughly. Sprinkle a thin layer of product over affected area twice daily (morning and night) or as directed by a doctor. Supervise children in the use of this product. For athlete's foot, pay special attention to the spaces between the toes; wear well-fitting, ventilated shoes and change shoes and socks at least once daily. For athlete's foot and ringworm use daily for 4 weeks; for jock itch use daily for 2 weeks. If condition persists longer, consult a doctor. This product is not effective on the scalp or nails.

Store between 2° and 30° C (36° and 86°F).

How Supplied: LOTRIMIN® AF Athlete's Foot Spray Powder, Spray Deodorant Powder and Jock Itch Spray Powder—3.5 oz. cans. LOTRIMIN® AF Spray Liquid—4 oz. can. LOTRIMIN® AF Powder—3 oz. plastic bottle.

Shown in Product Identification Guide, page 523

**FACED WITH AN
Rx SIDE EFFECT?**
Turn to the
Companion Drug Index
(Green Pages)
for products that
provide symptomatic
relief.

Shire US
**7900 TANNERS GATE DR.
FLORENCE, KY 41042**

Direct Inquiries to:
Customer Service Department:
(800) 828-2088
FAX: 859-372-7684

For Medical Emergencies Contact:
Medical Information Department
(800) 992-9306

COLACE®
[*kōlās*]
**docusate sodium,
Capsules • Syrup• Liquid (Drops)**

Description: Colace® (docusate sodium) is a stool softener. Colace® Capsules, 50 mg, contain the following inactive ingredients: D&C Red No. 33, FD&C Red No. 40, Polyethylene Glycol, Propylene Glycol, Sorbitol, Gelatin, and Glycerin.
Colace® Capsules, 100 mg, contain the following inactive ingredients: D&C Red No. 33, FD&C Red No. 40, FD&C Yellow No. 6, Polyethylene Glycol, Propylene Glycol, Sorbitol, Gelatin, Titanium Dioxide, Methylparaben, Propylparaben, and Glycerin.
Colace® Liquid, 1%, (10 mg/mL), contains the following inactive ingredients: Citric Acid, D&C Red No. 33, Methylparaben, Poloxamer, Polyethylene Glycol, Propylene Glycol, Propylparaben, Sodium Citrate, Vanillin, and Purified Water.
Colace® Syrup, 20 mg/5 mL, contains the following inactive ingredients: alcohol (not more than 1%), Citric Acid, D&C Red No. 33, FD&C Red No. 40, Flavor (natural), Menthol, Methylparaben, Peppermint Oil, Poloxamer, Polyethylene Glycol, Propylparaben, Sodium Citrate, Sucrose, and Purified Water.

Actions and Uses: Colace®, a surface-active agent, helps to keep stools soft for easy, natural passage and is not a laxative, thus, not habit forming. Useful in constipation due to hard stools, in painful anorectal conditions, in cardiac and other conditions in which maximum ease of passage is desirable to avoid difficult or painful defecation, and when peristaltic stimulants are contraindicated.

Note: When peristaltic stimulation is needed due to inadequate bowel motility, see Peri-Colace® (laxative and stool softener).

Contraindications: There are no known contraindications to Colace®.

Warning: As with any drug, pregnant or nursing women should seek the advice of a health professional before using this product. Keep this and all medication out of the reach of children.

Side Effects: The incidence of side effects—none of a serious nature—is ex-

---

ceedingly small. Bitter taste, throat irritation, and nausea (primarily associated with the use of the syrup and liquid) are the main side effects reported. Rash has occurred.

Administration and Dosage: *Orally*—Suggested daily Dosage: *Adults and older children:* 50 to 200 mg. *Children 6 to 12:* 40 to 120 mg. *Children 3 to 6:* 20 to 60 mg. *Infants and children under 3:* 10 to 40 mg. The higher doses are recommended for initial therapy. Dosage should be adjusted to individual response. The effect on stools is usually apparent 1 to 3 days after the first dose. Colace® liquid or syrup must be given in a 6 oz. to 8 oz. glass of milk or fruit juice or in infant's formula to prevent throat irritation. In *enemas*—Add 50 to 100 mg Colace® (5 to 10 mL Colace® liquid) to a retention or flushing enema.

How Supplied: Colace® capsules, 50 mg
  NDC 54092-052-11 Packages of 10
  NDC 54092-052-30 Bottles of 30
  NDC 54092-052-60 Bottles of 60
Colace® capsules, 100 mg
  NDC 54092-053-11 Packages of 10
  NDC 54092-053-30 Bottles of 30
  NDC 54092-053-60 Bottle of 60
  NDC 54092-053-02 Bottles of 250

Note: Colace® capsules should be stored at controlled room temperature (59°–86°F or 15°–30°C)
Colace® liquid, 1% solution; 10 mg/mL (with calibrated dropper)
  NDC 54092-414-30 Bottles of 30 mL
Colace® syrup, 20 mg/5 mL teaspoon; contains not more than 1% alcohol
  NDC 54092-415-16 Bottles of 16 fl oz
Manufactured for
Shire US Consumer Products Division

PERI-COLACE® Capsules • Syrup
(casanthranol and docusate sodium)

Description: Peri-Colace® is a combination of the mild stimulant laxative Casanthranol, and the stool-softener Colace® (docusate sodium).

Each capsule contains 30 mg of Casanthranol and 100 mg of Colace®; the syrup contains 30 mg of Casanthranol and 60 mg of Colace® per 15-mL tablespoon (10 mg of Casanthranol and 20 mg of Colace® per 5-mL teaspoon) and 10% alcohol.

Peri-Colace® Capsules contain the following inactive ingredients: FD&C Red No. 40, FD&C Blue No. 1, Polyethylene Glycol, Propylene Glycol, Sorbitol, Titanium Dioxide, Methylparaben, Propylparaben, Glycerin, and Gelatin.

Continued on next page

Peri-Colace—Cont.

Peri-Colace® Syrup contains the following inactive ingredients: Alcohol (10% v/v), Citric Acid, Flavors, Methyl Salicylate, Methylparaben, Poloxamer, Polyethylene Glycol, Propylparaben, Sodium Citrate, Sorbitol Solution, Sucrose, and Purified Water.

Action and Uses: Peri-Colace® provides gentle peristaltic stimulation and helps to keep stools soft for easier passage. Bowel movement is induced gently—usually overnight or in 8 to 12 hours. Nausea, griping, abnormally loose stools, and constipation rebound are minimized. Useful in management of chronic or temporary constipation.

Note: To prevent hard stools when laxative stimulation is not needed or undesirable, see Colace® (stool softener).

Warnings: Do not use when abdominal pain, nausea, or vomiting is present. Frequent or prolonged use of this preparation may result in dependence on laxatives.

As with any drug, pregnant or nursing women should seek the advice of a health professional before using this product.

Keep this and all medication out of the reach of children.

Side Effects: The incidence of side effects—none of a serious nature—is exceedingly small. Nausea, abdominal cramping or discomfort, diarrhea, and rash are the main side effects reported.

Administration and Dosage: *Adults* —1 or 2 capsules, or 1 or 2 tablespoons syrup at bedtime, or as indicated. In severe cases, dosage may be increased to 2 capsules or 2 tablespoons twice daily, or 3 capsules at bedtime. *Children* —1 to 3 teaspoons of syrup at bedtime, or as indicated. Peri-Colace® syrup must be given in a 6 oz. to 8 oz. glass of milk or fruit juice or in infant's formula to prevent throat irritation.

Overdosage: In addition to symptomatic treatment, gastric lavage, if timely, is recommended in cases of large overdosage.

How Supplied: Peri-Colace® Capsules

NDC 54092-054-11 Packages of 10
NDC 54092-054-30 Bottles of 30
NDC 54092-054-60 Bottles of 60
NDC 54092-054-02 Bottles of 250

Note: Peri-Colace® capsules should be stored at controlled room temperatures (59°–86°F or 15°–30°C).
Peri-Colace® Syrup
NDC 54092-418-16 Bottles of 16 fl oz
Manufactured for
Shire US Consumer Products Division

SmithKline Beecham Consumer Healthcare, L.P.

POST OFFICE BOX 1467
PITTSBURGH, PA 15230

For Medical Information Contact:
(800) 245-1040 (Consumer Inquiries)
(800) 378-4055 (Healthcare Professional Inquiries)

Direct Healthcare Professional Sample Requests to:
(800) BEECHAM

ABREVA™
Cold Sore/Fever Blister Treatment Cream
Docosanol 10% Cream

Uses:
- Treats cold sore/fever blisters on the face or lips
- Shortens healing time and duration of symptoms: tingling, pain, burning, and/or itching

Active Ingredient: **Purpose:**
Docosanol 10% ... Cold sore/fever blister treatment

Inactive Ingredients: Benzyl alcohol, light mineral oil, propylene glycol, purified water, sucrose distearate, sucrose stearate.

Directions:
- **adults and children 12 years or over:**
  - wash hands before and after applying cream
  - apply to affected area on face or lips at the first sign of cold sore/fever blister (tingle). Early treatment ensures the best results.
  - rub in gently but completely
  - use 5 times a day until healed
- **children under 12 years:** ask a doctor

Warnings:
For external use only.
Do not use
- if you are allergic to any ingredient in this product

When using this product
- apply only to affected areas
- do not use in or near the eyes
- avoid applying directly inside your mouth
- do not share this product with anyone. This may spread infection.

Stop use and ask a doctor if
- your cold sore gets worse or the cold sore is not healed within 10 days
- **Keep out of reach of children.** If swallowed, get medical help or contact a poison control center right away.

Other Information:
- store at 20°–25°C (68°–77°F)
- do not freeze

How Supplied: Abreva Cream is supplied in 2.0 g [.07 oz] tubes.
Question? Call 1-877-709-3539

Orange Flavor
CITRUCEL®
[sĭt 'rə-sĕl]
(Methylcellulose)
Bulk-forming Fiber Laxative

Description: Each 19 g adult dose (approximately one heaping measuring tablespoonful) contains Methylcellulose 2 g. Each 9.5 g child's dose (one-half the adult dose) contains Methylcellulose 1 g. Methylcellulose is a nonallergenic fiber. Also contains: Citric Acid, FD&C Yellow No. 6, Orange Flavors (natural and artificial), Potassium Citrate, Riboflavin, Sucrose, and other ingredients. Each adult dose contains approximately 3 mg of sodium and contributes 60 calories from Sucrose.

Actions: Promotes elimination by providing additional fiber (bulk) to the diet. This product generally produces bowel movement in 12 to 72 hours.

Indications: For relief of constipation (irregularity). May also be used for relief of constipation associated with other bowel disorders such as irritable bowel syndrome, diverticular disease, and hemorrhoids as well as for bowel management during postpartum, postsurgical, and convalescent periods when recommended by a physician.

Contraindications: Intestinal obstruction, fecal impaction, known hypersensitivity to formula ingredients.

Warnings: Patients should be instructed to consult their physician before using any laxative if they have noticed a sudden change in bowel habits which persists for two weeks. Unless directed by a physician, patients should be advised not to use laxative products when abdominal pain, nausea, or vomiting is present. Patients should also be advised to discontinue use and consult a physician if rectal bleeding or failure to have a bowel movement occurs after use of any laxative product. Unless recommended by a physician, patients should not exceed the recommended maximum daily dose. Patients should not use laxative products for a period longer than one week unless directed by a physician. **TAKING THIS PRODUCT WITHOUT ADEQUATE FLUID MAY CAUSE IT TO SWELL AND BLOCK YOUR THROAT OR ESOPHAGUS AND MAY CAUSE CHOKING. DO NOT TAKE THIS PRODUCT IF YOU HAVE DIFFICULTY IN SWALLOWING. IF YOU EXPERIENCE CHEST PAIN, VOMITING, OR DIFFICULTY IN SWALLOWING OR BREATHING AFTER TAKING THIS PRODUCT, SEEK IMMEDIATE MEDICAL ATTENTION. KEEP THIS AND ALL DRUGS OUT OF THE REACH OF CHILDREN.**

Dosage and Administration: Adult Dose: dissolve one leveled scoop (one heaping tablespoon – 19g) in 8 ounces of cold water up to three times daily at the first sign of constipation. Children age 6

to 12 years of age: *one-half the adult dose* stirred briskly in 8 ounces of cold water, once daily at the first sign of constipation. The mixture should be administered promptly and drinking another glass of water is highly recommended (see warnings). Children under 6 years of age: *Use only as directed by a physician.* Continued use for 12 to 72 hours may be necessary for full benefit.

TAKE THIS PRODUCT (CHILD OR ADULT DOSE) WITH AT LEAST 8 OZ. (A FULL GLASS) OF WATER OR OTHER FLUID. TAKING THIS PRODUCT WITHOUT ENOUGH LIQUID MAY CAUSE CHOKING. SEE WARNINGS.

How Supplied: 16 oz., 30 oz., and 50 oz. containers.
Boxes of 20-single-dose packets.
Store below 86°F (30°C). Protect contents from humidity; keep tightly closed.
Shown in Product Identification Guide, page 523

Sugar Free Orange Flavor
CITRUCEL®
[sĭt 'rə-sĕl]
(Methylcellulose)
Bulk-forming Fiber Laxative

Description: Each 10.2 g adult dose (approximately one rounded measuring tablespoonful) contains Methylcellulose 2 g. Each 5.1 g child's dose (one-half the adult dose) contains Methylcellulose 1 g. Methylcellulose is a nonallergenic fiber. Also contains: Aspartame, Dibasic Calcium Phosphate, FD&C Yellow No. 6, Malic Acid, Maltodextrin, Orange Flavors (natural and artificial), Potassium Citrate, and Riboflavin. Each 10.2 g dose contains approximately 3 mg of sodium and contributes 24 calories from Maltodextrin.

Actions: Promotes elimination by providing additional fiber (bulk) to the diet. This product generally produces bowel movement in 12 to 72 hours.

Indications: For relief of constipation (irregularity). May also be used for relief of constipation associated with other bowel disorders such as irritable bowel syndrome, diverticular disease, and hemorrhoids as well as for bowel management during postpartum, postsurgical, and convalescent periods when recommended by a physician.

Contraindications and Warnings: See entry for "Orange Flavor Citrucel".

Phenylketonurics: CONTAINS PHENYLALANINE 52 mg per adult dose. Individuals with phenylketonuria and other individuals who must restrict their intake of phenylalanine should be warned that each 10.2 g adult dose contains aspartame which provides 52 mg of phenylalanine.

Dosage and Administration: Adult Dose: dissolve one leveled scoop (one rounded measuring tablespoon – 10.2 g)

in 8 ounces of cold water up to three times daily at the first sign of constipation. Children age 6 to 12 years of age: *one-half the adult dose* stirred briskly into at least 8 ounces of cold water, once daily at the first sign of constipation. The mixture should be administered promptly and drinking another glass of water is highly recommended (see warnings). Children under 6 years of age: *Use only as directed by a physician.* Continued use for 12 to 72 hours may be necessary for full benefit.

TAKE THIS PRODUCT (CHILD OR ADULT DOSE) WITH AT LEAST 8 OZ. (A FULL GLASS) OF WATER OR OTHER FLUID. TAKING THIS PRODUCT WITHOUT ENOUGH LIQUID MAY CAUSE CHOKING. SEE WARNINGS.

How Supplied:
8.6 oz, 16.9 oz, and 32 oz containers.
Boxes of 20 single-dose packets.
Store below 86°F (30°C). Protect contents from humidity; keep tightly closed.
Shown in Product Identification Guide, page 523

Citrucel®
Soluble Fiber Caplet
Nonprescription Drugs Methylcellulose Fiber Therapy

Uses: Helps restore and maintain regularity. Helps relieve constipation. Also useful in treatment of constipation (irregularity) associated with other bowel disorders when recommended by a physician. This product generally produces a bowel movement in 12 to 72 hours.

Active Ingredient: Each caplet contains 500mg Methylcellulose.

Inactive Ingredients: Crospovidone, Dibasic Calcium Phosphate, FD&C Yellow No. 6 Aluminum Lake, Magnesium Stearate, Maltodextrin, Povidone, Sodium Lauryl Sulfate.

Directions: Adult dose: Take two caplets as needed with 8 ounces of liquid, up to six times daily. Children (6–12 years): Take one caplet with 8 ounces of liquid, up to six times per day. The dosage requirement may vary according to the severity of constipation. Children under 6 years: consult a physician. **TAKE THIS PRODUCT (CHILD OR ADULT DOSE) WITH AT LEAST 8 OUNCES (A FULL GLASS) OF WATER OR OTHER FLUID. TAKING THIS PRODUCT WITHOUT ENOUGH LIQUID MAY CAUSE CHOKING. SEE WARNINGS.**

Directions for Use: Take each dose with 8oz. of liquid.

Warnings: Consult a physician before using any laxative product if you have noticed a sudden change in bowel habits which persists for two weeks. Unless di

Age	Dose	Daily Maximum
Adults & Children over 12 years	2 Caplets	Up to 6 times daily*
Children (6 to 12 years)	1 Caplet	Up to 6 times daily*
Children under 6 years	Consult a physician	

*Refer to directions below. rected by a physician, do not use laxative products when abdominal pain, nausea, or vomiting are present. Discontinue use and consult a physician if rectal bleeding or failure to produce a bowel movement occurs after use of any laxative product. Unless recommended by a physician, do not exceed recommended maximum daily dose. Laxative products should not be used for a period longer than a weak unless directed by a physician. If sensitive to any of the ingredients, do not use. **TAKING THIS PRODUCT WITHOUT ADEQUATE FLUID MAY CAUSE IT TO SWELL AND BLOCK YOUR THROAT OR ESOPHAGUS AND MAY CAUSE CHOKING. DO NOT TAKE THIS PRODUCT IF YOU HAVE DIFFICULTY IN SWALLOWING. IF YOU EXPERIENCE CHEST PAIN, VOMITING, OR DIFFICULTY IN SWALLOWING OR BREATHING AFTER TAKING THIS PRODUCT, SEEK IMMEDIATE MEDICAL ATTENTION. KEEP THIS AND ALL DRUGS OUT OF THE REACH OF CHILDREN.**

Store at room temperature 15–30°C (59–86°F). Protect contents from moisture.
Tamper evident feature: Bottle sealed with printed foil under cap. Do not use if foil is torn or broken.

How Supplied: Bottles of 100 caplets
Questions or comments?
Call toll-free 1-800-897-6081 weekdays.
Patents Pending
The various Citrucel Logos and design elements of the packaging are Registered Trademarks of SmithKline Beecham.
©2000 SmithKline Beecham
Distributed by:
SmithKline Beecham
SmithKline Beecham Consumer Healthcare, L.P.
Pittsburgh, PA 15230, Made in Canada.

CONTAC® Non-Drowsy
Decongestant
12 Hour Cold Caplets

Product Information: Each Maximum Strength Contac 12 Hour Cold Caplet provides up to 12 hours of relief. Part of the caplet goes to work right away for fast relief; the rest is released gradually

Continued on next page

Contac—Cont.

to provide up to 12 hours of prolonged relief. With just one caplet in the morning and one at bedtime, you feel better all day, sleep better at night, breathing freely without congestion or sinus pressure.

Indications: Temporarily relieves nasal congestion due to the common cold, hay fever or other upper respiratory allergies and associated with sinusitis. Helps decongest sinus openings and passages; temporarily relieves sinus congestion and pressure.

Directions: Adults and children over 12 years of age: One caplet every 12 hours, not to exceed 2 caplets in 24 hours, or as directed by a doctor. Children under 12 years of age: consult a doctor.

TAMPER-EVIDENT PACKAGING FEATURES FOR YOUR PROTECTION:
Each caplet is encased in a plastic cell with a foil back; do not use if cell or foil is broken.

Warnings: Do not exceed the recommended dosage. If nervousness, dizziness, or sleeplessness occur, discontinue use and consult a doctor. If symptoms do not improve within 7 days or are accompanied by high fever, consult a doctor. Do not take this product, unless directed by a doctor, if you have heart disease, high blood pressure, thyroid disease, diabetes, glaucoma or difficulty in urination due to enlargement of the prostate gland.
KEEP THIS AND ALL DRUGS OUT OF REACH OF CHILDREN. IN CASE OF ACCIDENTAL OVERDOSE, SEEK PROFESSIONAL ASSISTANCE OR CONTACT A POISON CONTROL CENTER IMMEDIATELY. As with any drug, if you are pregnant or nursing a baby, seek the advice of a health professional before using this product.

Drug Interaction Precaution: Do not use this product if you are now taking a prescription monoamine oxidase inhibitor (MAOI) (certain drugs for depression, psychiatric or emotional conditions, or Parkinson's disease), or for 2 weeks after stopping the MAOI drug. If you are uncertain whether your prescription drug contains an MAOI, consult a health professional before taking this product.

Active Ingredient: Pseudoephedrine Hydrochloride 120 mg.

Store at 15° to 25°C (59° to 77°F) in a dry place and protest from light.

Each Caplet Also Contains: Carnauba Wax, Colloidal Silicon Dioxide, Dibasic Calcium Phosphate, Hydroxypropyl Methylcellulose, Magnesium Stearate, Microcrystalline Cellulose, Polyethylene Glycol, Polysorbate 80, Titanium Dioxide.

How Supplied: Consumer packages of 10 and 20 caplets.

Note: There are other CONTAC products. Make sure this is the one you are interested in. See the table below for all of the products in the CONTAC line.
Shown in Product Identification Guide, page 523

Contac® Non-Drowsy Timed Release-Maximum Strength 12 Hour Cold Caplets

Indications: For the temporary relief of nasal congestion due to the common cold, hay fever or other upper respiratory allergies, and nasal congestion associated with sinusitis. Promotes nasal and/or sinus drainage; temporarily relieves sinus congestion and pressure. Temporarily restores freer breathing through the nose.
Each Maximum Strength Contac 12-Hour Cold caplet provides up to 12 hours of relief. Part of the caplet goes to work right away for fast relief; the rest is released gradually to provide up to 12 hours of prolonged relief. With just one caplet in the morning and one at bedtime, you feel better all day, sleep better at night, breathing freely without congestion or sinus pressure.

Active Ingredient: Each coated extended-release caplet contains Pseudoephedrine Hydrochloride 120 mg.

Inactive Ingredients: carnauba wax, collodial silicon dioxide, dibasic calcium phosphate, hydroxypropyl methylcellulose, magnesium stearate, microcrystalline cellulose, polyethylene glycol, polysorbate 80, titanium dioxide.

Directions: Adults and children 12 years of age and over – One caplet every 12 hours, not to exceed two caplets in 24 hours. This product is not recommended for children under 12 years of age.

Warnings: Do not exceed recommended dosage. If nervousness, dizziness, or sleeplessness occur, discontinue use and consult a doctor. If symptoms do not improve within 7 days or are accompanied by fever, consult a doctor. Do not take this product if you have heart disease, high blood pressure, thyroid disease, diabetes, or difficulty in urination due to enlargement of the prostate gland unless directed by a doctor. As with any drug, if you are pregnant or nursing a baby, seek the advice of a health professional before using this product.

Drug Interaction Precaution: Do not use this product if you are now taking a prescription monoamine oxidase inhibitor (MAOI) (certain drugs for depression, psychiatric or emotional conditions, or Parkinson's disease), or for 2 weeks after stopping the MAOI drug. If you are uncertain whether your prescription contains an MAOI, consult a health professional before taking this product.
KEEP THIS AND ALL DRUGS OUT OF THE REACH OF CHILDREN. In case of ac-

cidental overdose, seek professional assistance or contact a Poison Control Center immediately.

Store at 15° to 25°C (59° to 77°F) in a dry place and protect from light.

How Supplied: Packets of 10 and 20 Caplets
U.S. Patent No. 5,895,663
Comments or questions?
Call toll-free 1-800-245-1040 weekdays.

CONTAC®
Severe Cold and Flu
Caplets Maximum Strength
Analgesic• Decongestant
Antihistamine• Cough Suppressant
CONTAC®
Severe Cold and Flu
Caplets Non-Drowsy
Nasal Decongestant • Analgesic•
Cough Suppressant

Active Ingredients: Each *Non-Drowsy Caplet* contains Acetaminophen 325 mg, Psudoephedrine HCl 30 mg and Dextromethorphan Hydrobromide 15 mg.
Each *Maximum Strength Caplet* contains Acetaminophen 500 mg, Dextromethorphan Hydrobromide 15 mg, Pseudoephedrine HCl 30 mg and chlorpheniromine Maleate 2 mg.

Product Information: Two caplets every 6 hours to help relieve the discomforts of severe colds with flu-like symptoms.

Indications: *Non-Drowsy & Maximum Strength Caplets:* Temporarily relieves nasal congestion & coughing due to the common cold. Provides temporary relief of fever, sore throat, headache & minor aches associated with the common cold or the flu.
Maximum Strength Caplets: Temporarily relieves runny nose, sneezing, itchy and watery eyes due to the common cold.

Directions: Adults (12 years and older): Two caplets every 6 hours, not to exceed 8 caplets in any 24-hour period, or as directed by a doctor. Children under 12 years of age: consult a doctor.
TAMPER-EVIDENT PACKAGING FEATURES FOR YOUR PROTECTION:
Caplets are encased in a plastic cell with a foil back; do not use if cell or foil is broken. The letters ND SCF for non-drowsy and SCF for maximum strength appear on each caplet; do not use this product if these letters are missing.

Warnings: For *Non-Drowsy and Maximum Strength Caplets:* Do not exceed recommended dosage. If nervousness, dizziness, or sleeplessness occur, discontinue use and consult a doctor. If symptoms do not improve or are accompanied by fever that lasts for more than 3 days, or if new symptoms occur, consult a doctor. If sore throat is severe, persists for more than 2 days, is accom-

PDR For Nonprescription Drugs

	CONTAC Non-Drowsy 12 Hour Cold Caplets	CONTAC 12 Hour Cold Capsules	CONTAC Severe Cold and Flu Caplets Maximum Strength (each 2 caplet dose)	CONTAC Severe Cold and Flu Non-Drowsy Caplets (each 2 caplet dose)	CONTAC Day & Night Cold & Flu Day Caplets	CONTAC Day & Night Cold & Flu Night Caplets
Phenylpropanolamine HCl	—	75.0 mg	—	—	—	—
Chlorpheniramine Maleate	120 mg	8.0 mg	4.0 mg	—	—	—
Pseudoephedrine HCl	—	—	60 mg	60.0 mg	60.0 mg	60.0 mg
Acetaminophen	—	—	1000.0 mg	650.0 mg	650.0 mg	650.0 mg
Dextromethorphan Hydrobromide	—	—	30.0 mg	30.0 mg	30.0 mg	—
Diphenhydramine HCl	—	—	—	—	—	50.0 mg

panied or followed by fever, headache, rash, nausea, or vomiting, consult a doctor promptly. A persistent cough may be a sign of a serious condition. If cough persists for more than 7 days, tends to recur, or is accompanied by rash, persistent headache, fever that lasts for more than 3 days, or if new symptoms occur, consult a doctor. Do not take this product for persistent or chronic cough such as occurs with smoking, asthma, emphysema, or if cough is accompanied by excessive phlegm (mucus) unless directed by a doctor. Do not take this product if you have heart disease, high blood pressure, thyroid disease, diabetes, glaucoma or difficulty in urination due to enlargement of the prostate gland unless directed by a doctor. **Alcohol Warning:** If you consume 3 or more alcoholic drinks every day, ask your doctor whether you should take acetaminophen or other pain relievers/fever reducers. Acetaminophen may cause liver damage. **KEEP THIS AND ALL DRUGS OUT OF THE REACH OF CHILDREN.** Prompt medical attention is critical for adults as well as for children even if you do not notice any signs or symptoms. In case of accidental overdose, seek professional assistance or contact a Poison Control Center immediately. As with any drug, if you are pregnant or nursing a baby, seek the advice of a health professional before using this product.

Additional Warnings for Maximum Strength Caplets: May cause excitability especially in children. Do not take this product, unless directed by a doctor, if you have a breathing problem such as emphysema or chronic bronchitis. May cause marked drowsiness: alcohol, sedatives, and tranquilizers may increase the drowsiness effect. Avoid taking alcoholic beverages while taking this product. Do not take this product if you are taking sedatives or tranquilizers, without first consulting your doctor. Use caution when driving a motor vehicle or operating machinery.

Drug Interaction Precaution: Do not use this product if you are now taking a prescription monoamine oxidase inhibitor (MAOI) (certain drugs for depres-sion, psychiatric or emotional conditions, or Parkinson's disease), or for 2 weeks after stopping the MAOI drug. If you are uncertain whether your prescription drug contains an MAOI, consult a health professional before taking this product.

Inactive Ingredients: Each **Non-Drowsy and Maximum Strength Caplet** contains: Carnauba Wax, Colloidal Silicon Dioxide, Hydroxypropyl Methylcellulose, Magnesium stearate, Microcrystalline Cellulose, Polyethylene Glycol, Polysorbate 80, Starch, Stearic Acid, Titanium Dioxide.
Each **Maximum Strength Caplet** also contains: FD&C Blue #1 Al Lake.

Avoid storing at high temperature (greater than 100°F).

How Supplied: Non-Drowsy: Consumer packages of 16.
Maximum Strength: Consumer packages of 16 & 30.
Shown in Product Identification Guide, page 523
Product Change: Maximum Strength Caplets now with new decongestant (pseudoephedrine HCl).

Note: There are other CONTAC products. Make sure this is the one you are interested in. See the table below for all of the products in the CONTAC line.
[See table above]

DEBROX® Drops
Ear Wax Removal Aid

Description: Carbamide peroxide 6.5%. Also contains citric acid, glycerin, propylene glycol, sodium stannate, water, and other ingredients.

Actions: DEBROX®, used as directed, cleanses the ear with sustained microfoam. DEBROX Drops foam on contact with earwax due to the release of oxygen (there may be an associated crackling sound). DEBROX Drops provide a safe, nonirritating method of softening and removing ear wax.

Indications: For occasional use as an aid to soften, loosen, and remove excessive earwax.

Directions: FOR USE IN THE EAR ONLY. Adults and children over 12 years of age: tilt head sideways and place 5 to 10 drops into ear. Tip of applicator should not enter ear canal. Keep drops in ear for several minutes by keeping head tilted or placing cotton in the ear. Use twice daily for up to four days if needed, or as directed by a doctor. Any wax remaining after treatment may be removed by gently flushing the ear with warm water, using a soft rubber bulb ear syringe. Children under 12 years of age: consult a doctor.

Warnings: Do not use if you have ear drainage or discharge, ear pain, irritation or rash in the ear, or are dizzy; consult a doctor. Do not use if you have an injury or perforation (hole) of the eardrum or after ear surgery unless directed by a doctor. Do not use for more than four days. If excessive earwax remains after use of this product, consult a doctor. Avoid contact with the eyes.

Cautions: Avoid exposing bottle to excessive heat and direct sunlight. Keep tip on bottle when not in use. Keep this and all drugs out of the reach of children. In case of accidental ingestion, seek professional assistance or contact a poison control center immediately.

How Supplied: DEBROX Drops are available in $1/2$- or 1-fl-oz (15 or 30 ml) plastic squeeze bottles with applicator spouts.
Shown in Product Identification Guide, page 523

ECOTRIN
Enteric-Coated Aspirin
Antiarthritic, Antiplatelet
COMPREHENSIVE PRESCRIBING INFORMATION

Description: Ecotrin enteric coated aspirin (acetylsalicylic acid) tablets available in 81mg, 325mg and 500 mg tablets for oral administration. The 325 mg and 500 mg tablets contain the following inactive ingredients: Carnuba

Continued on next page

Ecotrin—Cont.

Wax, Colloidal Silicon Dioxide, FD&C Yellow No. 6, Hydroxypropyl Methylcellulose, Methacrylic Acid Copolymer, Microcrystalline Cellulose, Pregelatinized Starch, Propylene Glycol, Simethicone, Sodium Starch Glycolate, Stearic Acid, Talc, Titanium Dioxide, and Triethyl Citrate. The 81 mg tablets contain Carnuba Wax, Corn Starch, D&C Yellow No. 10, FD&C Yellow No. 6, Hydroxypropyl Methylcellulose, Methacrylic Acid Copolymer, Microcrystalline Cellulose, Propylene Glycol, Simethicone, Stearic Acid, Talc and Triethyl Citrate.

Aspirin is an odorless white, needle-like crystalline or powdery substance. When exposed to moisture, aspirin hydrolyzes into salicylic and acetic acids, and gives off a vinegary-odor. It is highly lipid soluble and slightly soluble in water.

Clinical Pharmacology: Mechanism of Action: Aspirin is a more potent inhibitor of both prostaglandin synthesis and platelet aggregation than other salicylic acid derivatives. The differences in activity between aspirin and salicylic acid are thought to be due to the acetyl group on the aspirin molecule. This acetyl group is responsible for the inactivation of cyclooxygenase via acetylation.

PHARMACOKINETICS

Absorption: In general, immediate release aspirin is well and completely absorbed from the gastrointestinal (GI) tract. Following absorption, aspirin is hydrolyzed to salicylic acid with peak plasma levels of salicylic acid occurring within 1–2 hours of dosing (see Pharmacokinetics—Metabolism). The rate of absorption from the GI tract is dependent upon the dosage form, the presence or absence of food, gastric pH (the presence or absence of GI antacids or buffering agents), and other physiologic factors. Enteric coated aspirin products are erratically absorbed from the GI tract.

Distribution: Salicylic acid is widely distibuted to all tissues and fluids in the body including the central nervous system (CNS), breast milk, and fetal tissues. The highest concentrations are found in the plasma, liver, renal cortex, heart, and lungs.

The protein binding of salicylate is concentration-dependent, i.e., non-linear. At low concentrations (< 100 mcg/mL) approximately 90 percent of plasma salicylate is bound to albumin while at higher concentrations (> 400 mcg/mL), only about 75 percent is bound. The early signs of salicylic overdose (salicylism), including tinnitus (ringing in the ears), occur at plasma concentrations approximating 200 mcg/mL. Severe toxic effects are associated with levels > 400 mcg/mL (See Adverse Reactions and Overdosage.)

Metabolism: Aspirin is rapidly hydrolyzed in the plasma to salicylic acid such that plasma levels of aspirin are essentially undetectable 1–2 hours after dosing. Salicylic acid is primarily conjugated in the liver to form salicyluric acid, a phenolic glucuronide, an acyl glucuronide, and a number of minor metabolites. Salicylic acid has a plasma half-life of approximately 6 hours. Salicylate metabolism is saturable and total body clearance decreases at higher serum concentrations due to the limited ability of the liver to form both salicyluric acid and phenolic glucuronide. Following toxic doses (10–20 grams (g)), the plasma half-life may be increased to over 20 hours.

Elimination: The elimination of salicylic acid follows zero order pharmacokinetics; (i.e., the rate of drug elimination is constant in relation to plasma concentration). Renal excretion of unchanged drug depends upon urine pH. As urinary pH rises above 6.5, the renal clearance of free salicylate increases from < 5 percent to > 80 percent. Alkalinization of the urine is a key concept in the management of salicylate overdose. (See Overdosage.) Following therapeutic doses, approximately 10 percent is found excreted in the urine as salicylic acid, 75 percent as salicyluric acid, as the phenolic and acyl glucuronides, respectively.

Pharmacodynamics: Aspirin affects platelet aggregation by irreversibly inhibiting prostaglandin cyclo-oxygenase. This effect lasts for the life of the platelet and prevents the formation of the platelet aggregating factor thromboxane A2. Non-acetylated salicylates do not inhibit this enzyme and have no effect on platelet aggregation. At somewhat higher doses, aspirin reversibly inhibits the formation of prostaglandin 1_2 (prostacyclin), which is an arterial vasodilator and inhibits platelet aggregation.

At higher doses aspirin is an effective anti-inflammatory agent, partially due to inhibition of inflammatory mediators via cyclooxygenase inhibition in peripheral tissues. In vitro studies suggest that other mediators of inflammation may also be suppressed by aspirin administration, although the precise mechanism of action has not been elucidated. It is this non-specific suppression of cyclooxygenase activity in peripheral tissues following large doses that leads to its primary side effect of gastric irritation. (See Adverse Reactions.)

Clinical Studies: Ischemic Stroke and Transient Ischemic Attack (TIA): In clinical trials of subjects with TIA's due to fibrin platelet emboli or ischemic stroke, aspirin has been shown to significantly reduce the risk of the combined endpoint of stroke or death and the combined endpoint of TIA, stroke, or death by about 13–18 percent.

Suspect Acute Myocardial Infarction (MI): In a large, multi-center study of aspirin, streptokinase, and the combination of aspirin and streptokinase in 17,187 patients with suspected acute MI, aspirin treatment produced a 23-percent reduction in the risk of vascular mortality. Aspirin was also shown to have an additional benefit in patients given a thrombolytic agent.

Prevention of Recurrent MI and Unstable Angina Pectoris: These indications are supported by the results of six large, randomized, multi-center, placebo-controlled trials of predominantly male post-MI subjects and one randomized placebo-controlled study of men with unstable angina pectoris. Aspirin therapy in MI subjects was associated with a significant reduction (about 20 percent) in the risk of the combination endpoint of subsequent death and/or nonfatal reinfarction in these patients. In aspirin-treated unstable angina patients the event rate was reduced to 5 percent from the 10 percent rate in the placebo group.

Chronic Stable Angina Pectoris: In a randomized, multi-center, double-blind trial designed to assess the role of aspirin for prevention of MI in patients with chronic stable angina pectoris, aspirin significantly reduced the primary combined endpoint of nonfatal MI, fatal MI, and sudden death by 34 percent. The secondary endpoint for vascular events (first occurrence of MI, stroke, or vascular death) was also significantly reduced (32 percent).

Revascularization Procedures: Most patients who undergo coronary artery revascularization procedures have already had symptomatic coronary artery disease for which aspirin is indicated. Similarly, patients with lesions of the carotid bifurcation sufficient to require carotid endarterectomy are likely to have had a precedent event. Aspirin is recommended for patients who undergo revascularization procedures if there is a preexisting condition for which aspirin is already indicated.

Rheumatologic Diseases: In clinical studies in patients with rheumatoid arthritis, juvenile rheumatoid arthritis, ankylosing spondylitis and osteoarthritis, aspirin has been shown to be effective in controlling various indices of clinical disease activity.

Animal Toxicology: The acute oral 50 percent lethal dose in rats is about 1.5 g/kg and in mice 1.1 g/kg. Renal papillary necrosis and decreased urinary concentrating ability occur in rodents chronically administered high doses. Dose-dependent gastric mucosal injury occurs in rats and humans. Mammals may develop aspirin toxicosis associated with GI symptoms, circulatory effects, and central nervous system depression. (See Overdosage.)

Indications and Usage: Vascular Indications (Ischemic Stroke, TIA, Acute MI, Prevention of Recurrent MI, Unstable Angina Pectoris, and Chronic Stable Angina Pectoris): Aspirin is indicated to: (1) Reduce the combined risk of death and nonfatal stroke in patients who have had ischemic stroke of transient ischemia of the brain due to fibrin platelet emboli, (2) reduce the risk of vascular mortality in patients with a suspected acute MI, (3) reduce the combined risk of death and nonfatal MI in patients with a previous MI or unstable angina pectoris,

and (4) reduce the combined risk of MI and sudden death in patients with chronic stable angina pectoris.

Revascularization Procedures (Coronary Artery Bypass Graft (CABG), Percutaneous Transluminal Coronary Angioplasty (PTCA), and Carotid Endarterectomy): Aspirin is indicated in patients who have undergone revascularization procedures (i.e., CABG, PTCA, or carotid endarterectomy) when there is a preexisting condition for which aspirin is already indicated.

Rheumatologic Disease Indications (Rheumatoid Arthritis, Juvenile Rheumatoid Arthritis, Spondyloarthropathies, Osteoarthritis, and the Arthritis and Pleurisy of Systemic Lupus Erythematosus (SLE)): Aspirin is indicated for the relief of the signs and symptoms of rheumatoid arthritis, juvenile rheumatoid arthritis, osteoarthritis, spondyloarthropathies, and arthritis and pleurisy associated with SLE.

Contraindications: Allergy: Aspirin is contraindicated in patients with known allergy to nonsteroidal anti-inflammatory drug products and in patients with the syndrome of asthma, rhinitis, and nasal polyps. Aspirin may cause severe urticaria, angioedema, or bronchospasm (asthma).

Reye's Syndrome: Aspirin should not be used in children or teenagers for viral infections, with or without fever, because of the risk of Reye's syndrome with concomitant use of aspirin in certain viral illnesses.

Warnings: Alcohol Warning: Patients who consume three or more alcoholic drinks every day should be counseled about the bleeding risks involved with chronic, heavy alcohol use while taking aspirin.

Coagulation Abnormalities: Even low doses of aspirin can inhibit platelet function leading to an increase in bleeding time. This can adversely affect patients with inherited (hemophilia) or acquired (liver disease or vitamin K deficiency) bleeding disorders.

GI Side Effects: GI side effects include stomach pain, heartburn, nausea, vomiting, and gross GI bleeding. Although minor upper GI symptoms, such as dyspepsia, are common and can occur anytime during therapy, physicians should remain alert for signs of ulceration and bleedings, even in the absence of previous GI symptoms. Physicians should inform patients about the signs and symptoms of GI side effects and what steps to take if they occur.

Peptic Ulcer Disease: Patients with a history of active peptic ulcer disease should avoid using aspirin, which can cause gastric mucosal irritation and bleeding.

Precautions
General
Renal Failure: Avoid aspirin in patients with severe renal failure (glomerular filtration rate less than 10 mL/minute).

Hepatic Insufficiency: Avoid aspirin in patients with severe hepatic insufficiency.

Sodium Restricted Diets: Patients with sodium-retaining states, such as congestive heart failure or renal failure, should avoid sodium-containing buffered aspirin preparations because of their high sodium content.

Laboratory Tests: Aspirin has been associated with elevated hepatic enzymes, blood urea nitrogen and serum creatinine, hyperkalemia, proteinuria, and prolonged bleeding time.

Drug Interactions
Angiotensin Converting Enzyme (ACE) Inhibitors: The hyponatremic and hypotensive effects of ACE inhibitors may be diminished by the concomitant administration of aspirin due to its direct effect on the renin-angiotensin conversion pathway.

Acetazolamide: Concurrent use of aspirin and acetazolamide can lead to high serum concentrations of acetazolamide (and toxicity) due to competition at the renal tubule for secretion.

Anticoagulant Therapy (Heparin and Warfarin): Patients on anticoagulation therapy are at increased risk for bleeding because of drug-drug interactions and the effect on platelets. Aspirin can displace warfarin from protein binding sites, leading to prolongation of both the prothrombin time and the bleeding time. Aspirin can increase the anticoagulant activity of heparin, increasing bleeding risk.

Anticonvulsants: Salicylate can displace protein-bound phenytoin and valproic acid, leading to a decrease in the total concentration of phenytoin and an increase in serum valproic acid levels.

Beta Blockers: The hypotensive effects of beta blockers may be diminished by the concomitant administration of aspirin due to inhibition of renal prostaglandins, leading to decreased renal blood flow, and salt and fluid retention.

Diuretics: The effectiveness of diuretics in patients with underlying renal or cardiovascular disease may be diminished by the concomitant administration of aspirin due to inhibition of renal prostaglandins, leading to decreased renal blood flow and salt and fluid retention.

Methotrexate: Salicylate can inhibit renal clearance of methotrexate, leading to bone marrow toxicity, especially in the elderly or renal impaired.

Nonsteroidal Anti-inflammatory Drugs (NSAID's): The concurrent use of aspirin with other NSAID's should be avoided because this may increase bleeding or lead to decreased renal function.

Oral Hypoglycemics: Moderate doses of aspirin may increase the effectiveness of oral hypoglycemic drugs, leading to hypoglycemia.

Uricosuric Agents (Probenecid and Sulfinpyrazone): Salicylates antagonize the uricosuric action of uricosuric agents.

Carcinogenesis, Mutagenesis, Impairment of Fertility: Administration of as-

pirin for 68 weeks at 0.5 percent in the feed of rats was not carcinogenic. In the Ames Salmonella assay, aspirin was not mutagenic; however, aspirin did induce chromosome aberrations in cultured human fibroblasts. Aspirin inhibits ovulation in rats. (See Pregnancy.)

Pregnancy: Pregnant women should only take aspirin if clearly needed. Because of the known effects of NSAID's on the fetal cardiovascular system (closure of the ductus arteriosus), use during the third trimester of pregnancy should be avoided. Salicylate products have also been associated with alterations in maternal and neonatal hemostasis mechanisms, decreased birth weight, and with perinatal mortality.

Labor and Delivery: Aspirin should be avoided 1 week prior to and during labor and delivery because it can result in excessive blood loss at delivery. Prolonged gestation and prolonged labor due to prostaglandin inhibition have been reported.

Nursing Mothers: Nursing mothers should avoid using aspirin because salicylate is excreted in breast milk. Use of high doses may lead to rashes, platelet abnormalities, and bleeding in nursing infants.

Pediatric Use: Pediatric dosing recommendations for juvenile rheumatoid arthritis are based on well-controlled clinical studies. An initial dose of 90–130 mg/kg/day in divided doses, with an increase as needed for anti-inflammatory efficacy (target plasma salicylate levels of 150–300 mcg/mL) are effective. At high doses (i.e., plasma levels of greater than 200 mg/mL), the incidence of toxicity increases.

Adverse Reactions: Many adverse reactions due to aspirin ingestion are dose-related. The following is a list of adverse reactions that have been reported in the literature. (See Warnings.)

Body as a Whole: Fever, hypothermia, thirst.

Cardiovascular: Dysrhythmias, hypotension, tachycardia.

Central Nervous System: Agitation, cerebral edema, coma, confusion, dizziness, headache, subdural or intracranial hemorrhage, lethargy, seizures.

Fluid and Electrolyte: Dehydration, hyperkalemia, metabolic acidosis, respiratory alkalosis.

Gastrointestinal: Dyspepsia, GI bleeding, ulceration and perforation, nausea, vomiting, transient elevations of hepatic enzymes, hepatitis, Reye's Syndrome, pancreatitis.

Hematologic: Prolongation of the prothrombin time, disseminated intravascular coagulation, coagulopathy, thrombocytopenia.

Hypersensitivity: Acute anaphylaxis, angioedema, asthma, bronchospasm, laryngeal edema, urticaria.

Musculoskeletal: Rhabdomyolysis.

Continued on next page

Ecotrin—Cont.

Metabolism: Hypoglycemia (in children), hyperglycemia.

Reproductive: Prolonged pregnancy and labor, stillbirths, lower birth weight infants, antepartum and postpartum bleeding.

Respiratory: Hyperpnea, pulmonary edema, tachypnea.

Special Senses: Hearing loss, tinnitus. Patients with high frequency hearing loss may have difficulty perceiving tinnitus. In these patients, tinnitus cannot be used as a clinical indicator of salicylism.

Urogenital: Interstitial nephritis, papillary necrosis, proteinuria, renal insufficiency and failure.

Drug Abuse and Dependence: Aspirin is non-narcotic. There is no known potential for addiction associated with the use of aspirin.

Overdosage: Salicylate toxicity may result from acute ingestion (overdose) or chronic intoxication. The early signs of salicylic overdose (salicylism), including tinnitus (ringing in the ears), occur at plasma concentrations approaching 200 mcg/mL. Plasma concentrations of aspirin above 300 mcg/mL are clearly toxic. Severe toxic effects are associated with levels above 400 mcg/mL. (See Clinical Pharmacology.) A single lethal dose of aspirin in adults is not known with certainty but death may be expected at 30 g. For real or suspected overdose, a Poison Control Center should be contacted immediately. Careful medical management is essential.

Signs and Symptoms: In acute overdose, severe acid-base and electrolyte disturbances may occur and are complicated by hyperthermia and dehydration. Respiratory alkalosis occurs early while hyperventilation is present, but is quickly followed by metabolic acidosis.

Treatment: Treatment consists primarily of supporting vital functions, increasing salicylate elimination, and correcting the acid-base disturbance. Gastric emptying and/or lavage is recommended as soon as possible after ingestion, even if the patient has vomited spontaneously. After lavage and/or emesis, administration of activated charcoal, as a slurry, is beneficial, if less than 3 hours have passed since ingestion. Charcoal adsorption should not be employed prior to emesis and lavage.

Severity of aspirin intoxication is determined by measuring the blood salicylate level. Acid-base status should be closely followed with serial blood gas and serum pH measurements. Fluid and electrolyte balance should be maintained.

In severe cases, hyperthermia and hypovolemia are the major immediate threats to life. Children should be sponged with tepid water. Replacement fluid should be administered intravenously and augmented with correction of acidosis. Plasma electrolytes and pH should be monitored to promote alkaline diuresis

of salicylate if renal function is normal. Infusion of glucose may be required to control hypoglycemia.

Hemodialysis and peritoneal dialysis can be performed to reduce the body drug content. In patients with renal insufficiency or in cases of life-threatening intoxication, dialysis is usually required. Exchange transfusion may be indicated in infants and young children.

Dosage and Administration: Each dose of aspirin should be taken with a full glass of water unless patient is fluid restricted. Anti-inflammatory and analgesic dosages should be individualized. When aspirin is used in high doses, the development of tinnitus may be used as a clinical sign of elevated plasma salicylate levels except in patients with high frequency hearing loss.

Ischemic Stroke and TIA: 50–325 mg once a day. Continue therapy indefinitely.

Suspected Acute MI: The initial dose of 160–162.5 mg is administered as soon as an MI is suspected. The maintenance dose of 160–162.5 mg a day is continued for 30 days post infarction. After 30 days, consider further therapy based on dosage and administration for prevention of recurrent MI.

Prevention of Recurrent MI: 75–325 mg once a day. Continue therapy indefinitely.

Unstable Angina Pectoris: 75–325 mg once a day. Continue therapy indefinitely.

Chronic Stable Angina Pectoris: 75–325 mg once a day. Continue therapy indefinitely.

CABG: 325 mg daily starting 6 hours post-procedure. Continue therapy for 1 year post-procedure.

PTCA: The initial dose of 325 mg should be given 2 hours pre-surgery. Maintenance dose is 160–325 mg daily. Continue therapy indefinitely.

Carotid Endarterectomy: Doses of 80 mg once daily to 650 mg twice daily, started presurgery, are recommended. Continue therapy indefinitely.

Rheumatoid Arthritis: The initial dose is 3 g a day in divided doses. Increase as needed for anti-inflammatory efficacy with target plasma salicylate levels of 150–300 mcg/mL. At high doses (i.e., plasma levels of greater than 200 mg/mL), the incidence of toxicity increases.

Juvenile Rheumatoid Arthritis: Initial dose is 90–130 mg/kg/day in divided doses. Increase as needed for anti-inflammatory efficacy with target plasma salicylate levels of 150–300 mcg/mL. At high doses (i.e., plasma levels of greater than 200 mg/mL), the incidence of toxicity increases.

Spondyloarthropathies: Up to 4 g per day in divided doses.

Osteoarthritis: Up to 3 g per day in divided doses.

Arthritis and Pleurisy of SLE: The initial dose is 3 g a day in divided doses. Increase as needed for anti-inflammatory efficacy with target plasma salicyl-

ate levels of 150–300 mcg/mL. At high doses (i.e., plasma levels of greater than 200 mg/mL), the incidence of toxicity increases.

How Supplied: 81 mg convex orange film coated tablet with ECOTRIN LOW printed in black ink on one side of the tablet. Available as follows

NDC 0108-0117-82 Bottle of 36 tablets
NDC 0108-0117-83 Bottle of 120 tablets
325 mg convex orange film coated tablet with ECOTRIN REG printed in black ink on one side of the tablet. Available as follows:

NDC 0108-0014-26 Bottle of 100 tablets
NDC 0108-0014-29 Bottle of 250 tablets
500 mg convex orange film coated tablet with ECOTRIN MAX printed in black ink on one side of the tablet. Available as follows:

NDC 0108-0016-23 Bottle of 60 tablets
NDC 0108-0016-27 Bottle of 150 tablets
Store in a tight container at 25°C (77° F); excursions permitted to 15–30° C (59–86° F).

Shown in Product Identification Guide, page 524

GAVISCON® Regular Strength Antacid Tablets
[găv 'ĭs-kŏn]

Composition: Each chewable tablet contains the following active ingredients:
Aluminum hydroxide dried gel... 80 mg
Magnesium trisilicate .... 20 mg
and the following inactive ingredients: alginic acid, calcium stearate, flavor, sodium bicarbonate, starch (may contain corn starch), and sucrose.

Actions: Unique formulation produces soothing foam which floats on stomach contents. Foam containing antacid precedes stomach contents into the esophagus when reflux occurs to help protect the sensitive mucosa from further irritation. GAVISCON® acts locally without neutralizing entire stomach contents to help maintain integrity of the digestive process. Endoscopic studies indicate that GAVISCON Antacid Tablets are equally as effective in the erect or supine patient.

Indications: GAVISCON is specifically formulated for the temporary relief of heartburn (acid indigestion) due to acid reflux. GAVISCON is not indicated for the treatment of peptic ulcers.

Directions: Chew 2 to 4 tablets four times a day or as directed by a physician. Tablets should be taken after meals and at bedtime or as needed. For best results follow by a half glass of water or other liquid. DO NOT SWALLOW WHOLE.

Warnings: Do not take more than 16 tablets in a 24-hour period or 16 tablets daily for more than 2 weeks, except under the advice and supervision of a physician. Do not use this product except under the advice and supervision of a phy-

sician if you are on a sodium-restricted diet. Each GAVISCON Tablet contains approximately 0.8 mEq sodium.

Drug Interaction Precaution: Antacids may interact with certain prescription drugs. If you are presently taking a prescription drug, do not take this product without checking with your physician or other health professional. Store at a controlled room temperature in a dry place.

Keep this and all drugs out of the reach of children. In case of accidental overdose, seek professional assistance or contact a poison control center immediately.

How Supplied: Bottles of 100 tablets and in foil-wrapped 2s in boxes of 30 tablets.

Shown in Product Identification Guide, page 524

GAVISCON® EXTRA STRENGTH
Antacid Tablets
[găv ′ĭs-kŏn]

Composition: Each chewable tablet contains the following active ingredients:
Aluminum hydroxide .... 160 mg
Magnesium carbonate .... 105 mg
and the following inactive ingredients: alginic acid, calcium stearate, flavor, sodium bicarbonate, and sucrose. May contain stearic acid. Contains sorbitol or mannitol. May contain starch.

Actions: Gavison's unique antacid foam barrier neutralizes stomach acid.

Indications: For the relief of heartburn, sour stomach, acid indigestion and upset stomach associated with these conditions.

Directions: Chew 2 to 4 tablets four times a day or as directed by a physician. Tablets should be taken after meals and at bedtime or as needed. For best results follow by a half glass of water or other liquid. DO NOT SWALLOW WHOLE.

Warnings: Do not take more than 16 tablets in a 24-hour period or 16 tablets daily for more than 2 weeks, except under the advice and supervision of a physician. Do not use this product except under the advice and supervision of a physician if you are on a sodium-restricted diet. Each Extra Strength Gaviscon tablet contains approximately 1.3 mEq sodium.

Drug Interaction Precaution: Antacids may interact with certain prescription drugs. If you are presently taking a prescription drug, do not take this product without checking with your physician or other health professional.

Store at a controlled room temperature in a dry place.

Keep this and all drugs out of the reach of children. In case of accidental overdose, seek professional assistance or contact a poison control center immediately.

How Supplied: Bottles of 100 tablets and in foil-wrapped 2s in boxes of 6 and 30 tablets.

Shown in Product Identification Guide, page 524

GAVISCON® EXTRA STRENGTH
Liquid Antacid
[găv ′ĭs-kŏn]

Composition: Each 2 teaspoonfuls (10 mL) contains the following active ingredients:
Aluminum hydroxide .... 508 mg
Magnesium carbonate .... 475 mg
and the following inactive ingredients: Benzyl alcohol, edetate disodium, flavor, glycerin, saccharin sodium, simethicone emulsion, sodium alginate, sorbitol solution, water, and xanthan gum.

Actions: Gaviscon's unique antacid foam barrier neutralizes stomach acid.

Indications: For the relief of heartburn, sour stomach, acid indigestion and upset stomach associated with these conditions.

Directions: SHAKE WELL BEFORE USING. Take 2 to 4 teaspoonfuls four times a day or as directed by a physician. GAVISCON Extra Strength Liquid should be taken after meals and at bedtime. Dispense product only by spoon or other measuring device.

Warnings: Except under the advice and supervision of a physician, do not take more than 16 teaspoonfuls in a 24-hour period or 16 teaspoonfuls daily for more than 2 weeks. May have laxative effect. Do not use this product if you have a kidney disease. Do not use this product if you are on a sodium-restricted diet except under the advice and supervision of a physician. Each teaspoonful contains approximately 0.9 mEq sodium.

Keep this and all drugs out of the reach of children. In case of accidental overdose, seek professional assistance or contact a poison control center immediately.

Drug Interaction Precaution: Antacids may interact with certain prescription drugs. If you are presently taking a prescription drug, do not take this product without checking with your physician or other health professional.

Keep tightly closed. Avoid freezing. Store at a controlled room temperature.

How Supplied: 12 fl oz (355 mL) bottles.

Shown in Product Identification Guide, page 524

GAVISCON® Regular Strength
Liquid Antacid
[găv ′ĭs-kŏn]

Composition: Each tablespoonful (15 ml) contains the following active ingredients:
Aluminum hydroxide .... 95 mg
Magnesium carbonate .... 358 mg
and the following inactive ingredients: Benzyl alcohol, D&C Yellow #10, edetate disodium, FD&C Blue #1, flavor, glycerin, saccharin sodium, sodium alginate, sorbitol solution, water, and xanthan gum.

Actions: Gaviscon's unique antacid foam barrier neutralizes stomach acid.

Indications: For the relief of heartburn, sour stomach, acid indigestion and upset stomach associated with these conditions.

Directions: SHAKE WELL BEFORE USING. Take 1 or 2 tablespoonfuls four times a day or as directed by a physician. GAVISCON Regular Strength Liquid should be taken after meals and at bedtime. Dispense product only by spoon or other measuring device.

Warnings: Except under the advice and supervision of a physician, do not take more than 8 tablespoonfuls in a 24-hour period or 8 tablespoonfuls daily for more than 2 weeks. May have laxative effect. Do not use this product if you have a kidney disease. Do not use this product if you are on a sodium-restricted diet except under the advice and supervision of a physician. Each tablespoonful of GAVISCON Regular Strength Liquid contains approximately 1.7 mEq sodium.

Keep this and all drugs out of the reach of children. In case of accidental overdose, seek professional assistance or contact a poison control center immediately.

Drug Interaction Precaution: Antacids may interact with certain prescription drugs. If you are presently taking a prescription drug, do not take this product without checking with your physician or other health professional.

Keep tightly closed. Avoid freezing. Store at a controlled room temperature.

How Supplied: 12 fluid oz (355 ml) bottles.

Shown in Product Identification Guide, page 524

GLY–OXIDE® Liquid

Description/Active Ingredient: GLY-OXIDE® Liquid contains carbamide peroxide 10%.

Actions: GLY-OXIDE® Liquid has an oxygen-rich formula that works to relieve the pain of canker sores by cleaning and debriding damaged tissue so natural healing can occur. GLY-OXIDE Liquid's dense oxygenating microfoam helps destroy odor-forming germs and flushes out food particles that ordinary brushing can miss.

Indications For Temporary Use: Gly-Oxide liquid is for temporary use in cleansing canker sores and minor wound

Continued on next page

Gly-Oxide—Cont.

or gum inflammation resulting from minor dental procedures, dentures, orthodontic appliances, accidental injury, or other irritations of the mouth and gums. Gly-Oxide can also be used to guard against the risk of infections in the mouth and gums.

Everyday Uses: Gly-Oxide may be used routinely to improve oral hygiene as an aid to regular brushing or when regular brushing is inadequate or impossible such as total care geriatrics, etc. Gly-Oxide kills germs to reduce mouth odors and/or odors on dental appliances. Gly-Oxide penetrates between teeth and other areas of the mouth to flush out food particles ordinary brushing can miss. This can be especially useful when brushing is made more difficult by the presence of orthodontics or other dental appliances. Plus, Gly-Oxide helps remove stains on dental appliances to improve appearance.

Directions For Temporary Use: Do not dilute. Replace tip on bottle when not in use. **Adults and children 2 years of age and older:** Apply several drops directly from bottle onto affected area; spit out after 2 to 3 minutes. Use up to four times daily after meals and at bedtime or as directed by dentist or doctor. OR place 10 drops on tongue, mix with saliva, swish for several minutes, and then spit out. Use by children under 12 years of age should be supervised. **Children under 2 years of age:** Consult a dentist or doctor.

Directions For Everyday Use: The product may be used following the temporary use directions above. OR apply Gly-Oxide to the toothbrush (it will sink into the brush), cover with toothpaste, brush normally, and spit out.

Warnings: Severe or persistent oral inflammation, denture irritation, or gingivitis may be serious. If sore mouth symptoms do not improve in 7 days, or if irritation, pain, or redness persists or worsens, or if swelling, rash, or fever develops, discontinue use of product and see your dentist or doctor promptly. Avoid contact with eyes. **KEEP THIS AND ALL DRUGS OUT OF THE REACH OF CHILDREN.** In case of accidental overdose, seek professional assistance or contact a poison control center immediately.

Inactive Ingredients: Citric Acid, Flavor, Glycerin, Propylene Glycol, Sodium Stannate, Water, and Other Ingredients.

Protect from excessive heat and direct sunlight.

How Supplied: GLY-OXIDE® Liquid is available in $1/2$-fl-oz and 2-fl-oz plastic squeeze bottles with applicator spouts.

Comments or Questions? Call Toll-free 1-800-245-1040 Weekdays

SmithKline Beecham Consumer Healthcare, L.P.

Pittsburgh, PA 15230   Made in U.S.A.
Shown in Product Identification Guide, page 524

MASSENGILL® Douches, Towelettes and Cleansing Wash
[mas 'sen-gil]

PRODUCT OVERVIEW

Key Facts: Massengill is the brand name for a line of feminine hygiene products which are recommended for routine cleansing and for temporary relief of minor vaginal itching and irritation. Massengill disposable douches are available in two Vinegar & Water formulas (Extra Mild and Extra Cleansing), and other cosmetic solutions (Country Flowers, Fresh Baby Powder Scent, Fresh Mountain Breeze, and Spring Rain Freshness), and a Medicated formula (with povidone-iodine). Massengill also has products specially designed to safely and gently cleanse the external vaginal area: Baby Powder Soft Cloth Towelettes, Medicated Soft Cloth Towelettes and Feminine Cleansing Wash.

Major Uses: Massengill's Vinegar & Water, and other cosmetic douches are recommended for routine douching, or for cleansing following menstruation, prescribed use of vaginal medication or use of contraceptive creams or jellies. Massengill Medicated is recommended in a seven day regimen for the symptomatic relief of minor vaginal itching and irritation associated with vaginitis due to Candida albicans, Trichomonas vaginalis, and Gardnerella vaginalis. Massengill Feminine Cleansing Wash is a gentle soapfree way to clean the external vaginal area. Massengill Non-medicated Soft Cloth Towelettes are a convenient and portable way to cleanse the external vaginal area and wash odor away. Massengill Medicated Soft Cloth Towelettes provide temporary relief of minor external itching associated with irritation or skin rashes.

Safety Information: Do not douche during pregnancy unless directed by a physician. Douching does not prevent pregnancy. Do not use this product and consult your physician if you are experiencing any of the following symptoms: unusual vaginal discharge, vaginal bleeding, painful and/or frequent urination, lower abdominal/pelvis pain, nausea or fever, or you or your sex partner have genital sores or ulcers.

If vaginal dryness or irritation occurs, discontinue use.

Massengill Medicated — Women with iodine-sensitivity should not use this product. If symptoms persist after seven days, or if redness, swelling or pain develop, consult a physician. Do not use while nursing unless directed by a physician.

PRODUCT INFORMATION
MASSENGILL®
[mas 'sen-gil]
Disposable Douches

Ingredients: DISPOSABLES: Extra Mild Vinegar and Water—Purified Water, Sodium Citrate, Citric Acid, and Vinegar.

Extra Cleansing Vinegar and Water—Purified Water, Sodium Citrate, Citric Acid, Vinegar, Diazolidinyl Urea, Octoxynol-9, Cetylpyridinium Chloride, Edetate Disodium.

Fresh Baby Powder Scent—Purified Water, Sodium Citrate, Citric Acid, SD Alcohol 40, Diazolidinyl Urea, Octoxynol-9, Fragrance, Cetylpyridinium Chloride, Edetate Disodium, FD&C Blue #1.

Country Flowers—Purified Water, Sodium Citrate, Citric Acid, SD Alcohol 40, Diazolidinyl Urea, Octoxynol-9, Fragrance, Cetylpyridinium Chloride, Edetate Disodium, D&C Red #28, FD&C Blue #1.

Fresh Mountain Breeze—Purified Water, SD Alcohol 40, Diazolindinyl Urea, Citric Acid, Sodium Citrate, Octoxynol-9, Fragrance, Cetylpyridinium Chloride, Edetate Disodium, FD&C Blue #1, D&C Yellow #10.

Spring Rain Freshness—Purified Water, SD Alcohol 40, Diazolidinyl Urea, Citric Acid, Sodium Citrate, Octoxynol-9, Fragrance, Cetylpyridinium Chloride, Edetate Disodium.

Indications: Recommended for routine cleansing, at the end of menstruation, after use of contraceptive creams or jellies (check the contraceptive package instructions first) or to rinse out the residue of prescribed vaginal medication (as directed by physician).

Actions: The buffered acid solutions of Massengill Douches can be valuable adjuncts to specific vaginal therapy following the prescribed use of vaginal medication or contraceptives and in feminine hygiene.

Directions: DISPOSABLES: Twist off flat tab from bottle containing premixed solution, attach nozzle supplied and use. The unit is completely disposable.

Warning: Douching does not prevent pregnancy. Do not use during pregnancy except under the advice and supervision of your physician. If vaginal dryness or irritation occurs, discontinue use. Use this product only as directed for routine cleansing. You should douche no more than twice a week except on the advice of your doctor.

An association has been reported between douching and pelvic inflammatory disease (PID), a serious infection of your reproductive system which can lead to sterility and/or ectopic (tubal) pregnancy. PID requires immediate medical attention.

PID's most common symptoms are pain and/or tenderness in the lower part of the abdomen and pelvis. You may also experience a vaginal discharge, vaginal bleeding, nausea or fever. Other sexually transmitted dis-

eases (STDs) have similar symptoms and/or frequent urination, genital sores, or ulcers. Douches should not be used for the self treatment of any STDs or PID. If you suspect you have one of these infections or PID, stop using this product and see your doctor immediately.

See the enclosed insert for important health information concerning sexually transmitted diseases and PID.

How Supplied: Disposable—6 oz. plastic bottle.

MASSENGILL®
[*mas 'sen-gil*]
Baby Powder Scent Soft Cloth Towelette

Ingredients: Purified Water, Lactic Acid, Sodium Lactate, Potassium Sorbate, Octoxynol-9, Disodium EDTA, Cetylpyridinium Chloride, and Fragrance.

Indications: For cleansing and refreshing the external vaginal area.

Actions: Massengill Baby Powder Scent Soft Cloth Towelette safely cleanse the external vaginal area. The towelette delivery system makes the application soft and gentle.

Directions: Remove towelette from foil packet, unfold, and gently wipe from front to back. Throw away towelette after it has been used once. Safe to use daily. For external use only.

How Supplied: Sixteen individually wrapped, disposable towelettes per carton.

MASSENGILL Feminine Cleansing Wash, Floral
[*mas 'sen-gil*]

Ingredients: Purified Water, sodium laureth sulfate, magnesium laureth sulfate, sodium laureth-8 sulfate, magnesium laureth-8 sulfate, sodium oleth sulfate, magnesium oleth sulfate, lauramidopropyl betaine, myristamine oxide, lactic acid, PEG-120 methyl glucose dioleate, fragrance, sodium methylparaben, sodium ethylparaben, sodium propylparaben, methylchloroisothiazolinone, methylisothiazolinone, D&C Red #33.

Indications: For cleansing and refreshing of external vaginal area.

Actions: Massengill feminine cleansing wash safely and gently cleanses the external vaginal area.

Directions: Pour small amount into palm of hand or wash cloth and lather into wet skin. Rinse clean. Safe to use daily. For external use only.

How Supplied: 8 fl. oz plastic flip-top bottle.

MASSENGILL® Medicated
[*mas 'sen-gil*]
Disposable Douche

Active Ingredient: Povidone-iodine: When mixed as directed a 0.30% solution is formed (Cepticin™).

Indications: For symptomatic relief of minor vaginal irritation or itching associated with vaginitis due to Candida albicans, Trichomonas vaginalis, and Gardnerella vaginalis.

Action: Povidone-iodine is widely recognized as an effective broad spectrum microbicide against both gram negative and gram positive bacteria, fungi, yeasts and protozoa. While remaining active in the presence of blood, serum or bodily secretions, it possesses virtually none of the irritating properties of iodine.

Warning: Douching does not prevent pregnancy. Do not use during pregnancy or while nursing except under the advice and supervision of your physician. If vaginal dryness or irritation occurs discontinue use. Use this product only as directed. Do not use this product for routine cleansing.

An association has been reported between douching and pelvic inflammatory disease (PID), a serious infection of your reproductive system, which can lead to sterility and/or ectopic (tubal) pregnancy. PID requires immediate medical attention.
PID's most common symptoms are pain and/or tenderness in the lower part of the abdomen and pelvis. You may also experience a vaginal discharge, vaginal bleeding, nausea or fever. Other sexually transmitted diseases (STDs) have similar symptoms and/or frequent urination, genital sores, or ulcers. Douches should not be used for self-treatment of any STDs or PID. If you suspect you have one of these infections or PID, stop using this product and see your doctor immediately.
See the enclosed insert for important health information concerning sexually transmitted diseases and PID.
Women with iodine sensitivity should not use this product.
Keep out of the reach of children.
Avoid storing at high temperature (greater than 100°F).
Protect from freezing.

Dosage and Administration: Dosage is provided as a single unit concentrate to be added to 6 oz. of sanitized water supplied in a disposable bottle. A specially designed nozzle is provided. After use, the unit is discarded. Use one bottle a day for seven days. Although symptoms may be relieved earlier, for maximum relief, treatment should be continued for the full seven days.

How Supplied: 6 oz. bottle of sanitized water with 0.17 oz. vial of povidone-iodine and nozzle.

Shown in Product Identification Guide, page 524

MASSENGILL® Medicated
[*mas 'sen-gil*]
Soft Cloth Towelette

Active Ingredient: Hydrocortisone (0.5%).

Inactive Ingredients: Diazolidinyl Urea, DMDM Hydantoin, Isopropyl Myristate, Methylparaben, Polysorbate 60, Propylene Glycol, Propylparaben, Purified Water, Sorbitan Stearate, Steareth-2, Steareth-21.
Also available in non-medicated (Baby Powder Scent) to freshen and cleanse the external vaginal area.

Indications: For temporary, soothing relief of minor external feminine itching or other itching associated with minor skin irritations, and rashes. Other uses of this product should be only under the advice and supervision of a physician.

Action: Massengill Medicated Soft Cloth Towelettes contain hydrocortisone, a proven anti-inflammatory, anti-pruritic ingredient. The towelette delivery system makes the application soothing, soft, and gentle.

Warnings: For external use only. Avoid contact with eyes. If condition worsens, or if symptoms persist for more than seven days or symptoms recur within a few days, do not use this or any other hydrocortisone product unless you have consulted a physician. Do not use if you are experiencing a vaginal discharge, see a physician. Do not use this product for the treatment of diaper rash, see a physician.
Keep this and all drugs out of the reach of children. As with any drug, if you are pregnant or nursing a baby, seek the advice of a health professional before using this product. In case of accidental ingestion, seek professional assistance or contact a Poison Control Center immediately.

Directions: Adults and Children two years of age and older—apply to the affected area not more than four times daily. Remove towelette from foil packet and gently wipe from front to back. Throw away towelette after it has been used once. Children under 2 years of age: DO NOT USE.

How Supplied: Ten individually wrapped, disposable towelettes per carton.

EDUCATIONAL MATERIAL

"The facts about Vaginal Infections and STDs"
A guide for women on vaginal infections and sexually transmitted diseases (STDs).

Continued on next page

Free to physicians, pharmacists and patients in limited quantities by writing SmithKline Beecham Consumer Healthcare, L.P. PO Box 1469, Pittsburgh, PA 15230 or calling 1-800-233-2426.

NICODERM® CQ®
Nicotine Transdermal System/Stop Smoking Aid

Formerly available only by prescription
Available as:

Step 1 - 21 mg/24 hours
Step 2 - 14 mg/24 hours
Step 3 - 7 mg/24 hours

If you smoke:
More than 10 cigarettes per Day: Start with Step 1
10 Cigarettes a Day or Less: Start with Step 2
WHAT IS THE NICODERM CQ PATCH AND HOW IS IT USED?
NicoDerm CQ is a small, nicotine containing patch. When you put on a NicoDerm CQ patch, nicotine passes through the skin and into your body. NicoDerm CQ is very thin and uses special material to control how fast nicotine passes through the skin. Unlike the sudden jolts of nicotine delivered by cigarettes, the amount of nicotine you receive remains relatively smooth throughout the 24 or 16 hours period you wear the NicoDerm CQ patch. This helps to reduce cravings you may have for nicotine.

Active Ingredient: Nicotine

Purpose: Stop Smoking Aid

Use: reduces withdrawal symptoms, including nicotine craving, associated with quitting smoking

Directions:
- **if you are under 18 years of age, ask a doctor before use**
- before using this product, read the enclosed user's guide for complete directions and other information
- stop smoking completely when you begin using the patch
- **if you smoke more than 10 cigarettes per day,** use according to the following 10 week schedule:

STEP 1	STEP 2	STEP 3
Use one 21 mg patch/day	Use one 14 mg patch/day	Use one 7 mg patch/day
Weeks 1–6	Weeks 7–8	Weeks 9–10

- if you smoke **10 or less cigarettes per day,** do not use **STEP 1 (21 mg)**. Start with **STEP 2 (14 mg)** for 6 weeks, then **STEP 3 (7 mg)** for two weeks and then stop.
- steps 2 and 3 allow you to gradually reduce your level of nicotine. Completing the full program will increase your chances of quitting successfully.
- apply one new patch every 24 hours on skin that is dry, clean and hairless
- remove backing from patch and immediately press onto skin. Hold for 10 seconds.

- wash hands after applying or removing patch. Throw away the patch in the enclosed disposal tray. See enclosed user's guide for safety and handling.
- you may wear the patch for 16 or 24 hours
- if you crave cigarettes when you wake up, wear the patch for 24 hours
- if you have vivid dreams or other sleep disturbances, you may remove the patch at bedtime and apply a new one in the morning
- the used patch should be removed and a new one applied to a different skin site at the same time each day
- do not wear more than one patch at a time
- do not cut patch in half or into smaller pieces
- do not leave patch on for more than 24 hours because it may irritate your skin and loses strength after 24 hours
- stop using the patch at the end of 10 weeks. If you started with **STEP 2,** stop using the patch at the end of 8 weeks. If you still feel the need to use the patch talk to your doctor.

Warnings:
Do Not Use
- if you continue to smoke, chew tobacco, use snuff, or use a nicotine gum or other nicotine containing products

Ask a doctor before use if you have
- heart disease, recent heart attack, or irregular heartbeat. Nicotine can increase your heart rate.
- high blood pressure not controlled with medication. Nicotine can increase your blood pressure.
- an allergy to adhesive tape or skin problems because you are more likely to get rashes

Ask a doctor or pharmacist before use if you are
- using a non-nicotine stop smoking drug
- taking a prescription medication for depression or asthma. Your prescription dose may need to be adjusted.

Stop use and ask a doctor if
- skin redness caused by the patch does not go away after four days, or if skin swells, or you get a rash
- irregular heartbeat or palpitations occur
- you get symptoms of nicotine overdose such as nausea, vomiting, dizziness, weakness and rapid heartbeat

If pregnant or breast feeding, ask a health professional before use. Nicotine can increase your baby's heart rate. First try to stop without the nicotine patch.

Keep out of reach of children and pets. Used patches have enough nicotine to poison children and pets. If swallowed, get medical help or contact a Poison Control Center right away. Dispose of the used patches by folding sticky ends together and inserting in disposal tray in this box.

When using this product
- do not smoke even when not wearing the patch. The nicotine in your skin will still be entering your blood stream for several hours after you take off the patch.
- if you have vivid dreams or other sleep disturbances remove this patch at bedtime

READ THE LABEL
Read the carton and the User's Guide before using this product. Keep the carton and User's Guide. They contain important information.

Inactive Ingredients: Ethylene vinyl acetate-copolymer, polyisobutylene and high density polyethylene between pigmented and clear polyester backings. Store at 20–25°C (68–77°F)

TO INCREASE YOUR SUCCESS IN QUITTING:
1. You must be motivated to quit.
2. Complete the full treatment program, applying a new patch every day.
3. Use with a support program as described in the Users Guide.

NicoDerm CQ User's Guide
KEYS TO SUCCESS
1) You must really want to quit smoking for **NicoDerm® CQ®** to help you.
2) Complete the full program, applying a new patch every day.
3) **NicoDerm CQ** works best when used together with a support program
4) If you have trouble using **NicoDerm CQ**, ask your doctor or pharmacist or call SmithKline Beecham at 1-800-834-5895 weekdays (10:00 am 4:30 pm EST).

SO, YOU'VE DECIDED TO QUIT.
Congratulations. Your decision to stop smoking is one of the most important things you can do to improve your health. Quitting smoking is a two-part process that involves:
1) overcoming your physical need for nicotine, and
2) breaking your smoking habit.
NicoDerm CQ helps smokers quit by reducing nicotine withdrawal symptoms. Many NicoDerm CQ users will be able to stop smoking for a few days but often will start smoking again. Most smokers have to try to quit several times before they completely stop.
Your own chances of quitting smoking depend on how strongly you are addicted to nicotine, how much you want to quit, and how closely you follow a quitting plan like the one that comes with NicoDerm CQ.

QUITTING SMOKING IS HARD!
If you find you cannot stop or if you start smoking again after using NicoDerm CQ please talk to a health care professional who can help you find a program that may work better for you. Breaking this addiction doesn't happen overnight.
Because NicoDerm CQ provides some nicotine, the NicoDerm CQ patch will help you stop smoking by reducing nicotine withdrawal symptoms such as nicotine craving, nervousness and irritability.
This User's Guide will give you support as you become a non-smoker. It will answer common questions about NicoDerm CQ and give tips to help you stop smoking, and should be referred to often.

WHERE TO GET HELP.
You are more likely to stop smoking by using NicoDerm CQ with a support program that helps you break your smoking habit. There may be support groups in your area for people trying to quit. Call

your local chapter of the American Lung Association, American Cancer Society or American Heart Association for further information. Toll free phone numbers are printed on the wallet card on the back cover of this User's Guide.

If you find you cannot stop smoking or if you start smoking again after using NicoDerm CQ, remember breaking this addiction doesn't happen overnight. You may want to talk to a health care professional who can help you improve your chances of quitting the next time you try NicoDerm CQ or another method.

LET'S GET ORGANIZED.

Your reason for quitting may be a combination of concerns about health, the effect of smoking on your appearance, and pressure from your family and friends to stop smoking. Or maybe you're concerned about the dangerous effect of second-hand smoke on the people you care about.

All of these are good reasons. You probably have others. Decide your most important reasons, and write them down on the wallet card inside the back cover of this User's Guide. Carry this card with you. In difficult moments, when you want to smoke, the card will remind you why you are quitting.

WHAT YOU'RE UP AGAINST.

Smoking is addictive in two ways. Your need for nicotine has become both physical and mental. You must overcome both addictions to stop smoking. So while NicoDerm CQ will lessen your body's craving for nicotine, you've got to want to quit smoking to overcome the mental dependence on cigarettes. Once you've decided that you're going to quit, it's time to get started. But first, there are some important cautions you should consider.

SOME IMPORTANT WARNINGS.

This product is only for those who want to stop smoking.

Do not use

- if you continue to smoke, chew tobacco, use snuff or use a nicotine gum or other nicotine products.

Ask a doctor before use if you have:

- heart disease, recent heart attack, or irregular heartbeat. Nicotine can increase your heart rate.
- high blood pressure not controlled with medication. Nicotine can increase your blood pressure.
- an allergy to adhesive tape or have skin problems because you are more likely to get rashes.

Ask a doctor or pharmacist before use if you are

- using a non-nicotine stop smoking drug
- taking a prescription medication for asthma or depression. Your prescription dose may need to be adjusted.

When using this product:

- do not smoke even when not wearing the patch. The nicotine in your skin will still be entering your bloodstream for several hours after you take off the patch.
- you have vivid dreams or other sleep disturbances remove this patch at bedtime.

Stop use and ask a doctor if:

- skin redness caused by the patch does not go away after four days, or if your skin swells or you get a rash.
- irregular heartbeat or palpitations occur
- you get symptoms of nicotine overdose, such as nausea, vomiting, dizziness, weakness and rapid heartbeat.

If pregnant or breast-feeding, ask a health professional before use. Nicotine can increase your baby's heart rate. First try to stop smoking without the nicotine patch.

Keep out of reach of children and pets. Used patches have enough nicotine to poison children and pets. If swallowed, get medical help or contact a Poison Control Center right away. Dispose of the used patches by folding sticky ends together and inserting in the disposal tray in this box.

LET'S GET STARTED.

If you are under 18 years of age, ask a doctor before use.

Becoming a non-smoker starts today. Your first step is to read through this entire User's Guide carefully.

First, check that you bought the right starting dose.

If you smoke more than 10 cigarettes a day, begin with Step 1 (21 mg). As the carton indicates, people who smoke 10 or less cigarettes per day should not use Step 1 (21 mg). They should start with Step 2 (14 mg). Throughout this User's Guide we will give specific instructions for people who smoke 10 or less cigarettes per day.

Next, set your personalized quitting schedule.

Take out a calendar that you can use to track your progress. Pick a quit date, and mark this on your calendar using the stickers in the middle of this User's Guide, as described below.

DIRECTIONS: FOR PEOPLE WHO SMOKE MORE THAN 10 CIGARETTES PER DAY

STEP 1. (Weeks 1–6). Your quit date (and the day you'll start using NicoDerm CQ patch).

Choose your quit date (it should be soon).

This is the day you will quit smoking cigarettes entirely and begin using NicoDerm CQ to reduce your cravings for nicotine. Place the Step 1 sticker on this date. For the first six weeks, you'll use the highest-strength (21 mg) NicoDerm CQ patches. Be sure to follow the directions on page 10.

Completing the full program will increase your chances of quitting successfully. This is done by changing over to the Step 1 (14mg) patch for 2 weeks followed by a final 2 weeks with the Step 3 (7mg) patch. The Step 2 and Step 3 treatment periods allow you to gradually reduce the amount of nicotine you get, rather than stopping suddenly, and will increase your chances of quitting.

STEP 2. (Weeks 7–8). The day you'll start reducing your use of NicoDerm CQ patch.

Switching to Step 2 (14mg) patches after 6 weeks begins to gradually reduce your nicotine usage. Place the Step 2 sticker on this date (the first day of week seven). Use the 14mg patches for two weeks.

STEP 3. (Weeks 9–10). The day you'll further start reducing your use of Nico-Derm CQ patch.

After eight weeks, nicotine intake is further reduced by moving down to Step 3 (7mg) patches. Place the Step 3 sticker on this date (the first day of week nine). Use the 7 mg patches for two weeks.

THE NICODERM CQ PROGRAM

STEP 1	STEP 2	STEP 3
Use one	Use one	Use one
21 mg patch/day	14 mg patch/day	7 mg patch/day
Weeks 1–6	Weeks 7–8	Weeks 9–10

STOP USING NICODERM CQ AT THE END OF WEEK 10. If you still feel the need to use the patch after Week 10, talk with your doctor or health professional.

DIRECTIONS: FOR PEOPLE WHO SMOKE 10 OR LESS CIGARETTES PER DAY

Do not use Step 1 (21 mg).

Begin with STEP 2 – Initial Treatment Period (Weeks 1–6): 14mg patches.

Choose our quit date (it should be soon). This is the Day you will quit smoking cigarettes entirely and begin using NicoDerm CQ to reduce your cravings for nicotine. Place the Step 2 sticker on this date. For the first six weeks, you'll use the Step 2 (14mg) NicoDerm CQ patches. Be sure to follow the directions on page 10.

Continue with STEP 3 – Step Down Treatment Period (Weeks 7–8): 7mg patches.

Completing the full program will increase your chances of quitting successfully. This is done by changing over to the Step 3 (7mg) patches for 2 weeks. The two week step down treatment period allows you to gradually reduce the amount of nicotine you get, rather than stopping suddenly, and will increase your chances of quitting. Place the Step 3 sticker on the first day of week seven. Use the 7mg patches for two weeks. People who smoke 10 or less cigarettes per day should not use NicoDerm CQ for longer than 8 weeks. If you still feel the need to use NicoDerm CQ after 8 weeks, talk with your doctor.

PLAN AHEAD.

Because smoking is an addiction, it is not easy to stop. After you've given up nicotine, you may still have a strong urge to smoke. Plan ahead NOW for these times, so you're not tempted to start smoking again in a moment of weakness. The following tips may help:

- Keep the phone numbers of supportive friends and family members handy.
- Keep a record of your quitting process. Track whether you feel a craving for cigarettes. In the event that you slip, immediately stop smoking and resume your quit attempt with the NicoDerm

Continued on next page

Nicoderm CQ—Cont.

CQ patch. If you smoke at all, write down what you think caused the slip.
- Put together an Emergency Kit that includes items that will help take your mind off occasional urges to smoke. You might include cinnamon gum or lemon drops to suck on, a relaxing cassette tape, and something for your hands to play with, like a smooth rock, rubber band or small metal balls.
- Set aside some small rewards, like a new magazine or a gift certificate from your favorite store, which you'll "give" yourself after passing difficult hurdles.
- Think now about the times when you most often want a cigarette, and then plan what else you might do instead of smoking. For instance, you might plan to take your coffee break in a new location, or take a walk right after dinner, so you won't be tempted to smoke.

HOW NICODERM CQ WORKS.

NicoDerm CQ patches provide nicotine to your system. They work as a temporary aid to help you quit smoking by reducing nicotine withdrawal symptoms, including nicotine craving. NicoDerm CQ provides a lower level of nicotine to your blood than cigarettes, and allows you to gradually do away with your body's need for nicotine.

Because NicoDerm CQ does not contain the tar or carbon monoxide of cigarette smoke, it does not have the same health dangers as tobacco. However, it still delivers nicotine, the addictive part of cigarette smoke. Nicotine can cause side effects such as headache, nausea, upset stomach, and dizziness.

HOW TO USE NICODERM CQ PATCHES.

Read all the following instructions, and the instructions on the outer carton, before using NicoDerm CQ. Refer to them often to make sure you're using NicoDerm CQ correctly. Please refer to the audio tape for additional help.
1) Stop smoking completely before you start using NicoDerm CQ.
2) To reduce nicotine craving and other withdrawal symptoms, use NicoDerm CQ according to the directions on pages 6–8.
3) Insert used NicoDerm CQ patches in the child resistant disposal tray provided in the box – safely away from children and pets.

When to apply and remove NicoDerm CQ patches.

Each day apply a new patch to a different place on skin that is dry, clean and hairless. **You can wear a NicoDerm CQ patch for either 16 or 24 hours.** If you crave cigarettes when you wake up, wear the patch for 24 hours. If you begin to have vivid dreams or other disruptions of your sleep while wearing the patch 24 hours, try taking the patch off at bedtime (after about 16 hours) and putting on a new one when you get up the next day.

Do not smoke even when you are not wearing the patch.

Remove the used patch and put on a new patch at the same time every day. Applying the patch at about the same time

PLACE THESE STICKERS ON YOUR CALENDAR

STEP 1	STEP 2
A new 21 mg patch every day AT THE BEGINNING OF WEEK #1 (QUIT DAY)	A new 14 mg patch every day AT THE BEGINNING OF WEEK #7

For people who smoke 10 or less cigarettes per day: Do not use STEP 1 (21 mg). Use STEP 2 (14 mg) at the beginning of week #1 and STEP 3 (7 mg) at the beginning of week #7.

PLACE THESE STICKERS ON YOUR CALENDAR

STEP 3	EX-SMOKER
A new 7 mg patch every day AT THE BEGINNING OF WEEK #9	WHEN YOU HAVE COMPLETED YOUR QUITTING PROGRAM

each day (first thing in the morning, for instance) will help you remember when to put on a new patch. Do not leave the same NicoDerm CQ patch on for more than 24 hours because it may irritate your skin and because it loses strength after 24 hours.

Do not use NicoDerm CQ continuously for more than 10 weeks (8 weeks for people who smoke 10 or less cigarettes per day).

How to apply a NicoDerm CQ patch.

1. Do not remove the NicoDerm CQ patch from its sealed protective pouch until you are ready to use it. NicoDerm CQ patches will lose nicotine to the air if you store them out of the pouch.
2. Choose a non-hairy, clean, dry area of skin. Do not put a NicoDerm CQ patch on skin that is burned, broken out, cut, or irritated in any way. Make sure your skin is free of lotion and soap before applying a patch.
3. A clear, protective liner covers the sticky back side of the NicoDerm CQ patch—the side that will be put on your skin. The liner has a slit down the middle to help you remove it from the patch. With the sticky back side facing you, pull half the liner away from the NicoDerm CQ patch starting at the middle slit, as shown in the illustration above. Hold the NicoDerm CQ patch at one of the outside edges (touch the sticky side as little as possible), and pull off the other half of the protective liner.

Place this liner in the slot in the disposable tray provided in the NicoDerm CQ package where it will be out of reach of children and pets.
4. Immediately apply the sticky side of the NicoDerm CQ patch to your skin. **Press the patch firmly on your skin with the heel of your hand for at least 10 seconds.** Make sure it sticks well to your skin, especially around the edges.
5. Wash your hands when you have finished applying the NicoDerm CQ patch. Nicotine on your hands could get into your eyes and nose, and cause stinging, redness, or more serious problems.
6. After 24 or 16 hours, remove the patch you have been wearing. Fold the used

NicoDerm CQ patch in half with the sticky side together. Carefully dispose of the used patch in the slot of the disposal tray provided in the NicoDerm CQ package where it will be out of the reach of children and pets. Even used patches have enough nicotine to poison children and pets. Wash your hands.
7. Chose a different place on your skin to apply the next NicoDerm CQ patch and repeat Steps 1 to 6. Do not apply a new patch to a previously used skin site for at least one week.

If your NicoDerm CQ patch gets wet during wearing.

Water will not harm the NicoDerm CQ patch you are wearing if applied properly. You can bathe, swim, or shower for short periods while you are wearing the NicoDerm CQ patch.

If your NicoDerm CQ patch comes off while wearing.

NicoDerm CQ patches generally stick well to most people's skin. However, a patch may occasionally come off. If your NicoDerm CQ patch falls off during the day, put on a new patch, making sure you select a non-hairy, non-irritated area of the skin that is clean and dry.

If the soap you use has lanolin or moisturizers, the patch may not stick well. Using a different soap may help. Body creams, lotions and sunscreens can also cause problems with keeping your patch on. Do not apply creams or lotions to the place on your skin where you will put the patch.

If you have followed the directions and the patch still does not stick to you, try using medical adhesive tape over the patch.

Disposing of NicoDerm CQ patches.

Fold the used patch in half with the sticky side together.

Carefully dispose of the patch in the disposal slot of the tray provided in the NicoDerm CQ package where it will be out of the reach of children and pets. Small amounts of nicotine, even from a used patch, can poison children and pets.

Keep all nicotine patches away from children and pets. Wash your hands after disposing of the patch.

If your skin reacts to the NicoDerm CQ patch.

When you first put on a NicoDerm CQ patch, mild itching, burning, or tingling is normal and should go away within an hour. After you remove a NicoDerm CQ patch, the skin under the patch might be somewhat red. Your skin should not stay red for more than a day after removing the patch. **Stop use and ask a doctor if skin redness caused by the patch does not go away after four days, or if your skin swells, or you get a rash. Do not put on a new patch.**

Storage Instructions

Keep each NicoDerm CQ patch in its protective pouch, unopened, until you are ready to use it, because the patch will lose nicotine to the air if it's outside the pouch.

Store NicoDerm CQ patches at 20–25 C (68–77 F) because they are sensitive to heat. Remember, the inside of your car can reach temperatures much higher

than this. A slight yellowing of the sticky side of the patch is normal. Do not use NicoDerm CQ patches stored in pouches that are open or torn.

TIPS TO MAKE QUITTING EASIER.

Within the first few weeks of giving up smoking, you may be tempted to smoke for pleasure, particularly after completing a difficult task, or at a party or bar. Hear are some tips to help get you through the important first stages of becoming a nonsmoker:

On Your Quit Date:

Ask your family, friends and co-workers to support you in your efforts to stop smoking.
- Throw away all your cigarettes, matches, lighters, ashtrays, etc.
- Keep busy on your quit day. Exercise. Go to a movie. Take a walk. Get together with friends.
- Figure out how much money you'll save by not smoking. Most ex-smokers can save more than $1,000 a year on the price of cigarettes alone.
- Write down what you will do with the money you save.
- Know your high risk situations and plan ahead how you will deal with them.
- Visit your dentist and have your teeth cleaned to get rid of the tobacco stains.

Right after Quitting:

- During the first few days after you've stopped smoking, spend as much time as possible at places where smoking is not allowed.
- Drink large quantities of water and fruit juices.
- Try to avoid alcohol, coffee and other beverages you associate with smoking.
- Remember that temporary urges to smoke will pass, even if you don't smoke a cigarette.
- Keep your hands busy with something like a pencil or a paper clip.
- Find other activities that help you relax without cigarettes. Swim, jog, take a walk, play basketball.

Don't worry too much about gaining weight. Watch what you eat, take time for daily exercise, and change your eating habits if you need to.
- Laughter helps. Watch or read something funny

WHAT TO EXPECT.

The First Few Days.

Your body is now coming back into balance. During the first few days after you stop smoking, you might feel edgy and nervous and have trouble concentrating. You might get headaches, feel dizzy and a little out of sorts, feel sweaty or have stomach upsets. You might even have trouble sleeping at first. These are typical nicotine withdrawal symptoms that will go away with time. Your smoker's cough will get worse before it gets better. But don't worry, that's a good sign. Coughing helps clear the tar deposits out of your lungs.

After A Week Or Two.

By now you should be feeling more confident that you can handle those smoking urges. Many of your nicotine withdrawal symptoms have left by now, and you should be noticing some positive

signs: less coughing, better breathing and an improved sense of taste and smell, to name a few.

After A Month.

You probably have the urge to smoke much less often now. But urges may still occur, and when they do, they are likely to be powerful ones that come out of nowhere. Don't let them catch you off guard. Plan ahead for these difficult times.

Concentrate on the ways non-smokers are more attractive than smokers. Their skin is less likely to wrinkle. Their teeth are whiter, cleaner. Their breath is fresher.

Their hair and clothes smell better. That cough that seems to make even a laugh sound more like a rattle is a thing of the past. Their children and others around them are healthier, too.

What To Do About Relapse.

What should you do if you slip and start smoking again? The answer is simple. A lapse of one or two or even a few cigarettes should not spoil your efforts! Throw away your cigarettes, forgive yourself and continue with the program. Listen to the Audio Tape again and re-read the User's Guide to ensure that you're using NicoDerm CQ correctly and following the other important tips for dealing with the mental and social dependence on nicotine. Your doctor, pharmacist or other health professional can also provide useful counseling on the importance of stopping smoking. You should consider them partners in your quit attempt.

What To Do About Relapse After a Successful Quit Attempt.

If you have taken up regular smoking again, don't be discouraged. Research shows that the best thing you can do is try again, since several quitting attempts may be needed before you're successful. And your chances of quitting successfully increase with each quit attempt.

The important thing is to learn from your last attempt.
- Admit that you've slipped, but don't treat yourself as a failure.
- Try to identify the "trigger" that caused you to slip, and prepare a better plan for dealing with this problem next time.
- Talk positively to yourself – tell yourself that you have learned something from this experience.
- Make sure you used NicoDerm CQ patches correctly
- Remember that it takes practice to do anything, and quitting smoking is no exception.

WHEN THE STRUGGLE IS OVER.

Once you've stopped smoking, take a second and pat yourself on your back. Now do it again. You deserve it. Remember now why you decided to stop smoking in the first place. Look at your list of reasons. Read them again. And smile.

Now think about all the money you are saving and what you'll do with it. All the non-smoking places you can go, and what you might do there. All those years

you may have added to your life, and what you'll do with them. Remember that temptation may not be gone forever. However, the hard part is behind you so look forward with a positive attitude, and enjoy your new life as a non-smoker.

QUESTIONS & ANSWERS

1. How will I feel when I stop smoking and start using NicoDerm CQ?

You'll need to prepare yourself for some nicotine withdrawal symptoms. These begin almost immediately after you stop smoking, and are usually at their worst during the first three or four days. Understand that any of the following is possible:
- craving for nicotine
- anxiety, irritability, restlessness, mood changes, nervousness
- disruptions of your sleep
- drowsiness
- trouble concentrating
- increased appetite and weight gain headaches, muscular pain, constipation, fatigue.

NicoDerm CQ reduces nicotine withdrawal symptoms such as irritability and nervousness, as well as the craving for nicotine you used to satisfy by having a cigarette.

2. Is NicoDerm CQ just substituting one form of nicotine for another?

NicoDerm CQ does contain nicotine. The purpose of NicoDerm CQ is to provide you with enough nicotine to reduce the physical withdrawal symptoms so you can deal with the mental aspects of quitting.

3. Can I be hurt by using NicoDerm CQ?

For most adults, the amount of nicotine delivered from the patch is less than from smoking. If you believe you may be sensitive to even this amount of nicotine, you should not use this product without advice from your doctor. There are also some important warnings in this User's Guide (See page 4).

4. Will I gain weight?

Many people do tend to gain a few pounds the first 8–10 weeks after they stop smoking. This is a very small price to pay for the enormous gains that you will make in your overall health and attractiveness. If you continue to gain weight after the first two months, try to analyze what you're doing differently. Reduce your fat intake, choose healthy snacks, and increase your physical activity to burn off the extra calories. Drink lots of water. This is good for your body and skin, and also helps to reduce the amount you eat.

5. Is NicoDerm CQ more expensive than smoking?

The total cost of NicoDerm CQ program is similar to what a person who smokes one and a half packs of cigarettes a day would spend on cigarettes for the same period of time. Also, use of NicoDerm CQ is only a short-term cost, while the cost of smoking is a long-term cost, including the health problems smoking causes.

6. What if I slip up?

Discard your cigarettes, forgive yourself and then get back on track. Don't con-

Continued on next page

Nicoderm CQ—Cont.

sider yourself a failure or punish yourself. In fact, people who have already tried to quit are more likely to be successful the next time.

GOOD LUCK!

WALLET CARD

My most important reasons to quit smoking are:

WALLET CARD

Where to call for Help:

American Lung Association	American Cancer Society	American Heart Association
800-586-4872	800-227-2345	800-242-8721

For people who smoke more than 10 cigarettes per day:

STEP 1	STEP 2	STEP 3
Use one	Use one	Use one
21 mg	14 mg	7 mg
patch/day	patch/day	patch/day
Weeks 1–6	Weeks 7–8	Weeks 9–10

People who smoke 10 or less cigarettes per day. Do not use STEP 1 (21 mg). Use STEP 2 (14 mg) for six weeks and STEP 3 (7 mg) for two weeks and then stop.

Copyright © 1999 SmithKline Beecham

For your family's protection, NicoDerm CQ patches are supplied in child resistant pouches. Do not use if individual pouch is open or torn.

Manufactured by ALZA Corporation, Mountain View, CA 94043 for SmithKline Beecham Consumer Healthcare, L.P.

Comments or Questions? Call 1–800–834–5895 Weekdays. (10 a.m.–4:30 p.m. EST).

- **Not for sale to those under 18 years of age.**
- **Proof of age required.**
- **Not for sale in vending machines or from any source where proof of age cannot be verified.**

Available as

NicoDerm CQ Step 1 (21 mg/24 hours)–7 Patches*

NicoDerm CQ Step 1 (21 mg/24 hours)–14 Patches*

NicoDerm 7 mg, 14 patches

NicoDerm CQ Step 2 (14 mg/24 hours)–7 Patches*

NicoDerm CQ Step 2 (14 mg/24 hours)–14 Patches

NicoDerm 14 mg, 14 patches

NicoDerm CQ Step 3 (7 mg/24 hours)–7 Patches**

NicoDerm CQ Step 3 (7 mg/24 hours)–14 Patches

NicoDerm 21 mg, 14 patches

* User's Guide, Audio Tape & Child Resistant Disposal Tray

** User's Guide, & Child Resistant Disposal Tray

Shown in Product Identification Guide, page 524

NICORETTE®
Nicotine Polacrilex Gum/Stop Smoking Aid
Available in Original 2mg and 4mg Strengths,
Mint 2mg and 4mg Strengths and Orange 2mg and 4mg Strengths

If you smoke:

UNDER 25 CIGARETTES A DAY: Use 2 mg

OVER 24 CIGARETTES A DAY: Use 4 mg

Action: Stop Smoking Aid

Use:
- To reduce withdrawal symptoms, including nicotine craving, associated with quitting smoking.

Directions:
- Stop smoking completely when you begin using Nicorette.
- Read the enclosed User's Guide before using Nicorette.
- Use properly as directed in the User's Guide.
- Don't eat or drink for 15 minutes before using Nicorette or while chewing a piece.
- Use according to the following 12 week schedule:

Weeks 1 to 6	Weeks 7 to 9	Weeks 10 to 12
1 piece every 1 to 2 hours	1 piece every 2 to 4 hours	1 piece every 4 to 8 hours

- Do not exceed 24 pieces a day.
- Stop using Nicorette at the end of week 12. If you still feel the need for Nicorette, talk with your doctor.

Warnings:
- Keep this and all drugs out of the reach of children and pets. In case of accidental overdose, seek professional assistance or contact a poison control center immediately.
- Nicotine can increase your baby's heart rate; if you are pregnant or nursing a baby, seek the advice of a health professional before using this product.

DO NOT USE IF YOU
- Continue to smoke, chew tobacco, use snuff, or use a nicotine patch or other nicotine containing products.

ASK YOUR DOCTOR BEFORE USE IF YOU
- Are under 18 years of age.
- Have heart disease, recent heart attack, or irregular heartbeat. Nicotine can increase your heart rate.
- Have high blood pressure not controlled with medication. Nicotine can increase blood pressure.
- Have stomach ulcer or take insulin for diabetes.
- Take prescription medicine for depression or asthma. Your prescription dose may need to be adjusted.

STOP USE AND SEE YOUR DOCTOR IF YOU HAVE:
- Mouth, teeth or jaw problems.
- Irregular heartbeat, palpitations.
- Symptoms of nicotine overdose such as nausea, vomiting, dizziness, weakness and rapid heartbeat.

READ THE LABEL

Read the carton and the User's Guide before taking this product. Do not discard carton or User's Guide. They contain important information.

Original [2 mg] Inactive Ingredients: Flavors, glycerin, gum base, sodium carbonate, sorbitol, sodium bicarbonate.

Original [4 mg] Inactive Ingredients: Flavors, glycerin, gum base, sodium carbonate, sorbitol, D&C Yellow 10.

Mint 2 mg Inactive Ingredients: Gum base, magnesium oxide, menthol, peppermint oil, sodium bicarbonate, sodium carbonate, xylitol.

Mint 4 mg Inactive Ingredients: Gum base, magnesium oxide, menthol, peppermint oil, sodium carbonate, xylitol, D&C yellow #10.

Do not store above 86°F (30°C). Protect from light.

Orange [2 mg] Inactive Ingredients: Flavor, gum base, magnesium oxide, sodium bicarbonate, sodium carbonate, xylitol

Orange [4 mg] Inactive Ingredients: Flavor, gum base, magnesium oxide, sodium carbonate, xylitol, D&C Yellow #10 AL. lake

TO INCREASE YOUR SUCCESS IN QUITTING:
1. **You must be motivated to quit.**
2. **Use Enough** —Chew **at least 9 pieces** of Nicorette per day during the first six weeks.
3. **Use long enough** —Use Nicorette for the full 12 weeks.
4. **Use with a support program** as described in the enclosed User's Guide.

USER'S GUIDE:
HOW TO USE NICORETTE TO HELP YOU QUIT SMOKING
KEYS TO SUCCESS:
1) You must really want to quit smoking for Nicorette to help you.
2) You can greatly increase your chances for success by using at least 9 to 12 pieces every day when you start using Nicorette.
3) You should continue to use Nicorette as explained in the User's Guide for 12 full weeks.
4) Nicorette works best when used together with a support program.
5) If you have trouble using Nicorette, ask your doctor or pharmacist or call SmithKline Beecham at 1-800-419-4766 weekdays (10:00am–4:30pm EST).

SO YOU DECIDED TO QUIT

Congratulations. Your decision to stop smoking is an important one. That's why you've made the right choice in choosing Nicorette gum. Your own chances of quitting smoking depend on how much you want to quit, how strongly you are addicted to tobacco, and how closely you follow a quitting program like the one that comes with Nicorette.

QUITTING SMOKING IS HARD!

If you've tried to quit before and haven't succeeded, don't be discouraged! Quitting isn't easy. It takes time, and most people try a few times before they are successful. The important thing is to try again until you succeed. This User's Guide will give you support as you become a non-smoker. It will answer com-

mon questions about Nicorette and give tips to help you stop smoking, and should be referred to often.

WHERE TO GET HELP

You are more likely to stop smoking by using Nicorette with a support program that helps you break your smoking habit. There may be support groups in your area for people trying to quit. Call your local chapter of the American Lung Association (1-800-586-4872), American Cancer Society (1-800-227-2345) or American Heart Association (1-800-242-8721) for further information. If you find you cannot stop smoking or if you start smoking again after using Nicorette, remember breaking this addiction doesn't happen overnight. You may want to talk to a health care professional who can help you improve your chances of quitting the next time you try Nicorette or another method.

LET'S GET ORGANIZED

Your reason for quitting may be a combination of concerns about health, the effect of smoking on your appearance, and pressure from your family and friends to stop smoking. Or maybe you're concerned about the dangerous effect of second-hand smoke on the people you care about. All of these are good reasons. You probably have others. Decide your most important reasons, and write them down on the wallet card inside the back cover of the User's Guide. Carry this card with you. In difficult moments, when you want to smoke, the card will remind you why you are quitting.

WHAT YOU'RE UP AGAINST

Smoking is addictive in two ways. Your need for nicotine has become both physical and mental. You must overcome both addictions to stop smoking. So while Nicorette will lessen your body's physical addition to nicotine, you've got to want to quit smoking to overcome the mental dependence on cigarettes. Once you've decided that you're going to quit, it's time to get started. But first, there are some important cautions you should consider.

SOME IMPORTANT CAUTIONS

This product is only for those who want to stop smoking. Do not smoke, chew tobacco, use snuff or nicotine patches while using Nicorette. If you have heart disease, a recent heart attack, irregular heartbeats, palpitations, high blood pressure not controlled with medication, stomach ulcer, or take insulin for diabetes, ask your doctor whether you should use Nicorette. As with any drug, if you are pregnant or nursing a baby, seek the advice of a health professional before using this product. If you take a prescription medication for asthma or depression, be sure your doctor knows you are quitting smoking. Your prescription medication dose may need to be adjusted. Those under 18 should use this product under a doctor's care. Symptoms of nicotine overdose may include vomiting and diarrhea. Young children are more likely to have additional symptoms, including weakness. Also, seizures have been seen in children who swallowed cigarettes. Keep this and all drugs out of the reach of children. In case of accidental overdose, seek professional assistance or contact a poison control center immediately.

LET'S GET STARTED

Becoming a non-smoker starts today. Your first step is to read through the entire User's Guide carefully. **Next, set your personalized quitting schedule.** Take out a calendar that you can use to track your progress, and identify four dates, using the stickers in the User's Guide.

STEP 1: Your quit date (and the day you'll start using Nicorette gum). Choose your quit date (it should be soon). This is the day you will quit smoking cigarettes entirely and begin using Nicorette to satisfy your craving for nicotine. For the first six weeks, you'll use a piece of Nicorette every hour or two. Be sure to follow the directions on pages 8 and 11 of the User's Guide. Place the Step 1 sticker on this date.

STEP 2: The day you'll start reducing your use of Nicorette. After six weeks, you'll begin gradually reducing your Nicorette usage to one piece every two to four hours. Place the Step 2 sticker on this date (the first day of week seven).

STEP 3: The day you'll further reduce your use of Nicorette. Nine weeks after you begin using Nicorette, you will further reduce your nicotine intake by using one piece every four to eight hours. Place the Step 3 sticker on this date (the first day of week ten). For the next three weeks, you'll use a piece of Nicorette every four to eight hours. **End of treatment: The day you'll complete Nicorette therapy.** Nicorette should not be used for longer than twelve weeks. Identify the date thirteen weeks after the date you chose in Step 1 and place the "EX-Smoker" sticker on your calendar.

PLAN AHEAD

Because smoking is an addiction, it is not easy to stop. After you've given up cigarettes, you will still have a strong urge to smoke. Plan ahead NOW for these times, so you're not defeated in a moment of weakness. The following tips may help:

- Keep the phone numbers of supportive friends and family members handy.
- Keep a record of your quitting process. Track the number of Nicorette pieces you use each day, and whether you feel a craving for cigarettes. If you smoke at all, write down what you think caused the slip.
- Put together an Emergency Kit that includes items that will help take your mind off occasional urges to smoke. Include cinnamon gum or lemon drops to suck on, a relaxing cassette tape and something for your hands to play with, like a smooth rock, rubber band or small metal balls.
- Set aside some small rewards, like a new magazine or a gift certificate from your favorite store, which you'll 'give' yourself after passing difficult hurdles.
- Think now about the times when you most often want a cigarette, and then plan what else you might do instead of smoking. For instance, you might plan to take your coffee break in a new location, or take a walk right after dinner, so you won't be tempted to smoke.

HOW NICORETTE GUM WORKS

Nicorette's sugar-free chewing pieces provide nicotine to your system—they work as a temporary aid to help you quit smoking by reducing nicotine withdrawal symptoms. Nicorette provides a lower level of nicotine to your blood than cigarettes, and allows you to gradually do away with your body's need for nicotine. Because Nicorette does not contain the tar or carbon monoxide of cigarette smoke, it does not have the same health dangers as tobacco. However, it still delivers nicotine, the addictive part of cigarette smoke. Nicotine can cause side effects such as headache, nausea, upset stomach and dizziness.

HOW TO USE NICORETTE GUM

Before you can use Nicorette correctly, you have to practice! That sounds silly, but it isn't.

Nicorette isn't like ordinary chewing gum. It's a medicine, and must be chewed a certain way to work right. Chewed like ordinary gum, Nicorette won't work well and can cause side effects. An overdose can occur if you chew more than one piece of Nicorette at the same time, or if you chew many pieces one after another. Read all the following instructions before using Nicorette. Refer to them often to make sure you're using Nicorette gum correctly. If you chew too fast, or do not chew correctly, you may get hiccups, heartburn, or other stomach problems.

1. Stop smoking completely before you start using Nicorette.
2. To reduce craving and other withdrawal symptoms, use Nicorette according to the dosage schedule on page 11 of the User's Guide.
3. Chew each Nicorette piece <u>very slowly several times.</u>
4. Stop chewing when you notice a peppery taste, or a slight tingling in your mouth. (This usually happens after about 15 chews, but may vary from person to person.)
5. "PARK" the Nicorette piece between your cheek and gum and leave it there.
6. When the peppery taste or tingle is almost gone (in about a minute), start to chew a few times slowly again. When the taste or tingle returns, stop again.
7. Park the Nicorette piece again (in a different place in your mouth).
8. Repeat steps 3 to 7 (chew, chew, park) until most of the nicotine is gone from the Nicorette piece (usually happens in about half an hour; the peppery taste or tingle won't return).
9. Throw away the used Nicorette piece, safely away from children and pets.

See the chart in the **"DIRECTIONS"** section above for the recommended usage schedule for Nicorette.

To improve your chances of quitting, use at least 9 pieces of Nicorette a day. Heavier smokers may need more pieces to reduce their cravings. Don't eat or

Continued on next page

Nicorette—Cont.

drink for 15 minutes before using Nicorette or while chewing a piece. The effectiveness of Nicorette may be reduced by some foods and drinks, such as coffee, juices, wine or soft drinks.

HOW TO REDUCE YOUR NICORETTE USAGE

The goal of using Nicorette is to slowly reduce your dependence on nicotine. The schedule for using Nicorette will help you reduce your nicotine craving gradually. Here are some tips to help you cut back during each step:

- After a while, start chewing each Nicorette piece for only 10 to 15 minutes, instead of half an hour. Then gradually begin to reduce the number of pieces used.
- Or, try chewing each piece for longer than half an hour, but reduce the number of pieces you use each day.
- Substitute ordinary chewing gum for some of the Nicorette pieces you would normally use. Increase the number of pieces of ordinary gum as you cut back on the Nicorette pieces.

STOP USING NICORETTE AT THE END OF WEEK 12. If you still feel the need to use Nicorette after Week 12, talk with your doctor.

TIPS TO MAKE QUITTING EASIER

Within the first few weeks of giving up smoking, you may be tempted to smoke for pleasure, particularly after completing a difficult task, or at a party or bar. Here are some tips to help get you through the important first stages of becoming a non-smoker:

On your Quit Date:

- Ask your family, friends, and co-workers to support you in your efforts to stop smoking.
- Throw away all your cigarettes, matches, lighters, ashtrays, etc.
- Keep busy on your quit day. Exercise. Go to a movie. Take a walk. Get together with friends.
- Figure out how much money you'll save by not smoking. Most ex-smokers can save more than $1,000 a year.
- Write down what you will do with the money you save.
- Know your high risk situations and plan ahead how you will deal with them.
- Keep Nicorette gum near your bed, so you'll be prepared for any nicotine cravings when you wake up in the morning.
- Visit your dentist and have your teeth cleaned to get rid of the tobacco stains.

Right after Quitting:

- During the first few days after you've stopped smoking, spend as much time as possible at places where smoking is not allowed.
- Drink large quantities of water and fruit juices.
- Try to avoid alcohol, coffee and other beverages you associate with smoking.
- Remember that temporary urges to smoke will pass, even if you don't smoke a cigarette.
- Keep your hands busy with something like a pencil or a paper clip.
- Find other activities which help you relax without cigarettes. Swim, jog, take a walk, play basketball.

- Don't worry too much about gaining weight. Watch what you eat, take time for daily exercise, and change your eating habits if you need to.
- Laughter helps. Watch or read something funny.

WHAT TO EXPECT

Your body is now coming back into balance. During the first few days after you stop smoking, you might feel edgy and nervous and have trouble concentrating. You might get headaches, feel dizzy and a little out of sorts, feel sweaty or have stomach upsets. You might even have trouble sleeping at first. These are typical withdrawal symptoms that will go away with time. Your smoker's cough will get worse before it gets better. But don't worry, that's a good sign. Coughing helps clear the tar deposits out of your lungs.

After a Week or Two.

By now you should be feeling more confident that you can handle those smoking urges. Many of your withdrawal symptoms have left by now, and you should be noticing some positive signs: less coughing, better breathing and an improved sense of taste and smell, to name a few.

After a Month.

You probably have the urge to smoke much less often now. But urges may still occur, and when they do, they are likely to be powerful ones that come out of nowhere. Don't let them catch you off guard. Plan ahead for these difficult times. Concentrate on the ways non-smokers are more attractive than smokers. Their skin is less likely to wrinkle. Their teeth are whiter, cleaner. Their breath is fresher. Their hair and clothes smell better. That cough seems to make even a laugh sound more like a rattle is a thing of the past. Their children and others around them are healthier, too.

What To Do About Relapse.

What should you do if you slip and start smoking again? The answer is simple. A lapse of one or two or even a few cigarettes has not spoiled your efforts! Discard your cigarettes, forgive yourself and try again. If you start smoking again, keep your box of Nicorette for your next quit attempt. If you have taken up regular smoking again, don't be discouraged. Research shows that the best thing you can do is to try again. The important thing is to learn from your last attempt.

- Admit that you've slipped, but don't treat yourself as a failure.
- Try to identify the 'trigger' that caused you to slip, and prepare a better plan for dealing with this problem next time.
- Talk positively to yourself—tell yourself that you have learned something from this experience.
- Make sure you used Nicorette gum correctly over the full 12 weeks to reduce your craving for nicotine.
- Remember that it takes practice to do anything, and quitting smoking is no exception.

WHEN THE STRUGGLE IS OVER

Once you've stopped smoking, take a second and pat yourself on the back. Now do

it again. You deserve it. Remember now why you decided to stop smoking in the first place. Look at your list of reasons. Read them again. And smile. Now think about all the money you are saving and what you'll do with it. All the non-smoking places you can go, and what you might do there. All those years you may have added to your life, and what you'll do with them. Remember that temptation may not be gone forever. However, the hard part is behind you, so look forward with a positive attitude and enjoy your new life as a non-smoker.

QUESTIONS & ANSWERS

1. How will I feel when I stop smoking and start using Nicorette? You'll need to prepare yourself for some nicotine withdrawal symptoms. These begin almost immediately after you stop smoking, and are usually at their worst during the first three to four days. Understand that any of the following is possible:

- craving for cigarettes
- anxiety, irritability, restlessness, mood changes, nervousness
- drowsiness
- trouble concentrating
- increased appetite and weight gain
- headaches, muscular pain, constipation, fatigue.

Nicorette can help provide relief from withdrawal symptoms such as irritability and nervousness, as well as the craving for nicotine you used to satisfy by having a cigarette.

2. Is Nicorette just substuting one form of nicotine for another? Nicorette does contain nicotine. The purpose of Nicorette is to provide you with enough nicotine to help control the physical withdrawal symptoms so you can deal with the mental aspects of quitting. During the 12 week program, you will gradually reduce your nicotine intake by switching to fewer pieces each day. Remember, don't use Nicorette together with nicotine patches or other nicotine containing products.

3. Can I be hurt by using Nicorette? For most adults, the amount of nicotine in the gum is less than from smoking. Some people will be sensitive to even this amount of nicotine and should not use this product without advice from their doctor. Because Nicorette is a gum-based product, chewing it can cause dental fillings to loosen and aggravate other mouth, tooth and jaw problems. Nicorette can also cause hiccups, heartburn and other stomach problems especially if chewed too quickly or not chewed correctly.

4. Will I gain weight? Many people do tend to gain a few pounds in the first 8–10 weeks after they stop smoking. This is a very small price to pay for the enormous gains that you will make in your overall health and attractiveness. If you continue to gain weight after the first two months, try to analyze what you're doing differently. Reduce your fat intake, choose healthy snacks, and increase your physical activity to burn off the extra calories.

5. Is Nicorette more expensive than smoking? The total cost of Nicorette for the twelve week program is about equal to what a person who smokes one and a half packs of cigarettes a day would spend on cigarettes for the same period of time. Also use of Nicorette is only a

short-term cost, while the cost of smoking is a long-term cost, because of the health problems smoking causes.

6. What if I slip up? Discard your cigarettes, forgive yourself and then get back on track. Don't consider yourself a failure or punish yourself. In fact, people who have already tried to quit are more likely to be successful the next time.

GOOD LUCK!

[End User's Guide]
Copyright © 1999 SmithKline Beecham

To remove the gum, tear off a single unit.
Peel off backing starting at corner with loose edge.
Push gum through foil.

Blister packaged for your protection. Do not use if individual seals are broken.
Manufactured by Pharmacia & Upjohn AB, Stockholm, Sweden for SmithKline Beecham Consumer Healthcare, LP Pittsburgh, PA 15230
Comments or Questions? Call 1-800-419-4766 weekdays.
(10 a.m.–4:30 p.m. EST).

• **Not for sale to those under 18 years of age.**
• **Proof of age required.**
• **Not for sale in vending machines or from any source where proof of age cannot be verified.**

Nicorette Original, Mint, and Orange are available in:
 2 mg or 4 mg Starter kit*—108 pieces
 2 mg or 4 mg Refill—48 pieces
*User's Guide and Audio Tape included in kit

Shown in Product Identification Guide, page 524

SINGLET® For Adults
Nasal Decongestant/Antihistamine/Analgesic (pain reliever)/Antipyretic (fever reducer)

Indications: For temporary relief of nasal congestion and sinus and headache pain associated with sinusitis or due to a cold, hay fever or other upper respiratory allergies. Also temporarily relieves nasal congestion, sinus headache, runny nose, sneezing, itching of the nose or throat, and itchy, watery eyes due to hay fever or other upper respiratory allergies. Also temporarily relieves fever due to the common cold.

Directions: Adults (12 years and older): 1 caplet every 4 to 6 hours, **not to exceed 4 caplets in any 24-hour period,** or as directed by a doctor. Children under 12 years of age: Consult a doctor.

Warnings: Do not exceed recommended dosage. If nervousness, dizziness, or sleeplessness occur, discontinue use and consult a doctor. Do not take this product for more than 10 days. If symptoms do not improve or are accompanied by fever that lasts for more than 3 days, or if new symptoms occur, consult a doctor. Do not take this product, unless directed by a doctor, if you have a breathing problem such as emphysema or chronic bronchitis, or if you have heart disease, high blood pressure, thyroid disease, diabetes, glaucoma or difficulty in urination due to enlargement of the prostate gland. May cause excitability especially in children. May cause drowsiness; alcohol, sedatives, and tranquilizers may increase the drowsiness effect. Avoid alcoholic beverages while taking this product. Do not take this product if you are taking sedatives or tranquilizers, without first consulting your doctor. Use caution when driving a motor vehicle or operating machinery. **KEEP THIS AND ALL DRUGS OUT OF THE REACH OF CHILDREN.** Prompt medical attention is critical for adults as well as for children even if you do not notice any signs or symptoms. In case of accidental overdose, seek professional assistance or contact a Poison Control Center immediately. As with any drug, if you are pregnant or nursing a baby, seek the advice of a health professional before using this product.

Alcohol Warning: If you consume 3 or more alcoholic drinks every day, ask your doctor whether you should take acetaminophen or other pain reliever/fever reducers. Acetaminophen may cause liver damage.

Drug Interaction Precaution: Do not use this product if you are now taking a prescription monoamine oxidase inhibitor (MAOI) (certain drugs for depression, psychiatric or emotional conditions, or Parkinson's disease), or for 2 weeks after stopping the MAOI drug. If you are uncertain whether your prescription drug contains an MAOI, consult a health professional before taking this product.

Active Ingredients: Each caplet contains: Pseudoephedrine Hydrochloride 60 mg, Chlorpheniramine Maleate 4 mg, Acetaminophen 650 mg.

Inactive Ingredients: D&C Red 27, D&C Yellow 10, FD&C Blue 1, Hydroxypropyl Cellulose, Hydroxypropyl Methylcellulose, Magnesium Stearate, Microcrystalline Cellulose, Polyethylene Glycol, Pregelatinized Corn Starch, Sodium Starch Glycolate, Sucrose and Titanium Dioxide.
Store at room temperature (59°–86°F). Avoid excessive heat and humidity.
Comments or Questions? Call toll-free 1-800-245-1040 weekdays
Distributed by: SmithKline Beecham Consumer Healthcare, L.P.
Pittsburgh, PA 15230. Made in U.S.A.

SOMINEX Original Formula
Nighttime Sleep Aid
Doctor-preferred sleep ingredient

Indications: Helps to reduce difficulty falling asleep.

Directions: Adults and children 12 years and over: Take 2 tablets at bedtime if needed, or as directed by a doctor. For best results, take recommended dose. This will provide approximately six to eight hours of restful sleep.

Warnings: Do not give to children under 12 years of age. If sleeplessness persists continually for more than 2 weeks, consult your doctor. Insomnia may be a symptom of serious underlying medical illness. Do not take this product, unless directed by a doctor, if you have a breathing problem such as emphysema or chronic bronchitis, or if you have glaucoma or difficulty in urination due to enlargement of the prostate gland. Avoid alcoholic beverages while taking this product. Do not take this product if you are taking sedatives or tranquilizers, without first consulting your doctor. As with any drug, if you are pregnant or nursing a baby, seek the advice of a health professional before using this product. **Keep this and all drugs out of the reach of children.** In case of accidental overdose, seek professional assistance or contact a poison control center immediately.

Active Ingredients: Each tablet contains 25 mg Diphenhydramine HCl.

Inactive Ingredients: Dibasic Calcium Phosphate, FD&C Blue #1, Magnesium Stearate, Microcrystalline Cellulose, Silicon Dioxide, Starch.
Tamper Evident Feature: Individually sealed in foil for your protection. Do not use if foil or plastic bubble is torn or punctured.
Store at room temperature, avoid excessive heat (greater than 100°F) or humidity.

How Supplied: Consumer Packages of 16, 32 and 72 tablets
Also Available in Maximum Strength and Pain Relief Formulas.
Comments or Questions? Call Toll-Free 1-800-245-1040 Weekdays.
SmithKline Beecham Consumer Healthcare, L.P.
Pittsburgh, PA 15230. Made in U.S.A.

TAGAMET HB® 200
Cimetidine Tablets 200 mg/
Acid Reducer

Tagamet HB® 200 relieves and prevents heartburn, acid indigestion and sour stomach when used as directed. It contains the same ingredient found in prescription strength Tagamet. Tagamet HB 200 reduces the production of stomach acid.

Active Ingredient: Cimetidine, 200 mg.

Inactive Ingredients: cellulose, cornstarch, hydroxypropyl methylcellulose, magnesium stearate, polyethylene glycol, polysorbate 80, povidone, sodium lauryl sulfate, sodium starch glycolate, titanium dioxide.

continued on next page

Tagamet HB 200—Cont.

Uses:
- For relief of heartburn associated with acid indigestion and sour stomach.
- For prevention of heartburn associated with acid indigestion and sour stomach brought on by eating or drinking certain food and beverages.

Directions:
- For **relief** of symptoms, swallow 1 tablet with a glass of water.
- For **prevention** of symptoms, swallow 1 tablet with a glass of water **right before or anytime up to 30 minutes before** eating food or drinking beverages that cause heartburn.
- Tagamet HB 200 can be used up to twice daily (up to 2 tablets in 24 hours).
- This product should not be given to children under 12 years old unless directed by a doctor.

Warnings:
Allergy Warning: Do not use if you are allergic to Tagamet HB 200 (cimetidine) or other acid reducers.
Ask a Doctor Before Use If You are Taking:
- theophylline (oral asthma medicine)
- warfarin (blood thinning medicine)
- phenytoin (seizure medicine)

If you are not sure whether your medication contains one of these drugs or have any other questions about medicines you are taking, call our consumer affairs specialist at 1-800-482-4394.
- Do not take the maximum daily dosage for more than 2 weeks continuously except under the advice and supervision of a doctor.
- If you have trouble swallowing, or persistent abdominal pain, see your doctor promptly. You may have a serious condition that may need a different treatment.
- As with any drug, if you are pregnant or nursing a baby, seek the advice of a health professional before using this product.
- Keep this and all medications out of the reach of children.
- In case of accidental overdose, seek professional assistance or contact a poison control center immediately.

Read The label
Read the directions and warnings before taking this medication.
Store at 15°–30°C (59°–86°F).
Comments or questions? Call Toll-Free 1-800-482-4394 weekdays.

Pharmacokinetic Interactions:
Cimetidine at prescription doses is known to inhibit various P450 metabolizing isoenzymes, which could affect metabolism of other drugs and increase their blood concentration. Investigation of pharmacokinetic interactions at the recommended OTC doses of cimetidine have thus far shown only small effects. A pharmacokinetic study conducted in 26 normal male subjects (mean age, 38 years) at steady state using the maximum recommended OTC dose level (200 mg twice a day), showed that Tagamet HB 200, on average, increased the 24 hour AUC of theophylline by 14% and increased peak theophylline levels by 15%.

This interaction should be borne in mind in advising patients on the use of Tagamet HB 200. At the prescription doses of cimetidine, clinically significant pharmacokinetic interactions between cimetidine and warfarin, phenytoin, and theophylline have been reported. At prescription doses, pharmacokinetic interactions have been reported for a number of other drugs as well, such as with dihydropyridine calcium channel blockers or some short acting benzodiazepines. At the maximum recommended OTC dose level (200 mg twice a day), a pharmacokinetic study conducted in 21 normal male subjects (mean age, 38 years) showed that Tagamet HB 200, on average, increased the total AUC of triazolam by 26–28% and increased peak triazolam levels by 11–23%. Tagamet HB 200 did not alter the apparent terminal elimination half-life of triazolam.

This labeling information is current as of October 30, 1999.

How Supplied: Tagamet HB 200 (Cimetidine Tablets 200 mg) is available in boxes of blister packs in 6, 12, 18, 30, 50, 70 & 80 tablet sizes.

Shown in Product Identification Guide, page 525

TAGAMET HB® 200
Cimetidine Suspension 200 mg
Acid Reducer

Tagamet HB® 200 relieves and prevents heartburn, acid indigestion and sour stomach. When used as directed. It contains the same ingredient found in prescription strength Tagamet. Tagamet HB® 200 reduces the production of stomach acid.

Active Ingredient: Cimetidine, 200 mg.

Uses:
- relieves heartburn associated with acid indigestion and sour stomach
- prevents heartburn associated with acid indigestion and sour stomach brought on by eating or drinking certain food and beverages.

Warnings
Allergy alert: Do not use if you are allergic to cimetidine or other acid reducers.
Do not use
- in children under 12 years (see **Directions**)
- if you have trouble swallowing
- with other acid reducers
Ask a doctor or pharmacist before use if you are taking
- **theophylline (oral asthma medicine)**
- **warfarin (blood thinning medicine)**
- **phenytoin (seizure medicine)**
If you are not sure you are taking one of these medicines, talk to your doctor or pharmacist.
Stop use and ask a doctor if
- stomach pain continues
- you need to take this product for more than 14 days
If pregnant or breast-feeding, ask a health professional before use.
Keep out of reach of children.

In case of overdose, get medical help or contact a Poison Control Center right away.

Directions:
- shake well
- adults and children 12 years and over:
  - to **relieve** symptoms, take 4 teaspoons (20 mL) in pre-measured dose cup provided, with a glass of water
  - to **prevent** symptoms, take 4 teaspoons (20 mL) in pre-measured dose cup provided, with a glass of water **right before or any time up to 30 minutes before** eating food or drinking beverages that cause heartburn
  - do not take more than 4 teaspoons twice in 24 hours
  - children under 12 years: **not for use in children under 12. The safety and effectiveness for use in children under 12 has not been proven.**

Other Information:
- store at 20–30°C (68–86°F)

Inactive Ingredients butylparaben, FD&C blue #1, flavors, microcrystalline cellulose and carboxymethylcellulose sodium, propylene glycol, propylparaben, purified water, saccharin sodium, sucrose, xanthan gum

Pharmacokinetic Interactions Cimetidine at prescription doses is known to inhibit various P450 metabolizing isoenzymes, which could affect metabolism of other drugs and increase their blood concentration. Investigation of pharmacokinetic interactions at the recommended OTC does of cimetidine have thus far shown only small effects. A pharmacokinetic study conducted in 26 normal male subjects (mean age, 38 years) at steady state using the maximum recommended OTC dose level (200 mg twice a day), on average, increased the 24 hour AUC of theophylline by 14% and increased peak theophylline levels by 15%. This interaction should be borne in mind in advising patients on the use of Tagamet HB 200. At the prescription doses of cimetidine, clinically significant pharmacokinetic interactions between cimetidine and warfarin, phenytoin, and theophylline have been reported. At prescription doses, pharmacokinetic interactions have been reported for a number of other drugs as well, such as with dihydropyridine calcium channel blockers or some short acting benzodiazepines. At the maximum recommended OTC dose level (200 mg twice a day), a pharmacokinetic study conducted in 21 normal male subjects (mean age, 38 years) showed that Tagamet HB 200, on average, increased the total AUC of triazolam by 26–28% and increased peak triazolam levels by 11–23%. The apparent terminal elimination half life of triazolam was not altered at this dosage.

Shown in Product Identification Guide, page 525

TUMS® Regular Antacid/Calcium Supplement Tablets
TUMS E–X® and TUMS E–X® Sugar Free Antacid/Calcium Supplement Tablets
TUMS ULTRA® Antacid/Calcium Supplement Tablets

Professional Labeling: Indicated for the symptomatic relief of hyperacidity associated with the diagnosis of peptic ulcer, gastritis, peptic esophagitis, gastric hyperacidity, and hiatal hernia.

Indications: For fast relief of acid indigestion, heartburn, sour stomach, and upset stomach associated with these symptoms.

Active Ingredient:
Tums, Calcium Carbonate 500 mg
Tums E-X, Calcium Carbonate 750 mg
Tums ULTRA, Calcium Carbonate 1000 mg

Actions: Tums provides rapid neutralization of stomach acid. Each Tums tablet has an acid-neutralizing capacity (ANC) of 10 mEq. Each Tums E-X tablet has an ANC of 15 mEq and each Tums ULTRA tablet, an ANC of 20 mEq. This high neutralization capacity makes Tums tablets an ideal antacid for management of conditions associated with hyperacidity. It effectively neutralizes free acid yet does not cause systemic alkalosis in the presence of normal renal function. A double-blind placebo-controlled clinical study demonstrated that calcium carbonate taken at a dosage of 16 Tums tablets daily for a two-week period was non-constipating/non-laxative.

Warnings: Tums: Do not take more than 15 tablets in a 24-hour period or use the maximum dosage of this product for more than 2 weeks, except under the advice and supervision of a physician. If symptoms persist for 2 weeks, stop using this product and see a physician. Keep this and all drugs out of the reach of children.
Tums E-X: Do not take more than 10 tablets in a 24-hour period or use the maximum dosage of this product for more than two weeks, except under the advice and supervision of a physician. If symptoms persist for two weeks, stop using this product and see a physician. Keep this and all drugs out of the reach of children.
Additionally, for Tums E-X Sugar Free: Phenylketonurics: Contains phenylalanine, less than 1 mg per tablet.
Tums ULTRA: Do not take more than 7 tablets in 24-hour period or use the maximum dosage of this product for more than two weeks, except under the advice and supervision of a physician. If symptoms persist for two weeks, stop using and see a physician. Keep this and all drugs out of the reach of children.

Drug Interaction Precaution: Antacids may interact with certain prescription drugs. If you are presently taking a prescription drug, do not take this product without checking with your physician or other health professional.

Supplement Facts

	Tums	Tums E-X	Tums E-X Sugar Free	Tums Ultra
Serving Size	2 Tablets	2 Tablets	2 Tablets	2 Tablets
Amount Per Serving				
Calories	5	10	5	10
Sorbitol (g)	—	—	1	—
Sugars (g)	1	2	—	3
Calcium (mg)	400	600	600	800
% Daily Value	40	60	60	80
Sodium (mg)	—	5	—	10
% Daily Value	—	<1%	—	<1%

Dosage and Administration:
Tums: Chew 2-4 tablets as symptoms occur. Repeat hourly if symptoms return, or as directed by physician.
Tums E-X: Chew 2-4 tablets as symptoms occur. Repeat hourly if symptoms return, or as directed by a physician.
Tums ULTRA: Chew 2-3 tablets as symptoms occur. Repeat hourly if symptoms return, or as directed by a physician.

AS A DIETARY SUPPLEMENT: Calcium Supplement Directions
Tums, Tums E-X, & Tums ULTRA:
USES: As a daily source of extra calcium. Tums is recommended by the National Osteoporosis Foundation.

IMPORTANT INFORMATION ON OSTEOPOROSIS: Research shows that certain ethnic, age and other groups are at higher risk for developing osteoporosis, including Caucasian and Asian teen and young adult women, menopausal women, older persons and those persons with a family history of fragile bones. **A balanced diet with enough calcium and regular exercise throughout life will help you to build and maintain healthy bones and may reduce your risk of developing osteoporosis.** Adequate calcium intake is important, but daily intakes above 2,000 mg are not likely to provide any additional benefit.

DIRECTIONS: Chew 2 tablets twice daily.
[See table above]

Ingredients (all variants except sugar free): Sucrose, Corn Starch, Talc, Mineral Oil, Flavors (natural and/or artificial), Sodium Polyphosphate. May also contain 1% or less of Adipic Acid, Blue 1 Lake, Yellow 6 Lake, Yellow 5 Lake, Red 40 Lake.

Ingredients (Sugar Free): Sorbitol, Acacia, Natural and Artificial Flavors, Calcium Stearate, Adipic Acid, Yellow 6 Lake, Aspartame.

How Supplied:
Tums: Peppermint flavor is available in 12-tablet rolls, 3-roll wraps, and bottles of 75, 150, and 180. **Assorted Flavors** (Cherry, Lemon, Orange, and Lime), are available in 12-tablet rolls, 3-roll wraps, and bottles of 75, 150, 180, and 400.
Tums E-X: Wintergreen 3-roll wraps and bottles of 48, 96, and 116.

Tums E-X: Assorted Fruit, Assorted Tropical Fruit, and Assorted Berries, Fresh Blend 8 tablet rolls, 3-roll wraps, 6-roll wraps, and bottles of 48, 96, and 116. Assorted Tropical Fruit and Assorted Berries are also available in bottles of 250 tablets.
Tums EX Sugar Free: Orange Cream; bottles of 48 and 96 tablets.
Tums ULTRA: Assorted Berries, and **Spearmint** bottles of 160 tablets. **Assorted Fruit** and **Assorted Mint** bottles of 36, 72, and 86 tablets. Assorted Fruit also available in bottles of 160 tablets. **Tropical Fruit** bottles of 160 tablets.
Shown in Product Identification Guide, page 525

VIVARIN Tablets & Caplets Alertness Aid with Caffeine Maximum Strength

Each Tablet or Caplet Contains 200 mg. Caffeine, Equal to About Two Cups of Coffee
Take Vivarin for a safe, fast pick up anytime you feel drowsy and need to be alert. The caffeine in Vivarin is less irritating to your stomach than coffee, according to a government appointed panel of experts.

FDA APPROVED USES: Helps restore mental alertness or wakefulness when experiencing fatigue or drowsiness.

Active Ingredients: Caffeine 200 mg.

Inactive Ingredients: Tablet: Colloidal Silicon Dioxide, D&C Yellow #10 Al. Lake, Dextrose, FD&C Yellow #6 Al. Lake, Magnesium Stearate, Microcrystalline Cellulose, Starch.
Caplet: Carnauba Wax, Colloidal Silicon Dioxide, D&C Yellow #10 Al Lake, Dextrose, FD&C Yellow #6 Al Lake, Hydroxypropyl Methylcellulose, Magnesium Stearate, Microcrystalline Cellulose, Polyethylene Glycol, Polysorbate 80, Starch, Titanium Dioxide.

Directions: Adults and children 12 years and over: Take 1 tablet (200 mg) not more often than every 3 to 4 hours.

Warnings: The recommended dose of this product contains about as much caf-

Continued on next page

Vivarin—Cont.

feine as two cups of coffee. Limit the use of caffeine containing medications, foods, or beverages while taking this product because too much caffeine may cause nervousness, irritability, sleeplessness, and occasionally, rapid heartbeat. For occasional use only. Not intended for use as a substitute for sleep. If fatigue or drowsiness persists or continues to recur, consult a doctor. Do not give to children under 12 years of age. As with any drug, if you are pregnant or nursing a baby, seek the advice of a health professional before using this product. In case of accidental overdose, seek professional assistance or contact a poison control center immediately. Keep this and all drugs out of the reach of children.

Tamper Evident Feature: Individually sealed in foil for your protection. Do not use if foil or plastic bubble is torn or punctured.

Store at room temperature, avoid excessive heat (greater than 100°F) or humidity.

How Supplied:
Tablets: Consumer packages of 16, 40 and 80 tablets
Caplets: Consumer packages of 24 and 48 caplets

Comments or Questions? Call Toll-Free 1-800-245-1040 Weekdays.
SmithKline Beecham Consumer Healthcare, L.P.
Pittsburgh, PA 15230. Made in U.S.A.

©1996 SmithKline Beecham
Shown in Product Identification Guide, page 525

Standard Homeopathic Company
**210 WEST 131st STREET
BOX 61067
LOS ANGELES, CA 90061**

Direct Inquiries to:
Jay Borneman
(800) 624-9659 x20

HYLAND'S ARNISPORT™

Formula: Arnica Montana 30X HPUS, Hypericum Perefoliatium 6X HPUS, Ruta Graveolens 6X HPUS, Ledum Palustre 6X HPUS, Bellis Perennis 6X HPUS, plus Hyland's Bioplasma™ in a base of Lactose, N.F.
Hyland's Bioplasma™ contains: Calcarea Fluorica 6X HPUS, Calcarea Phosphorica 3X HPUS, Calcarea Sulphurica 3X HPUS, Ferrum Phosphoricum 3X HPUS, Kali Muriaticum 3X HPUS, Kali

Phosphoricum 3X HPUS, Kali Sulphuricum 3X HPUS, Magnesia Phosphorica 3X HPUS, Natrum Muriaticum 6X HPUS, Natrum Phosphoricum 3X HPUS, Natrum Sulphuricum 3X HPUS, Silicea 6X HPUS.

Indications: Natural relief for muscle pain and soreness from overexertion.

Directions: Adults: Dissolve 3–4 tablets in mouth every 2 hours until relieved. Children 2 years or older: Dissolve 1–2 tablets in mouth every 2 hours until relieved.

Warnings: Do not use if imprinted cap band is broken or missing. If symptoms persist for more than 7 days or worsen, contact a licensed health care professional. As with any drug, if you are pregnant or nursing a baby, consult a licensed health care professional before using this or any other medication. Keep this and all medications out of the reach of children. In case of accidental overdose, contact a poison control center immediately. In case of emergency, the manufacturer may be contacted 24 hours a day, 7 days a week by calling 800/624-9659.

How Supplied: Bottles of 50 three-grain sublingual tablets (NDC 54973-0232-01). Store at room temperature.

HYLAND'S BACKACHE WITH ARNICA

Active Ingredients: BENZOICUM ACIDUM 3X HPUS, COLCHICUM AUTUMNALE 3X HPUS, SULPHUR 3X HPUS, ARNICA MONTANA 6X HPUS.

Inactive Ingredients: Lactose, N.F.

Indications: A homeopathic medicine for the temporary relief of symptoms of low back pain due to strain or overexertion.

Directions: Adults and children over 12 years of age: Take 1–2 caplets with water every 4 hours or as needed.

Warnings: Do not use if imprinted cap band is broken or missing. If symptoms persist for more than seven days or worsen, contact a licensed health care professional. As with any drug, if you are pregnant or nursing a baby, seek the advice of a licensed health care professional before using this product. Keep this and all medications out of the reach of children. In case of accidental overdose, contact a poison control center immediately. In case of emergency, the manufacturer may be reached 24 hours a day, 7 days a week at 800/624-9659.

How Supplied: Bottles of 40 5.5 grain caplets (NDC 54973-2965-2). Store at room temperature.

HYLAND'S BUMPS 'N BRUISES™ TABLETS

Active Ingredients: Arnica Montana 6X HPUS, Hypericum Perforatum 6X HPUS, Bellis Perennis 6X HPUS, Ruta Graveolens 6X HPUS.

Inactive Ingredients: Lactose, N.F.

Indications: A homeopathic medicine for the temporary relief of symptoms of bruising and swelling from falls, trauma or overexertion. Easy to take soft tablets dissolve instantly in the mouth.

Directions: For over 1 year of age: Dissolve 3–4 tablets in a teaspoon of water or on the tongue at the time of injury. May be repeated as needed every 15 minutes until relieved.

Warnings: Do not use if imprinted cap band is broken or missing. If symptoms persist for more than 7 days or worsen, consult a licensed health care professional. As with any drug, if you are pregnant or nursing a baby, consult a health care professional before using this product. Keep this and all medications out of the reach of children. In case of accidental overdose, contact a poison control center immediately. In case of emergency, the manufacturer may be reached 24 hours a day, 7 days a week at 800/624-9659.

How Supplied: Bottles of 125 1-grain sublingual tablets (NDC 54973-7508-1). Store at room temperature.

HYLAND'S CALMS FORTÉ™

Active Ingredients: *Passiflora* (Passion Flower) 1X triple strength HPUS, *Avena Sativa* (Oat) 1X double strength HPUS, *Humulus Lupulus* (Hops) 1X double strength HPUS, *Chamomilla* (Chamomile) 2X HPUS, *Calcarea Phosphorica* (Calcium Phosphate) 3X HPUS, *Ferrum Phosphorica* (Iron Phosphate) 3X HPUS, *Kali Phosphoricum* (Potassium Phosphate) 3X HPUS, *Natrum Phosphoricum* (Sodium Phosphate) 3X HPUS, *Magnesia Phosphoricum* (Magnesium Phosphate) 3X HPUS.

Inactive Ingredients: Lactose, N.F.

Indications: Temporary symptomatic relief of simple nervous tension and sleeplessness.

Directions: Adults: As a relaxant: Swallow 1–2 tablets with water as needed, three times daily, preferably before meals. For insomnia: 1 to 3 tablets ½ to 1 hour before retiring. Repeat as needed without danger of side effects. Children: As a relaxant: Swallow 1 tablet with water as needed, three times daily, preferably before meals. For insomnia: 1 to 2 tablets ½ to 1 hour before retiring. Repeat as needed without danger of side effects.

Warning: Do not use if imprinted cap band is broken or missing. If symptoms persist for more than seven days or worsen, consult a licensed health care professional. As with any drug, if you are pregnant or nursing a baby, seek the advice of a licensed health care professional before using this product. Keep this and all medications out of the reach of chil-

dren. In case of accidental overdose, contact a Poison Control Center immediately. In case of emergency, the manufacturer may be reached 24 hours a day, 7 days a week by calling 800/624-9659.

How Supplied: Bottles of 100 4-grain tablets (NDC 54973-1121-02), 50 4-grain tablets (NDC 54973-1121-01) and 32 5.5-grain caplets (NDC 54973-1121-48). Store at room temperature.

HYLAND'S COLD TABLETS WITH ZINC

Active Ingredients: Aconitum Napellus 6X, HPUS; Allium Cepa 6X, HPUS; Gelsemium Sempervirens 6X, HPUS; Zinc Gluconate 2X, HPUS.

Inactive Ingredients: Lactose, NF

Indications: Temporary symptomatic treatment for the relief of the common cold.

Directions: Take 2 – 3 quick dissolving tablets under the tongue every 4 hours or as needed. Children 6 to 12 years old: ½ adult dose.

Warnings: Do not use if imprinted cap band is broken or missing. If symptoms persist for more than seven days or worsen, contact a licensed health care professional. Discontinue if symptoms are accompanied by a high fever (over 101 °F) and contact a licensed health care professional. As with any drug, if you are pregnant or nursing a baby, seek the advice of a licensed health care professional before using this product. Keep this and all medications out of the reach of children. In case of accidental overdose, contact a poison control center immediately. In cases of emergency, the manufacturer may be contacted 24 hours a day, 7 days a week at 800/624-9659.

How Supplied: Bottles of 50 three-grain sublingual tablets (NDC 54973-3010-01). 60 three grain sublingual tablets (NDC 54973-2952-01). Store at room temperature.

HYLAND'S COLIC TABLETS

Active Ingredients: *Disocorea* (Wild Yam) 3X HPUS, *Chamomilla* (Chamomile) 3X HPUS, *Colocynthinum* (Bitter Apple) 3X HPUS.

Inactive Ingredients: Lactose N.F.

Indications: A homeopathic combination for the temporary relief of symptoms of colic and gas pains caused by irritating food, feeding too quickly, swallowing air and similar conditions during teething, colds and other minor upset periods in children.

Directions: For children up to 2 years of age: Dissolve 2 tablets under the tongue every 15 minutes for up to 8 doses until relieved; then every 2 hours as re-

quired. If you prefer, tablets may first be dissolved in a teaspoon of water and then given to the child. Children over 2 years: Dissolve 3 tablets under the tongue as above; or as recommended by a licensed health care professional. Colic Tablets are very soft and dissolve almost instantly under the tongue. If your baby has been crying or has been very upset, your baby may fall asleep after using this product. This is because pain has been relieved and your child can rest.

Warnings: Do not use if imprinted cap band is broken or missing. If symptoms persist for more than seven days or worsen, consult a licensed health care professional. As with any drug, if you are pregnant or nursing a baby, seek the advice of a licensed health care professional before using this product. Keep this and all medications out of the reach of children. In case of accidental overdose, contact a poison control center immediately. In cases of emergency, the manufacturer may be contacted 24 hours a day, 7 days a week at 800/624-9659

How Supplied: Bottles of 125—one grain sublingual tablets (NDC 54973-7502-1). Store at room temperature.

HYLAND'S EARACHE TABLETS

Active Ingredients: Pulsatilla (Wind Flower) 30C, HPUS; Chamomilla (Chamomile) 30C, HPUS; Sulphur 30C, HPUS; Calcarea Carbonica (Carbonate of Lime) 30C, HPUS; Belladonna 30C, HPUS; $(3 \times 10^{-60} \%$ Alkaloids) and Lycopodium (Club Moss) 30C, HPUS.

Inactive Ingredients: Lactose NF

Indications: For the relief of symptoms of fever, pain, irritability and sleeplessness associated with earaches in children after diagnosis by a physician. If symptoms persist for more than 48 hours or if there is a discharge from the ear, discontinue use and contact your health care professional.

Directions: Dissolve 4 tablets under the tongue 3 times per day for 48 hours or until symptoms subside. If you prefer, tablets may be dissolved in a teaspoon of water and then given to the child. Earache Tablets are very soft and dissolve almost instantly under the tongue.

Warnings: Do not use if imprinted blisters are broken or damaged. If symptoms persist for more than 48 hours, or if there is a discharge from the ear, discontinue use and consult a licensed health care professional. As with any drug, if you are pregnant or nursing a baby, seek the advice of a licensed health care professional before using this product. Keep this and all medications out of the reach of children. In case of accidental overdose, contact a poison control center immediately. In cases of emergency, the manufacturer may be contacted 24 hours a day, 7 days a week at 800/624-9659.

How Supplied: Blister pack of 40 tablets (NDC 54973-7507-1). Store at room temperature.

HYLAND'S LEG CRAMPS WITH QUININE

Active Ingredients: Cinchona Officinalis 3X, HPUS (Quinine), Viscum Album 3X, HPUS; Gnaphalium Polycephalum 3X, HPUS; Rhus Toxicodendron 6X, HPUS; Aconitum Napellus 6X, HPUS; Ledum Palustre 6X, HPUS; Magnesia Phosphorica 6X, HPUS.

Inactive Ingredients: Lactose, N.F.

Indications: Hyland's Leg Cramps is a traditional homeopathic formula for the relief of symptoms of cramps and pains in lower back and legs often made worse by damp weather. Working without contraindications or side effects, Hyland's Leg Cramps stimulates your body's natural healing response to relieve symptoms. Hyland's Leg Cramps is safe for adults and can be used in conjuction with other medications.

Directions: Adults: Dissolve 2–3 tablets under tongue every 4 hours as needed.

Warnings: Do not use if imprinted cap band is missing or broken. If symptoms persist for more than seven days or worsen, contact a licensed health care professional. As with any drug, if you are pregnant or nursing a baby, seek the advice of a licensed health care professional before using this product. Do not use if pregnant, sensitive to quinine or under 12 years of age. Keep this and all medications out of the reach of children. In case of accidental overdose, contact a poison control center immediately. In case of emergency, the manufacturer may be reached 24 hours a day, 7 days a week at 800-624-9659.

How Supplied: Bottles of 100 three-grain sublingual tablets (NDC 54973-2956-02), Bottles of 50 three-grain sublingual tablets (NDC 54973-2956-01), Bottles of 40 5.5 grain caplets (NDC 54973-2956-68). Store at room temperature.

HYLAND'S MENOCALM™

Ingredients: AMYL NITROSUM 6X HPUS, SANGUINARIA CAN. 3X HPUS, LACHESIS MUTA 12X HPUS, CIMICIFUGA RACEMOSA 10MG RHIZOME (AS 40 MG CIMIPURE STANDARDIZED TO PROVIDE 4 MG TRITERPENE GLYCOSIDES DAILY), CALCIUM CITRATE USP 953 MG (TO PROVIDE 800MG CALCIUM PER DAY) EXCIPIENTS 5% (CELLULOSE, CROSCARMELLOSE SODIUM, VEGETABLE

Continued on next page

Hyland's MenoCalm—Cont.

STEARIC ACID, SILICA, VEGETABLE MAGNESIUM STEARATE WITH A CELLULOSE COATING.)

Indications: Symptomatic relief for hot flashes, moodiness and irritability associated with menopause.

Directions: Take 2 tablets two times per day. Due to the calcium in MenoCalm™, the tablets are large. You may break the tablets along the score line without affecting the product's effectiveness. If symptoms persist for more than 14 days, discontinue use and contact your health care provider.

Warnings: Do not use if imprinted cap band is broken or missing. If symptoms persist for more than 14 days or worsen, consult a licensed health care practitioner. Do not use this product if your are pregnant or nursing. Keep this and all medications out of the reach of children. In case of accidental overdose, contact a poison control center immediately. In cases of emergency, the manufacturer may be contacted 24 hours a day, 7 days a week at 800/624-9659.

How Supplied: Bottles of 84 seven-grain tablets (NDC 54973-6056-1). Store at room temperature.

HYLAND'S NERVE TONIC

Active Ingredients: Calcarea Phosphorica (Calcium Phosphate) 3X HPUS; Ferrum Phosphorica (Iron Phosphate) 3X HPUS; Kali Phosphoricum (Potassium Phosphate) 3X HPUS; Natrum Phosphoricum (Sodium Phosphate) 3X HPUS; Magnesia Phosphoricum (Magnesium Phosphate) 3X HPUS.

Inactive Ingredients: Lactose, N.F.

Indications: Temporary symtomatic relief of simple nervous tension and stress.

Directions: Adults take 2–6 tablets before each meal and at bedtime. Children: 2 tablets. In severe cases take 3 tablets every 2 hours.

Warnings: Do not use if imprinted cap band is broken or missing. If symptoms persist for more than seven days or worsen, contact a licensed health care professional. As with any drug, if you are pregnant or nursing a baby, seek the advice of a licensed health care professional before using this product. Keep this and all medications out of the reach of children. In case of accidental overdose, contact a poison control center immediately. In cases of emergency, the manufacturer may be contacted 24 hours a day, 7 days a week at 800/624-9659.

How Supplied: Bottles of 32 caplets (NDC 54973-1129-68), Bottles of 500 tablets (NDC 54973-1129-1), Bottles of 1000 tablets (NDC 54973-1129-2)

SMILE'S PRID®

Contains: Acidum Carbolicum 2X HPUS, Ichthammol 2X HPUS, Arnica Montana 3X HPUS, Calendula Off 3X HPUS, Echinacea Ang 3X HPUS, Sulphur 12X HPUS, Hepar Sulph 12X HPUS, Silicea 12X HPUS, Rosin, Beeswax, Petrolatum, Stearyl Alcohol, Methyl & Propyl Paraben.

Indications: Temporary topical relief of pain symptoms associated with boils, minor skin eruptions, redness and irritation. Also aids in relieving the discomfort of superficial cuts, scratches and wounds.

Directions: Wash affected parts with hot water, dry and apply PRID® twice daily on clean bandage or gauze. Do not squeeze or pressure irritated skin area. After irritation subsides, repeat application once a day for several days. Children under two years: consult a physician. CAUTION: If symptoms persist for more than seven days or worsen, or if fever occurs, contact a licensed health care professional. Do not use on broken skin. Keep out of reach of children. In case of accidental ingestion, seek professional assistance or contact a poison control center. For external use only. Avoid contact with eyes.

How Supplied: 20GM tin (NDC 0619-4202-54). Keep in a cool dry place.

HYLAND'S TEETHING GEL

Active Ingredients: Calcarea Phosphorica (Calcium Phosphate) 12X, HPUS; Chamomilla (Chamomile) 6X, HPUS; Coffea Cruda (Coffee) 6X, HPUS; and Belladonna 6X, HPUS (Alkaloids 0.0000003%)

Inactive Ingredients: Deionized water, Vegetable Glycerin, Hydroxyethyl Cellulose, Methyl Paraben and Propyl Paraben.

Indications: A homeopathic combination for the temporary relief of symptoms of simple restlessness and wakeful irritability due to cutting teeth.

Directions: Apply to gums as necessary. If symptoms persist for more than seven days or worsen, discontinue use and contact your health care professional. Please note, if your baby has been crying or has been very upset, your baby may fall asleep after using this product because the pain has been relieved and your child can rest.

Warnings: Do not use if tube tip is broken or missing. If symptoms persist for more than seven days or if irritation persists, inflammation develops or fever or infection develop, discontinue use and consult a licensed health care professional. As with any drug, if you are pregnant or nursing a baby, seek the advice of a licensed health care professional before using this product. Keep this and all medications out of the reach of children.

In case of accidental overdose, contact a poison control center immediately. In case of emergency, the manufacturer may be contacted 24 hours a day, 7 days a week at 800/624-9659.

How Supplied: Tubes of 1/3 OZ. (NDC 54973-7504-3). Store at room temperature.

HYLAND'S TEETHING TABLETS

Active Ingredients: *Calcarea Phosphorica* (Calcium Phosphate) 3X HPUS, *Chamomilla* (Chamomile) 3X HPUS, *Coffea Cruda* (Coffee) 3X HPUS, *Belladonna* 3X HPUS (Alkaloids 0.0003%).

Inactive Ingredients: Lactose N.F.

Indications: A homeopathic combination for the temporary relief of symptoms of simple restlessness and wakeful irritability due to cutting teeth.

Directions: Dissolve 2 to 3 tablets under the tongue 4 times per day. If you prefer, tablets may first be dissolved in a teaspoon of water and then given to the child. If the child is restless or wakeful, 2 tablets every hour for 6 doses or as recommended by a licensed health care professional. Teething Tablets are very soft and dissolve almost instantly under the tongue. Please note, if your baby has been crying or has been very upset, your baby may fall asleep after using this product because the pain has been relieved and your child can rest.

Warning: Do Not use if imprinted cap band is broken or missing. If symptoms persist for more than seven days, or if irritation persist, inflammation develops or fever or infection develop, discontinue use and consult a licensed health care professional. As with any drug, if you are pregnant or nursing a baby, seek the advice of a health care professional before using this product. Keep this and all medications out of the reach of children. In case of accidental overdose, contact a poison control center immediately. In case of emergency, the manufacturer may be contacted 24 hours a day, 7 days a week at 800/624-9659.

How Supplied: Bottles of 125—one grain sublingual tablets (NDC 54973-7504-01). Store at room temperature.

EDUCATIONAL MATERIAL

Booklets—Brochures
"Homeopathy—What it is, How it Works," A Consumer's Guide to Homeopathic Medicine, Free
"Homeopathy—A Guide for Pharmacists," An ACPE (0.2 CEU) program on the basic principles of homeopathy.

UAS Laboratories
**5610 ROWLAND RD #110
MINNETONKA, MN 55343**

Direct Inquiries To:
Dr. S.K. Dash: (612) 935-1707
Fax: (612) 935-1650

Medical Emergency Contact:
Dr. S.K. Dash: (612) 935-1707
Fax: (612) 935-1650

DDS®-ACIDOPHILUS
Capsule, Tablet & Powder free of dairy products, corn, soy, and preservatives

Description: DDS®-Acidophilus is the source of a special strain of Lactobacillus acidophilus free of dairy products, corn, soy and preservatives. Each capsule or tablet contains one billion viable DDS-1 L.acidophilus at the time of manufacturing. One gram of powder contains two billion viable DDS®- L.acidophilus.

Indications and Usages: An aid in implanting the gut with beneficial Lactobacillus acidophilus under conditions of digestive disorders, acne, yeast infections, and following antibiotic therapy.

Administration: One to two capsules or tablets twice daily before meals. One-fourth teaspoon powder can be substituted for two capsules or tablets.

How Supplied: Bottles of 100 capsules or tablets. 12 bottles per case. Powder is available in 2 oz. bottle; 12 bottles per case.

Storage: Keep refrigerated under 40°F.

EDUCATIONAL MATERIAL

DDS-Acidophilus
Booklet describing superior-strain Acidophilus without dairy products, corn, soy, or preservatives. Two billion viable DDS-L. acidopohilus per gram.

UNKNOWN DRUG?
Consult the
Product Identification Guide
(Gray Pages)
for full-color photos of
leading over-the-counter
medications

Upsher-Smith Laboratories, Inc.
**14905 23rd AVENUE N.
PLYMOUTH, MN 55447**

Direct inquiries to:
Professional Services
(763) 475-3023
Fax (763) 475-3410

AMLACTIN® 12% Moisturizing Lotion and Cream
[ăm-lăk-tĭn]
Cosmetic Lotion and Cream

Description: AMLACTIN® Moisturizing Lotion and Cream are special formulations of 12% lactic acid neutralized with ammonium hydroxide to provide a lotion or cream pH of 4.5–5.5. Lactic acid, an alpha-hydroxy acid, is a naturally occurring humectant for the skin. AMLACTIN® moisturizes and softens rough, dry skin.

How Supplied: 225g (8oz) plastic bottle: List No. 0245-0023-22
400g (14oz) plastic bottle: List No. 0245-0023-40
140g (4.9oz) tube: List No. 0245-0024-14

Wallace Laboratories
**P.O. BOX 1001
HALF ACRE ROAD
CRANBURY, NJ 08512**

Direct Inquiries to:
Wallace Laboratories
Div. of Carter-Wallace, Inc.
P.O. Box 1001
Cranbury, NJ 08512
609-655-6000

**For Medical Information, Contact:
Generally:
Professional Services**
800-526-3840

After Hours and Weekend Emergencies
609-655-6474

MALTSUPEX®
**(malt soup extract)
Powder, Liquid, Tablets**

Composition: MALTSUPEX is a non-diastatic extract from barley malt, which is available in powder, liquid, and tablet form. Each MALTSUPEX product has a gentle laxative action and promotes soft, easily passed stools.
Tablet: Each tablet contains 750 mg of Malt Soup Extract. Other ingredients: D&C Yellow No. 10, FD&C Red No. 40, flavor (artificial), hydroxypropyl methylcellulose, methylparaben, polyethylene glycol, povidone, propylparaben, simethicone emulsion, stearic acid, talc, tita-

nium dioxide. Sodium content: Each tablet contains approximately 1 mg of sodium.
Powder: Each level scoop provides approximately 8 g of Malt Soup Extract. Sodium content: Each scoopful contains approximately 5 mg of sodium.
Liquid: Each tablespoonful ($^1/_2$ fl. oz.) contains approximately the equivalent of 16 g Malt Soup Extract Powder. Other ingredients: Potassium sorbate and sodium propionate. Sodium content: Each tablespoon contains approximately 36 mg of sodium.

EFFECTIVE, NON-HABIT-FORMING

Indications: For relief of occasional constipation. This product generally produces a bowel movement in 12 to 72 hours.

Warnings: Do not use laxative products when abdominal pain, nausea or vomiting are present unless directed by a physician. If constipation persists, consult a physician.
If you have noticed a sudden change in bowel habits that persists over a period of 2 weeks, consult a physician before using a laxative.
Keep this and all medications out of the reach of children. In case of accidental overdose, seek professional assistance or contact a poison control center immediately.
Laxative products should not be used for a period longer than one week unless directed by a physician. Rectal bleeding or failure to have a bowel movement after use of a laxative may indicate a serious condition. Discontinue use and consult a physician.
As with any drug, if you are pregnant or nursing a baby, seek the advice of a health professional before using this product.
MALTSUPEX Liquid only—Do not use this product if you are on a sodium-restricted diet unless directed by a physician. Maltsupex Liquid contains approximately 1.58 mEq (36 mg) of sodium per tablespoon.
Maltsupex Tablets contain approximately 0.02 mEq (0.46 mg) of sodium per tablet.
Each scoop of Maltsupex Powder contains approximately 0.22 mEq (5 mg) of sodium per scoop.
Note: Allow for carbohydrate content in diabetic diets and infant formulas.
Liquid: (67%, 14 g/tablespoon, or 56 calories/tablespoon)
Powder: (83%, 6 g or 24 calories per scoop)
Tablets: (Approximately 83%, 0.5 g or 2.5 calories per tablet)

Directions: General—Drink a full glass (8 ounces) of liquid with each dose. The recommended daily dosage of MALTSUPEX may vary. Use the smallest dose that is effective and lower dosage as improvement occurs.

Continued on next page

Maltsupex—Cont.

MALTSUPEX Powder—Each bottle contains a scoop. Each scoopful (which is the equivalent of a standard measuring tablespoon) should be levelled with a knife.

MALTSUPEX Tablets: Adult Dosage: Start with four tablets (3 g) four times daily (with meals and at bedtime) and adjust dosage according to response, not to exceed 48 tablets (36 g) daily. Drink a full glass (8 oz.) of liquid with each dose.

Usual Dosage—Powder:
[See table below]

Usual Dosage—Liquid:
[See table below]

Preparation Tips: Powder—Add dosage to milk, water, or fruit juice and stir until dissolved. Mixing is easier if added to warm milk or warm water. May be flavored with vanilla or cocoa to make "malteds." Excellent with warm milk at bedtime. Also available in tablet and liquid forms.

Note: Although shade, texture, taste, and height of contents may vary between bottles, action remains the same.

Liquid: Mixing is easier if MALTSUPEX Liquid is added to an ounce or two of warm water and stirred. Then add milk, water, or fruit juice and stir until dissolved. May be flavored with vanilla or cocoa to make "malteds." Excellent with warm milk at bedtime. Also available in tablet and powder forms.

Professional Labeling: The dosage for children under 2 years of age is:

Powder: 2 to 3 level measuring teaspoonfuls, 3 to 4 times per day, in water, fruit juice, or formula.

Liquid: 1 to 2 measuring teaspoonfuls, 2 to 3 times per day, in water, fruit juice, or formula.

How Supplied: MALTSUPEX is supplied in 8 ounce (NDC 0037-9101-12) and 16 ounce (NDC 0037-9101-08) jars of MALTSUPEX Powder; 8 fluid ounce (NDC 0037-9051-12) and 1 pint (NDC 0037-9051-08) bottles of MALTSUPEX Liquid; and in bottles of 100 MALTSUPEX Tablets (NDC 0037-9201-01).

Storage: Store at controlled room temperature 20°–25°C (68°–77°F). Protect MALTSUPEX powder and tablets from moisture.

MALTSUPEX **Powder** and **Liquid** are

Distributed by
WALLACE LABORATORIES
Division of Carter-Wallace, Inc.
Cranbury, New Jersey 08512

MALTSUPEX **Tablets** are

Manufactured by
WALLACE LABORATORIES
Division of Carter-Wallace, Inc.
Cranbury, New Jersey 08512

Rev. 8/97

Shown in Product Identification Guide, page 525

MALTSUPEX Powder

AGE	CORRECTIVE*	MAINTENANCE
12 years to ADULTS	Up to 4 scoops twice a day (Take a full glass [8 oz.] of liquid with each dose.)	2 to 4 scoops at bedtime
CHILDREN 6–12 years of age	Up to 2 scoops twice a day (Take a full glass [8 oz.] of liquid with each dose.)	
CHILDREN 2–6 years of age	1 scoop twice a day (Take a full glass [8 oz.] of liquid with each dose.)	
INFANTS under 2 years of age	Consult a doctor.	

* Full corrective dosage should be used for 3 or 4 days or until relief is noted. Then continue on maintenance dosage as needed. Use a clean, dry scoop to remove powder. Replace cover tightly to keep out moisture.

MALTSUPEX Liquid

AGE	CORRECTIVE*	MAINTENANCE
12 years to ADULTS	2 tablespoonfuls twice a day (Take a full glass [8 oz.] of liquid with each dose.)	1 to 2 tablespoonfuls at bedtime
CHILDREN 6–12 years of age	1 tablespoonful twice a day (Take a full glass [8 oz.] of liquid with each dose.)	
CHILDREN 2–6 years of age	$1/_2$ tablespoonful twice a day (Take a full glass [8 oz.] of liquid with each dose.)	
INFANTS under 2 years of age	Consult a doctor.	

* Full corrective dosage should be used for 3 or 4 days or until relief is noted. Then continue on maintenance dosage as needed. Use a clean, dry spoon to remove liquid. Replace cover tightly after use.

RYNA®
(Liquid)
RYNA–C®
(Liquid)

Ⓒ

Description:
RYNA® (Liquid)—Each 5 mL (one teaspoonful) contains:
Chlorpheniramine maleate .... 2 mg
Pseudoephedrine hydrochloride .. 30 mg
Other ingredients: flavor (artificial), glycerin, malic acid, purified water, sodium benzoate, sorbitol in a clear, colorless to slightly yellow-colored, lemon-vanilla flavored demulcent base containing no sugar, dyes, or alcohol.
RYNA-C® (Liquid)—Each 5 mL (one teaspoonful) contains, in addition:
Codeine phosphate .... 10 mg
(WARNING: May be habit-forming)
Other ingredients: flavor (artificial), glycerin, malic acid, purified water, saccharin sodium, sodium benzoate, sorbitol in a clear, colorless to slightly yellow, cinnamon flavored demulcent base containing no sugar, dyes, or alcohol.

Actions:
Chlorpheniramine maleate in RYNA and RYNA-C is an antihistamine that antagonizes the effects of histamine.
Codeine phosphate in RYNA-C is a centrally-acting antitussive that relieves cough.
Pseudoephedrine hydrochloride in RYNA and RYNA-C is a sympathomimetic nasal decongestant that acts to shrink swollen mucosa of the respiratory tract.

Indications:
RYNA: For the temporary relief of nasal congestion due to the common cold, hay fever, or other upper respiratory allergies. Temporarily relieves runny nose, and alleviates sneezing, itching of the nose or throat, and itchy, watery eyes due to hay fever, or other respiratory allergies such as allergic rhinitis.
RYNA-C: For the temporary relief of nasal congestion due to the common cold, hay fever, or other upper respiratory allergies. Temporarily relieves runny nose and alleviates sneezing, itching of the nose or throat, and itchy, watery eyes due to the common cold, hay fever, or other upper respiratory allergies. Temporarily relieves cough due to minor throat and bronchial irritation as may occur with a cold. Temporarily helps to control the cough reflex that causes coughing. Temporarily reduces the intensity of coughing. Controls the impulse to cough to help you sleep. Calms the cough control center and relieves coughing.

Warnings:
For RYNA: Do not give this product to children taking other medication or to children under 6 years except under the advice and supervision of a doctor. **Do not exceed the recommended dosage.** If nervousness, dizziness or sleeplessness occur, discontinue use and call a doctor. If symptoms do not improve

within 7 days or are accompanied by fever, consult a doctor. Do not take this product, unless directed by a doctor, if you have a breathing problem such as emphysema or chronic bronchitis, or if you have glaucoma, heart disease, high blood pressure, thyroid disease, diabetes, or difficulty in urination due to enlargement of the prostate gland. May cause excitability, especially in children. May cause drowsiness; alcohol, sedatives, and tranquilizers may increase drowsiness effect. Avoid alcoholic beverages while taking this product. Do not take this product if you are taking sedatives or tranquilizers, without first consulting your doctor. Use caution when driving a motor vehicle or operating machinery. As with any drug, if you are pregnant or nursing a baby, seek the advice of a health care professional before taking this product.

For RYNA-C: Adults and children who have a chronic pulmonary disease or shortness of breath, or children who are taking other drugs, should not take this product unless directed by a doctor. Do not give this product to children under 6 years of age except under the advice and supervision of a doctor. A persistent cough may be a sign of a serious condition. If cough persists for more than one week, tends to recur, or is accompanied by fever, rash or persistent headache, consult a doctor. Do not take this product for persistent or chronic cough such as occurs with smoking, asthma, or emphysema, or if cough is accompanied by excessive phlegm (mucus) unless directed by a doctor. Do not take this product unless directed by a doctor if you have a breathing problem such as emphysema or chronic bronchitis, or if you have glaucoma, heart disease, high blood pressure, thyroid disease, diabetes, or difficulty in urination due to enlargement of the prostate gland. May cause or aggravate constipation. May cause marked drowsiness; alcohol, sedatives, and tranquilizers may increase the drowsiness effect. Avoid alcoholic beverages while taking this product. Do not take this product if you are taking sedatives or tranquilizers without first consulting your doctor. Use caution when driving a motor vehicle or operating machinery. May cause excitability, especially in children. **Do not exceed recommended dosage.** If nervousness, dizziness or sleepiness occur, discontinue use and consult a doctor. If symptoms do not improve within 7 days or are accompanied by a fever, consult a doctor. This product contains an ingredient (codeine phosphate) known to cause birth defects or other reproductive harm. As with any drug, if you are pregnant or nursing a baby, seek the advice of a health professional before using this drug.

For RYNA and RYNA-C:

Drug Interaction Precaution:

Do **not** use this product if you are now taking a prescription monoamine oxidase inhibitor (MAOI) (certain drugs for depression, psychiatric or emotional conditions, or Parkinson's disease), or for 2 weeks after stopping the MAOI drug. If you are uncertain whether your prescription drug contains an MAOI, consult a health professional before taking this product.

Dosage and Administration:
Adults and children 12 years of age and over: 2 teaspoonfuls every 4 to 6 hours, not to exceed 8 teaspoonfuls in 24 hours, or as directed by a doctor.
Children 6 to under 12 years: 1 teaspoonful every 4 to 6 hours, not to exceed 4 teaspoonfuls in 24 hours, or as directed by a doctor.
Children under 6 years of age: Consult a doctor.
RYNA-C:
A special measuring device should be used to give an accurate dose of this product to children under 6 years of age. Giving a higher dose than recommended by a doctor could result in serious side effects for the child.

How Supplied:
RYNA: bottles of 4 fl oz (NDC 0037-0638-66).
RYNA-C: bottles of 4 fl oz (NDC 0037-0522-66) and one pint (NDC 0037-0522-68).

TAMPER-EVIDENT BAND ON CAP PRINTED "WALLACE LABORATORIES." DO NOT USE IF BAND IS MISSING OR BROKEN.

Storage:
RYNA: Store at controlled room temperature 20°–25°C (68°–77°F).
RYNA-C: Store at controlled room temperature 20°–25°C (68°–77°F). Dispense in a tight, light-resistant container.

KEEP THESE AND ALL DRUGS OUT OF THE REACH OF CHILDREN. IN CASE OF ACCIDENTAL OVERDOSE, SEEK PROFESSIONAL ASSISTANCE OR CONTACT A POISON CONTROL CENTER IMMEDIATELY.

WALLACE LABORATORIES
Division of Carter-Wallace, Inc.
Cranbury, New Jersey 08512

Rev. 4/99
RYNA-C
Shown in Product Identification Guide, page 525

FACED WITH AN Rx SIDE EFFECT?
Turn to the Companion Drug Index (Green Pages) for products that provide symptomatic relief.

Wellness International Network, Ltd.
5800 DEMOCRACY DRIVE
PLANO, TX 75024

Direct Inquiries to:
Product Coordinator
(972) 312-1100
FAX: (972) 943-5250

BIO-COMPLEX 5000™
Gentle Foaming Cleanser

Uses: BIO-COMPLEX 5000™ Gentle Foaming Cleanser, with alpha-hydroxy acids, aloe vera and botanical infusions, is an advanced cleansing gel designed for all skin types. BIO-COMPLEX 5000 Gentle Foaming Cleanser protects the skin and works to restore elasticity while gently removing surface impurities, make-up and pollution.

Ingredients: Aloe Vera Gel, Infusion of Sage, Infusion of Chamomile, Ammonium Lauryl Sulfate, Lauramidopropyl Betaine, Glycerin, Lauramide DEA, Cetyl Betaine, Tocopherol (Vitamin E), Citric Acid, Lactic Acid, Malic Acid, Ascorbic Acid (Vitamin C), Methylchloroisothiazolinone, Methylisothiazolinone, Propylparaben, Methylparaben.

Directions: Splash warm water onto face. Place a small amount of gel on fingertips. Apply evenly to face and neck in circular motions, massaging skin gently but thoroughly. Rinse completely and pat dry with a soft towel.

How Supplied: 8 fluid ounce/236 ml. bottle.

BIO-COMPLEX 5000™
Revitalizing Conditioner

Uses: BIO-COMPLEX 5000™ Revitalizing Conditioner, with vitamins, antioxidants, and sunscreen, helps restore moisture to dried-out, heat-styled hair. This advanced conditioner contains silkening agents which enhance the hair as well as detangle it after shampooing. Hair is left clean, soft, manageable, and protected against styling aids and environmental elements. BIO-COMPLEX 5000 Revitalizing Conditioner is excellent for all hair types, especially damaged or over-processed hair.

Ingredients: Water, Stearyl Alcohol, Propylene Glycol, Stearamidopropyl Dimethylamine, Cyclomethicone, Polyquaternium - 11, Stearalkonium Chloride, Cetearyl Alcohol, PEG - 40 Hydrogenated Castor Oil, Citric Acid, Tocopherol (Vitamin E), Ascorbic Acid (Vitamin C), Retinyl Palmitate (Vitamin A), Octyl Methoxycinnamate, Awapuhi

Continued on next page

Bio-Complex 5000 Cond—Cont

Fragrance, Ceteth - 20, Soluble Animal Keratin, Imidazolidinyl Urea, Propylparaben, Methylparaben.

Directions: After shampooing with BIO-COMPLEX 5000™ Revitalizing Shampoo, apply to wet hair. Massage through hair, paying special attention to the ends. Leave on 2–3 minutes. Rinse thoroughly. Towel dry and style as usual.

How Supplied: 12 fluid ounce bottle.

BIO-COMPLEX 5000™
Revitalizing Shampoo

Uses: BIO-COMPLEX 5000™ Revitalizing Shampoo, with vitamins, antioxidants, and sunscreen, cleanses and moisturizes hair for excellent manageability. Specially formulated with the essence of awapuhi, a Hawaiian ginger plant extract known for its healing qualities, this formula contains the mildest blend of surfactants and a wealth of natural conditioning ingredients to provide body, luster and healthier-looking hair.

Ingredients: Water, Ammonium Lauryl Sulfate, Tea Lauryl Sulfate, Cetyl Betaine, Lauramide DEA, Cocamidopropyl Betaine, Glycerin, Ascorbic Acid (Vitamin C), Tocopherol (Vitamin E), Retinyl Palmitate (Vitamin A), Citric Acid, Hydrolyzed Wheat Protein, Awapuhi Fragrance, Octyl Methoxycinnamate, PEG - 7 Glyceryl Cocoate, Methylchloroisothiazolinone, Methylisothiazolinone, Caramel.

Directions: Apply a small amount to wet hair and massage gently into scalp, creating a generous lather. Rinse and repeat if necessary. To further intensify this reconstructive process, follow with BIO-COMPLEX 5000™ Revitalizing Conditioner.

How Supplied: 12 fluid ounce bottle.

STEPHAN™ BIO-NUTRITIONAL
Daytime Hydrating Creme

Uses: Hypo-allergenic STEPHAN™ BIO-NUTRITIONAL Daytime Hydrating Creme hydrates the skin and preserves the moisture level of the upper layers of the epidermis. It is an excellent day cream for both men and women who wish to combat the visible signs of aging skin, the appearance of wrinkles or lines, and the inelastic look of facial features and contours. These light emulsions are absorbed rapidly, leaving an invisible protective film which hydrates the epidermis, regulates moisture levels and leaves skin feeling supple and soft.

Ingredients: Purified Water, Stearic Acid, Isodecyl Neopentanoate, Isostearyl Stearoyl Stearate, DEA-Cetyl Phosphate, C12-15 Alkyl Benzoate, Tocoph-

erol (Vitamin E), Aloe Barbadensis Gel, Squalane, Cetyl Esters, Benzophenone-3, Dimethicone, Fragrance, Carbomer, Triethanolamine, Imidazolidinyl Urea, Propylparaben, Methylparaben, Annatto.

Directions: Apply evenly on a completely cleansed face and neck. May be used around the eye area, avoiding direct contact with the eyes. Suitable for all skin types. For best results, use in conjunction with the complete STEPHAN BIO-NUTRITIONAL Skin Care line.

Warnings: For external use only. Avoid contact with eyes.

How Supplied: Net Wt. 1.75 oz.

STEPHAN™ BIO-NUTRITIONAL
Eye-Firming Concentrate

Uses: Hypo-allergenic STEPHAN™ BIO-NUTRITIONAL Eye-Firming Concentrate is specially formulated to revitalize the delicate area around the eyes. This non-oily fluid pampers sensitive eyes while reducing the look of puffiness and dark circles, and smoothing and softening the appearance of fine lines in the eye area.

Ingredients: Purified Water, Cornflower Extract, Methylsilanol Hydroxyproline Aspartate, Methyl Gluceth-20, Dimethicone Copolyol, PEG-30 Glyceryl Laurate, Horsetail Extract, Panthenol, Propylene Glycol, Carbomer, Disodium EDTA, Triethanolamine, Xanthan Gum, Diazolidinyl Urea, Methylparaben, Propylparaben.

Directions: Apply in the morning, or any time of the day, in small quantities to the skin around the eyes with light, tapping motions, avoiding direct contact with the eyes. In the evening, apply gently to the entire eye contour area. For best results, use in conjunction with the complete STEPHAN BIO-NUTRITIONAL Skin Care line.

Warnings: For external use only. Avoid direct contact with eyes.

How Supplied: 1 fl. oz.

STEPHAN™ BIO-NUTRITIONAL
Nightime Moisture Creme

Uses: Hypo-allergenic STEPHAN™ BIO-NUTRITIONAL Nightime Moisture Creme is a heavier, richer cream for mature, dry or sun-damaged skin. This advanced formula is excellent for dehydrated skin, promoting suppleness and moisture, while improving the appearance of fine lines and wrinkles.

Ingredients: Purified Water, Caprylic/Capric Triglyceride, Propylene, Glycol/Dicaprylate/Dicaprate, Stearic Acid, Polysorbate 60, Cetyl Alcohol, Octyl Palmitate, Beeswax, Sorbitan Stearate, Canola Oil, Avocado Oil, Safflower Oil, Squalane, Lecithin (Liposomes), Soluble

Collagen, Dimethicone, Bisabolol, Aloe Barbadensis Gel, Fragrance, C12–15 Alkyl Benzoate, Hydroxyethylcellulose, Octyl Methoxycinnamate, Disodium EDTA, Sodium Borate, Benzophenone-3, Allantoin, Potassium Sorbate, Phenoxyethanol, Methylparaben, Propylparaben, Butylparaben, Ethylparaben, D&C Yellow No. 10, Caramel.

Directions: In the evening, apply by lightly massaging onto a thoroughly cleansed face and neck. Avoid direct contact with eyes. For drier skin, it may be used during the day as a moisturizer, under make-up or after sun bathing. For best results, use in conjunction with the complete STEPHAN BIO-NUTRITIONAL Skin Care line.

Warning: For external use only. Avoid contact with eyes.

How Supplied: Net Wt. 1.75 oz.

STEPHAN™ BIO-NUTRITIONAL
Refreshing Moisture Gel

Uses: Hypo-allergenic STEPHAN™ BIO-NUTRITIONAL Refreshing Moisture Gel is specially formulated to refine pores and promote a clear, clean and smooth-looking complexion. It is designed to deeply cleanse and super-stimulate the skin. This gel is suitable for all skin types, especially problem areas. A quick "pick-me-up," STEPHAN BIO-NUTRITIONAL Refreshing Moisture Gel immediately restores the radiant, firm and youthful appearance of the face while acting as a cumulative, revitalizing beauty treatment.

Ingredients: Water, Propylene Glycol, Glycerin, Hydroxyethylcellulose, Sugar Cane Extract, Citrus Extract, Apple Extract, Green Tea Extract, Hydrolyzed Wheat Protein, Tissue Respiratory Factors, Panthenol, Aloe Vera Gel, Laureth-4, Magnesium Aluminum Silicate, Tetrasodium EDTA, Benzophenone-3, Imidazolidinyl Urea, Methylchloroisothiazolinone, Methylisothiazolinone, Methylparaben, Propylparaben, Phenethyl Alcohol, FD&C Yellow No. 10, FD&C Red No. 40, FD&C Yellow No. 5.

Directions: After thoroughly cleansing in the morning or evening, apply a liberal layer to the face, neck and eye area, avoiding eye contact. Remove after 20–30 minutes with warm water. Suitable for all skin types. For best results, use in conjunction with the complete STEPHAN BIO-NUTRITIONAL Skin Care line.

Warnings: For external use only. Avoid contact with eyes.

How Supplied: Net Wt. 1.75 oz.

STEPHAN™ BIO-NUTRITIONAL
Ultra Hydrating Fluid

Uses: Hypo-allergenic STEPHAN™ BIO-NUTRITIONAL Ultra Hydrating

Fluid is a complete treatment formulated to soften fine lines and preserve youthful-looking, radiant skin. By utilizing ingredients focused on revitalization, STEPHAN BIO-NUTRITIONAL Ultra Hydrating Fluid possesses a progressive firming effect, helping to combat the aged look of skin due to external negative conditions.

Ingredients: Purified Water, Methyl Gluceth-20, Dimethicone Copolyol, Peg-30 Glyceryl Laurate, Panthenol Sugar Cane Extract, Citrus Extract, Apple Extract, Green Tea Extract, Live Yeast Cell Derivative, Laureth-4, Plant Pseudocollagen, Hydrolyzed Wheat Protein, Methylchloroisothiazolinone, Methylisothiazolinone, Methylsilanol Hydroxyproline Aspartate, Phenethyl Alcohol, 2-Bromo-2-Nitropropane-1, 3-Diol, Xanthan Gum, Disodium EDTA, Methylparaben, Propylparaben.

Directions: Gently apply all over the face, neck and eye contour area, preferably in the morning. Use as a part of a regular daily skin care routine or as an occasional preventive treatment. For best results, use in conjunction with the complete STEPHAN BIO-NUTRITIONAL Skin Care line.

Warnings: For external use only. Avoid direct contact with eyes.

How Supplied: 1 fl. oz.

Whitehall-Robins Healthcare American Home Products Corporation

**FIVE GIRALDA FARMS
MADISON, NJ 07940**

Direct Inquiries to:
Whitehall Consumer Product Information 800-322-3129
Robins Consumer Product Information 800-762-4672

ADVIL®
[ad 'vil]
**Ibuprofen Tablets, USP
Ibuprofen Caplets (Oval-Shaped Tablets)
Ibuprofen Gel Caplets (Oval-Shaped Gelatin Coated Tablets)
Ibuprofen Liqui-Gel Capsules**

Active Ingredient: Each tablet, caplet, or liquigel capsule contains ibuprofen 200 mg

Inactive Ingredients:
Tablets and Caplets: Acetylated Monoglyceride, Beeswax and/or Carnauba Wax, Croscarmellose Sodium, Iron Oxides, Lecithin, Methylparaben, Microcrystalline Cellulose, Pharmaceutical Glaze, Povidone, Propylparaben, Silicon Dioxide, Simethicone, Sodium Benzoate, Sodium Lauryl Sulfate, Starch, Stearic Acid, Sucrose, Titanium Dioxide.
Gel Caplets: Croscarmellose Sodium, FD&C Red 40, FD&C Yellow 6, Gelatin, Glycerin Hydroxypropyl Methylcellulose, Iron Oxides, Lecithin, Pharmaceutical Glaze, Propyl Gallate, Silicon Dioxide, Simethicone, Sodium Lauryl Sulfate, Starch, Stearic Acid, Titanium Dioxide, Triacetin.
Liqui-Gels: FD&C Green No. 3, Gelatin, Pharmaceutical Ink, Polyethylene Glycol, Potassium Hydroxide, Purified Water, Sorbitan, Sorbitol.

Indications: temporarily relieves minor aches and pains due to common cold, headache, toothache, muscular aches, backache, minor pain of arthritis, menstrual cramps; and temporarily reduces fever.

Dosage and Administration:
Directions—Do not take more than directed
Adults:
* take 1 tablet, caplet, gelcap or liquigel capsule every 4 to 6 hours while symptoms occur
* if pain or fever does not respond to 1 tablet, caplet, gelcap, or liquigel capsule, 2 tablets, caplets, gelcaps or liquigel capsules may be used, but do not exceed 6 tablets, caplets, gelcaps or liquigel capsules in 24 hours, unless directed by a doctor
* the smallest effective dose should be used
Children: do not give to children under 12 unless directed by a doctor

Warnings
Allergy alert: ibuprofen may cause a severe allergic reaction which may include:
* hives
* facial swelling
* asthma (wheezing)
* shock
Alcohol warning: if you consume 3 or more alcoholic drinks every day, ask your doctor whether you should take ibuprofen or other pain relievers/fever reducers. Ibuprofen may cause stomach bleeding.
Do not use if you have ever had an allergic reaction to any other pain reliever/fever reducer
Ask a doctor before use if you have had problems or side effects with any pain reliever/fever reducer
Ask a doctor or pharmacist before use if you are
* under a doctor's care for any continuing medical condition
* taking other drugs on a regular basis
* taking any other product containing ibuprofen, or any other pain reliever/fever reducer
Stop use and ask a doctor if
* an allergic reaction occurs. Seek medical help right away.
* fever gets worse or lasts more than 3 days
* pain gets worse or lasts more than 10 days
* stomach pain occurs with the use of this product
* the painful area is red or swollen
* any new or unexpected symptoms occur

If pregnant or breast-feeding, ask a health professional before use. It is especially important not to use ibuprofen during the last 3 months of pregnancy unless definitely directed to do so by a doctor because it may cause problems in the unborn child or complications during delivery.
Keep out of reach of children. In case of overdose, get medical help or contact a Poison Control Center right away.

How Supplied:
Coated tablets in bottles of 6, 8, 24, 50, 72 (non-child resistant E-Z open cap), 100, 165, and 250. Coated caplets in bottles of 24, 50, 72 (non-child resistant E-Z Cap) 100, 165, and 250.
Gel caplets in bottles of 24, 50, 100, 165 and 250.
Liqui-Gels in bottles of 20, 40, 80, 135 and 200.
Storage: Store at 20–25°C (68–77°F)
Avoid excessive heat 40°C (above 104°F)

ADVIL® COLD and SINUS
**Ibuprofen/Pseudoephedrine HCl Caplets* and Tablets
Pain Reliever/Fever Reducer/Nasal Decongestant**

***Oval-Shaped tablets**

Active Ingredients: Each caplet contains ibuprofen 200 mg and pseudoephedrine HCl 30 mg

Inactive Ingredients: Carnauba or Equivalent Wax, Croscarmellose Sodium, Iron Oxides, Methylparaben, Microcrystalline Cellulose, Propylparaben, Silicon Dioxide, Sodium Benzoate, Sodium Lauryl Sulfate, Starch, Stearic Acid, Sucrose, Titanium Dioxide

Indications:
Temporarily relieves the following symptoms associated with the common cold, sinusitis or flu: nasal congestion, headache; fever; body aches and pains

Dosage and Administration:
Directions—Do not take more than directed
Adults: take 1 caplet/tablet every 4 to 6 hours as needed while symptoms persist
* If symptoms do not respond to 1 caplet/tablet, 2 caplets/tablets may be used. Do not take more than 6 caplets/tablets in any 24-hour period, unless directed by a doctor
* the smallest effective dose should be used
Children: Do not give to children under 12 unless directed by a doctor.

Warnings:
Allergy alert: ibuprofen may cause a severe allergic reaction which may include; hives; facial swelling; asthma (wheezing); shock.

Alcohol warning: If you consume 3 or more alcoholic drinks every day, ask your

Continued on next page

Advil Cold/Sinus—Cont.

doctor whether you should take ibuprofen or other pain relievers/fever reducers. Ibuprofen may cause stomach bleeding.

Do not use:
- if you have ever had an allergic reaction to any other pain reliever/fever reducer
- if you are now taking a prescription monoamine oxidase inhibitor (MAOI) (certain drugs for depression, psychiatric, or emotional conditions, or Parkinson's disease), or for 2 weeks after stopping the MAOI drug. If you do not know if your prescription drug contains an MAOI, ask a doctor or pharmacist before taking this product

Ask a doctor before use if you have:
- heart disease
- high blood pressure
- thyroid disease
- diabetes
- trouble urinating due to an enlarged prostate gland
- any serious condition for which you are under a doctor's care or any condition which requires you to take prescription drugs
- had any problems or serious side effects from taking any pain reliever/fever reducer

Ask a doctor or pharmacist before use if you are:
- taking other drugs on a regular basis
- using other non-prescription pain relievers or ibuprofen-containing product

When using this product do not use more than directed.

Stop use and ask a doctor if:
- an allergic reaction occurs. Seek medical help right away.
- you get nervous, dizzy, or sleepless
- you need to use more than 7 days for a cold or 3 days for a fever
- symptoms do not improve, get worse, or are accompanied by a fever that lasts for more than 3 days
- cold or fever persists or gets worse or if new symptoms occur. These could be signs of a serious illness.
- stomach pain occurs with use of this product
- you experience any symptoms which are unusual or seem unrelated to the condition for which you took this product

If pregnant or breast-feeding, ask a health professional before use. It is especially important not to use this product during the last 3 months of pregnancy unless definitely directed to do so by a doctor because it may cause problems in the unborn child or complications during delivery.

Keep out of the reach of children. In case of accidental overdose, seek professional assistance or contact a poison control center right away.

How Supplied: Advil® Cold and Sinus is an oval-shaped, tan-colored caplet, or tan-colored tablet. The caplet is supplied in blister packs of 20 and 40. The tablet is available in blister packs of 20.

Storage: Store at 20–25°C (68–77°F); avoid excessive heat 40°C, (above 104°F).

ADVIL® FLU & BODY ACHE Caplets

Uses:
- temporarily relieves these symptoms associated with the common cold, sinusitis, or flu
  - headache
  - fever
  - nasal congestion
  - body aches and pains

Active Ingredients (In each caplet): — **Purpose:**
Ibuprofen 200 mg .... Pain reliever/fever reducer
Pseudoephedrine HCl 30 mg .... Nasal decongestant

Inactive Ingredients: Carnauba or equivalent wax, croscarmellose sodium, iron oxide, methylparaben, microcrystalline cellulose, propylparaben, silicon dioxide, sodium benzoate, sodium lauryl sulfate, starch, stearic acid, sucrose, titanium dioxide

Directions:
- Adults and children 12 years of age and over: Take 1 caplet every 4 to 6 hours while symptoms persist. If symptoms do not respond to 1 caplet, 2 caplets may be used.
- do not use more than 6 caplets in any 24-hour period unless directed by a doctor
- the smallest effective dose should be used
- Children under 12 years of age: consult a doctor

Warnings:

Allergy alert: ibuprofen may cause a severe allergic reaction which may include: • hives • facial swelling • asthma (wheezing) • shock

Alcohol warning: if you consume 3 or more alcoholic drinks every day, ask your doctor whether you should take ibuprofen or other pain relievers/fever reducers. Ibuprofen may cause stomach bleeding.

Do not use:
- if you have ever had an allergic reaction to any other pain reliever/fever reducer
- if you are now taking a prescription monoamine oxidase inhibitor (MAOI) (certain drugs for depression, psychiatric, or emotional conditions, or Parkinson's disease), or for 2 weeks after stopping the MAOI drug. If you do not know if your prescription drug contains an MAOI, ask a doctor or pharmacist before taking this product.

Ask a doctor before use if you have:
- heart disease
- high blood pressure
- thyroid disease
- diabetes
- trouble urinating due to an enlarged prostate gland
- any serious condition for which you are under a doctor's care or any condition which requires you to take prescription drugs
- had any problems or serious side effects from taking any pain reliever/fever reducer

Ask a doctor or pharmacist before use if you are:
- taking other drugs on a regular basis
- using other non-prescription pain relievers or ibuprofen-containing product

When using this product do not use more than directed.

Stop use and ask a doctor if:
- an allergic reaction occurs. Seek medical help right away.
- you get nervous, dizzy, or sleepless
- you need to use more than 7 days for a cold or 3 days for a fever
- symptoms do not improve, get worse, or are accompanied by a fever that lasts for more than 3 days
- cold or fever persists or gets worse or if new symptoms occur. These could be signs of a serious illness
- stomach pain occurs with use of this product
- you experience any symptoms which are unusual or seem unrelated to the condition for which you took this product

If pregnant or breast-feeding, ask a health professional before use. It is especially important not to use this product during the last 3 months of pregnancy unless definitely directed to do so by a doctor because it may cause problems in the unborn child or complications during delivery.

Keep out of reach of children. In case of overdose, get medical help or contact a Poison Control Center right away.
- store at room temperature 20–25°C (68–77°F); avoid excessive heat (40°C, 104°F)

How Supplied:
Blister packs of 20 caplets.

ADVIL® MIGRAINE LiquiGels

Use: Treats migraine

Active Ingredient: Each brown, oval capsule contains solubilized ibuprofen equal to 200 mg ibuprofen (present as the free acid and potassium salt)

Inactive Ingredients: D&C yellow no. 10, FD&C green no. 3, FD&C red no. 40, gelatin, light mineral oil, pharmaceutical ink, polyethylene glycol, potassium hydroxide, purified water, sorbitan, sorbitol

Directions:

Adults:	• take 2 capsules with a glass of water
	• if symptoms persist or worsen, ask your doctor
	• do not take more than 2 capsules in 24 hours, unless directed by a doctor
Under 18 years of age:	• ask a doctor

Warnings:

Allergy alert: Ibuprofen may cause a severe allergic reaction which may include:
- hives
- facial swelling
- asthma (wheezing)
- shock

Alcohol warning: If you consume 3 or more alcoholic drinks every day, ask your doctor whether you should take ibuprofen or other pain relievers/fever reducers. Ibuprofen may cause stomach bleeding.

Do not use if you have ever had an allergic reaction to any other pain reliever/fever reducer

Ask a doctor before use if you have:
- never had migraines diagnosed by a health professional
- a headache that is different from your usual migraines
- the worse headache of your life
- fever and stiff neck
- headaches beginning after, or caused by head injury, exertion, coughing or bending
- experienced your first headache after the age of 50
- daily headaches
- a migraine so severe as to require bed rest
- problems or serious side effects from taking pain relievers or fever reducers stomach pain

Ask a doctor or pharmacist before use if you are:
- under a doctor's care for any continuing medical condition
- taking other drugs on a regular basis
- taking another product containing ibuprofen, or any other pain reliever/fever reducer

Stop use and ask a doctor if:
- an allergic reaction occurs. Seek medical help right away.
- migraine headache pain is not relieved or gets worse after first dose
- stomach pain occurs with the use of this product
- new or unexpected symptoms occur

If pregnant or breast-feeding, ask a health professional before use. It is especially important not to use ibuprofen during the last 3 months of pregnancy unless definitely directed to do so by a doctor because it may cause problems in the unborn child or complications during delivery.

Keep out of reach of children. In case of overdose, get medical help or contact a Poison Control Center right away.

Other information:
- read all directions and warnings before use. Keep carton.
- store at 20–25°C (68–77°F)
- avoid excessive heat 40°C (above 104°F)

How Supplied: Bottles of 20, 40, & 80 liquigels.

Children's Advil Suspension

WEIGHT (lb.)	AGE (yr.)	DOSE (tsp.)
Under 24	Under 2	Consult a Doctor
24-35	2-3	1 tsp.
36-47	4-5	1 $\frac{1}{2}$tsp.
48-59	6-8	2 tsp.
60-71	9-10	2 $\frac{1}{2}$ tsp.
72-95	11	3 tsp.

Junior Strength Advil

WEIGHT (lb.)	AGE (yr.)	DOSE (Tablets)
Under 48	Under 6	Ask a Doctor
48-71	6-10	2
72-95	11	3

CHILDREN'S ADVIL®
Oral Suspension
JUNIOR STRENGTH ADVIL Tablets
JUNIOR STRENGTH ADVIL
Chewable Tablets
CHILDREN'S ADVIL Chewable Tablets
INFANTS' ADVIL Drops
[ad ' vil]
Ibuprofen

Description: Children's Advil® Ibuprofen Oral Suspension is an alcohol-free, fruit-flavored or grape-flavored liquid specially developed for children. Each 5 mL (teaspoon) contains ibuprofen 100 mg. Each Junior Strength Advil Coated Tablet contains 100 mg ibuprofen. Each Chewable Tablet contains 50 or 100 mg ibuprofen. Each 1.25 mL of Infants' Advil Drops contains ibuprofen 50 mg.

Inactive Ingredients (Children's Advil Oral Suspension, Infants' Advil Drops): Artificial flavors, Caroboxymethylcellulose Sodium, Citric Acid, Edetate Disodium, FD&C Red No. 40, FD&C Blue No.1 (grape flavor only), Glycerin, Microcrystalline Cellulose, Polysorbate 80, Purified Water, Sodium Benzoate, Sorbitol Solution, Sucrose, Xanthan Gum.

Inactive Ingredients (Junior Strength Advil Tablets): Acetylated Monoglycerides, Carnauba Wax, Colloidal Silicon Dioxide, Croscarmellose Sodium, Iron Oxides, Methylparaben, Microcrystalline Cellulose, Povidone, Pregelatinized Starch, Propylene Glycol, Propylparaben, Shellac, Sodium Benzoate, Starch, Stearic Acid, Sucrose, and Titanium Dioxide.

Inactive Ingredients (Junior Strength Advil Chewable Tablets): Artificial flavor, Aspartame, Cellulose Acetate Phthalate, D&C Red #30 Lake (grape only), D&C Red No. 27 Lake (fruit only), FD&C Blue #2 Lake (grape only), FD&C Red No. 40 Lake (fruit only), Gelatin, Magnasweet, Magnesium Stearate, Mannitol, Microcrystalline Cellulose, Natural Flavors (fruit only), Silicon Dioxide, Sodium Starch Glycolate.

Indications: Children's Advil® Ibuprofen Oral Suspension, Junior Strength Advil Tablets, Junior Strength Advil Chewable Tablets, Children's Advil Chewable Tablets, and Infants' Advil Drops are indicated for the temporary relief of fever and minor aches and pains due to the common cold, flu, sore throat (for all products except Infants' Drops), headaches and toothaches. One dose lasts 6–8 hours.

Warnings:

Allergy Alert: Ibuprofen may cause a severe allergic reaction which may include hives, asthma (wheezing), facial swelling, shock.

Sore throat warning: severe or persistent sore throat or sore throat accompanied by high fever, headache, nausea, and vomiting may be serious. Consult doctor promptly. Do not use more than 2 days or administer to children under 3 years of age unless directed by doctor.

Do Not Use:
- if the child has ever had an allergic reaction to any pain reliever/fever reducer

Ask a doctor before use if the child has
- not been drinking fluids
- lost a lot of fluid due to continued vomiting or diarrhea
- stomach pain
- problems or serious side effects from taking fever reducers or pain relievers

Ask a doctor or pharmacist before use if the child is
- under a doctor's care for any serious condition
- taking any other drug
- taking any other product that contains ibuprofen or any other pain reliever/fever reducer

When using this product give with food or milk if upset stomach occurs.

Stop use and ask a doctor if
- an allergic reaction occurs. Seek medical help right away.
- fever or pain gets worse or lasts more than 3 days.
- the child does not get any relief within first day (24 hours) of treatment
- stomach pain or upset gets worse or lasts
- redness or swelling is present in the painful area
- any new symptoms appear

Continued on next page

Children's Advil—Cont.

Keep out of reach of children. In case of overdose, seek professional assistance or contact a poison control center immediately.

Directions (Children's Advil Oral Suspension): Do not give more than directed. Shake well before using. Use this product only with chart provided. Find right dose on chart. If possible, use weight to dose; otherwise, use age. Measure dose with cup provided. Do not discard the measuring cup. Repeat dose every 6–8 hours, if needed. Do not use more than 4 times a day.

[See table at top of previous page]

Directions (Junior Strength Advil Tablets): Do not give more than directed. Use this product only with chart provided. Find right dose on chart below. If possible, use weight to dose; otherwise use age. Repeat dose every 6–8 hours, if needed.

Do not use more than 4 times a day.

[See table at top of previous page]

Directions (Infants' Advil Drops): Do not give more than directed. Shake well before using. Find the right dose on chart below. This product is intended for use in children ages 6 to 23 months of age. If possible, use weight to dose. Otherwise, use age. Measure dose with the dosing device provided. Do not use with any other device. Repeat dose every 6–8 hours, if needed. Do not use more than 4 times a day.

[See table below]

Directions (Junior Strength Advil Chewable Tablets): Do not give more than directed. Use this product only with chart provided. Find right dose on chart. If possible, use weight to dose. Otherwise, use age. Repeat dose every 6–8 hours, if needed. Do not use more than 4 times a day. If stomach upset occurs while taking this product, give with food or milk.

[See table below]

How Supplied: Children's Advil Oral Suspension: bottles of 2 fl. oz. and 4 fl. oz. in grape and fruit flavors.

Junior Strength Advil: Coated Tablets in bottles of 24. Chewable Tablets: bottles of 24 (fruit and grape flavors)
Infants' Advil Drops: bottles of $1/2$ fl. oz. in grape and fruit flavors.
Children's Advil Chewable Tablets: blister of 24 (fruit and grape flavors)
Store at 20–25°C (68–77°F)
Phenylketonurics:
Junior Strength Advil Chewable Tablets contains Phenylalanine, 4.2 mg per tablet.
Children's Advil Chewable Tablets contain Phenylalanine, 2.1 mg per tablet.

MAXIMUM STRENGTH
ANBESOL® Gel and Liquid
[an 'ba-sol ″]
Oral Anesthetic

ANBESOL JUNIOR® Gel
Oral Anesthetic Gel

BABY ANBESOL®
Grape Flavor
Oral Anesthetic Gel

Description: Anbesol is an oral anesthetic which is available in a Maximum Strength gel and liquid. Anbesol Junior, available in a gel, is an oral anesthetic. Baby Anbesol, available in a grape-flavored gel, is an oral anesthetic and is alcohol-free.
The Maximum Strength formulations contain Benzocaine 20%.
The Anbesol Junior Gel contains Benzocaine 10%.
The Baby Anbesol Gels contain Benzocaine 7.5%.

Indications: Maximum Strength Anbesol is indicated for the temporary relief of pain associated with toothache, canker sores, minor dental procedures, sore gums, braces, and dentures. Anbesol Junior is indicated for the temporary relief of braces, sore gums, canker sores, toothaches, and minor dental procedures. Baby Anbesol Gel is indicated for the temporary relief of sore gums due to teething in infants and children 4 months of age and older.

Warnings: **Allergy alert:** Do not use this product if you have a history of allergy to local anesthetics such as procaine, butacaine, benzocaine, or other "caine" anesthetics.

Do not use to treat fever and nasal congestion. These are not symptoms of teething and may indicate the presence of infection. If these symptoms persist, consult your doctor.
When using this product
• avoid contact with the eyes
• do not exceed recommended dosage
• do not use for more than 7 days unless directed by a doctor/dentist
Stop use and ask a doctor if
• sore mouth symptoms do not improve in 7 days
• irritation, pain, or redness persists or worsens
• swelling, rash, or fever develops
Keep out of reach of children. If more than used for pain is accidentally swallowed, get medical help or contact a Poison Control Center right away.

Dosage and Administration: Maximum Strength Anbesol:
Gel
• to open tube, cut tip of the tube on score mark with scissors
• adults and children 2 years of age and older: apply to the affected area up to 4 times daily or as directed by a doctor/dentist
• children under 12 years of age: adult supervision should be given in the use of this product
• children under 2 years of age: consult a doctor/dentist
• for denture irritation:
  • apply thin layer to the affected area
  • do not reinsert dental work until irritation/pain is relieved
  • rinse mouth well before reinserting
Liquid
• adults and children 2 years of age and older:
  • wipe liquid on with cotton, or cotton swab, or fingertip
  • apply to the affected area up to 4 times daily or as directed by a doctor/dentist
• children under 12 years of age: adult supervision should be given in the use of this product
• children under 2 years of age; consult a doctor/dentist
Anbesol Junior:
• to open tube, cut tip of the tube on score mark with scissors
• adults and children 2 years of age and older: apply to the affected area up to 4 times daily or as directed by a doctor/dentist
• children under 12 years of age: adult supervision should be given in the use of this product
• children under 2 years of age: consult a doctor/dentist
Grape Baby Anbesol:
• to open tube, cut tip of the tube on score mark with scissors
• children 4 months of age and older: apply to the affected area not more than 4 times daily or as directed by a doctor/dentist
• infants under 4 months of age: no recommended treatment except under the advice and supervision of a doctor/dentist

Infants' Advil Drops

WEIGHT (lb.)	AGE (mo.)	DOSE (mL)
	under 6 mo	Ask a Doctor
12-17	6-11	1.25
18-23	12-23	1.875

Children's Advil Chewable Tablets

WEIGHT (lb.)	AGE (yr.)	DOSE (tablets)	
		50 mg	100 mg
Under 24	Under 2	Ask a Doctor	Ask a Doctor
24-35	2-3	2	Ask a Doctor
36-47	4-5	3	Ask a Doctor
48-59	6-8	4	2
60-71	9-10	5	$2 1/2$
72-95	11	6	3

Inactive Ingredients:
Maximum Strength Gel: Carbomer 934P, D&C Yellow No. 10, FD&C Blue No. 1, FD&C Red No. 40, Flavor, Glycerin, Methylparaben, Phenylcarbinol, Polyethylene Glycol, Propylene Glycol, Saccharin.
Maximum Strength Liquid: D&C Yellow No. 10, FD&C Blue No. 1, FD&C Red No. 40, Flavor, Methylparaben, Phenylcarbinol, Polyethylene Glycol, Propylene Glycol, Saccharin.
Junior Gel: Artificial flavor, benzyl alcohol, carbomer 934P, D&C red no. 33, glycerin, methylparaben, polyethylene glycol, potassium acesulfame
Grape Baby Gel: Benzoic acid, carbomer 934P, D&C red no. 33, edetate disodium, FD&C blue no. 1, flavor, glycerin, methylparaben, polyethylene glycol, propylparaben, saccharin, water

How Supplied: All Gels in .25 oz (7.1 g) tubes, Maximum Strength Liquid in .31 fl oz (9 mL) bottle. Store at 20–25°C (68–77°F)
Safety Sealed Tube. Do Not Use if tube tip is cut prior to opening

---

DIMETAPP COLD AND FEVER
Suspension
[dī 'mĕ-tap]
Nasal Decongestant, Antihistamine, Pain Reliever/Fever Reducer
Alcohol-Free

Active Ingredients (in each 5 mL tsp):
Acetaminophen, USP .... 160 mg
Brompheniramine maleate, USP .. 1 mg
Pseudoephedrine HCl, USP .... 15 mg

Inactive Ingredients: Carboxymethylcellulose Sodium, Citric Acid, D&C Red No. 33, Edetate Disodium, FD&C Blue No. 1, Flavors, Glycerin, High Fructose Corn Syrup, Maltol, Methylparaben, Microcrystalline Cellulose, Polysorbate 80, Potassium Sorbate, Propylene Glycol, Propylparaben, Sorbitol, Sucrose, Water, Xanthan Gum.

Uses:
- temporarily relieves these symptoms associated with a cold: headache, nasal congestion, sore throat, fever, minor aches and pains, and muscular aches
- temporarily relieves minor aches, pains, and headache as well as these symptoms due to hay fever or other upper respiratory allergies: runny nose, sneezing, itching of the nose or throat, and itchy, watery eyes
- temporarily relieves minor aches, pains, headache and nasal congestion associated with sinusitis

Warnings:
Sore throat warning: if sore throat is severe, persists for more than 2 days, is accompanied or followed by fever, headache, rash, nausea, or vomiting, consult a doctor promptly.
Do not use in a child who is taking a prescription monoamine oxidase inhibitor (MAOI) (certain drugs for depression, psychiatric, or emotional conditions, or Parkinson's disease), or for 2 weeks after stopping the MAOI drug. If you do not know if your child's prescription drug contains an MAOI, ask a doctor or pharmacist before giving this product.
Ask a doctor before use if your child has:
- heart disease
- high blood pressure
- thyroid disease
- diabetes
- a breathing problem such as chronic bronchitis
- glaucoma
Ask a doctor or pharmacist before use if your child is taking sedatives or tranquilizers.
When using this product:
- do not give more than directed
- drowsiness may occur
- sedatives and tranquilizers may increase drowsiness
- excitability may occur, especially in children
Stop use and ask a doctor if:
- your child gets nervous, dizzy, or sleepless
- new symptoms occur
- redness or swelling is present
- symptoms do not get better, get worse, or are accompanied by fever more than 3 days
- your child needs to use for more than 5 days
Keep out of reach of children. In case of overdose, get medical help or contact a Poison Control Center right away. Quick medical attention is critical even if you do not notice any signs or symptoms.

Directions:
- shake well before using
- do not give more than 4 doses in any 24-hour period
- children 6 to under 12 years: 2 teaspoonfuls every 4 hours
- children under 6 years: ask a doctor
Storage: Store at 20°C and 25°C (68°F and 77°F).

How Supplied: 4 oz bottle with dosage cup.

DIMETAPP® Infant Drops
Decongestant
[dī 'mĕ-tap]

Description: Nasal Decongestant (Pseudoephedrine Hydrochloride)
Alcohol-Free

Active Ingredients: Each 0.8 mL (1 dropperful) contains: 7.5 mg Pseudoephedrine Hydrochloride, USP.

Inactive Ingredients: caramel, citric acid, D&C red no. 33, FD&C blue no. 1, flavors, glycerin, high fructose corn syrup, maltol, menthol, polyethylene glycol, propylene glycol, sodium benzoate, sorbitol, sucrose, water

Indications: For temporary relief of nasal congestion due to the common cold, hay fever, other upper respiratory allergies, or associated with sinusitis.

Warnings:
Do not use in a child who is taking a prescription monoamine oxidase inhibitor (MAOI) (certain drugs for depression, psychiatric, or emotional conditions, or Parkinson's disease), or for 2 weeks after stopping the MAOI drug. If you do not know if your child's prescription drug contains an MAOI, ask a doctor or pharmacist before giving this product.
Ask a doctor before use if your child has:
- heart disease
- high blood pressure
- thyroid disease
- diabetes
When using this product:
- do not use more than directed
- give by mouth only; not for nasal use
Stop use and ask a doctor if:
- your child gets nervous, dizzy, or sleepless
- symptoms do not get better within 7 days or are accompanied by fever
Keep out of reach of children. In case of overdose, get medical help or contact a Poison Control Center right away.

Directions:
- do not give more than 4 doses in any 24-hour period
- children 2 to 3 years: 2 dropperfuls (1.6 mL) every 4 to 6 hours or as directed by a physician
- children under 2 years: ask a doctor
Storage: Store at Controlled Room Temperature, between 20°C and 25°C (68°F and 77°F).

How Supplied: ¼ oz (8 mL) bottle with dropper.

DIMETAPP® DM COLD & COUGH
Elixir
[dī 'mĕ-tap]
Nasal Decongestant, Antihistamine, Cough Suppressant

Description: Each 5 mL (1 teaspoonful) of DIMETAPP DM Elixir contains:

Brompheniramine
Maleate, USP .... 1 mg
Pseudoephedrine
Hydrochloride .... 15 mg
Dextromethorphan
Hydrobromide, USP .... 5 mg

Inactive Ingredients: artificial flavor, citric acid, FD&C blue no. 1, FD&C red no. 40, glycerin, high fructose corn syrup, propylene glycol, saccharin sodium, sodium benzoate, sorbitol, water

Uses:
- temporarily relieves cough due to minor throat and bronchial irritation occurring with a cold, and nasal congestion due to the common cold, hay fever or other upper respiratory allergies, or associated with sinusitis
- temporarily relieves these symptoms due to hay fever (allergic rhinitis):
  - runny nose
  - sneezing
  - itchy, watery eyes
  - itching of the nose or throat
- temporarily restores freer breathing through the nose

Indications:
Temporarily relieves cough due to minor throat and bronchial irritation occur

Continued on next page

Dimetapp DM/C&C—Cont.

with a cold, and nasal congestion due to the common cold, hay fever or other upper respiratory allergies, or associated with sinusitis. Temporarily relieves runny nose, sneezing, itching of the nose or throat and itchy, watery eyes due to allergic rhinitis (hay fever). Temporarily restores freer breathing through the nose.

Warnings:
Do not use if you are now taking a prescription monoamine oxidase inhibitor (MAOI) (certain drugs for depression, psychiatric, or emotional conditions, or Parkinson's disease), or for 2 weeks after stopping the MAOI drug. If you do not know if your prescription drug contains an MAOI, ask a doctor or pharmacist before taking this product.
Ask a doctor before use if you have
• heart disease
• high blood pressure
• thyroid disease
• diabetes
• trouble urinating due to an enlarged prostate gland
• glaucoma
• cough that occurs with too much phlegm (mucus)
• a breathing problem or persistent or chronic cough that lasts or as occurs with smoking, asthma, chronic bronchitis, or emphysema
Ask a doctor or pharmacist before use if you are taking sedatives or tranquilizers.
When using this product:
• **do not use more than directed**
• marked drowsiness may occur
• avoid alcoholic beverages
• alcohol, sedatives, and tranquilizers may increase drowsiness
• be careful when driving a motor vehicle or operating machinery
• excitability may occur, especially in children
Stop use and ask a doctor if:
• you get nervous, dizzy, or sleepless
• symptoms do not get better within 7 days or are accompanied by fever
• cough lasts more than 7 days, comes back, or is accompanied by fever, rash, or persistent headache. These could be signs of a serious condition
If pregnant or breast-feeding, ask a health professional before use.
Keep out of reach of children. In case of overdose, get medical help or contact a Poison Control Center right away.

Directions:
• do not take more than 4 doses in any 24-hour period

Age	Dose
adults and children 12 years and over	4 tsp every 4 hours
children 6 to under 12 years	2 tsp every 4 hours
children under 6 years	ask a doctor

Store at Controlled Room Temperature, Between 20°C and 25°C (68°F and 77°F)

How Supplied (DIMETAPP DM ELIXIR): Red, grape-flavored liquid in bottles of 4 fl oz, 8 fl oz and 12 fl oz. Not a USP Elixir. Dosage cup provided.

DIMETAPP®
Infant Drops Decongestant Plus Cough
Nasal decongestant/cough suppressant
Alcohol-Free/non-staining

Active Ingredients: Each 0.8 mL (1 dropperful) contains: 7.5 mg Pseudoephedrine Hydrochloride, USP; 2.5 mg Dextromethorphan Hydrobromide, USP.
Inactive Ingredients: Citric Acid, Flavors, Glycerin, High Fructose Corn Syrup, Maltol, Menthol, Polyethylene Glycol, Propylene Glycol, Sodium Benzoate, Sorbitol, Sucrose, Water.

Indications: Temporarily relieves cough occurring with the common cold and temporarily relieves nasal congestion due to a cold, hay fever, or other upper respiratory allergies.

Warnings:
Do not use in a child who is taking a prescription monoamine oxidase inhibitor (MAOI) (certain drugs for depression, psychiatric, or emotional conditions, or Parkinson's disease), or for 2 weeks after stopping the MAOI drug. If you do not know if your child's prescription drug contains an MAOI, ask a doctor or pharmacist before giving this product.
Ask a doctor before use if your child has:
• heart disease
• high blood pressure
• thyroid disease
• diabetes
• cough that occurs with too much phlegm (mucus)
• cough that lasts or is chronic such as occurs with asthma
When using this product:
• **do not use more than directed**
• give by mouth only; not for nasal use
Stop use and ask a doctor if:
• your child gets nervous, dizzy, or sleepless
• symptoms do not get better within 7 days or are accompanied by fever
• cough lasts more than 7 days, comes back, or is accompanied by fever, rash, or persistent headache. These could be signs of a serious condition.
Keep out of reach of children. In case of overdose, get medical help or contact a Poison Control Center right away.

Directions: do not give more than 4 doses in any 24-hour period

Age	Dose
children 2-3 years	2 dropperfuls (1.6 mL) every 4 hours or as directed by a physician
children under 2 years	ask a doctor

Storage: Store at Controlled Room Temperature, between 20°C and 25°C (68°F and 77°F).

How Supplied: Infant Drops ¼ fl oz (8mL). Oral Dropper Enclosed

---

DIMETAPP®
NIGHTTIME FLU SYRUP

Uses: Temporarily relieves these symptoms associated with a cold or flu: headache, sore throat, fever, muscular aches, minor aches and pains. Temporarily relieves nasal congestion, and cough due to minor throat and bronchial irritation occurring with a cold. Temporarily relieves these symptoms due to hay fever or other respiratory allergies: sneezing; itching of the nose or throat; itchy, watery eyes, runny nose. Temporarily restores freer breathing through the nose.

Active Ingredients:

(in each 5 mL tsp):	Purpose:
Acetaminophen, USP 160 mg	Pain reliever/fever reducer
Brompheniramine maleate, USP 1 mg	Antihistamine
Dextromethorphan, HBr, USP 5 mg	Cough suppressant
Pseudoephedrine HCl, USP 15 mg	Nasal decongestant

Inactive Ingredients: citric acid, FD&C red no. 40, flavor, glycerin, high fructose corn syrup, polyethylene glycol, povidone, saccharin sodium, sodium benzoate, sodium citrate, sorbitol, water.

Directions:
• do not use more than 4 doses in any 24-hour period

Age	Dose
adults and children 12 years and over	4 teaspoonfuls every 4 hours
children 6 to under 12 years	2 teaspoonfuls every 4 hours
children under 6 years	consult a doctor

Warnings:
Alcohol warning: if you consume 3 or more alcoholic drinks every day, ask your doctor whether you should take acetaminophen or other pain relievers/fever reducers. Acetaminophen may cause liver damage.
Sore throat warning: if sore throat is severe, persists for more than two days, is accompanied or followed by fever, headache, rash, nausea, or vomiting, consult a doctor promptly.
Do not use if you are now taking a prescription monoamine oxidase inhibitor (MAOI) (certain drugs for depression, psychiatric, or emotional conditions, or Parkinson's disease), or for 2 weeks after stopping the MAOI drug. If you do not know if your prescription drug contains an MAOI, ask a doctor or pharmacist before taking this product.
Ask a doctor before use if you have:
• heart disease

- high blood pressure
- thyroid disease
- diabetes
- trouble urinating due to an enlarged prostate gland
- glaucoma
- cough that occurs with too much phlegm (mucus)
- a breathing problem or persistent or chronic cough that lasts or as occurs with smoking, asthma, chronic bronchitis, or emphysema

Ask a doctor or pharmacist before use if you are taking sedatives or tranquilizers.

When using this product:
- do not use more than directed
- marked drowsiness may occur
- avoid alcoholic beverages
- alcohol, sedatives, and tranquilizers may increase drowsiness
- be careful when driving a motor vehicle or operating machinery
- excitability may occur, especially in children

Stop use and ask a doctor if:
- you get nervous, dizzy, or sleepless
- new symptoms occur
- you need to use for more than 7 days (adults) or 5 days (children)
- symptoms do not get better, get worse, or are accompanied by fever more than 3 days
- redness or swelling is present
- cough lasts more than 7 days, comes back, or is accompanied by fever, rash, or persistent headache. These could be signs of a serious condition.

If pregnant or breast-feeding, ask a health professional before use. **Keep out of reach of children.** In case of overdose, get medical help or contact a Poison Control Center right away. Quick medical attention is critical for adults as well as for children, even if you do not notice any signs or symptoms.

Other information:
- store at 20–25°C (68–77°F)
- not USP. Meets specifications when tested with a validated non-USP assay method.

How Supplied: 4 oz bottle with dosage cup.

DIMETAPP®
NON-DROWSY FLU Syrup

Uses: Temporarily relieves these symptoms associated with a cold, or flu: headache, sore throat, fever, muscular aches, minor aches and pain Temporarily relieves nasal congestion, and cough due to minor throat and bronchial irritation occurring with a cold. Temporarily restores freer breathing through the nose

Active Ingredients:

(in each 5 mL tsp):	Purpose:
Acetaminophen, USP	
160 mg	Pain reliever/fever reducer
Dextromethorphan HBr, USP	
5 mg	Cough suppressant
Pseudoephedrine HCl, USP	
15 mg	Nasal decongestant

Inactive Ingredients: Citric acid, FD&C red no. 40, FD&C yellow no. 6, flavor, glycerin, high fructose corn syrup, polyethylene glycol, povidone, saccharin sodium, sodium benzoate, sodium citrate, sorbitol, water.

Directions:
- do not use more than 4 doses in any 24-hour period

Age	Dose
adults and children 12 years and over	4 tsp every 4 hours
children 6 to under 12 years	2 tsp every 4 hours
children 2 to under 6 years	1 tsp every 4 hours
children under 2 years	consult a doctor

Warnings:
Alcohol warning: if you consume 3 or more alcoholic drinks every day, ask your doctor whether you should take acetaminophen or other pain relievers/fever reducers. Acetaminophen may cause liver damage.
Sore throat warning: if sore throat is severe, persists for more than two days, is accompanied or followed by fever, headache, rash, nausea, or vomiting, consult a doctor promptly.
Do not use if you are now taking a prescription monoamine oxidase inhibitor (MAOI) (certain drugs for depression, psychiatric, or emotional conditions, or Parkinson's disease), or for 2 weeks after stopping the MAOI drug if you do not know if your prescription drug contains an MAOI, ask a doctor or pharmacist before taking this product.
Ask a doctor before use if you have: heart disease, high blood pressure, thyroid disease, diabetes, trouble urinating due to an enlarged prostate gland, cough that occurs with too much phlegm (mucus), or cough that lasts or is chronic such as occurs with smoking, asthma, or emphysema.
When using this product do not use more than directed.
Stop use and ask a doctor if: you get nervous, dizzy, or sleepless; new symptoms occur; you need to use for more than 7 days (adults) or 5 days (children); symptoms do not get better, get worse, or are accompanied by fever more than 3 days; if redness or swelling is present; or if cough lasts more than 7 days, comes back, or is accompanied by fever, rash, or persistent headache These could be signs of a serious condition.
If pregnant or breast-feeding, ask a health professional before use. **Keep out of reach of children.** In case of overdose, get medical help or contact a Poison Control Center right away Quick medical attention is critical for adults as well as for children, even if you do not notice any signs or symptoms.

Other information:
- store at 20–25°C (68–77°F)

- not USP. Meets specifications when tested with a validated non-USP assay method

How Supplied: 4 oz bottle with dosage cup.

DIMETAPP® Elixir
Nasal Decongestant, Antihistamine

Active Ingredients:
Each 5 mL (1 teaspoonful) contains:
Brompheniramine
   Maleate, USP .... 1 mg
Pseudoephedrine
   Hydrochloride .... 15 mg

Inactive ingredients: Artificial Flavor, Citric Acid, FD&C Blue No. 1, FD&C Red No. 40, Glycerin, High Fructose Corn Syrup, Propylene Glycol, Saccharin Sodium, Sodium Benzoate, Sorbitol, Water

Uses:
- temporarily relieves nasal congestion due to the common cold, hay fever or other upper respiratory allergies, or associated with sinusitis
- temporarily relieves these symptoms due to hay fever (allergic rhinitis):
  - runny nose
  - sneezing
  - itchy, watery eyes
  - itching of the nose or throat
- temporarily restores freer breathing through the nose

Warnings:
Do not use if you are now taking a prescription monoamine oxidase inhibitor (MAOI) (certain drugs for depression, psychiatric, or emotional conditions, or Parkinson's disease), or for 2 weeks after stopping the MAOI drug. If you do not know if your prescription drug contains an MAOI, ask a doctor or pharmacist before taking this product.
Ask a doctor before use if you have:
- heart disease
- high blood pressure
- thyroid disease
- diabetes
- trouble urinating due to an enlarged prostate gland
- glaucoma
- a breathing problem such as emphysema or chronic bronchitis
Ask a doctor or pharmacist before use if you are taking sedatives or tranquilizers.
When using this product:
- do not use more than directed
- drowsiness may occur
- avoid alcoholic beverages
- alcohol, sedatives, and tranquilizers may increase drowsiness
- be careful when driving a motor vehicle or operating machinery
- excitability may occur, especially in children
Stop use and ask a doctor if:
- you get nervous, dizzy, or sleepless
- symptoms do not get better within 7 days or are accompanied by fever
If pregnant or breast-feeding, ask a health professional before use.

Continued on next page

Dimetapp—Cont.

Keep out of reach of children. In case of overdose, get medical help or contact a Poison Control Center right away.

Directions:
- do not take more than 4 doses in any 24-hour period

AGE	DOSE
adults and children 12 years and over	4 tsp every 4 hours
children 6 to under 12 years	2 tsp every 4 hours
children under 6 years	ask a doctor

Storage: Store at Controlled Room Temperature, between 20°C and 25°C (68°F and 77°F).

How Supplied: Purple, grape-flavored liquid in bottles of 4 fl oz, 8 fl oz, and 12 fl oz. Not a USP elixir.

ORUDIS® KT™

[*Orūdĭs*]

Description: Pain Reliever/Fever Reducer.

Active Ingredients: Each tablet contains ketoprofen 12.5 mg.

Inactive Ingredients: Cellulose, D&C Yellow No. 10 Lake, FD&C Blue No. 1 Lake, FD&C Yellow No. 5 Lake (Tartrazine), Iron Oxide, Pharmaceutical Glaze, Povidone, Silica, Sodium Benzoate, Sodium Lauryl Sulfate, Starch, Stearic Acid, Sugar, Titanium Dioxide, Wax.

Indications: Temporarily relieves minor aches and pains due to common cold, headache, toothache, muscular aches, backache, minor pain of arthritis and menstrual cramps. Temporarily reduces fever.

Warnings:
Allergy alert: ketoprofen may cause a severe allergic reaction which may include:
- hives
- facial swelling
- asthma (wheezing)
- shock

Alcohol warning: if you consume 3 or more alcoholic drinks every day, ask your doctor whether you should take ketoprofen or other pain relievers/fever reducers. Ketoprofen may cause stomach bleeding.

Do not use if you ever had an allergic reaction to any other pain reliever/fever reducer

Ask a doctor before use if you have had problems or side effects with any pain reliever/fever reducer

Ask a doctor or pharmacist before use if you are:
- under a doctor's care for any continuing medical condition

- taking other drugs on a regular basis
- taking any other product containing ketoprofen, or any other pain reliever/fever reducer

Stop use and ask a doctor if:
- an allergic reaction occurs. Seek medical help right away.
- fever gets worse or lasts more than 3 days
- pain gets worse or lasts more than 10 days
- stomach pain occurs with use of this product
- the painful area is red or swollen
- any new or unexpected symptoms occur

If you are pregnant or breast-feeding, ask a health professional before use. It is especially important not to use ketoprofen during the last 3 months of pregnancy unless definitely directed to do so by a doctor because it may cause problems in the unborn child or complications during delivery.

Keep out of reach of children. In case of overdose, get medical help or contact a Poison Control Center right away.

Directions:
- do not take more than directed
- take with a full glass of water or other liquid
- adults, take 1 tablet *or* caplet every 4 to 6 hours
- if pain or fever does not get better in 1 hour, you may take 1 more tablet *or* caplet
- with experience, some people may find they need 2 tablets *or* caplets for the first dose
- the smallest effective dose should be used
- do not take more than 2 tablets *or* caplets in any 4 to 6 hour period
- do not take more than 6 tablets *or* caplets in any 24 hour period
- children: do not give to children under age 16 unless directed by a doctor

How Supplied: Coated tablets in bottles of 24, 50, 100
ORUDIS is a registered trademark of RHONE-POULENC. KT and the appearance of the green ORUDIS KT tablet are trademarks of WHITEHALL-ROBINS HEALTHCARE.

Storage: Store at 20–25°C (68–77°F). Avoid excessive heat 40°C (above 104°F)

PREPARATION H®

[*prep-e 'rā-shen-āch*]
Hemorrhoidal Ointment and Cream
PREPARATION H®
Hemorrhoidal Suppositories
PREPARATION H®
Hemorrhoidal Cooling Gel

Description: Preparation H is available in ointment, cream, gel, and suppository product forms. The **Ointment** contains Petrolatum 71.9%, Mineral Oil 14%, Shark Liver Oil 3% and Phenylephrine HCl 0.25%.
The **Cream** contains Petrolatum 18%, Glycerin 12%, Shark Liver Oil 3% and Phenylephrine HCl 0.25%.
The **Suppositories** contain Cocoa Butter 85.5%, Shark Liver Oil 3%, and Phenylephrine HCL 0.25%.

The **Cooling Gel** contains Phenylephrine HCl 0.25% and Witch Hazel 50%.

Indications: Preparation H Ointment, Cream, and Suppositories help:
- relieve the local itching and discomfort associated with hemorrhoids
- temporarily shrink hemorrhoidal tissue and relieve burning
- temporarily provide a coating for relief of anorectal discomforts
- temporarily protect the inflamed, irritated anorectal surface to help make bowel movements less painful
Cooling Gel helps:
- relieve the local itching and discomfort associated with hemorrhoids
- temporarily relieves irritation and burning
- temporarily shrinks hemorrhoidal tissue
- aids in protecting irritated anorectal areas

Warnings:
Ask a doctor before use if you have:
- heart disease
- high blood pressure
- thyroid disease
- diabetes
- difficulty in urination due to enlargement of the prostate gland
Ask a doctor or pharmacist before use if you are presently taking a prescription drug for high blood pressure or depression.
When using this product do not exceed the recommended daily dosage unless directed by a doctor.
Cream/Cooling Gel: Do not put into the rectum by using fingers or any mechanical device or applicator. For external use only.
Stop use and ask a doctor if:
- bleeding occurs
- condition worsens or does not improve within 7 days
Ointment: Stop use and ask a doctor if introduction of applicator into the rectum causes additional pain. For external and/or intrarectal use only.
Suppositories: For rectal use only.
If pregnant or breast-feeding, ask a health professional before use.
Keep out of reach of children. If swallowed, get medical help or contact a Poison Control Center right away.

Dosage and Administration:
Ointment—
- adults: when practical, cleanse the affected area by patting or blotting with an appropriate cleansing wipe. Gently dry by patting or blotting with a tissue or a soft cloth before applying ointment.
- when first opening the tube, puncture foil seal with top end of cap
- apply to the affected area up to 4 times daily, especially at night, in the morning or after each bowel movement
- intrarectal use:
  - remove cover from applicator, attach applicator to tube, lubricate applicator well and gently insert applicator into the rectum
  - thoroughly cleanse applicator after each use and replace cover
- also apply ointment to external area
- regular use provides continual therapy for relief of symptoms
- children under 12 years of age: ask a doctor

Tamper-Evident: Do Not Use if tube seal under cap embossed with "H" is broken or missing.

Cream—

- adults: when practical, cleanse the affected area by patting or blotting with an appropriate cleansing wipe. Gently dry by patting or blotting with a tissue or a soft cloth before applying cream.
- when first opening the tube, puncture foil seal with top end of cap
- apply externally or in the lower portion of the anal canal only
- apply externally to the affected area up to 4 times daily, especially at night, in the morning or after each bowel movement
- for application in the lower anal canal: remove cover from dispensing cap. Attach dispensing cap tube. Lubricate dispensing cap well, then gently insert dispensing cap partway into the anus.
- thoroughly cleanse dispensing cap after each use and replace cover
- children under 12 years of age: ask a doctor

Tamper-Evident: Do Not Use if tube seal under cap embossed with "H" is broken or missing.

Suppositories—

- adults: when practical, cleanse the affected area by patting or blotting with an appropriate cleansing wipe. Gently dry by patting or blotting with a tissue or a soft cloth before insertion of this product
- detach one suppository from the strip; remove the foil wrapper before inserting into the rectum as follows:
  - hold suppository with rounded end up
  - as shown, carefully separate foil tabs by inserting tip of fingernail at end marked "peel down"
  - slowly and evenly peel apart (do not tear) foil by pulling tabs down both sides, to expose the suppository
  - remove exposed suppository from wrapper
  - insert one suppository into the rectum up to 4 times daily, especially at night, in the morning or after each bowel movement
- children under 12 years of age: ask a doctor

Tamper-Evident: Individually quality sealed for your protection. Do Not Use if foil imprinted "PREPARATION H" is torn or damaged (appears on end flap)

Cooling Gel—

- adults: when practical, cleanse the affected area by patting or blotting with an appropriate cleansing wipe. Gently dry by patting or blotting with a tissue or a soft cloth before applying gel.
- when first opening the tube, puncture foil seal with top end of cap
- apply externally to the affected area up to 4 times daily, especially at night, in the morning or after each bowel movement
- children under 12 years of age: ask a doctor

Tamper-Evident: Do Not Use if tube seal under cap embossed with "H" is broken or missing.

Inactive Ingredients: Ointment— Beeswax, Benzoic Acid, BHA, Corn Oil, Glycerin, Lanolin, Lanolin Alcohol, Methylparaben, Paraffin, Propylparaben, Thyme Oil, Tocopherol, Water.

Cream—BHA, Carboxymethylcellulose Sodium, Cetyl Alcohol, Citric Acid, Edetate Disodium, Glyceryl Oleate, Glyceryl Stearate, Lanolin, Methylparaben, Propyl Gallate, Propylene Glycol, Propylparaben, Simethicone, Sodium Benzoate, Sodium Lauryl Sulfate, Stearyl Alcohol, Tocopherol, Water, Xanthan Gum.

Suppositories—Methylparaben, Propylparaben, Starch.

Cooling Gel—Alcohol (7.5%), Benzophenone-4, Edetate Disodium, Hydroxyethyl Cellulose, Methylparaben, Propylene Glycol, Propylparaben, Purified Water, Sodium Citrate.

How Supplied: Ointment: Net Wt. 1 oz and 2 oz **Cream:** Net Wt. 0.9 oz and 1.8 oz **Suppositories:** 12's, 24's and 48's. **Cooling Gel:** Net Wt. 0.9 oz and 1.8 oz

Storage: Cream, Gel, Suppositories: Store at room temperature or in cool place but not over 80° F.

Ointment: Store at 20–25°C (68–77°F).

PREPARATION H®
MEDICATED WIPES

Uses:

- helps relieve the local itching and discomfort associated with hemorrhoids
- temporary relief of irritation and burning
- aids in protecting irritated anorectal areas
- hygenic wipe: medicated wipes are effective for everyday personal hygienic use on outer rectal and vaginal areas. Used in place of toilet tissue, **Preparation H® Medicated Wipes** gently and thoroughly remove irritation-causing matter. They are especially handy during menstrual periods.
- Moist Compress: For additional relief, can be folded and used as a compress on inflamed tissue.

Active Ingredients: Soft pads are pre-moistened with a solution containing Witch Hazel 50%.

Inactive ingredients: Aloe barbadensis gel, capryl/capramidopropyl betaine, citric acid, diazolidinyl urea, glycerin, methylparaben, propylene glycol, propylparaben, purified water, sodium citrate.

Directions:

- remove tab on right side of wipes pouch label and peel back to open
- grab the top wipe at the edge of the center fold and pull out of pouch
- carefully reseal label on pouch after each use to retain moistness
- adults: unfold wipe and cleanse the area by gently wiping, patting or blotting. If necessary, repeat until all matter is removed from the area.
- use up to 6 times daily or after each bowel movement and before applying topical hemorrhoidal treatments
- children under 12 years of age: consult a doctor

Warnings:
For external use only
When using this product

- do not exceed the recommended daily dosage unless directed by a doctor
- do not put this product into the rectum by using fingers or any mechanical device or applicator

Stop use and ask a doctor if.

- bleeding occurs
- condition worsens or does not improve within 7 days

If pregnant or breast-feeding, ask a health professional before use. **Keep out of reach of children.** If swallowed, get medical help or contact a Poison Control Center right away.

- store at 20–25°C (68–77°F)
- for best results, flush only one or two wipes at a time

How Supplied: Containers of 48 wipes.

PRIMATENE®
[prīm 'a-tēn]
Mist
(Epinephrine Inhalation Aerosol Bronchodilator)

Description: Primatene Mist contains Epinephrine 5.5 mg/mL. Each inhalation delivers 0.22 mg of epinephrine.

FDA approved uses.

Indications: For temporary relief of shortness of breath, tightness of chest, and wheezing due to bronchial asthma. Eases breathing for asthma patients by reducing spasms of bronchial muscles.

Directions:

- adults and children 4 years of age and older: start with one inhalation, then wait 1 minute If not relieved, use once more Do not use again for at least 3 hours
- children under 4 years of age: consult a doctor
- the use of this product by children should be supervised by an adult
- see insert for mouthpiece use and care instructions

Warnings:
For inhalation only
Do not use:

- unless a diagnosis of asthma has been made by a doctor
- if you are now taking a prescription monoamine oxidase inhibitor (MAOI) (certain drugs for depression, psychiatric, or emotional conditions, or Parkinson's disease), or for 2 weeks after stopping the MAOI drug If you do not know if your prescription drug contains an MAOI, ask a doctor or pharmacist before taking this product

Ask a doctor before use if you have:

- heart disease
- thyroid disease
- diabetes
- high blood pressure
- ever been hospitalized for asthma
- trouble urinating due to an enlarged prostate gland

Ask a doctor or pharmacist before use if you are taking any prescription drug for asthma

When using this product:

- do not use more often or at higher doses than recommended unless directed by a doctor

Continued on next page

Primatene Mist—Cont.

- excessive use may cause nervousness and rapid heart beat, and, possibly, adverse effects on the heart
- do not continue to use, but seek medical assistance immediately if symptoms are not relieved within 20 minutes or become worse
- do not tamper with, puncture or throw container into incinerator Contents under pressure
- using or storing near open flame or heating above 120°F (49°C) may cause bursting

Contains CFC 12, 114, substances which harm public health and environment by destroying ozone in the upper atmosphere.

If pregnant or breast-feeding, ask a health professional before use

Keep out of reach of children. In case of overdose, get medical help or contact a Poison Control Center right away

Directions For Use of Mouthpiece:

The Primatene Mist mouthpiece, which is enclosed in the Primatene Mist 15 mL size (not the refill size), should be used for inhalation only with Primatene Mist.
1. Take plastic cap off mouthpiece. (For refills, use mouthpiece from previous purchase.)
2. Take plastic mouthpiece off bottle.
3. Place other end of mouthpiece on bottle.
4. Turn bottle upside down. Place thumb on bottom of mouthpiece over circular button and forefinger on top of vial. Empty the lungs as completely as possible by exhaling.
5. Place mouthpiece in mouth with lips closed around opening. Inhale deeply while squeezing mouthpiece and bottle together. Release immediately and remove unit from mouth. Complete taking the deep breath, drawing the medication into your lungs and holding breath as long as comfortable.
6. Exhale slowly keeping lips nearly closed. This helps distribute the medication in the lungs.
7. Replace plastic cap on mouthpiece.

Care of the Mouthpiece:

The Primatene Mist mouthpiece should be washed once daily with soap and hot water, and rinsed thoroughly. Then it should be dried with a clean, lint-free cloth.

If the unit becomes clogged and fails to spray, please send the clogged unit to:

Whitehall Laboratories

5 Giralda Farms

Madison, N.J. 07940

Inactive Ingredients: Alcohol 34%, Ascorbic Acid, Fluorocarbons (Propellant), Water. Contains No Sulfites.

Storage: Store at room temperature, between 15–25°C (59–77°F).

How Supplied:

$\frac{1}{2}$ Fl oz (15 mL) With Mouthpiece.

$\frac{1}{2}$ Fl oz (15 mL) Refill

$\frac{3}{4}$ Fl oz (22.5 mL) Refill

PRIMATENE®
[prīm 'a-tēn]
Tablets

Description: Primatene Tablets contain Ephedrine Hydrochloride USP, 12.5 mg, Guaifenesin, USP 200 mg.

Indications: For temporary relief of shortness of breath, tightness of chest, and wheezing due to bronchial asthma. Eases breathing for asthma patients by reducing spasms of bronchial muscles. Helps loosen phlegm (mucus) and thin bronchial secretions to rid bronchial passageways of bothersome mucus, and to make coughs more productive.

Warnings:
Do not use
- unless a diagnosis of asthma has been made by a doctor
- if you are now taking a prescription monoamine oxidase inhibitor (MAOI) (certain drugs for depression, psychiatric, or emotional conditions, or Parkinson's disease), or for 2 weeks after stopping the MAOI drug If you do not know if your prescription drug contains an MAOI, ask a doctor or pharmacist before taking this product

Ask a doctor before use if you have:
- heart disease
- high blood pressure
- thyroid disease
- diabetes
- trouble urinating due to an enlarged prostate gland
- ever been hospitalized for asthma
- cough that occurs with too much phlegm (mucus)
- cough that lasts or is chronic such as occurs with smoking, asthma, chronic bronchitis, or emphysema

Ask a doctor or pharmacist before use if you are taking any prescription drug for asthma

When using this product some users may experience nervousness, tremor, sleeplessness, nausea, and loss of appetite

Stop use and ask a doctor if:
- symptoms are not relieved within 1 hour or become worse
- nervousness, tremor, sleeplessness, nausea, and loss of appetite persist or become worse
- cough lasts more than 7 days, comes back, or occurs with fever, rash, or persistent headache These could be signs of a serious condition

If pregnant or breast-feeding, ask a health professional before use

Keep out of reach of children. In case of overdose, get medical help or contact a Poison Control Center right away.

Directions:
- do not use more than dosage below unless directed by a doctor
- adults and children 12 years and over: take 2 tablets initially, then 2 tablets every 4 hours, as needed, not to exceed 12 tablets in 24 hours
- children under 12 years: ask a doctor

Inactive Ingredients: crospovidone, D&C yellow No. 10 aluminum lake, FD&C yellow No. 6 aluminum lake, magnesium stearate, microcrystalline cellulose, povidone, silicon dioxide (colloidal)

How Supplied: Available in 24 and 60 tablet thermoform blister cartons. Store at room temperature, between 20°C and 25°C (68°F to 77°F).

ROBITUSSIN® COLD COLD & CONGESTION SOFTGELS, CAPLETS
[ro "bĭ-tuss 'ĭn]
Nasal Decongestant, Expectorant, Cough Suppressant

Active Ingredients
(in each Softgel, caplet):

Dextromethorphan HBr, USP	10 mg
Guaifenesin, USP	200 mg
Pseudoephedrine HCl, USP	30 mg

Inactive Ingredients: Softgels: FD&C Blue No. 1, FD&C Red No. 40, Gelatin, Glycerin, Mannitol, Pharmaceutical Glaze, Polyethylene Glycol, Povidone, Propylene Glycol, Sorbitan, Sorbitol, Titanium Dioxide, Water.

Inactive Ingredients: Caplets: Calcium Stearate, Croscarmellose Sodium, FD&C Red No. 40 Aluminum Lake, Hydroxypropyl Methylcellulose, Maltodextrin, Microcrystalline Cellulose, Polydextrose, Polyethylene Glycol, Povidone, Pregelatinized Starch, Silicon Dioxide, Stearic Acid, Titanium Dioxide, Triacetin.

Indications:
- temporarily relieves nasal congestion, and cough due to minor throat and bronchial irritation occurring with the common cold
- helps loosen phlegm (mucus) and thin bronchial secretions to make coughs more productive
- temporarily relieves nasal congestion associated with hay fever or other upper respiratory allergies, or associated with sinusitis

Warnings:
Do not use if you are now taking a prescription monoamine oxidase inhibitor (MAOI) (certain drugs for depression, psychiatric, or emotional conditions, or Parkinson's disease), or for 2 weeks after stopping the MAOI drug. If you do not know if your prescription drug contains an MAOI, ask a doctor or pharmacist before taking this product.

Ask a doctor before use if you have:
- heart disease
- high blood pressure
- thyroid disease
- diabetes
- trouble urinating due to an enlarged prostate gland
- cough that occurs with too much phlegm (mucus)
- cough that lasts or is chronic such as occurs with smoking, asthma, chronic bronchitis, or emphysema

When using this product do not use more than directed.

Stop use and ask a doctor if:
- you get nervous, dizzy, or sleepless
- symptoms do not get better within 7 days or are accompanied by fever

- cough lasts more than 7 days, comes back, or is accompanied by fever, rash, or persistent headache. These could be signs of a serious condition.

If pregnant or breast-feeding, ask a health professional before use.

Keep out of reach of children. In case of overdose, get medical help or contact a Poison Control Center right away.

Directions: Follow dosage below: Do Not Exceed 4 Doses in a 24-Hour Period. Adults and children 12 years of age and over: 2 softgels or caplets every 4 hours. Children 6 to under 12 years: 1 softgel or caplet every 4 hours. Children under 6: Ask a doctor.

How Supplied: Softgels in consumer packages of 12 and 20 (individually packaged). Red caplets imprinted CC in consumer packages of 20 (individually packaged).

Storage: Store at Controlled Room Temperature, between 20°C and 25°C (68°F and 77°F)

ROBITUSSIN® COLD MULTI-SYMPTOM COLD& FLU SOFTGELS, CAPLETS

[ro "bĭ-tuss 'ĭn]

Pain Reliever, Fever Reducer, Cough Suppressant, Nasal Decongestant, Expectorant

Active Ingredients Softgels:

Acetaminophen, USP .... 250 mg
Guaifenesin, USP .... 100 mg
Pseudoephedrine HCL, USP .... 30 mg
Dextromethorphan HBr, USP ..... 10 mg

Active Ingredients Caplets:

Acetaminophen, USP .... 325 mg
Guaifenesin, USP .... 200 mg
Pseudoephedrine HCL, USP .... 30 mg
Dextromethorphan HBr, USP ..... 10 mg

Inactive Ingredients Softgels: D&C Yellow No. 10, FD&C Red No. 40, Gelatin, Glycerin, Iron Oxides, Lecithin, Mannitol, Pharmaceutical Glaze, Polyethylene Glycol, Povidone, Propylene Glycol, Simethicone, Sorbitan, Sorbitol, Water.

Inactive Ingredients Caplets: Calcium Stearate, Croscarmellose Sodium, D&C Yellow No. 10 Aluminum Lake, FD&C Yellow No. 6 Aluminum Lake, Hydroxypropyl Methylcellulose, Maltodextrin, Microcrystalline Cellulose, Polydextrose, Polyethylene Glycol, Povidone, Pregelatinized Starch, Silicon Dioxide, Stearic Acid, Titanium Dioxide, Triacetin.

Indications: For the temporary relief of minor aches and pains, headache, muscular aches and sore throat associated with cold or flu, and to reduce fever. Temporarily relieves cough due to minor throat and bronchial irritation and nasal congestion as may occur with a cold. Helps loosen phlegm (mucus) and thin bronchial secretions to make coughs more productive.

Warnings:

Alcohol warning: if you consume 3 or more alcoholic drinks every day, ask your doctor whether you should take acetaminophen or other pain relievers/fever reducers. Acetaminophen may cause liver damage.

Sore throat warning: if sore threat is severe, persists for more than two days, is accompanied or followed by fever, headache, rash, nausea, or vomiting, consult a doctor promptly.

Do not use if you are now taking a prescription monoamine oxidase inhibitor (MAOI) (certain drugs for depression, psychiatric, or emotional conditions, or Parkinson's disease), or for 2 weeks after stopping the MAOI drug. If you do not know if your prescription drug contains an MAOI, ask a doctor or pharmacist before taking this product.

Ask a doctor before use if you have:

- heart disease
- high blood pressure
- thyroid disease
- diabetes
- trouble urinating due to an enlarged prostate gland
- cough that occurs with too much phlegm (mucus)
- cough that lasts or is chronic such as occurs with smoking, asthma, chronic bronchitis, or emphysema

When using this product do not use more than directed.

Stop use and ask a doctor if:

- you get nervous, dizzy, or sleepless
- new symptoms occur
- you need to use for more than 7 days
- symptoms do not get better, get worse, or are accompanied by fever more than 3 days
- redness or swelling is present
- cough lasts more than 7 days, comes back, or is accompanied by fever, rash, or persistent headache. These could be signs of a serious condition.

If pregnant or breast-feeding, ask a health professional before use.

Keep out of reach of children. In case of overdose, get medical help or contact a Poison Control Center right away. Quick medical attention is critical for adults as well as for children, even if you do not notice any signs or symptoms.

Directions: Multi-Symptom Cold & Flu **Softgels:** Follow dosage below: Do not exceed 4 doses in a 24-hour period. Adults and children 12 yrs. and over: 2 softgels every 4 hrs.

Children under 12 years: Ask a doctor.

Directions: Multi-Symptom Cold & Flu **Caplets: Follow dosage below: Do not exceed 4 doses in a 24-hour period.**

Adults and children 12 years and over: 2 caplets every 4 hours. Children 6 to under 12 years: 1 caplet every 4 hours. Children under 6 years: Ask a doctor.

How Supplied: Blister Packs of 12's and 20's.

Storage: Store at Controlled Room Temperature, between 20°C and 25°C (68°F and 77°F).

ROBITUSSIN® COUGH DROPS

[ro "bĭ-tuss 'ĭn]

Menthol Eucalyptus, Cherry, and Honey-Lemon Flavors

Active Ingredients: Each cough drop contains:

Menthol Eucalyptus:

Menthol, USP .... 10 mg

Cherry and Honey-Lemon:

Menthol, USP .... 5 mg

Inactive Ingredients:

Menthol Eucalyptus: Corn Syrup, Eucalyptus Oil, Flavor, Sucrose.

Cherry: Corn Syrup, FD&C Red #40, Flavor, Methylparaben, Propylparaben, Sodium Benzoate, Sucrose.

Honey-Lemon: Citric Acid, Corn Syrup, D&C Yellow #10, FD&C Yellow #6, Honey, Lemon Oil, Methylparaben, Povidone, Propylparaben, Sodium Benzoate, Sucrose.

Indications: Temporarily relieves coughs and occasional minor irritation, pain, sore mouth, and sore throat due to colds or inhaled irritants.

Warnings:

Sore throat warning: severe or persistent sore throat or sore throat accompanied by high fever, headache, nausea, and vomiting may be serious. Consult a doctor right away. Do not use more than 2 days or give to children under 3 years of age unless directed by a doctor

Ask a doctor before use if you have:

- cough that occurs with too much phlegm (mucus)
- cough that lasts or is chronic such as occurs with smoking, asthma, or emphysema

Stop use and ask a doctor if:

- cough lasts more than 7 days, comes back, or is accompanied by fever, rash, or persistent headache. These could be signs of a serious condition.

If pregnant or breast-feeding, ask a health professional before use.

Keep out of reach of children.

Directions:

- adults and children 4 years and over: allow 1 drop to dissolve slowly in the mouth
  - for sore throat: may be repeated every 2 hours, as needed, or as directed by a doctor
  - for cough: may be repeated every hour, as needed, or as directed by a doctor
- children under 4 years of age: ask a doctor

How Supplied: All 3 flavors of Robitussin Cough Drops are available in bags of 25 drops.

Storage: Store at 20–25°C (68–77°F).

Continued on next page

ROBITUSSIN®-PE SYRUP
ROBITUSSIN® COLD SEVERE CONGESTION SOFTGELS

[ro "bĭ-tuss 'ĭn]
Nasal Decongestant, Expectorant Alcohol-Free Cough Formula

Active Ingredients:
Each teaspoonful of Robitussin-PE (5 mL) contains:

Guaifenesin, USP .... 100 mg
Pseudoephedrine Hydrochloride, USP .... 30 mg

Inactive Ingredients:
Robitussin-PE: Citric Acid, FD&C Red No. 40, Flavors, Glucose, Glycerin, High Fructose Corn Syrup, Maltol, Menthol, Propylene Glycol, Saccharin Sodium, Sodium Benzoate, Water.

Indications: Temporarily relieves nasal congestion due to a cold. Helps loosen phlegm (mucus) and thin bronchial secretions to make coughs more productive.

Active Ingredients:
Each Robitussin Severe Congestion Softgel contains:

Guaifenesin, USP .... 200 mg
Pseudoephedrine Hydrochloride, USP .... 30 mg

Inactive Ingredients:
Robitussin Severe Congestion Softgels: FD&C Green No. 3, Gelatin, Glycerin, Mannitol, Pharmaceutical Glaze, Polyethylene Glycol, Povidone, Propylene Glycol, Sorbitan, Sorbitol, Titanium Dioxide, Water.

Indications: For the temporary relief of nasal congestion due to the common cold, hay fever or other upper respiratory allergies, or associated with sinusitis. Helps loosen phlegm (mucus) and thin bronchial secretions to make coughs more productive.

Warnings:
Do not use if you are now taking a prescription monoamine oxidase inhibitor (MAOI) (certain drugs for depression, psychiatric, or emotional conditions, or Parkinson's disease), or for 2 weeks after stopping the MAOI drug. If you do not know if your prescription drug contains an MAOI, ask a doctor or pharmacist before taking this product.
Ask a doctor before use if you have:
• heart disease
• high blood pressure
• thyroid disease
• diabetes
• trouble urinating due to an enlarged prostate gland
• cough that occurs with too much phlegm (mucus)
• cough that lasts or is chronic such as occurs with smoking, asthma, chronic bronchitis, or emphysema
When using this product
• do not use more than directed.
Stop use and ask a doctor if:
• you get nervous, dizzy, or sleepless
• symptoms do not get better within 7 days or are accompanied by fever
• cough lasts more than 7 days, comes back, or is accompanied by fever, rash, or persistent headache. These could be signs of a serious condition.
If pregnant or breast-feeding, ask a health professional before use.

Keep out of reach of children. In case of overdose, get medical help or contact a Poison Control Center right away.

Directions: Robitussin-PE: Dosage cup provided.

Follow dosage below:
Do Not Exceed 4 Doses in a 24-Hour Period.
ADULT DOSE (and children 12 years and over): 2 teaspoonfuls every 4 hrs.
CHILD DOSE
6 yrs. to under 12 yrs. 1 teaspoonful every 4 hrs.
2 yrs. to under 6 yrs. 1/2 teaspoonful every 4 hrs.
Under 2—Ask a Doctor.

Directions: Robitussin Severe Congestion Softgels: Do Not Exceed 4 Doses in a 24-Hour Period. Adults and children 12 years of age and over: 2 softgels every 4 hours. Children 6 to under 12 years: 1 softgel every 4 hours. Children under 6, ask a doctor.

How Supplied: Robitussin-PE (orangered) in bottles of 4 fl oz, and 8 fl oz. Softgels in consumer packages of 12 and 20 (individually packaged).

Storage: Store at Controlled Room Temperature, between 20°C and 25°C (68°F and 77°F).

ROBITUSSIN COUGH & COLD INFANT DROPS

[ro "bĭ-tuss 'ĭn]
Nasal Decongestant, Cough Suppressant, Expectorant Alcohol-Free Cough & Cold Formula

Active Ingredients:
Each half teaspoonful (2.5 mL) contains:
Guaifenesin, USP .... 100 mg
Pseudoephedrine HCl, USP .... 15 mg
Dextromethorphan HBr, USP .... 5 mg

Inactive Ingredients: Citric Acid, FD&C Red No. 40, Flavors, Glycerin, High Fructose Corn Syrup, Maltitol, Maltol, Polyethylene Glycol, Providone, Propylene Glycol, Saccharin Sodium, Sodium Benzoate, Sodium Citrate, Water.

Indications: Temporarily relieves cough due to minor throat and bronchial irritation, and nasal congestion due to a cold. Helps loosen phlegm (mucus) and thin bronchial secretions to make coughs more productive.

Warnings:
Do not use in a child who is taking a prescription monoamine oxidase inhibitor (MAOI) (certain drugs for depression, psychiatric, or emotional conditions, or Parkinson's disease), or for 2 weeks after stopping the MAOI drug. If you do not know if your child's prescription drug contains an MAOI, ask a doctor or pharmacist before giving this product.
Ask a doctor before use if your child has:
• heart disease
• high blood pressure

• thyroid disease
• diabetes
• cough that occurs with too much phlegm (mucus)
• cough that lasts or is chronic such as occurs with asthma
When using this product do not use more than directed.
Stop use and ask a doctor if:
• your child gets nervous, dizzy, or sleepless
• symptoms do not get better within 7 days or are accompanied by fever
• cough lasts more than 7 days, comes back, or is accompanied by fever, rash, or persistent headache. These could be signs of a serious condition.
Keep out of reach of children. In case of overdose, get medical help or contact a Poison Control Center right away.

Directions: Follow dosage below. Oral dosing syringe provided. Do not use more than 4 doses in any 24-Hour Period. Repeat every 4 hours.

Dosage: Choose by weight. (If weight is not known, choose by age):

Age	Weight	Dose
Under 2yrs.	Under 24 lbs.	Consult doctor
2 to under 6 yrs.	24–47 lbs.	2.5 mL

How Supplied: 1 fluid oz bottle with dosing syringe.
Storage: Store at 20°C–25°C (68°F and 77°F).

ROBITUSSIN®

[ro "bĭ-tuss 'ĭn]
Alcohol-Free Cough Formula Expectorant

Active Ingredients: Each teaspoonful (5 mL) contains:
Guaifenesin, USP .... 100 mg

Inactive Ingredients: Caramel, Citric Acid, FD&C Red No. 40, Flavors, Glucose, Glycerin, High Fructose Corn Syrup, Menthol, Saccharin Sodium, Sodium Benzoate, Water.

Indications: Helps loosen phlegm (mucus) and thin bronchial secretions to make coughs more productive.

Warnings:
Ask a doctor before use if you have
• cough that occurs with too much phlegm (mucus)
• cough that lasts or is chronic such as occurs with smoking, asthma, chronic bronchitis, or emphysema
Stop use and ask a doctor if cough lasts more than 7 days, comes back, or is accompanied by fever, rash, or persistent headache. These could be signs of a serious condition.
If pregnant or breast-feeding, ask a health professional before use.
Keep out of reach of children. In case of overdose, get medical help or contact a Poison Control Center right away.

Directions: Follow dosage below. Dosage cup provided (except for the 16 oz size).

Do not take more than 6 doses in any 24-hour period.

ADULT DOSE (and children 12 years and over): 2–4 teaspoonsfuls every 4 hrs.

CHILD DOSE

6 yrs. to under 12 yrs. 1–2 teaspoonfuls every 4 hrs.

2 yrs. to under 6 yrs. 1/2–1 teaspoonful every 4 hrs.

Under 2 years: ask a doctor.

How Supplied: Robitussin (wine-colored) in bottles of 4 fl oz, 8 fl oz, 16 fl oz. Store at 20°C–25°C (68°F and 77°F).

ROBITUSSIN®–CF

[ro "bĭ-tuss 'ĭn]

Alcohol-Free Cough Formula
Nasal Decongestant, Cough
Suppressant, Expectorant

Active Ingredients: Each teaspoonful (5 mL) contains:
Guaifenesin, USP .... 100 mg
Pseudoephedrine
 Hydrochloride, USP .... 30 mg
Dextromethorphan
 Hydrobromide, USP .... 10 mg

Inactive Ingredients: Citric Acid, FD&C Red No. 40, Flavors, Glycerin, Propylene Glycol, Saccharin Sodium, Sodium Benzoate, Sorbitol, Water.

Indications: Temporarily relieves cough due to minor throat and bronchial irritation and nasal congestion as may occur with a cold. Helps loosen phlegm (mucus) and thin bronchial secretions to make coughs more productive.

Warnings:
Do not use if you are now taking a prescription monoamine oxidase inhibitor (MAOI) (certain drugs for depression, psychiatric, or emotional conditions, or Parkinson's disease), or for 2 weeks after stopping the MAOI drug. If you do not know if your prescription drug contains an MAOI, ask a doctor or pharmacist before taking this product.

Ask a doctor before use if you have:
• heart disease
• high blood pressure
• thyroid disease
• diabetes
• trouble urinating due to an enlarged prostate gland
• cough that occurs with too much phlegm (mucus)
• cough that lasts or is chronic such as occurs with smoking, asthma, chronic bronchitis or emphysema

When using this product do not use more than directed.

Stop use and ask a doctor if:
• you get nervous, dizzy, or sleepless
• symptoms do not get better within 7 days or are accompanied by fever
• cough lasts more than 7 days, comes back, or is accompanied by fever, rash, or persistent headache. These could be signs of a serious condition.

If pregnant or breast-feeding, ask a health professional before use.

Keep out of reach of children. In case of overdose, get medical help or contact a Poison Control Center right away.

Directions: Follow dosage below. Dosage cup provided. Do not take more than 4 doses in any 24-hour period.

ADULT DOSE (and children 12 years and over): 2 teaspoonfuls every 4 hrs.

CHILD DOSE

6 yrs. to under 12 yrs.
1 teaspoonful every 4 hrs.

2 yrs. to under 6 yrs.
$^1/_2$ teaspoonful every 4 hrs.

Under 2: Ask a doctor.

How Supplied: Robitussin-CF (red-colored) in bottles of 4 fl oz, 8 fl oz, and 12 fl oz.
Store at 20°C–25°C (68°F and 77°F).

ROBITUSSIN®-DM
ROBITUSSIN DM INFANT DROPS

[ro "bĭ-tuss 'ĭn]

Cough suppressant, Expectorant

Active Ingredients: Each teaspoonful of **Robitussin DM** (5 mL) contains:
Dextromethorphan Hydrobromide,
 USP .... 10 mg
Guaifenesin, USP .... 100 mg

Inactive Ingredients (Robitussin DM): Citric Acid, FD&C Red No. 40, Flavors, Glucose, Glycerin, High Fructose Corn Syrup, Menthol, Saccharin Sodium, Sodium Benzoate, Water.

Active Ingredients:
Each 2.5 mL ($^1/_2$ teaspoonful) of **Robitussin DM Infant Drops** contains:
Dextromethorphan Hydrobromide,
 USP .... 5 mg
Guaifenesin, USP .... 100 mg
Alcohol-Free Cough Formula

Inactive Ingredients (Robitussin DM Infant Drops):

Inactive Ingredients: Citric Acid, FD&C Red No. 40, Flavors, Glycerin, High Fructose Corn Syrup, Malitol, Maltol, Polyethylene Glycol, Povidone, Propylene Glycol, Saccharin Sodium, Sodium Benzoate, Sodium Chloride, Sodium Citrate, Water.

Indications: Temporarily relieves cough due to minor throat and bronchial irritation as may occur with a cold and helps loosen phlegm (mucus) and thin bronchial secretions to make coughs more productive.

Warnings:
Do not use if you or child are now taking a prescription monoamine oxidase inhibitor (MAOI) (certain drugs for depression, psychiatric, or emotional conditions, or Parkinson's disease), or for 2 weeks after stopping the MAOI drug. If you do not know if you or your child's prescription drug contains an MAOI, ask a doctor or pharmacist before taking this product.

Ask a doctor before use if you have:
• cough that occurs with too much phlegm (mucus)
• cough that lasts or is chronic such as occurs with smoking, asthma, chronic bronchitis, or emphysema

---

Stop use and ask a doctor if:
• cough lasts more than 7 days, comes back, or is accompanied by fever, rash, or persistent headache. These could be signs of a serious condition.

If pregnant or breast-feeding, ask a health professional before use.

Keep out of reach of children. In case of overdose, get medical help or contact a Poison Control Center right away.

Directions Robitussin DM: Follow dosage below or use as directed by a doctor. Dosage cup provided (except for the 16 oz size). Do not exceed 6 doses in a 24-hour period. Adults and children 12 years and over: 2 teaspoonfuls every 4 hours; children 6 years to under 12 years, 1 teaspoonful every 4 hours; children 2 years to under 6 years, $^1/_2$ teaspoonful every 4 hours; children under 2 years: ask a doctor.

Directions Robitussin DM Infant Drops: Oral dosing syringe provided. Do not use more than 6 doses in any 24-hour period. Repeat every 4 hours. Choose by weight (if weight not known, choose by age). 2 years to under 6 years (24–47 lbs.) 2.5 mL; under 2 yrs (under 24 lbs.): ask a doctor.

How Supplied: Robitussin-DM (cherry-colored) in bottles of 4 fl oz, 8 fl oz, 12 fl oz, 16 fl oz and single doses: premeasured doses—$^1/_3$ fl oz each.

How Supplied (Robitussin DM Infant Drops): (berry flavor) in 1 fl oz bottles with oral syringe.

Storage: Store at 20°C–25°C (68°F and 77°F).

ROBITUSSIN®
HONEY CALMERS THROAT
DROPS (BERRY)

Use: Temporarily relieves occasional minor irritation, pain, sore mouth, and sore throat.

Active ingredient
(in each drop):   **Purpose:**
Menthol,
USP, 1 mg .... Oral pain reliever

Inactive Ingredients: Carmine, citric acid, cochineal extract, corn syrup, glycerin, natural flavor blend, natural grade A wildflower honey, sucrose.

Directions:
• adults and children 4 years and over: allow 2 drops to dissolve slowly in the mouth. May be repeated every 2 hours, as needed, or as directed by a doctor.
• children under 4 years of age: ask a doctor

Warnings:
Sore throat warning: severe or persistent sore throat or sore throat accompanied by high fever, headache, nausea, and vomiting may be serious. Consult a doctor right away. Do not use more than 2 days or give to children under 3 years of age unless directed by a doctor.

Continued on next page

Robitussin—Cont.

If pregnant or breast-feeding, ask a health professional before use. **Keep out of reach of children.**

Storage: Store at 20–25°C (68–77°F)

How Supplied: Packages of 25 drops.

ROBITUSSIN®
HONEY COUGH™
Non-drowsy formula
Alcohol-Free Cough Formula
Cough Suppressant

Active Ingredient:
Each teaspoonful (5 mL) contains:
Dextromethorphan HBr, USP ..... 10 mg

Inactive Ingredients: Flavors, Glucose, Glycerin, Honey, Maltol, Methylparaben, Propylene Glycol, Sodium Benzoate, Water.

Indications: Temporarily relieves cough due to minor throat and bronchial irritation as may occur with a cold.

Directions: Follow dosage below. Dosage cup provided. Do not take more than 4 doses in any 24-hour period.

AGE	DOSE
adults and children 12 years and older	3 teaspoonfuls every 6 to 8 hours
children 6 to under 12 years	1.5 teaspoonfuls every 6 to 8 hours
children under 6 years	not recommended

Warnings:
Do not use if you are now taking a prescription monoamine oxidase inhibitor (MAOI) (certain drugs for depression, psychiatric, or emotional conditions, or Parkinson's disease), or for 2 weeks after stopping the MAOI drug. If you do not know if your prescription drug contains an MAOI, ask a doctor or pharmacist before taking this product.
Ask a doctor before use if you have:
• cough that occurs with too much phlegm (mucus)
• cough that lasts or is chronic such as occurs with smoking, asthma, or emphysema
Stop use and ask a doctor if: cough lasts more than 7 days, comes back, or is accompanied by fever, rash, or persistent headache. These could be signs of a serious condition
If pregnant or breast-feeding, ask a health professional before use.
Keep out of reach of children. In case of overdose, get medical help or contact a Poison Control Center right away.

How Supplied: Bottle of 4 fl. oz. (118 mL)
Storage: Store at 20–25°C (68°–77°F).

ROBITUSSIN®
HONEY COUGH Drops
Honey-Lemon Tea, Honey Citrus, and Natural Honey Center

Uses:
• Temporarily relieves:
 • occasional minor irritation, pain, sore mouth, and sore throat
 • cough associated with a cold or inhaled irritants

Active Ingredients:
Each cough drop contains:
Natural Honey Center and *Honey-Lemon Tea*:
Menthol 5mg
Honey Citrus:
Menthol 2.5mg

Inactive Ingredients:
Natural Honey Center: Caramel, corn syrup, glycerin, high fructose corn syrup, honey, natural herbal flavor, sorbitol, sucrose
Honey Lemon Tea: Caramel, citric acid, corn syrup, honey, natural flavor, sucrose, tea extract
Herbal Honey Citrus: Citric acid, corn syrup, flavors, honey, sucrose

Directions:
• adults and children 4 years and over:
 • for sore throat: allow 1 drop to dissolve slowly in the mouth. May be repeated every 2 hours, as needed, or as directed by a doctor.
 • for cough: *Honey-Lemon Tea and Natural Honey Center*—allow 1 drop to dissolve slowly in mouth. *Honey Citrus*—allow 2 drops to dissolve slowly in mouth.
Maybe repeated every hour, as needed, or as directed by a doctor.
• children under 4 years: ask a doctor

Warnings:
Sore throat warning: severe or persistent sore throat or sore throat accompanied by high fever, headache, nausea, and vomiting may be serious. Consult a doctor right away. Do not use more than 2 days or give to children under 3 years of age unless directed by a doctor.
Ask a doctor before use if you have:
• cough that occurs with too much phlegm (mucus)
• cough that lasts or is chronic such as occurs with smoking, asthma, or emphysema
Stop use and ask a doctor if:
• cough lasts more than 7 days, comes back, or is accompanied by fever, rash, or persistent headache. These could be signs of a serious condition.
If pregnant or breast-feeding, ask a health professional before use. **Keep out of reach of children.**
Storage: Store at 20–25°C (68–77°F).

How Supplied: Packages of 20 drops.

ROBITUSSIN® MAXIMUM
STRENGTH COUGH
SUPPRESSANT
ROBITUSSIN® PEDIATRIC
COUGH SUPPRESSANT
[ro "bĭ-tuss 'ĭn]

Active Ingredients:
Robitussin Maximum Strength Cough Suppressant: Each teaspoonful [5 mL] contains Dextromethorphan Hydrobromide, USP .... 15 mg
Robitussin Pediatric Strength Cough Suppressant: Each teaspoonful [5 mL] contains Dextromethorphan Hydrobromide, USP .... 7.5 mg

Inactive Ingredients (Robitussin Maximum Strength Cough Suppressant): Alcohol, Citric Acid, FD&C Red No. 40, Flavors, Glucose, Glycerin, High Fructose Corn Syrup, Menthol, Saccharin Sodium, Sodium Benzoate, Water.

Inactive Ingredients (Robitussin Pediatric Cough Suppressant): Citric Acid, FD&C Red No. 40, Flavor, Glycerin, High Fructose Corn Syrup, Saccharin Sodium, Sodium Benzoate, Sodium Chloride, Sodium Citrate, Water.

Indications: Temporarily relieves cough due to minor throat and bronchial irritation as may occur with a cold.

Warnings:
Do not use if you are now taking a prescription monoamine oxidase inhibitor (MAOI) (certain drugs for depression, psychiatric, or emotional conditions, or Parkinson's disease), or for 2 weeks after stopping the MAOI drug. If you do not know if your prescription drug contains an MAOI, ask a doctor or pharmacist before taking this product.
Ask a doctor before use if you have:
• cough that occurs with too much phlegm (mucus)
• cough that lasts or is chronic such as occurs with smoking, asthma, or emphysema
Stop use and ask a doctor if: cough lasts more than 7 days, comes back, or is accompanied by fever, rash, or persistent headache　These could be signs of a serious condition.
If pregnant or breast-feeding, ask a health professional before use.
Keep out of reach of children. In case of overdose, get medical help or contact a Poison Control Center right away.

Directions: Follow dosage below. Dosage cup provided. Do not exceed 4 doses in any 24-hour period. **Robitussin Maximum Strength Cough Suppressant ADULT DOSE** (and children 12 yrs. and over): 2 teaspoonfuls every 6–8 hours, in dosage cup. **CHILD DOSE** (under 12 yrs.): Ask a doctor.
Robitussin Pediatric Cough Suppressant Repeat every 6 to 8 hours. Dosage: choose by weight, if known; if weight is not known, choose by age.

[See table at top of next page]

How Supplied: Robitussin Maximum Strength (dark red-colored) in bottles of 4 and 8 fl oz. Store at 20–25°C (68–77°F).

How Supplied: Robitussin Pediatric (cherry-colored) in bottles of 4 fl oz.

Storage: Store at 20–25°C (68–77°F).

Age	Weight	Dose
Under 2 yrs.	Under 24 lbs.	Ask a doctor
2 to under 6 yrs.	24–47 lbs.	1 Teaspoonful
6 to under 12 yrs.	48–95 lbs.	2 Teaspoonfuls
12 yrs. and older	96 lbs. and over	4 Teaspoonfuls

ROBITUSSIN® MAXIMUM STRENGTH COUGH & COLD
ROBITUSSIN® PEDIATRIC COUGH & COLD FORMULA
[ro"bĭ-tuss 'ĭn]
Cough Suppressant, Nasal Decongestant

Active Ingredients: Each teaspoonful (5 mL) of Robitussin Maximum Strength Cough & Cold contains:
Dextromethorphan Hydrobromide, USP .... 15 mg
Pseudoephedrine Hydrochloride, USP .... 30 mg

Active Ingredients: Each teaspoonful (5 mL) of Robitussin Pediatric Cough & Cold Formula contains:
Dextromethorphan Hydrobromide, USP .... 7.5 mg
Pseudoephedrine Hydrochloride, USP .... 15 mg

Inactive Ingredients (Robitussin Maximum Strength Cough & Cold): Alcohol, Citric Acid, FD&C Red No. 40, Flavors, Glycerin, High Fructose Corn Syrup, Menthol, Saccharin Sodium, Sodium Benzoate, Water.

Inactive Ingredients (Robitussin Pediatric Cough & Cold Formula): Citric Acid, FD&C Red No. 40, Flavor, Glycerin, High Fructose Corn Syrup, Saccharin Sodium, Sodium Benzoate, Sodium Chloride, Sodium Citrate, Water.

Indications: Temporarily relieves cough due to minor throat and bronchial irritation and nasal congestion as may occur with a cold.

Warnings:
Do not use if you are now taking a prescription monoamine oxidase inhibitor (MAOI) (certain drugs for depression, psychiatric, or emotional conditions, or Parkinson's disease), or for 2 weeks after stopping the MAOI drug. If you do not know if your prescription drug contains an MAOI, ask a doctor or pharmacist before taking this product.
Ask a doctor before use if you have:
• heart disease
• high blood pressure
• thyroid disease
• diabetes

Age	Weight	Dose
Under 2 yrs.	Under 24 lbs.	Ask a doctor
2 to under 6 yrs.	24–47 lbs.	1 Teaspoonful
6 to under 12 yrs.	48–95 lbs.	2 Teaspoonfuls
12 yrs. and older	96 lbs. and over	4 Teaspoonfuls

• trouble urinating due to an enlarged prostate gland
• cough that occurs with too much phlegm (mucus)
• cough that lasts or is chronic such as occurs with smoking, asthma, or emphysema
When using this product do not use more than directed.
Stop use and ask a doctor if:
• you get nervous, dizzy, or sleepless
• symptoms do not get better within 7 days or are accompanied by fever
• cough lasts more than 7 days, comes back, or is accompanied by fever, rash, or persistent headache. These could be signs of a serious condition.
If pregnant or breast-feeding, ask a health professional before use.
Keep out of reach of children. In case of overdose, get medical help or contact a Poison Control Center right away.

Directions: Follow dosage (dosage cup provided). Do Not Exceed 4 Doses in any 24-Hour Period. **Robitussin Maximum Strength Cough & Cold.** Adults and children 12 years and over: 2 teaspoonfuls every 6 hours, as needed. Children under 12 years: Ask a doctor.
Robitussin Pediatric Cough & Cold Formula Repeat every 6 hours. Dosage: choose by weight, if known; if weight is not known, choose by age. [See table below]

How Supplied Robitussin Maximum Strength Cough & Cold: Red syrup in bottles of 4 fl oz and 8 fl oz.
How Supplied: Robitussin Pediatric Cough & Cold formula (bright red) in bottles of 4 fl oz and 8 fl oz.
Storage: Store at 20°C–25°C (68°F and 77°F).

ROBITUSSIN® MULTI SYMPTOM HONEY FLU™
Non-Drowsy Cough Formula
Cough Suppressant, Nasal Decongestant, Pain Reliever/Fever Reducer

Active Ingredients:
Each teaspoonful (5 mL) contains:
Acetaminophen, USP .... 166.6 mg
Dextromethorphan HBr, USP .... 6.6 mg
Pseudoephedrine HCl, USP .... 20 mg

Inactive Ingredients: Citric Acid, Flavors, Glucose, Glycerin, High Fructose Corn Syrup, Menthol, Natural Grade A Honey, Polyethylene Glycol, Propylene Glycol, Saccharin Sodium, Sodium Benzoate, Water.

Indications For the temporary relief of these symptoms associated with a cold or flu: nasal congestion, minor aches and pains, sore throat, cough, fever, headache, muscular aches.

Directions: Do not take more than 4 doses in any 24-hour period. Follow dosage below. Dosage cup provided.
Adults and children over 12 years of age: Take 3 teaspoons every 4 hours, as needed.
Children: Children under 12 years: not recommended. Do not use in children under 2 years of age.

Warnings:
Alcohol warning: if you consume 3 or more alcoholic drinks every day, ask your doctor whether you should take acetaminophen or other pain relievers/fever reducers. Acetaminophen may cause liver damage.
Sore throat warning: if sore throat is severe, persists for more than two days, is accompanied or followed by fever, headache, rash, nausea, or vomiting, consult a doctor promptly.
Do not use if you are now taking a prescription monoamine oxidase inhibitor (MAOI) (certain drugs for depression, psychiatric, or emotional conditions, or Parkinson's disease), or for 2 weeks after stopping the MAOI drug. If you do not know if your prescription drug contains an MAOI, ask a doctor or pharmacist before taking this product.
Ask a doctor before use if you have:
• heart disease
• high blood pressure
• thyroid disease
• diabetes
• trouble urinating due to an enlarged prostate gland
• cough that occurs with too much phlegm (mucus)
• a breathing problem or chronic cough that lasts or as occurs with smoking, asthma, or emphysema
When using this product
• do not use more than directed
Stop use and ask a doctor if:
• you get nervous, dizzy, or sleepless
• new symptoms occur
• you need to use for more than 7 days
• symptoms do not get better, get worse, or are accompanied by fever more than 3 days
• redness or swelling is present
• cough lasts more than 7 days, comes back, or is accompanied by fever, rash, or persistent headache. These could be signs of a serious condition.
If pregnant or breast-feeding, ask a health professional before use.
Keep out of reach of children. In case of overdose, get medical help or contact a Poison Control Center right away. Quick medical attention is critical for adults as well as for children, even if you do not notice any signs or symptoms.

Continued on next page

Robitussin Honey Flu—Cont.

How Supplied: Bottle of 4 fl. oz. (118 mL).
Not labeled USP due to microbial content of natural honey.

Storage: Store at 20–25°C (68–77°F).

ROBITUSSIN® NIGHTTIME HONEY FLU™
Cough Suppressant, Nasal Decongestant, Pain Reliever/Fever Reducer, Antihistamine

Active Ingredients:
Each pouch (15 mL) contains:
Acetaminophen, USP .... 500 mg
Chlorpheniramine Maleate, USP .. 4 mg
Dextromethorphan HBr, USP ..... 20 mg
Pseudoephedrine HCl, USP .... 60 mg

Inactive Ingredients: Citric Acid, Flavors, Glucose, Glycerin, High Fructose Corn Syrup, Natural Grade A Honey, Polyethylene Glycol, Propylene Glycol, Saccharin Sodium, Sodium Benzoate, Water.

Indications: For the temporary relief of these symptoms associated with a cold, or flu, hay fever, or other respiratory allergies: cough, minor aches and pains, sore throat, headache, muscular aches, fever, nasal congestion, itching of the nose and throat, runny nose, itchy, watery eyes, sneezing.

Dosage:
Directions: Do not take more than 4 doses in any 24-hour period. Follow dosage below.
Adults and children over 12 years of age: Empty 1 entire pouch into a 4–6 oz cup of hot beverage (tea). Repeat every 4 hours, as needed.
Children: Children under 12 years: not recommended. Do not use in children under 2 years of age.

Warnings:
Alcohol warning: if you consume 3 or more alcoholic drinks every day, ask your doctor whether you should take acetaminophen or other pain relievers/fever reducers. Acetaminophen may cause liver damage.
Sore throat warning: if sore throat is severe, persists for more than two days, is accompanied or followed by fever, headache, rash, nausea, or vomiting, consult a doctor promptly.
Do not use if you are now taking a prescription monoamine oxidase inhibitor (MAOI) (certain drugs for depression, psychiatric, or emotional conditions, or Parkinson's disease), or for 2 weeks after stopping the MAOI drug. If you do not know if your prescription drug contains an MAOI, ask a doctor or pharmacist before taking this product.
Ask a doctor before use if you have:
• heart disease
• high blood pressure
• thyroid disease
• diabetes

• trouble urinating due to an enlarged prostate gland
• glaucoma
• cough that occurs with too much phlegm (mucus)
• a breathing problem or chronic cough that lasts or as occurs with smoking, asthma, chronic bronchitis, or emphysema
Ask a doctor or pharmacist before use if you are taking sedatives or tranquilizers.
When using this product:
• **do not use more than directed**
• marked drowsiness may occur
• avoid alcoholic drinks
• alcohol, sedatives, and tranquilizers may increase drowsiness
• be careful when driving a motor vehicle or operating machinery
• excitability may occur, especially in children
Stop use and ask a doctor if:
• you get nervous, dizzy, or sleepless
• new symptoms occur
• you need to use for more than 7 days
• symptoms do not get better, get worse, or are accompanied by fever more than 3 days
• redness or swelling is present
• cough lasts more than 7 days, comes back, or is accompanied by fever, rash, or persistent headache. These could be signs of a serious condition.
If pregnant or breast-feeding, ask a health professional before use.
Keep out of reach of children. In case of overdose, get medical help or contact a Poison Control Center right away. Quick medical attention is critical for adults as well as for children, even if you do not notice any signs or symptoms.

How Supplied:
Each box contains 6 honey syrup pouches (15 mL each).
Not labeled USP due to the microbial content of natural honey.
Storage: Store at 20°–25°C (68°–77°F).

ROBITUSSIN® SUGAR FREE Throat Drops
(Natural Citrus and Tropical Fruit Flavors)

Uses:
• temporarily relieves:
  • occasional minor irritation, pain, sore mouth, and sore throat
  • cough associated with a cold or inhaled irritants

Active ingredient
(in each drop): **Purpose:**
Menthol,
USP 2.5 mg .... Oral pain reliever/cough suppressant

Inactive Ingredients: Aspartame, canola oil, citric acid, D&C Yellow No. 10 aluminum lake (Natural Citrus only), FD&C blue No. 1 (Natural Citrus only), FD&C Yellow No. 6 (Tropical Fruit only), isomalt, mannitol, natural flavor.

Directions:
• adults and children 4 years and over: allow 2 drops to dissolve slowly in the mouth

• for sore throat: may be repeated every 2 hours, as needed, up to 9 drops per day, or as directed by a doctor
• for cough: may be repeated every hour, as needed, up to 9 drops per day, as or as directed by a doctor
• children under 4 years: ask a doctor

Warnings:
Sore throat warning: severe to persistent sore throat or sore throat accompanied by high fever, headache nausea, and vomiting may be serious. Consult a doctor right away. Do not use more than 2 days or give to children under 3 years of age unless directed by a doctor.
Ask a doctor before use if you have:
• cough that occurs with too much phlegm (mucus)
• cough that lasts or is chronic such as occurs with smoking, asthma, or emphysema
When using this product:
• excessive use may have a laxative effect
Stop use and ask a doctor if:
• cough lasts more than 7 days, comes back, or is accompanied by fever, rash, or persistent headache. These cough be signs of a serious condition.
If pregnant or breast-feeding, ask a health professional before use. **Keep out of reach of children.**

Other Information:
• each drop contains: **phenylalanine 3.37 mg**
• store at 20–25°C (68°–77°F)
• does not promote tooth decay
• product may be useful in a diabetic's diet on the advice of a doctor.
  Exchange information*:
  3 Drops = Free Exchange
  9 Drops = 1 Fruit
*The dietary exchanges are based on Exchange Lists for Meal Planning. Copyright 1995 by the American Diabetes Association Inc. and the American Dietetic Association.

How Supplied: Packages of 18 drops.

J.B. Williams Company, Inc.
**65 HARRISTOWN ROAD
GLEN ROCK, NJ 07452**

Address Inquiries to:
Consumer Affairs: (800) 254-8656
(201) 251-8100
FAX: (201) 251-8097

For Medical Emergency Contact:
(800) 254-8656

CĒPACOL®
[sē 'pə-cŏl]
Antiseptic Mouthwash/Gargle, Original and Mint Flavors

Ingredients: Cēpacol Original Antiseptic Mouthwash: Ceepryn® (cetylpyridinium chloride) 0.05%. Also contains: Alcohol 14%, Edetate Disodium, FD&C Yellow No. 5 (tartrazine) as a color

additive, Flavors, Glycerin, Polysorbate 80, Saccharin, Sodium Biphosphate, Sodium Phosphate, and Water.

Cēpacol Mint Antiseptic Mouthwash: Ceepryn® (cetylpyridinium chloride) 0.05%. Also contains: Alcohol 14.5%, D&C Yellow No. 10, FD&C Green No. 3, Flavor, Glucono Delta-Lactone, Glycerin, Poloxamer 407, Sodium Saccharin, Sodium Gluconate, and Water.

Actions: Cēpacol is an effective antiseptic mouthwash/gargle. It kills germs that cause bad breath for a fresher, cleaner mouth.
Cēpacol has a low surface tension, approximately $1/2$ that of water. This property is the basis of the spreading action in the oral cavity as well as its foaming action. Cēpacol leaves the mouth feeling fresh and clean and helps provide soothing, temporary relief of dryness and minor mouth irritations.

Uses: Recommended as a mouthwash and gargle for daily oral care; as an aromatic mouth freshener to provide a clean feeling in the mouth; as a soothing, foaming rinse to freshen the mouth.
Used routinely before dental procedures, helps give patient confidence of not offending with mouth odor. Often employed as a foaming and refreshing rinse before, during, and after instrumentation and dental prophylaxis. Convenient as a mouth-freshening agent after taking dental impressions. Helpful in reducing the unpleasant taste and odor in the mouth following gingivectomy.
Used in hospitals as a mouthwash and gargle for daily oral care. Also used to refresh and soothe the mouth following emesis, inhalation therapy, and intubations, and for swabbing the mouths of patients incapable of personal care.

Warning: In case of accidental ingestion seek professional assistance or contact a poison control center immediately. Do not use in children under 6 years of age. Children over 6 should be supervised when using Cēpacol. Keep out of reach of children.

Directions: Rinse vigorously before or after brushing or any time to freshen the mouth. Cēpacol leaves the mouth feeling refreshingly clean.
Use full strength every two or three hours as a soothing, foaming gargle, or as directed by a physician or dentist. May also be mixed with warm water.

Product label directions are as follows:
Rinse or gargle full strength before or after brushing or as directed by a physician or dentist.

How Supplied: Cēpacol Original/Cēpacol Mint Antiseptic Mouthwash: 12 oz, 24 oz, and 32 oz. Also available in 4 oz trial size.

Shown in Product Identification Guide, page 526

CĒPACOL®
[sē ′pə-cŏl]
Maximum Strength Sore Throat Spray; Cherry, Cool Menthol and Honey Lemon Flavors.

Active Ingredient:
Dyclonine Hydrochloride 0.1%.

Inactive Ingredients *Cherry:* Cetylpyridinium Chloride, D&C Red No. 33, Dibasic Sodium Phosphate, FD&C Yellow No. 6, Flavors, Glycerin, Phosphoric Acid, Poloxamer, Potassium Sorbate, Sorbitol, and Water.

Cool Menthol: Cetylpyridinium Chloride, Dibasic Sodium Phosphate, FD&C Blue No. 1, Flavors, Glycerin, Phosphoric Acid, Poloxamer, Potassium Sorbate, Polysorbate 20, Sodium Saccharin, Sorbitol and Water.

Honey Lemon: Caramel, Cetylpyridinium Chloride, Dibasic Sodium Phosphate, FD&C Yellow No. 6, Flavors, Glycerin, Phosphoric Acid, Poloxamer, Polysorbate 20, Potassium Sorbate, Sorbitol and Water.

Indications: For temporary relief of occasional minor sore throat pain and sore mouth. Also, for temporary relief of pain due to canker sores, minor irritation or injury to the mouth and gums, minor dental procedures, dentures or orthodontic appliances.

Directions: Adults: Spray 4 times into throat or affected area (children 2 to 12 years of age: spray 2–3 times) and swallow. Repeat as needed up to 4 times daily or as directed by a physician or dentist. Children 2 to 12 years of age should be supervised in product use. Children under 2 years: Consult physician or dentist.

Warnings: If sore throat is severe, persists for more than 2 days, is accompanied or followed by fever, headache, rash, nausea, or vomiting, consult a physician promptly. If sore mouth symptoms do not improve in 7 days, or if irritation, pain, or redness persists or worsens, see your dentist or physician promptly. Do not exceed recommended dosage. Keep this and all drugs out of the reach of children. In case of accidental overdose, seek professional assistance or contact a Poison Control Center immediately. As with any drug, if you are pregnant or nursing a baby, seek the advice of a health professional before using this product.

Store at room temperature. Do not freeze.

How Supplied: Available in Cherry, Cool Menthol, and Honey Lemon flavors in 4 fl. oz. (118 mL) plastic bottles with pump sprayer.

Shown in Product Identification Guide, page 526

CĒPACOL®
[sē ′pə-cŏl]
Sore Throat Lozenges
Regular Strength Original Mint,
Regular Strength Cherry,
Maximum Strength Mint,
Maximum Strength Cherry.
Sugar Free Maximum Strength Cool Mint
Sugar Free Maximum Strength Cherry
Oral Anesthetic

Ingredients: (per lozenge)
Regular Strength Original Mint: **Active Ingredient:** Menthol 2 mg. Also contains: Cetylpyridinium Chloride (Ceepryn®), D&C Yellow No. 10, FD&C Yellow No. 6, Flavor, Glucose, and Sucrose.

Regular Strength Cherry: **Active Ingredient:** Menthol 3.6 mg. Also contains: Cetylpyridinium Chloride (Ceepryn®), D&C Red No. 33, FD&C Red No. 40, Flavor, Glucose, and Sucrose.

Maximum Strength Mint: **Active Ingredients:** Benzocaine 10 mg., Menthol 2 mg. Also contains: Cetylpyridinium Chloride (Ceepryn®), D&C Yellow No. 10, FD&C Yellow No. 6, Flavor, Glucose, Simethicone, and Sucrose.

Maximum Strength Cherry: **Active Ingredients:** Benzocaine 10 mg., Menthol 3.6 mg. Also contains: Cetylpyridinium Chloride (Ceepryn®), D&C Red No. 33, FD&C Red No. 40, Flavor, Glucose, Simethicone, and Sucrose.

Sugar Free Maximum Strength Cool Mint: **Active Ingredients:** Benzocaine 10 mg., Menthol 2.5 mg. Also contains: Acesulfame Potassium, Cetylpyridinium Chloride (Ceepryn®), D&C Yellow No. 10, FD&C Yellow No. 6, Flavor, Isomalt, Maltitol, and Propylene Glycol.

Sugar Free Maximum Strength Cherry: **Active Ingredients:** Benzocaine 10 mg., Menthol 4.5 mg. Also contains: Acesulfame Potassium, Cetylpyridinium Chloride (Ceepryn®), D&C Red No. 33, FD&C Red No. 40, Flavor, Isomalt, Maltitol, and Propylene Glycol.

Actions: Menthol provides a mild anesthetic effect and cooling sensation for symptomatic relief of occasional minor sore throat pain and minor throat irritations. Benzocaine in the Maximum Strength lozenges provides an anesthetic effect for additional symptomatic relief of minor sore throat pain.

Indications: For temporary relief of occasional minor sore throat pain and dry, scratchy throat.

Warnings: If sore throat is severe, persists for more than 2 days, is accompanied or followed by fever, headache, rash, nausea, or vomiting, consult a physician promptly. Do not administer to children under 6 years of age unless directed by physician or dentist. Keep this and all

Continued on next page

Cepacol Lozenges—Cont.

drugs out of the reach of children. In case of accidental overdose, seek professional assistance or contact a Poison Control Center immediately. As with any drug, if you are pregnant or nursing a baby, seek the advice of a health professional before using this product.

Directions: Adults and children 6 years of age and older: Dissolve 1 lozenge in the mouth every 2 hours as needed or as directed by a physician or dentist. For children under 6 years, consult a physician or dentist.

How Supplied:

Trade package: 18 lozenges in 2 pocket packs of 9 each.
Sugar Free Maximum Strength: 16 lozenges in 2 pocket packs of 8 each.

Institutional package: Regular Strength Original Mint and Cherry, and Maximum Strength Mint: 648 lozenges in 72 blisters of 9 each.
Store at room temperature, below 86°F (30°C). Protect contents from humidity.
Shown in Product Identification Guide, page 526

CĒPACOL® VĪRACTIN®
[sē 'pə-cŏl] [vī 'rak-tin]
Cold Sore and Fever Blister Treatment; Gel and Cream Formulas

Ingredients:

Gel: Active Ingredient: Tetracaine HCl 2%. Also contains: Ethoxydiglycol, Eucalyptus Oil, Hydroxyethyl Cellulose, Maleated Soybean Oil, Methylparaben, Propylparaben, Sodium Lauryl Sulfate, Water.

Cream: Active Ingredient: Tetracaine 2%. Also contains: Chloroxylenol, Eucalyptus Oil, Hydrochloric Acid, Lauramide DEA, Methylparaben, Sodium Borate, Sodium Lauryl Sulfate, Steareth-2, Steareth-21, Stearic Acid, Water, White Wax.

Indications: For the temporary relief of pain and itching associated with cold sores and fever blisters.

Directions: Adults and children 2 years of age and older: apply to affected area not more than 3 to 4 times daily. Children under 2 years of age: Consult a doctor.

Warnings: For external use only. Avoid contact with eyes. If contact occurs, rinse

eyes thoroughly with water. If condition worsens, or symptoms persist for more than 7 days, or clear up and occur again within a few days, discontinue use of this product and consult a doctor. Do not use in large quantities, particularly over raw surfaces or blistered areas. Keep this and all drugs out of the reach of children. In case of accidental ingestion, seek professional assistance or contact a Poison Control Center immediately. Store at room temperature. Do not freeze.

How Supplied: Available in Gel and Cream formulas in 0.25 oz. (7.1 g) tubes.
Shown in Product Identification Guide, page 526

CHILDREN'S CĒPACOL® SORE THROAT FORMULA
[sē' pə-cŏl]
Pain Reliever, Nasal Decongestant, Fever Reducer
Grape and Cherry Flavor Liquids

Active Ingredients: Each teaspoon (5 mL) contains Acetaminophen USP 160 mg and Pseudoephedrine Hydrochloride USP 15 mg.

Inactive Ingredients: *Grape:* Benzoic Acid, Carboxymethyl Cellulose, Cetylpyridinium Chloride (Ceepryn®), Citric Acid, FD&C Blue No. 1, FD&C Red No. 40, Flavor, Glycerin, PEG-8, Polysorbate 20, Propylene Glycol, Purified Water, Saccharin Sodium, Sodium Benzoate, and Sorbitol.
Cherry: Benzoic Acid, Carboxymethyl Cellulose, Cetylpyridinium Chloride (Ceepryn®), Citric Acid, D&C Red No. 33, FD&C Red No. 40, Flavor, Glycerin, PEG-8, Polysorbate 20, Propylene Glycol, Purified Water, Saccharin Sodium, Sodium Benzoate, and Sorbitol.

Indications: For temporary relief of sore throat pain, other minor aches and pains, and nasal congestion due to a cold or flu. Promotes nasal and/or sinus drainage; temporarily relieves sinus congestion and pressure. Reduces fever.

Directions: Follow dosage recommendations below, or as directed by a doctor. Dosages may be repeated every 4–6 hours, not to exceed 4 doses in 24 hours. For accurate dosing, use the enclosed dosage cup.
SHAKE WELL BEFORE USING.
[See table below]
Store at room temperature.

Warnings: If sore throat is severe, persists for more than 2 days, is accompanied or followed by fever, headache, rash, nausea, or vomiting, consult a doctor

promptly. Do not take for pain or nasal congestion for more than 5 days or for fever for more than 3 days unless directed by a physician. If pain or fever persists or gets worse, if new symptoms occur, or if redness or swelling is present, consult a physician because these could be signs of a serious condition. Do not exceed recommended dosage. If nervousness, dizziness, or sleeplessness occur, discontinue use and consult a doctor. KEEP THIS AND ALL MEDICINES OUT OF THE REACH OF CHILDREN. Do not use with other products containing acetaminophen. In case of accidental overdose, contact a physician or poison control center immediately. Prompt medical attention is critical even if you do not notice any signs or symptoms.

Do not take product if you have heart disease, high blood pressure, thyroid disease, diabetes, or difficulty in urination due to enlargement of the prostate gland unless directed by a physician. As with any drug, if you are pregnant or nursing a baby, seek the advice of a health professional before using this product.

Drug Interaction Precaution: Do not take this product if you are now taking a prescription monoamine oxidase inhibitor (MAOI) (certain drugs for depression, psychiatric or emotional conditions, or Parkinson's disease), or for 2 weeks after stopping the MAOI drug. If you are uncertain whether your prescription drug contains an MAOI, consult a health professional before taking this product.

How Supplied: Available in Grape and Cherry flavors in 4 fl. oz. (118 mL) plastic bottles with dosage cup.

Wyeth-Ayerst Pharmaceuticals

Division of American Home Products Corporation
P.O. BOX 8299
PHILADELPHIA, PA 19101

Direct General Inquiries to:
(610) 688-4400

For Professional Services
(For example: Sales representative information, product pamphlets, educational materials):
800-395-9938

For Medical Product Information Contact:
Medical Affairs

Day: (800) 934-5556 (8:30 AM to 4:30 PM, Eastern Standard Time, Weekdays only)

Night: (610) 688-4400 (Emergencies only; non-emergencies should wait until the next day)

AGE (yr)	WEIGHT (lb)	DOSE (teaspoon)
Under 2	Under 24	Consult doctor
2–5	24–47	1
6–11	48–95	2
12 and Over	Over 95	4

Wyeth-Ayerst
Tamper-Resistant/Evident
Packaging

Statements alerting consumers to the specific type of Tamper-Resistant/Evident Packaging appear on the bottle labels and cartons of all Wyeth-Ayerst over-the-counter products. This includes plastic cap seals on bottles, individually wrapped tablets or suppositories, and sealed cartons. This packaging has been developed to better protect the consumer.

AMPHOJEL®
[am 'fo-jel]
Antacid
(aluminum hydroxide gel)
ORAL SUSPENSION

Composition: *Suspension—Peppermint flavored* —Each teaspoonful (5 mL) contains 320 mg aluminum hydroxide [Al(OH)$_3$] as a gel. The inactive ingredients present are calcium benzoate, glycerin, hydroxypropyl methylcellulose, mentholparaben, peppermint oil, propylparaben, saccharin, simethicone, sorbitol solution, and water. Good tasting Amphojel contains peppermint flavor.

Indications: For temporary relief of heartburn, upset stomach, sour stomach, and/or acid indigestion.

Directions: *Suspension* —Two teaspoonfuls (10 ml) to be taken five or six times daily, between meals and on retiring or as directed by a physician. Medication may be followed by a sip of water if desired.

Warnings: Do not take more than 12 teaspoonfuls (60 ml) of suspension in a 24-hour period or use this maximum dosage for more than two weeks except under the advice and supervision of a physician. May cause constipation. Prolonged use of aluminum-containing antacids in patients with renal failure may result in or worsen dialysis osteomalacia. Elevated tissue aluminum levels contribute to the development of dialysis encephalopathy and osteomalacia syndromes. Also, a number of cases of dialysis encephalopathy have been associated with elevated aluminum levels in the dialysate water. Small amounts of aluminum are absorbed from the gastrointestinal tract and renal excretion of aluminum is impaired in renal failure. Prolonged use of aluminum-containing antacids in such patients may contribute to increased plasma levels of aluminum. Aluminum is not well removed by dialysis because it is bound to albumin and transferrin, which do not cross dialysis membranes. As a result, aluminum is deposited in bone, and dialysis osteomalacia may develop when large amounts of aluminum are ingested orally by patients with impaired renal function.

As with any drug, if you are pregnant or nursing a baby, seek the advice of a health professional before using this product.

Drug Interaction Precaution: Antacids may interact with certain prescription drugs. Do not use this product if you are presently taking a prescription antibiotic containing any form of tetracycline. If you are presently taking a prescription drug, do not take this product without checking with your physician.
Keep tightly closed—store at room temperature, Approx. 77°F (25°C). Suspension should be shaken well before use. Avoid freezing.
Keep this and all drugs out of the reach of children.

How Supplied: *Suspension* —Peppermint flavored; bottles of 12 fluid ounces.
Manufactured by:
Wyeth Laboratories
A Wyeth-Ayerst Company
Philadelphia, PA 19101
　　Shown in Product Identification
　　Guide, page 528

Professional Labeling: Consult *2001 Physicians' Desk Reference.*
　　Shown in Product Identification
　　Guide, page 526

DONNAGEL®
[don 'nă-jel]
Liquid

Active Ingredients per Tablespoon (15 mL): Attapulgite Activated, USP 600 mg; Alcohol 1.4%.

Inactive Ingredients: Benzyl Alcohol, Carboxymethylcellulose Sodium, Citric Acid, FD&C Blue 1, Flavors, Magnesium Aluminum Silicate, Methylparaben, Phosphoric Acid, Propylene Glycol, Propylparaben, Saccharin Sodium, Sorbitol, Titanium Dioxide, Water, Xanthan Gum.

Indications: Donnagel is indicated for the symptomatic relief of diarrhea. It reduces the number of bowel movements, improves consistency of loose, watery bowel movements and relieves cramping.

Warnings: Patients are told that diarrhea may be serious. They are warned not to use this product for more than 2 days, or in the presence of fever, or in children under 6 years of age unless directed by a doctor.
This product should not be taken by patients who are hypersensitive to any of the ingredients. As with any drug, women who are pregnant or nursing a baby should seek the advice of a health professional before using this product.
KEEP THIS AND ALL DRUGS OUT OF THE REACH OF CHILDREN. IN CASE OF ACCIDENTAL OVERDOSE, SEEK PROFESSIONAL ASSISTANCE OR CONTACT A POISON CONTROL CENTER IMMEDIATELY.

Dosage and Administration: Full recommended dose should be administered at the first sign of diarrhea and after each subsequent bowel movement, NOT TO EXCEED 7 DOSES IN A 24-HOUR PERIOD.

Liquid

Adults	2 Tablespoons
Children	
12 years and over	2 Tablespoons
6 to under 12 years	1 Tablespoon
Under 6 years	Consult Physician

Liquid should be shaken well.

How Supplied: Donnagel Liquid (green suspension) in 4 fl. oz. (NDC 0008-0888-02), and 8 fl. oz. (NDC 0008-0888-04).
Store at controlled room temperature, between 20°C and 25°C (68°F and 77°F).
Manufactured by:
Wyeth Laboratories
A Wyeth-Ayerst Company
Philadelphia, PA 19101
　　Shown in Product Identification
　　Guide, page 526

MITROLAN®
[mĭt'rōw-lăn]
Stool Normalizer
(calcium polycarbophil)
Citrus/Vanilla Flavor
Chewable Tablets

Description: Each chewable tablet contains calcium polycarbophil (equivalent to 500 mg polycarbophil, USP). The inactive ingredients present are aminoacetic acid, corn starch, D&C yellow 10 aluminum lake, flavors, magnesium stearate, mannitol, povidone, sucrose.

Actions: Mitrolan (calcium polycarbophil) is a hydrophilic agent. As a bulk laxative, Mitrolan retains free water within the lumen of the intestine, and indirectly opposes dehydrating forces of the bowel, promoting well-formed stools. In diarrhea, when the intestinal mucosa is incapable of absorbing water at normal rates, Mitrolan absorbs free fecal water, forming a gel and producing formed stools. Thus, in both diarrhea and constipation, the drug works by restoring a more normal moisture level and providing bulk in the patient's intestinal tract.

Indications: For the treatment of constipation or diarrhea. Restores normal stool consistency by regulating its water and bulk content.

Contraindications: As with all hydrophilic bulking agents, calcium polycarbophil should not be used in patients with signs of gastrointestinal obstruction.

Warnings: WHEN USED FOR CONSTIPATION: If you have noticed a sudden change in bowel habits that persists

Continued on next page

Mitrolan—Cont.

over a period of 2 weeks, consult a physician before using. If the recommended use of this product for 1 week has had no effect, discontinue use and consult a physician. Do not use when abdominal pain, nausea, or vomiting are present except under the direction of a physician. WHEN USED FOR DIARRHEA: Unless directed by a physician, do not use for more than 2 days, or in the presence of high fever, or for children under 3 years of age. If diarrhea is associated with high fever, contact a physician.

As with any drug, if you are pregnant or nursing a baby, seek the advice of a health professional before using this product.

Adverse Reactions: Abdominal fullness may be noted occasionally. An adjustment of the dosage schedule with smaller doses given more frequently but spaced evenly throughout the day may provide relief of this symptom during continued use of Mitrolan.

Drug Interaction: Antacids containing aluminum, calcium or magnesium impair absorption of tetracycline. Although Mitrolan is not an antacid, it releases free calcium after ingestion and should not be used by any patient who is taking a prescription antibiotic drug containing any form of tetracycline.

Directions for Use:
CHEW TABLETS: DO NOT SWALLOW WHOLE.
Adults—Chew and swallow 2 tablets 4 times a day, or as needed. Do not exceed 12 tablets in a 24-hour period.
Children (6 to under 12 years)—Chew and swallow 1 tablet 3 times a day, or as needed. Do not exceed 6 tablets in a 24-hour period.
Children (3 to under 6 years)—Chew and swallow 1 tablet 2 times a day, or as needed. Do not exceed 3 tablets in a 24-hour period.
Children under 3 years: Consult a physician.

If necessary, for episodes of acute (short-term) diarrhea, the dose may be repeated every $1/2$ hour, but do not exceed the maximum daily dosage.

Dosage may be adjused according to individual response.
WHEN USING THIS PRODUCT FOR RELIEF OF CONSTIPATION DRINK A FULL GLASS (8 FL. OZ.) OF WATER OR OTHER LIQUID WITH EACH DOSE.

Sodium Content: Less than 0.02 mEq (0.46 mg) per tablet.

How Supplied: *Chewable Tablets*—cartons of 36 individually packaged blister units (NDC 0031-1535-57) and bottles of 100 (NDC 0031-1535-63).
Store at controlled room temperature, between 20°C and 25°C (68°F and 77°F).
Manufactured by:
Pharmaceutical Division
A.H. Robins Company

Richmond, Virginia 23220
Shown in Product Identification Guide, page 526

Zanfel Laboratories, Inc.
P.O. BOX 349
MORTON, IL 61550

Direct Inquiries to:
1-800-401-4002
Or visit our website:
www.zanfel.com

Zanfel™
Urushiol Wash

Use: Zanfel is a specially formulated lotion to cleanse and remove Urushiol from the skin. Urushiol is the toxin that causes the itching and rash associated with exposures to poison ivy, poison oak, poison sumac, poisonwood, mango, and related plants. The elimination of Urushiol from the body will, therefore, control the itching and rash associated with exposures to those plants.

Unlike soaps that must be used within 10–20 minutes of contact with Urushiol, or treatments that require continued use until the rash is gone (which can take up to 5 weeks), Zanfel washes away Urushiol at any stage of the body's reaction to the substance and often with only one washing. Some individuals with particularly severe reactions may require more than one use. Persons with poison oak and poisonwood typically require more than one washing. Most individuals experience relief from the itching within 30 seconds after Zanfel is used to wash the affected area. The rash will begin to subside within hours after washing.

Indications: Contact dermatitis resulting from exposure to Urushiol.

Ingredients: Polyethylene granules, sodium lauroyl sarcosinate, nonoxynol-9, C12-15 pareth-9, disodium EDTA, quatemium-15, carbomer 2%, triethanolamine, water.

Directions:
1. For best results, use Zanfel in a shower or other area where it is easy to thoroughly rinse off the product.
2. Wet the affected area.
3. Squeeze about an inch and a half of Zanfel onto the hands.
4. Wet both hands and rub the product into a paste. (Zanfel uses anti-foaming agents, and thus does not foam up.)
5. Rub hands directly on the affected area for 1 minute, working Zanfel into the skin.
6. Rinse thoroughly.
7. If any itch remains after rinsing, repeat steps 1–6 (only on the itching area) until all itching is gone. This is considered one application.

Warnings: In the case of a particularly severe reaction to Urushiol, a second

washing may be necessary a few hours after the first washing. The itch may return, usually in the same area, when imbedded Urushiol begins to surface. (Reapply as necessary, when itching returns.) In severe systemic cases where steroids are recommended but contraindicated for other reasons, it may require 3 to 5 days of washing with Zanfel. If symptoms persist, re-read the Q&A insert and see a physician. Note: For reactions having the appearance of thick leathery spots, further washings may be needed in those areas also. For external use only. As with most soaps, avoid contact with the eyes. If Zanfel gets into the eyes, rinse thoroughly with cold water until irritation subsides. If symptoms persist, consult a physician.

How Supplied: 1 oz. plastic tube.
Zanfel Laboratories, Inc.
Morton, IL 61615
For Information
Contact: 1-800-401-4002
©2001, Zanfel Laboratories, Inc.
Shown in Product Identification Guide, page 526

Zila Consumer Pharmaceuticals, Inc.
5227 NORTH 7th STREET
PHOENIX, AZ 85014-2800

Direct Inquiries to:
Carol Suich
Marketing Manager
(602) 266-6700
World Wide Web Address
www.zila.com

ZILACTIN® Oral Pain Reliever, Fever Blister/Cold Sore Treatment Gel
ZILACTIN®-L Liquid Fever Blister/ Cold Sore Treatment
ZILACTIN®-B Oral Pain Reliever Gel

Indication:
Zilactin Medicated Gel stops pain and speeds healing of canker sores, fever blisters and cold sores. Zilactin forms a tenacious, occlusive film which holds the medication in place while controlling pain. Intra-orally, the film can last up to 6 hours, usually allowing pain-free eating and drinking. Extra-orally, the film will last much longer.

Zilactin-L is a non film-forming liquid that treats and relieves the pain, itching and burning of developing and existing cold sores and fever blisters. Zilactin-L is specially formulated to treat the initial signs of tingling, itching or burning that signal an oncoming cold sore or fever blister.

Zilactin-B is a medicated gel containing benzocaine that forms a smooth, flexible and occlusive film on the oral mucosa. It's specially formulated to control pain

and shield the mouth sores, canker sores, cheek bites and gum sores that occur from dental appliances from the environment of the mouth. The film can last up to 6 hours. *Clinical studies on the effectiveness of Zila's products are available on request.*

Active Ingredients: Zilactin—Benzyl Alcohol (10%); **Zilactin-L**—Lidocaine (2.5%); **Zilactin-B**—Benzocaine (10%);

Directions:
Zilactin: FOR USE IN THE MOUTH AND ON LIPS. Apply every four hours for the first three days and then as needed. Dry the affected area. Apply a thin coat of Zilactin and allow 60 seconds for the gel to dry into a film. Outside the mouth, Zilactin forms a transparent film. Inside the mouth, the film is white.

Zilactin-L: FOR USE ON THE LIPS AND AROUND THE MOUTH. Moisten a cotton swab with several drops of Zilactin-L. Apply on lip area where symptoms are noted or directly on existing cold sore or fever blister and allow for 15 seconds. Do not apply more than 3 to 4 times daily. For optimal effectiveness use at first signs of tingling or itching.

Zilactin-B: FOR USE IN THE MOUTH. Apply every four hours for the first three days and then as needed. Dry the affected area. Apply a thin coat of Zilactin-B and allow 60 seconds for the gel to dry into a film.

Warning: A mild, temporary stinging sensation may be experienced when applying Zilactin, Zilactin-L or Zilactin-B to an open cut, sore or blister. This may be minimized by first applying ice for a minute before application of the medication. **Do not peel off protective film.** Attempting to peel off film may result in skin irritation or tenderness. To remove film, first apply another coat of Zilactin-B to film, and immediately wipe the area with a moist gauze pad or tissue. DO NOT USE IN OR NEAR EYES. In the event of accidental contact with the eye, flush with water immediately and continuously for ten minutes. Seek immediate medical attention if pain or irritation persists. For temporary relief only. As with all medications, keep out of the reach of children. Do not use Zilactin-L or Zilactin-B if you have a history of allergy to local anesthetics such as benzocaine, lidocaine or other "caine" anesthetics. If condition worsens, or if symptoms persist for more than 7 days or clear up and occur again within a few days, discontinue use of this product and consult a physician.

How Supplied: Zila products are nonprescription and carried by most drug wholesalers, retail chains and independent pharmacies. Each product is available to physicians and dentists directly from Zila in single use packages.
For further information call or write:

Zila Consumer Pharmaceuticals, Inc.
5227 N. 7th Street, Phoenix, AZ 85014-2800, (602) 266-6700

U.S. patent numbers 4,285,934; 4,381,296; and 5,081,158

ZILACTIN® BABY
Oral Pain Reliever Gel
Alcohol-Free

Indication:
Zilactin-Baby medicated gel is uniquely formulated to temporarily relieve sore gums caused by teething in infants and children 4 months of age and older. The extra strength level of medication in Zilactin-Baby begins relieving the discomfort of teething pain in seconds. This specially developed gel combines a pleasant grape flavor with an advanced ingredient that imparts a cooling sensation.

Active Ingredient: Benzocaine (10%)

Inactive Ingredients: PEG-8, PEG-75, Glycerin, Water, Potassium Acesulfame, Flavor, Menthyl Lactate, Glycine, Methylparaben, Propylparaben, Sorbic Acid.

Directions: Wash hands. Apply small amount to the affected gum area with fingertip or cotton applicator. Apply to affected area not more than 4 times daily or as directed by a dentist or physician. For infants under 4 months of age, there is no recommended dosage or treatment except under the advice and supervision of a physician.

Warning: DO NOT USE THIS PRODUCT FOR MORE THAN 7 DAYS UNLESS DIRECTED BY A DENTIST OR PHYSICIAN. If sore mouth symptoms do not improve in 7 days, or if irritation, pain, rash or fever develops, see a dentist or physician promptly. Do not exceed the recommended dosage. Do not use this product if there is a history of allergy to topical anesthetics such as procaine, butacaine, benzocaine or other "caine" anesthetics. Fever and nasal congestion are not symptoms of teething and may indicate the presence of infection. If these symptoms persist consult your physician. Keep this and all drugs out of the reach of children. In case of accidental overdose, seek professional assistance or contact a Poison Control Center immediately.

EDUCATIONAL MATERIAL

Samples and literature are available to medical professionals on request.

DIETARY SUPPLEMENT INFORMATION

This section presents information on natural remedies and nutritional supplements marketed under the Dietary Supplement Health and Education Act of 1994. It is made possible through the courtesy of the manufacturers whose products appear on the following pages. The information concerning each product has been prepared, edited, and approved by professional staff of the manufacturer.

Products to be found in this section include vitamins, minerals, herbs and other botanicals, amino acids, other substances intended to supplement the diet, and concentrates, metabolites, constituents, extracts, and combinations of these ingredients. The descriptions of these products are designed to provide all information necessary for informed use, including, when applicable, active ingredients, inactive ingredients, actions, warnings, cautions, interactions, symptoms and treatment of oral overdosage, dosage and directions for use, and how supplied.

Descriptions in this section must be in full compliance with the Dietary Supplement Health and Education Act, which permits claims regarding a product's effect on the structure or functioning of the body, but forbids claims regarding a product's ability to treat, diagnose, cure, or prevent any specific disease. Descriptions of products marketed under the act do not receive formal evaluation or approval from the Food and Drug Administration.

In compiling this section, the publisher has emphasized the necessity of describing products comprehensively. The descriptions seen here include all information made available by the manufacturer. The publisher does not warrant or guarantee any product described here, and does not perform any independent analysis of the information provided. Inclusion of a product in this book does not represent an endorsement, and the publisher does not necessarily advocate the use of any product listed.

A & Z Pharmaceutical Inc.

**180 OSER AVENUE, SUITE 300
HAUPPAUGE, NY 11788**

Direct Inquiries to:
Customer Service
(631) 952-3800
Fax: (631) 952-3900

D-CAL™
**Calcium Supplement with Vitamin D
Chewable Caplets**

Ingredients: Calcium Carbonate, Vitamin D, Sorbitol, Flavor, D&C Red #27 Lake, Magnesium Stearate. No sugar, No salt, No lactose, No preservative.

Supplement Facts

Serving Size One Caplet

Each Caplet Contains		% Daily Value
Calcium (as calcium carbonate)	300 mg	30%
Vitamin D	100 IU	25%

Recommended Intake: Take two caplets daily for adult and one caplet for child, or as directed by your physician.

Warnings: KEEP OUT OF REACH OF CHILDREN. Do not accept if safely seal under cap is broken or missing.

Actions: D-Cal™ provides a concentrated form of calcium to help build healthy bones. It contains Vitamin D to help the body absorb calcium. D-Cal™ can also help prevent osteoporosis. It is helpful to pregnant and nursing women, children's growth, and calcium deficiency at all ages.

How Supplied: Bottle of 60 caplets
Shown in Product Identification Guide, page 503

AdvoCare International, L.L.C.

**2727 REALTY ROAD
SUITE 134
CARROLLTON, TX 75006**

Direct inquiries to:
Medical/Scientific Advisory Board
(972) 478-4500
Fax: (972) 478-4751

ACTOTHERM

Uses: ActoTherm provides a gentle, cumulative rise in the metabolic production of heat, helping the body to effectively burn more calories.

ActoTherm's proprietary herbal concentrate, ThermoGen HC™, is based on the Chinese model of thermogenesis and includes herbs, vitamins and minerals. Antioxidants are also included to protect against free radical production associated with increased metabolism. Thermogenesis is central to metabolic nutrition. The production of heat and body energy greatly aids in boosting and fine-tuning metabolism. A heightened sense of energy also supports wise, healthy food and lifestyle choices.

Directions: Take one or two caplets twice a day, 30 minutes prior to a meal.

Warning: *Not recommended for pregnant or lactating women. Keep out of reach of children.*

Ingredients: *Each caplet contains ThermoGen HC™ (Extracts of gotu kola, cinnamon ramulus, peppermint, lemon verbena, chamomile, ginger, Chinese licorice root, sweet citrus peel and chicory), guarana extract (standardized), potassium phosphate, magnesium phosphate, niacin, capsicum extract (standardized), green tea extract (standardized) and beta carotene.*

How Supplied: Each bottle contains 180 caplets.

ADVANTIN

Uses: Advantin, a high-potency, all-natural mixture of standardized botanical extracts blended into a whole papaya base, is scientifically designed to support improved digestion and absorption of nutrients. With optimized digestion, energy levels increase, skin tone improves, joints move more smoothly and heartburn and other gastrointestinal discomforts subside.

With improved fat and protein digestion, more nutrients are absorbed from food, beverages and dietary supplements. Higher nutrient uptake helps people to eat less food and make better food choices, making Advantin an important part of a weight management program. Advantin supports the body's production and release of digestive enzymes. Standardized ginger extract is combined with natural digestive enzymes to help increase the efficiency of digestion. Curcumin is a revolutionary new botanical fraction loaded with powerful antioxidants to help protect the delicate intestinal cell lining from free radical damage.

Advantin is also beneficial in allowing the joints to move more smoothly. Boswellia extract, along with curcumin extract, contains powerful elements to help reduce inflammation and water build-up (edema).

Directions: Take one Advantin capsule immediately before a meal. For best results, take Advantin two or three times every day. Advantin is appropriate for anyone 12 years of age and older.

Ingredients: One capsule provides 200 mg of Ginger extract (standardized), 150 mg of Boswellia extract (standardized), 100 mg of Curcumin (standardized), 50 mg of whole Papaya powder, 50 mg of Papain and 50 mg of Bromelain.

How Supplied: One bottle contains 60 capsules.

ANTIOXIDANT BOOSTER

Uses: Antioxidant Booster helps protect against free radical damage and oxidation of LDL cholesterol.

Free radicals are extremely destructive chemical species in our bodies which are now strongly linked to an increased risk of a plethora of serious diseases, as well as premature aging. Oxidized LDL cholesterol has received a great deal of current biomedical research attention, and is thought to be one of the main factors contributing to increased risk of heart disease and strokes.

Because of the tremendously destructive action of free radicals, and the ability of antioxidants to neutralize these free radicals, antioxidant supplementation is now advocated by most leading nutrition and health authorities and government public health agencies. Over 80 percent of all nutritionists and physicians consume antioxidant supplementation. Antioxidant Booster gives a complete and potent profile of the many nutrients your body needs to best guard against free radical damage.

Antioxidant Booster's unique formulation provides essential minerals for the body's own internal antioxidant enzyme systems. The minerals zinc, manganese and selenium, are in highly bioavailable forms for maximum potency.

Antioxidant Booster contains a unique and scientifically based blend of phytochemicals to further protect body tissues against the hazards of free radical damage. These phytochemicals contain compounds known as "flavones", some of the most active of which are found in green tea, ginkgo biloba and silymarin. Antioxidant Booster contains natural vitamin E, beta-carotene and both water-and fat-soluble forms of vitamin C, thus giving a more complete spectrum of protection than products just containing ascorbic acid (vitamin C).

Directions: Take two caplets of Antioxidant Booster daily, with food, to enhance the body's protection against free radicals.

Ingredients: Two caplets provide the following: 250IU of Vitamin E (D-alpha tocopheryl succinate), 1000 mg of Vitamin C (ascorbic acid and ascorbyl palmitate), 15,000 IU of Beta-carotene, 35 mcg of Selenium (Selenomethionine), 5 mg of Zinc (OptiZinc), 1 mg of Manganese (Amino Acid Chelate), 50 mg of Green Tea Extract (Standardized), 50 mg of Silymarin (Standardized milk thistle extract) and 100 mg of Grape Seed Flavonoids (Activin).

How supplied: Each bottle contains 60 caplets.

BODYLEAN
Protein Mix

Uses: BodyLean is an exceptional source of high protein combined with muscle enhancing nutrients. BodyLean is designed to optimize muscle mass during times of intensive exercise such as weight lifting. BodyLean may also be used in a weight management program, or for anyone seeking to increase their protein intake.

When used for weight management, BodyLean is an easy way to balance a diet rich in carbohydrates, fruits and vegetables. Optimal protein intake is essential for healthy weight loss and to maintain body composition after body fat has been lost.

BodyLean provides a full 50 grams of partially predigested protein in each serving. The highest grade proteins available are used for easy digestion and maximum utilization by the body.

The exceptional protein profile of BodyLean is further enhanced with free-form branched chain amino acids (BCAAs). During intensive physical activity, muscles selectively lose BCAAs, and supplementation with BCAAs may help spare muscle breakdown and replenish muscle losses quickly.

During weight loss, protein is essential for muscle strength and to maintain muscle mass. Diets rich in carbohydrates and plant foods often lack enough protein to sustain muscle while losing body fat. Calorie restriction may also compromise muscle integrity, particularly causing a loss of BCAAs. BodyLean is a great way to ensure protein balance and to help maintain muscle while burning fat.

Directions: Blend or shake three heaping scoops of Body Lean powder into at least 16 fluid ounces of any beverage of choice.

For support of muscle-building, take BodyLean 90 minutes before exercise or 90 minutes after exercise.

For weight management, enjoy BodyLean with a meal to enhance your protein intake. The serving size of BodyLean can be tailored to individual body needs (i.e., smaller-bodied people may require less than larger-bodied people.)

Ingredients: Metabolically Balanced Protein Isolate™ (containing total milk protein, calcium sodium caseinate, whey protein concentrate, soy protein concentrate, branched chain amino acids [L-leucine, L-isoleucine, L-valine]), fructose, natural and artificial flavors, magnesium oxide, ascorbic acid, adrenal extract, acesultame potassium, pyridoxine hydrochloride, calcium pantothenate, niacin, manganese sulfate, papain, bromelain, thiamine hydrochloride, riboflavin, biotin and cyanocobalamin.

How Supplied: One can contains 10 servings of 75 grams each. One box contains 15 packets containing 37.5 grams each (25 grams of protein per serving).

BRITE-LIFE
Metabolic Nutrition

Uses: Brite-Life is a gentle yet powerful blend of standardized herbal extracts and vitamins designed to enhance a positive mood and feelings of well-being.

Brite-Life contains the important mood-boosting herb St. John's Wort. St. John's Wort has been found to help alleviate depression through its influence on brain serotonin levels. Serotonin is also involved in weight management. Higher serotonin levels are linked to appetite suppression. Lower serotonin levels are associated with obesity. Brite-Life uses the highest potency, standardized St. John's Wort extract to give brain chemistry maximum support.

Green orange extract provides an array of gentle energy – enhancing compounds. Vitamin B6 and German chamomile have been used traditionally to help calm and focus the mind and to support the body's own production of serotonin.

Positive feelings and a bright outlook on life are essential for vibrant health, abundant energy and lasting weight loss.

Directions: Take one caplet two times a day, 30 minutes before meals, as a natural dietary supplement.

Ingredients: One caplet contains 450 mg of St. John's Wort extract (standardized), 100 mg of Pyridoxine (HCl), 300 mg L-Tyrosine.

How Supplied: One bottle contains 60 caplets.

C-GRAMS

Uses: C-Grams is an advanced vitamin C product containing a balanced ratio of mineral ascorbates formulated to parallel the body's own proportions of vitamin C. This best maintains vitamin C levels in tissue and replenishes minerals lost with higher intake of vitamin C.

The antioxidant features of vitamin C are further enhanced by mixed citrus bioflavonoids and potent standardized bilberry extract.

The lysine contained in C-Grams is included to complement the positive role of vitamin C in cardiovascular health. This lysine-vitamin C connection represents the newest breakthrough in the science of nutrition.

Optimal vitamin C levels are necessary to promote and support metabolic nutrition, resulting in enhanced energy production, stronger immune responsiveness, heightened cardiovascular fitness, improved strength and elasticity of skin,

blood vessels and other body tissues, as well as an improved ability to respond to stress.

Directions: Take C-Grams daily as the ultimate source of vitamin C. Many leading nutrition and health experts suggest 2,000 to 10,000 mg. (2 to 10 grams) of vitamin C per day for optimal health and well-being.

Ingredients: Two caplets provide 100 mg of vitamin C (ascorbic acid), 560 mg of vitamin C (potassium ascorbate), 160 mg of vitamin C (magnesium ascorbate), 180 mg of vitamin C (calcium ascorbate), 100 mg of mixed citrus bioflavonoids, 10 mg of bilberry (standardized extract-anthocyanosides) and 300 mg L-lysine.

How supplied: One bottle contains 120 caplets.

CARDIOPTIMA

Uses: CardiOptima is a heart-healthy drink mix rich in the most potent blend of antioxidants, blood vessel protectors and cardiac tonics. This pleasant-tasting product provides nutritional support for the prevention and elimination of oxidized LDL cholesterol and sticky platelets, thereby dramatically decreasing the likelihood of cardiovascular disease.

CardiOptima contains a proprietary blend of antioxidant mineral ascorbates, vitamin E and ActiVin™ grape seed extract which work together to support cardiovascular function. Also features Coenzyme Q-10, taurine and selected amino acids to prevent LDL deposition on arterial walls.

Complementary vitamins, minerals and herbs also assist the body in clearing homocysteine, a metabolic by-product identified as a cardiovascular risk factor.

Directions: Drink one or more glasses of CardiOptima daily on an empty stomach any time of the day or night.

Ingredients: One serving of CardiOptima 100 mg L-methionine, 600 mg L-lysine, 400 mg Taurine, 100 mg L-proline, 10 mg Coenzyme Q-10, 20 mg L-carnitine and 100 mg Activin™ Grape Seed Extract as well as dextrose, fructose, 1000 mg vitamin C (potassium/calcium ascorbates), Krebs Cycle Mineralized Substrates™ (citric acid, magnesium citrate, calcium citrate), 300 IU D-alpha tocopheryl succinate (vitamin E), gum arabic, beet powder, food flavoring, magnesium sulfate, inositol hexanicotinate, pyridoxine hydrochloride, Phytocardia Complex™ (hibiscus flower powder, hawthorn berry powder, Golden Root extract), folic acid and cyanocobalamin.

How supplied: Each box contains 15 packets, with a total net weight of 13.75 ounces.

Continued on next page

CATALYST

Uses: Catalyst is a high-potency amino acid formulation designed to support muscle strength and structure, and to help boost mental energy and focus. Catalyst helps prevent muscle breakdown, an effect which is critical for beneficial weight loss and for athletic performance. Catalyst helps preserve muscle mass during times of calorie restriction.

Glutamine is also included in the Catalyst formula to buffer lactic acid production in muscle. Glutamine appears to be selectively drained from the muscles and other body systems during the early stages of exercise and of weight loss. Glutamine is also a neuroactive nutrient, and helps supply the brain with an essential building block and energy compound needed for proper mental functioning.

Directions: Take three Catalyst capsules between meals or immediately prior to exercise. Because food protein can interfere with the absorption and utilization of free-form amino acids such as those contained in Catalyst, you get maximum benefits when Catalyst is consumed on an empty stomach. For exercise enhancement, take Catalyst about 5 minutes prior to a workout or competition. This is designed to maximize the energy-boosting and the muscle-sparing effects of the formula.

Ingredients: Three capsules contain 1200 mg of L-glutamine, 450 mg of L-leucine, 225 mg of L-isoleucine and 225 mg of L-valine.

How Supplied: Each bottle contains 90 capsules.

COFFECCINO

Coffeccino is a pleasant-tasting beverage mix designed to curb the appetite for assistance in weight loss. It contains herbs and an outstanding mixture of nutrients formulated to provide mental energy.

Coffeccino is formulated with Garcinia cambogia extract, an all-natural fruit source which contains the appetite-suppressing compound—hydroxycitric acid, or HCA. HCA helps reduce the desire to eat high-calorie foods.

Directions: As a hot or cold breakfast beverage, Coffeccino has an energizing effect as well as helping to reduce appetite for high-calorie foods. Drink Coffeccino before lunch to help cut mid-day food cravings and facilitate wise food choices. Taken at mid-afternoon, Coffeccino can curb desire to over-eat in the evening.

Ingredients: Each serving contains 500 mg of Garcinia cambogia extract, 120 mg of caffeine and 800 mg L-tyrosine as well as fructose, sugar, polydextrose, canola oil, corn syrup solids, modified casein, coffee powder, cocoa powder, natural and artificial flavors, xanthan gum, ascorbic acid, calcium pantothenate, pyridoxine hydrochloride, chromium polynicotinate (ChromeMate™) and folic acid.

How Supplied: Each box of Coffeccino contains 15 packets, each having a net weight of 35 grams.

COLD SEASON NUTRITION BOOSTER

Uses: Cold Season Nutrition Booster is a potent immune-boosting formula designed to augment resistance to colds and flu. Cold Season Nutrition Booster contains large quantities of standardized herbal extracts, providing maximum efficacy for immune function.

Echinacea is widely known for its immune boosting properties, and the standardized extract contained in the product provides the most potent echinacea available. Echinacea is best used for short periods of time (e.g., 7 to 10 days) in an on-off pattern, rather than consumed daily. Golden seal extract complements the benefits of echinacea.

Astragalus is widely used in Chinese herbal medicine as an immune booster. Shiitake mushroom also enjoys great popularity in Asia as a major immune support. Elderberry extract, thymus and quercitin round out Cold Season Nutrition Booster and provide powerful synergy to give maximum strength and benefit.

Directions: Take Cold Season Nutrition Booster at the first sign of a cold or flu. Consume Cold Season Nutrition Booster for 7 to 10 days, then go off of the formula for 4 to 7 days. This on-off pattern helps ensure that the ingredients in Cold Season Nutrition Booster work at maximum potency and helps guard against the body getting used to the immune boosters in this maximum strength formula.

Ingredients: Each capsule contains 200 mg of echinacea extract (standardized), 50 mg astragalus extract (standardized), 25 mg golden seal extract (standardized), 100 mg shiitake mushroom extract (standardized), 10 mg elderberry extract (standardized), 50 mg thymus extract and 50 mg quercetin.

COREPLEX
Metabolic Nutrition

Uses: *CorePlex is a premier multi-nutrient supplement including vitamins, minerals and complementary pytochemicals.*

CorePlex supplies the body with all known essential vitamins and minerals (except iron) in a metabolically optimizing formula. CorePlex is nutritionally proportioned for maximum potency and support of metabolic nutrition, balancing each nutrient against the others for maximum absorption and utilization. CorePlex contains mineral chelates such as OptiZinc™ (zinc monomethionine), ChromeMate™, (niacin-bound chromium) and selenomethionine for highest bioavailability. Most leading multiple vitamin/mineral products contain ionic forms of minerals such as zinc oxide and chromium chloride, which are much more poorly absorbed than the chelated minerals used in CorePlex.

Directions: Take three CorePlex daily as the cornerstone of the AdvoCare nutrition program. Take CorePlex with food, either in the morning or at noon. For ease of use, take all tablets at once. Alternatively, you can spread out the intake and consume one tablet with each meal.

Warning: Keep out of reach of children.

Ingredients: Three capsules provide 2,500 IU of vitamin A (palmitate), 12,500 IU of vitamin A (beta carotene), 600 mg of vitamin C, 400 IU of vitamin D (ergocalciferol), 150 IU vitamin E (d-alpha tocopheryl succinate), 9 mg thiamine, 10.2 mg riboflavin, 20 mg niacin, 100 mg niacinamide, 40 mg panothenic acid, 12 mg pyridoxine (HCl), 36 mcg vitamin B-12 (cyanocobalamin), 400 mcg folic acid, 300 mcg biotin, 6 mg inositol, 60 mg choline, 150 mg calcium, 200 mg magnesium, 15 mg zinc, 150 mcg iodine (Kelp), 80 mg selenium (selenomethionine), 4 mg Manganese, 100 mcg Chromium (ChromeMate®), 50 mcg Molybdenum, 2 mg copper, 100 mg potassium, 300 mcg Boron, 50 mcg Vanadium (BMOV), 100 mg Phosphorus, 500 mcg silicon, 150 mcg coenzyme Q10, 2 mg Octacosanol, 2 mg RNA, 50 mg odorless garlic, 5 mg L-Glutathione, 5 mg Gamma Oryzanol, 100 mg Citrus Bioflavonoids, 5 mg red wine polyphenols (Standardized), 5 mg Milk Thistle extract (Standardized), 10 mg Ginkgo biloba (Standardized) and 100 mg L-Methionine.

FEMESSENCE

Uses: FemEssence provides nutritional support for female hormonal function. FemEssence contains a proprietary blend of high potency standardized herbs and essential nutrients which can help reduce symptoms of premenstrual syndrome and ease the tension of menopause.

The botanical extracts in FemEssence support the transitional effects of menopause, and helps moderate emotional mood swings. Mexican wild yam extract and Resveratrol are especially helpful in achieving balance.

Moomiyo, a rare herbal ingredient from central Asia, helps skin look soft and supple, as well as boosting the immune system. Moomiyo has been taken in supplement form for centuries as a natural beauty aid, as well as for PMS and menopause.

Cranberry extract and freeze-dried acidophilus help strengthen a woman's reproductive and urinary systems to defend against harmful bacteria and yeast infections. Raspberry leaf is a time-honored women's herb, and along with the other ingredients in FemEssence, helps overall toning and balance of the body and mind.

AdvoCare only uses standardized herbal extracts, which ensures the highest quality, highest potency, and most reliable formula to be found.

Directions: Take three capsules per day, preferably one half hour before a meal or at bedtime.

Ingredients: Three capsules contain 100 mg of Mexican wild yam extract, 500 mg glucosamine HCl, 60 mg saw palmetto extract, 30 mg vitamin B6 (pyridoxine HCl), 100 mg Moomiyo, 200 mg cranberry extract, 50 mg raspberry leaf extract, 13.5 mg iron (Ferrochel™), 200 MM Lactobacillus acidophilus, 5 mg Resveratrol, 20 mg niacin, and 75 mg Ginkgo biloba extract.

How Supplied: One bottle contains 90 capsules.

FIBER 10

Uses: Fiber 10 provides a full 10 grams of soluble and insoluble fibers formulated to boost intestinal function and reduce serum cholesterol. This unique mixture is created to optimize cleansing functions in the intestines, assist in the transport and removal of dietary fats, sterols and bile acids from the bloodstream and to aid in the elimination of other harmful physiological waste products. Fiber 10 also gives a feeling of fullness, which helps curb appetite. Inclusion of probiotic organisms further enhances the intesinal support provided by Fiber 10.

Regular use of Fiber 10 can help achieve the recommended 25 to 30 grams of dietary fiber intake suggested by leading health and nutrition experts and US government health agencies.

Directions: *Stir contents of one packet into 8 ounces of chilled water or fat-free beverage of choice two or three times daily, preferably before meals. Follow each serving with consumption of additional 8 ounces of water.*

Ingredients: One serving contains fiber blend (psyllium husk, guar gum, carboxymethyl cellulose, citrus pectin, butternut bark powder), fructose, beta-carotene, citric acid, natural and artificial flavors, acesulfame, papaya powder, prune powder, ascorbic acid, digestive enzyme complex (protease, lipase, cellulase), rhubarb root extract, black walnut hull extract, licorice root extract, Lactobacillus acidophilus, Bifidobacterium bifidus.

How Supplied: Each box contains thirty 0.7-ounce packets, each providing ten grams of fiber derived from the most effective sources.

INTELLEQ

Uses: IntelleQ is a formula providing nutritional support for mental alertness which contains a proprietary blend of biochemical building blocks.

Phospholipids are key to brain structure and function and are converted to the biochemicals used by nerve and brain cells. The standardized phospholipid complex contains a unique mixture of choline and phosphatidylserine, a most sophisticated mixture based on the latest breakthroughs in nutrition research. Ginkgo biloba has been used for over 5000 years as a mental tonic and is among the top selling herbal extracts in Europe. Most people in Germany over the age of 45 take Ginkgo, prescribed by their doctor, to help keep the mind sharp. The standardized extract used in IntelleQ insures the most potent, most reliable Ginkgo available anywhere in the world.

Rhodiola is a botanical widely used in eastern Europe, Asia and Tibet. Some studies have found that Rhodiola helps to increase memory in human subjects. Brahm IQ™ is a standardized extract of Bacopa monniera, shown in both human and animal studies to increase short-term and long-term memory.

The other ingredients in IntelleQ also serve to optimize metabolism, help to increase antioxidant protection, or are reported to enhance memory and thinking ability.

Directions: Take one (1) to two (2) capsules per day with a meal, preferably early in the day.

Ingredients: Two capsules contain 150 mg of phospholipid complex (standardized), 100 mg of Ginkgo biloba extract (standardized), 10 mg grape seed anthocyanidins (Activin™), 700 mcg boron (amino acid complex), 20 mg niacin, 1000 mcg RNA, 200 mg taurine, 100 mg choline (bitartrate), 60 mg vitamin C (potassium ascorbate), 500 mg Bacopa extract (Brahm IQ®).

LIPOTROL

Uses: LipoTrol contains hydroxycitric Acid (HCA), a naturally-derived fruit extract which helps reduce appetite and boost the burning of fat. Unlike harsh chemical appetite suppressants, use of HCA gives desired results in a safe and gentle manner.

LipoTrol also contains niacin-bound chromium (ChromeMate), which helps form Glucose Tolerance Factor, essential for proper metabolism of sugars and fats, and for support of muscle mass.

LipoTrol contains the BMOV form of vanadium, known to inhibit the buildup of cholesterol. BMOV is seven times more bioavailable and therefore more effective than vanadyl sulfate, the form typically used in many other brands of nutrition supplements.

LipoTrol contains a unique lipotropic complex of inositol and choline, included to help the body burn fat. LipoTrol also contains beta-sitosterol to help reduce the absorption of dietary cholesterol.

LipoTrol contains specific vitamins, minerals and phytochemicals (biologically active plant-based chemicals) included to boost optimal burning of body fat. The formula also contains gymnema, an extraordinary natural herb which may help reduce active sugar absorption.

Directions: Because of the important appetite suppressing effect of HCA, take LipoTrol 30 to 45 minutes before a meal, on an empty stomach.

Take LipoTrol at least twice a day. HCA has been shown to be seven times more effective in suppressing appetite when spread out in multiple small doses, compared to taking the same amount of HCA all at once. Therefore, taking two LipoTrol tablets before breakfast and two tablets prior to lunch and/or before dinner is recommended.

Ingredients: *Four caplets contain 2000 mg Garcinia extract, 50 mg Tulsi extract, 50 mg taurine, 25 mg L-carnitine, 25 mg beta sitosterol, 2 mg zinc (OptiZinc™), 10 mg gymnema sylvestre extract, 4 mg pyridoxine (HCl), 200 mcg vanadium (BMOV) and 100 mcg chromium (ChromeMate®).*

How Supplied: *One bottle contains 120 caplets.*

MACRO-MINERAL COMPLEX

Uses: Macro-Mineral Complex is a comprehensive formulation which incorporates the full spectrum of bone-building nutrients in highly bioavailable forms.

The chelated calcium complex offers absorption which is superior to typical calcium supplements (which use the relatively poorly absorbed calcium carbonate). The forms of magnesium and complementary trace elements in Macro-Mineral Complex are also in the chelated form, thus speeding these bone-building nutrients into the body at the highest absorption rate.

The balance between calcium and magnesium is critical. Taking calcium by itself can actually drain the body of magnesium, which could result in muscle cramps, irritability, depression and other serious conditions. Macro-Mineral Complex uses a 1 to 1 calcium to magnesium ratio to perfectly balance these two key minerals.

Calcium absorption is enhanced with vitamin D and potassium bicarbonate. Recent studies have found that potassium bicarbonate helps balance the body acid-base levels to better optimize calcium absorption and bone mineralization.

Directions: Take two to six caplets daily, preferably with meals or at bed-

Continued on next page

Macro-Mineral—Cont.

time. Since calcium and magnesium tend to calm and relax the body, taking Macro-Mineral Complex in the evening may be desirable.

Ingredients: *Two caplets contain 220 mg calcium (citrate and hydroxyapatite), 200 mg magnesium (amino acid chelate and magnesium ascorbate), 2 mg zinc (OptiZinc™), 300 mcg silicon (amino acid complex), 1 mg manganese (amino acid chelate), 200 mcg boron (amino acid complex), 200 mcg copper (amino acid chelate), 40 IU vitamin D (ergocalciferol), 60 mg vitamin C (magnesium ascorbate), 3 mg pyridoxine (HCl), 500 mg potassium bicarbonate, 50 mg shave grass extract, 50 mg green tea extract and 25 mg ginger extract.*

How Supplied: *One bottle contains 120 caplets.*

METABOLIC NUTRITION SYSTEM

Uses: *Metabolic Nutrition System Yellow*—Optimum foundational nutrients for metabolic support. Includes Acto-Therm which provides gentle support for thermogenesis and energy production. *Metabolic Nutrition System Gold*—Natural appetite suppression plus optimum levels of nutrients. Includes Thermo-G. *Metabolic Nutrition System Orange*—Weight management, energy and a heightened sense of well-being. Includes Thermo-E, which provides a proprietary combination of ephedra alkloids and other adrenergic boosting herbs for maximum thermogenesis and weight management.

Every ingredient in the components of Metabolic Nutrition has been specifically selected based on the latest, most advanced scientific research studies from around the world.

Each of the four versions of Metabolic Nutrition System contain the following components:

CorePlex™ is a premier multinutrient supplement containing the complete spectrum of vitamins, minerals, phytochemical antioxidants, and complementary herbal concentrates. (See complete list of ingredients for CorePlex in this section).

LipoTrol™ is a natural formula designed to help control appetite and encourage proper metabolism of fats. The formula contains standardized Garcinia extract, standardized Tulsi extract, taurine, L-carnitine, beta sitosterol, zinc (monomethionine-OptiZinc™), standardized Gymnema sylvestre extract, pyridoxine (HCl), vanadium (BMOV), chromium (polynicotinate-ChromeMate®).

OmegaPlex™ is an exceptional source of the omega-3 fatty acids, eicosapentaenoic acid (EPA) and docosahexaenoic acid (DHA) for maximum cardiovascular support.

MetaBoost™ is a blend of nutrients and phytochemicals formulated to support the endocrine system. The formula includes potassium/magnesium/sodium ascorbates, desiccated pituitary extract, desiccated adrenal extract, iodine, guarana extract and Siberian ginseng extract.

METABOOST

Uses: MetaBoost provides nutritional support for the endocrine system, helping boost energy levels and strength. MetaBoost also provides ascorbic acid metabolites designed to boost transport of critical energy-associated minerals into the cell to assist in the higher production of energy at the subcellular level.

Directions: Take two to four caplets a day.

Warning: This product is not recommended for pregnant or lactating women. Keep out of reach of children.

Ingredients: Two caplets provide 745 mg of potassium/magnesium/sodium ascorbates, 50 mg desiccated pitutary extract, 50 mg desiccated adrenal extract, 50 mcg iodine (potassium iodide), 150 mg guarana extract (standardized) and 50 mg Siberian ginseng extract (standardized).

How Supplied: One bottle contains 120 caplets.

PERFECT MEAL

Uses: Perfect Meal features a proprietary mixture of whole proteins, amino acids, peptides, digestive enzymes, and whole vegetable powders, as well as simple and complex carbohydrates, plus a full spectrum of vitamins and minerals. Easy-to-digest proteins and high-energy, easily absorbed peptides help build strong, powerful muscles and maximize metabolic function—essential for general well-being during weight loss.

A comprehensive blend of fibers, probiotics and digestive enzymes help maximize intestinal function, a key to elimination of toxins and excess dietary fat.

Directions: Perfect Meal is designed to replace a lunch or dinner meal as part of a comprehensive weight loss program which also includes sensible food choices, plenty of water and regular physical activity.

Ingredients: One 170-calorie serving provides PM Ultra Protein complex (modified casein, soy protein powder, whey protein concentrate, di-/tri-peptides), fructose, maltodextrin, cocoa powder, purified cellulose, canola oil, hydrolyzed guar gum, L-lysine monohydrochloride, potassium chloride, L-glutamine, calcium carbonate, magnesium oxide, soy lecithin, dicalcium phosphate, natural and artificial flavors, carrot powder, oat

grass powder, lactobacillus acidophilus, acesultame, medium chain triglycerides, papain, bromelain, rice syrup solids, choline citrate, ascorbic acid, vitamin E acetate, inositol, ferrous fumarate, niacinamide, zinc oxide, calcium pantothenate, vitamin A palmitate, copper sulfate, manganese sulfate, vitamin D, pyridoxine hydrochloride, riboflavin, thiamine mononitrate, chromium polynicotinate, folid acid, biotin, sodium selenite, sodium molybdate, potassium iodide, vitamin K and cyanocobalamin.

How Supplied: One can contains fourteen 45-gram servings. Also available in vanilla flavor.

PERFORMANCE GOLD

Uses: Performance Gold is an energy-enhancing formulation supplying key nutritional support for building muscle and for aerobic performance. The herbal extracts which comprise Performance Gold are called adaptogens. They help the body adapt to physical and mental stress. The enzyme-hydrolyzed whey protein is a source of easily absorbable peptides (protein fragments) which accelerate the positive benefits of the herbal extracts. One of the key herbal extracts is Golden Root. Research has shown that Golden Root helps bring oxygen to tissues, which is vital for optimal performance. During exercise, the muscles and the brain suffer from lowered oxygen status, which brings on fatigue. Golden Root helps oxygenate the body, allowing lengthier, more rigorous exercise as well as quicker recovery.

The benefits of Golden Root are enhanced dramatically when combined with Siberian Ginseng. Moomiyo also boosts the adaptogenic abilities of Performance Gold, especially when complexed with peptides. Inosine supports nucleic acid function and protein synthesis.

Performance Gold was formulated in consultation with Dr. Nikolai Volkov who pioneered studies in Russia on adaptogens and peptides in high-performance athletes.

Directions: Take one or two caplets 60 minutes before exercise or between meals.

Warning: This product is not intended for persons under 18, or for pregnant or lactating women.

Ingredients: Two caplets contain 100 mg of moomiyo, 25 mg of Golden Root extract (Standardized), 50 mg Siberian ginseng extract (Standardized), 500 mg of inosine and 1000 mg of enzyme-hydrolyzed whey protein.

PERFORMANCE OPTIMIZER SYSTEM

Uses: *Performance Optimizer System is a family of four interlocking nutri-*

tional formulas designed to enhance physical performance, promote peak muscle physiology and speed post-exercise recovery.

Peak physical performance depends on a series of physiological processes including body and muscle fueling, hydration, support of anabolic and energy systems, and proper rest and recovery. AdvoCare's Performance Optimizer System addresses the metabolic needs of the active person.

Performance Optimizer System 1 supports anabolic physiology, enhancing the production of muscle. Muscle production is essential to anyone seeking to lose weight and perform at top physical levels.

Performance Optimizer System 2 supports the body's ability to make muscle protein and heal micro-tears that occur in muscle fiber during physical exercise. The unique blend of high quality dietary proteins combined with sports-enhancing glucose polymers and other unique carbohydrates provides energy and structural support for building strength. The inclusion of branched chain amino acids (BCAAs), creatine, medium chain triglycerides and digestive enzymes results in a superior formulation.

Performance Optimizer System 3 is an advanced sports drink which includes B-vitamins to support aerobic and anaerobic body energy pathways, as well as coenzyme Q-10 and PAK, two natural energy compounds for extensive energy support for muscles, brain and body. By combining both quick-acting and "time-released" carbohydrates, the energy effects are both immediate and sustained. This beverage also contains glutamine, a key amino acid which helps buffer lactic acid buildup in muscles during exercise-and also supports keener mental function. Glutamine has also been shown to increase plasma bicarbonate which helps eliminate acids from the muscles and bloodstream. Isotonicity of POS 3 assures rapid gastric emptying for quick and effective rehydration and replenishment of electrolytes.

Performance Optimizer System 4 (Arginine Power) Arginine Power is a dynamic way to help boost muscle strength. Along with the other POS formulas, POS 4 is designed to provide the exercising body with the nutritional support it needs for optimal performance, quick recovery and lasting benefits.

Arginine Power is designed to support muscle strength in two ways. First, POS 4 keeps the level of arginine boosted during exercise, enabling longer, more vigorous exercise. Second, POS 4 provides nutritional support for the body's production of growth hormone, a key to repairing and strengthening tired muscles.

Arginine Power is also designed to support the body's production of nitric oxide. Increased nitric oxide levels typically result in improved blood flow to the sexual and reproductive system, as well as to the cardiovascular and immune system. So POS 4 can help produce more vigor as well as muscle strength.

Directions: Performance Optimizer System 1 is designed to be taken at bedtime, preferably on an empty stomach. Performance Optimizer System 2 should be used immediately after exercise to aid recovery and healing of muscles. Performance Optimizer System 3 should be consumed to provide rapid re-hydration as well as sustained energy during and after physical activity. Performance Optimizer System 4 should be taken at bedtime. Stir or blend one (1) rounded tablespoon of powder into 6 fluid ounces of chilled water or juice of your choice. Take on an empty stomach, at least thirty (30) minutes prior to consuming a meal. Take up to 3 servings a day for maximum effect.

Ingredients: Three caplets of Performance Optimizer System 1 contain 100 mg of moomiyo, 1200 mg of L-arginine, 600 mg of L-ornithine, 200 mg of oatgrass extract, 50 mg of nettles extract, 25 mg of Siberian ginseng extract, 50 mg of ashwaganda extract, 5 mg of zinc (OptiZinc™), 500 mcg of copper (amino acid chelate), 150 mg of magnesium (amino acid chelate), 200 mg vanadium (BMOV), 100 mg of saw palmetto extract, 20 mg of niacin, and 50 mg of wild yam extract.

One serving of Performance Optimizer System 2 contains glucose polymers, fructose, modified casein, soy protein powder, cocoa powder, soy lecithin, Myo-Force™ (creatine monohydrate, creatine phosphate, Siberian ginseng), carob powder, canola oil, dicalcium phosphate, corn syrup solids, branched chain amino acids (leucine, isoleucine, valine), natural and artificial flavors, medium chain triglycerides, magnesium oxide, calcium carbonate, DL-methionine, silicon dioxide, guar gum, xanthan gum, ascorbic acid, potassium chloride, rice syrup solids, fructooligosaccharides, citrus pectin, zinc gluconate, L-carnitine hydrochloride, calcium pantothenate, niacinamide, vitamin E succinate, beta carotene, manganese sulfate, ferrous fumarate, selenomethionine, calcium borate, copper gluconate, pyridoxine hydrochloride, riboflavin, thiamine hydrochloride, vanadyl sulfate, chromium polynicotinate (ChromeMate™), vitamin D, papain, bromelain, gamma oryzanol, folic acid, choline dihydrogen citrate, biotin, sodium molybdate, dibencozide, cyanocobalamin, potassium iodide. Also available in vanilla flavor.

One serving of Performance Optimizer System 3 contains fructose, glucose polymers, magnesium/sodium/potassium citrates, citric acid, dextrose, tricalcium phosphate, natural flavors, ascorbic acid, potassium chloride, pyridoxine alpha ketoglutarate, creatine monohydrate/creatine phosphate, beta carotene, salt, l-glutamine, niacinamide, calcium pantothenate, riboflavin, thiamine hydro-

chloride, chromium polynicotinate (ChromeMate®), l-glutathione, coenzyme Q-10.

One serving of Performance Optimizer System 4 contains fructose, citric acid, malic acid, fumaric acid, L-arginine, glycine, L-methionine, choline, calcium pantothenate, beta carotene, cyanocobalamin, folic acid, chromium polynicolinete, orange flavor, sucralose, silicon dioxide and sodium phosphate.

Ingredients: L-Arginine, Glycine, D, L-Methionine Choline (as bitartrate) Fructose, citric acid, malic acid, natural flavor, fumaric acid, acesulfame potassium, vitamins A, B-5, B-12, folic acid and chromium.

How Supplied: A bottle of Performance Optimizer System 1 contains 90 caplets.

One can of Performance Optimizer System 2 contains fifteen 60-gram servings. One can of Performance Optimizer System 3 contains thirty 15-gram servings. One bottle of Performance Optimizer System 4 contains thirty 20-gram servings.

PROBIOTIC RESTORE

Uses: Restore contains more than two billion freeze-dried, beneficial microflora, the consumption of which promotes optimal digestion, absorption of nutrients and elimination of wastes. Additionally, this product can ease constipation by supporting normal intestinal function.

Directions: Take one to three capsules per day with water, preferably on an empty stomach, 30 minutes or more before a meal. For children, capsules may be opened and contents mixed with water or fruit juice.

Ingredients: Lactobacillus acidophilus, Bifidobacterium bifidus, fructooligosaccharides, moomiyo, zinc monomethionine (OptiZinc™), vitamin A (beta-carotene and palmitate), aloe vera juice powder.

How Supplied: Each bottle contains 90 capsules

PROFORM

Uses: ProForm is a pleasant-tasting food bar which contains an ideal mixture of easily digested carbohydrates (21 g/bar) and proteins (8g/bar) to provide a timed-release fuel mix for physical performance. ProForm contains AdvoCare's exclusive NeuroActives™, a blend of natural amino acids and herbs, which provides nutritional support for mental clarity.

Directions: Consume a ProForm bar 60 minutes before physical activity to provide fuel for muscles and brain. As a

Continued on next page

ProForm—Cont.

complement to a weight management program, ProForm can function as a healthy snack.

Ingredients: One bar contains dark chocolate flavored coating [sugar, palm kernel oil, cocoa (processed with alkali), lactose, lecithin, natural flavor], fructose, maltodextrin, soy protein isolate, water, crisp rice (rice flour, malt extract, rice bran), whey protein concentrate, glycerine, guarana extract, L-glutamine, choline citrate, L-phenylalaline, L-lysine, partially defatted peanut flour, peanuts, kola nut extract, taurine, green tea extract, potassium chloride, ascorbic acid, caramel added for color, creatine monohydrate, calcium pantothenate, niacinamide, salt, D-alpha tocopheryl succinate, pyridoxine hydrochloride, L-carnitine, folic acid, riboflavin, thiamine hydrochloride, ginkgo biloba extract, beta-carotene, chromium polynicotinate (ChromeMate TM), biotin, cyanocobalamin.

How Supplied: One box contains eighteen 40-gram bars.
Available in two flavors: Chocolate Peanut and Fudge Brownie.

PROMOTION

Uses: ProMotion contains compounds that provides both lubrication and protection to the articular surfaces of the bone, promoting ease of motion. At the same time, ProMotion nourishes these tissues with the key biochemical building block for cartilage synthesis, essential for joint function.

ProMotion contains glucosamine HCl, a newly available and readily absorbed form of this vital biochemical. Glucosamine is one of the major building blocks of articular cartilage and of synovial fluid, the lubricating and cushioning material in joints. Glucosamine is found in high concentrations in hyaluronic acid and glycosaminoglycans, a group of compounds that are responsible for proper hydration and moisture retention throughout the body.

In several recent studies, glucosamine was shown to have a positive effect on both joint mobility and joint inflammatory conditions. In these studies, glucosamine relieved the most overt symptoms of osteoarthrosis, including tenderness, pain, and restricted movement, outperforming aspirin, ibuprofen, and naproxen in alleviating these symptoms. The glucosamine selected for ProMotion is a 100% pure, natural form for maximum bioactivity. Owing to its high solubility, it is readily absorbed from the gastrointestinal tract and actively taken up by an incorporated into articular cartilage.

ProMotion also contains grape proanthocyanidans, phytochemicals that posses powerful antioxidant activity as well as potent protection against breakdown of cartilage.

These polyphenols are a subclass of flavonoids which have been shown in scores of scientific studies to be anti-inflammatory, anti-allergic, and to increase capillary strength. Proanthocyanidins have a particular affinity for collagen, protecting it from free radical attack and the inflammation that often accompanies this errant process.
Recent research has also validated the ability of proanthocyanidins to inhibit hyaluronidase.
ProMotion contains a specially selected high potency wine grape extract that delivers a standardized concentration of proanthocyanidins. Manganese sulfate is included to assist in the endogenous production of glycosaminoglycans.

Directions: Take three (3) to six (6) capsules per day, preferably with meals. ProMotion can be taken all at once or divided throughout the day, as desired.

Ingredients: *Three capsules contain 1500 mg of glucosamine HCl, 25 mg, 25 mg proanthocyanidins (wine grape seed), and 25 mg manganese sulfate.*

How supplied: *One bottle contains 90 capsules.*

SECOND LOOK

Uses: Second Look provides nutritional support for the basic structural matrix of the skin, and increases moisture retention. Second Look helps strengthen collagen and elastin production, increasing the appearance of smoothness of skin.

Directions: Take one capsule twice each day—one in the morning and one in the evening. Maximum benefits will be achieved in approximately 90 days.

Ingredients: Manganese (as amino acid chelate), Silicon (as silicic acid), Shave Grass extract (herb-Equisetum arvense), MariPlex-PGTM (chondroitin sulfate, shark cartilage concentrate, l-pyroglutamic acid, n-acetyl glucosamine, ribonucleic acid) Silicon dioxide, magnesium stearate, gelatin, horsetail extract (standardized), and zinc (OptiZinc™).

How Supplied: One bottle contains 60 capsules.

SPARK!
Nutritional Beverage Mix

Uses: Spark is a stimulating powdered beverage mix containing neuroactives, which are natural promoters of brain biochemistry. An array of vitamins, minerals and other factors are presented for efficient production of neuro-energy. The neuroactives in Spark also work to help reduce appetite.
Unlike many other energy drinks, Spark does not over stimulate and overburden body energy systems, but rather supports their activities with specific nutrients and neuro-precursor compounds.

Spark provides endocrine support for energy without the let-down feeling often associated with non-nutritional artificial stimulants.

Directions: Blend one level scoop (15 grams) into 8 ounces of chilled or warm water or beverage of choice, 2 or 3 times a day or as desired.

Warning: Phenylketonurices: Contains phenylalanine. Children and pregnant or lactating women should consult a physician prior to use. Not for use by persons who are abnormally sensitive to caffeine or choline.

Ingredients: One serving contains 10 mg of L-carnitine, 200 mg of taurine, 50 mg of GABA, 100 mg of L-glycine, 500 mg of L-phenylalanine, 2 mg of RNA, 100 mcg of ubiquinone, 500 mg of choline, 120 mg of caffeine, as well as fructose, maltodextrin, citric acid, ascorbic acid, natural flavor, calcium pantothenate, vitamin A (beta carotene, palmitate), niacinamide, vitamin E succinate, Sucralose®, niacin, pyridoxine hydrochloride, zinc monomethionine (OptiZinc™), riboflavin, thiamine hydrochloride, copper amino acid chelate, ribonucleic acid, chromimum polynicotinate (ChromeMate™) and cyanocobalamin.

How Supplied: One can contains thirty 15-gram powdered servings.
Also available in individual packets, 30 servings per carton.

SYSTEM 3-4-3: Metabolic Cleansing System

Uses: System 3-4-3 is a ten-day routine formulated to cleanse and rejuvenate the internal system. System 3-4-3 helps rid the body of toxins, enhancing energy levels, improving skin tone and assisting in weight management.
The proprietary formulation of herbal concentrates, vitamins and minerals in the Herbal Cleanse Tablets help mobilize toxins from body tissues. Cleansing also involves the removal of these wastes and toxins in a gentle and safe manner. The unique components in the Restore Tablets help to replenish and restore tissue integrity and metabolic stability. The nutrients, herbal extracts and concentrated lactic microflora help to restore intestinal and epithelial cell health throughout the body.

Directions: Take the Herbal Cleanse Tablets for the first seven days, take Fiber-10 for the first three days and, subsequently, on days eight through ten, and take ProBiotic Restore on days four through ten.

Warning: System 3-4-3 is not intended for use by pregnant or breast-feeding women, or for children. If you are ill, consult a health care professional before starting System 3-4-3. This product contains senna. Read and follow directions carefully. Do not use if you have or de-

velop diarrhea, loose stools or abdominal pain. Consult your physician if you have frequent diarrhea. If you are taking medication, or have a medical condition, consult your physician before using this product.

The booklet enclosed with each System 3-4-3 box gives a day-by-day guide on how to use each component.

Because of the mobilization of toxins and their subsequent elimination, large amounts of clean, pure fluids (filtered water, herbal teas and diluted, fresh juices) and diluted vegetable broths are absolutely essential. Follow a diet plan which emphasizes light, healthy foods, and scrupulously avoid all fried foods, junk foods and fast foods.

Start System 3-4-3 at the beginning of a weekend. Or simply plan to take a restful three day home holiday while undergoing detoxification.

Ingredients: *FIBER 10—Fiber blend (psyllium husk, guar gum, carboxymethyl cellulose, citrus pectin, butternut bark powder), fructose, beta-carotene, citric acid, natural and artificial flavors, Sucralose®, Fructooligosaccharides, papaya powder, prune powder, ascorbic acid, digestive enzyme complex (protease, lipase, cellulase), rhubarb root extract, black walnut hull extract, licorice root extract, Lactobacillus acidophilus, Bifidobacterium bifidus.*

HERBAL CLEANSE—Three tablets contain: 3-4-3- Herbal Cleanse Complex (Green Kamut juice powder, Burdock Root extract, Cranberry juice powder, Senna extract, Astragalus extract, Echinacea extract, Odorless Garlic, Milk Thistle extract, Beet Root powder, Shisandra extract), Ascorbic Acid, Taurine, Niacin/Niacinamide, Pantothenic Acid, Zinc monomethionine, Pyridoxine, Riboflavin, Thiamine, Inositol, Folic Acid, Biotin, Vitamin B-12 (cyanocobalamin).

RESTORE—Two capsules contain: Lactobacillus acidophilus, Bifodobacterium bifidus, Fructooligosaccharides, Aloe vera powder, Moomiyo, Zinc Monomethionine, Beta-Carotene, Vitamin A (palmitate).

Use System 3-4-3:
- at the start of a healthy weight loss program
- if you are among the 80 million people who suffer from constipation
- after you have finished using antibiotics
- as part of a sports training and rehabilitation program
- if you have recurring colds or flus
- if you have fatigue, irritability, or experience mood swings
- if you have problems losing body fat
- as part of a comprehensive health promotion program

THERMO-E

Uses: Thermo-E is a unique blend of herbal extracts designed to stimulate thermogenesis (the production of heat and energy) and promote loss of excess weight. Also reduces appetite and heightens one's sense of energy.

Directions: Take one caplet of Thermo-E twice daily, 30 to 45 minutes prior to meals.

Warning: *This product contains ephedra. Do not use this product if you are under 18 years of age, if you are pregnant or lactating, or if you have high blood pressure, cardiovascular disease (especially cardiac arrhythmias), diabetes, prostatic hypertrophy, glaucoma, asthma, psychosis or thyroid disease. Do not use this product if you are taking any form of phenylpropanolamine, which may include weight loss products and decongestants or cold/allergy medications. Do not use this product within 14 days after taking MAO inhibitor medications such as certain anti-depressants. Consult your physician prior to use if you are taking prescription anorectic, anti-depressant, or cardiovascular medications. If symptoms of allergy develop, discontinue use.*

Ingredients: Each caplet contains ephedra extract (standardized), guarana extract, potassium (phosphate), magnesium (phosphate), niacin, green tea extract (standardized), beta-carotene and beet powder.

How Supplied: One bottle contains 180 caplets.

THERMO-G

Uses: Thermo-G is a unique blend of herbal extracts designed to stimulate thermogenesis (the production of heat and energy) and promote loss of excess weight. Also reduces appetite and heightens one's sense of energy.

Directions: Take one caplet of Thermo-G twice daily, 30 to 45 minutes prior to meals.

Ingredients: Each caplet contains Green Orange extract (standardized), Guarana extract (standardized), potassium (phosphate), magnesium (phosphate), niacin, green tea extract (standardized), beta-carotene and beet powder.

How Supplied: One bottle contains 180 caplets.

ZZZ

How does it work?

Zzz contains micro-multiphasic liposomes—microscopic droplets of nutrients and standardized herbal extracts—suspended in purified water. Liposomes are rapidly absorbed by the small blood vessels in the mouth, speeding the active ingredients into your body for quick results.

Zzz contains standardized kava kava extract, an herb which has been used for centuries for its calming, relaxing effect. Zzz also contains 5-hydroxytryptophan, a neuroactive nutrient building block which is converted into serotonin, a key brain compound associated with rest, relaxation and sleep. Synergistic nutrients are included in the Zzz liposomes, and a small amount of melatonin rounds out the Zzz formula. Melatonin is secreted by the brain in response to low light, and is helpful for inducing sleep. Melatonin is also very useful for helping to reset the body's internal timeclock when traveling through different time zones.

How to use Zzz?

At bedtime, spray one or two full pumps of Zzz liposome liquid under your tongue. Allow the liquid to remain under your tongue for 30 seconds, then swallow.

Benefits of Zzz are likely to be noticed in 10 to 15 minutes.

Ingredients: *Purified water, micro-multiphasic liposomes (vitamin B6, L-5 hydroxytryptophan, kava kava extract*, lecithin, melatonin, tocopheryl acetate, zinc gluconate), fructose, stevia extract*, natural mixed fruit flavor, potassium sorbate, polysorbate-20.*

*Standardized

AkPharma Inc.

P.O. BOX 111
PLEASANTVILLE, NJ
08232-0111

Direct Inquiries To:
Elizabeth Klein: (609) 645-5100
FAX: (609) 645-0767

Medical Emergency Contact:
Alan E. Kligerman: (609) 645-5100

PRELIEF®

PRODUCT OVERVIEW

Key Facts: Prelief is AkPharma's brand name for calcium glycerophosphate. It is used to remove acid from acidic foods and beverages when acidic foods are to be avoided for more tolerable ingestion. Prelief tablets are swallowed with the food or beverage. Prelief granulate is added to each serving of acidic food or beverage.

Major Uses: Takes acid out of acidic foods such as tomato sauce, citrus, fruit drinks, coffee, wine, beer and colas. Acid foods are now established as problematic for persons with Interstitial Cystitis, urinary urgency and are suspect in some intestinal irritation. Those with Interstitial Cystitis or incontinence, whose

Continued on next page

Prelief—Cont.

symptoms may be exacerbated by acidic foods, may particularly benefit.

Safety Information: Prelief is made from an FDA Generally Recognized as Safe (GRAS)[1] dietary supplement ingredient and is also listed as a food ingredient in the US Government Food Chemicals Codex (FCC)[2]

PRODUCT INFORMATION

Prelief®

Description: Prelief Tablets: Each tablet contains 333 mg of calcium glycerophosphate. The tablets also contain 0.5% magnesium stearate as a processing aid. Two or three tablets should be swallowed with the food or beverage. (See chart)

Prelief Granulate: Each packet contains 333 mg of calcium glycerophosphate. Add 2 packets of granulate to each serving of acidic food or beverage. Except for alcoholic beverages, the granulate dissolves rapidly in the acidic food or beverage. An additional 1–2 tablets or packets may be needed on foods that may be particularly high in acid. (See chart)

Each tablet or packet of granulate supplies 6% (65 mg) of the US Recommended Daily Allowance (USRDA) for calcium and 5% (50 mg) of the USRDA for phosphorus. Note: It is not clear if all or any of the phosphorus is biologically available or if it stays bound in its phosphate-glycerol bond. No sodium; no aluminum; no sugar.

[1]reference 21 CFR §184.1201
[2]reference Food Chemicals Codex, 3rd Edition, pp 51–52

Reasons for Use: Prelief is a dietary supplement for use with acidic foods and beverages. It is a dietary intervention used to take acid out of these ingestibles

for persons who identify acid discomfort with the ingestion of acidic foods and beverages.

Action: Prelief neutralizes the acid found in a large number of foods which many people find cause them discomfort. **See Table.**

Usage: 2 tablets or 2 granulate packets per serving of acidic food or beverage.

How Supplied: Prelief is supplied in both tablet form (30, 60 and 120 tablet bottle sizes and 24 tablets in 12–2 tablet packets), and granulate form (36 packets and 50 serving granulate shaker).

Kosher: Prelief is Kosher and Pareve.

Use Limitations: None, except as may apply below.

Adverse Reactions: None known

Toxicity: None known

Lead Content: Conforms with California Prop. 65 on lead content, to 15 tablets per day and 30 packets of granulate per day.

Interactions with Drugs: Calcium may interfere with efficacy of some medications. If a medication is being taken, check with physician, pharmacist or other health professional about the possible interactions of calcium with that medication. No other drug interactions known.

Precautions: People who have been advised by their physician not to take calcium, phosphorus or glycerin/glycerol should consult with their physician before using Prelief.

Prelief is classified as a dietary supplement, not a drug.

For more information and samples, please write or call toll-free 1-800-994-4711.

[See table below]

Shown in Product Identification Guide, page 503

Typical Food Acid Removal by Prelief

Product	1 Packet or 1 Tablet	2 Packets or 2 Tablets	3 Packets or 3 Tablets
Pepsi Cola® – 8 oz.	98%	99.8%	–
Mott's® 100% Apple Juice – 4 oz.	49.8%	74.9%	90%
Tropicana® Orange Juice – 4 oz.	20.6%	36.9%	60%
Coors Light® Beer – 12 oz.	80.1%	95%	96.8%
Monty's Hill® Chardonnay – 4 oz.	37%	60.1%	80%
Ireland® Coffee – 6 oz.	93.7%	96.8%	98%
Tetley® Iced Tea – 8 oz.	99%	99.5%	–
Seven Seas® Red Wine & Vinegar Salad Dressing – 31 gm	90%	95%	98%
Old El Paso® Thick'n Chunky Salsa Medium – 2 Tbsp.	80.1%	95%	97.5%
Heinz® Tomato Ketchup – 1 Tbsp.	68.4%	87.4%	92.1%
Kraft® Original Barbeque Sauce 2 Tbsp.	60.2%	80%	90%
Ragu® Old World Style Traditional Sauce – 125 gm	20.6%	36.9%	60.2%
Dannon® Strawberry Lowfat Yogurt (fully mixed) – 116 gm	49.9%	68.4%	80.1%
Grapefruit Sections – 150 gm	36.9%	50%	68.3%
Sauerkraut – 2 Tbsp.	60.3%	80%	92.1%
Red Cabbage – 130 gm	49.7%	68.3%	74.8%

Bayer Corporation Consumer Care Division

36 Columbia Road
P.O. Box 1910
Morristown, NJ 07962-1910

Direct Inquiries to:
Consumer Relations
(800) 331-4536
www.bayercare.com

For Medical Emergency Contact:
Bayer Corporation
Consumer Care Division
(800) 331-4536

FERGON®
Ferrous Gluconate
Iron Supplement

Directions: Adults: One tablet daily, with food.

	Amount Per Serving	% Daily Value
Iron	27 mg	150%

Ingredients: 240 mg Ferrous Gluconate equal to approximately 27 mg elemental Iron. **Also contains:** Sucrose, Corn Starch, Talc, Maltodextrin, Magnesium Stearate, Silicon Dioxide, Hydroxypropyl Methylcellulose, Titanium Dioxide, Polyethylene Glycol, FD&C Yellow #5 Aluminum Lake (Tartrazine), FD&C Blue #1 Aluminum Lake, Polysorbate 80, Carnauba Wax.

Warning: Accidental overdose of iron-containing products is a leading cause of fatal poisoning in children under 6. Keep this product out of the reach of children. In case of accidental overdose, call a doctor or poison control center immediately.

If you are pregnant or nursing, consult a health professional before using this product. AVOID EXCESSIVE HEAT.

How Supplied: Bottles of 100 Tablets.
Shown in Product Identification Guide, page 504

FLINTSTONES® Original Children's Chewable Multivitamin Supplement
BUGS BUNNY™ Plus Iron Chewable Children's Multivitamin Plus Iron Supplement
FLINTSTONES® Plus Iron Chewable Children's Multivitamin Plus Iron Supplement

Directions: Adults and children two years of age and older—**Chew** one tablet daily.

Amount Per Tablet

	% Daily Value for Children 2–3 Years of Age	% Daily Value for Adults and Children 4 Years of Age and older
Vitamin A 2500 IU	100%	50%
Vitamin C 60 mg	150%	100%
Vitamin D 400 IU	100%	100%
Vitamin E 15 IU	150%	50%
Thiamin (B$_1$) 1.05 mg	150%	70%
Riboflavin (B$_2$) 1.2 mg	150%	70%
Niacin 13.5 mg	150%	67%
Vitamin B$_6$ 1.05 mg	150%	52%
Folic Acid 300 mcg	150%	75%
Vitamin B$_{12}$ 4.5 mcg	150%	75%
*Iron (elemental) 15 mg	150%	83%

*FLINTSTONES® Original Children's Chewable Vitamins provide the same quantities of vitamins, but do not provide iron.

Ingredients:

Flintstones Original: Sucrose (a natural sweetener), Sodium Ascorbate, Stearic Acid, Invert Sugar, Artificial Flavors (including fruit acids), Gelatin, Vitamin E Acetate, Niacinamide, FD&C Red #40 Lake, FD&C Yellow #6 Lake, FD&C Blue #2 Lake, Pyridoxine Hydrochloride, Riboflavin, Thiamine Mononitrate, Vitamin A Acetate, Folic Acid, Beta Carotene, Vitamin D, Vitamin B$_{12}$.

Bugs Bunny Plus Iron: Sorbitol, Sodium Ascorbate, Ferrous Fumarate, Starch, Stearic Acid, Natural and Artificial Flavors (including fruit acids), Gelatin, Vitamin E Acetate, Niacinamide, FD&C Red #40 Lake, FD&C Yellow #6 Lake, FD&C Blue #2 Lake, Aspartame* (a sweetener), Pyridoxine Hydrochloride, Riboflavin, Thiamine Mononitrate, Vitamin A Acetate, Folic Acid, Beta Carotene, Vitamin D, Vitamin B$_{12}$.

Flintstones Plus Iron: Sucrose (a natural sweetener), Sodium Ascorbate, Ferrous Fumarate, Stearic Acid, Artificial Flavors (including fruit acids), Gelatin, Invert Sugar, Vitamin E Acetate, Niacinamide, FD&C Red #40 Lake, FD&C Yellow #6 Lake, FD&C Blue #2 Lake, Pyridoxine Hydrochloride, Riboflavin, Thiamine Mononitrate, Vitamin A Acetate, Folic Acid, Beta Carotene, Vitamin D, Vitamin B$_{12}$.

Warnings: For Bugs Bunny Only: PHENYLKETONURICS: CONTAINS PHENYLALANINE.

FOR IRON CONTAINING SUPPLEMENTS ONLY:

> WARNING: Accidental overdose of iron-containing products is a leading cause of fatal poisoning in children under 6. Keep this product out of the reach of children. In case of accidental overdose, call a doctor or poison control center immediately.

KEEP OUT OF THE REACH OF CHILDREN.

How Supplied: Flintstones are supplied in bottles of 60 and 100, Bugs Bunny in bottles of 60.
THE FLINTSTONES and all related characters and elements are trademarks of Hanna-Barbera © 2000.
LOONEY TUNES, characters, names and all related indicia are trademarks of Warner Bros. © 2000.
Shown in Product Identification Guide, page 504

FLINTSTONES® COMPLETE
Children's Chewable Multivitamin/ Multimineral Supplement

BUGS BUNNY™ COMPLETE
Children's Chewable Multivitamin/ Multimineral Supplement (Sugar Free)

Directions: 2 & 3 years of age—**Chew** one-half tablet daily. Adults and children 4 years of age and older—**Chew** one tablet daily.

Supplement Facts
Serving Size: $^1/_2$ tablet (2 & 3 years of age); 1 tablet (4 years of age and older)

Amount Per Tablet	% Daily Value for Children 2 & 3 Years of Age ($^1/_2$ Tablet)	% Daily Value for Adults and Children 4 Years of Age and older (1 Tablet)
Vitamin A 5000 IU	100%	100%
Vitamin C 60 mg	75%	100%
Vitamin D 400 IU	50%	100%
Vitamin E 30 IU	150%	100%
Thiamin (B$_1$ 1.5 mg)	107%	100%
Riboflavin (B$_2$) 1.7 mg	106%	100%
Niacin 20 mg	111%	100%
Vitamin B$_6$ 2 mg	143%	100%
Folic Acid 400 mcg	100%	100%
Vitamin B$_{12}$ 6 mcg	100%	100%
Biotin 40 mcg	13%	13%
Pantothenic Acid 10 mg	100%	100%
Calcium 100 mg	6%	10%
Iron (elemental) 18 mg	90%	100%
Phosphorus 100 mg	6%	10%
Iodine 150 mcg	107%	100%
Magnesium 20 mg	5%	5%
Zinc 15 mg	94%	100%
Copper 2 mg	100%	100%

Ingredients:
Bugs Bunny Complete: Dicalcium Phosphate, Sorbitol, Magnesium Phosphate, Sodium Ascorbate, Gelatin, Ferrous Fumarate, Natural and Artificial Flavors (including fruit acids), Starch, Stearic Acid, FD&C Red #40 Lake, Vitamin E Acetate, Carrageenan, Niacinamide, Magnesium Stearate, Hydrogenated Vegetable Oil, Zinc Oxide, FD&C Yellow #6 Lake, FD&C Blue #2 Lake, Calcium Pantothenate, Aspartame* (a sweetener), Cupric Oxide, Pyridoxine Hydrochloride, Vitamin A Acetate, Riboflavin, Thiamine Monoitrate, Beta Carotene, Folic Acid, Potassium Iodide, Vitamin D, Biotin, Magnesium Oxide, Vitamin B$_{12}$. * PHENYLKETONURICS: CONTAINS PHENYLALANINE

Flintstones Complete: Dicalcium Phosphate, Sorbitol, Magnesium Phosphate, Sodium Ascorbate, Gelatin, Ferrous Fumarate, Natural and Artificial Flavors (including fruit acids), Starch, Stearic Acid, Vitamin E Acetate, Carrageenan, Magnesium Stearate, Niacinamide, Zinc Oxide, Hydrogenated Vegetable Oil, Calcium Pantothenate, FD&C Red #40 Lake, FD&C Yellow #6 Lake, Xylitol, Aspartame* (a sweetener), FD&C Blue #2 Lake, Cupric Oxide, Pyridoxine Hydrochloride, Vitamin A Acetate, Riboflavin, Thiamine Mononitrate, Monoammonium Glycyrrhizinate, Beta Carotene, Folic Acid, Potassium Iodide, Vitamin D, Biotin, Magnesium Oxide, Vitamin B$_{12}$.
***PHENYLKETONURICS: CONTAINS PHENYLALANINE.**

> Warning: Accidental overdose of iron-containing products is a leading cause of fatal poisoning in children under 6. Keep this product out of the

Continued on next page

Flintstones/B. Bunny —Cont.

reach of children. In case of accidental overdose, call a doctor or poison control center immediately.

KEEP OUT OF THE REACH OF CHILDREN.

How Supplied: Bottles of 60s.
THE FLINTSTONES and all related characters and elements are trademarks of Hanna-Barbera © 2000.
LOONEY TUNES, characters, names and all related indicia are trademarks of Warner Bros. © 2000.

Shown in Product Identification Guide, page 504

FLINTSTONES® PLUS CALCIUM
Children's Chewable Multivitamin Plus Calcium Supplement

Directions: Adults and children 2 years of age and older—**Chew** one tablet daily.

Amount Per Tablet

	% Daily Value for Children 2–3 Years of Age	% Daily Value for Adults and Children 4 Years of Age and older
Vitamin A 2500 IU	100%	50%
Vitamin C 60 mg	150%	100%
Vitamin D 400 IU	100%	100%
Vitamin E 15 IU	150%	50%
Thiamin (B$_1$) 1.05 mg	150%	70%
Riboflavin (B$_2$) 1.2 mg	150%	70%
Niacin 13.5 mg	150%	67%
Vitamin B$_6$ 1.05 mg	150%	52%
Folic Acid 300 mcg	150%	75%
Vitamin B$_{12}$ 4.5 mcg	150%	75%
Calcium 200 mg	25%	20%

Ingredients: Calcium Carbonate, Sorbitol, Starch, Sodium Ascorbate, Natural and Artificial Flavors (including fruit acids), Stearic Acid, Gelatin, Magnesium Stearate, Vitamin E Acetate, Niacinamide, FD&C Red #40 Lake, FD&C Yellow #6 Lake, Aspartame* (a sweetener), FD&C Blue #2 Lake, Pyridoxine Hydrochloride, Riboflavin, Thiamine Mononitrate, Vitamin A Acetate, Monoammonium Glycyrrhizinate, Folic Acid, Beta Carotene, Vitamin D, Vitamin B$_{12}$.

Warning: *PHENYLKETONURICS: CONTAINS PHENYLALANINE
KEEP OUT OF THE REACH OF CHILDREN.

How Supplied: Bottles of 60 Tablets.
THE FLINTSTONES and all related characters and elements are trademarks of Hanna-Barbera © 2000.

Shown in Product Identification Guide, page 504

FLINTSTONES® Plus Extra C
Children's Chewable Multivitamin Supplement

BUGS BUNNY™ Plus Extra C
Children's Chewable Multivitamin Supplement
(Sugar Free)

Directions: Adults and children 2 years of age and older—**Chew** one tablet daily.

Amount Per Tablet

	% Daily Value for Children 2–3 Years of Age	% Daily Value for Adults and Children 4 Years of Age and older
Vitamin A 2500 IU	100%	50%
Vitamin C 250 mg	625%	417%
Vitamin D 400 IU	100%	100%
Vitamin E 15 IU	150%	50%
Thiamin (B$_1$) 1.05 mg	150%	70%
Riboflavin (B$_2$) 1.2 mg	150%	70%
Niacin 13.5 mg	150%	67%
Vitamin B$_6$ 1.05 mg	150%	52%
Folic Acid 300 mcg	150%	75%
Vitamin B$_{12}$ 4.5 mcg	150%	75%

Ingredients:
Flintstones: Sucrose (a natural sweetener), Sodium Ascorbate, Fructose, Ascorbic Acid, Microcrystalline Cellulose, Stearic Acid, Gelatin, Artificial Flavors (including fruit acids), Vitamin E Acetate, Invert Sugar, Niacinamide, FD&C Red #40 Lake, FD&C Yellow #6 Lake, FD&C Blue #2 Lake, Pyridoxine Hydrochloride, Riboflavin, Thiamine Mononitrate, Vitamin A Acetate, Folic Acid, Beta Carotene, Vitamin D, Vitamin B$_{12}$.
Bugs Bunny: Sorbitol, Sodium Ascorbate, Ascorbic Acid, Starch, Stearic Acid, Gelatin, Natural and Artificial Flavors (including fruit acids), Vitamin E Ace-

tate, FD&C Red #40 Lake, Niacinamide, FD&C Yellow #6 Lake, FD&C Blue #2 Lake, Aspartame* (a sweetener), Pyridoxine Hydrochloride, Riboflavin, Thiamine Mononitrate, Vitamin A Acetate, Folic Acid, Beta Carotene, Vitamin D, Vitamin B$_{12}$.

***Warning—For Bugs Bunny Only:**
PHENYLKETONURICS: CONTAINS PHENYLALANINE.
KEEP OUT OF THE REACH OF CHILDREN.

How Supplied: Flintstones in bottles of 60's & 100's, Bugs Bunny in bottles of 60.
THE FLINTSTONES and all related characters and elements are trademarks of Hanna-Barbera © 2000.
LOONEY TUNES, characters, names and all related indicia are trademarks of Warner Bros. © 2000.

Shown in Product Identification Guide, page 504

ONE-A-DAY® 50 PLUS
Multivitamin/Multimineral Supplement For Adults

Directions: Adults: One tablet daily with food.

VITAMINS	AMOUNT PER SERVING	% DAILY VALUE
Vitamin A	5000 IU	100%
Vitamin C	120 mg	200%
Vitamin D	400 IU	100%
Vitamin E	60 IU	200%
Vitamin K	20 mcg	25%
Thiamin (B$_1$)	4.5 mg	300%
Riboflavin (B$_2$)	3.4 mg	200%
Niacin	20 mg	100%
Vitamin B$_6$	6 mg	300%
Folic Acid	400 mcg	100%
Vitamin B$_{12}$	30 mcg	500%
Biotin	30 mcg	10%
Pantothenic Acid	15 mg	150%

MINERALS	AMOUNT PER SERVING	% DAILY VALUE
Calcium (elemental)	120 mg	12%
Iodine	150 mcg	100%
Magnesium	100 mg	25%
Zinc	22.5 mg	150%
Selenium	105 mcg	150%
Copper	2 mg	100%
Manganese	4 mg	200%
Chromium	180 mcg	150%
Molybdenum	90 mcg	120%
Chloride	34 mg	1%
Potassium	37.5 mg	1%

Ingredients: Calcium Carbonate, Magnesium Hydroxide, Niacinamide Ascorbate, Potassium Chloride, Ascorbic Acid, Gelatin, Vitamin E Acetate, Zinc Sulfate, Starch, Modified Cellulose Gum, Cellulose, Calcium Silicate, Dicalcium Phosphate, Citric Acid, Calcium Pantothenate, Titanium Dioxide, Dextrin, Zinc Oxide, Pyridoxine Hydrochloride, Cupric

Sulfate, Thiamine Mononitrate, Manganese Sulfate, Riboflavin, Vitamin A Acetate, Beta Carotene, FD&C Yellow #6 Lake, Folic Acid, Biotin, Potassium Iodide, FD&C Yellow #5 (Tartrazine) Lake, Chromium Chloride, Vitamin D, Sodium Selenate, Sodium Molybdate, Phytonadione, Vitamin B_{12}, FD&C Blue #2 Lake.

KEEP OUT OF REACH OF CHILDREN

How Supplied: Bottles of 50's and 80's with child-resistant caps.

Shown in Product Identification Guide, page 504

ONE-A-DAY® ANTIOXIDANT
Antioxidant Supplement

Directions: Adults: One softgel daily with food. To preserve quality and freshness, keep bottle tightly closed and store at room temperature.

VITAMINS	AMOUNT PER SERVING	% DAILY VALUE
Vitamin A (100% as beta-carotene)	5000 IU	100%
Vitamin C	250 mg	417%
Vitamin E	200 IU	667%

MINERALS	AMOUNT PER SERVING	% DAILY VALUE
Zinc	7.5 mg	50%
Selenium	15 mcg	21%
Copper	1 mg	50%
Manganese	1.5 mg	75%

Ingredients: Ascorbic Acid, dl-Alpha Tocopheryl Acetate, Gelatin, Glycerin, Soybean Oil, Selenium Yeast, Lecithin, Zinc Oxide, Vegetable Oil, Yellow Wax (Beeswax, Yellow) Manganese Sulfate, Beta Carotene, Cupric Oxide, Titanium Dioxide, FD&C Blue #1, FD&C Yellow #5 (Tartrazine), Silicon Dioxide.

KEEP OUT OF REACH OF CHILDREN

How Supplied: Bottle of 50 softgels.

Shown in Product Identification Guide, page 504

ONE-A-DAY® BEDTIME & REST
Step

Directions: Adults (18 years and older): Take 2 tablets one hour before bedtime.

Supplement Facts
Serving Size: 2 tablets
Servings Per Container: 15

	Amount Per Serving	% Daily Value
Calcium	450 mg	45%
Magnesium	80 mg	20%

Lecithin	20 mg	*
Kava Kava Standardized Extract (*Piper methysticum*) (root)	100 mg	*
Valerian Standardized Extract (*Valeriana officinalis*) (root)	200 mg	*
Rosemary Standardized Extract (*Rosmannus officinalis*) (leaf)	10 mg	*

* Daily Value not established

Ingredients: Calcium Carbonate, Cellulose, Magnesium Citrate, Calcium Citrate, Valerian Extract, Kava Kava Extract, Croscarmellose Sodium, Stearic Acid, Acacia, Crospovidone, Silicon Dioxide, Dextrin, Titanium Dioxide, Deoiled Lecithin, Hydroxypropyl Methylcellulose, Magnesium Stearate, Rosemary Extract, Polyethylene Glycol, Lecithin, FD&C Red #40 Lake, FD&C Yellow #6 Lake, FD&C Blue #1 Lake.

Warnings: Do not take continuously for more than 3 months without first consulting a health care professional. Do not take this product if you: suffer from depression; have an allergy to Kava Kava, Valerian Root, or Rosemary; have Parkinson's disease or liver disease. This product may cause drowsiness. Use caution when driving a motor vehicle or operating machinery.
Drug Interaction Precaution: If you are taking any prescription medication, consult your health care professional prior to taking this product. Kava Kava and Valerian Root may potentiate the effects of alcohol, sedatives and tranquilizers. Keep out of the reach of children.
In case of accidental overdose contact a Poison Control Center or your health care professional immediately.
Before any surgery ask your doctor about continued use of this product.
Do not use if pregnant or breast-feeding.

How Supplied: 30 tablets.
Shown in Product Identification Guide, page 505

ONE-A-DAY® CALCIUM PLUS
Calcium Supplement with Vitamin D and Magnesium

Directions: One to two chewable tablets daily (with food).

Each Tablet Contains

VITAMINS:	AMOUNT PER SERVING	% DAILY VALUE
Vitamin D	100 IU	25%

MINERALS:	AMOUNT PER SERVING	% DAILY VALUE
Calcium (elemental)	500 mg	50%
Magnesium (elemental)	50 mg	12.5%

Ingredients: Calcium Carbonate, Sorbitol, Magnesium Carbonate, Maltodextrin, Xylitol, Starch, Stearic Acid, Aspartame* (a sweetener), Natural and Artificial Flavors, Magnesium Stearate, Polyethylene Glycol, Gelatin, Polydextrose, Poloxamer 407, Docusate Sodium, Vitamin D_3.
*PHENYLKETONURICS: CONTAINS PHENYLALANINE.
Two tablets provide 1,000 mg of elemental calcium, 100% of the Recommended Daily Value for adults and children 12 years of age or older.
Special Note for Pregnant and Lactating Women: Three tablets provide 1,500 mg of elemental calcium (125% of the Recommended Daily Value).

KEEP OUT OF THE REACH OF CHILDREN

How Supplied: Bottles of 60 Chewable Tablets.
Shown in Product Identification Guide, page 505

ONE-A-DAY® CHOLESTEROL HEALTH
Dietary Supplement

Directions: Take two tablets daily, with food.

Two tablets of One-A-Day Cholesterol Health provides:

	AMOUNT PER SERVING	% DAILY VALUE
Vitamin E	200 IU	667%
Lecithin	100 mg	*
Garlic (*Allium sativum*) (freeze-dried) (bulb)	30 mg	*
Soy Standardized Extract (*Glycine max* or spp.) (bean)	140 mg	*

*Daily Value not established.

Ingredients: Dicalcium Phosphate, Cellulose, dl-alpha Tocopheryl Acetate, Soy Extract, Gelatin, Lecithin, Croscarmellose Sodium, Hydroxypropyl Methylcellulose, Polyethylene Glycol, Silicon Dioxide, Garlic Powder, Calcium Silicate, Magnesium Stearate, Titanium Dioxide, Hydroxypropyl Cellulose, FD&C Yellow #6 Lake, FD&C Red #40 Lake, FD&C Blue #1 Lake, Polysorbate 80.

Continued on next page

One-A-Day Cholesterol—Cont.

Warning: Before any surgery, ask your doctor about continued use of this product. **If pregnant or breast-feeding, ask a health professional before use. KEEP OUT OF THE REACH OF CHILDREN**

How Supplied: Bottles of 30.

Shown in Product Identification Guide, page 505

ONE-A-DAY® ENERGY FORMULA
Dietary Supplement

Directions: Take one tablet daily, with food.

One tablet of One-A-Day Energy Formula provides:

	AMOUNT PER SERVING	% DAILY VALUE
Thiamin (B₁)	2.25 mg	150%
Niacin	20 mg	100%
Vitamin B₆	3 mg	150%
Folic Acid	200 mcg	50%
Pantothenic Acid	10 mg	100%
Chromium (as Picolinate)	100 mcg	83%
American Ginseng Standardized Extract (Panax quinquefolius) (root)	200 mg	*

*Daily Value not established.

Ingredients: Calcium Carbonate, American Ginseng Extract, Cellulose, Maltodextrin, Hydroxypropyl Methylcellulose, Nicotinic Acid, Croscarmellose Sodium, d-Calcium Pantothenate, Crospovidone, Stearic Acid, Silicon Dioxide, Titanium Dioxide, Pyridoxine Hydrochloride, Magnesium Stearate, Starch, Thiamine Mononitrate, Hydroxypropyl Cellulose, Acacia, Polyethylene Glycol, FD&C Yellow #6 Lake, Chromium Picolinate, FD&C Blue #1 Lake, Folic Acid, Polysorbate 80.

Warnings: Seek the advice of a health professional before using it if you are taking medication for high blood pressure or anticoagulation (blood-thinning) or if you have diabetes. DO NOT USE IF PREGNANT OR BREAST-FEEDING. If using for more than 6 months, consult your doctor. Before any surgery, ask your doctor about continued use of this product. **KEEP OUT OF REACH OF CHILDREN.**

How Supplied: Bottles of 30.

Shown in Product Identification Guide, page 505

ONE–A–DAY® Essential
Multivitamin Supplement

Directions: Adults: One tablet daily, with food.

VITAMINS	AMOUNT PER SERVING		% DAILY VALUE
Vitamin A	5000	IU	100%
Vitamin C	60	mg	100%
Vitamin D	400	IU	100%
Vitamin E	30	IU	100%
Thiamin (B₁)	1.5	mg	100%
Riboflavin (B₂)	1.7	mg	100%
Niacin	20	mg	100%
Vitamin B₆	2	mg	100%
Folic Acid	400	mcg	100%
Vitamin B₁₂	6	mcg	100%
Pantothenic Acid	10	mg	100%

Ingredients: Calcium Carbonate, Ascorbic Acid, Gelatin, DL-Alpha Tocopheryl Acetate, Cellulose, Niacinamide, Maltodextrin, D-Calcium Pantothenate, Starch, Hydroxypropyl Methylcellulose, Croscarmellose Sodium, Sodium Starch Glycolate, FD&C Red #40 Lake, Hydroxypropyl Cellulose, Pyridoxine Hydrochloride, Polyethylene Glycol, Vitamin A Acetate, Silicon Dioxide, Magnesium Stearate, Riboflavin, Thiamine Mononitrate, Polysorbate 80, Resin, Folic Acid, Titanium Dioxide, Povidone, Beta Carotene, Ergocalciferol, Cyanocobalamin.

KEEP OUT OF THE REACH OF CHILDREN.

How Supplied: Bottles of 75's and 130's.

Shown in Product Identification Guide, page 504

ONE-A-DAY® GARLIC SOFTGELS
Garlic Supplement

Directions: One softgel daily with a meal, alone or with a One-A-Day Multivitamin. Swallow whole with liquid to ensure maximum strength and fresh breath. To preserve quality and freshness, keep bottle tightly closed and store at room temperature.

	Amount Per Serving	% Daily Value
Garlic Oil Macerate	600 mg	*

* Daily Value not established

Other Ingredients: Gelatin, Glycerin, Sorbitol, Xylose.

KEEP OUT OF THE REACH OF CHILDREN

How Supplied: Bottles of 45 softgels

Shown in Product Identification Guide, page 505

ONE-A-DAY® Joint Health

Dietary Supplement

Directions: Adults (18 years and older): Take 1 tablet 3 times daily, with food.

Supplement Facts
Serving Size: 1 tablet

	Amount Per Serving	% Daily Value
Vitamin C	30 mg	50%
Vitamin E	30 IU	100%
Manganese	1.5 mg	75%
Lecithin	10 mg	*
Glucosamine Sulfate Powder (Includes 125 mg of Potassium Cl)	500 mg	*
Devil's Claw Standardized Extract (Harpagophytum procumbens)(root)	134 mg	*

* Daily Value not established

Ingredients: Calcium Carbonate, Glucosamine Sulfate, Devil's Claw Extract, Potassium Chloride, Cellulose, Croscarmellose Sodium, Ascorbic Acid, dl-alpha Tocopheryl Acetate, Gelatin, Stearic Acid, Methylcellulose, Maltodextrin, Crospovidone, Manganese Gluconate, Silicon Dioxide, Dextrin, Titanium Dioxide, Deoiled Lecithin, Hydroxypropyl Methylcellulose, Magnesium Stearate, Acacia, Polyethylene Glycol, Starch, Lecithin, Caramel Color, Dextrose.

Warnings: Do not take this product if you: are pregnant or nursing a baby, have allergies to glucosamine preparations or Devil's Claw, have diabetes, ulcers, stomach problems or heart problems. Stop using this product and consult your health care professional if you develop stomach problems while taking this product. **KEEP OUT OF THE REACH OF CHILDREN.** In case of accidental overdose contact a Poison Control Center or your health care professional immediately.

This product contains herbal ingredients, which have a distinct natural odor.

How Supplied: 30 tablets

Shown in Product Identification Guide, page 505

ONE-A-DAY® KIDS COMPLETE™
MULTIVITAMIN/MULTIMINERAL SUPPLEMENT

Directions for Use: For kids 4 years of age and older, **chew** one tablet daily.

Supplement Facts

Serving Size: One tablet.

	Amount Per Serving	% Daily Value
Vitamin A	5000 IU	100%
Vitamin C	60 mg	100%
Vitamin D	400 IU	100%
Vitamin E	30 IU	100%
Thiamin (B₁)	1.5 mg	100%
Riboflavin (B₂)	1.7 mg	100%
Niacin	20 mg	100%
Vitamin B₆	2 mg	100%
Folic Acid	400 mcg	100%
Vitamin B₁₂	6 mcg	100%
Biotin	40 mcg	13%
Pantothenic Acid	10 mg	100%
Calcium (elemental)	100 mg	10%
Iron	18 mg	100%
Phosphorus	100 mg	10%
Iodine	150 mcg	100%
Magnesium	20 mg	5%
Zinc	15 mg	100%
Copper	2 mg	100%

Ingredients: Dicalcium Phosphate, Sorbitol, Magnesium Phosphate, Sodium Ascorbate, Gelatin, Ferrous Fumarate, Natural & Artificial Flavors (including fruit acids), Starch, Stearic Acid, Vitamin E Acetate, Carrageenan, Magnesium Stearate, Niacinamide, Zinc Oxide, Hydrogenated Vegetable Oil, FD&C Red #40 Lake, FD&C Yellow #6 Lake, FD&C Blue #2 Lake, Calcium Pantothenate, Aspartame* (a sweetener), Cupric Oxide, Pyridoxine Hydrochloride, Vitamin A Acetate, Riboflavin, Thiamine Mononitrate, Monoammonium Glycyrrhizinate, Beta Carotene, Folic Acid, Potassium Iodide, Vitamin D, Biotin, Magnesium Oxide, Vitamin B₁₂.

*PHENYLKETONURICS: CONTAINS PHENYLALANINE

USP One-A-Day Kids Complete formula meets the USP standards for strength, quality, and purity for Oil- and Water-soluble Vitamins with Minerals Tablets.†

WARNING: Accidental overdose or iron-containing products is a leading cause of fatal poisoning in children under 6. Keep this product out of the reach of children. In case of accidental overdose, call a doctor or poison control center immediately.

†Complies with USP Method 2: Vitamins A, D, E, Ascorbic Acid, Biotin, B₁₂, Thiamin, Riboflavin, Niacin and B₆; Method 3: Pantothenic Acid

How Supplied: 50 Fruit Flavored Chewable Tablets
Shown in Product Identification Guide, page 505

ONE-A-DAY® MAXIMUM
Multivitamin/Multimineral Supplement

Directions: Adults: One tablet daily, with food.

VITAMINS	AMOUNT PER SERVING		% DAILY VALUE
Vitamin A	5000	IU	100%
Vitamin C	60	mg	100%
Vitamin D	400	IU	100%
Vitamin E	30	IU	100%
Vitamin K	25	mcg	31%
Thiamin (B₁)	1.5	mg	100%
Riboflavin (B₂)	1.7	mg	100%
Niacin	20	mg	100%
Vitamin B₆	2	mg	100%
Folic Acid	400	mcg	100%
Vitamin B₁₂	6	mcg	100%
Biotin	30	mcg	10%
Pantothenic Acid	10	mg	100%

MINERALS	AMOUNT PER SERVING		% DAILY VALUE
Calcium (elemental)	162	mg	16%
Iron	18	mg	100%
Phosphorus	109	mg	11%
Iodine	150	mcg	100%
Magnesium	100	mg	25%
Zinc	15	mg	100%
Selenium	20	mcg	29%
Copper	2	mg	100%
Manganese	3.5	mg	175%
Chromium	65	mcg	54%
Molybdenum	160	mcg	213%
Chloride	72	mg	2%
Potassium	80	mg	2%
Boron	150	mcg	*
Nickel	5	mcg	*
Silicon	2	mg	*
Tin	10	mcg	*
Vanadium	10	mcg	*

*Daily Value not established

Ingredients: Dicalcium Phosphate, Magnesium Hydroxide, Potassium Chloride, Cellulose, Ferrous Fumarate, Zinc Sulfate, Calcium Carbonate, Niacinamide Ascorbate, Gelatin, Vitamin E Acetate, Ascorbic Acid, Modified Cellulose Gum, Hydroxypropyl Methylcellulose, Citric Acid, Tablet Lubricant, Manganese Sulfate, Calcium Pantothenate, Niacinamide, Cupric Sulfate, FD&C Red #40 Lake, Pyridoxine Hydrochloride, Titanium Dioxide, Vitamin A Acetate, Riboflavin, Sodium Borate, Thiamine Mononitrate, Beta Carotene, Folic Acid, Sodium Molybdate, Chromium Chloride, FD&C Blue #2 Lake, Biotin, Potassium Iodide, Vitamin D, Sodium Metasilicate, Sodium Selenate, Phytonadione, Sodium Metavanadate, Nickelous Sulfate, Stannous Chloride, Vitamin B₁₂.

Warning: Accidental overdose of iron-containing products is a leading cause of fatal poisoning in children under 6. Keep this product out of the reach of children. In case of accidental overdose, call a doctor or poison control center immediately. **If pregnant or breast-feeding, ask a health professional before use.**

KEEP OUT OF THE REACH OF CHILDREN.

How Supplied: Bottles of 60 and 100.
Shown in Product Identification Guide, page 504

ONE-A-DAY® MEMORY & CONCENTRATION
Dietary Supplement

Directions: Adults (18 years and older): Take one to two tablets daily, with food.

One tablet of One-A-Day Memory & Concentration provides:

	AMOUNT PER SERVING	% DAILY VALUE
Vitamin B6	1 mg	50%
Vitamin B12	3 mcg	50%
Choline	60 mg	*
Ginkgo Standardized Extract (*Ginkgo biloba*) (Leaf)	60 mg	*

*Daily Value not established.

Ingredients: Calcium Carbonate, Choline Bitartrate, Cellulose, Ginkgo Biloba Leaf Extract, Maltodextrin, Hydroxypropyl Methylcellulose, Polyethylene Glycol, Silicon Dioxide, Croscarmellose Sodium, Magnesium Stearate, Acacia, Crospovidone, Titanium Dioxide, FD&C Yellow #5 Lake (Tartrazine), Starch, Pyridoxine Hydrochloride, Hydroxypropyl Cellulose, Resin, FD&C Yellow #6 Lake, Polysorbate 80, Cyanocobalamin.

Warnings: Do not take this product, without first consulting a health professional, if you are taking medication for anticoagulation (thinning the blood). If

Continued on next page

One-A-Day Memory—Cont.

you are pregnant or nursing a baby, seek the advice of a health professional before using this product. **KEEP OUT OF THE REACH OF CHILDREN.**

How Supplied: Bottles of 30.
Shown in Product Identification Guide, page 505

ONE-A-DAY® MENOPAUSE HEALTH
Dietary Supplement

Directions: Adults: Take one to two tablets daily, with food.

One tablet of One-A-Day Menopause provides:

	AMOUNT PER SERVING	% DAILY VALUE
Vitamin E	15 IU	50%
Calcium (precipitated)	250 mg	25%
Lecithin	15 mg	*
Black Cohosh Standardized Extract (*Cimicifuga racemosa*) (root)	10 mg	*
Soy Standardized Extract (*Glycine max* or spp.) (bean)	42 mg	*

*Daily Value not established.

Ingredients: Calcium Carbonate, Starch, Cellulose, Soy Extract, Maltodextrin, Hydroxypropyl Methylcellulose, Talc, dl-alpha Tocopheryl Acetate, Gelatin, Polyethylene Glycol, Lecithin, Croscarmellose Sodium, Black Cohosh Extract, Titanium Dioxide, Acacia, Magnesium Stearate, Silicon Dioxide, Pharmaceutical Glaze, Hydroxypropyl Cellulose, Polysorbate 80, FD&C Yellow #6 Lake, FD&C Yellow #5 Lake (Tartrazine).

Warnings: If you are taking blood pressure medication, consult your doctor before using this product. **If pregnant or breast-feeding, ask a health professional before use.**
If using for more than six months, consult your doctor. **KEEP OUT OF THE REACH OF CHILDREN.**

How Supplied: Bottles of 30.
Shown in Product Identification Guide, page 505

ONE-A-DAY® MEN'S MULTIVITAMIN/MULTIMINERAL SUPPLEMENT

Directions: Adults: One tablet daily with food.

VITAMINS	AMOUNT PER SERVING	% DAILY VALUE
Vitamin A	5000 IU	100%
Vitamin C	90 mg	150%
Vitamin D	400 IU	100%
Vitamin E	45 IU	150%
Thiamin (B$_1$)	2.25 mg	150%
Riboflavin (B$_2$)	2.55 mg	150%
Niacin	20 mg	100%
Vitamin B$_6$	3 mg	150%
Folic Acid	400 mcg	100%
Vitamin B$_{12}$	9 mcg	150%
Pantothenic Acid	10 mg	100%

MINERALS	AMOUNT PER SERVING	% DAILY VALUE
Iodine	150 mcg	100%
Magnesium	100 mg	25%
Zinc	15 mg	100%
Selenium	87.5 mcg	125%
Copper	2 mg	100%
Manganese	3.33 mg	167%
Chromium	150 mcg	125%
Molybdenum	75 mcg	100%
Chloride	34 mg	1%
Potassium	37.5 mg	1%

Ingredients: Magnesium Hydroxide, Niacinamide Ascorbate, Potassium Chloride, Zinc Sulfate, Gelatin, Vitamin E Acetate, Ascorbic Acid, Modified Cellulose Gum, Cellulose, Dicalcium Phosphate, Calcium Silicate, Calcium Pantothenate, Citric Acid, Povidone, Dextrin, Cupric Sulfate, Titanium Dioxide, Pyridoxine Hydrochloride, Manganese Sulfate, Riboflavin, Thiamine Mononitrate, Vitamin A Acetate, FD&C Yellow #6, Lake, Beta Carotene, Folic Acid, FD&C Yellow #5 Lake (Tartrazine), Potassium Iodide, Chromium Chloride, Vitamin D, Sodium Selenate, Sodium Molybdate, Vitamin B$_{12}$.

KEEP OUT OF REACH OF CHILDREN

How Supplied: Bottles of 60's & 100's.
Shown in Product Identification Guide, page 504

ONE-A-DAY® PROSTATE HEALTH
Dietary Supplement

Directions: Take two softgels daily, with food.

Two softgels of One-A-Day Prostate Health provides:

	AMOUNT PER SERVING	% DAILY VALUE
Zinc	15 mg	100%
Pumpkin Seed Oil Standardized Extract	80 mg	*
Saw Palmetto Standardized Extract (*Serenoa repens*) (berry)	320 mg	*

*Daily Value not established.

Ingredients: Saw Palmetto Berry Extract, Gelatin, Glycerin, Zinc Gluconate, Pumpkin Seed Oil Extract, Vegetable Oil, Beeswax, Lecithin, Titanium Dioxide, FD&C Red #40 Lake, FD&C Yellow #6 Lake, FD&C Blue #1 Lake, FD&C Yellow #5 Lake (Tartrazine)

Warnings: If you are experiencing urinary problems, or are being treated for prostate problems, consult your doctor. **KEEP OUT OF THE REACH OF CHILDREN.**

How Supplied: Bottles of 30.
Shown in Product Identification Guide, page 505

ONE-A-DAY® TENSION & MOOD
Dietary Supplement

Directions: Adults (18 years and older): Take one to two tablets daily with food.
One tablet of One-A-Day Tension & Mood provides:

	AMOUNT PER SERVING	% DAILY VALUE
Vitamin C	60 mg	100%
Thiamin (B1)	1.125 mg	75%
Niacin	10 mg	50%
Folic Acid	100 mcg	25%
Pantothenic Acid	5 mg	50%
Lecithin	15 mg	*
Kava Kava Standardized Extract (*Piper methysticum*) (rhizome and root)	100 mg	*
St. John's Wort Standardized Extract (*Hypericum perforatum*) (leaves and flowers)	225 mg	*

*Daily Value not established.

Ingredients: Dicalcium Phosphate, St. John's Wort Extract, Cellulose, Kava Kava Extract, Ascorbic Acid, Croscarmellose Sodium, Hydroxypropyl Methylcellulose, Lecithin, Stearic Acid, Niacin, Silicon Dioxide, Magnesium Stearate, d-Calcium Pantothenate, Titanium Dioxide, Pharmaceutical Glaze, Polyethylene Glycol, Thiamine Mononitrate, Starch, Hydroxypropyl Cellulose, FD&C Yellow #5 Lake (Tartazine), FD&C Yellow #6 Lake, Polysorbate 80, Folic Acid, FD&C Blue #1 Lake, FD&C Red #40 Lake.

Warnings: Ask a doctor before use if you are presently or have been taking a monoamine oxidase inhibitor (MAOI) (certain drugs for depression, psychiatric or emotional conditions, or Parkinson's disease) in the past 2 weeks, or if you are taking any other prescription drug. May cause drowsiness. Alcohol, sedatives and tranquilizers may increase the drowsiness effect. Avoid use with alcohol. Use caution when driving a motor vehicle or operating machinery.

Before any surgery ask your doctor about continued use of this product. **Do not use if pregnant or breast-feeding. KEEP OUT OF THE REACH OF CHILDREN.**

How Supplied: Bottles of 30.

Shown in Product Identification Guide, page 505

ONE-A-DAY® WOMEN'S
Multivitamin/Multimineral Supplement

Directions: Adults: One tablet daily with food.

VITAMINS	AMOUNT PER SERVING		% DAILY VALUE
Vitamin A	5000	IU	100%
Vitamin C	60	mg	100%
Vitamin D	400	IU	100%
Vitamin E	30	IU	100%
Thiamine (B$_1$)	1.5	mg	100%
Riboflavin (B$_2$)	1.7	mg	100%
Niacin	20	mg	100%
Vitamin B$_6$	2	mg	100%
Folic Acid	400	mcg	100%
Vitamin B$_{12}$	6	mcg	100%
Pantothenic Acid	10	mg	100%

MINERALS	AMOUNT PER SERVING		% DAILY VALUE
Calcium	450	mg	45%
Iron	27	mg	150%
Zinc	15	mg	100%

Ingredients: Calcium Carbonate, Starch, Ferrous Fumarate, Ascorbic Acid, Gelatin, Vitamin E Acetate, Modified Cellulose Gum, Niacinamide, Zinc Oxide, Titanium Dioxide, Calcium Pantothenate, Pyridoxine Hydrochloride, Vitamin A Acetate, Riboflavin, Thiamine Mononitrate, Beta Carotene, Folic Acid, Vitamin D, Vitamin B$_{12}$, FD&C Yellow #5 (Tartrazine) Lake, FD&C Yellow #6 Lake, FD&C Blue #2 Lake.

> **Warning:** Accidental overdose of iron-containing products is a leading cause of fatal poisoning in children under 6. Keep this product out of the reach of children. In case of accidental overdose, call a doctor or poison control center immediately.

KEEP OUT OF THE REACH OF CHILDREN

How Supplied: Bottles of 60 and 100.

Shown in Product Identification Guide, page 504

Beach Pharmaceuticals
Division of Beach Products, Inc.
5220 SOUTH MANHATTAN AVE.
TAMPA, FL 33611

Direct Inquiries to:

Richard Stephen Jenkins, Exec. V.P.:
(813) 839-6565

BEELITH Tablets
MAGNESIUM SUPPLEMENT with PYRIDOXINE HCL

Description: Each tablet contains magnesium oxide 600 mg and pyridoxine hydrochloride (Vitamin B$_6$) 25 mg equivalent to Vitamin B$_6$ 20 mg.

Supplement Facts
Serving Size: 1 Tablet

	Amount Per Tablet	% Daily Value
Magnesium	362 mg	90%
Vitamin B$_6$	20 mg	1000%

Inactive Ingredients: D&C Yellow No. 10, FD&C Yellow No. 6 (Sunset Yellow), hydroxypropylmethylcellulose, magnesium stearate, microcrystalline cellulose, polyethylene glycol, sodium starch glycolate, titanium dioxide, and water.

Indications: As a dietary supplement for patients with magnesium and/or Vitamin B$_6$ deficiencies resulting from malnutrition, alcoholism, magnesium depleting drugs, chemotherapy, and inadequate nutritional intake or absorption. Also, increases urinary magnesium levels.

Dosage: One tablet daily or as directed by a physician.

Warnings: Do not take this product if you are presently taking a prescription drug without consulting your physician or other health professional. If you have kidney disease, take only under the supervision of a physician. Excessive dosage may cause laxation. If pregnant or breast-feeding, ask a health professional before use. **KEEP OUT OF THE REACH OF CHILDREN.**

How Supplied: Golden yellow, film-coated tablet with the letters **BP** and the number **132** imprinted on each tablet. Packaged in bottles of 100 (NDC 0486-1132-01) tablets.

Block Drug Company, Inc.
257 CORNELISON AVENUE
JERSEY CITY, NJ 07302

Direct Inquiries to:
Consumer Affairs/Block
(201) 434-3000 Ext. 1308

For Medical Emergencies Contact:
Consumer Affairs/Block
(201) 434-3000 Ext. 1308

BEANO®
[*bēan ō*]
Food Enzyme Dietary Supplement

PRODUCT INFORMATION

Description:
Beano drops: each 5 drop dosage follows Food Chemical Codex (FCC) standards for activity and contains 150 GalU (galactosidase units) of alpha-D-galactosidase derived from *Aspergillus niger* mold. The enzyme is in a liquid carrier of water and xylitol. Add about 5 drops on the first bite of food serving, but remember a normal meal has 2-3 servings of the problem foods.
Beano tablets: each tablet follows Food Chemical Codex (FCC) standards for activity and contains 150 GalU (galactosidase units) of alpha-D-galactosidase derived from *Aspergillus niger* mold. The enzyme is in a carrier of cellulose gel, mannitol, invertase, potato starch, magnesium stearate, gelatin (fish), colloidal silica. 3 tablets swallowed, chewed, or crumbled onto food should be enough for a normal meal of 3 servings of problem foods (1 tablet per serving). Beano® will hydrolyze complex sugars, raffinose, stachyose and verbascose, into the simple sugars - glucose, galactose and fructose, and the easily digestible disaccharide, sucrose. (Sucrose hydrolysis happens simultaneously with normal digestion.) In some cases, more enzyme than 5 drops or 3 tablets will be required, and this is a function of the quantity of food eaten, the levels of alpha-linked sugars in the food, and the gas-producing propensity of the person.

Action: Hydrolysis converts raffinose, stachyose and verbascose into their monosaccharide components: glucose, galactose, fructose and sucrose. Raffinose yields sucrose + galactose; stachyose yields sucrose + galactose; verbascose yields glucose + fructose + galactose.

Indications: Helps prevent flatulence and/or bloat from a variety of grains, cereals, nuts, seeds, and vegetables containing the sugars raffinose, stachyose and/or verbascose. This includes all or most legumes and all or most cruciferous vegetables. Examples of such foods are

Continued on next page

Beano—Cont.

oats, wheat, beans of all kinds, chick-peas, peas, lentils, peanuts, soy-content foods, broccoli, brussel sprouts, cabbage, carrots, corn, leeks, onions, parsnips, squash. Note: Most vegetables and beans also contain fiber, which is gas productive in some people, but usually far less so than the alpha-linked sugars. Beano® has no effect on fiber.

Usage: About 5 drops per food serving or 3 tablets per meal (1 tablet per serving) of 3 servings of problem foods; higher levels depending on symptoms.

Adverse Reactions: Reports to date include gastroenterological symptoms, such as cramping and diarrhea as well as allergic-type reactions including rash and pruritus. Rare reports of more serious allergic reactions have been received.

Precautions: If you are pregnant or nursing, ask your doctor before product use. Galactosemics should not use without physician's advice, since one of the breakdown sugars is galactose.

How Supplied: Beano® is supplied in both a liquid form (30 and 75 serving sizes, at 5 drops per serving), and a tablet form (30, 60, and 100 tablet sizes as well as 24 tablets in packets of 3). These statements have not been evaluated by the Food and Drug Administration. This product is not intended to diagnose, treat, cure or prevent any disease. For more information and free samples, please write or call toll-free 1-800-257-8650 or visit www.beano.net.

Body Wise International Inc

2802 DOW AVENUE
TUSTIN, CA 92780

For direct inquiries contact:
Wellness Research Center:
Phone# (714) 505-6121
Fax# (714) 832-7247
Email: wellness@bodywise.com

PRODUCT LISTING:

BETA-C™

BIOLAX®

CARBO ENERGY BAR™

CHITO-MAXX™

CoENZYME Q10+™

ELECTRO ALOE®

FUTURE PERFECT®

MEM X²™

OXY-G²®

SUPER RESHAPE FORMULA®

St. JOHN'S COMPLEX™

SUPER CELL™

TIGER VITES™

WORKOUT FORMULA™

XTREME™

AG-Immune Capsules

Description: A normally functioning immune system is necessary for good health. A key marker for an ineffective immune system is a low, natural killer (NK) cell activity. These cells primarily attack and destroy diseased cells. The NK cells must be "activated" in order to be effective and this is achieved through a complex communication network within the body. When used in clinical studies, products containing the patented Antigen Infused Extract such as the Body Wise **AG-Immune,** supported by healthy NK cell activity consistently produce very large increases in NK cell activity.

Highlighted Ingredients:
Arabinogalactin
Arabinogalactin dramatically increases the macrophage activity and, along with it, inhibits bacteria from attaching to cells. This amazing nutrient has also proven to be more powerful in its effects on the immune system than the popular herb Echinacea. It has friendly pro-biotic activity and increases good bacteria, such as lactobacillus and bifidobacteria.

AIE-10

Description: Antigenically Infused Dialyzable Bovine Colostrum/Whey Extract (AIE-10) is a complex extract that requires highly controlled conditions in order to attain the desired product. The fruit of nearly fifty years of research, it is utilized as a "trigger" to turn-on and direct the immune system. In conjunction with a healthy lifestyle, which includes a good nutritional basis, AIE-10 seeks to modulate your immune system and support your overall health.

Method of Action: Jesse A. Stoff, M.D. has conducted extensive clinical research illustrating that AIE-10 when used in conjunction with other nutrients will produce dramatic increases in the immune system's natural killer (NK) activity. These NK cells are the body's fore-most protection against the daily attack of viruses and cancer cells that reach it. Stoff notes a unique "Spreading Effect" that occurs with the use of AIE-10. AIE-10 contains numerous immune system factors that are all valuable. Within AIE-10, the presence of certain transfer factors, cytokines, defensins, and other immunological co-factors create a vast and strong influence on the immune system, which facilitates improved immune function and aids in raising NK cell function. Due to this effect, AIE-10 can be used as both a preventive measure and as an aid to the treatment of certain health conditions. Currently, research has shown that using AIE-10 increased NK cell function in numerous patients suffering from the following conditions: Weakened Immune Function, Irritable Bowel Syndrome, Chronic Fatigue, Candida, Arthritis and Rheumatism, Infection, Hepatitis C, Colds and Flu, Sinusitis, HIV/AIDS, Lupus and Cancer.

Safety Factors: When taken as directed, there are no known side effects of AIE-10. Some individuals experience moderate cold-like, detoxing symptoms usually alleviated within a few days. Although derived from a dairy source, no milk proteins remain in AIE-10 and it is considered safe for those with a dairy allergy.

References: Stoff, J, M.D. The Ultimate Nutrient. Tucson, Arizona: Insight Consulting Services, 2000

Astragalus: Astragalus is a perennial plant that western herbalists believe can help stimulate the immune system. The polysaccharides in this herb have been known to generally strengthen the body, speed up metabolism, promote tissue regeneration, and increase energy. Recent studies in China led researchers to report that astragalus can be part of an effective treatment for supporting the immune systems of cancer patients.

Maitake Mushroom: Studies on the health benefits of mushrooms for humans have focused on immune enhancement properties. The complex sugars and their derivatives are able to stimulate a higher level of cytokine production. Some common cytokines include interleukins, interferon, natural killer cells (NK cells) activating factors, and tumor necrosis factors. The maitake mushroom is also rich in host defense potentiators.

Ingredients: (Each 2 Capsules contain):

Arabanogalactan	300mg
Ai/E10	100mg
Astragalus Root	50mg
Maitake Mushroom Extract 4:1	50mg

Directions: Take one capsule two times per day, can take up to 8 a day for a severely compromised immune system.

How Supplied: Bottles of 60 Capsules.

Beta-C Tablets

Description:
Beta-C is your sunshine connection! Its remarkable nutrient matrix is composed of beta carotene, an antioxidant and immune system modulator, plus an exclusive, more-easily digested form of vitamin C. We've also added the nutritional benefits of cruciferous vegetables, bilberry and garlic—a powerful combination of life-affirming nutrients!

Highlighted Ingredients:
Vitamin C
Essential for collagen formation, this vitamin aids in immune system functioning.
Natural Mixed Carotenoids
Plant-based compounds which fight free radicals and promote a strong immune system.
Cruciferous Vegetables
Rich in antioxidants and a great source of fiber.
Garlic
Shown to have cholesterol lowering properties and promote cardiovascular health.

Beta-C
Supplement facts

Serving Size 4 Tablets

Amount per 4 Tablets		% Daily Value
Beta Carotene (Dunaliella salina algae)	3 mg	
Equivalent to Vitamin A	5000 IU	100%

Contains other naturally occurring carotenoids in D. salina; Alpha Carotene, Cryptoxanthin, Zeaxanthin and Lutein.

Vitamin C (Esterified)	2000 mg	3333%
Calcium (from Dicalcium Phosphate)	96 mg	10%
Cruciferous Vegetable Concentrate	500 mg	*
Deodorized Garlic Bulb	400 mg	*
Mixed Bioflavonoid Complex	200 mg	*
Bilberry Fruit Extract 4:1	100 mg	*
Acerola Cherry Fruit Extract 4:1	40 mg	*
Rose Hips	40 mg	*
Grapefruit Bioflavonoid Complex	40 mg	*
Hesperidin Fruit Citrus Complex	40 mg	*
Red Clover Blossoms	40 mg	*
Rutin Flower Buds	40 mg	*

*Daily Value not established.

Directions: As a dietary supplement, adults take four tablets daily with food.
How Supplied: Bottles of 120 Tablets.

Relief™
Natural Immune System Booster Nasal & Throat Spray

General Description: **Relief** is a homeopathic nasal and throat spray that triggers your immune system to jump into action and fight off your body's natural enemies.
Safe for adults, as well as children, **Relief** is an effective way to give your immune system the boost it needs to fight off bacteria, viruses, parasites, germs, and other microscopic invaders. It is designed to work on contact in the upper respiratory tract where your body first comes in contact with germ-laden air.
Ingredients in **Relief** have been clinically proven to relieve symptoms associated with the following illnesses:
• Common Cold
• Influenza
• Tonsillitis
• Sore Throat
• Earache
• Cough
• Headache
• Fever
• Nasal Discharge
• Sinus Congestion
• Cold Sores
There is only one immune system trigger in the entire nutritional marketplace, one that provides the exact coded information that tells your immune system how to get back into action and fight these invaders. **Relief** contains this tigger, Ai/E.[10] Produced using patented and proprietary technology, it simply can't be found in your local health food store. It's the most important health benefit you could possibly have.

A Natural Immune System Modulator
Body Wise International announces it's newest product—**Relief**—a new homeopathic nasal and throat spray that is designed to work on contact in the upper respiratory tract where your body first comes in contact with germ laden air. Ingredients in **Relief** have been clinically proven to relieve symptoms associated with influenza and the common cold.

Active Ingredient: Relief contains the same ingredient Ai/E10 that is found in the highly successful Body Wise formula, **AG-Immune.** Ai/E10 is an immune system trigger that provides the exact coded information that tells your immune system how to fight off the foreign invaders that attack our bodies on a daily basis. And, it is only available through Body Wise!

Inactive Ingredients: Benzalkonium chloride, 2-deoxy-d-glucose, disodium EDTA, eucalyptus oil, filtered water, sodium hydroxide, thimerosal.

SUPPLEMENT FACTS
Active Homeopathic Ingredients:

Bushmaster (Lachesis mutus)	12	X	HPUS*
Quicksilver (Mercurius vivus)	12	X	HPUS
Liver of sulfer (Hepar sulphuris calcareum)	8	X	HPUS
Belladonna	4	X	HPUS

*Homeopathic Pharmacopoeia of the United States

Directions: (Adults and Children over 3): Keep head upright, spray 1 to 4 times in each nostril and/or throat 1 to 6 times daily as needed. Shake well before using.

RIGHT CHOICE® A.M. MULTI FORMULA

Description: Body Wise Right Choice® A.M. Formula contains a wide range of vitamins that focus on microcellular nutrition and essential metabolic functions.

Each three caplets contain:

	Amount	%RDA
Vitamins		
Beta Carotene (Dunaliella salina algae)	6 mg	
equivalent to Vitamin A	10,000 IU	200
(contains other naturally occurring carotenoids in D. salina: Alpha Carotene, Cryptoxanthin, Zeaxanthin, Lutein and Lycopene)		
Vitamin A (palmitate)	5,000 IU	100
Vitamin C	1,000 mg	1667
Ascorbyl Palmitate	50 mg	**
Vitamin B1 (thiamine mononitrate)	25 mg	1667
Vitamin B2 (riboflavin)	15 mg	882
Niacinamide	50 mg	250
Vitamin B6 (pyridoxine HCL)	25 mg	1250
Folic Acid	800 mcg	200
Vitamin B12 (cobalamin concentrate)	200 mcg	3333
Pantothenic Acid (d-cal pantothenate)	50 mg	500
Biotin	300 mcg	100

Right Choice A.M.—Cont.

Vitamin E Complex

Vitamin E	200 IU	667
(d-alpha tocopherol acid succinate and mixed tocopherols beta, gamma and delta)		

PhytoNutrients/Food Factors

Green Barley	50 mg	**
Chlorella	50 mg	**
Spirulina	50 mg	**
Lemon Bioflavonoid Complex	50 mg	**

Additional Constituents

Chromium***	100 mcg	**
L-Glutamine	50 mg	**
Alpha Ketoglutarate	200 mg	**
Ginkgo Biloba	50 mg	**
Orchard Blend	100 mg	**

**No nutritional requirement established.
***Krebs Cycle Chelate.

Inactive Ingredients: Cellulose, vegetable stearine, magnesium stearate, silicon dioxide, and aqueous base white filmcoat.

Recommended Adult Use: As a dietary supplement, take three caplets with your morning meal.

How Supplied/Availability: Supplied in bottles of 90 or 270. Available through Body Wise International.

Studies/References:
1. Levin. *NEJM*, 1986.
2. Steinberg. *The Herb Quarterly*, 1994.
3. Reynolds. *Journal of Neuroimmunol*, 1992.

*These Statements have not been evaluated by the U.S. FDA. This product is not intended to diagnose treat, cure or prevent any disease.

RIGHT CHOICE® P.M. MULTI FORMULA

Description: Body Wise Right Choice* P.M. includes minerals and other nutrients essential for maintenance of the skeletal system.

Each three caplets contain:

	Amount	%RDA
Minerals		
Calcium**	500 mg	50
Magnesium**	250 mg	63
Zinc**	15 mg	100
Copper**	2 mg	100
Manganese**	25 mg	1250
Chromium**	100 mcg	83
Selenium (1-selenomethionine)	50 mcg	71
Molybdenum**	100 mcg	133
Vanadium**	50 mcg	***
Potassium**	99 mg	***
Trace Mineral Complex**	250 mg	***
Lipotropic Complex		
Inositol	50 mg	
Betaine HCl	100 mg	****

Choline (bitartrate)	50 mg	****
Amino Acid/Antioxidant		
L-Glutathione	15 mg	****
PhytoNutrients/Food Factors		
Green Barley	50 mg	****
Chlorella	50 mg	****
Spirulina	50 mg	****
Additional Constituents		
Vitamin D3 (ergocalciferol)	400 IU	100
Iodine (kelp)	150 mcg	100

**Krebs Cycle Chelated* Mineral Replenishment Factors are uniquely formulated with Citrates, Aspartates, Fumarates, Succinates and Malates.
***Determined to be essential nutrient but actual requirements have not been established.
****No nutritional requirement established.

Inactive Ingredients: Cellulose, vegetable stearine, magnesium stearate, silicon dioxide, and an aqueous base green film coating.

Recommended Adult Use: As a dietary supplement, take three caplets with your evening meal.

How Supplied/Availability: Supplied in bottles of 90 or 270. Available through Body Wise International.

Studies/References:
1. Hendler. *Doctor's Vitamin & Mineral Encyclopedia*, 1990.
2. Heaney. *Clin Invest Med*, 1981.
3. Rude, et al. *J. Clin Endo Metabol*, 1985.

---

*These Statements have not been evaluated by the U.S. FDA. This product is not intended to diagnose treat, cure or prevent any disease.

Cooke Pharma

**1404 OLD COUNTRY ROAD
BELMONT, CA 94002**

Direct Inquiries to:
Customer Service Dept.
(888) 808-6838

HEARTBAR®
**L-arginine-enriched
Medical Food**

Description: The HeartBar® is a medical food for the dietary management of cardiovascular disease. These ingredients are placed in a convenient and pleasant-tasting nutrition bar. The major active ingredient in the HeartBar is L-arginine, which is an amino acid required for the production of nitric oxide (NO). Each 50g bar contains L-arginine (3 g) and other amino acids, folate (200 μcg) and other B-complex vitamins, antioxidant vitamins E (200 IU) and C (250 mg), niacin (25 mg) and phytoestrogens. These nutrients are combined in a fruit, fiber, and soy protein-based nutrition bar. One HeartBar contains 13 g of protein (10g of soy protein), 27 g of carbohydrate (20 g of sugars, 3 g of fiber), 2.5 g of fat (no saturated fat, 0 mg of cholesterol), and 190 calories. HeartBar does not require a prescription but is to be used under the supervision of a health care professional.

Composition (original flavor): High fructose corn syrup, soy protein isolate, fructose, toasted soy pieces, raisins, vanilla cookie pieces (including wheat flour), L-arginine HCl, natural and artificial flavors, oat fiber, D-alpha-tocopherol acetate, sodium ascorbate, dipotassium phosphate, niacinamide, pyridoxine hydrochloride, folic acid, cyanocobalamin.

Clinical Background: The major active ingredient of the HeartBar, L-arginine, is a semi-essential amino acid, and is the precursor for endothelium-derived nitric oxide (NO). NO is a potent vasodilator, and a major regulator of vasomotion and blood pressure. In addition, NO inhibits platelet aggregation, vascular smooth muscle proliferation and adherence of leukocytes to the vessel wall, key processes in atherosclerosis and restenosis.

Endothelium-derived NO activity is reduced in patients with cardiovascular disease; this abnormality contributes to insufficient blood flow, elevated blood pressure, as well as progression of disease. L-arginine has been shown to enhance the synthesis of NO. In humans, L-arginine improves vasodilation, enhances coronary and peripheral blood flow, and inhibits platelet aggregation.

The usual dietary intake of L-arginine is about 3 to 5 g/day, which in some cardiovascular conditions, may not be sufficient intake to maintain healthy NO levels. Two HeartBars/day provides an additional 6 g of L-arginine. The other active ingredients of the HeartBar contribute to the production of, or help prevent the breakdown of NO further augmenting the activity of NO.

The HeartBar has been tested clinically in several patient populations and shown to be effective in improving blood flow. In two separate studies of individuals with total cholesterol over 230 mg/dl (n=41 & n=39), two HeartBars/day restored flow-mediated vasodilation to normal within one and two weeks respectively (compared to no change with placebo).

In patients with peripheral arterial disease secondary to atherosclerosis (n=39), 2 HeartBars/day for 2 weeks improved pain-free walking distance by 66% (compared to placebo of 18%). In addition to this improvement in physical function, these patients experienced an improvement in quality of life scores as measured by the SF-36 Medical Outcomes Survey.

In patients with stable angina (n=36), 2 HeartBars/day for 2 weeks improved

flow-mediated vasodilation. This was associated with a 22% increase in exercise time, 43% increase in work performance and a significant improvement in quality of life as measured by SF-36 and Seattle Angina Questionnaire scores.

In a study of diabetic patients (n =10), there was no change in pre- and post-prandial serum glucose measures or glycosylated hemoglobin during 3 months of HeartBar use at 2 bars/day.

Pharmacokinetics: Following the administration of 1 HeartBar, plasma arginine levels rise from 68 ± 27 µM/L to a peak of 119 ± 48 µM/L within one hour of ingestion. Arginine levels are maintained above those of individuals on an arginine-free diet for at least 8 hours after ingestion. A similar pattern of arginine levels is observed following the ingestion of a single HeartBar after a week of b.i.d. use. After 2 weeks, trough L-arginine levels are 42% higher than levels before HeartBar use. These arginine levels compare favorably with L-arginine administration by capsular form.

Precautions:
Diabetics
Each HeartBar is equal to 2 carbohydrate exchanges. Although there was no effect of regular use on daily fasting and post-prandial serum glucose or gylcosylated hemoglobin measures, diabetics should monitor their blood glucose carefully while initiating regular use of the HeartBar. The effect of L-arginine on retinopathy is not known, therefore, those with diabetic retinopathy should not use HeartBar.
Renal Failure Patients
The HeartBar contains 13 g of protein. This amount of protein should be considered when determining total daily protein load.
Allergies
The base of the bar is of soy protein, which is generally considered hypoallergenic. The original flavor also contains a small amount of wheat flour, is low in gluten but not gluten-free. Therefore, individuals with allergies to wheat products or gluten intolerance should be cautious.
Sepsis
The hypotension associated with sepsis is, in-part, mediated by excessive NO production. Such patients should not be given HeartBar.

Adverse Reactions: No serious adverse reactions have been demonstrated or reported in clinical trials or in the HeartBar Safety-In-Use study of over 2 years duration.

Minor adverse reactions are infrequent, generally related to gastrointestinal disturbances and appear unrelated to the L-arginine in the bar (Adverse events were just as common in the group given placebo bar). In a two-week study of the HeartBar, 4 of 41 individuals reported increased flatulence that resolved after several days of bar use. One of 41 individuals complained of increased frequency of bowel movements and soft stools. In a 10-week study of the HeartBar, 2 of 41 individuals reported dry mouth. A change in bowel habits was reported by 1 individual in each of the placebo and HeartBar groups. Use of HeartBar has not been associated with increased incidence of herpes cold sore formation.

The HeartBar is not indicated for individuals with co-existing conditions of diabetic retinopathy or neoplastic disease because the effect of L-arginine on the progression of these disorders is unknown.

Administration:
Symptomatic or high-risk population
One HeartBar twice daily
At-risk population
One HeartBar daily

How Supplied: Individually wrapped bars, cartons of 16 and cases of 64. Also available in 20g trial size.
Original Flavor
Individual Bars   NDC 63535-10102
By Carton   NDC 63535-10103
By Case   NDC 63535-10104
Cranberry Flavor
Individual Bars   NDC 63535-10302
By Carton   NDC 63535-10303
By Case   NDC 63535-10304
Peanut Butter Flavor
Individual Bars   NDC 63535-10502
By Carton   NDC 63535-10503
By Case   NDC 63535-10504

References:
J. P. Cooke, V. J. Dzau, *Annu. Rev. Med.* **48**, 489–509 (1997).
A. J. Maxwell, J. P. Cooke, *Curr Opin Nephrol Hypertens* **7**, 63–70 (1998).
A. J. Maxwell, B. A. Anderson, M. P. Zapien, J. P. Cooke, *CV Drugs & Therapy* **14**, 357–364 (2000).
A. J. Maxwell, B. A. Anderson, J. P. Cooke, *Vascular Med* **5**, 11–19 (2000).
A. J. Maxwell, *Nutrition & MD* **25**, 1–4 (1999).
A. J. Maxwell, M. P. Zapien, B. A. Anderson, P. H. Stone, *J Am Coll Cardiol* **35**, 408A (2000).
Cooke Pharma
1404 Old County Road
Belmont, CA 94002-3928
Direct Inquiries to:
Customer Service Dept.
(888) 808-6838

Covex
SECTOR OFICIOS 33, 1-3
28760 TRES CANTOS
MADRID SPAIN

For direct inquiries contact:
+34-91-804-4545
Fax +34-91-804-3030
vinpocetin@covex.es

INTELECTOL® MEMORY ENHANCER
VINPOCETINE TABLETS COVEX

Description: Intelectol® is a powerful memory enhancer. Scientific studies have shown that its ingredient vinpocetine helps the body to maintain healthy circulation in the brain by decreasing cerebral vascular resistance, improving cerebral blood flow and cerebral oxygen and glucose utilization, and that vinpocetine increases the concentration of some neurotransmitters involved in the process of memory formation. Intelectol® can be taken for enhancing the following cognitive functions: memory, attention, orientation, perception, information fixation, judgment. Clinical studies have also shown that vinpocetine helps to maintain healthy microcirculation in the inner ear and eyes.

Active ingredients: Vinpocetine 5mg (No U.S. RDA established)

Inactive ingredients: Lactose, Hydropropylcellulose, Magnesium Stearate, Talc.

Recommended Use: 1 to 2 tablets × 3 times daily with meals.

Warning: Keep out of reach of children. Do not take if you are pregnant or lactating. If you have hemophilia or are on blood thinning medication, please consult your physician before taking this product.

Interactions: Not known.

How Supplied: packs of 50 tablets.
Availability: Available at Web Site http://www.intelectol.com, http://www.the-memory-pill.com, toll free number 1 888 613 9920.

References/Function Claim:
Visit Web Site http://www.intelectol.com
Shown in Product Identification Guide, page 507

Fleming & Company
1600 FENPARK DR.
FENTON, MO 63026

Direct Inquiries to:
Tom Fleming
636 343-8200
FAX (636) 343-9865
e-mail: info@flemingcompany.com

MAGONATE® Tablets

MAGONATE® Liquid

MAGONATE NATAL Liquid
Magnesium Gluconate (Dihydrate), USP
(Dietary Supplement)

Description: Each 2 tablets contain magnesium 54 mgs (from 1000 mg magnesium gluconate dihydrate) calcium 175 mg and phosphorous 182 mg (from 752 mg dibasic calcium phosphate dihydrate). Each 5 mL of MAGONATE® liquid contains magnesium (elemental) 54 mgs. (Each 5 mL contains the same amount of magnesium as contained in 1000 mgs of magnesium gluconate dihydrate). Each mL of MAGONATE NATAL Liquid (magnesium gluconate) contains 3.52 mg (0.29 mEq) of magnesium as the gluconate in a sugarless and flavor free isotonic base.

Suggested Uses: Magonate® Tablets and Liquid are indicated to maintain magnesium levels when the dietary intake of magnesium is inadequate or when excretion and loss are excessive. Magonate® is recommended during and for three weeks after a course in chemotherapy, then monitored regularly. MAGONATE NATAL Liquid is indicated for newborns with magnesium deficiency and for the restoration of magnesium in infants.

Precautions: Excessive dosage may cause loose stools.

Contraindications: Patients with kidney disease should not take magnesium supplements without the supervision of a physician.

Dosages And Administration: Two Magonate® tablets or 1 teaspoon Magonate® Liquid three times a day (mid-morning, mid-afternoon and bedtime) on an empty stomach with a glass of water. MAGONATE Natal Liquid usual dose is 1 mL per kg of body weight daily, divided into two doses of 10 drops per kg twice a day.

How Supplied: Magonate® Tablets are orange scored, and supplied in bottles of 100 (NDC 258-0172-01), and 1000 (NDC 256-0172-02) tablets. Magonate® Liquid is supplied in pints, (NDC 256-0184-01). MAGONATE NATAL Liquid is supplied in 90 mL bottles.

Rev. 7/00

4Life Research™, LC
9850 SOUTH 300 WEST
SANDY, UT 84070

Direct Inquiries to:
(801) 562-3600
FAX: (801) 562-3670
www.4-life.com

TRANSFER FACTOR™
Advanced Immune System Support
Exclusive • Patented

Description: 4Life Transfer™ is one of the most exciting, new discoveries in immune system support in decades! A well-regulated immune system helps promote optimum health, strength, energy, stamina, and quality of life.*
Transfer factors are small molecules (MW 3,000–10,000) that help strengthen and regulate our immune systems.* These special "response messenger compounds" are naturally found in the immune rich portion of cow's milk, called colostrum. Through special patented techniques, (licensed to 4Life Research™) *transfer factors* are isolated and concentrated from bovine colostrum for human consumption.

*These statements have not been evaluated by the Food and Drug Administration. This product is not intended to diagnose, treat, cure, or prevent any disease.

Directions: Take one (1) capsule three times daily, for a total of three (3) capsules per day. For best results, 4Life Transfer Factor™ should be taken with 8 oz. of water.

Supplement Facts
Serving Size: One (1) Capsule
Servings Per Container: 90

Amount Per Serving	% Daily Value*
Transfer Factor XF™ (A proprietary concentrated extract of bovine colostrum containing *transfer factors* and other natural components)	200 mg

*Daily Value not established

KEEP OUT OF REACH OF CHILDREN. 4LIFE TRANSFER FACTOR™ SHOULD BE STORED IN THE REFRIGERATOR, OR OTHER COOL, DRY PLACES TO MAINTAIN SHELF LIFE.

How Supplied: Bottles of 90 Capsules.
Distributed by:
4Life Research™, LC
Sandy, UT 84070
www.4-life.com
Item #24001

Protected by US Patent 4,816,563
Shown in Product Identification Guide, page 526

Lederle Consumer Health
A Division of Whitehall-Robins Healthcare
FIVE GIRALDA FARMS
MADISON, NJ 07940

Direct Inquiries to:
Lederle Consumer Product Information
(800) 282-8805

CALTRATE® 600
CALTRATE® 600 + D
CALTRATE® 600 + SOY
[căl-trāte]

Description: CALCIUM DIETARY SUPPLEMENT WITHOUT/WITH VITAMIN D, NATURE'S MOST CONCENTRATED FORM OF CALCIUM® NO SALT, NO LACTOSE, NO PRESERVATIVES; TABLET SHAPE SPECIALLY DESIGNED FOR EASIER SWALLOWING
CALTRATE 600 + SOY CONTAINS SOY ISOFLAVONES

SUPPLEMENT FACTS
Serving Size 1 Tablet

AMOUNT PER SERVING		% DAILY VALUE
CALTRATE® 600	Calcium 600 mg	60%
CALTRATE® 600 + D	Vitamin D 200 IU	50%
	Calcium 600 mg	60%
CALTRATE® 600 + SOY	Vitamin D 200 IU	50%
	Calcium 600 mg	60%
	Soy Isoflavones 25 mg	*

*Daily Value Not Established

Ingredients: *CALTRATE® 600:* Calcium Carbonate, Maltodextrin, Cellulose, Mineral Oil, Hydroxypropyl Methylcellulose, Titanium Dioxide, Light Mineral Oil, Polysorbate 80, Sodium Lauryl Sulfate, Carnauba Wax, Crospovidone, Magnesium Stearate, Stearic Acid.
CALTRATE® 600 + D: Calcium Carbonate, Maltodextrin, Cellulose, Hydroxypropyl Methylcellulose, Mineral Oil, Titanium Dioxide, Polysorbate 80, Polyethylene Glycol, Gelatin, Sucrose, Corn Starch, Canola Oil, Carnauba Wax, FD&C Yellow #6 Aluminum Lake, Crospovidone, Magnesium Stearate, Stearic Acid, Cholecalciferol (Vit. D3), dl-Alpha Tocopherol (Vit. E).
CALTRATE® 600 + SOY: Calcium Carbonate, Maltodextrin, Soy Isoflavones

Extract, Cellulose, Mineral Oil, Soy Polysaccharides, Hydroxypropyl Methylcellulose, Gelatin, Sucrose, Corn Starch, Polyethylene Glycol, Canola Oil, Carnauba Wax, Crospovidone, Magnesium Stearate, Stearic Acid, Cholecalciferol (Vit. D3), dl-Alpha Tocopherol (Vit. E).

Warnings: KEEP OUT OF REACH OF CHILDREN.

Suggested Use: Take two tablets daily (one tablet twice a day) with food or as directed by your physician.
Bottle is sealed with printed foil under cap. Do not use if foil is torn.

How Supplied: Caltrate 600, Bottle of 60 tablets
Caltrate 600 + D, Bottles of 60, 120 tablets
Caltrate 600 + SOY, Bottle of 60 tablets
Storage: Store at room temperature. Keep tightly closed.
© 1999

CALTRATE® 600 PLUS™ Tablets, CALTRATE® 600 PLUS™ Chewables
[căl-trāte]
Calcium Carbonate

Calcium Dietary Supplement With Vitamin D & Minerals
No Salt, No Lactose, No Preservatives

SUPPLEMENT FACTS
Serving Size: 1 Tablet
AMOUNT PER
SERVING: % Daily Value†

Vitamin D	200 IU	50%
Calcium	600 mg	60%
Magnesium	40 mg	10%
Zinc	7.5 mg	50%
Copper	1 mg	50%
Manganese	1.8 mg	90%
Boron	250 mcg	*

Chewables only:
Calories 10		
Total		
Carbohydrate	2 g	<1%†
Sugars	2 g	*

* Daily Value not established.
† Percent daily value is based on a 2000 calorie diet.

Suggested Use: Take two tablets daily (one tablet twice a day) with food or as directed by your physician.

Warnings: Keep out of the reach of children. Bottle is sealed with printed foil under cap. Do not use if foil is torn.

Ingredients (Tablets): Calcium Carbonate, Maltodextrin, Magnesium Oxide, Cellulose, Hydroxypropyl Methylcellulose, Mineral Oil, Zinc Oxide, Soy Polysaccharides, Titanium Dioxide, Manganese Sulfate, Polysorbate 80, Sodium Borate, Cupric Oxide, Polyethylene Glycol, Gelatin, Sucrose, FD&C Yellow No. 6 Aluminum Lake, Corn Starch,

Canola Oil, Carnauba Wax, FD&C Red No. 40 Aluminum Lake, FD&C Blue No. 1 Aluminum Lake, Crospovidone, Magnesium Stearate, Stearic Acid, Cholecalciferol (Vit. D3), dl-Alpha Tocopherol (Vit. E).

Ingredients (Chewables): Assorted Fruit Flavors (• Cherry • Orange • Fruit Punch): Dextrose, Calcium Carbonate, Maltodextrin, Magnesium Stearate, Magnesium Oxide, Adipic Acid, Cellulose, Mineral Oil, Zinc Oxide, Manganese Sulfate, Sodium Borate, Natural and Artificial Flavors, FD&C Red #40 Lake, Cupric Oxide, FD&C Yellow #6 Lake, FD&C Blue #2 Lake, Gelatin, Sucrose, Cornstarch, Vegetable Oil, Hydroxypropyl Methylcellulose, dl-Alpha Tocopherol, Vitamin D, Crospovidone

How Supplied: Bottles of 60 with Assorted Fruit Flavors
Storage: Store at Room Temperature. Keep tightly closed.
© 1999

CENTRUM®
[sĕn-trŭm]
High Potency Multivitamin-Multimineral Dietary Supplement, Advanced Formula From A to Zinc®

Supplement Facts:
Serving Size 1 Tablet

Each Tablet Contains	**% DV**
Vitamin A 5000 IU (20% as Beta Carotene)	100%
Vitamin C 60 mg	100%
Vitamin D 400 IU	100%
Vitamin E 30 IU	100%
Vitamin K 25 mcg	31%
Thiamin 1.5 mg	100%
Riboflavin 1.7 mg	100%
Niacin 20 mg	100%
Vitamin B6 2 mg	100%
Folic Acid 400 mcg	100%
Vitamin B12 6 mcg	100%
Biotin 30 mcg	10%
Pantothenic Acid 10 mg	100%
Calcium 162 mg	16%
Iron 18 mg	100%
Phosphorus 20 mg	2%
Iodine 150 mcg	100%
Magnesium 100 mg	25%
Zinc 15 mg	100%
Selenium 20 mcg	29%
Copper 2 mg	100%
Manganese 2 mg	100%
Chromium 120 mcg	100%
Molybdenum 75 mcg	100%
Chloride 72 mg	2%
Potassium 80 mg	2%
Boron 150 mcg	*
Nickel 5 mcg	*
Silicon 2 mg	*
Tin 10 mcg	*
Vanadium 10 mcg	*
Lutein 250 mcg	*

*Daily Value (%DV) not established.

Suggested Use: Adults, 1 tablet daily with food.

Warning: Accidental overdose of iron-containing products is a leading cause of fatal poisoning in children under 6. Keep this product out of reach of children. In case of accidental overdose, call a doctor or a Poison Control Center immediately.

Ingredients: Calcium Carbonate, Magnesium Oxide, Potassium Chloride, Microcrystalline Cellulose, Dibasic Calcium Phosphate, Ascorbic Acid (Vit. C), Ferrous Fumarate, Starch, dl-Alpha Tocopheryl Acetate (Vit. E), Gelatin, Crospovidone, Niacinamide, Zinc Oxide, Calcium Pantothenate, Manganese Sulfate, Silicon Dioxide, Pyridoxine Hydrochloride (Vit. B6), Cupric Oxide, Vitamin A Acetate, Riboflavin (Vit. B2), Thiamin Mononitrate (Vit. B1), Borates, Beta Carotene, Chromium Chloride, Folic Acid, Lutein, Potassium Iodide, Sodium Molybdate, Sodium Selenate, Phytonadione (Vit. K), Biotin, Sodium Metavanadate, Nickelous Sulfate, Stannous Chloride, Ergocalciferol (Vit. D2), Cyanocobalamin (Vit. B12). Contains less than 2% of the following ingredients: Acacia Gum, Ascorbyl Palmitate, Butylated Hydroxytoluene (BHT), Calcium Stearate, Citric Acid, FD&C Yellow No. 6 Aluminum Lake, Hydroxypropyl Methylcellulose, Magnesium Stearate, Polysorbate 80, Potassium Sorbate, Sodium Aluminum Silicate, Sodium Ascorbate (Vit. C), Sodium Benzoate, Sodium Citrate, Sorbic Acid, Sucrose, Titanium Dioxide, Triethyl Citrate, May also contain the following ingredient: Lactose.

How Supplied: Light peach, engraved CENTRUM C1.
Bottles of 60, 130, 180, and 250 tablets
Liquid in bottles of 8 oz.
Storage: Store at Room Temperature. Keep bottle tightly closed.
Bottle sealed with printed foil under cap. Do not use if foil is torn.

CENTRUM® FOCUSED FORMULAS BONE HEALTH TABLETS
Dietary Supplement

Supplement Facts:
Serving Size: 2 Tablets

Amount Per Serving		**% DV**
Vitamin D	200 IU	50%
Calcium (Citrate)	500 mg	50%
Magnesium	40 mg	10%
Zinc	7.5 mg	50%
Copper	1 mg	50%
Manganese	1.8 mg	90%
Boron	250 mcg	*

*Daily Value (% DV) not established

Ingredients: Calcium Citrate, Magnesium Oxide, Talc, Sodium Starch Glyco-

Continued on next page

Centrum Bone Health—Cont.

late, Magnesium Stearate, Zinc Oxide, Hydroxypropyl Methylcellulose, Manganese Sulfate, Sodium Borate, Cupric Oxide, Titanium Dioxide, Light Mineral Oil, Gelatin, Sucrose, Polysorbate 80, Polyethylene Glycol, Starch, Canola Oil, Carnauba Wax, Cholecalciferol, dl-Alpha Tocopherol.

Directions: (Adults) Take two tablets two times daily with a glass of water. Take each day for best results.

Precautions: Use only as directed. Do not exceed recommended dose. As with any supplement, if you are taking a prescription product, or if you are pregnant or are nursing a baby, contact your physician before taking this product. STORE IN A COOL DRY PLACE. KEEP BOTTLE TIGHTLY CLOSED.

How Supplied: Bottles of 120 tablets.

CENTRUM® FOCUSED FORMULAS ENERGY TABLETS
Dietary Supplement

Supplement Facts:
Serving Size 1 Tablet

Amount Per Tablet		% DV
Thiamin	3 mg	200%
Riboflavin	0.85 mg	50%
Niacin	10 mg	50%
Vitamin B6	1 mg	50%
Vitamin B12	3 mcg	50%
Biotin	15 mcg	5%
Pantothenic Acid	5 mg	50%
Taurine	100 mg	*
Ginseng Standardized Root Extract *Panax ginseng*	62.5 mg	*

*Daily Value (%DV) not established.

Ingredients: Dibasic Calcium Phosphate, Taurine, Microcrystalline Cellulose, Ginseng Standardized Root Extract *Panax ginseng,* Hydroxypropyl Methylcellulose, Crospovidone, Maltodextrin, Niacinamide, Calcium Pantothenate, Magnesium Stearate, Thiamin Mononitrate, Polyethylene Glycol, Titanium Dioxide, Pyridoxine Hydrochloride, Polysorbate 80, FD&C Yellow #6 Aluminum Lake, Riboflavin, Starch, Biotin, Citric Acid, Sodium Citrate, Silicon Dioxide, Cyanocobalamin, Sodium Benzoate, Sorbic Acid.

Directions: (Adults) Take one tablet two times daily with a glass of water. Take each day for best results.

Precautions: Use only as directed. Do not exceed recommended dose. As with any supplement, if you are taking a prescription product, or if you are pregnant or are nursing a baby, contact your physician before taking this product.

How Supplied: Bottles of 60 tablets.

CENTRUM FOCUSED FORMULAS HEART TABLETS
Dietary Supplement

Ingredients: Garlic Bulb Powder *Allium sativum,* dl-Alpha Tocopheryl Acetate, Microcrystalline Cellulose, Dibasic Calcium Phosphate, Gelatin, Taurine, Croscarmellose Sodium, Hydroxypropyl Methylcellulose, Starch, Calcium Silicate, Magnesium Stearate, Silicon Dioxide, Pyridoxine Hydrochloride, Coenzyme Q10, Titanium Dioxide, Polyethylene Glycol, Manganese Sulfate, Polysorbate 80, Sodium Citrate, Citric Acid, FD&C Red #40 Aluminum Lake, FD&C Blue #2 Aluminum Lake, Folic Acid, Cyanocobalamin, Sodium Benzoate, Sodium Selenate, Sorbic Acid.

Supplement Facts
Serving Size 1 Tablet

Amount Per Tablet		% DV
Vitamin E	200 IU	667%
Vitamin B6	5 mg	250%
Folic Acid	200 mcg	50%
Vitamin B12	200 mcg	3,333%
Selenium	25 mcg	36%
Manganese	1 mg	50%
Garlic Bulb Powder *Allium sativum*	300 mg	*
Taurine	33 mg	*
Coenzyme Q10	4 mg	*

*Daily Value (%DV) not established.

Directions: (Adults) Take one tablet two times daily with a glass of water. Take each day for best results.

Precautions: Use only as directed. Do not exceed recommended dose. As with any supplement, if you are taking a prescription product, or if you are pregnant or are nursing a baby, contact your physician before taking this product. KEEP THIS AND ALL DIETARY SUPPLEMENTS OUT OF THE REACH OF CHILDREN.

How Supplied: Bottles of 50 tablets.

CENTRUM FOCUSED FORMULAS MENTAL CLARITY TABLETS
Dietary Supplement

Ingredients: Dibasic Calcium Phosphate, Microcrystalline Cellulose, Ginkgo Biloba Standardized Leaf Extract *Ginkgo biloba,* dl-Alpha Tocopheryl Acetate, Choline Bitartrate, Hydroxypropyl Methylcellulose, Crospovidone, Niacinamide, Zinc Oxide, Calcium Pantothenate, Gelatin, Magnesium Stearate, Polyethylene Glycol, Silicon Dioxide, Calcium Silicate, FD&C Blue #2 Aluminum Lake, FD&C Red #40 Aluminum Lake, FD&C Yellow #6 Aluminum Lake, Polysorbate 80, Titanium Dioxide, Pyridoxine Hydrochloride, Riboflavin, Thiamin Mononitrate, Folic Acid, Starch, Citric Acid, Sodium Citrate, Cyanocobalamin, Sodium Benzoate, Sorbic Acid.

Supplement Facts:
Serving Size 1 Tablet

Amount Per Tablet		% DV
Vitamin E	20 IU	67%
Thiamin	0.55 mg	37%
Riboflavin	0.85 mg	50%
Niacin	10 mg	50%
Vitamin B6	1 mg	50%
Folic Acid	200 mg	50%
Vitamin B12	3 mcg	50%
Pantothenic Acid	5 mg	50%
Zinc	7.5 mg	50%
Ginkgo Biloba Standardized Leaf Extract *Ginkgo biloba*	60 mg	*
Choline	8 mg	*

*Daily Value (%DV) not established.

Directions: (Adults) Take one tablet two times daily with a glass of water. Take each day for best results.

Warnings: KEEP THIS AND ALL DIETARY SUPPLEMENTS OUT OF THE REACH OF CHILDREN. STORE IN A COOL DRY PLACE. KEEP BOTTLE TIGHTLY CLOSED.

How Supplied: Bottles of 60 tablets.

CENTRUM® FOCUSED FORMULA PROSTATE SOFTGELS
Dietary Supplement

Supplement Facts
Serving Size 1 Softgel

Amount Per Softgel		% DV
Vitamin A (as beta-carotene)	5,000 IU	100%
Lycopene	1.5 mg	*
Saw Palmetto Standard Lipophilic Fruit Extract *Serenoa repens*	160 mg	*

*Daily Value (%DV) not established.

Ingredients: Softgel Shell (Gelatin, Glycerin, Purified Water, Colors: Caramel, Titanium Dioxide, Carmine), Vege-

table Oil, Saw Palmetto Standardized Lipophilic Fruit Extract *Serenoa repens,* Tomato Oleoresin (providing Lycopene), Corn Oil, Beta-Carotene, dl-Alpha Tocopherol.

Directions: (Adult Males) Take one softgel two times daily with a glass of water. Take each day for best results.

Precautions: Use only as directed. Do not exceed recommended dose. On rare occasions, mild stomach upset may occur. If this happens, try taking with food. If you are taking a prescription product or undergoing medical treatment for the prostate or are experiencing a prostate problem, contact a physician before taking this product.
STORE IN A COOL DRY PLACE. KEEP BOTTLE TIGHTLY CLOSED.

How Supplied: Bottles of 50 softgels.

CENTRUM® HERBALS:
CENTRUM ECHINACEA
CENTRUM GINKGO BILOBA
CENTRUM GINSENG
CENTRUM SAW PALMETTO
CENTRUM ST. JOHN'S WORT

See Whitehall-Robins Healthcare

CENTRUM® KIDS™ COMPLETE
[sĕn-trŭm]
Rugrats®
Children's Chewable
Vitamin/Mineral Formula

[See table above]

Suggested Use: Children 2 and 3 years of age, chew approximately ½ tablet daily with food. Adults and children 4 years of age and older, chew 1 tablet daily with food.

Contains Aspartame. **Phenylketonurics: Contains Phenylalanine.

> **Warning:** Accidental overdose of iron-containing products is a leading cause of fatal poisoning in children under 6. Keep this product out of reach of children. In case of accidental overdose, call a doctor or poison control center immediately.

Ingredients: Sucrose, Dibasic Calcium Phosphate, Mannitol, Calcium Carbonate, Stearic Acid, Starch, Magnesium Oxide, Ascorbic Acid (Vit. C), Microcrystalline Cellulose, dl-Alpha Tocopheryl Acetate (Vit. E), Niacinamide, Zinc Oxide, Ferronyl Iron, Calcium Pantothenate, Manganese Sulfate, Pyridoxine Hydrochloride (Vit. B_6), Vitamin A Acetate, Cupric Oxide, Riboflavin (Vit. B_2), Thiamin Mononitrate (Vit. B_1), Beta Carotene, Folic Acid, Potassium Iodide, Chromium Chloride, Sodium Molybdate, Biotin, Ergocalciferol (Vit. D_2), Phytonadione (Vit. K_1), Cyanocobalamin (Vit. B_{12}). Contains less than 2% of the following: Acacia Gum, Ascorbyl Palmitate, Aspartame**, Butylated Hydroxytoluene (BHT), Carra-

Supplement Facts:

Serving Size	½ Tablet	1 Tablet
Amount Per Tablet	%DV for Children 2 and 3 Years (1/2Tablet)	%DV for Adults and Children 4 and Older (1Tablet)
Total Carbohydrate <1g	†	<1%*
Vitamin A 5000 IU (20% as Beta Carotene)	100%	100%
Vitamin C 60 mg	75%	100%
Vitamin D 400 IU	50%	100%
Vitamin E 30 IU	150%	100%
Vitamin K 10 mcg	†	13%
Thiamin 1.5 mg	107%	100%
Riboflavin 1.7 mg	106%	100%
Niacin 20 mg	111%	100%
Vitamin B_6 2 mg	143%	100%
Folic Acid 400 mcg	100%	100%
Vitamin B_{12} 6 mcg	100%	100%
Biotin 45 mcg	15%	15%
Pantothenic Acid 10 mg	100%	100%
Calcium 108 mg	7%	11%
Iron 18 mg	90%	100%
Phosphorous 50 mg	3%	5%
Iodine 150 mcg	107%	100%
Magnesium 40 mg	10%	10%
Zinc 15 mg	94%	100%
Copper 2 mg	100%	100%
Manganese 1 mg	†	50%
Chromium 20 mcg	†	17%
Molybdenum 20 mcg	+	27%

†Daily Value (%DV) not established.
*Percent Daily Values are based on a 2,000 calorie diet.

geenan, Citric Acid, dl-Alpha Tocopherol, FD&C Blue #2 Aluminum Lake, FD&C Red #40 Aluminum Lake, FD&C Yellow #6 Aluminum Lake, Gelatin, Glucose, Guar Gum, Lactose, Magnesium Stearate, Malic Acid, Maltodextrin, Mono and Diglycerides, Natural and Artificial Flavors, Potassium Sorbate, Silicon Dioxide, Sodium Aluminum Silicate, Sodium Ascorbate, Sodium Benzoate, Sodium Citrate, Sorbic Acid, Tribasic Calcium Phosphate, Vanillin, Water. May also contain less than 2% of the following: Dextrose, Fructose.

How Supplied: Assorted Flavors—Uncoated Tablet—Bottle of 60 tablets
Also available as: Centrum® Kids™ + Extra C (250 mg); and as: **Centrum® Kids™ + Extra Calcium** (200 mg). Storage: Store at Room Temperature. Keep bottle tightly closed.
© 1999

CENTRUM® PERFORMANCE MULTIVITAMIN-MULTIMINERAL Tablets

Dietary Supplement with Ginseng and Gingko Biloba

Supplement Facts
Serving Size 1 Tablet

Each Tablet Contains	%DV
Vitamin A 5000 IU (20% as Beta Carotene)	100%
Vitamin C 120 mg	200%
Vitamin D 400 IU	100%
Vitamin E 60 IU	200%
Vitamin K 25 mcg	31%

Centrum Performance—Cont.

Thiamin 4.5 mg		300%
Riboflavin 5.1 mg		300%
Niacin 40 mg		200%
Vitamin B₆ 6 mg		300%
Folic Acid 400 mcg		100%
Vitamin B₁₂ 18 mcg		300%
Biotin 40 mcg		13%
Pantothenic Acid 10 mg		100%
Calcium 100 mg		10%
Iron 18 mg		100%
Phosphorus 48 mg		5%
Iodine 150 mcg		100%
Magnesium 40 mg		10%
Zinc 15 mg		100%
Selenium 70 mcg		100%
Copper 2 mg		100%
Manganese 4 mg		200%
Chromium 120 mcg		100%
Molybdenum 75 mcg		100%
Chloride 72 mg		2%
Potassium 80 mg		2%
Ginseng Root (Panax ginseng) 50 mg Standardized Extract		*
Ginkgo Biloba Leaf (Ginkgo biloba) 60 mg Standardized Extract		*
Boron 60 mcg		*
Nickel 5 mcg		*
Silicon 4 mg		*
Tin 10 mcg		*
Vanadium 10 mcg		*

*Daily Value (%DV) not established.

Ingredients: Dibasic Calcium Phosphate, Potassium Chloride, Ascorbic Acid (Vit. C), Microcrystalline Cellulose, Calcium Carbonate, dl-Alpha Tocopheryl Acetate (Vit. E), Magnesium Oxide, Ginkgo Biloba Leaf (*Ginkgo biloba*) Standardized Extract, Gelatin, Ginseng Root (*Panax ginseng*) Standardized Extract, Ferrous Fumarate, Niacinamide, Crospovidone, Starch, Zinc Oxide, Calcium Pantothenate, Silicon Dioxide, Manganese Sulfate, Pyridoxine Hydrochloride (Vit B₆), Riboflavin (Vit. B₂), Thiamin Mononitrate (Vit. B₁), Cupric Oxide, Vitamin A Acetate, Beta Carotene, Chromium Chloride, Folic Acid, Potassium Iodide, Sodium Selenate, Sodium Molybdate, Boron, Biotin, Phytonadione (Vit K₁), Sodium Metavanadate, Nickelous Sulfate, Stannous Chloride, Cyanocobalamin (Vit. B₁₂), Ergocalciferol (Vit. D₂). Contains less than 2% of the following: Acacia Gum, Ascorbyl Palmitate, Butylated Hydroxytoluene (BHT), Citric Acid, dl-Alpha Tocopherol (Vit. E), FD&C Red No. 40 Aluminum Lake, FD&C Yellow No. 6 Aluminum Lake, Glucose, Hydroxypropyl Methylcellulose, Lactose, Magnesium Stearate, Polyethylene Glycol, Polysorbate 80, Potassium Sorbate, Sodium Aluminum Silicate, Sodium Ascorbate, Sodium Benzoate, Sodium Citrate, Sorbic Acid, Sucrose, Titanium Dioxide, Tribasic Calcium Phosphate, Water. May also contain Maltodextrin.

Suggested Use: Adults—One tablet daily with food.

Warning: Accidental overdose of iron-containing products is a leading cause of fatal poisoning in children under 6. Keep this product out of reach of children. In case of accidental overdose, call a doctor or poison control center immediately.

Precaution: As with any supplement, if you are taking a prescription medication, or if you are pregnant or nursing a baby, contact your physician before using this product.
Store at room temperature. Keep bottle tightly closed. Bottle sealed with printed foil under cap. Do not use if foil is torn.

How Supplied: Bottles of 75, 120, & 180 Tablets.

CENTRUM® SILVER®
Multivitamin/Multimineral Dietary Supplement for Adults 50+ From A to Zinc®

**Supplement Facts
Serving Size 1 Tablet**

Each Tablet Contains	%DV
Vitamin A 5000 IU (20% as Beta Carotene)	100%
Vitamin C 60 mg	100%
Vitamin D 400 IU	100%
Vitamin E 45 IU	150%
Vitamin K 10 mcg	12%
Thiamin 1.5 mg	100%
Riboflavin 1.7 mg	100%
Niacin 20 mg	100%
Vitamin B₆ 3 mg	150%
Folic Acid 400 mcg	100%
Vitamin B₁₂ 25 mcg	417%
Biotin 30 mcg	10%
Pantothenic Acid 10 mg	100%
Calcium 200 mg	20%
Phosphorus 20 mg	2%
Iodine 150 mcg	100%
Magnesium 100 mg	25%
Zinc 15 mg	100%
Copper 2 mg	100%
Potassium 80 mg	2%
Selenium 20 mcg	29%
Manganese 2 mg	100%
Chromium 150 mcg	125%
Molybdenum 75 mcg	100%
Chloride 72 mg	2%
Nickel 5 mcg	*
Silicon 2 mg	*
Vanadium 10 mcg	*
Boron 150 mcg	*
Lutein 250 mcg	*

*Daily Value (% DV) not established.

Recommended Intake:
Adults, 1 tablet daily with food.

Warning: Keep out of the reach of children.

Ingredients: Calcium Carbonate, Magnesium Oxide, Potassium Chloride, Microcrystalline Cellulose, Dibasic Calcium Phosphate, Ascorbic Acid (Vit. C), Starch, dl-Alpha Tocopheryl Acetate (Vit. E), Gelatin, Crospovidone, Niacinamide, Zinc Oxide, Calcium Pantothenate, Silicon Dioxide, Manganese Sulfate, Pyridoxine Hydrochloride (Vit. B₆), Cupric Oxide, Vitamin A Acetate, Riboflavin (Vit. B₂), Thiamin Mononitrate (Vit. B₁), Chromium Chloride, Borates, Beta Carotene, Folic Acid, Lutein, Potassium Iodide, Sodium Molybdate, Sodium Selenate, Biotin, Cyanocobalamin (Vit. B₁₂), Sodium Metavanadate, Nickelous Sulfate, Phytonadione (Vit. K), Ergocalciferol (Vit. D₂). Contains less than 2% of the following: Acacia Gum, Ascorbyl Palmitate, Butylated Hydroxytoluene (BHT), Calcium Stearate, Citric Acid, FD&C Blue No. 2 Aluminum Lake, FD&C Red No. 40 Aluminum Lake, FD&C Yellow No. 6 Aluminum Lake, Hydroxypropyl Methylcellulose, Magnesium Stearate, Polysorbate 80, Potassium Sorbate, Sodium Aluminum Silicate, Sodium Ascorbate, Sodium Benzoate, Sodium Citrate, Sorbic Acid, Sucrose, Titanium Dioxide, Triethyl Citrate. May also contain: Lactose.

How Supplied: Bottles of 50, 100, 150, and 220 tablets
Storage: Store at Room Temperature. Keep bottle tightly closed. Bottle is sealed with printed foil under cap. Do not use if foil is torn.
© 1999

Legacy® for Life
P.O. BOX 2522
MELBOURNE, FL 32902-2522

Direct Inquiries to:
1.800.557.8477
www.legacyusa.com

BIOCHOICE
BIOCHOICE IMMUNE²⁶
BIOCHOICE IMMUNE SUPPORT

Description: BioChoice® is a powdered, pure egg product derived from hens hyperimmunized with >26 killed enteric pathogens of human origin. (Organisms such as: *Shigella, Staphylococcus, Escherichia coli, Salmonella, Pseu-*

domonas, *Klebsiella pneumoniae, Haemophilis,* and *Streptococcus* are included in the inoculum.)

Clinical Background: Upon oral administration, BioChoice's specific immunoglobulins and immunomodulatory factors are passively transferred.

BioChoice has the following *documented* structure and function claims: • Balances and supports the immune system • Helps the body modulate autoimmune responses • Helps maintain digestive tract health • Helps maintain flexible and healthy joints • Helps maintain cardiovascular function, a healthy circulatory system and healthy levels of cholesterol • Helps increase energy levels.

How Supplied: BioChoice is available as BioChoice Immune[26] ("hyperimmune" egg) in powder and capsule form and as BioChoice Immune Support when enriched with minerals, and 100% of the daily value of more than 13 essential vitamins.

Precautions: Those with known allergies to eggs should consult with a health practitioner before consuming this product.

Note: BioChoice is not intended to diagnose, treat, cure, or prevent any disease. These statements have not been evaluated by the Food and Drug Administration.

Shown in Product Identification Guide, page 508

Mannatech, Inc.

**600 S. ROYAL LANE
SUITE 200
COPPELL, TX 75019**

For Medical Professional Inquiries Contact:
Kia Gary, RN LNCC
(972) 471-8189
Kgary@mannatech.com

Direct Inquiries to:
Customer Service
(972) 471-8111

Product Information:
www.mannatech.com

Ingredient Information:
www.glycoscience.com

Ambrotose®
A Glyconutritional Dietary Supplement

Supplement Facts:
Serving Size 0.44 g (approx. ¼ teaspoon)
Powder canister: 100 g or 50 g

Amount Per Serving	% Daily Value
0.44 g	*

Ambrotose powder
(patent pending)
Arabinogalactan (*Larix decidua*) (gum), Rice starch, Aloe vera extract, (inner leaf gel) - Manapol® powder, Ghatti (*Anogeissus latifolia*)(gum), Glucosamine HCl, Tragacanth (*Astragalus gummifer*) (gum).

*Daily Values not established.

Ambrotose capsules

Supplement Facts:
Serving Size: one to two capsules
Capsules per container: 60

Amount Per Serving	% Daily Value
1–2 capsules	*

Ambrotose capsules
(patent pending)
Arabinogalactan (*Larix decidua*) (gum), Rice starch, Aloe vera extract, (inner leaf gel) - Manapol® powder, Ghatti (*Anogeissus latifolia*)(gum), Tragacanth (*Astragalus gummifer*) (gum).

*Daily Values not established.

Ambrotose® with Lecithin

Supplement Facts:
Serving Size: one to two capsules
Capsules per container: 60

Amount Per Serving	% Daily Value
1–2 capsules	*

Ambrotose with Lecithin capsules
(patent pending)
Arabinogalactan (*Larix decidua*) (gum), Rice starch, Aloe vera extract, (inner leaf gel) - Manapol® powder, Ghatti (*Anogeissus latifolia*)(gum), Tragacanth (*Astragalus gummifer*) (gum).
Other ingredients: Calcium, lecithin powder

*Daily Values not established.

For additional information on ingredients, visit www.glycoscience.com

Use: Ambrotose complex is a proprietary formula designed to help provide saccharides used in glycoconjugate synthesis** to promote proper cellular communication and immune support. Consumers who are healthy may notice improved concentration, more energy, better sleep, improved athletic performance, and a greater sense of well-being. Those who have health challenges may discern improvements in specific signs and symptoms.

Directions: The recommended intake of Ambrotose powder is ¼ teaspoon one or two times a day; the recommended intake of Ambrotose capsules or Ambrotose with Lecithin is one or two capsules two to three times a day. Begin by taking the lowest amount recommended on the labels. If well tolerated, you may take larger amounts. As a blend of plant saccharides, Ambrotose complex is safe in amounts well in excess of the label recommendations. Children between the ages of 12 and 48 months with growth/nutritional problems (failure to thrive) have been given 1 tablespoon a day of Ambrotose powder for 3 months with no adverse effects. Individuals have reported taking as much as 10 tablespoons of Ambrotose powder (approx. 50 grams) each day for several months with no adverse effects. The amount needed by each individual may vary with time, age, genetic makeup, metabolic rate, and activities, stress level, current dietary intake, and health challenges of the moment. A health care professional experienced with use of Ambrotose complex may be helpful.

Warning: Anyone who is taking medication may wish to advise his/her physician. Diabetics who take Ambrotose complex should regularly monitor glucose levels and make necessary adjustments to their diabetes medications accordingly. One teaspoon of Ambrotose powder (equivalent to 12 Ambrotose capsules) contains the amount of glucose equivalent to $1/25$ teaspoon of sucrose (table sugar).

KEEP BOTTLE TIGHTLY CLOSED. STORE IN A COOL, DRY PLACE.

How Supplied: Bottle of 3.50 oz (100 g) powder. Bottle of 1.75 oz (50 g) powder. Bottle of 60 (150 mg) capsules.

**This statement has not been evaluated by the Food and Drug Administration. This product is not intended to diagnose, treat, cure or prevent any disease.

Mannatech Inc.
600 S. Royal Lane, Suite 200
Coppell, Texas 75019
www.mannatech.com
Shown in Product Identification Guide, page 508

PhytAloe® with Ambrotose® Complex
A Dietary Supplement of Dried Fruits and Vegetables

Supplement Facts
Serving size: 1 capsule or ¼ teaspoon
Capsules per container: 60 capsules
Powder canister: 3.5 oz. (100 g)

Amount Per Serving:	% Daily Value
PhytAloe 490 mg	*
Ambrotose complex 50 mg	*

Broccoli, Brussels sprout, cabbage, carrot, cauliflower, garlic, kale, onion, tomato, turnip, papaya, pineapple.
Ambrotose complex, naturally occurring plant polysaccharides including freeze-dried Aloe vera (inner leaf gel extract) - Manapol® powder.

* Percent Daily Values not established.

Other ingredients: Magnesium stearate.

This product contains no sugar, starch, preservatives, synthetic colorants or chemical stabilizers.

Use: PhytAloe is a blend of dehydrated fruits and vegetables in combination

Continued on next page

Phytaloe—Cont.

with Ambrotose complex for immune system support.** PhytAloe contains no synthetic additives and is supplied as powder and as capsules.

Directions: The recommended intake of PhytAloe powder is ¼ teaspoon twice a day; the recommended intake of PhytAloe capsules is one capsule twice a day. PhytAloe can be taken in amounts in excess of that recommended on the label.

Warnings: If any one of the fruits or vegetables in PhytAloe has caused stomach upset or any other adverse reaction in the past, start at the lowest recommended amount and gradually increase as tolerated. Individuals who are undergoing radiation therapy may wish to consult with their physicians.
KEEP BOTTLE TIGHTLY CLOSED. STORE IN A COOL, DRY PLACE.

How Supplied: Bottle of 60 capsules. Bottle of 3.5 oz. (100 g) powder.

> ****This statement has not been evaluated by the Food and Drug Administration. This product is not intended to diagnose, treat, cure or prevent any disease.**

Shown in Product Identification Guide, page 508

PLUS with Ambrotose® Complex Dietary Supplement Caplets

Supplement Facts
Serving Size - 1 Caplet

	Amount per Serving	% Daily Value
Iron	1 mg	5
Wild Yam (root)	200 mg	*
Standardized for	25 mg phytosterols	
L-Glutamic acid	200 mg	*
L-Glycine	200 mg	*
L-Lysine	200 mg	*
L-Arginine	100 mg	*
Beta Sitosterol	25 mg	*
Ambrotose® Complex (patent pending)	2.5 mg	*

Naturally occurring plant polysaccharides including freeze-dried Aloe vera inner gel extract-Manapol®powder.

Other ingredients: Microcrystalline cellulose, silicon dioxide, croscarmellose sodium, magnesium stearate, titanium dioxide coating.

* Daily value not established

For additional information on ingredients, visit www.glycoscience.com

Use: PLUS caplets provide nutrients to help support the endocrine system's natural production and balance of hormones. A well-functioning endocrine system works in harmony with the body's immune system, helps support the efficient metabolism of fat, and supports natural recovery from physical or emotional stress.** The functional components of PLUS caplets are wild yam extract, amino acids, and beta sitosterol. PLUS caplets contain no hormones.

Directions: The recommended intake of PLUS caplets is one to three caplets per day. Start with one caplet a day for a week. For many people, this is enough. Others may want to increase to two or three a day. Some people take as many as five or six caplets a day, and some take twice that amount. As with all dietary supplements, pay attention to how you feel as you increase intake of PLUS. Take the amount that gives you the best response.

Warning: After an extensive review of the literature, no documented evidence was found linking the ingredients in PLUS caplets with any form of human cancer or with any problems associated with pregnancy. However, as with all supplements, you should consult your health care professional if you are pregnant.
KEEP BOTTLE TIGHTLY CLOSED. STORE IN A COOL, DRY PLACE.

How Supplied: Bottle of 90 caplets.

> ****This statement has not been evaluated by the Food and Drug Administration. This product is not intended to diagnose, treat, cure or prevent any disease.**

Shown in Product Identification Guide, page 508

Matol Botanical International, Ltd.

**1111, 46th AVENUE
LACHINE QUEBEC,
CANADA H8T 3C5**

Direct Inquiries to:
Ph: (800) 363-3890
website: www.matol.com

BIOMUNE OSF™ PLUS
Dietary supplement for immune system support

Description: Biomune OSF™ Plus is an immune system support product for all ages. Biomune OSF™ Plus is a combination of a special extract of antigen infused colostrum and whey with the herb Astragalus. The exclusive colostrum/whey extract (Ai/E^{10}™) is prepared using patented and proprietary process unique to the nutritional industry. Astragalus is a traditional Chinese herb that is known for its immune enhancing properties. Clinical studies show that Biomune OSF™ Plus is effective in consistently and dramatically increasing Natural Killer cell activity. Medical research has shown that low NK cell activity is present in most illness. A double blind study with antigen infused dialyzable bovine colostrum/whey shows its effectiveness as an immune system modulator.

Summary of clinical studies:
The Use of Dialyzable Bovine Colostrum/Whey Extract in Conjunction with a Holistic Treatment Model for Natural Killer Cell Stimulation in Chronic Illness by Jesse A. Stoff, MD
This clinical study consists of 107 patients with an average treatment time of 13.2 months. The average initial Natural Killer (NK) cell activity was 18 Lytic Units (LU) and the average final NK cell activity 246 LU. All patients in the study greatly improved, went into remission or recovered.
Conclusions: The Study Group demonstrated that increased NK activity paralleled restored resistance to illness and recovery from illness.
An Examination of Immune Response Modulation in Humans by Antigen Infused Dialyzable Bovine Colostrum/Whey Extract Utilizing a Double Blind Study by Jesse A. Stoff, MD.
This study provides double blind evidence that the cytokines, peptide neurohormones and other informational molecules in Antigen Infused Dialyzable Bovine Colostrum/Whey Extract modulate and normalize immune function. Further, Antigen Infused Dialyzable Bovine Colostrum/Whey Extract demonstrates its effectiveness as a Biological Immune Response Modulator for increasing the protective functions of the immune system.
Both studies are available from Matol Botanical International, Ltd. upon request.

Use: Dietary Supplement

Directions for Use: Take one capsule daily for maintenance and one or two capsules every 2–3 hours when additional immune support is needed. The product can be taken daily for maintenance or as above for extended periods of time. There is no known toxicity.

How Supplied: One bottle contains 30 capsules.
Shown in Product Identification Guide, page 508

Mayor Pharmaceutical Laboratories

**2401 S. 24TH ST.
PHOENIX, AZ 85034**

Direct Inquiries to:
Medical Director
(602) 244-8899

www.vitamist.com

VITAMIST® Intra-Oral Spray
[vīt '-ə-mĭst]
Nutraceuticals/Dietary Supplements

DESCRIPTION
VitaMist® products are patented, intra-oral sprays for the delivery of vitamins, minerals, and other nutritional supplements, directly into the oral cavity. A 55 microliter spray delivers high concentrations of nutrients directly onto the mouth's sensitive tissue. The buccal mucosa transfers the nutrients into the bloodstream. (U.S. Patent 4,525,341—Foreign patents issued and pending.)

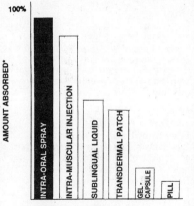

METHOD OF DELIVERY

*Representative of the product class.

Benefits:
- Spray supplementation provides an absorption rate approximately nine times greater than that of pills.
- Once the formula is sprayed into the mouth, the nutrients reach the bloodstream within minutes.
- No fillers or binders are added; the body receives only pure ingredients.
- An alternative method of supplementation for those that cannot take pills, or simply do not enjoy swallowing pills.
- Convenient administration; no water needed.

PRODUCT OVERVIEW
Multiple: vitamins and minerals in three separate formulations: adult, children's, and prenatal.
C+Zinc: with vitamin E and the amino acids L-lysine and glycine.
B12: contains 1000% of the US RDI of vitamin B12.
Stress: herbal formula with B vitamins.
St. John's Wort: St. John's wort extract with vitamin B12, ginkgo biloba, kava kava and folic acid.

E+Selenium: contains vitamin E and selenomethionine.
Anti-Oxidant: with vitamins A, C, E, niacin, folate, and beta-carotene.
VitaSight®: with vitamins A, C and E, beta-carotene, zinc, selenium, bilberry, lutein, and ginkgo biloba.
Colloidal Minerals: more than 70 trace and essential minerals from natural sources.
Smoke-Less™: herbal combination with additional nutrients designed to reduce cravings.
PMS and LadyMate: supplementation for the nutritional needs of pre-menstrual syndrome.
Folacin: vitamins B6 and B12 added to folate (folic acid).
Slender-Mist®: dietary snack supplements containing a combination of B vitamins, hydroxy-citric acid, L-carnitine and chromium. Four different flavors.
Blue-Green Sea Spray: spirulina extract, additional omega 3 fatty acids from flaxseed oil, and vitamin E.
Re-Leaf: a blend of more than 10 herbs that are recommended for minor discomfort, anxiety, and stress.
Osteo-CalMag: herbal supplement with additional vitamin D, calcium and magnesium.
Pine Bark and Grape Seed: powerful proanthocyanidins (anti-oxidants) from natural sources, with additional B vitamins.
1-Before, 2-During, 3-After: three performance sprays designed for the needs of physical activity.
CardioCare™: with vitamins C and E, the amino acids L-lysine and L-proline, coenzyme Q10 and additional herbal extracts.
Melatonin: a natural hormone that is effective in re-establishing sleep patterns.
DHEA: dehydroepiandrosterone in both men's and women's formulations.
Revitalizer®: high levels of B vitamins, as well as vitamins A and E, the amino acids L-cysteine and glycine, and selenium.
GinkgoMist™: with ginkgo biloba, vitamin B12, acetyl-L-carnitine, choline, inositol, phosphatidylserine and niacin.
ArthriFlex™: with chondroitin sulfate, glucosamine sulfate, vitamins C and D, calcium, manganese, boron and dong quai.
VitaMotion-S™: dimenhydrinate with ginger and vitamin B6.
Echinacea +G: stimulation for the immune system provided from echinacea, goldenseal and garlic extracts, together with honey and lemon.
Ex. O: powerful blend of cayenne and peppermint with additional herbs recommended for allergy control.

HOW SUPPLIED
VitaMist dietary supplements are supplied in sealed containers fitted with a natural pump. Each container provides a 30-day supply.

RECOMMENDED DOSAGE
Two sprays, four times per day, for a total dosage of eight sprays per day.

McNeil Consumer Healthcare

**Division of McNeil-PPC, Inc.
FORT WASHINGTON, PA 19034**

Direct Inquiries to:
Consumer Relationship Center
Fort Washington, PA 19034
(215) 273-7000

AFLEXA™ Glucosamine Tablets

Description: Aflexa is a dietary supplement containing glucosamine a natural building block of healthy cartilage. Each *AFLEXA™ Tablet* contains 340 mg of glucosamine (300 mg glucosamine sulfate and 200 mg glucosamine hydrochloride).

Actions: Taken daily, *AFLEXA™* offers a number of valuable benefits:
- Helps maintain lubricating fluid in joints*
- Promotes joint flexibility and range of motion*
- Provides a natural building block of healthy cartilage*
- Promotes comfortable joint function*

Uses: *AFLEXA™* is intended to help maintain healthy cartilage in people whose joints may be affected by the natural aging process.

Precautions: Do not use if you are allergic to shellfish. If you are pregnant or breast-feeding, ask your doctor before use. Use only as directed. Keep out of reach of children.

Directions: Take one tablet three times a day. Benefits may begin within 2–4 weeks of daily use.

Ingredients: GLUCOSAMINE SULFATE, GLUCOSAMINE HYDROCHLORIDE, CELLULOSE, HYDROXYPROPYL METHYLCELLULOSE, POLYETHYLENE GLYCOL, SILICON DIOXIDE, PROPYLENE GLYCOL, CROSPOVIDONE, HYDROXYPROPYL CELLULOSE, TITANIUM DIOXIDE, MAGNESIUM STEARATE, POLYSORBATE 80, POVIDONE.

How Supplied: *AFLEXA™* is available in bottles of 50, 110 and 250.
Store at room temperature.
DO NOT USE IF CARTON IS OPENED OR IF NECK WRAP OR FOIL INNER SEAL IS BROKEN OR MISSING.

---

* These Statements Have Not Been Evaluated By The Food & Drug Administration. This Product Is Not Intended To Diagnose, Treat, Cure Or Prevent Any Disease.

Shown in Product Identification Guide, page 508

Continued on next page

LACTAID® Original Strength Caplets
(lactase enzyme)
LACTAID® Extra Strength Caplets
(lactase enzyme)
LACTAID® Ultra Caplets and Chewable Tablets
(lactase enzyme)

Description: Each *LACTAID® Original Strength Caplet* contains 3000 FCC (Food Chemical Codex) units of lactase enzyme (derived from *Aspergillus oryzae*).
Each *LACTAID® Extra Strength Caplet* contains 4500 FCC units of lactase enzyme (derived from *Aspergillus oryzae*).
Each *LACTAID® Ultra Caplet* contains 9000 FCC units of lactase enzyme (derived from *Aspergillus oryzae*).
Each *LACTAID® Ultra Chewable Tablet* contains 9000 FCC units of lactase enzyme (derived from *Aspergillus oryzae*).
LACTAID® is the original lactase dietary supplement that makes milk and dairy foods more digestible. *LACTAID®* lactase enzyme hydrolyzes lactose into two digestible simple sugars: glucose and galactose. *LACTAID® Caplets* are taken orally for *in vivo* hydrolysis of lactose.

Actions: *LACTAID® Caplets/Chewable Tablets* work to naturally replenish lactase enzyme that aids in dairy food digestion. Lactase enzyme hydrolyzes lactose sugar (a double sugar) into its simple sugar components, glucose and galactose.

Uses: Lactaid contains a natural enzyme that helps your body break down lactose, the complex sugar found in dairy foods. If not properly digested, lactose can cause gas, bloating, cramps or diarrhea.*

*This statement has not been evaluated by the Food and Drug Administration. This product is not intended to diagnose, treat, cure, or prevent any disease.

Directions: Original Strength: Swallow or chew 3 caplets with the first bite of dairy food. For best results, you may have to adjust the number of caplets up or down. **Extra Strength:** Swallow or chew 2 caplets with first bite of dairy food. For best results, you may have to adjust the number of caplets up or down. **Ultra Caplets:** Swallow 1 caplet with the first bite of dairy food. If you suffer from severe digestive discomfort, you may have to take more than one caplet, but no more than two at a time. **Ultra Chewables:** Chew and swallow 1 chewable tablet with your first bite of dairy food. If you suffer from severe digestive discomfort, you may have to take more than one tablet but no more than two at a time. Don't be discouraged if at first Lactaid does not work to your satisfaction. Because the degree of enzyme deficiency naturally varies from person to person and from food to food, you may have to adjust the number of caplets/chewable tablets up or down to find your own level

of comfort. Since Lactaid Caplets/Chewable Tablets work only on the food as you eat it, use them every time you enjoy dairy foods.

Warnings: Consult your doctor if you experience any symptoms which are unusual or seem unrelated to the condition for which you took this product. **Do not use if carton is open or if printed plastic neckwrap is broken or if single serve packet is open.**
LACTAID® Ultra Chewable Tablets: Contains Phenylalanine 0.49 mg/tablet

Ingredients: *LACTAID® Original Strength Caplets:* Mannitol, Cellulose, Lactase Enzyme (3,000 FCC Lactase units/Caplet), Dextrose, Sodium Citrate, Magnesium Stearate.
LACTAID® Extra Strength Caplets: Lactase Enzyme (4,500 FCC Lactase units/Caplet), Mannitol, Cellulose, Dextrose, Sodium Citrate, Magnesium Stearate.
LACTAID® Ultra Caplets: Cellulose, Lactase Enzyme (9,000 FCC Lactase units/Caplet), Dextrose, Sodium Citrate, Magnesium Stearate, Colloidal Silicon Dioxide. *LACTAID® Ultra Chewable Tablets:* Mannitol, Cellulose, Lactase Enzyme (9,000 FCC Lactase units/tablet), Sodium Citrate, Dextrose, Magnesium Stearate, Flavor, Citric Acid, Acesulfame K, Aspartame.

How Supplied: *LACTAID® Original Strength Caplets* are available in bottles of 120 count. Store at or below room temperature (below 77°F) but do not refrigerate. Keep away from heat. *LACTAID® Extra Strength Caplets* are available in bottles of 50 count. Store at or below room temperature (below 77°F) but do not refrigerate. *LACTAID® Ultra Caplets* are available in single serve packets in 12, 32, 60 and 90 count packages. Store at or below room temperature (below 77°F) but do not refrigerate. *LACTAID® Ultra Chewable Tablets* are available in bottles of 12 and 32 counts. Store at or below room temperature (below 77°F), but do not refrigerate. Keep away from heat and moisture.
LACTAID® Caplets and *LACTAID® Ultra Chewable Tablets* are certified kosher from the Orthodox Union.
Also available: 70% lactose-reduced Lactaid Milk and 100% lactose-reduced Lactaid Milk.

Shown in Product Identification Guide, page 509

LACTAID® Drops
(lactase enzyme)

Description:
LACTAID® is the original dairy digestive supplement that makes milk more digestible. *LACTAID® Drops* may be added to milk for *in vitro* hydrolysis of lactose.
LACTAID® Drops contain sufficient lactase enzyme (derived from *Kluyveromyces lactis*) to hydrolyze lactose in milk.

Actions:
LACTAID® Drops are a liquid form of the natural lactase enzyme that makes

milk more digestible. The lactase enzyme hydrolyzes the lactose sugar (a double sugar) into its simple sugar components, glucose and galactose.

Uses:
Lactaid contains a natural enzyme that helps break down lactose, the complex sugar found in dairy foods. If not properly digested, lactose can cause gas, bloating, cramps or diarrhea.*

*This statement has not been evaluated by the Food and Drug Administraiton. This product is not intended to diagnose, treat, cure, or prevent any disease.

Directions:
Add 5–7 drops of *LACTAID® Drops* to a quart of milk, shake gently and refrigerate for 24 hours. Because sensitivity to lactose can vary, you may have to adjust the number of drops you use. If you are still experiencing discomfort after consuming milk with 5–7 *LACTAID® Drops* per quart, you may want to add 10 or even 15 drops per quart. Lactaid may be used with any kind of milk: whole, 1%, 2%, non-fat, skim, powdered and chocolate milk.

Warnings:
Consult your doctor: If you experience any symptoms which are unusual or seem unrelated to the condition for which you took this product. **Do not use if carton is opened, or if bottle wrap imprinted "Safety Seal®" is broken or missing.**

Ingredients:
Glycerin, Water, Lactase Enzyme.

How Supplied:
LACTAID® Drops are available in .22 fl. oz. (7 mL), (30 quart supply). Store at or below room temperature (below 77°F). Refrigerate after opening.
Lactaid Drops are certified kosher from the Orthodox Union.
Also available: 70% lactose-reduced Lactaid Milk and 100% lactose-reduced Lactaid Milk.

Shown in Product Identification Guide, page 509

Probiotica
Daily Dietary Supplement
(Lactobacillus reuteri)

Description: Each Probiotica Tablet contains 100 million cells of Lactobacillus reuteri.

Actions: Probiotica is intended to help people maintain gastrointestinal balance and promotes digestive function.* Probiotica helps maintain digestive health and balance by delivering "friendly" bacteria to the digestive system.
Taken daily, Probiotica offers many healthful benefits:
• Provides natural support for digestive health and function.*
• Helps maintain a healthy balance of bacteria in the digestive system.*
• Promotes digestive functioning and gastrointestinal health.*

* These statements have not been evaluated by the Food & Drug Administration. This product is not intended to diagnose, treat, cure or prevent any disease.

Uses: Probiotica is a dietary supplement containing Lactobacillus reuteri, a naturally occurring healthful bacteria that promotes digestive health, balance, and function.* Helps maintain a healthy balance of "friendly" bacteria in the digestive tract.*

Precautions: If you are pregnant or nursing a baby, ask your doctor before use. This product is not intended for use in children under the age of 2 years. Keep out of reach of children.

Directions: Take one tablet per day. Chew thoroughly before swallowing. Store in a cool, dry place. Use only as directed.

Ingredients: Lactobacillus reuteri, mannitol, xylitol, lactulose, mono- and diglycerides, malic acid, natural lemon flavor, zein (corn protein), riboflavin phosphate (for color).

How Supplied: Bottles of 60 and 90.
Shown in Product Identification Guide, page 510

Meyenberg Goat Milk Products

**P.O BOX 934
TURLOCK, CA 95381**

Direct Inquiries to:
209-667-2019
Toll Free: 800-343-1185
www.meyenberg.com
Medical professionals contact:
Carol Jones 209-667-2019

MEYENBERG GOAT MILK

Description: MEYENBERG GOAT MILK is natural milk that can often alleviate symptoms of cow and/or soymilk allergy due to its differences in protein and fatty acid structures. Goat milk is free of the controversial bovine growth hormone (BGH) used to increase milk production in dairy cows.

Uses: Adults and children with weak digestive systems and/or cow milk sensitivity. Goat milk is not a complete infant formula.

Ingredients: Goats milk, folic acid, vitamins A & D_3, disodium phosphate (ingredients vary by product form).

Directions: Evaporated goat milk—dilute with equal parts water; Powdered goat milk—mix 4 level Tbs. (2 scoops) powder to 8 ounces water; Aseptic, Fresh whole and 1% goat milk is ready to drink. These are *whole* milks. Special dilutions are needed for babies prior to weaning.

Warnings: Consult your medical professional if you have medically diagnosed cow milk allergy because goat milk and cow milk have many components in common to which you may be allergic. Do not feed to a baby under the age of 1 unless diluted and supplemented under the direction of a medical professional.

How Supplied: Evaporated in 12 fl. oz. cans; Powdered in 12 oz. cans; Aseptic, Whole and 1% in quart cartons. Refrigerate after opening
Kosher: Scroll K
For Information:
Meyenberg Goat Milk Products
(Jackson-Mitchell Inc.)
P.O. Box 934
Turlock, CA 95381
(209) 667-2019
TOLL FREE: (800) 343-1185
www.meyenberg.com
Medical professionals contact:
Carol Jones (209) 667-2019

Mission Pharmacal Company

**10999 IH 10 WEST
SUITE 1000
SAN ANTONIO, TX 78230-1355**

Direct Inquiries to:
PO Box 786099
San Antonio, TX 78278-6099
TOLL FREE: (800) 292-7364
(210) 696-8400
FAX: (210) 696-6010
**For Medical Information Contact:
In Emergencies:**
George Alexandrides
(830) 249-9822
FAX: (830) 816-2545

CITRACAL® Ⓤ
[sit'ra-cal]
Ultradense™ Calcium Citrate Dietary Supplement

Ingredients: Calcium (as Ultradense™ calcium citrate) 200 mg, polyethylene glycol, croscarmellose sodium, HPMC, color added, magnesium silicate, magnesium stearate.

Sensitive Patients: CITRACAL® contains no wheat, barley, yeast or rye; is sugar, dairy and gluten free and contains no artificial colors.

Directions: Take 1 to 2 tablets twice daily or as recommended by a physician, pharmacist or health professional.

Warning: Keep out of reach of children.

How Supplied: CITRACAL® is supplied as white, rectangular (nearly oval), coated tablets in bottles of 100 UPC 0178-0800-01, and bottles of 200 UPC 0178-0800-20.
Store at room temperature.
Ⓤ=Kosher Parvae approved by Orthodox Union.

CITRACAL® 250 MG + D
[sit 'ra-cal]
Ultradense™ Calcium Citrate-Vitamin D Dietary Supplement

Ingredients: Each tablet contains: calcium (as Ultradense™ calcium citrate) 250 mg., polyethylene glycol, citric acid, microcrystalline cellulose, HPMC, croscarmellose sodium, color added, magnesium silicate, magnesium stearate vitamin D_3 (62.5 IU).

How Supplied: CITRACAL® 250 MG + D is available in bottles of 150 tablets, UPC 0178-0837-15.

CITRACAL® Caplets + D
[sit ' ra-cal]
Ultradense™ Calcium Citrate-Vitamin D Dietary Supplement

CITRACAL® Caplets + D are supplied in an ultra-dense caplet formulation, each containing Vitamin D_3 (as cholecalciferol) 200 IU, and Calcium (as Ultradense™ calcium citrate) 315 mg.

Ingredients: calcium citrate, polyethylene glycol, croscarmellose sodium, HPMC, color added, magnesium silicate, magnesium stearate, vitamin D_3.

Directions: Take 1 to 2 caplets two times daily or as recommended by a physician, pharmacist or health professional.

Warning: Keep out of reach of children.

How Supplied: CITRACAL® Caplets + D are available in bottles of 60 UPC 0178-0815-60, and bottles of 120 UPC 0178-0815-12.
Store at room temperature.

CITRACAL® LIQUITAB® Ⓤ
[sit ´ ra-cal]
Calcium Citrate Effervescent Calcium Dietary Supplement

Ingredients: CITRACAL® LIQUITAB® is supplied as effervescent tablets each containing calcium (as calcium citrate) 500 mg, citric acid, adipic acid, saccharin sodium, orange flavor, cellulose gum, aspartame.
**This product contains NutraSweet®.
Phenylketonurics: Contains 6 mg phenylalanine per tablet.**

Directions: Take 1 tablet dissolved in a glass of water, one to two times daily, or as recommended by a physician, pharmacist or health professional.

Warning: Keep out of reach of children.

How Supplied: CITRACAL® LIQUITAB® is available in bottles of 30 tablets. UPC 0178-0811-30.
Store at room temperature.
Ⓤ=Kosher Parvae approved by Orthodox Union.

Continued on next page

CITRACAL® PLUS
[sit 'ra-cal]
Ultradense™ Calcium Citrate-Vitamin D-multimineral Dietary Supplement

Ingredients: Each tablet contains: calcium (as Ultradense™ calcium citrate) 250 mg., polyethylene glycol, magnesium oxide, povidone, croscarmellose sodium, HPMC, color added, pyridoxine hydrochloride, zinc oxide, sodium borate, manganese gluconate, copper gluconate, magnesium stearate, magnesium silicate, maltodextrin, carnauba wax, vitamin D$_3$ (125 IU).

How Supplied: CITRACAL® PLUS is available in bottles of 150 tablets, UPC 0178-0825-15.

Novartis Consumer Health, Inc.
**560 MORRIS AVE.
SUMMIT, NJ 07901-1312**

Direct Product Inquiries to:
Consumer & Professional Affairs
(800) 452-0051
Fax: (800) 635-2801

Or write to above address.

ReSource® Wellness ALLERPRO™ Allergy Formula Capsules
Dietary Supplement

Description: For Whom? People looking to moderate their body's reactions to external allergens.*
To Do What? Helps lessen discomfort commonly associated with allergies.*
Featured Ingredients:
Xanthium sibiricum, gardinia jasminoides, chrysanthemum morifolium Natural fruit and flower extracts that help moderate discomforts commonly associated with allergies*
Scutellaria baicalensis: Natural root extract that helps improve the body's defenses against irritating allergies*

Other ingredients: Gelatin, Maltodextrin, Magnesium Stearate, Silicon Dioxide, Sodium Lauryl Sulfate, Polysorbate 80

Directions: Take 2 or 3 Capsules once per day.

Warnings: FOR ADULTS ONLY. Keep out of reach of children. Consult your health professional before using if you are pregnant, nursing a baby, or are taking any precription medications. Do not use if you have an ulcer. May cause photosensitivity.

How Supplied: Bottles of 60 Capsules.

* These statements have not been evaluated by the Food and Drug Administration. This product is not in-tended to diagnose, treat, cure or prevent any disease.

Call toll-free 1-877-939-3556
8AM-5PM E.T.
Or visit www.resourcewellness.com
Store at controlled room temperature 20–25°C (68–77°F).
Distributed by: **Novartis Consumer Health, Inc.,** Summit, NJ 07901-1312
Shown in Product Identification Guide, page 514

ReSource® Wellness CALCIWISE™ Bone Health Soft Chews
Dietary Supplement

Description: Builds and maintains strong healthy bones.*

Supplement Facts
Serving Size: 1 Chew

Amount Per Serving		% Daily Value**
Calories	15	
Calories from Fat	5	
Total Fat	0.5 g	<1%
Total Carbohydrate	3 g	1%
Sugars	2 g	†
Vitamin A	1000 IU	20%
Vitamin D	200 IU	50%
Vitamin K	40 mcg	50%
Riboflavin	0.8 mg	50%
Calcium	600 mg	60%
Sodium	10 mg	<1%

**Percent Daily Values are based on a 2,000 calorie diet.
† Daily value not established.

Ingredients: Calcium Carbonate, Corn Syrup, High Fructose Corn Syrup, Sweetened Condensed Skim Milk, Chocolate Liquor, Sugar, High Oleic Sunflower Oil, Cocoa (Processed with Alkali), Glycerol Monostearate, Salt, Artificial Flavor, Soy Lecithin, Riboflavin, Vitamin A Palmitate, Phytonadione (Vitamin K$_1$), Cholecalciferol (Vitamin D$_3$)

Directions: Take 1 Chew up to 2 times per day preferably with meals.

How Supplied: Packages of 60 Chews. Store at controlled room temperature 20–25°C (68–77°F).

* These statements have not been evaluated by the Food and Drug Administration. This product is not intended to diagnose, treat, cure or prevent any disease.

Call toll-free 1-877-939-3556
8AM–5PM E.T.
Or visit www.resourcewellness.com

Distributed by: **Novartis Consumer Health, Inc.,** Summit, NJ 07901-1312
Shown in Product Identification Guide, page 514

ReSource® Wellness ENVIGOR™ Energy Enhancement Caplets
Dietary Supplement

Description: For whom? People looking to increase energy and stamina.*
To Do What? Help your body generate the energy it needs.*
Featured Ingredients:
Standardized Ginseng Extract Improves overall well-being and energy levels*
Standardized Ginkgo Biloba Extract An antioxidant that promotes blood flow circulation*
Vitamin B Complex: Essential B Vitamins involved in energy metabolism*
Vitamins C & E: Antioxidants that help protect the body's cells*

Supplement Facts
Serving Size: 1 Caplet (1.4 g)
Servings Per Container: 30

Amount Per Serving		% Daily Value**
Vitamin C	60 mg	100%
Vitamin E	30 IU	100%
Thiamin	1.5 mg	100%
Riboflavin	1.7 mg	100%
Niacin	20 mg	100%
Vitamin B$_6$	2 mg	100%
Vitamin B$_{12}$	6 mcg	100%
Biotin	300 mcg	100%
Pantothenic Acid	10 mg	100%
Calcium	260 mg	26%
Standardized Ginkgo Biloba Extract (Leaves)	120 mg	†
Standardized Panax Ginseng Extract (Root)	200 mg	†

**Percent Daily Values are based on a 2,000 calories diet.
† Daily Value not established.

Other ingredients: Dicalcium Phosphate, Microcrystalline Cellulose, Ascorbic Acid (Vitamin C), Croscarmellose Sodium, Vitamin E Acetate, Niacinamide, Calcium Silicate, Stearic Acid, Magnesium Stearate, Calcium Pantothenate, Pyridoxine HCl (Vitamin B$_6$), Riboflavin, Thiamine Mononitrate, Biotin, Cyanocobalamin (Vitamin B$_{12}$), Hydroxy-

propyl Methylcellulose, Hydroxypropyl Cellulose, Polyethylene Glycol

Directions: Take 1 Caplet daily.

Warnings: FOR ADULTS ONLY. Keep out of reach of children. Consult your health professional before using if you are pregnant, nursing a baby, or are taking any prescription medications. Do not take if using steroids, hormone drugs, MAOI's, aspirin, or any other anticoagulants. Do not use for more than three months at a time.

How Supplied: Bottles of 60 Caplets.

* These statements have not been evaluated by the Food and Drug Administration. This product is not intended to diagnose, treat, cure or prevent any disease.

Store at controlled room temperature 20–25°C (68–77°F).
Call toll-free 1-877-939-3556
8AM–5PM E.T.
Or visit www.resourcewellness.com
Distributed by: **Novartis Consumer Health, Inc.,** Summit, NJ 07901-1312
Shown in Product Identification Guide, page 514

ReSource® Wellness
FLEXTEND™ Joint Health Caplets
Dietary Supplement

Description: For Whom? People looking for improved joint function.*
To Do What? Helps improve mobility and joint comfort.*

Featured Ingredients:
Glucosamine Sulfate: A form of amino glucose that helps build healthy cartilage*
Vitamin C & E: Antioxidants that help maintain joint health*

Supplement Facts
Serving Size: 3 Caplets (5.3 g)
Servings Per Container: 20

Amount Per Serving		% Daily Value**
Calories	10	
Total Carbohydrate	2 g	1%
Vitamin C	180 mg	300%
Vitamin E	60 IU	200%
Iron	0.78 mg	4%
Sodium	160 mg	6%
Glucosamine Sulfate (sodium salt)	1.5 g	†

**Percent Daily Values are based on a 2,000 calorie diet.
† Daily Value not established.

Other Ingredients: Microcrystalline Cellulose, Maltodextrin, Ascorbic Acid

(Vitamin C), Croscarmellose Sodium, Stearic Acid, Vitamin E Acetate, Magnesium Stearate, Silicon Dioxide, Hydroxypropyl Methylcellulose, Titanium Dioxide, Polyethylene Glycol, Caramel, Polysorbate 80

Directions: Take 3 Caplets daily.

Warnings: FOR ADULTS ONLY. Keep out of reach of children. Consult your health professional before using if you are pregnant, nursing a baby, or are taking any prescription medications. Diabetics must consult with their health professional before taking this supplement. Store at controlled room temperature 20–25°C (68–77°F).

How Supplied: Bottles of 60 Caplets.

* These statements have not been evaluated by the Food and Drug Administration. This product is not intended to diagnose, treat, cure or prevent any disease.

Call toll-free 1-877-939-3556
8AM–5PM E.T.
Or visit www.resourcewellness.com
Distributed by: **Novartis Consumer Health, Inc.,** Summit, NJ 07901-1312
Shown in Product Identification Guide, page 514

ReSource® Wellness
FORSIGHT™ Eye Health Caplets
Dietary Supplement

Description: For Whom? People wanting to maintain healthy eye function.*
To Do What? Help maintain macular and retinal health.*

Featured Ingredients: Lutein/Zeaxanthin, Beta & Alpha Carotenes: Offer antioxidant protection to help maintain macular health*
Vitamins C & E: Offer antioxidant support to help maintain retinal health*
Standardized Grape Seed Extract Provides antioxidant properties that help promote healthy eye function*

Supplement Facts
Serving Size: 3 Caplets (4.3 g)
Servings Per Container: 20

Amount Per Serving		% Daily Value**
Calories	10	
Total Carbohydrate	2 g	<1%
Dietary Fiber	<1 g	2%
Vitamin A (89% as Beta Carotene)	15,000 IU	300%
Vitamin C	300 mg	500%
Vitamin E	400 IU	1330%
Calcium	650 mg	65%
Iron	0.74 mg	4%
Sodium	10 mg	<1%
Lutein/Zeaxanthin	6 mg	†
Alpha Carotene	2 mg	†
Standard Grape Seed Extract	50 mg	†

**Percent Daily Values are based on a 2,000 calories diet.
† Daily Value not established.

Other ingredients: Dicalcium Phosphate, Vitamin E Acetate, Ascorbic Acid (Vitamin C), Microcrystalline Cellulose, Croscarmellose Sodium, Calcium Silicate, Magnesium Stearate, Stearic Acid, Hydroxypropyl Methylcellulose, Propylene Glycol, Polyethylene Glycol, Titanium Dioxide, FD&C Yellow No.6 Lake, FD&C Red No. 40 Lake, FD&C Blue No. 2 Lake

Directions: Take 3 Caplets daily.

Warnings: FOR ADULTS ONLY. Keep out of reach of children. Consult your health professional before using if you are pregnant, nursing a baby, or are taking any prescription medications. Do not use if taking anticoagulants.
Store at controlled room temperature 20–25°C (68–77°F).

How Supplied: Bottles of 60 Caplets.

* These statements have not been evaluated by the Food and Drug Administration. This product is not intended to diagnose, treat, cure or prevent any disease.

Call toll-free 1-877-939-3556
8AM-5PM E.T.
Or visit www.resourcewellness.com
Distributed by: **Novartis Consumer Health, Inc.,** Summit, NJ 07901-1312
Shown in Product Identification Guide, page 514

ReSource® Wellness
MEMORABLE™ Mental Enhancement Softgels
Dietary Supplement

Description: For Whom? People seeking to minimize absent-mindedness or mild memory problems associated with aging.*
To Do What? Helps to improve mental alertness and performance.*

Featured Ingredients:
Standardized Ginkgo Biloba Extract

Continued on next page

Information on Novartis Consumer Health, Inc., products appearing on these pages is effective as of November 2000.

Memorable—Cont.

An antioxidant that enhances blood circulation throughout the body*

Lecithin: Contains phosphotidyl choline, an essential component of brain cell membranes*

Vitamins B$_6$ & B$_{12}$: Vitamins important for brain cell function*

Supplement Facts
Serving Size: 2 Softgels (2.7 g)
Servings Per Container: 30

Amount Per Serving		% Daily Value**
Calories	10	
Calories from Fat	5	
Total Carbohydrate	1 g	<1%
Dietary Fiber	<1 g	3%
Vitamin B$_6$	2 mg	100%
Vitamin B$_{12}$	6 mcg	100%
Standardized Ginkgo Biloba Extract (Leaves)	120 mg	†
Lecithin	1200 mg	†

**Percent Daily Values are based on a 2,000 calorie diet.
† Daily Value not established.

Other ingredients: Gelatin, Soybean Oil, Glycerin, Beeswax, Titanium Dioxide, FD&C Yellow No. 6, FD&C Red No. 40, FD&C Blue No. 1, Pyridoxine HCl (Vitamin B$_6$), Cyanocobalamin (Vitamin B$_{12}$)

Directions: Take 2 Softgels daily.

Warnings: FOR ADULTS ONLY. Keep out of reach of children. Consult your health professional before using if you are pregnant, nursing a baby, or are taking any prescription medications. Do not take it using anticoagulants, including aspirin.

Store at controlled room temperature 20–25°C (68–77°F).

How Supplied: Bottles of 60 Softgels.

* These statements have not been evaluated by the Food and Drug Administration. This product is not intended to diagnose, treat, cure or prevent any disease.

Call toll-free 1-877-939-3556
8AM–5PM E.T.
Or visit www.resourcewellness.com
Distributed by: **Novartis Consumer Health, Inc.,** Summit, NJ 07901-1312
Shown in Product Identification Guide, page 514

ReSource® Wellness RESISTEX™ Immune Health Capsules
Dietary Supplement

Description: For Whom? People wanting to maintain a healthy immune system.*
To Do What? Help improve your body's resistance and support normal immune function.*

Featured Ingredients:
Echinacea and epimedium
Supports a healthy immune system*
Panax ginseng extract
Improves overall well-being*
Siberian ginseng extract
Increases overall energy levels*

Other ingredients: Maltodextrin, Gelatin, Magnesium Stearate, Silicon Dioxide, Sodium Lauryl Sulfate, Polysorbate 80

Directions: Take 2 Capsules once a day before or between meals.

Warnings: FOR ADULTS ONLY. Keep out of reach of children. Consult your health professional before using if you are pregnant, nursing a baby, or are taking any prescription medications. Do not take if you have high blood pressure or are using anticoagulants, other heart medications or immunosuppressants. Do not use for more than three months at a time.
Store at controlled room temperature 20–25°C (68–77°F).

How Supplied: Bottles of 60 Capsules.

* These statements have not been evaluated by the Food and Drug Administration. This product is not intended to diagnose, treat, cure or prevent any disease.

Call toll-free 1-877-939-3556
8AM–5PM E.T.
Or visit www.resourcewellness.com
Distributed by: **Novartis Consumer Health, Inc.,** Summit, NJ 07901-1312
Shown in Product Identification Guide, page 514

ReSource® Wellness 2ndWIND™ Stamina & Muscle Recovery Capsules
Dietary Supplement

Description:
For Whom? People wanting to speed muscle recovery and improve stamina.*
To Do What? Helps muscles recover faster from physical exertion and improves stamina so you can work out harder and longer.*

Featured Ingredients:
Flammulina velutipes: Improves lactic acid clearance for faster recovery of muscle strength and improves stamina*

Siberian ginseng extract: Improves overall energy levels to help you work out longer*

Panax ginseng extract: Helps improve stamina needed for vigorous exercise or physical exertion*

Other ingredients: Gelatin, Maltodextrin, Magnesium Stearate, Silicon Dioxide, Sodium Lauryl Sulfate, Polysorbate 80

Directions: Take 2 Capsules once per day.

Warnings: FOR ADULTS ONLY. Keep out of reach of children. Consult your health professional before using if you are pregnant, nursing a baby, or are taking any prescription medications. Do not take if you have high blood pressure or are using anticoagulants or other heart medications. Do not use for more than three months at a time.
Store at controlled room temperature 20–25°C (68–77°F)

How Supplied: Bottles of 60 Capsules.

* These statements have not been evaluated by the Food and Drug Administration. This product is not intended to diagnose, treat, cure or prevent any disease.

Call toll-free 1-877-939-3556
8AM–5PM E.T.
Or visit www.resourcewellness.com
Distributed by: **Novartis Consumer Health, Inc.,** Summit, NJ 07901-1312
Shown in Product Identification Guide, page 514

ReSource® Wellness STAYCALM™ Stress Management Caplets
Dietary Supplement

Description: For Whom? People wanting to improve their mood and enhance their ability to manage stress.*

To Do What? Supports a positive outlook by helping you relax and cope with stress.*

Featured Ingredients:

Standardized St. John's Wort Extract: An herb that helps support a positive sense of well-being and mood improvement*

Standardized Valerian Extract: An herb traditionally used to calm and relax*

B Vitamins (Thiamin, Vitamins B$_6$ & B$_{12}$): B Vitamins that help your body cope with stress and regulate mood*

Supplement Facts
Serving Size: 1 Caplet (1.1 g)
Servings Per Container: 60

Amount Per Serving		% Daily Value**
Vitamin C	10 mg	17%
Thiamin	0.25 mg	17%
Vitamin B$_6$	0.33 mg	17%
Vitamin B$_{12}$	1 mcg	17%
Calcium	190 mg	19%
Standardized St. John's Wort Extract (Aerial Parts)	300 mg	†
Standardized Valerian Extract (Root)	50 mg	†

**Percent Daily Values are based on a 2,000 calorie diet.
† Daily Value not established.

Other ingredients: Dicalcium Phosphate, Microcrystalline Cellulose, Croscarmellose Sodium, Magnesium Stearate, Stearic Acid, Ascorbic Acid (Vitamin C), Maltodextrin, Silicon Dioxide, Hydroxypropyl Methylcellulose, Hydroxypropyl Cellulose, Polyethylene Glycol, Cyanocobalamin (Vitamin B$_{12}$), Pyridoxine HCl (Vitamin B$_6$), Thiamine Mononitrate

Directions: Take 1 Caplet 3 times daily.

Warnings: FOR ADULTS ONLY. Keep out of reach of children. Consult your health professional before using if you are pregnant, nursing a baby, or are taking any prescription medications. Do not take if using protease inhibitors, cyclosporines, MAOI's, or antidepressants. Do not take while driving a car or operating heavy machinery. Avoid taking with alcohol or other sedatives. May cause drowsiness.

Store at controlled room temperature 20–25°C (68–77°F).

How Supplied: Bottles of 60 Caplets.

* These statements have not been evaluated by the Food and Drug Administration. This product is not intended to diagnose, treat, cure or prevent any disease.

Call toll-free 1-877-939-3556

8AM–5PM E.T.

Or visit www.resourcewellness.com

Distributed by: **Novartis Consumer Health, Inc.,** Summit, NJ 07901-1312

Shown in Product Identification Guide, page 514

ReSource® Wellness VEINTAIN™ Vein Health Caplets
Dietary Supplement

Description: For Whom? People wanting to maintain good vein health.*
To Do What? Maintains leg vein health by enhancing blood circulation.*

Featured Ingredients:
Standardized Horse Chestnut Extract: Helps improve blood circulation and strengthens vein walls*
Standardized Grape Seed Extract & Vitamin C: Antioxidants essential for protection of collagen, an important structural component in vein health*
Vitamin A: An essential nutrient for healthy skin*

Supplement Facts
Serving Size: 1 Caplet (1.1 g)
Servings Per Container: 60

Amount Per Serving		% Daily Value**
Vitamin A	250 IU	5%
Vitamin C	30 mg	50%
Calcium	175 mg	17%
Standardized Grape Seed Extract	25 mg	†
Standardized Horse Chestnut Extract	250 mg	†

**Percent Daily Values are based on a 2,000 calorie diet.
† Daily value not established.

Other ingredients: Dicalcium Phosphate, Microcrystalline Cellulose, Ascorbic Acid (Vitamin C), Croscarmellose Sodium, Stearic Acid, Magnesium Stearate, Silicon Dioxide, Hydroxypropyl Methylcellulose, Hydroxypropyl Cellulose, Polyethylene Glycol, Vitamin A Acetate

Directions: Take 1 Caplet 2 times daily.

Warnings: FOR ADULTS ONLY. Keep out of reach of children. Consult your health professional before using if you are pregnant, nursing a baby, or are taking any prescription medications. Do not take if using anticoagulants. Take with food.
Store at controlled room temperature 20–25°C (68–77°F)

How Supplied: Bottles of 60 Caplets.

* These statements have not been evaluated by the Food and Drug Administration. This product is not intended to diagnose, treat, cure or prevent any disease.

Call toll-free 1-877-939-3556
8AM–5PM E.T.
Or visit www.resourcewellness.com
Distributed by: **Novartis Consumer Health, Inc.,** Summit, NJ 07901-1312
Shown in Product Identification Guide, page 514

SLOW FE®
Slow Release Iron Tablets

Description: SLOW FE supplies ferrous sulfate for the treatment of iron deficiency and iron deficiency anemia with a significant reduction in the incidence of the common side effects of oral iron preparations. The wax matrix delivery system of SLOW FE is designed to maximize the release of ferrous sulfate in the duodenum and the jejunum where it is best tolerated and absorbed. SLOW FE has been clinically shown to be associated with a lower incidence of constipation, diarrhea and abdominal discomfort when compared to an immediate release iron tablet[1] and a leading sustained release iron capsule.[2]

Formula: Each tablet contains: Active Ingredient: 160 mg. dried ferrous sulfate USP, equivalent to 50 mg. elemental iron. Inactive Ingredients: cetostearyl alcohol, FD&C Blue No. 2 aluminum lake, hydroxypropyl methylcellulose, lactose, magnesium stearate, polysorbate 80, talc, titanium dioxide, yellow iron oxide.

Dosage: ADULTS—one or two tablets daily or as recommended by a physician. A maximum of four tablets daily may be taken. CHILDREN—one tablet daily. Tablets must be swallowed whole.

Warning: Accidental overdose of iron-containing products is a leading cause of fatal poisoning in children under 6. Keep this product out of reach of children. In case of accidental overdose, call a doctor or poison control center immediately.

Warning: The treatment of any anemic condition should be under the advice and supervision of a physician. As oral iron products interfere with absorption of oral tetracycline antibiotics, these products should not be taken within two hours of each other. As with any drug, if you are pregnant or nursing a baby, seek the advice of a health professional before using this product.
Blister packaged for your protection. Do not use if individual seals are broken.

How Supplied: Child-resistant blister packages of 30, 60, and 90.
Do Not Store Above 30°C (86°F). Protect From Moisture.
Tablets made in Great Britain
Novartis Consumer Health, Inc.
Summit, NJ 07901–1312

References
1. Brock C et al. Adverse effects of iron supplementation: A comparative trial of a wax-matrix iron preparation and conventional ferrous sulfate tablets. *Clin Ther.* 1985; 7:568-573.

Continued on next page

Information on Novartis Consumer Health, Inc., products appearing on these pages is effective as of November 2000.

Slow Fe—Cont.

2. Brock C, Curry H. Comparative incidence of side effects of a wax-matrix and a sustained-release iron preparation. *Clin Ther.* 1985; 7:492-496.
Shown in Product Identification Guide, page 514

SLOW FE® WITH FOLIC ACID
(Slow Release Iron, Folic Acid)
Dietary Supplement

Description: Slow Fe + Folic Acid delivers 50 mg. elemental iron (160 mg. dried ferrous sulfate) plus 400 mcg. folic acid using the unique wax matrix delivery system described above (for SLOW FE® Slow Release Iron Tablets).
Provides women of childbearing potential with the daily target level of folic acid to reduce the risk of neural tube birth defects. These birth defects are rare, but serious, and occur within 28 days of conception, often before a woman knows she's pregnant.

Formula: Each tablet contains: 160 mg. dried ferrous sulfate, USP (equivalent to 50 mg. elemental iron) and 400 mcg. folic acid.
Other Ingredients: lactose, hydroxypropyl methylcellulose, talc, magnesium stearate, cetostearyl alcohol, polysorbate 80, titanium dioxide, yellow iron oxide.

Dosage: ADULTS—One or two tablets once a day or as recommended by a physician. A maximum of two tablets daily may be taken. CHILDREN UNDER 12—Consult a physician. Tablets must be swallowed whole.

Warning: The treatment of any anemic condition should be under the advice and supervision of a physician. As oral iron products interfere with absorption of oral tetracycline antibiotics, these products should not be taken within two hours of each other. Intake of folic acid from all sources should be limited to 1000 mcg. per day to prevent the masking of Vitamin B_{12} deficiencies. Should you become pregnant while using this product, consult a physician as soon as possible about good prenatal care and the continued use of this product. If you are already pregnant or nursing a baby, seek the advice of a health care professional before using this product.

Warning: Accidental overdose of iron-containing products is a leading cause of fatal poisoning in children under 6. Keep this product out of reach of children. In case of accidental overdose, call a doctor or poison control center immediately.

How Supplied: Blister packages of 20 supplied in Child-Resistant packaging. Do not store above 30°C (86°F). Protect from moisture.

Tablets made in Great Britain
Novartis Consumer Health, Inc.
Shown in Product Identification Guide, page 514

Numark Laboratories, Inc.
164 NORTHFIELD AVENUE
EDISON, NJ 08837

Direct Inquiries to:
Consumer Services
Phone (800) 331-0221
Fax (732) 225-0066

LIPOFLAVONOID® Nutritional Supplement
with Eriodictyol Glycoside, Vitamin B Complex, and Lemon Bioflavonoids

Suggested Use: Nutritional Supplement for improved circulation in the inner ear.

Three Caplets daily provide:		% U.S RDA*
Vitamin C	300 mg	500%
Thiamine (B1)	1 mg	67%
Riboflavin (B2)	1 mg	59%
Niacin (Niacinamide)	10 mg	50%
Vitamin B6 (Pyridoxine HCl)	1 mg	50%
Vitamin B12 (Cyanocobalamin)	5 mcg	83%
Panthothenic Acid	5 mg	50%
Choline	334 mg	**
Bioflavonoids***	300 mg	**
Inositol	334 mg	**

* Percentage of U.S. Recommended Daily Allowance for Adults.
** U.S. RDA has not been established.
***Contains the flavor Eridictyol Glycoside.

Ingredients: Choline Bitartrate, Dibasic Calcium Phosphate, Microcystalline Cellulose, Inositol, Ascorbic Acid, Lemon Bioflavonoids complex, Croscarmellose Sodium, Stearic Acid, Niacinamide, Calcium Pantothenate, Silica, Ethyl Vanillin, Pyridoxine HCl, Thiamine Mononitrate, Riboflavin, Cyanocobalamin, Pharmaceutical Glaze, Hydroxypropyl Methylcellulose, Methylcellulose, FD&C Red #40 Lake, FD&C Blue #1 Lake, FD&C Yellow #6 Lake (Sunset Yellow), and Titanium Dioxide.

Recommended Intake: Three caplets daily. For best results use for at least six (6) months.

Caution: If you are pregnant or nursing a baby, seek the advice of a health professional before using this product. **Keep out of reach of children.**

Pharmaton Natural Health Products Division of Boehringer Ingelheim Pharmaceuticals, Inc.
900 RIDGEBURY ROAD
RIDGEFIELD, CT 06877

Direct Inquiries to:
Consumer Affairs
(800) 451-6688
FAX: (203) 798-5771

For Medical Emergency Contact:
David Morrison
203-775-7826

GINKOBA®
[gĭn-kō-bă]
ORIGINAL STANDARDIZED GINKGO BILOBA EXTRACT
The Thinking Person's Supplement.™

What is GINKOBA®?
- **America's #1 supplement for memory and concentration.**
- **The herbal supplement proven to help sharpen mental focus, improve memory, and enhance concentration.**
- **The supplement that's clinically shown to increase the flow of oxygen to the brain.**
- **The #1 doctor recommended brand of Ginkgo biloba.**

Why GINKOBA?
GINKOBA is a supplement that safely enhances memory and concentration by improving blood circulation to the brain.• It is believed that improved blood circulation increases the flow of oxygen, resulting in positive effects on mental performance.
With more than 30 years of clinical support, GINKOBA contains the most extensively tested Ginkgo biloba extract in the world and is made using a patented (U.S. Patent No. 5,399,348) standardization process that guarantees every tablet contains a consistent amount of active components. This means you can trust GINKOBA to help deliver improved mental sharpness—consistently and safely.• Most other ginkgo brands can't guarantee that.

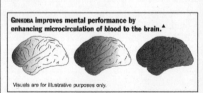

GINKOBA improves mental performance by enhancing microcirculation of blood to the brain.▲

Visuals are for illustrative purposes only.

Over 20 million people worldwide have used the all-natural extract in GINKOBA, so you can count on it to be safe. Additionally, GINKOBA contains no sugar, caffeine, or other stimulants.
GINKOBA works gradually. You'll begin to see results after taking it as directed for four weeks. Take it every day to help sharpen mental focus.•

Standardized for Reliability.

The natural herbal extract in GINKOBA is unlike that found in other Ginkgo biloba products. GINKOBA is produced using strict pharmaceutical company standards. It is prepared using a patented standardization process that ensures every tablet contains a consistent amount of active components. This is important, because unlike most other ginkgo brands, GINKOBA has been shown to meet the strict standards of reliability necessary to produce clinical proof of effectiveness. In fact, with more than 30 years of clinical research, GINKOBA contains the most extensively tested ginkgo extract in the world.

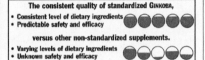

The consistent quality of standardized GINKOBA,
* Consistent level of dietary ingredients
* Predictable safety and efficacy

versus other non-standardized supplements.
* Varying levels of dietary ingredients
* Unknown safety and efficacy

Current research suggests that a ginkgo product should provide 24% ginkgo flavone glycosides and 6% terpene lactones for optimal effectiveness. GINKOBA is guaranteed to provide these active components in their clinically proven ratios in every tablet.

A History of Quality.

You can feel confident choosing GINKOBA because it is marketed by Pharmaton Natural Health Products. Pharmaton is the natural health care division of Boehringer Ingelheim Pharmaceuticals, Inc., a leading pharmaceutical company.

Frequently Asked Questions About GINKOBA®.

How does GINKOBA work?

GINKOBA has been clinically shown to help improve memory, concentration, and mental focus by safely increasing the flow of oxygen to the brain—so you can be more productive and feel more confident.•

What's the difference between GINKOBA and other Ginkgo biloba products?

The patented GINKOBA manufacturing process is rigorously controlled to bring you the highest-quality standardized extract of the Ginkgo biloba leaf. Since every tablet contains the same amount of active constituents, GINKOBA's effects have been proven reliable in clinical studies.

GINKOBA contains the most extensively tested Ginkgo biloba extract in the world.

How long before I feel the results?

GINKOBA is an herbal supplement, which means it works with your body. GINKOBA takes about four weeks of continuous use to reach its effectiveness.

Are there any side effects?

Adverse reactions with GINKOBA are very rare and generally mild: headaches, mild gastrointestinal disturbances, and mild allergic skin rashes.

Can I take GINKOBA with other supplements and vitamins or prescription drugs?

Yes. You can take GINKOBA with any other vitamin, mineral, or herbal supplement. If you are taking a prescription medicine, such as an anticoagulant agent, or any other blood-thinning agents, it is recommended that you inform your doctor before taking any Ginkgo biloba product. You should take your prescription medications either an hour before or an hour after daily supplements.

Will GINKOBA raise my blood pressure?

GINKOBA is not known to raise blood pressure. It is recommended that you let your doctor know that you are taking GINKOBA and monitor your blood pressure daily. If you notice any changes, stop taking GINKOBA and request a refund from Pharmaton Natural Health Products.

Other Questions About GINKOBA?

To receive more information about GINKOBA, call toll free 1-800-451-6688 or visit our Web site at http://www.ginkoba.com.

Recommended Adult Intake:

Adults should take one tablet with water three times daily at mealtimes. Research on doses above 120 mg per day does not substantiate any better effectiveness. GINKOBA is not a stimulant, so it works gradually over time and should be taken as part of an ongoing healthy daily regimen. Optimal effectiveness has been shown after 4 weeks of continuous uninterrupted use. GINKOBA is not intended for use by children 12 and under.

Precautions:

As with other vitamins and supplements, please keep this product out of the reach of children.

No serious side effects have been reported to date. However, as with any supplement, if you are taking a prescription medicine, such as an anticoagulant agent, are pregnant, or are lactating, please contact your doctor before taking any Ginkgo biloba product. In case of accidental ingestion/overdosage, seek the advice of a healthcare professional immediately.

* These statements have not been evaluated by the Food and Drug Administration. This product is not intended to diagnose, treat, cure, or prevent any disease

Pharmaton Quality Guarantee: This product has been proven safe and effective in well-controlled clinical studies and is manufactured according to the highest-quality standards.

PHARMATON
NATURAL HEALTH PRODUCTS
900 Ridgebury Road,
Ridgefield, CT 06877
A Division of Boehringer Ingelheim

GINKOBA M/E™ Mental Energy™
Clinically Proven
MENTAL PERFORMANCE DIETARY SUPPLEMENT
Unique Standardized Formula GK501™
Ginkgo Biloba/G115® Ginseng

GINKOBA M/E™ is Mental Energy™*

To get more out of life requires you to get more out of your brain. That's that spirit behind GINKOBA M/E, the daily supplement for Mental Energy.*

GINKOBA M/E is the only clinically proven formula shown to promote fast, accurate thinking and reduce mental fatigue. GINKOBA M/E is unique because each Suppli-Cap™ capsule contains a standardized formula of GK501™ Ginkgo biloba extract and G115® ginseng extract, to safely enhance the circulation of oxygen to the brain.*

Measuring the Effectiveness of GINKOBA M/E

In order to measure the effects of the herbal formula in GINKOBA M/E, scientists have employed a battery of standardized cognitive tests to determine its impact on key measures of mental performance. Among other measures, GINKOBA M/E has been shown to enhance
* Short-term or working memory (for performing tasks at hand)*
* Secondary or long-term memory (important in organizing, planning, relating)*
* Choice reaction time (decision making)*
* Simple reaction time (alertness, attention)*

Importantly, these positive results were seen even after several hours of demanding mental activity, indicating that GINKOBA M/E can help enhance mental endurance.*

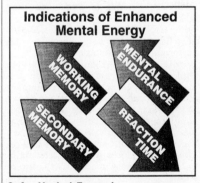

Indications of Enhanced Mental Energy

WORKING MEMORY　MENTAL ENDURANCE　SECONDARY MEMORY　REACTION TIME

Safe, Herbal Formula

GINKOBA M/E does not contain caffeine, sugar, or artificial stimulants. Its standardized herbal formula enhances mental performance by safely improving blood circulation and oxygen supply to the brain.* Its herbal ingredients have been used worldwide for decades, so you can trust the long-term safety of GINKOBA M/E.

Recommended Adult Intake: Research suggests that adults should take

Continued on next page

Ginkoba M/E—Cont.

one GINKOBA M/E Suppli-Cap™ capsule with water twice daily. Optimal results have been shown after 4 weeks of continuous daily use. Like most herbal supplements, it works gradually over time and should be taken regularly as part of an ongoing healthy regimen to achieve optimum benefits.

Precautions: As with other vitamins and supplements, please keep this product out of the reach of children. No serious side effects have been reported to date. As with any supplement, if you are taking a prescription medicine, such as an anticoagulant agent, are pregnant, or are lactating, please contact your doctor before taking this product. In case of accidental ingestion/overdosage, seek the advice of a healthcare professional immediately.

> ***These statements have not been evaluated by the Food and Drug Administration. This product is not intended to diagnose, treat, cure, or prevent any disease.**

Frequently Asked Questions
How does GINKOBA M/E work?
GINKOBA M/E contains a unique formula of GK501™ Ginkgo biloba and G115® ginseng. Research has shown that these herbal substances can enhance blood flow to the brain, thereby delivering oxygen and other nutrients more efficiently.* It is important to note that GINKOBA M/E is not a stimulant. It does not contain caffeine, sugar, or artificial stimulants.

What's the difference between GINKOBA M/E and regular GINKOBA?
Both GINKOBA and GINKOBA M/E have been shown to help improve mental performance safely and effectively.*
Regular GINKOBA contains a unique Ginkgo biloba extract that has been clinically shown to help improve memory and concentration.* GINKOBA is one of the world's most widely used herbal supplements. Research suggests that many people who use GINKOBA are those concerned about normal age-related forgetfulness who want to maintain their memory and ability to concentrate.
GINKOBA M/E is a unique formula of GK501™ Ginkgo biloba (a different ginkgo extract than that found in GINKOBA) and G115® ginseng. When combined in this formula, these two specific extracts have been shown to help enhance mental processing speed and accuracy, information retention, and mental endurance.* These benefits may have specific appeal to active-minded people looking to enhance their cognitive function to help them be more effective, efficient, better organized, and have greater mental stamina.

What is a Suppli-Cap™?
GINKOBA M/E is sold in a special capsule form called a "Suppli-Cap™". A Suppli-Cap™ is a soft gelatin capsule uniquely shaped with a snapping feature for better safety than traditional hard shell capsules.

Is GINKOBA M/E a "standardized" supplement?
Actually, GINKOBA M/E is two standardized herbal extracts combined in a standardized formula, which means each GINKOBA M/E Suppli-Cap™ capsule contains the same level of proven active components in their proven ratios. GK501™ is standardized at 24% ginkgo flavone glycosides and 6% terpene lactones. G115® is standardized at 4% across the full range of eight ginsenosides. This is very important because the standardized formula in GINKOBA M/E has been shown to meet the strict standards of reliability necessary to produce clinical proof of effectiveness.

How many weeks until I feel the results?
Optimal results have been seen after 4 weeks of continuous daily use at the recommended dosage of 2 Suppli-Caps per day. Like most herbal supplements, GINKOBA M/E works gradually over time and should be taken regularly as part of an on-going healthy regimen to achieve optimum benefits.

Are there any side effects?
No serious side effects have been reported to date. If any side effects occur, discontinue use and consult your health care professional.

Can I take GINKOBA M/E with other supplements and vitamins or prescription drugs?
Yes. You can take GINKOBA M/E with any other vitamin, mineral or herbal supplement. As with any supplement, if you are taking a prescription medicine, such as an anticoagulant agent, are pregnant, or are lactating, please contact your doctor before taking this product.

Other questions about GINKOBA M/E?
To receive more information about GINKOBA M/E, call toll free 1-800-451-6688 or visit us at our web site at http://www.ginkoba.com.

> *** These statements have not been evaluated by the Food and Drug Administration. This product is not intended to diagnose, treat, cure, or prevent any disease.**

Pharmaton Quality Guarantee:
This product has been proven safe and effective in well controlled clinical studies and is manufactured according to the highest quality standards.
Distributed by: **PHARMATON** NATURAL HEALTH PRODUCTS 900 Ridgebury Road, Ridgefield, CT 06877
G115 and GK501 are trademarks of Pharmaton Ltd., Switzerland.

GINKOBA M/E, Mental Energy and Suppli-Caps are trademarks of Pharmaton Natural Health Products, Division of Boehringer Ingelheim Pharmaceuticals, Inc., Ridgefield, CT 06877
© Copyright Boehringer Ingelheim Pharmaceuticals, Inc. 1999.
All rights reserved.   8B4580 001
Shown in Product Identification Guide, page 521

GINSANA®
G115 Ginseng Extract
[Gin-sa-na]

GINSANA Capsules — Standardized G115® Ginseng Extract (4%).
GINSANA Chewy Squares—Standardized G115® Ginseng Extract.
No other ginseng extract meets the quality standards of the one in GINSANA. Over 25 years of extensive research has shown that GINSANA is a safe and beneficial way to supplement your diet.

NUTRITION FACTS:
Serving Size: 1 capsule
Each Capsule contains:
Calories: 5   Calories from Fat 0

	% Daily Value*
Total Fat 0g	0%
Cholesterol 0mg	0%
Sodium 0mg	0%
Total Carbohydrate 0g	0%
Protein 0g	0%

---

* Percent Daily Values are based on a 2,000 calorie diet.

Supplement Facts
Serving Size: 1 Square
Amount Per Square: Standardized G115® Ginseng Extract (Panax Ginseng, C.A. Meyer) (root) 50 mg*
* Daily Value not established

Ingredients: Each GINSANA capsule contains 100 mg of highly standardized, concentrated ginseng extract from the roots of the highest quality Korean Panax Ginseng, C.A. Meyer. This special standardization insures a consistent level of the eight most effective ginsenosides in their proven ratios.

Also contains: Sunflower oil, gelatin, glycerin, lecithin, beeswax, chlorophyll.

Ingredients: Each GINSANA Chewy Square contains 50 mg of highly standardized, concentrated ginseng extract from the roots of the highest quality Korean Panax Ginseng, C.A. Meyer.

Also contains: Sucrose, glucose, palm kernel oil, gelatin, citric acid, ascorbic acid, lecithin, natural flavoring and coloring.

Suggested Use: When taken as directed, GINSANA is a natural way to enhance your physical endurance by improving your body's ability to utilize oxygen more efficiently. GINSANA will help you maintain your natural energy and an overall feeling of healthy well-being.

Recommended Adult Intake/Capsules: Adults over 12 years old should take two soft gelatin capsules, swallowed whole, with water in the morning or one capsule in the morning and one in the afternoon. Research on doses above 200 mg per day does not substantiate any better effectiveness. Optimal effectiveness has been shown with 4 weeks of continuous use.

Recommended Adult Intake/Chewy Squares: Adults over 12 years old should take up to four GINSANA Chewy Squares daily.

Precautions: As with other vitamins and supplements, please keep this product out of the reach of children. No serious or significant adverse reactions or drug interactions have been reported to date. However, as with any supplement, contact your doctor if you are taking a prescription medicine, are pregnant or lactating. There have been rare reports of mild allergic skin reactions with the use of the extract in this product. In case of accidental overdose, seek the advice of a professional immediately.

The statements presented on this package have not been evaluated by the Food and Drug Administration. This product is not intended to diagnose, treat, cure or prevent any disease.
Store at room temperature and avoid excess heat above 40°C (104°F) to maintain optimal freshness.

Shown in Product Identification Guide, page 521

GINSANA® Sport
DAILY ENERGIZING DIETARY
SUPPLEMENT
ORIGINAL STANDARDIZED G115®
GINSENG EXTRACT

Why take GINSANA® SPORT?
These days, professional athletes aren't the only ones looking to enhance their physical performance. To stay on top of life, it takes a healthy, active lifestyle that includes an ample supply of work and play. That's why there is GINSANA SPORT; the unique daily supplement for active people whose health and fitness are important to them. Whether you work out every day or you're more of a "weekend warrior", GINSANA SPORT may help you get more out of your workouts and more out of life.

Convenient Once A Day Dosage
Each capsule of GINSANA SPORT contains the maximum proven daily dose of G115® ginseng, so one soft gelatin capsule each day as recommended is all you

need to realize the benefits of GINSANA SPORT. And because you only have to take GINSANA SPORT once a day, it easily fits your busy lifestyle.

Proven Safe and Effective
G115® is a natural standardized ginseng extract that contains the full range of active ginseng constituents called ginsenosides. This extract helps your body use oxygen more efficiently.▲ Each GINSANA SPORT capsule is standardized, so it contains an equal and optimum amount of G115®, one of the most extensively researched ginseng extracts available.

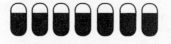

GINSANA is standardized:
- **Consistent level of dietary ingredients**
- **Predictable safety and efficacy**

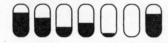

Non-standardized supplements:
- **Level of dietary ingredients varies**
- **Unknown safety and efficacy**

▲These statements have not been evaluated by the Food and Drug Administration. This product is not intended to diagnose, treat, cure, or prevent any disease.

GINSANA SPORT will take time to reach its maximum effect. Take it regularly for four weeks and you'll see results. Make it part of a healthy regimen to play harder, go longer, and help you to be at your best.

Helps Maintain Aerobic Capacity During Workouts
The G115® in GINSANA SPORT works with your body to improve endurance.▲ Objective measurements of oxygen absorption, serum lactate levels, heart rate and blood chemistry changes are known to be important factors in measuring physical work performance and increased endurance. Clinical studies have shown that G115® can lower serum lactate levels and heart rate.▲ This means that GINSANA SPORT can help you perform work and physical activity more efficiently over longer periods of time.▲

Promotes Efficient Oxygen Utilization
The human body needs an ample supply of oxygen to function properly. However, the body cannot store oxygen, making it imperative that the body is able to ab-

sorb and utilize oxygen as efficiently as possible. Oxygen absorption is regarded as important for peak performance and endurance. Clinical studies have shown that the unique G115® in GINSANA SPORT can improve oxygen absorption and utilization.▲ Efficient use of oxygen can play a role in shortening recovery time after exercise.

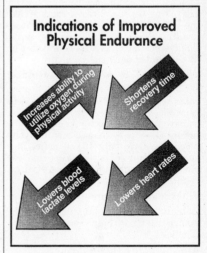

Indications of Improved Physical Endurance

Increases ability to utilize oxygen during physical activity
Shortens recovery time
Lowers blood lactate levels
Lowers heart rates

Long Term Safety
GINSANA SPORT® contains the same natural extract found in GINSANA®, one of the most widely used natural supplements in the world. With over 25 years of international GINSANA experience, you can trust the long-term safety of GINSANA SPORT. Unlike many workout supplements, GINSANA SPORT contains no caffeine, sugar or artificial stimulants.

Frequently Asked Questions
How does GINSANA SPORT work?
GINSANA SPORT's G115® ginseng extract is clinically shown to increase your body's oxygen uptake to help make the most of your natural, healthy energy.▲ GINSANA SPORT energizes naturally without sugar, caffeine or artificial stimulants.▲

What's the difference between GINSANA SPORT and other ginseng products?
GINSANA SPORT contains G115®, the same standardized ginseng extract made with the premium-quality Panax Ginseng, C.A. Meyer available in GINSANA. This unique extract delivers a consistent level of ginsenosides (the active element of the root). Since GINSANA is a world leader supported by decades of clinical research, you can rely on the safety and efficacy of GINSANA SPORT.

How long until I feel the results?
GINSANA SPORT is an herbal supplement, which means it works with your body.▲ Because of this mode of action, it takes at least four weeks of continuous use to reach its optimal effect.

Can I take GINSANA SPORT with other supplements and vitamins or prescription drugs?

Continued on next page

Ginsana Sport—Cont.

Yes. You can take GINSANA SPORT with any other vitamin, mineral or herbal supplement. You should also be able to take GINSANA SPORT with your prescription medications as no serious or significant drug interactions have been reported, but, as with any supplement, it is recommended that you inform your doctor you are taking GINSANA SPORT if you are taking prescription drugs, are pregnant or lactating. You should take your prescription medications either an hour before or an hour after daily supplements.

Will GINSANA SPORT raise may blood pressure?

GINSANA SPORT is not commonly known to raise blood pressure. It is recommended that you let your doctor know you are taking GINSANA SPORT and monitor your blood pressure daily. If you notice any changes, stop taking GINSANA and request a refund form Pharmaton Natural Health Products.

What is an adaptogen?

GINSANA SPORT is an adaptogen, a substance that can help normalize body functions.▲

Are there any side effects?

Many studies have been completed on the unique formulation of GINSANA SPORT and have shown only rare, mild adverse reactions: occasional headaches and gastrointestinal disturbances like gas, cramps, diarrhea and nausea. There have been reports of mild allergic skin reactions with the use of the extract in the product. Some consumers have reported that taking the product has caused drowsiness or sleeplessness.

Other Questions About GINSANA SPORT?

To receive more information about GINSANA SPORT, call toll free 1-800-451-6688 or visit us at our web site at http://www.ginsana.com.

Directions for Use

Recommended Adult Intake: Adults over 12 years old should take one 200 mg soft gelatin capsule with water each morning. Research on doses above 200 mg per day does not substantiate any better effectiveness. Optimal results have been shown with 4 weeks of continuous use, taken as directed.

Precautions: As with vitamins and other supplements, please keep this product out of the reach of children. No serious or significant adverse reactions or drug interactions have been reported to date. However, as with any supplement, contact your doctor if you are taking a prescription medicine, are pregnant or lactating. There have been rare reports of mild allergic skin reactions with the use of the extract in this product. In case of accidental overdose, seek the advice of a professional immediately.

▲These statements have not been evaluated by the Food and Drug Administration. This product is not intended to diagnose, treat, cure, or prevent any disease.

Pharmaton Quality Guarantee:
This extract has been proven safe and effective in well controlled clinical studies and is manufactured according to the highest quality standards.
PHARMATON
NATURAL HEALTH PRODUCTS
900 Ridgebury Road, Ridgefield, CT 06877
A Division of Boehringer Ingelheim
©1999 All rights reserved
                                                8B2945
Shown in Product Identification Guide, page 521

MOVANA™
[mō-vă-nă]
Clinically Proven
Advanced St. John's Wort
Hyperforin-Rich Formula
Dietary Supplement For Mood Support

St. John's Wort extract is clinically proven to enhance emotional well-being by promoting normal levels of neurotransmitters responsible for maintaining positive emotions. However, all St. John's Wort products are not alike. Researchers have identified a component of St. John's Wort called hyperforin that is a key ingredient responsible for its effectiveness. Hyperforin can degrade rapidly, often compromising a product's efficacy. But in MOVANA the hyperforin is stabilized to ensure potency and effectiveness. This process is such a breakthrough that the extract in MOVANA (WS-5572) has patents pending around the world. MOVANA is safe and there are no sedative side effects.

Suggested Use: Use MOVANA™ regularly, as directed below, to maintain normal emotional balance, a healthy good mood and a sense of well-being even during times of stress, and low-light seasons. MOVANA™ helps maintain a healthy motivation and a positive outlook on life.

Recommended Adult Intake: Adults (12 years and older) should take one tablet 3 times per day. Like most herbal supplements, MOVANA™ takes time to work; optimal effectiveness has been shown in as little as 2 weeks with continued use. Doses above 900 mg per day have not shown any greater effectiveness.

Precautions: As with vitamins and other supplements, please keep this product out of the reach of children. No serious side effects have been reported to date. However, as with any supplement, consult a healthcare professional if you are taking a prescription medicine, are pregnant or lactating. St. John's Wort may reduce the effect of an-

---

ticoagulant medication (Coumadin). Irregular menstrual cycles have been observed in some women taking both oral contraceptives and St. John's Wort. If you have fair and sensitive skin avoid prolonged direct sunlight, as photosensitivity may occur. There have been rare reports (<1%) of gastrointestinal disturbances, allergic reactions, or fatigue. In case of accidental overdose, seek the advice of a healthcare professional immediately.

These statements have not been evaluated by the Food and Drug Administration. This product is not intended to diagnose, treat, cure, or prevent any disease.

Questions about Movana?
For more information about MOVANA™, visit us at our web site http://www.Movana.com or write to:
Pharmaton Natural Health Products
900 Ridgebury Road
Ridgefield, CT 06877

How Supplied:

SUPPLEMENT FACTS:
Serving Size: 1 Tablet
Amount Per Tablet
Standardized WS-5572 St. John's Wort Extract (flower & leaves)   300mg*
*Daily value not established

Other Ingredients: Microcrystalline Cellulose, Corn Starch, Croscarmellose Sodium, Hydroxypropyl Methylcellulose, PEG-4000, Magnesium Stearate, Silicon Dioxide, Ascorbic Acid, Synthetic Iron Oxide, Titanium Dioxide, Talc, Vanillin. Contains no artificial stimulants, caffeine, or sugar.
Store in a cool dry place. Avoid excessive moisture and heat (above 86° F).
Shown in Product Identification Guide, page 521

PROSTATONIN®
Dietary Supplement for Urinary & Prostate Health

The *PROSTATONIN* regimen
PROSTATONIN is a proven dietary supplement for men whose health and lifestyle are important to them. When taken as directed in the morning and evening, *PROSTATONIN* safely and effectively helps promote normal urinary patterns and manages frequent urination during the day and night.*
PROSTATONIN has been used throughout Europe for over 10 years to help men maintain urinary & prostate health*. It is the safe, effective and natural way to help manage frequent and urgent trips to the bathroom both day & night, and to help promote normal urinary patterns.*
Over its many years of use, no serious side-effects have been reported.*

Clinically Proven Safe and Effective

PROSTATONIN works to help maintain a normal hormonal balance.* It has been proven safe & effective in controlled clinical studies. In fact, over 18 studies have been conducted on each of the individual extracts and on *PROSTATONIN*. Among the findings, these studies reported that daily use of *PROSTATONIN* for 6 weeks resulted in: a decrease in nighttime and daytime frequency of urination, a reduction in residual urine, and an increase in urine flow.* You can call us toll-free at 1-800-451-6688 and ask to receive these clinicals to read yourself or share with your doctor.

How does *PROSTATONIN* work?

While the mechanism of action is not fully understood yet, there is evidence that a decrease in testosterone levels is associated with an increase in the activity of an enzyme called 5-alpha-reductase. *PROSTATONIN* inhibits the activity of 5-alpha-reductase and thereby helps inhibit prostate growth because it functions as a "blocker" of the key enzymes that can affect the prostate.* This is one of the mechanisms thought to be responsible for the beneficial effects of *PROSTATONIN*.

PROSTATONIN – a unique combination of P. africanum and Nettle Extracts

PROSTATONIN contains two clinically proven herbal extracts: Pygeum africanum (PY 102) and Urtica dioica (UR 102). Clinical studies on *PROSTATONIN* suggest that its unique combination of P. africanum and Urtica dioica work in a complementary or synergistic fashion.* This means that the combination of these two herbs works better than the individual herbs alone. The Pygeum africanum extract (PY102) is derived from the bark of the African Prune tree; a tall forest tree native to the mountains of tropical Africa. Pygeum africanum has been widely used in Europe for many years as a prostate health supplement. Urtica dioica, or Nettle as it is more commonly known, belongs to the urticacea plant family and is found throughout the world. The extract used in *PROSTATONIN*, Urtica dioica (UR102), is derived from the root of the Nettle plant. Both of the extracts in *PROSTATONIN* are standardized extracts which means that you can be sure that you will receive a consistent amount of *PROSTATONIN's* active constituents in every softgel capsule.

Directions for Use:

Recommended Adult Intake: Adult males should take one softgel capsule twice a day with water (in the morning and evening with meals). *PROSTATONIN* works gradually over time to help balance testosterone levels and therefore should be taken as part of an on-going daily regimen.

Optimal effectiveness has been shown after 6 weeks with continuous uninterrupted use.

Cautions: As with other vitamins and supplements, please keep this product out of the reach of children. In case of accidental overdose, seek the advice of a professional immediately. If you are receiving medical treatment and/or taking medication for a prostate problem, or experiencing symptoms of a prostate problem such as painful, frequent or difficult urination, consult your physician.

Frequently Asked Questions About *PROSTATONIN®*

Can I take *PROSTATONIN* with other supplements and vitamins or prescription drugs?

Yes. You can take *PROSTATONIN* with any other vitamin, mineral or herbal supplement. You should also be able to take *PROSTATONIN* with your prescription medications as no serious or significant drug interactions have been reported. However, as with any supplement, it is recommended that you inform your doctor you are taking *PROSTATONIN* if you are taking prescription drugs.

Are all herbs clinically proven?

No. You should be careful what you buy because many herbal supplements currently in the marketplace are not clinically proven. When you purchase *PROSTATONIN* you can be sure that the herbal extracts, its quantity, and its recommended dose have been proven in controlled clinical trials.

Are there any side effects?

In the 18 clinical studies that have been conducted on *PROSTATONIN* there have been no reports of any significant side-effects associated with its use. Rare reports of mild gastrointestinal symptoms have been noted at the beginning of consumption, but gradually disapear with time. In addition, both of the extracts in *PROSTATONIN* have been used for over 20 years to help safely maintain prostate health.

What does standardization mean?

Standardization refers to the process of manufacturing herbal extracts which guarantees a consistent amount of the herb's active constituents. Due to many factors such as the quality or quantity of sunshine, the elevation or location of the plant, and seasonal variations, the composition of a plant can vary with every harvest. We standardize our products to account for this natural variability so each softgel provides the benefit you seek.

Are Standardized Herbs a better value?

Yes. Standardized herbs are more reliable and a better value than Whole herbs because they take into account the natural variability of a plant's active constituents. Whole herbs do not account for this variability – most simply contain ground up parts of plant including many inactive components such as cellulose. With a standardized product like *PROSTATONIN*, you get your money's worth because you get a consistent product that is clinically proven safe and effective.

Other questions about *PROSTATONIN?*

To receive more information about *PROSTATONIN*, call toll free 1-800-451-6688 or visit us at our web site at http://www.pharmaton.com.

If this product fails to meet your satisfaction, call Pharmaton at 1-800-451-6688 for a refund.

PHARMATON
NATURAL HEALTH PRODUCTS
900 Ridgebury Road, Ridgefield, CT 06877
A Division of Boehringer Ingelheim
©1999 All rights reserved   8B3890
Prostatonin is a registered trademark of Pharmaton SA.
Product of Switzerland

> ***These statements have not been evaluated by the Food and Drug Administration. This product is not intended to diagnose, treat, cure, or prevent any disease.**

Shown in Product Identification Guide, page 521

VENASTAT®
[vē-nă-stăt]
Leg Health Dietary Supplement
VENASTAT—Backed by Decades of Clinical Research and Worldwide Experience

The all-natural horse chestnut seed extract in VENASTAT is one of the most researched natural health supplements in the world. A patented extraction process delivers the standardized horse chestnut seed extract (HCE50™) unique only to VENASTAT. The international research on HCE50 includes over 40 clinical trials. This research, combined with years of worldwide patient experience, has demonstrated that VENASTAT is a safe way to supplement your dietary regimen.

VENASTAT—Sustained Release Standardized Extract HCE50 50mg (16%). The HCE50 used in VENASTAT is Aesculin free and has been shown through extensive research to be a safe and beneficial way to supplement your diet and promote leg vein health. The HCE50 in VENASTAT has been used by more than 10 million patient years around the world with no serious side effects.

Suggested Use: When taken as directed, VENASTAT is a natural way to promote leg vein health and protect against lower leg swelling by maintaining the circulation in the leg veins. VENASTAT stops the process that breaks down vein wall membranes and seals the vessels to protect against swelling, thereby maintaining good venous blood flow in your legs.

Recommended Adult Intake: Adults over 12 years old should take one Suppli-

Continued on next page

Venastat—Cont.

Cap™ every 12 hours swallowed whole with water. Research shows that effectiveness is reached after 4 to 6 weeks of use and sustained with continuous use.

Precautions: As with other vitamins and supplements, please keep this product out of the reach of children. Rare and mild reactions with VENASTAT include stomach irritation and nausea. Discontinue use and see a physician if gastric irritation, nausea or rapid heartbeat occurs. If you have had a stroke, heart disease or are pregnant or nursing a baby, see a doctor before using this product.

SUPPLEMENT FACTS:
Serving Size: 1 Suppli-Cap™ Capsule
Amount per Suppli-Cap:
Sustained Release Pellets of Standardized Horse Chestnut Seed Extract (seed) 300 mg* as Triterpene glycosides calculated as Escin (16%)
*Daily value not established

Other Ingredients: Dextrin, gelatin, copolyvidone, talc, polymethacrylic acid derivitives, titanium dioxide, dibutyl phthalate, synthetic iron oxide.

The statements presented on this package have not been evaluated by the Food and Drug Administration. This product is not intended to diagnose, treat, cure or prevent any disease.

Store at room temperature and avoid excessive heat above 40°C (104°F) to maintain optimal freshness.

Shown in Product Identification Guide, page 521

VITASANA™
DAILY DIETARY SUPPLEMENT

VITASANA is the first scientifically formulated and clinically tested ginseng multivitamin combination. VITASANA is a unique formula of essential vitamins and minerals you need for good nutrition, plus GINSANA's exclusive G115 ginseng extract for the vitality that's an integral part of your total health. VITASANA is the first multivitamin/ginseng supplement in an easy to swallow Gelcap dosage form.

Recommended Adult Intake: Adults over 12 years old should take two Gelcaps in the morning or one gelcap in the morning and one in the afternoon. Optimal effectiveness has been clinically seen after 4 weeks of continuous use.

The statements presented on this package have not been evaluated by the Food and Drug Administration. This product is not intended to diagnose, treat, cure or prevent any disease.

Supplement Facts
Serving Size 2 Gelcaps

Each Serving Contains			% Daily Value
Vitamin A (as beta carotene)	4000	IU	80%
Vitamin C (as ascorbic acid)	120	mg	200%
Vitamin D (as cholecalciferol)	400	IU	100%
Vitamin E (as dl-alpha tocopherol)	30	IU	100%
Vitamin B1 (as thiamine mononitrate)	2.4	mg	160%
Vitamin B2 (riboflavin)	3.4	mg	200%
Vitamin B3 (niacinamide)1	30	mg	50%
Vitamin B6 (as pyridoxine HCl)	4	mg	200%
Folic Acid	400	mcg	100%
Vitamin B12 (as cobalamin conc.)	2	mcg	33%
Calcium (as calcium phosphate)	200	mg	20%
Iron (as ferrous sulfate)	18	mg	100%
Phosphorus (as calcium phosphate)	160	mg	16%
Magnesium (as magnesium oxide)	20	mg	5%
Zinc (as zinc sulfate)	2	mg	13.3%
Copper (as copper sulfate)	2	mg	100%
Manganese (as manganese sulfate)	2	mg	100%
Potassium (as potassium chloride)	16	mg	0.5%

Standardized G115 Ginseng Extract 80 mg (from Panax Ginseng C.A. Meyer) (root)*

*Daily Value not established

Other Ingredients: Microcrystalline Cellulose, Povidone, Croscarmellose Sodium, Magnesium Stearate, Colloidal Silica, Hydroxypropyl mentyl cellulose, Ethylcellulose, Dibutyl Sebecate, Vanillin powder, Polyethylene Glycol.

Warning: Close tightly and keep out of reach of children. Contains iron, which can be harmful or fatal to children in large doses. In case of accidental overdose, seek professional assistance or contact a Poison Control Center Immediately.

Store at room temperature and avoid excessive heat above 40° C (104° F) to maintain optimal freshness.

Shown in Product Identification Guide, page 521

Procter & Gamble
P. O. BOX 5516
CINCINNATI, OH 45201

Direct Inquiries to:
Charles Lambert
(800) 358-8707

For Medical Emergencies:
Call Collect: (513) 636-5107

METAMUCIL® DIETARY FIBER SUPPLEMENT
[met uh-mū sil]
(psyllium husk)
*Also see **Metamucil Fiber Laxative** in Nonprescription Drugs section*

Description: Metamucil contains psyllium husk (from the plant *Plantago ovata*), a concentrated source of soluble fiber which can be used to increase one's dietary fiber intake. When used as part of a diet low in saturated fat and cholesterol, 7g per day of soluble fiber from psyllium husk (the amount in 3 doses of Metamucil) may reduce the risk of heart disease by lowering cholesterol. Each dose contains approximately 3.4 grams of psyllium husk (or 2.4 grams of soluble fiber). A listing of ingredients and nutrition information is available in the listing of Metamucil Fiber Laxative in the Nonprescription Drug section. Metamucil Smooth Texture Sugar-Free Regular Flavor contains no sugar and no artifical sweeteners. Metamucil Smooth Texture Sugar-Free Orange Flavor contains aspartame (phenylalanine content of 25 mg per dose). Metamucil powdered products are gluten-free.

Actions: Metamucil Dietary Fiber Supplement can be used as a concentrated source of soluble fiber to increase the dietary intake of fiber. Diets low in saturated fat and cholesterol that include 7g per day of soluble fiber from psyllium husk, as in Metamucil, may reduce the risk of heart disease by lowering cholesterol.

Claims: Clinical studies have shown that 7 grams of soluble fiber from psyllium husk, the amount in three doses of Metamucil, may help reduce the risk of heart disease when part of a diet low in saturated fat and cholesterol. For laxative indications and directions for use, see **Metamucil Fiber Laxative** in the Nonprescription Drugs Section.

Contraindications: Intestinal obstruction, fecal impaction, allergy to any component.

Warnings: Patients are advised they should consult a doctor before using this product if they have abdominal pain, nausea, vomiting or rectal bleeding, if they have noticed a sudden change in bowel habits that persists over a period of two weeks, or if they are considering use of Metamucil as part of a cholesterol-

lowering program. If taking Metamucil for contipation relief, patients are advised to consult a physician if constipation persists for longer than one week, as this may be a sign of a serious medical condition. **Patients are cautioned that taking this product without adequate fluid may cause it to swell and block the throat or esophagus and may cause choking. They should not take the product if they have difficulty in swallowing. If they experience chest pain, vomiting, or difficulty in swallowing or breathing after taking this product, they are advised to seek immediate medical attention.** Psyllium products may cause allergic reaction in people sensitive to inhaled or ingested psyllium. Keep out of the reach of children. In case of accidental overdose, seek professional assistance or contact a poison control center immediately.

Precaution: Notice to Health Care Professionals: To minimize the potential for allergic reaction, health care professionals who frequently dispense powdered psyllium products should avoid inhaling airborne dust while dispensing these products. Handling and Dispensing: To minimize generating airborne dust, spoon product from the canister into a glass according to label directions.

Dosage and Administration: The usual adult dosage is one rounded teaspoon, or tablespoon, depending on the product version. Some versions are available in single-dose packets. For children under 12 consult a docutor. The appropriate dose should be mixed with 8 oz. of liquid (e.g., cool water, fruit juice, milk) following the label instructions. **The product should be taken with at least 8 oz. (a full glass) of water or other fluid. Taking this product without enough liquid may cause choking (see warnings).** Metamucil can be taken three times per day.

This product, like other bulk fibers, may affect how well medicines work. If you are taking a prescription medicine by mouth, take this product at least 2 hours before or 2 hours after the prescribed medicine. As your body adjusts to increased fiber intake, you may experience changes in bowel habits or minor bloating.

How Supplied: Powder: canisters and cartons of single-dose packets. For complete ingredients and sizes for each version, see Metamucil Table 1, page 722, Nonprescription Drug section.
Shown in Product Identification Guide, page 521

IF YOU SUSPECT AN INTERACTION. . .
The 1,800-page
PDR Companion Guide™ can help.
Use the order form
in the front of this book.

Shire Pharmaceuticals US Consumer Products Division

7900 TANNERS GATE DRIVE FLORENCE, KY 41042

Direct Inquiries to:
Customer Service Department
Phone: 800-828-2088
Fax: 859-372-7684

For Medical Emergencies Contact:
Medical Information Department
Phone: 800-536-7878

SLOW-MAG®
MAGNESIUM CHLORIDE

Description: SLOW-MAG® is enteric coated Magnesium Chloride available in tablet form in a dosage unit of 64mg magnesium per tablet. Magnesium is an essential mineral of a healthy diet and may help to maintain the functions of the heart, muscles and nervous system.
SLOW-MAG® is a dietary supplement that provides a Magnesium Chloride formulation that is enteric coated to avoid the stomach upset and diarrhea commonly associated with oral magnesium supplements.

Ingredients: Each tablet contains Magnesium Chloride Hexahydrate, Calcium Carbonate, Povidone, Talc, Magnesium Stearate, Cellulose Acetate Phthalate, Diethyl Phthalate, Titanium Dioxide, Hydroxypropyl Cellulose, FD&C Blue No. 2 Lake.

Directions For Use: As a dietary supplement, take 2 tablets daily or as directed by a physician. Two 64mg tablets contain 32% of the recommended daily allowance for magnesium.

How Supplied: Bottles of 60 tablets. Do not use if the inner seal or protective band around the cap is broken or missing.
Manufactured for
Shire US Consumer Products Division

UNKNOWN DRUG?
Consult the
Product Identification Guide
(Gray Pages)
for full-color photos of
leading over-the-counter
medications

Sigma-Tau Consumer Products

A division of Sigma-Tau
Pharmaceuticals, Inc.
GAITHERSBURG, MARYLAND 20877

Direct Medical Inquiries to:
Toll Free: (877) PROXEED (776–9333)
Or: (301) 948–5450
Fax: (301) 948–5452
Email: proxeed@sigmatau.com

Direct Product Orders to:
Toll Free: (877) PROXEED (776–9333)
Web: www.proxeed.com

PROXEED™
[prox'-ēde]
Dietary Supplement
Promotes optimum sperm quality*

Description: PROXEED is a dietary supplement specifically formulated to optimize sperm quality. Sperm quality refers to motility, rapid linear progression, count, concentration and morphology.*

Suggested Use: To optimize sperm quality.*

Active Ingredients: L-carnitine fumarate, fructose, acetyl-L-carnitine HCl, citric acid.

Levocarnitine (L-carnitine) is a carrier molecule for medium- and long-chain fatty acids and is essential in the transportation of these fatty acids into the mitochondria where they can be utilized for β-oxidation. Levocarnitine is a component of both seminal plasma and sperm cells, and it plays a critical role in sperm maturation and potential sperm motility.[1-3]*

Fructose is one of the major energy-yielding substrates present in seminal fluid.[4]*

Acetyl-L-carnitine is the acetyl ester of levocarnitine and occurs naturally in the body. When converted to acetyl-CoA, it can enter the Krebs Cycle, be converted to acetoacetate (a ketone body) or be used for fatty acid synthesis. Additionally, acetyl-L-carnitine is important for membrane stabilization, is the most prominent form of carnitine in sperm,[5-7] serves as a circulating energy source for sperm,[5-7] plays an important role in sperm maturation and metabolism[5-7] and provides the primary fuel for sperm motility.[4-5, 8]*

Citric acid is a key intermediate in the Kreb's Cycle.*

Inactive Ingredients: mannitol, polyethylene glycol, artificial flavorings, povidone, silicon dioxide.

Continued on next page

Proxeed—Cont.

Supplement Facts:
Serving Size 1 Packet
Servings Per Container 30

	Amount Per Packet	% Daily Value
Calories	10	<1%*
Total Carbohydrates	2g	<1%*
Sugars	2g	‡
L-carnitine fumarate	1g	‡
Acetyl-L-carnitine HCl	0.5g	‡

* Percent Daily Values based on a 2,000 calorie diet.
‡ Daily Value not established.

Clinical Findings*: Among healthy couples taking longer than expected to conceive, poor sperm quality is a contributing factor for nearly 40% of all cases.[5] PROXEED'S primary ingredients are levocarnitine and acetyl-L-carnitine. In 12 clinical trials, levocarnitine and acetyl-L-carnitine have been proven to provide the nutritional support needed for sperm's production of energy and optimum sperm quality.[2–3, 5, 8–16] Supplementation with the ingredients in PROXEED significantly improved percent motile sperm.[2, 3, 8–16]

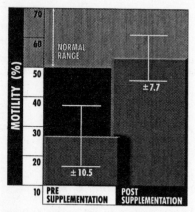

Mean (± SD) percent motile sperm was normalized after 3 months of supplementation with L-carnitine.[2] [p-not reported]*
[See graphic at top of next column]
Mean (± SEM) percent rapid linear progression showed a greater than 60% improvement after 4 months of supplementation with L-carnitine.[8] [p>0.001]*
[See graphic at top of next column]
Mean (±SEM) sperm count increased 14.7% after 4 months of supplementation with L-carnitine.[8] [p <0.001]*

Sperm concentration also improved after 3–4 months of supplementation.[2, 8, 10, 12, 16]

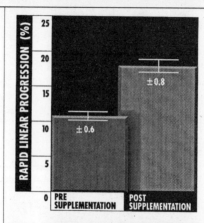

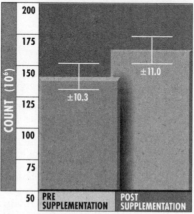

There has been only limited data on whether the ingredients in PROXEED have a measurable effect on sperm morphology.

Bioavailability/Pharmacokinetics:* Levocarnitine and acetyl-L-carnitine have bioavailabilities of between 5 and 15% in healthy adults. Clinical studies have shown that oral doses of 3 g per day (total) of carnitines are appropriate to optimize sperm quality.[2, 8, 12, 16] To achieve the appropriate dose, it is necessary for PROXEED to be provided as a powder formulation.
The oral half-lives of L-carnitine and acetyl-L-carnitine are approximately 3–4 hours. As a result, the total daily dose should be divided b.i.d., and spaced 8 or more hours apart to maintain elevated blood levels of L-carnitine and acetyl-L-carnitine.

Precautions: As with all supplements, please keep this product out of the reach of children, and consult with your physician before use if you are taking any medications.

Contraindications: None known.

Drug Interactions: None known.

Dosage & Administration: For Adult Males: Take two packets of PROXEED per day, one packet in the morning and one packet in the evening. Mix each packet with at least 4 ounces (120 ml) of juice or other beverage. Initial results should be seen within 3 months and con-

tinued improvement-leading to optimum results-within 6 months.* Patients who miss a dose should continue with the next dose. Double dosing is not necessary.
PROXEED is designed for long-term administration and should be taken for as long as attempting to conceive.*

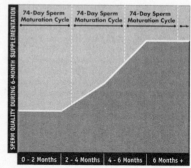

On average, sperm require 74 days to mature, and up to 30 additional days to become capable of fertilization. Initial results should be seen within 3 months and continued improvement-leading to optimum results-within 6 months.

How Supplied: PROXEED is available in single dose packets packaged 30 per box. PROXEED's powder formulation allows for the necessary ingredients in the amounts shown to be effective in clinical trials.

To order PROXEED, visit the web site, www.proxeed.com or call toll-free, (877) PROXEED (776–9333).

PROXEED is manufactured for Sigma-Tau Pharmaceuticals, Inc., Gaithersburg, Maryland 20877. Product of Italy. PROXEED™ is a trademark of Sigma-Tau HealthScience S.p.A. U.S. Patent #5,863,940. All rights reserved.

References:
1. Jeulin, C, et al, Role of Free L-carnitine and Acetyl-L-carnitine in Post-Gonadal Maturation of Mammalian Spermatozoa. *Human Reproduction Update* 1996; 2(2): 87–102
2. Vitali, G, et al, Carnitine Supplementation in Human Idiopathic Asthenospermia: Clinical Results. *Drugs Experimental Clinical Research* 1995; 21(4): 157–159
3. Loumbakis, P, et al, Effect of L-carnitine in Patients with Asthenospermia; 12th Congress of the European Association of Urology, Sept. 1–4, 1996. *Paris in European Urology* 1996; 30(2): 225, Abstract 954
4. Golan, R, et al, Influence of Various Substrates on the Acetylcarnitine: Carnitine Ratio in Motile and Immotile Human Spermatozoa. *Reproduction and Fertility* 1986; 78: 287–293
5. Moncada, ML, et al, Effect of Acetylcarnitine Treatment in Oligoasthenospermic Patients. *Acta Europaea Fertilitatis* 1992; 23(5): 221–224
6. Bartellini, M, et al, L-carnitine and Acetylcarnitine in Human Sperm with Normal and Reduced Motility. *Acta Europaea Fertilitatis* 1987; 19(1): 29–31

7. Kohengkul, S, *et al*, Levels of L-carnitine and L-0-acetylcarnitine in Normal and Infertile Human Semen: A Lower Level of L-0-acetylcarnitine in Infertile Semen. *Fertility and Sterility* 1977; 28(12): 1333–1336

8. Costa, M, *et al*, L-carnitine in Idiopathic Asthenozoospermia: A Multicenter Study. *Andrologia* 1994; 26: 155–159

9. Campaniello, E, *et al*, Carnitine Administration in Asthenospermia; 4th International Congress of Andrology, Firenze, May 14–18, 1989. Abstract

10. Muller-Tyl, E, *et al*, Effects of Carnitine on Sperm Count and Motility. *Fertilitat* 1988; 4(1): 1–4

11. Micic, S, *et al*, Does L-carnitine Administered In Vivo Improve Sperm Motility? *ARTA* 1995; 7: 127–130

12. Micic, S, Effects of L-carnitine on Sperm Motility and Number in Infertile Men; 16th World Congress on Fertility and Sterility, San Francisco, Oct. 4–9, 1998. Abstract

13. Vicari, E, Effectiveness of Short-Term Anti-Oxidant High-Dose Therapy of IVF Program Outcome in Infertile Male Patients with Previous Excessive Antimicrobials Administered for Epididymitis: Preliminary Results. *Infertility and Assisted Reproductive Technology: From Research to Therapy*, Ambrosini, A, *et al*, Monduzzi Editore, Bologna, 1997; 93–97

14. Vicari, E, *et al*, Effectiveness of Single and Combined Antioxidant Therapy in Patients with Asthenonecrozoospermia from Non-Bacterial Epididymitis: Effects after Acetyl-L-carnitine or Levocarnitine. Italian Andrology Association, 12th National Conference, Copanello (CZ), June 9–12, 1999. Abstract

15. Vicari, E, *et al*, Production of Oxygen Free Radicals in Varicocele: Pre- and Post-Treatment Evaluation and Observations after Pharmacological Trial. Italian Andrology Association, 12th National Conference, Copanello (CZ), June 9–12, 1999. Abstract

16. Micic, S, *et al*, Carnitine Therapy of Oligospermic Men. 25th Annual Meeting of the American Society of Andrology. Boston, 2000. Abstract

pxd-papi-4 ©2000 Sigma-Tau Consumer Products 9/00

Sigma-Tau Consumer Products a division of Sigma-Tau Pharmaceuticals, Inc. Gaithersburg, Maryland 20877

---

* These statements have not been evaluated by the Food and Drug Administration. This product is not intended to diagnose, treat, cure or prevent any disease.

Shown in Product Identification Guide, page 523

SmithKline Beecham Consumer Healthcare, L.P.

POST OFFICE BOX 1467
PITTSBURGH, PA 15230

For Medical Information Contact:
(800) 245-1040 (Consumer Inquiries)
(800) 378-4055 (Healthcare Professional Inquiries)

Direct Healthcare Professional Sample Requests to:
(800) BEECHAM

Alluna™ Sleep
Herbal Supplement Tablet

Use: **Alluna Sleep** is an herbal supplement that can relieve occasional sleeplessness.* It works by helping you relax, so you can drift off to sleep naturally.*

Alluna Sleep has been clinically tested and shown to be effective in actually promoting your body's own natural sleep pattern – safely and gently.* This is a natural process. Depending upon your particular circumstances, benefits are typically seen within a few nights with more consistent results within two weeks.

Alluna Sleep is not habit forming and is safe to take over time. You can expect to wake up refreshed, with no groggy side effects, because you experience a natural, healthy sleep through the night.*

Supplement Facts:
Serving Size: 2 Tablets
Servings Per Container: 28

	Amount Per 2 Tablets	% Daily Value
Calories	5	
Valerian Root Extract	500 mg	†
Hops Extract	120 mg	†

†Daily Value Not Established

Other Ingredients: microcrystalline cellulose, soy polysaccharide, hydrogenated castor oil, hydroxypropyl methylcellulose. Contains less than 2% of titanium dioxide, propylene glycol, magnesium stearate, silica, polyethylene glycol (400, 6,000 and 20,000), blue 2 lake, artificial flavoring.

Directions: Take **two** (2) tablets one hour before bedtime with a glass of water.

Warning: As with all dietary supplements, contact your doctor before use if you are pregnant or lactating. Keep this and all dietary supplements out of the reach of children. Driving or operating machinery while using this product is not recommended. Chronic insomniacs should consult their doctor before using this product.

Please Note: The herbs in this product have a distinct natural aroma.
Tamper Evident Packaging. Tablets are sealed in blisters.
Do not use if seal is cut, torn, or broken. Illustrations and overall packaging design elements are trademarked.
Store in a cool, dry place. Avoid temperatures above 86°F.

How Supplied: Packets of 28 and 56 Tablets
Visit us at www.allunasleep.com
Comments or Questions?
Call Toll-Free 1-877-7ALLUNA Weekdays
Distributed by:
SmithKline Beecham
Consumer Healthcare, L.P.
Pittsburgh, PA 15230
Made in Switzerland
©2000 SmithKline Beecham

FEOSOL® Caplets
Hematinic
Iron Supplement

Description: FEOSOL Caplets contain pure iron micro particles called carbonyl iron. Replacing FEOSOL Capsules, this advanced formula is specially designed to be well absorbed, gentle on the stomach and offers enhanced safety in the event of an accidental overdose. Each FEOSOL carbonyl iron caplet delivers 45 mg of pure elemental iron, the same amount of elemental iron contained in the 225 mg ferrous sulfate capsule. At equivalent doses, carbonyl iron and ferrous sulfate were shown to be equally efficacious in correcting hemoglobin, hematocrit and serum iron levels in iron-deficient patients[1].

Safety: According to the American Association of Poison Control Centers, iron containing supplements are the leading cause of pediatric poisoning deaths for children under six in the United States[2]. Widely used as a food additive, carbonyl iron must be gastrically solubilized before it can be absorbed, giving it lower toxicity and enhancing its safety versus any of the ferrous salts[3]. As a result, carbonyl iron presents less chance of harm from accidental overdose. In addition, at equivalent doses, carbonyl iron side effects are no greater than those experienced with ferrous sulfate[4].

Warnings: Do not exceed recommended dosage. The treatment of any anemic condition should be under the advice and supervision of a physician. Since oral iron products interfere with absorption of oral tetracycline antibiotics, these products should not be taken within two hours of each other. Occasional gastrointestinal discomfort (such as nausea) may

Continued on next page

Feosol Caplets—Cont.

be minimized by taking with meals. Iron containing medication may occasionally cause constipation or diarrhea. If you are pregnant or nursing a baby, seek the advice of a health professional before using this product.

WARNING: Accidental overdose of iron-containing products is a leading cause of fatal poisoning in children under 6. Keep this product out of reach of children. In case of accidental overdose, call a doctor or poison control center immediately.

SUPPLEMENT FACTS

Serving Size: 1 caplet

Amount per Tablet	% Daily Value
Iron 45 mg	250%

Ingredients: Lactose, Sorbitol, Carbonyl Iron, Hydroxypropyl Methylcellulose. Contains 1% or less of the following ingredients: Carnauba Wax, Crospovidone, FD&C Blue #2 A1 Lake, FD&C Red #40 A1 Lake, FD&C Yellow #6 A1 Lake, Magnesium Stearate, Polydextrose, Polyethylene Glycol, Polyethylene Glycol 8000 (Powder), Stearic Acid, Titanium Dioxide, Triacetin.

Directions: Adults—one caplet daily or as directed by a physician. Children under 12 years: Consult a physician.

Tamper-Evident Feature: Each caplet is encased in a plastic cell with a foil back; do not use if cell or foil is broken.

References: [1]Devasthali SD, Gordeuk VR, Brittenham GM, et al, "Bioavailability of Carbonyl Iron: A randomized, double-blind study." Eur J Haematology, 1991; 46:272–278.

[2]FDA Consumer; March 1996:7.

[3]Heubers, JA, Brittenham GM, Csiba E and Finch CA. "Absorption of carbonyl iron." J Lab Clin Med 1986; 108:473–78.

[4]Devasthali SD, Gordeuk VR, Brittenham GM, et al, "Bioavailability of a Carbonyl Iron: A randomized, double-blind study." Eur J Haematology, 1991; 46:272–278.

Store at room temperature, avoid excessive heat (greater than 100°F) or humidity.

How Supplied: Boxes of 30 and 60 caplets in blisters. Also available in single unit packages of 100 caplets intended for institutional use.

Also available: FEOSOL Tablets.

Comments or Questions? Call Toll-Free 1-800-245-1040 Weekdays.

SmithKline Beecham Consumer Healthcare, L.P.

Pittsburgh, PA 15230   Made in USA

Shown in Product Identification Guide, page 524

FEOSOL® TABLETS
Hematinic
Iron Supplement

Description: Feosol tablets provide the body with ferrous sulfate—an iron supplement for iron deficiency and iron deficiency anemia when the need for such therapy has been determined by a physician.

SUPPLEMENT FACTS

Serving Size: 1 Tablet

Amount per Tablet	% Daily Value
Iron 65 mg	360%

Ingredients: Dried ferrous sulfate 200 mg (65 mg of elemental iron) equivalent to 325 mg of ferrous sulfate USP per tablet. Lactose, Sorbitol, Crospovidone, Magnesium Stearate, Carnauba Wax. Contains 2% or less of the following ingredients: FD&C Blue #1, FD&C Yellow #6, Hydroxypropyl Methylcellulose, Polydextrose, Polyethylene Glycol, Titanium Dioxide, Triacetin.

Directions: Adults and children 12 years and over—One tablet daily or as directed by a physician. Children under 12 years—Consult a physician.

Tamper-Evident Feature: Each tablet is encased in a plastic cell with a foil back; do not use if cell or foil is broken.

Warnings: Do not exceed recommended dosage. The treatment of any anemic condition should be under the advice and supervision of a physician. Since oral iron products interfere with absorption of oral tetracycline antibiotics, these products should not be taken within two hours of each other. Occasional gastrointestinal discomfort (such as nausea) may be minimized by taking with meals. Iron containing medication may occassionally cause constipation or diarrhea.

If you are pregnant or nursing a baby, seek the advice of a health professional before using this product.

WARNING: Accidental overdose of iron-contraining products is a leading cause of fatal poisoning in children under 6. Keep this product out of reach of children. In case of accidental overdose, call a doctor, or poison control center immediately.

Store at room temperature (59–86°F).

Not USP for dissolution.

How Supplied: Cartons of 100 tablets in child-resistant blisters.

Previously packaged in bottles.

Also available: FEOSOL caplets.

**Comments or Questions?
Call toll-free 800-245-1040 weekdays.**

SmithKline Beecham Consumer Healthcare, L.P.

Pittsburgh, PA 15230   Made in USA

Shown in Product Identification Guide, page 524

OS-CAL® CHEWABLE
Calcium Supplement

Description: Calcium supplement to help reduce the risk of osteoporosis. Osteoporosis affects middle-aged and older persons, especially Caucasian and Asian women, and those whose families tend to have fragile bones in later years. A lifetime of regular exercise and eating a healthful diet that includes enough calcium, especially during teen and early adult years, builds and maintains good bone health and may reduce the risk of osteoporosis in later life. Adequate calcium intake is important, but daily intakes above 2000 mg are not likely to provide any additional benefit.

Supplement Facts:
Serving Size: 1 Tablet

Amount Per Tablet	% Daily Value
Calories 5	
Calcium 500 mg	50%

Ingredients: Calcium carbonate, dextrose monohydrate, maltodextrin, microcrystalline cellulose, magnesium stearate, artificial flavors, sodium chloride.

Directions: One tablet two to three times a day with meals, or as recommended by your physician.

How Supplied: Bottle of 60 tablets
Store at room temperature.
Keep out of reach of children.

Shown in Product Identification Guide, page 525

OS-CAL® 250 + D
Calcium with Vitamin D Supplement

Description: Calcium supplement to help reduce the risk of osteoporosis (see below*). Also contains Vitamin D.

Supplement Facts:
Serving Size: 1 Tablet

Amount Per Tablet	% Daily Value
Vitamin D 125 IU	31%
Calcium 250 mg	25%

Ingredients: Oyster shell powder, talc, corn syrup solids, hydroxypropyl methylcellulose, corn starch. Contains less than 1% of calcium stearate, polysorbate 80, titanium dioxide, polyethylene glycol, Vitamin D, propylparaben and methylparaben (preservative), simethicone, yellow 5 lake, blue 1 lake, carnauba wax, edetate sodium.

Directions: One tablet three times a day with meals, or as recommended by your physician.

How Supplied: Bottle of 100 and 240 tablets.
Store at room temperature.
Keep out of reach of children.

*Osteoporosis affects middle-aged and older persons, especially Caucasian and Asian women, and those whose families tend to have fragile bones in later years. A lifetime of regular exercise and eating a healthful diet that includes enough calcium, especially during teen and early adult years, builds and maintains good bone health and may reduce the risk of osteoporosis in later life.

Adequate calcium intake is important, but daily intakes above 2000 mg are not likely to provide any additional benefit.

Shown in Product Identification Guide, page 525

OS-CAL® 500
Calcium Supplement

Description: Calcium supplement to help reduce the risk of osteoporosis. Osteoporosis effects middle-aged and older persons, especially Caucasian and Asian women, and those whose families tend to have fragile bones in later years. A lifetime of regular exercise and eating a healthful diet that includes enough calcium, especially during teen and early adult years, builds and maintains good bone health and may reduce the risk of osteoporosis in later life.

Adequate calcium intake is important, but daily intakes above 2000 mg are not likely to provide any additional benefit.

Supplement Facts:
Serving Size: 1 Tablet

Amount Per Tablet	% Daily Value
Calcium 500 mg	50%

Ingredients: Oyster shell powder, talc, corn syrup solids, hydroxypropyl methylcellulose, corn starch. Contains less than 1% of sodium starch glycolate, calcium stearate, polysorbate 80, titanium dioxide, polyethylene glycol, propylparaben and methylparaben (preservative), polydextrose, triacetin, yellow 5 lake, blue 1 lake, carnauba wax.

Directions: One tablet two to three times a day with meals, or as recommended by your physician.

How Supplied: Bottles of 75 and 160 tablets.
Store at room temperature.
Keep out of reach of children.

Shown in Product Identification Guide, page 525

OS-CAL® 500 + D
Calcium with Vitamin D Supplement

Description: Calcium supplement to help reduce the risk of osteoporosis (see below*). Also contains Vitamin D.

Supplement Facts:
Serving Size: 1 Tablet

Amount Per Tablet	% Daily Value
Vitamin D 200 IU	50%
Calcium 500 mg	50%

Ingredients: Oyster shell powder, talc, corn syrup solids, hydroxypropyl methylcellulose, corn starch. Contains less than 1% of sodium starch glycolate, calcium stearate, polysorbate 80, titanium dioxide, polyethylene glycol, Vitamin D, propylparaben and methylparaben (preservative), polydextrose, triacetin, yellow 5 lake, blue 1 lake, carnauba wax.

Directions: One tablet two to three times a day with meals, or as recommended by your physician.

How Supplied: Bottle of 75 and 160 tablets
Store at room temperature.
Keep out of reach of children.

*Osteoporosis affects middle-aged and older persons, especially Caucasian and Asian women, and those whose families tend to have fragile bones in later years. A lifetime of regular exercise and eating a healthful diet that includes enough calcium, especially during teen and early adult years, builds and maintains good bone health and may reduce the risk of osteoporosis in later life.

Adequate calcium intake is important, but daily intakes above 2000 mg are not likely to provide any additional benefit.

Shown in Product Identification Guide, page 525

REMIFEMIN Menopause
Drug Free
Herbal Supplement
A safe, natural, effective way to help ease the physical and emotional symptoms of menopause*

Remifemin Menopause is a unique, natural formula. For over 40 years in Europe, it has helped reduce the unpleasant physical and emotional symptoms associated with menopause, such as hot flashes, night sweats and mood swings. Clinically shown to be safe and effective. Not a drug.
Remifemin Menopause helps you approach menopause with confidence – naturally.*

Ingredients:	Amount Per Tablet:	% Daily Value:
Black Cohosh Extract (Root and Rhizome) Equivalent to	20 mg	†

†Daily Value Not Established.

Other Ingredients: Lactose, Cellulose, Potato Starch, Magnesium Stearate, and Natural Peppermint Flavor.

Standardized to be equivalent to 20 mg Black Cohosh (*Cimicifuga racemosa*) root and rhizome.
Contains no salt, yeast, wheat, gluten, corn, soy, coloring, or preservatives.

Directions: Take one tablet in the morning and one tablet in the evening, with water. You can expect to notice improvements within a few weeks with full benefits after using Remifemin twice a day for 4 to 12 weeks. This product is intended for use by women who are experiencing menopausal symptoms. Does not contain estrogen. Remifemin is not meant to replace any drug therapy.

Warnings: This product should not be used by women who are pregnant or considering becoming pregnant or are nursing. As with any dietary supplement, always keep out of reach of children. For a few consumers, gastric discomfort may occur but should not be persistent. If gastric discomfort persists, discontinue use and see your health care practitioner. As part of an overall good health care program, we encourage you to see your health care practitioner on a regular basis.

SEE PACKAGE INSERT BELOW FOR FURTHER INFORMATION ON HOW TO APPROACH MENOPAUSE WITH CONFIDENCE – NATURALLY.
Making Sense Out of Menopause with Remifemin Menopause
Today, women are leading very dynamic and diverse lifestyles. Despite this diversity, there is one constant. They are all experiencing physiological changes. They will all experience menopause. The time when you have menopausal symptoms is a multiphasic period. Technically, the change or transitional process of menopause is known as the *"Climacteric"*. There are different phases of the climacteric that a woman experiences:

1. Perimenopause is the transitional phase when hormone levels begin to drop. This phase lasts typically 3 to 5 years but can last up to 10 years. This gradual decline in estrogen levels causes the troublesome effects of menopause.

2. Menopause is the permanent cessation of menstruation. The average age at menopause is 51, but there is considerable variation in this timing among women. Menopause is medically defined as one year without menstruation.

3. Postmenopause is the phase following menopause. During this phase, your body gets used to the loss of estrogen and eventually the symptoms such as hot flashes go away.
Some Commonly Asked Questions Regarding Remifemin Menopause
1. What is Remifemin Menopause?
Remifemin Menopause is a uniquely formulated natural herbal supplement derived from the black cohosh plant. It is formulated to work with your body to promote physical and emotional balance during menopause. Over 40 years of clinical research has shown Remifemin Menopause helps reduce hot flashes, night sweats, related occasional sleep-

Continued on next page

Remifemin—Cont.

lessness, irritability and mood swings. In a recent clinical study, on average, women experienced the following overall improvements:

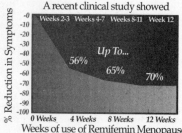

A recent clinical study showed

Up To...
56%
65%
70%

% Reduction in Symptoms

Weeks of use of Remifemin Menopause

2. What makes Remifemin Menopause so special? Remifemin Menopause contains an **exclusive** extract of black cohosh. It is developed with specific modern analytical techniques which produce a standardized extract of the black cohosh root and rhizome.

3. With so many products out there claiming to be "natural," how can I be sure that this product is safe and effective? Remifemin's Menopause formulation is supported by over 40 years of clinical research, and millions of women in Europe have safely used it. Remifemin Menopause is drug free and estrogen free. And it is brought to you from a world-renowned health care company.

4. How does Remifemin Menopause work? Remifemin Menopause contains a proprietary standardized extract taken from the rootstock of the black cohosh plant. Studies have shown that the compounds found within this standardized herbal extract seem to interact with certain hormone receptors – without influencing hormone levels.*

5. How long does it take for Remifemin Menopause to work? Remifemin Menopause is a natural herbal supplement, not a drug. It will take time for your body's cycles to respond to its gentle onset. Personally, you may notice improvements within a few weeks. But for some women, it may take 4 to 12 weeks to benefit fully from Remifemin Menopause. Since the effects of Remifemin Menopause increase after extended twice daily use, we recommend that you take Remifemin Menopause for at least 12 weeks. If you do not find any difference in your well being after 12 weeks, please consult your physician to discuss other options.

6. Can I take it over a long period of time, since the menopausal period lasts for years? We recommend that you take Remifemin Menopause twice daily for up to 6 months continuously. If, after discontinuing use, your symptoms return, you may start taking Remifemin Menopause again. Keep in mind that Remifemin Menopause is a natural herbal supplement that supports a natural change that may take you years to go through.* As part of an overall good health care program, we encourage you to see your health care practitioner on a regular basis.

e there any known side effects? used properly following the pack-

age directions, Remifemin Menopause has few side effects, if any. In clinical research, there was a small percentage of gastric discomfort complaints. If you have been taking Remifemin Menopause and find that this or any other condition develops and persists, please discontinue use and see your physician.

8. Is there a certain time of the day when I should take this product? Do I need to take it with food? You can take Remifemin Menopause with or without food. We recommend that you take one tablet in the morning with your breakfast and one tablet in the evening with water for relief from day and nighttime effects of menopause.

9. Can I chew a tablet? While they do have a mild peppermint flavor, Remifemin Menopause tablets are purposely made to be swallowed with water. They could be chewed, but some women may find the taste unpleasant.

10. Can I take my herbal tea, vitamins, or other dietary supplements with Remifemin Menopause? Typically, dietary supplements can be taken with other dietary supplements. Always follow package directions. If you should notice any undesirable effects, discontinue taking them together.

Expiration and Storage Information
The expiration date of this package is printed on the side panel flap of the outer carton as well as on the blister packs. Do not use this product after this date.
Store this product in a cool, dry place. Keep out of the reach of children. Avoid storing at temperatures above 86°F.

These statements have not been evaluated by the Food and Drug Administration. This product is not intended to diagnose, treat, cure, or prevent any disease.

Questions or Comments? Call toll-free 1-800-965-8804 weekdays, or visit www.remifemin.com anytime.

Remifemin ® is a trademark of Schaper & Brümmer GmbH & Co. KG, licensed to SmithKline Beecham.
© 2000 SmithKline Beecham 59175XA

FACED WITH AN Rx SIDE EFFECT?
Turn to the Companion Drug Index (Green Pages) for products that provide symptomatic relief.

Strategic Science & Technologies, Inc.
**PO BOX 395
NEWTON CENTER, MA 02459**

Direct Inquires to:
Consumer Product Information Center
1-888-408-6262

Doctor Ginsberg's PSORIA RID Cream™

Description: Intensive Tea Tree Oil therapy with vitamins E and C to relieve skin itching, scaling or redness due to psoriasis, and related disorders.

Suggested Use: Use as often as needed to relieve itching and scaling of psoriasis and dry scaling skin conditions. Apply directly to the affected area by gently rubbing the cream into the skin. May also be applied to the scalp. To remove, wash with water.

Active Ingredients: Tea tree oil, vitamins E & C.

Other Ingredients: Water, Tea Tree Oil, White Oil, Glyceryl Stearate SE, Squalane, Cetyl Alcohol, Propylene Glycol Stearate SE, Wheat Germ Oil, Glyceryl Stearate, Isopropyl Myristate, Stearyl Stearate, Polysorbate-60, Propylene Glycol, Oleic Acid, Tocopheryl Acetate, Collagen, Sorbitan Stearate, Vitamin A, C & D, Triethanolamine, Aloe Vera Extract, Imidazolidinyl Urea, Methylparaben, Propylparaben, BHA

Direct Inquires to:
Consumer Product Information Center
1-888-408-6262
**Strategic Science & Technologies, Inc.
PO BOX 395
Newton Center, MA 02459**

These statements have not been evaluated by the Food and Drug Administration. This product is not intended to diagnose, treat, cure, or prevent any disease.

Shown in Product Identification Guide, page 525

Natural AROUSAL™

Description: Natural AROUSAL™ is a patented transdermal preparation of L-Arginine in a pleasant cream base. It is used topically to increase the concentration of nitric oxide, derived from L-Arginine in the tissue of the corpus cavernosum of the penis, improving the erectile response. The erectile response begins within 3–5 minutes.

Suggested Use: Apply gently to the flacid or semi-erect penis. Rub in tenderly for 3–5 minutes. For best results apply regularly morning and evening as

well as a few minutes before sexual activity. Repeat as often as needed. To remove wash with water.

Active Ingredient: L-Arginine

Other Ingredients: Water, Choline Chloride, Sodium Chloride, Magnesium Chloride, White Oil, Glyceryl Stearate SE, Squalane, Cetyl Alcohol, Propylene Glycol Stearate SE, Wheat Germ Oil, Glyceryl Stearate, Isopropyl Myristate, Stearyl Stearate, Polysorbate-60, Propylene Glycol, Oleic Acid, Tocopheryl Acetate, Collagen, Sorbitan Stearate, Vitamin A & D, Triethanolamine, Aloe Vera Extract, Imidazolidinyl Urea, Methylparaben, Propylparaben, BHA

Direct Inquires to:
Consumer Product Information Center
1-888-408-6262
Strategic Science & Technologies, Inc.
PO Box 395
Newton Center, MA 02459

These statements have not been evaluated by the Food and Drug Administration. This product is not intended to diagnose, treat, cure, or prevent any disease.

Shown in Product Identification Guide, page 525

NATURAL SENSATION™

Description: Natural SENSATION™ is a patented transdermal preparation of L-Arginine in a pleasant cream base. It is used topically to increase the concentration of nitric oxide, derived from L-Arginine, in the female genital tissue, especially the clitoris, improving sensitivity and therefore the ability to reach satisfactory orgasm. The increased sensitivity begins within 2–4 minutes.

Active Ingredient: L-Arginine

Other Ingredients: Water, Choline Chloride, Sodium Chloride, Magnesium Chloride, White Oil, Glyceryl Stearate SE, Squalane, Cetyl Alcohol, Propylene Glycol Stearate SE, Wheat Germ Oil, Glyceryl Stearate, Isopropyl Myristate, Stearyl Stearate, Polysorbate-60, Propylene Glycol, Oleic Acid, Tocopheryl Acetate, Collagen, Sorbitan Stearate, Vitamin A & D, Triethanolamine, Aloe Vera Extract, Imidazolidinyl Urea, Methylparaben, Propylparaben, BHA

Suggested Use: Apply gently to the labia, clitoris and outer area of the vagina. Rub in tenderly for 3–5 minutes. The effect begins at once. Repeat as often as needed. To remove, wash with water.

These statements have not been evaluated by the Food and Drug Administration. This product is not intended to diagnose, treat, cure, or prevent any disease.

Nature's Own PAIN EXPELLER™

Description: Nature's Own PAIN EXPELLER™ is a patented transdermal preparation of L-Arginine and oleoresin capsicum in a pleasant cream base that relieves pain, naturally by providing
L-Arginine in the tissue for the synthesis of the natural pain controlling substance, kyotorphin. In addition, components of oleoresin capsicum are known to deplete the pain transmitting agent, substance P in nerve fibers. Repeated use increases effectiveness.

Suggested Use: Apply liberally to the area of joint or muscle pain. Rub in completely for 3–5 minutes. Pain relief begins in 5–30 minutes. Repeat as needed. Repeated application lengthens the duration of the pain free period. To remove, wash with water.

Active Ingredients: L-Arginine and Oleoresin Capsicum.

Other Ingredients: Water, Choline Chloride, Sodium Chloride, Magnesium Chloride, White Oil, Glyceryl Stearate SE, Squalane, Cetyl Alcohol, Propylene Glycol Stearate SE, Wheat Germ Oil, Glyceryl Stearate, Isopropyl Myristate, Stearyl Stearate, Polysorbate-60, Propylene Glycol, Oleic Acid, Tocopheryl Acetate, Collagen, Sorbitan Stearate, Vitamin A & D, Triethanolamine, Aloe Vera Extract, Imidazolidinyl Urea, O. Capsicum, Methylparaben, Propylparaben, BHA

Caution: Avoid eyes, mucus membranes and open cuts.

Direct Inquires to:
Consumer Product Information Center
1-888-408-6262
Strategic Science & Technologies, Inc.
PO Box 395
Newton Center, MA 02459

These statements have not been evaluated by the Food and Drug Administration. This product is not intended to diagnose, treat, cure, or prevent any disease.

WARM CREAM™

Description: Warm Cream™ is a patented transdermal preparation of L-Arginine in a pleasant cream base. It is used topically to restore the bodies own warmth to cold hands and feet by increasing the concentration of nitric oxide derived from L-Arginine in the tissue of the hands and feet.

Suggested Use: Apply liberally to cold area. For hands, rub all over including back of hands and fingers. For feet, rub all over including tops of the feet. Rub in for three to five minutes. Warming begins within 30 minutes.

Active Ingredient: L-Arginine

Other Ingredients: Water, Choline Chloride, Sodium Chloride, Magnesium Chloride, White Oil, Glyceryl Stearate SE, Squalane, Cetyl Alcohol, Propylene Glycol Stearate SE, Wheat Germ Oil, Glyceryl Stearate, Isopropyl Myristate, Stearyl Stearate, Polysorbate-60, Propylene Glycol, Oleic Acid, Tocopheryl Acetate, Collagen, Sorbitan Stearate, Vitamin A & D, Triethanolamine, Aloe Vera Extract, Imidazolidinyl Urea, O. Capsicum Methylparaben, Propylparaben, BHA

Caution: Avoid eyes and mucus membranes and open cuts. To remove, wash with water.

Direct Inquires to:
Consumer Product Information Center
1-888-408-6262
Strategic Science & Technologies, Inc.
PO Box 395
Newton Center, MA 02459

These statements have not been evaluated by the Food and Drug Administration. This product is not intended to diagnose, treat, cure, or prevent any disease.

Shown in Product Identification Guide, page 525

Sunpower Nutraceutical Inc.

18003 SKY PARK CIRCLE
SUITE G
IRVINE, CA 92614

Direct Inquiries to:
Ph: (949) 833-8899

PRODUCT LISTING

Descriptions: Sunpower Nutraceutical System combined vitamins, minerals, special formulated herbs, Pycnogenol® and proprietary Traditional Chinese Medicines (TCM) from S.P. Pharmaceutical Inc. (S.P.) which manufactured at GMP facility and under FDA Act and U.S. Pharmacopeia quality, purity and potency standards.
Time-released, Double-layered tablets are made by advanced manufacturing techniques which allows nutrients to be released slowly for better absorption during digestion.

Sunpower Product Overview:
Sun Liver™: contains vitamins, minerals, Pycnogenol® and S.P. Pro-Liver Formula to help to fight free radical damage, and provide nutrients essential for healthy liver function.

Shown in Product Identification Guide, page 523

Continued on next page

Sunpower Product—Cont.

Sun Cardio™: contains CoQ10, OPC, Ginkgo Biloba, Red Wine Extract and S.P. Pro-Cardio Formula to help maintain normal cardiovascular system.

Power Circulation™: contains Ginkgo Biloba, Barley Grass, Lecithin and S.P. Pro-Circulation Formula to help maintain a healthy blood circulatory system.

Sun Joint™: contains Glucosamine, Chondroitin, Wild Yam, Bee Propolis and S.P. Pro-Connection Formula to provide essential nutrients for bone, joint, ligament and cartilage function.

Power Lasting™: contains Yohimbe, Damiana, Saw Palmetto, Pumpkin Seed, Sarsaparilla Root, and S.P. Pro-Long Formula to help maintain normal kidney and sexual function and enhance endurance.

Sun Beauty™ 1: Formulated for women ages 14–28 contains Alfalfa, St. John's Wort, Cranberry, Royal Jelly, and S.P. Beauty I Formula to help establish healthy hormonal rhythms and basic immunity.

Sun Beauty™ 2: Formulated for women ages 29–42 contains Alfalfa, Selenium, Green Tea, Uva Ursi Leaves, Cranberry, and S.P. Beauty II Formula to support and balance a woman's vitality and healthy immunity during the menstrual cycle.

Sun Beauty™ 3: Formulated for women ages over 43 contains chromium, Burdock Root, Fo-Ti, Black Cohoshe, Red Clover, Chaste Tree Berries, and S.P. Beauty III Formula to support general well-being during menopause and postmenopause.

Shown in Product Identification Guide, page 525

Wellness International Network, Ltd.

**5800 DEMOCRACY DRIVE
PLANO, TX 75024**

Direct Inquiries to:
Product Coordinator
(972) 312-1100
FAX: (972) 943-5250

BIOLEAN®
Herbal & Amino Acid Dietary Supplement

Uses: BIOLEAN® is a unique combination of Chinese herbal extracts and pharmaceutical-grade amino acids specifically designed to help raise overall health, participate in individual life extension programs, and enhance athletic performance. It has been shown to be extremely effective in promoting the healthy loss of excess body fat while helping to maintain lean body mass and potent energy levels. BIOLEAN, when used as a daily nutritional supplement, has also been shown to stimulate immune function in individuals with blunted sympathetic nervous systems, especially overweight and obese persons. It acts as a positive stimulator to immune functions involved in protection from environmental and dietary carcinogens. Components in BIOLEAN are known to cause fat loss through thermogenic activity and altered fuel metabolism resulting from sympathomimetic response to stimulation of beta receptors in adipose and muscle cells. The positive immune response, though not completely understood, is at least partially attributable to beta stimulation in adipocytes and the adaptogenic and tonifying activity of certain of the herbal extracts. This has been demonstrated in their long history of use in traditional Chinese herbal medicine as well as current scientific research which points to, among other possibilities, the extremely potent antioxidant properties found in some of the component plants, most notably in Green Tea and Schizandrae extracts. BIOLEAN may increase athletic performance and endurance through three pathways: 1) increased oxygen uptake in the lungs as a result of expanding bronchial passages; 2) enhanced mental acuity and response resulting from sympathetic nervous system stimulus; and 3) increasing the employment of fatty acids as fuel in muscle mitochondria while simultaneously sparing muscle glycogen and nitrogen.

The herbal extracts in BIOLEAN are produced in a unique and exclusive process which is proprietary to this product. Instead of creating extracts based on a set quantity of one particular active within many which may be present in any particular plant, BIOLEAN components are concentrated to maintain the natural and complete spectrum of biologically active factors, in the same ratio presented by the unprocessed plant.

Directions: AM Serving – Adults take one capsule and two tablets with low calorie food. PM Serving – Adults may take one tablet with low calorie food. If using BIOLEAN dietary supplement for the first time, limit daily intake to one capsule and one tablet on days one and two, and one capsule and two tablets on day three. Needs vary with each individual. This product has a maximum of 25mg concentrated ephedrine group alkaloids per serving in the form of herbal extracts.

Warnings: Not for use by children under the age of 18. If you are pregnant or nursing, if you have heart disease, thyroid disease, diabetes, high blood pressure, depression or other psychiatric condition, glaucoma, difficulty urinating, prostate enlargement, or seizure disorder, if you are using a monoamine oxidase inhibitor (MAOI) or any other prescription drug or over-the-counter drug containing ephedrine, pseudoephedrine or phenylpropanolamine (ingredients found in certain allergy, asthma, cough/cold and weight control products), consult a health professional before using this product. Exceeding recommended serving may cause serious adverse effects. Taking this product with other stimulants such as caffeine may cause serious side effects. Discontinue use and call a health professional immediately if you experience rapid heartbeat, dizziness, severe headache, shortness of breath, or other similar symptoms. Phenylketonurics: Contains phenylalanine. The maximum recommended daily dosage of ephedrine for a healthy, human adult is 100 mg, for not more than 12 weeks.

Ingredients: Calcium, Ephedra Alkaloids (as ma haung), Caffeine (as green tea leaf), Schizandrae berry, Rehmannia root, Hawthorne berry, Jujube seed, Alisma root, Angelicae dahuricae root, Epemidium, Poria Cocos, Rhizoma rhei, Stephania root, Angelicae sinensis root, Codonopsis root, Euconium bark, Notoginseng root, L-phenylalanine, L-tyrosine, L-carnitine, Cellulose, Stearic acid, Starch, Sodium lauryl sulfate, Hydroxypropyl cellulose, Magnesium stearate, Crosscarmelose sodium and Silicon dioxide and alfalfa.

How Supplied: One box contains 28 packets (28 daily servings), with one capsule and three tablets per packet.

BIOLEAN Accelerator™
Herbal & Amino Acid Formulation

Uses: BIOLEAN Accelerator™ is a unique combination of Chinese herbal extracts and pharmaceutical grade amino acids specifically designed to complement both BIOLEAN® and BIOLEAN Free® by extending and accelerating their actions. BIOLEAN and BIOLEAN Free are, in the traditional view of Chinese herbal medicine, strong Yang blends. This means that they are energy or heat-producing at their core. The addition of the amino acids and certain of the herbal components lends a very definite restorative or Yin element, as well. BIOLEAN Accelerator is a strong Yin herbal formula, intended to augment the lesser replenishing Yin elements of the other two herbal and amino acid supplements. Though the physiological actions of many herbs are complex and not totally understood, the formula in BIOLEAN Accelerator extends the adaptogenic, thermogenic, restorative and detoxifying results experienced with BIOLEAN and BIOLEAN Free, with an emphasis on the restorative and adaptogenic effects. The herbal formula is a combination of tonifiers traditionally used in China for the lungs, liver and kidneys.

Directions: For maximum effectiveness, use in conjunction with original

BIOLEAN or BIOLEAN Free. (Do not consume BIOLEAN and BIOLEAN Free on the same day.) Take one tablet in the morning with original BIOLEAN or BIOLEAN Free. BIOLEAN Accelerator™ may also be taken in the afternoon with or without additional BIOLEAN or BIOLEAN Free if desired. Maximum absorption will be attained if taken with low-calorie food.

Warnings: Phenylketonurics: Contains Phenylalanine. Not for use by children. Consult your physician before using this product if you are taking appetite suppressing drugs or antidepressants, or if you are pregnant or lactating. If symptoms of allergy develop, discontinue use.

Ingredients: Each tablet contains 250 mg. herbal mix (Microcrystalline Cellulose Black Sesame Seed, Raw Chinese Foxglove Root, Chinese Wolfberry Fruit, Achyranthes Root, Cornelian Cherry Fruit, Chinese Yam, Eclipta Herb, Rose Hips, Privet Fruit, Mulberry Fruit-Spike, Polygonati Rhizome, Cooked Chinese Foxglove Root, Poria Cocos, Cuscuta Seed, Foxnut Seed, Alisma Rhizome, Moutan Bark, Phellodendron Bark, Anemarrhena Rhizome, Schisandra Berry, Royal Jelly), L-Tyrosine, L-Phenylalanine, Calcium Carbonate, Calcium Phosphate Dibasic, Partially Hydrogenated Vegetable Oil, Hydroxypropyl Cellulose, Croscarmelose Sodium, Magnesium Stearate, Silicon Dioxide and Sodium Lauryl Sulfate.

How Supplied: One bottle contains 56 tablets.

BIOLEAN Free®
Herbal & Amino Acid Dietary Supplement

Uses: BIOLEAN Free® is a strategic blend of herbs, spices, vitamins, minerals and amino acids specifically formulated to enhance fat utilization and energy production through various metabolic pathways. It has been shown to reduce body fat through its thermogenic effects and to enhance both physical and mental performance.

Thermogenesis refers to the body's ability to convert substrates such as proteins, fats and carbohydrates into heat energy. This is carried out most efficiently in the Brown Adipose Tissue of our body which uses fatty acids as its preferred fuel. Other fat cells, namely White Adipose Tissue, are concerned primarily with the storage of fat rather than its conversion to energy. The thermogenic pathway is complex and relies upon a series of reactions to occur. BIOLEAN Free utilizes many compounds which act at various locations in this pathway to ensure the maximum efficiency of the thermogenic process. Quebracho is one of these very special compounds. This South American plant contains quebrachine, aspidiospermine and other alkaloids that possess the ability

to block alpha-2 adrenergic receptors in the body. This produces an enhanced sympathetic nervous system effect which, in turn, increases lipolysis (fat breakdown) within fat cells. The fatty acids released by this process can then be transported into the mitochondria to be used as a fuel. Ginger, cinnamon, horseradish, turmeric, cayenne and mustard are spices that stimulate thermogenesis in different ways. Some stimulate lipid mobilization in adipose tissue; others raise the resting metabolic rate; and some increase cAMP levels by inducing more beta receptors on fat cells and by increasing the concentration of adenylate cyclase. cAMP increases the breakdown of triglycerides to free fatty acids which are later used as fuel by the mitochondria in the cell. Methylxanthines (such as those found in green tea and yerba maté) also increase cAMP levels, but do this by inhibiting the enzyme, phosphodiesterase. These compounds have been noted to increase mental alertness, improve vitality, satisfy the appetite and increase energy. In addition to its methylxanthine content, green tea has recently been shown to possess strong antioxidant properties. Yerba maté is a plant that has been shown to produce the positive effects above without causing the insomnia seen with other methylxanthine-containing plants (such as coffee and kola nut). BIOLEAN Free also contains vitamin B-3 (niacin), vitamin B-6 (pyridoxine), chromium and vanadium, which aid in the proper metabolism of fats, proteins and carbohydrates. L-tyrosine also aids in metabolism and promotes satiety through hypothalamic release of CCK. Methionine is a precursor of L-carnitine which aids in the transport of fatty acids into the mitochondria for thermogenesis. Other herbs have been utilized in BIOLEAN Free. Ginseng and ho shou wu possess adaptogenic properties. Adaptogens help the body adapt to physiological and environmental stresses. Ginseng accomplishes this through its stabilizing effect on the hypothalamic-pituitary-adrenal-sympathetic nervous system. It can mediate an increased adrenal response to stress.

Ho shou wu has a stabilizing effect on the endocrine system and has restorative properties. It is also an antioxidant with a high flavonoid content. *Centella asiatica* contains asiaticoside and has been shown to increase activity levels and ease the body's ability to overcome fatigue when taken with ginseng and cayenne. Individually, *centella* has been shown to increase memory and mental acuity in studies abroad. Uva ursi contains the glycoside arbutin and promotes urinary health and body strength through its purifying effects. Ginkgo biloba is a tree whose leaves have been used for centuries as an herbal medicine. It contains flavonoids and is therefore a strong antioxidant. It reduces the tendency of platelets to stick together by inhibiting Platelet Activating Factor. It has been shown to increase blood flow to the heart, brain and other organs.

Directions: Adults (18 years and older) may take 4 tablets in the mid to late morning with a low-calorie food. Needs may vary with each individual. Some persons may require less than 4 caplets, or may prefer taking 3 tablets mid morning and 1 additional tablet mid afternoon to achieve optimum results. Do not exceed recommended daily amounts. It is recommended that you drink at least eight glasses of water daily.

Warnings: Not for use by children, pregnant women or lactating women. Consult your physician before using this product if you are taking appetite suppressing drugs or cardiovascular medication. Consult your physician if you have hypertension, heart disease, arrhythmias, prostatic hypertrophy, glaucoma, liver disease, renal disease or diabetes. Do not use if you have hyperthyroidism, psychosis, Parkinson's Disease, or are taking Monoamine oxidase inhibitors. BIOLEAN Free should not be taken on the same day as original BIOLEAN®. It is recommended that you minimize your caffeine intake while consuming this product. If allergic symptoms develop, discontinue use. Store in a cool, dry place. Keep out of reach of children.

Ingredients: Niacin (as niacinamide), Vitamin B6 (as pyridoxine HCI), Chromium (as chromium Chelavite® dinicotinate glycinate), Potassium (as potassium citrate), Green tea leaf extract, Yerba mate leaf extract, Korean ginseng root extract, Uva ursi leaf, Guarana seed, Quebracho bark extract, Gotu kola leaf, Ceylon cinnamon bark, Chinese horseradish root, Jamaican ginger root, Turmeric rhizome, Nigerian cayenne pepper, English mustard seed, Ho shou wu root, Ginkgo biloba leaf, L-Tyrosine, DL-Methionine, Vanadium, Dicalcium phosphate, Cellulose, Cellulose gum, Vegetable stearic acid, Silica, Vegetable magnesium stearate and vegetable resin glaze.

How Supplied: One box contains 28 packets, four tablets per packet.

BIOLEAN LipoTrim™
All-Natural Dietary Supplement

Uses: LipoTrim™ is a highly active, synergistic combination of garcinia cambogia extract and chromium polynicotinate specifically created for use with the other products in the BIOLEAN® System. The method of action is by inhibition of lipogenesis and regulation of blood glucose levels. Serum glucose derived from dietary carbohydrates and not immediately converted to energy or glycogen tends to be converted into fat stores and cholesterol. In individuals with excess body fat stores or slow basal metabolism, this tendency is thought to be higher. The garcinia cambogia extract present in LipoTrim is verified by HPLC analysis to be no less that 50%(-) hy-

Continued on next page

Biolean LipoTrim—Cont.

droxycitrate (HCA). HCA inhibits ATP-citrate lyase which retards Acetyl CoA synthesis, severely restricting conversion of excess glucose into fatty acids and cholesterol. Animal studies have shown a post-meal fatty acid synthesis reduction of 40–80% for an 8–12 hour period. When glucose to fat/cholesterol conversion is retarded, glycogen conversion continues, increasing liver stores and causing satiety signals to be sent to the brain resulting in appetite suppression. In situations of intense physical exercise, increased glycogen stores have been shown to result in enhanced endurance and recovery. By restricting the activity of insulin, chromium has been shown to exhibit a regulating effect on blood glucose levels thus extending the benefits of HCA.

Directions: As a dietary supplement, take one capsule three times daily, 30 minutes before each meal. LipoTrim should be used in conjunction with a healthy diet and exercise plan.

Warnings: Do not consume if you are pregnant or lactating. Not for use by young children. Consult your physician before using this product if your diet consists of less than 1,000 calories per day.

Ingredients: Garcinia Cambogia (as CitriMax™* supplying naturally occuring hydroxycitrate), Chromium Polynicotinate (as Chromemate®* supplying elemental chromium, gelatin, calcium sulfate, talc, magnesium stearate, silicon dioxide).

How Supplied: One bottle contains 84, easy-to-swallow capsules.

---

*CitriMax™ is a trademark of Inter-Health.
ChromeMate® is a registered trademark of InterHealth.

FOOD FOR THOUGHT™
Choline-Enriched Nutritional Drink

Uses: By utilizing scientifically established "smart nutrients," Food For Thought™ is a great-tasting citrus beverage ideal for work, school or anytime peak mental performance is desired.
Choline, a member of the B-complex family, is determined to be one of the few substances that possesses the ability to penetrate the blood-brain barrier—a protectant of the brain from the onslaught of chemicals taken into the body each day—and go directly into the brain cells to produce acetylcholine.
The most abundant neurotransmitter in the body, acetylcholine is the primary neurotransmitter between neurons and muscles. It is vital because of its role in motor behavior (muscular movement) and memory. Acetylcholine helps control muscle tone, learning, and primitive drives and emotions, while also controlling the release of the pituitary hormone

vasopressin—which is involved in learning and in the regulation of urine output. Studies show that low levels of acetylcholine can contribute to lack of concentration and forgetfulness, and may interfere with sleep patterns.
Food For Thought further enhances its effectiveness through the utilization of essential vitamins—required for promoting the synthesis of brain neurotransmitters—with a unique blend of minerals. The brain uses vitamins B3 (niacin) and B6 (pyridoxine), to convert the amino acid L-tryptophan into the mood- and sleep-regulating neurotransmitter serotonin, while vitamins B1 (thiamin), B5 (pantothenic acid), B6 (pyridoxine), and C and the minerals zinc and calcium are required for the production of acetylcholine.

Directions: Add 6 ounces of chilled water or fruit juice to one packet of mix. Stir briskly. Consume 1–2 times per day. Keep in a cool, dry place. For maximum results, combine this product with one serving of Winrgy™.

Warnings: Not for use by children, pregnant or lactating women. Persons taking medications should seek medical advice before taking this product. Persons with ulcers or a history of ulcers should consult their physician before using a choline supplement. Do not consume more than four servings per day. Avoid the use of antacids containing aluminum with this product.

Ingredients: Carbohydrates, Sugars, Vitamin C (as ascorbic acid), Vitamin E (as alpha tocopherol acetate), Thiamin (as thiamin mononitrate), Riboflavin, Niacin (as niacinamide), Vitamin B6 (as pyridoxine hydrochloride), Vitamin B12 (as cyanocobalamin), Pantothenic Acid (as calcium pantothenate), Calcium (as calcium pantothenate), Zinc (as zinc gluconate), Copper (as copper gluconate), Chromium (as chromium aspartate), Choline (as choline bitartrate), Glycine, Lysine (as L-lysine hydrochloride), Fructose, Natural Flavors, Silicon Dioxide and Magnesium Gluconate.

How Supplied: One box contains 28 packets of drink mix. Serving size equals one packet.

STEPHAN Clarity™
Nutritional Supplement

Uses: STEPHAN Clarity™, designed for use by both men and women, contains selected tissue proteins in the form of nutrients important to memory and concentration.
This is achieved by utilizing such ingredients as lecithin and glutamic acid. Lecithin is a popular supplement widely embraced for the treatment and prevention of memory loss. Known for properties that have been scientifically proven to increase the firing of neurons in the nervous system, glutamic acid is an amino

acid which influences the body by serving as brain fuel. It also metabolizes sugars and fats, as well as detoxifies.
Ginkgo biloba, a third primary ingredient in STEPHAN Clarity™, is a special additive which increases the flow of blood to the brain and is noted for improving concentration and learning ability. Recently, a study published in the *Journal of the American Medical Association* demonstrated that ginkgo biloba extract improves mental performance in dementias for individuals with Alzheimer's disease and multi-infarct dementia. It was also reported to stabilize and – in 20% of the cases – improve the subjects' functioning for periods of six months to a year.
Together with the support of carefully selected vitamins, minerals, amino acids, and herbs, STEPHAN Clarity™ is a natural and effective way to better one's health.

Directions: Take one to two capsules per day.

Warnings: Phenylketonurics: Contains Phenylalanine.

Ingredients: Vitamin A (as acetate), Vitamin C (as ascorbic acid), Vitamin D (as cholecalciferol), Vitamin E (as DL-alpha tocopheryl acetate), Thiamin (as thiamin HCl), Riboflavin, Niacin (as niacinamide), Vitamin B6 (as pyridoxine HCl), Folic Acid, Vitamin B12 (as cyanocobalamin), Biotin, Pantothenic Acid (as D-calcium pantothenic acid), Lecithin, Bee Pollen, Glutamic Acid (as L-glutamic acid), Ribonucleic Acid (RNA), Ginkgo Biloba 8:1 extract (leaf), Aspartic Acid (as L-aspartic acid) Leucine (as L-leucine), Arginine (as L-arginine), Lysine (as L-lysine), Phenylalanine (as L-phenylalanine), Serine (as L-serine), Proline (as L-proline), Valine (as L-valine), Isoleucine (as L-isoleucine), Alanine (as L-alanine), Glycine (as L-glycine), Threonine (as L-threonine), Tyrosine (as L-tyrosine), Histidine (as L-histidine), Methionine (as L-methionine), Adenosine Triphosphate Cysteine (as L-cysteine), Talc, Ethylcellulose and Silicon Dioxide.

How Supplied: One bottle contains 60 easy-to-swallow capsules.

DHEA Plus™
Pharmaceutical-Grade Formulation

Uses: By utilizing the latest and most advanced breakthrough applications in age management, DHEA Plus™ uniquely combines dehydroepiandrosterone (DHEA), Bioperine® and ginkgo biloba leaf to safely and effectively aid the body.
These age management factors are mainly attributed to the properties of DHEA, a natural substance obtained from the barbasco root, also known as Mexican Wild Yam, which is synthesized in a pharmaceutical laboratory to be utilized for specific health applications.

Once supplemental DHEA is orally consumed, it is quickly absorbed into the bloodstream through the intestines and binds to a sulfate compound which creates DHEA-S. DHEA-S is the ultimate substance for which the body uses to manufacture hormones. Natural DHEA levels, abundant in the bloodstream and present at an even higher level in the tissues of the brain, are known to decline with age in both sexes. Scientific research proves that adequate levels of DHEA in the body can actually slow the aging process. Further studies have shown that it often prevents, improves and, many times, reverses conditions such as cancer, heart disease, memory loss, obesity and osteoporosis.

Bioperine, a pure piperine extract, enhances the body's natural thermogenic activity and is another important ingredient in DHEA Plus. Thermogenesis is the metabolic process that generates energy at the cellular level. While thermogenesis plays an integral role in our body's ability to properly utilize daily foods and nutrients in the body, it also sets in motion the mechanisms that lead to digestion and subsequent gastrointestinal absorption.

Known for possessing antioxidant activity, or flavonoid effects, ginkgo biloba proves to decrease platelet aggregation and increase vasodilation which appears to extend blood flow to the peripheral arteries and the brain. Some improvement in cognitive abilities has been noted as well as inhibition of lipid peroxidation, thereby stabilizing the cell wall against free-radical attack.

Directions: Adults take one capsule daily with food.

Warnings: This product should only be consumed by adults and is not intended for use by children. Do not consume if you are pregnant or lactating. Consult your physician before using this product if you are taking prescription medications. Persons with a history of prostate cancer should seek medical advice before using this product.

Ingredients: Dihydroxyepiandrosterone (DHEA), Ginkgo Biloba leaf, Bioperine, Calcium Phosphate Dibasic, Partially Hydrogenated Vegetable Oil, Talc, Magnesium Stearate, Silicon Dioxide and Croscarmellose Sodium.

How Supplied: One bottle contains 60 capsules.

---

*Bioperine is a registered trademark of Sabinsa Corporation.

MASS APPEAL™
Amino Acid & Mineral Workout Supplement

Uses: Utilizing natural compounds which mimic the beneficial effects of anabolic steroids, Mass Appeal™ is specifically formulated to enhance athletic performance without the harmful side effects of steroids.

Among Mass Appeal's scientifically researched and proven ingredients is creatine, a naturally occurring substance which functions as a storage molecule for high-energy phosphate – the ultimate source of muscular energy known as adenosine triphosphate, or ATP. More than 95 percent of the body's total amount of creatine is contained within the muscles, with type II muscle fibers (fibers that generate large amounts of force) possessing greater initial levels and higher rates of utilization. Unlike other artificial aids used to enhance performance, creatine monohydrate saturates the muscle cells and causes a muscle "cell volumizing" effect by beneficially forcing water molecules inside the muscle cell. This promotes an increase in muscle growth by helping muscles form new proteins faster while slowing down the destructive breakdown of muscle cells during exercise. Studies show that creatine loading not only improves performance during short-duration, high intensity and intermittent exercises, but it accelerates energy recovery and reduces muscle fatigue by reducing lactic acid build-up as well.

Found in high concentrations within muscle cells and proteins throughout the body, the branched chain amino acids (BCAAs) L-leucine, L-valine and L-isoleucine are also incorporated into Mass Appeal's scientifically engineered formulation. BCAAs increase protein synthesis and can be oxidized inside muscle cells as ATP, a protein-sparing effect which indirectly increases anabolism by reducing the muscle's need to burn its own proteins during bodybuilding or strenuous exercise. When dietary intake of these amino acids is inadequate, muscle protein is broken down into its individual amino acid constituents and utilized in other essential metabolic reactions within the body. Through supplementation, the catabolic breakdown of muscle can be minimized and the muscle tissue preserved.

Alpha-ketoglutaric acid and the amino acid L-glutamine also protect against muscle catabolism by assisting muscle protein synthesis and preserving the body's natural stores of glutamine in the muscle.

Another major contributor to the Mass Appeal™ formulation is the amino acid inosine. By increasing hemoglobin's affinity for binding oxygen within red blood cells, inosine supplementation enables red blood cells to carry more oxygen as they travel from the lungs to the muscles.

Vanadyl sulfate, known for its vasodilator effects, has been shown to markedly increase the blood flow to muscle cells. Researchers also believe that this mineral not only contributes to increased efficiency in the metabolic pathways controlled by the body's insulin, but also triggers certain glucose transporters much in the same way insulin does. This results in increased glucose transport into the muscle tissue, in-

creased glycogen storage, and decreases the breakdown of muscle protein as an energy source.

Directions: Adults (18 years and older) may take a loading dose of 3 packets in the morning and 2 packets in the late afternoon for one week. This dose may be repeated every three months. Following one week of the loading dose, begin the maintenance dose of 1 packet daily two hours after exercise. Needs may vary with each individual.

For individuals desiring enhanced effects, increase the loading dose to 3 to 4 packets, three times per day (morning, afternoon and evening). Following one week of this enhanced loading dose, begin the enhanced maintenance dose of 2 packets in the morning and 2 packets in the late afternoon. It is recommended that one maintain a low-fat, high-protein diet; drink at least eight glasses of water per day; and engage in 30 to 60 minutes of aerobic and anaerobic exercise three to four times per week. For optimal effects, take in conjunction with Phyto-Vite®, Pro-Xtreme™ and Sure2Endure™.

Warning: Not for use by children, pregnant women or lactating women. Consult your physician before using this product if you have any medical conditions. Do not take if you have kidney disease, muscle disease or are on a protein-restricted diet. Discontinue immediately if allergic symptoms develop. Keep out of the reach of children. Store in a cool, dry place.

Ingredients: Creatine Monohydrate, Inosine (phosphate-bonded), L-leucine, L-valine, L-isoleucine, Alpha-Ketoglutaric acid, KIC (calcium keto-isocaproate), L-glutamine, Vanadyl Sulfate, Dicalcium phosphate, Microcrystalline Cellulose, Stearic Acid, Croscarmellose Sodium, Silica, Magnesium Stearate and film coating (hydroxypropyl methylcellulose, hydroxypropyl cellulose, polyethylene glycol, titanium dioxide and propylene glycol).

How Supplied: One box contains 28 packets, four tablets per packet.

PRO-XTREME™
Dietary Supplement

Uses: The need for protein in the human diet has been increasingly studied, especially in the last decade. As a result of this research, several factors regarding the optimal daily requirements and sources of protein have become very clear. Even the current government published RDIs, which are based solely on minimal needs for survival, have increased to .6–.8 grams per kilogram of body weight per day.

Current clinical findings however indicate that an RDI necessary to maintain

Continued on next page

Protein Xtreme—Cont.

optimum health for even a sedentary adult are closer to double that. Circumstances including illness, fat-loss diets, regular exercise, accelerated adolescent growth, or chronic mental or emotional stress indicate requirements 2–3 times that. Competitive or strength athletes, post surgical patients or any situation causing wasting disease such as chemotherapy, HIV, burn trauma or radiation therapy can increase the metabolic need for protein by a factor of up to 6 times the official government RDIs.

Furthermore, these figures represent protein which has been absorbed and made available to the tissues of the body and *not* merely that which has been consumed. This is a distinction current clinical research has recognized as *critical* to proper understanding of the need for protein in the human diet.

Before protein can be absorbed and utilized it must first be digested. Following digestion the free amino acids and di and tripeptides that result from protein breakdown are absorbed at the surface of the small intestine. The process of digestion and absorption requires several steps and is most efficient in the upper portion or proximal section of the jejunum (small intestine). In order for absorption of dietary protein to occur, it must first be reduced from larger oligo and polypeptides to di and tripeptides, the smallest protein fragments consisting of only two or three peptide-bonded amino acids, and free amino acids. Di and tripeptides have been clearly shown to be preferential over free forms. This process must occur fast enough and at a rate high enough to take advantage of the proximal transporters, those that specialize in di and tripeptides and which are in abundance only in this short section of upper intestinal bowel. Once protein has passed this lumenal area, relatively no further protein breakdown or absorption occurs. The balance moves on relatively unchanged into the colon, where it is definitely a negative health factor causing minimal gas and gastrointestinal distress, and when experienced chronically, can lead to colon disease and malignancy. It is now generally believed to be the number one factor responsible for the world's highest rate of colon cancer experienced in the U.S.

Pro-Xtreme™ is specifically engineered based on a new profile for protein in optimum human metabolism arising from these new clinical findings. With an exceptionally high protein content of 40 percent, Pro-Xtreme™ not only promotes increased nitrogen retention—thereby minimizing the negative effects of increased protein intake or reduced caloric intake—but it works in harmony with natural gastrointestinal activity to produce maximum absorption as well.

Because of the fat content and the density of the bolus, meals containing tissue-source protein are released from the stomach and travel through the intestines at a rate which is naturally slower and more conducive to efficient digestion and absorption. The problems begin when too much tissue protein is consumed or the process of digestion and absorption is incomplete. It is estimated that at best only 30–35% of the protein consumed in an average protein-containing meal is absorbed allowing the balance of now detrimental undigested protein to pass into the colon.

In the case of liquid protein supplements, the problem is one not only of excessive amounts of protein being consumed but also the speed at which the bolus travels throughout the jejunum. Liquid meals, especially those with insufficient soluble fiber, have decreased transit time, leaving less time for digestion and absorption. Consequently, even in individuals with normal gastrointestinal function, liquid forms of whole proteins generally result in equally incomplete and oftentimes less absorption than their tissue food counterparts.

Pro-Xtreme™ utilizes sequentially hydrolyzed whey protein isolates of the highest quality to insure complete and rapid absorption of the highest levels of essential and branched-chain amino acids (BCAAs) in the preferred smallest peptide bonded form. These features, coupled with its industry-leading lowest average molecular weight, soluble-fiber content and delicious vanilla-cappuccino flavor, offer a primary source of protein that may be used any time a protein supplement is desired.

The combination and sequencing of amino acids in whey protein also results in increased tissue storage of glutathione, a stable tripeptide whose antioxidant activity is known to improve immune function. And, although whey protein naturally contains 5 to 7 percent of glutamine, the formula for Pro-Xtreme™ incorporates additional gram amounts of L-glutamine to its list of highly evolved ingredients as well. This extra step is designed to promote anticatabolic effects in skeletal muscle while focusing on gastrointestinal and immune function improvement. Glutamine and the critical BCAA leucine are deemed indispensable for the healthy functioning of other tissues and metabolic processes. By maintaining a rich supply of BCAAs, Pro-Xtreme™ proves protein sparing within muscle and offers the highest biological value possible.

Pro-Xtreme™ is formulated specifically for use with the other products in the BIOLEAN® System.

Directions: Add 1 packet (40 grams) Pro-Xtreme™ to 1 cup (8 ounces) cold water and stir. There is no need for blending or shaking. Pro-Xtreme™ may also be mixed with lowfat or nonfat milk, milk substitutes or blended with ice for a delicious and nourishing dessert.

Warning: Phenylketonurics: Contains phenylalanine.

Ingredients: Calcium, Iron, Magnesium, Chloride, Sodium, Potassium, Branched Chain Amino Acid Proprietary Blend, Glutamic Acid (as whey protein hydrolysate & L-glutamine), Leucine, Aspartic Acid, Lysine, Threonine, Isoleucine, Proline, Valine, Alanine, Serine, Cysteine, Phenylalanine, Tyrosine, Arginine, Methionine, Glycine, Histidine, Tryptophan, Maltodextrin, Natural & Artificial Flavorings, Fructose, Cocoa, Salt and Sucralose.

How Supplied: One box contains 14 packets. Serving size equals one packet.

SATIETE®
Herbal and Amino Acid Supplement

Uses: With its synergistic blend of herbs and amino acids, Satiete® addresses many of today's health concerns by ensuring maximum nutritional support.

One such ingredient is 5-HTP (5-Hydroxytryptophan). 5-HTP is an amino acid derivative and the immediate precursor to serotonin, a neurotransmitter involved in regulating mood, sleep, appetite, energy level and sensitivity to pain. Like drugs known as selective serotonin reuptake inhibitors (SSRI's), 5-HTP enhances the activity of serotonin, a hormone produced by the brain that is involved in mood, sleep, and appetite. Low levels of serotonin are associated with depression, anxiety, and sleep disorders. SSRI's prevent the brain cells from using up serotonin too quickly, thereby causing a deficiency. 5-HTP increases the cell's production of serotonin, which boosts serotonin levels.

L-5-HTP is a standardized extract of Griffonia simplicifolia (containing greater than 95% anhydrous 5-HTP), and the focus of an ABC *Prime Time Live* report that aired on June 17, 1998. The news segment explored claims that 5-HTP can help alleviate the effects of a variety of conditions, including depression, anxiety, insomnia, and obesity.

The diverse physiological functions of serotonin in the body include actions as a neurotransmitter, a regulator of smooth muscle function in the cardiovascular and gastrointestinal system, and a regulator of platelet function. Serotonin is involved in numerous central nervous system actions such as regulating mood, sleep and appetite. In the gastrointestinal system, serotonin stimulates gastric motility. Serotonin also stimulates platelet aggregation.

As a precursor to serotonin, 5-HTP helps to normalize serotonin activity in the body. Considerable research has been conducted regarding the activity of 5-HTP. Some of the clinical studies are summarized below:

Mood—Dysregulation of serotonin metabolism in the central nervous system has been shown to affect mood. 5-HTP helps to normalize serotonin levels and,

thereby, positively affect mood. In a double-blind study using objective assessments of mood, researchers in Zurich reported significant improvements in mood with 5-HTP. Likewise, in a double-blind, multi-center study in Germany, researchers reported significant improvements in both objective and self-assessment indices of mood.

Sleep—Many studies have shown that depletion of serotonin results in insomnia, which is reversed by administration of 5-HTP. Likewise, Soulairac and Lambinet reported that 100 mg of 5-HTP resulted in significant improvement for people who complained of trouble sleeping. Futhermore, serotonin is metabolized to the hormone melatonin, which is known to help regulate the sleep cycle; by increasing serotonin levels with 5-HTP, melatonin levels are also increased.

Appetite—Food intake is thought to suppress appetite through the production of serotonin from the amino acid tryptophan. Because it is an intermediary in the conversion process of tryptophan to serotonin, 5-HTP may reduce appetite in a similar manner as food intake, but without the calories. In a recent double-blind placebo-controlled study, subjects taking 5-HTP lost significant weight compared to control subjects. A reduction in carbohydrate intake and early satiety were seen in the 5-HTP group.

Another key ingredient in the Satiete formulation is Gymnema sylvestre, whose active ingredient "gymnemic acid" affects the taste buds in the oral cavity as the acid prevents the taste buds from being activated by any sugar molecules in the food; and the absorptive surface of the intestines where the acid prevents the intestine from absorbing sugar molecules. Practically speaking, this creates a reduced appetite for sweet tasting food, as well as reducing the metabolic effect of sugar by reducing its digestion in the intestines thus reducing the blood sugar level. In experimental and clinical trials, Gymnema sylvestre has been successful in treating both insulin-dependent and non-insulin dependent diabetics without reducing the blood sugar level to below the normal blood sugar levels, an effect seen with the use of insulin oral hypoglycemic sulphony lurea compounds. Due to its non-toxic nature and sweetness-suppression activity, Gymnema sylvestre can play a role in treating conditions caused by excessive sugar intake. Not only may diabetics benefit from it, conditions like obesity, hypoglycemia, anemia and osteoporosis can also be treated using Gymnema sylvestre.

Vanadyl sulfate, because of its insulin-like properties and its ability to improve cell responsiveness, is being used by progressive alternative physicians and natural healers to treat diabetes. Studies show that vanadyl is very effective in normalizing blood sugar levels and controlling conditions such as insulin resistance, or Type II diabetes.

Magnesium, malic acid and St. John's Wort are also combined in Satiete's proven formulation. Magnesium is a key mineral cofactor for many anaerobic as well as aerobic reactions that generate energy, and has an oxygen-sparing effect. It is essential for the cell's mitochondria "powerhouses" to function normally, being involved in both the production and utilization of ATP.

Malic Acid has an oxygen-sparing effect and there are a number of indications that malic acid is a very critical molecule in controlling mitochondrial function. Malate is a source of energy from the Krebs cycle and is the only metabolite of the cycle which falls in concentration during exhaustive physical activity. Depletion of malate has also been linked to physical exhaustion. By giving malic acid and magnesium as dietary supplements, flexibility to use aerobic and anaerobic energy sources can be enhanced and energy production can be boosted. Lab studies show that many patients with fibromyalgia (or with chronic fatigue) have low magnesium levels. Magnesium supplementation enhances the treatment of both conditions. Its benefits appear to result, at least in part, from its positive impact on serotonin function.

Combining 5-HTP with St. John's Wort Extract (0.3% hypericin context), malic acid, and magnesium, is part of an overall fibromyalgia treatment plan providing excellent results, due in large measure to its improvement of sleep quality and mood.

Directions: Start by taking one hypoallergenic tablet three times per day 30 to 60 minutes before meals. If needed after two weeks of use, increase the dosage to two tablets, three times per day. Do not exceed nine tablets daily without medical supervision.

Warning: If you are taking MAO inhibitor drugs, tricyclic antidepressants, SSRI antidepressants (Prozac, Paxil, Zoloft) or prescription diet drugs, do not take this product without medical supervision. If you suffer from liver or kidney disease, serious gastrointestinal disorders or carcinoid syndrome, do not take this product without medical supervision. If gastrointestinal upset develops and persists, reduce dosage, take only with large meals or discontinue use. As with any product, pregnant or lactating women should first consult their doctor.

Ingredients: Thiamin (as thiamin HCl), Riboflavin, Niacin (as niacinamide), Vitamin B6 (as pyridoxine HCl), Folic Acid, Vitamin B12 (as cyanocobalamin), Magnesium (as magnesium oxide), Malic Acid, St. John's Wort herb extract, Griffonia Simplicifolia seed extract, Gymnema Sylvestris Leaf, Ginkgo Biloba leaf extract, Vanadyl Sulfate, Adenoside Triphosphate (ATP), Ribonucleic Acid (RNA), Microcrystalline Cellulose, Stearic Acid, Croscarmellose Sodium, Magnesium Stearate, Silicon Dioxide, Ethylcellulose and Hydroxypropylcellulose.

How Supplied: One bottle contains 84 tablets.

STEPHAN™ Elasticity®
Nutritional Supplement

Uses: A nutritional food supplement for men and women, STEPHAN™ Elasticity® contains a scientifically balanced mixture of specific tissue proteins established as important for skin tone and texture.

Utilizing such scientifically respected ingredients as vitamin A and selenium, STEPHAN Elasticity is also supported by various other vitamins, minerals and amino acids dedicated to epidermal appearance.

Due to its antioxidant properties, vitamin A has been dubbed the "skin vitamin." It is commonly used as a means of preventing premature aging of the skin. In addition, synthetic derivatives of vitamin A are often used to treat acne and psoriasis.

Selenium is also considered beneficial to the skin. It was recently reported that low blood selenium in the context of low blood vitamin A increases the risk for certain types of skin cancer.

Directions: Take one to two capsules per day.

Warning: Accidental overdose of iron-containing products is a leading cause of fatal poisoning in children under 6. Keep this product out of the reach of children. In case of accidental overdose, call a doctor or poison control center immediately. Phenylketonurics: Contains Phenylalanine.

Ingredients: Vitamin A (as acetate), Vitamin C (as ascorbic acid), Vitamin E (as DL-alpha tocopheryl acetate), Calcium (as calcium amino acid chelate), Iron (as iron amino acid chelate), Magnesium (as magnesium amino acid chelate), Zinc (as zinc amino acid chelate), Selenium (as selenium acid chelate), Manganese (as manganese amino acid chelate), Chromium (as chromium amino acid chelate), Horsetail (Equisetum arvense), Fucus Vesiculosus, Glutamic Acid (as L-glutamic acid), Ribonucleic Acid (RNA), Aspartic Acid (as L-aspartic acid), Leucine (as L-leucine), Arginine (as L-arginine HCl), Lysine (as Lysine HCl), Serine (as L-serine), Phenylalanine (as L-phenylalanine), Proline (as L-proline), Valine (as L-valine), Isoleucine (as L-isoleucine), Alanine (as L-alanine), Glycine (as L-glycine), Threonine (as L-threonine), Tyrosine (as L-tyrosine), Histidine (as L-histidine), Methionine (as L-methionine), Adenosine Triphosphate, Cysteine (as L-cysteine HCl), Talc, Ethylcellulose, Food Glaze and Silicon Dioxide.

How Supplied: One bottle contains 60 easy-to-swallow capsules.

Continued on next page

STEPHAN Elixir®
Nutritional Supplement

Uses: Formulated with an exclusive blend of specific proteins, STEPHAN Elixir® is ideal for both men and women. These tissue proteins are supported by vitamins, minerals, amino acids and herbs recognized as important for general health and well-being.

Among the scientifically researched and proven ingredients utilized in STEPHAN Elixir are vitamin E and cysteine. Vitamin E protects against the ravages of aging in several ways. It is essential for the normal functioning of the body and is especially important for normal neurological functions in humans. It also serves as a potent antioxidant and has been dubbed the body's "first line of defense" against free-radical attack by helping to guard against free radicals, the type of cellular damage that has been linked to the initiation of cancer and heart disease.

Cysteine has also been found to inactivate free radicals and thus protect and preserve the cells. This sulfur-containing amino acid is a precursor of glutathione, a tripeptide, that is claimed to safeguard the body against various toxins and pollutants, therefore extending the life span.

Directions: Take one to two capsules per day.

Warnings: Accidental overdose of iron-containing products is a leading cause of fatal poisoning in children under 6. Keep this product out of the reach of children. In case of accidental overdose, call a doctor or poison control center immediately. Phenylketonurics: Contains phenylalanine.

Ingredients: Vitamin A (as vitamin A acetate), Vitamin C (as ascorbic acid), Vitamin D (as cholecalciferol), Vitamin E (as D-alpha tocopheryl acetate), Thiamin (as thiamin HCl), Riboflavin, Niacin (as niacinamide), Vitamin B6 (as pyridoxine HCl), Folic Acid, Vitamin B12 (as cyanocobalamin), Biotin, Pantothenic Acid (as D-calcium pantothenate), Calcium (as D-calcium pantothenate), Iron (as amino acid chelate), Zinc (as zinc amino acid chelate), Selenium (as selenium amino acid chelate), Bee Pollen, Glutamic Acid (as isolated soy protein), Citric Acid, Ginkgo Biloba 4:1 extract (leaf), Malic Acid, Yeast (RNA), Aspartic Acid, Leucine, Arginine, Lysine, Phenylalanine, Serine, Proline, Valine, Isoleucine, Alanine, Glycine, Threonine, Tyrosine, Histidine, Methionine, Cysteine, Tryptophan, Adenosine Triphosphate, Ribonucleic Acid (RNA), Starch, Talc and Silicon Dioxide.

How Supplied: One bottle contains 60 easy-to-swallow capsules.

STEPHAN Essential®
Nutritional Supplement

Uses: STEPHAN Essential® is a nutritional food supplement which contains specific tissue proteins supported by vitamins, minerals, herbs and amino acids that are proactive to cardiovascular and circulatory management. L-carnitine, vitamin E and linoleic acid are only some of these very important components.

Scientifically researched and a major contributor to the effects of STEPHAN Essential, L-carnitine is necessary for the transport of long-chain fatty acids into the mitochondria, the metabolic furnaces of the cells. These fatty acids prove a major source for the production of energy in the heart and skeletal muscles, structures that are particularly vulnerable to L-carnitine deficiency. Appropriate levels of L-carnitine in the body have been shown to protect against cardiovascular disease, muscle disease, diabetes and kidney disease.

While vitamin E has proven beneficial in serving to boost the immune system and protect against cardiovascular disease, it has also been established as an important therapy for disorders related to neurologic symptoms. Omega 3–Oil, another important addition to STEPHAN Essential, can lower serum cholesterol levels and decrease platelet stickiness, proving beneficial in the prevention of coronary heart disease.

STEPHAN Essential may be consumed by both men and women.

Directions: Take one to two capsules per day.

Warnings: Phenylketonurics: Contains Phenylalanine.

Ingredients: Vitamin E (as D-alpha tocopheryl succinate), Magnesium (as magnesium amino acid chelate), Selenium (as selenium amino acid chelate), Bee Pollen, Carnitine (as L-carnitine bitartrate), Fish Oil (as omega 3 fatty acids), Glutamic Acid, Yeast (RNA), Aspartic Acid, Leucine, Arginine, Lysine, Phenylalanine, Serine, Proline, Valine, Isoleucine, Alanine, Glycine, Threonine, Tyrosine, Histidine, Adenosine Triphosphate, Methionine, Cysteine, Tryptophan, Talc and Silicon Dioxide.

How Supplied: One bottle contains 60 easy-to-swallow capsules.

STEPHAN Feminine®
Nutritional Supplement

Uses: Specifically designed for women, STEPHAN Feminine® contains selected tissue proteins supported by vitamins, minerals and amino acids regarded as important to the ever-changing female body. This is achieved through such scientifically researched ingredients as magnesium and boron.

STEPHAN Feminine utilizes magnesium as an important ingredient responsible for regulating the flow of calcium between cells. Studies reveal that women with high-calcium diets report fewer PMS symptoms including less irritability and depression, as well as fewer headaches, backaches and cramps. Magnesium thus ensures individuals are receiving maximum benefits from calcium intake.

Researchers also report many promising results on the effects of dietary boron. Conclusions show that supplementary boron markedly reduces the excretion of both calcium and magnesium while increasing production of an active form of estrogen and testosterone.

Directions: Take one to two capsules per day.

Warnings: Phenylketonurics: Contains Phenylalanine.

Ingredients: Vitamin E (as DL-alpha tocopheryl acetate), Selenium (as selenium amino acid chelate), Magnesium Oxide, Glutamic Acid, Ribonucleic Acid (RNA), Aspartic Acid, Leucine, Arginine, Lysine, Phenylalanine, Serine, Proline, Valine, Isoleucine, Alanine, Glycine, Threonine, Tyrosine, Histidine, Methionine, Cysteine, Tryptophan, Adenosine Triphosphate, Boron (as boron amino acid chelate), Talc and Silicon Dioxide.

How Supplied: One bottle contains 60 easy-to-swallow capsules.

STEPHAN™ Flexibility®
Nutritional Supplement

Uses: A nutritional supplement for both men and women, STEPHAN™ Flexibility® is rich with exclusive proteins which are supported by vitamins, minerals and amino acids recognized as beneficial to the health of joint and soft tissues.

Glycine, an amino acid, is one very significant ingredient utilized in STEPHAN Flexibility. In a pilot study investigating the possibility of glycine's effect on spastic control, a 25% improvement was noted on subjects with chronic multiple sclerosis. Furthermore, all patients benefited to some degree, and no toxicity or other adverse side effects were noted.

Another important amino acid in STEPHAN Flexibility is L-histidine. Reports suggest that supplementary L-histidine may actually boost the activity of suppressor T cells. Because rheumatoid arthritis is one of the many autoimmune diseases in which T-cell activity is subnormal, these conclusions lend further support that L-histidine may prove beneficial in its treatment.

Vitamin E can also be found in STEPHAN Flexibility because of its ability to relieve muscular cramps. According to one popular study, supplemental vitamin E caused remarkable relief from persistent nocturnal leg and foot cramps in 82% of the 125 patients tested.

Directions: Take one to two capsules per day.

Warnings: Phenylketonurics: Contains Phenylalanine.

Ingredients: Vitamin A (as vitamin A palmitate), Vitamin C (as ascorbic acid), Vitamin D (as cholecalciferol), Vitamin E (as DL-alpha tocopheryl acetate), Thiamin (as thiamin HCl), Riboflavin, Niacin (as niacinamide), Vitamin B6, (as pyridoxine HCl), Folic Acid, Vitamin B12 (as cyanocobalamin), Biotin, Pantothenic Acid (as D-calcium pantothenate), Calcium (as calcium amino acid chelate), Zinc (as zinc amino acid chelate), Selenium (as selenium amino acid chelate), Glutamic Acid (as L-glutamic acid), Ribonucleic Acid (RNA), Aspartic Acid (as L-aspartic acid), Leucine (as L-leucine), Arginine (as L-arginine), Lysine (as L-lysine), Bee Pollen, Phenylalanine (as L-phenylalanine), Serine (as L-serine), Proline (as L-proline), Valine (as L-valine), Isoleucine (as L-isoleucine), Alanine (as L-alanine), Glycine (as L-glycine), Threonine (as L-threonine), Tyrosine (as L-tyrosine), Histidine (as L-histidine), Methionine (as L-methionine), Adenoside Triphosphate, Boron (as boron amino acid chelate), Cysteine (as L-cysteine), Talc, Whey, Magnesium Stearate, Silicon Dioxide and Cellulose.

How Supplied: One bottle contains 60 easy-to-swallow capsules.

STEPHAN Lovpil™
Nutritional Supplement

Uses: STEPHAN Lovpil™ is a nutritional food supplement for men and women of all ages that is formulated with vitamins, minerals, herbs, amino acids and selected proteins recognized as important for general health and sexual vitality.

Damiana, typically thought of as an aphrodisiac by those who are familiar with its effects, is an important ingredient utilized in STEPHAN Lovpil. A major herbal remedy in Mexican medical folklore, damiana is often used for the treatment of both impotency and sterility. However, its proven stimulating properties of male virility and libido make it an ideal addition to STEPHAN Lovpil's formulation.

A number of scientific studies have shown a direct relationship between low sperm count and diets deficient in arginine. Well established as being significant to normal sperm production, arginine is, therefore, an important contributor to STEPHAN Lovpil.

A third imperative ingredient is vitamin C. Scientific studies have uncovered that ascorbic acid may actually protect human sperm from oxidative DNA damage, which could in turn help prevent birth defects.

Directions: Take one to two capsules per day.

Warnings: Phenylketonurics: Contains Phenylalanine.

Ingredients: Vitamin A (as vitamin A acetate), Vitamin C (as ascorbic acid), Vitamin D (as cholecalciferol), Folic Acid, Vitamin B12 (as cyanocobalamin), Calcium (as calcium carbonate), Zinc (as zinc amino acid chelate), Selenium (as selenomethionine), Manganese (as manganese amino acid chelate), Damiana (leaf), Isolated Soybean Protein, Ribonucleic Acid (RNA), Adenosine Triphosphate, Talc, Magnesium, Stearate and Silicon Dioxide.

How Supplied: One bottle contains 60 easy-to-swallow capsules.

STEPHAN Masculine®
Nutritional Supplement

Uses: A nutritional food supplement formulated for the adult male, STEPHAN Masculine® contains a special blend of nutrients with vitamins, minerals, herbs and amino acids.

Scientifically researched ingredients have been carefully selected to help ensure STEPHAN Masculine's effectiveness. Zinc is one such ingredient. Proven to be closely interrelated with the male sex hormone, testosterone, zinc deficiency often results in regression of the male sex glands, decreased sexual interest, mental lethargy, emotional problems and even poor appetite. It has been found that in males with only a mild zinc deficiency, zinc supplementation was accompanied by increased sperm count and plasma testosterone.

Directions: Take one to two capsules per day.

Ingredients: Calcium (as calcium carbonate), Magnesium (as magnesium amino acid chelate), Zinc (as zinc amino acid chelate), Histidine (as L-histidine), Bee Pollen, Parsley (leaf), Ribonucleic Acid (RNA), Adenosine Triphosphate Talc and Magnesium Stearate.

How Supplied: One bottle contains 60 easy-to-swallow capsules.

PHYTO-VITE®
Advanced Antioxidant, Vitamin and Mineral Supplement

Uses: Phyto-Vite® is a state-of-the-art nutritional supplement providing chelated minerals, vitamins and a diverse group of antioxidants. It was formulated to meet the nutritional needs of our society where studies estimate only 9% consume foods in the quantities necessary to protect against the oxidative damage caused by free radicals.

The antioxidant coverage provided by Phyto-Vite is both comprehensive and diverse. First, it includes optimal amounts of vitamins A, C, and E as well as the pro-vitamins alpha and beta carotene. Vitamin A, in addition to its antioxidant capabilities, is also felt to improve immune function, protein synthesis, RNA synthesis and steroid hormone synthesis. In this product, vitamin A is derived from two sources: retinyl palmitate and lemongrass. Additional vitamin A activity is provided by the alpha and beta carotene found in *Dunaliella salina*. These carotenoids are strong antioxidants in their own right; however, they can also be converted to vitamin A. This occurs only when the body is deficient in this vitamin. Consequently, vitamin A toxicity cannot be caused by alpha or beta carotene. Vitamin C has long been associated with wound healing, collagen formation, and maintaining the structural integrity of capillaries, cartilage, dentine and bone. Its antioxidant effects are felt to play a major role in the prevention of cardiovascular disease and some cancers. Phyto-Vite utilizes esterified vitamin C which has been shown to provide a quicker uptake and a decreased rate of excretion when compared with conventional vitamin C. This allows for higher, more sustained levels of this vitamin in the body. Phyto-Vite also contains 400 I.U. of vitamin E, from natural sources. The antioxidant effects of vitamin E have been shown to stabilize cell membranes, increase HDL cholesterol, and decrease platelet aggregation.

Many flavonoids are incorporated into Phyto-Vite. These substances possess antioxidant activity themselves and also potentiate the effects of vitamins C and E. This later effect is produced by decreasing the degradation of vitamin C and E into inactive metabolites. Ginkgo biloba has flavonoid activity as well as other significant effects. Among these are a decrease in platelet aggregation and an increase in vasodilation which appears to increase blood flow to the peripheral arteries and the brain. Some improvement in cognitive abilities has been noted. It also helps to inhibit lipid peroxidation, thereby stabilizing the cell wall against free radical attack.

A phytonutrient blend has been incorporated into Phyto-Vite to further enhance its antioxidant effects. Phytonutrient is a term given to the thousands of chemical compounds found in fruits and vegetables. Some of these compounds, including sulforaphane in broccoli and isothiocyanate in cabbage, have been shown to inhibit cancer in laboratory animals and human cell cultures. Others have shown great promise in aiding the cardiovascular system. Currently, much research is ongoing to isolate and identify more of these compounds, but it has already been clearly established that phytonutrients work best when the entire plant source is used rather than just the isolated compound. The phytonutrients found in Phyto-Vite are obtained from alfalfa (lutein), broccoli (indoles), cabbage (isothiocyanates), cayenne (capsanthin and capsorubin), green onion (thioallyl compounds), parsley (chlorophyll), spirulina (gamma linolenic acid), tomato (lycopene), soy isoflavones (genistein, lecithin and daidzein), aged garlic concentrate, and Pure-Gar-A-8000™ (allicin).

Continued on next page

Phyto-Vite—Cont.

The antioxidant minerals copper, zinc, manganese and selenium have also been incorporated into Phyto-Vite. These minerals have been chelated via a patented process in which the mineral is wrapped within an amino acid. Once inside the body, the minerals can then be utilized in the millions of metabolic reactions that take place in the body. With this process, overall mineral absorption can approach 95% instead of the 5 to 10% absorption seen with other mineral supplements.

Phyto-Vite also provides two antioxidant enzymes (catalase and peroxidase). These help to reduce the body's free radical burden by neutralizing free radicals in the pharynx or stomach.

There are three other features that make Phyto-Vite unique among supplements. First, a small amount of canola oil was included to aid in the proper absorption of fat soluble vitamins, even on an empty stomach. Canola oil also provides essential fatty acids. Second, the product is formed into prolonged-release tablets which allow flexibility in dosing frequency. It can be taken all at once or staggered throughout the day. Dissolution testing has been performed to insure that the product will dissolve properly. Lastly, Phyto-Vite tablets are covered with a Betacoat™. This is a beta carotene coating that is designed to provide antioxidant coverage to the tablet itself. This helps to protect the integrity and activity of the product.

Directions: As a dietary supplement take six tablets per day with eight ounces of liquid. Tablets may be taken all at once or staggered throughout the day.

Warnings: If pregnant or lactating, consult physician before using. Accidental overdose of iron-containing products is a leading cause of fatal poisoning in children under 6. Keep this product out of reach of children. In case of accidental overdose, call a doctor or poison control center immediately. This hypoallergenic formula is free of dairy, yeast, wheat, sugar, starch, animal products, dyes, preservatives, artificial flavors and pesticide residues.

Ingredients: Vitamin A (as retinyl palmitate and 80% as beta-carotene and mixed carotenoids from D. salina algae), Vitamin C (as calcium ascorbate), Vitamin D (as cholecalciferol), Vitamin E (as D-alpha-tocopheryl succinate), Vitamin K (as phylloquinone), Thiamin (as thiamin mononitrate), Riboflavin, Niacin (as niacinamide), Vitamin B6 (as pyridoxine HCl), Folate (as folic acid), Vitamin B12 (as cyanocobalamin), Biotin, Pantothenic Acid (as D-calcium pantothenate), Calcium (as dicalcium phosphate, calcium carbonate, citrate and lactate), Iron (as Ferrochel® iron bisglycinate), Phosphorus (as dicalcium phosphate), Iodine [from kelp (Ascophyllum nodosum)], Magnesium (as magnesium oxide, mag-

nesium amino acid chelate and magnesium citrate), Zinc (as zinc Chelazome® glycinate), Selenium (as L-selenomethionine), Copper (as copper Chelazome glycinate), Manganese (as manganese Chelazome glycinate), Chromium (as chromium Chelavite® glycinate), Potassium (as potassium citrate), Alfalfa leaf, Aged garlic bulb concentrate, Pur-Gar® A-10,000 odorless garlic bulb, Soy protein isolate, Broccoli floret, Cabbage leaf, Cayenne pepper fruit, Green onion bulb, Parsley leaf, Tomato, Spirulina algae, Canola oil concentrate, Citrus bioflavonoid complex, Rutin and quercetin dihydrate, Choline (as choline bitartrate), Inositol, PABA, Ginkgo biloba leaf standardized extract (24% ginkgo flavone glycosides and 6% terpene lactones), Bilberry fruit standardized extract (25% antihocyanosides), Catalase enzymes, Grape seed proanthocyanidins, Red grape skin extract (14–18% total polyphenols), Boron (as boron citrate), Microcrystalline cellulose, stearic acid, silica, magnesium stearate, croscarmellose sodium and pharmaceutical glaze with vanillin.

How Supplied: One bottle contains 180 Betacoat™ tablets.

STEPHAN Protector®
Nutritional Supplement

Uses: STEPHAN Protector® is a nutritional food supplement that combines specific proteins, vitamins, minerals and amino acids recognized as important for the health of areas associated with the human immune system.

Among these specially selected and scientifically researched ingredients are astragalus, kelp and arginine. Known for its strengthening effects of both the immune and digestive systems, astragalus can be combined with other herbs to increase phagocytosis, interferon production and the number of macrophages. It, in combination, enhances T-cell transformation and functions as an adaptogen to relieve stress-induced immune system suppression.

Research clearly indicates that kelp supplies dozens of important nutrients for improved cardiovascular health and is used to balance the thyroid gland. Arginine stimulates the thymus gland and promotes production of lymphocytes, crucial for immunity, in that gland. The arginine lymphocytes are not only produced in better quantity, but they have also proven more active and effective in fighting illness.

STEPHAN Protector may be used by men and women of all ages.

Directions: Take one to two capsules per day.

Warnings: Phenylketonurics: Contains Phenylalanine.

Ingredients: Bee Pollen, Astragalus, Kelp, Glutamic Acid, Ribonucleic Acid,

Aspartic Acid, Leucine, Arginine, Lysine, Phenylalanine, Serine, Proline, Valine, Isoleucine, Alanine, Glycine, Threonine, Tyrosine, Histidine, Methionine, Cysteine, Adenosine Triphosphate, Cellulose, Talc, Magnesium Stearate and Silicon Dioxide.

How Supplied: One bottle contains 60 easy-to-swallow capsules.

STEPHAN Relief®
Nutritional Supplement

Uses: Designed for both men and women, STEPHAN Relief® has been formulated with a special combination of nutrients, vitamins, minerals, amino acids and herbs which are recognized as important to the digestive and excretory systems.

Parsley, one of the ingredients found in STEPHAN Relief and a member of the carrot family, can be used as a carminative and an aid to digestion. While the root has a mild diuretic property, parsley has also been reported, in large doses, to lower blood pressure.

A second important ingredient in STEPHAN Relief is psyllium. This gel-forming fiber is used in many bulk laxatives to promote bowel regularity. In recent years, because of its ability to lower cholesterol, psyllium has gained widespread popularity and can be found in some ready-to-eat cereals.

Directions: Take one to two capsules per day.

Ingredients: Pantothenic Acid (as D-calcium pantothenate), Fucus Vesiculosus 5:1 extract (leaf), Parsley 4:1 extract (leaf), Plantago Ovata Seed (psyllium), Isoleucine (as L-isoleucine), Leucine (as L-leucine), Valine (as L-valine), Bee Pollen, Ribonucleic Acid (RNA), Adenosine Triphosphate, Ethylcellulose, Talc and Silicon Dioxide.

How Supplied: One bottle contains 60 easy-to-swallow capsules.

SLEEP-TITE™
Herbal Sleep Aid

Uses: Sleep-Tite™ is a non-addicting herbal sleep aid formulated to promote a deeper, more restorative sleep without the use of pharmaceutically synthesized hormones. With the body's overall health, and proper functioning, dependent upon efficient sleep patterns in order to achieve cellular, organ, tissue and emotional repair, this powerful tool's primary function is to rejuvenate and restore by assisting the body in initiating and maintaining sleep.

Sleep-Tite is a blend of 10 highly effective, all-natural herbs. California poppy, passion flower, valerian, kava kava and skullcap have been used for centuries as a remedy for insomnia because of their

calming effects and ability to relieve muscle tension. Hops and celery seed produce a generalized calming effect and are especially helpful for indigestion, gastrointestinal and smooth muscle relaxation. Chamomile also has a relaxing effect on the body and the gastrointestinal tract, but with the added benefit of producing anti-inflammatory effects on joints. Feverfew has been used as a treatment for fever, migraines and arthritic complaints dating back to ancient Greece. A study published in **Lancet** demonstrated that feverfew inhibited the body's production of prostaglandin and serotonin. These biochemicals can cause inflammation, fever and the vasoactive response that triggers migraine headaches.

By utilizing this unique blend of herbs to aid in the effective initiation and maintenance of sleep patterns, Sleep-Tite can be consumed by adults, thereby promoting physical and emotional well-being in a safe, active manner.

Directions: Adults (18 years and older) may take two Sleep-Tite caplets approximately 30 to 60 minutes prior to bedtime. Needs may vary with each individual. Some persons may require less than two caplets to achieve optimum results. Do not exceed recommended nightly amounts.

Warnings: Not for use by children, pregnant women or lactating women. Consult your physician before using this product if you have any medical condition or are taking antidepressant, sedative or hypnotic medications. Do not take this product if using Monoamine Oxidase (M.A.O.) Inhibitors. This product may cause drowsiness and should not be taken with alcohol or while operating a vehicle or other machinery. If allergic symptoms develop, discontinue use. Store in a cool, dry place. Keep out of reach of children.

Ingredients: European Valerian Root 4:1 extract, Celery Seed 4:1 extract, Hops Strobile 4:1 extract, Passion Flower 4:1 extract (whole plant), California Poppy 5:1 extract (aerial parts), Chamomile Flower 5:1 extract, Chinese Fu Ling 5:1 extract (Poria Cocos), Kava Kava Root 5:1 extract, Feverfew 5:1 extract (aerial parts), Skullcap (aerial parts), Dicalcium Phosphate, Microcrystalline Cellulose, Croscarmellose Sodium, Stearic Acid, Silica, Magnesium Stearate and Sugar Coat (calcium sulfate, sucrose, kaolin, talc, gelatin, shellac, titanium dioxide, anise oil, beeswax and carnauba wax).

How Supplied: One box contains 28 packets. Two caplets per packet.

STEPHAN Tranquility™
Nutritional Supplement

Uses: Designed for both men and women, STEPHAN Tranquility™ is a nutritional food supplement which con-

tains a blend of vitamins, minerals and amino acids recognized as important to areas involved in stress management. Myo-Inositol is among these specially researched ingredients. It has long been claimed to lower blood concentrations of triglycerides and cholesterol, as well as to generally protect against cardiovascular disease. In addition, Myo-Inositol intake can influence the phosphatidylinositol levels in the membranes of brain cells. Compounds derived from this process could conceivably have some beneficial effect on insomnia and anxiety proving a safer alternative than most to treat these common problems.

Another key ingredient used in STEPHAN Tranquility is valerian root, a folk remedy used throughout the years for several disorders including insomnia, hysteria, palpitations, nervousness and menstrual problems. Valerian root contains valepotriates which are said to be the source of its sedative effects. Studies reveal that valeranon, an essential oil component of this herb, produces a pronounced smooth-muscle effect on the intestine.

Directions: Take one to two capsules per day.

Warnings: Phenylketonurics: Contains Phenylalanine.

Ingredients: Vitamin A (as vitamin A palmitate), Vitamin C (as ascorbic acid), Vitamin D (as cholecalciferol), Vitamin E (as DL-alpha tocopheryl acetate), Thiamin (as thiamin HCI), Riboflavin, Niacin (as niacinamide), Vitamin B6 (as pyridoxine HCI), Folic Acid, Vitamin B12 (as cyanocobalamin), Biotin, Pantothenic Acid (as D-calcium pantothenate), Calcium (as calcium amino acid chelate), Magnesium (as magnesium amino acid chelate), Glutamic Acid, Choline Bitartrate, Inositol, Lecithin, Ribonucleic Acid (RNA), Valerian root 4:1 extract (Valerian officianalis), Aspartic Acid, Leucine, Arginine, Lysine, Phenylalanine, Serine, Proline, Valine, Isoleucine, Alanine, Glycine, Threonine, Tyrosine, Histidine, Methionine, Adenosine Triphosphate, Cysteine, Talc, Silicon Dioxide and Hydroxypropyl Cellulose.

How Supplied: One bottle contains 60 easy-to-swallow capsules.

SURE2ENDURE™
Herbal, Vitamin & Mineral Workout Supplement

Uses: Attaining peak physical and athletic performance can be an elusive and time-consuming endeavor. It requires a conditioning process whereby the body's endurance, stamina and ability to recover are enhanced. Sure2Endure™ is formulated to aid in this process through an innovative blend of herbs, vitamins and minerals.

Among these specially selected ingredients is ciwujia (*Radix Acanthopanax*

senticosus). Used in traditional Chinese medicine for almost 1,700 years to treat fatigue and boost the immune system, ciwujia has been shown to improve overall performance in aerobic exercise, endurance activities and weight lifting without any stimulant effects. According to a recent study, ciwujia increases fat metabolism during exercise by shifting toward the use of fat as an energy source instead of carbohydrates. In addition, the caffeine-free herb improves endurance by reducing lactic acid build-up in the muscles. This process delays the muscle fatigue which often leads to muscle pain and cramps.

Sure2Endure™ also provides antioxidant coverage and enzyme cofactors. Vitamins C and E address the otherwise high levels of free radicals generated from the oxidation of fuel substrates during exercise, while vitamins B1 (thiamin), B2 (riboflavin), B6 (pyridoxine), and B12 (cyanocobalamin) aid in proper carbohydrate metabolism and serve as cofactors in numerous biochemical reactions in the body. Ciwujia has been credited with antioxidant properties as well. Since tissue stress and damage are often the result of strenuous exercise, it is important to maintain proper integrity and recovery of connective tissue. Glucosamine, one of the basic constituents making up joint cartilage, is another special additive to Sure2Endure™. This substance enhances the synthesis of cartilage cells and protects against destructive enzymes. It stabilizes cell membranes and intercellular collagen thereby protecting cartilage during rest, exercise and recovery.

The anti-inflammatory activities of bromelain and boswellia further prove beneficial to the health of joint and soft tissues.

Directions: Adults (18 years and older) take 3 tablets one hour prior to exercise. Needs may vary with each individual. For optimum performance, use in conjunction with BIOLEAN® or BIOLEAN Free® one hour before exercise. Phyto-Vite® may be taken with this product to maximize the antioxidant effect necessary with exercise. ProXtreme™ and Mass Appeal™ may also be consumed for maximum effectiveness.

Warning: Not for use by children, pregnant women or lactating women. Consult your physician before using this product if you have any medical conditions. Discontinue immediately if allergic symptoms develop. Keep out of the reach of children. Store in a cool, dry place.

Ingredients: Vitamin C (as ascorbic acid), Vitamin E (as d-alpha tocopheryl succinate), Thiamin (as thiamin mononitrate), Riboflavin, Vitamin B6 (as pyridoxine hydrochloride), Vitamin B12 (as cyanocobalamin), Chromium (as patented Chelavite® chromium dinicotinate glycinate), Ciwujia root standardized extract (0.8% eleutherosides) (Acantho-

Continued on next page

Sure2Endure—Cont.

panax senticosus), Magnesium L-aspartate, Potassium L-aspartate, Boswellia Serrata standardized extract (40% boswellic acids (as gum resins), Bromelain (600 GDU/g), Glucosamine hydrochloride, Dicalcium Phosphate, Microcrystalline Cellulose, Croscarmellose Sodium, Stearic Acid, Silica, Magnesium Stearate and Sugar Coat (calcium sulfate, sucrose, kaolin, talc, gelatin, shellac, titanium dioxide, wintergreen oil, FD&C yellow #5, FD&C blue #1, beeswax and carnauba wax).

How Supplied: One box contains 28 packets, three tablets per packet.

WINRGY™
Nutritional Drink with Vitamin C

Uses: Through nutrients in the diet, nerves are able to send signals throughout the body called neurotransmitters. One such neurotransmitter, noradrenaline, provides individuals with the necessary alertness and energy required in day-to-day activity. A unique blend of vitamins and minerals important to the creation of noradrenaline has been incorporated into Winrgy™, making it a delicious, nutritional alternative to coffee and cola.

Studies reveal that vitamin B2 (riboflavin) helps the body release energy from protein, carbohydrates and fat, while vitamin B12 (cobalamin) is given to combat fatigue and alleviate neurological problems, including weakness and memory loss. Another important component of Winrgy, vitamin B3 (niacin), works with both thiamin and riboflavin in the metabolism of carbohydrates and is essential for providing energy for cell tissue growth. Niacin has also proven to dilate blood vessels and thereby increase the blood flow to various organs of the body, sometimes resulting in a blush of the skin and a healthy sense of warmth. Unlike caffeine, Winrgy offers the raw materials necessary to continue the production of noradrenaline and is ideal for anytime performance is required.

Directions: Add 6 ounces of chilled water or fruit juice to one packet of mix. Stir briskly. Consume 1–2 times per day. Keep in a cool, dry place. For maximum results, combine this product with one serving size of Food For Thought.™

Warnings: Phenylketonurics: Contains Phenylalanine. Not for use by children, pregnant or lactating women. Persons taking medications should seek medical advice before taking this product. Do not consume more than four servings per day. Avoid the use of antacids containing aluminum with this product.

Ingredients: Vitamin C (as ascorbic acid), Vitamin E (as alpha tocopherol acetate), Thiamin (as thiamin mononitrate), Riboflavin, Niacin (as niacinamide), Vitamin B6 (as pyridoxine hydrochloride), Folic Acid, Vitamin B12, Pantothenic Acid (as calcium pantothenate), Zinc (as zinc gluconate), Copper (as copper gluconate), Manganese (as manganese aspartate), Chromium (as chromium aspartate), Potassium (as potassium aspartate), Phenylalanine (as L-phenylalanine), Taurine, Glycine, Caffeine, Fructose, Natural Flavor, Citric Acid and Silicon Dioxide.

How Supplied: One box contains 28 packets. Serving size equals one packet.

Whitehall-Robins Healthcare
American Home Products Corporation
FIVE GIRALDA FARMS
MADISON, NJ 07940

Direct Inquiries to:
Whitehall-Robins (and) Lederle Consumer Product Information 800-322-3129

CENTRUM ECHINACEA

This natural product is derived from the flowers and the root of the echinacea, or purple coneflower, plant which is native to North America. It is traditionally used during the winter months and has been shown in numerous clinical studies to:
• Help support immune system function and the body's natural defenses.*

Supplement Facts	
Serving Size: 2 Softgels	
Amount Per Serving	
Echinacea Extract - Standardized to at least 4% Total Phenols (*Echinacea purpurea*) Aerial Part & Root (*Echinacea angustifolia*) Root	250 mg†
†Daily Value not established.	

Other Ingredients: Soybean Oil, Gelatin, Yellow Wax, Glycerin, Sorbitol, Dibasic Calcium Phosphate, Lecithin, Water, Titanium Dioxide, FD&C Yellow #6, FD&C Blue #1, FD&C Red #40, Propylene Glycol, Hydroxypropyl Methylcellulose.

Directions: Adults—Take two softgels 2–3 times daily with a full glass of water. For best results, take consistently each day, when needed, for a maximum of eight weeks.

Precautions: Use only as directed. Do not exceed recommended dosage. If you suspect or have a known allergy to the daisy family (Asteraceae) do not use this product. Individuals with auto-immune disease should consult their healthcare practitioner before use. As with any supplement, if you are taking a prescription product, or if you are pregnant or are nursing a baby, contact your physician before taking this product.
STORE AT ROOM TEMPERATURE. AVOID TEMPERATURES ABOVE 86°F (30°C). KEEP BOTTLE TIGHTLY CLOSED.
KEEP THIS AND ALL DIETARY SUPPLEMENTS OUT OF THE REACH OF CHILDREN.

> *** These (this) statement(s) have (has) not been evaluated by the Food and Drug Administration. This product is not intended to diagnose, treat, cure or prevent any disease.**

CENTRUM GINKGO BILOBA

This natural product is derived from the leaves of the Ginkgo Biloba tree. It has been shown in clinical studies to:
• Help maintain normal mental alertness, concentration, and memory.*

Supplement Facts	
Serving Size: 1 Softgel	
Amount Per Softgel	
Ginkgo Biloba Extract - Standardized to 24% ginkgo flavone glycosides (*Ginkgo biloba*) Leaf	40 mg†
†Daily Value not established.	

Other Ingredients: Soybean Oil, Gelatin, Yellow Wax, Glycerin, Sorbitol, Water, Lecithin, Polysorbate 80, Annatto Oil Concentrate, Titanium Dioxide, FD&C Yellow #6, FD&C Red #40, FD&C Blue #1, Propylene Glycol, Hydroxypropyl Methylcellulose.

Directions: Adults—Take one softgel three times daily with a full glass of water. Take consistently each day for at least four weeks for best results.

Precautions: Use only as directed. Do not exceed recommended dosage. On rare occasions, mild headache or stomach upset may occur. Usually these go away. If they persist, discontinue use. As with any supplement, if you are taking a prescription product, or if you are pregnant or are nursing a baby, contact your physician before taking this product.
STORE AT ROOM TEMPERATURE. AVOID TEMPERATURES ABOVE 86°F (30°C). KEEP BOTTLE TIGHTLY CLOSED.
KEEP THIS AND ALL DIETARY SUPPLEMENTS OUT OF THE REACH OF CHILDREN.

CENTRUM GINSENG

This natural product is derived from the root of the ginseng plant. It has been shown in clinical studies to:
• Help your body generate the energy it needs and may enhance physical performance.*

Supplement Facts	
Serving Size: 1 Softgel	
Amount Per Softgel	
Ginseng Extract - Standardized to 7% Total Ginsenosides (Panax ginseng) Root	100 mg†
† Daily Value not established.	

Other Ingredients: Soybean Oil, Gelatin, Yellow Wax, Glycerin, Sorbitol, Lecithin, Glucose, Water, Polysorbate 80, Titanium Dioxide, FD&C Red #40, FD&C Blue #1, FD&C Yellow #6, Propylene Glycol, Hydroxypropyl Methylcellulose.

Directions: Adults—Take one softgel two times daily with a full glass of water. Take consistently each day for best results.

Precautions: Use only as directed. Do not exceed recommended dosage. As with any supplement, if you are taking a prescription product, or if you are pregnant or are nursing a baby, contact your physician before taking this product.
STORE AT ROOM TEMPERATURE. AVOID TEMPERATURES ABOVE 86°F (30°C). KEEP BOTTLE TIGHTLY CLOSED.
KEEP THIS AND ALL DIETARY SUPPLEMENTS OUT OF THE REACH OF CHILDREN.

CENTRUM SAW PALMETTO

This natural product is derived from the berries of the saw palmetto plant, native to North America. It has been shown in clinical studies to:
• Help maintain prostate health and normal urine flow.*

Supplement Facts	
Serving Size: 1 Softgel	
Amount Per Softgel	
Saw Palmetto Extract - Standardized to not less than 80% free fatty acids (Serenoa repens) Fruit	160 mg†
† Daily Value not established.	

Other Ingredients: Soybean Oil, Gelatin, Glycerin, Sorbitol, Water, Annatto Oil Concentrate, Titanium Dioxide, Propylene Glycol, Hydroxypropyl Methylcellulose.

Directions: Adult Males—Take one softgel two times daily with a full glass of water. Take consistently each day for at least four weeks for best results.

Precautions: Use only as directed. Do not exceed recommended dosage. On rare occasions, mild stomach upset may occur. If this happens, try taking with food. If you are taking a prescription product or undergoing medical treatment for the prostate or are experiencing a prostate problem, contact a physician before taking this product.
STORE AT ROOM TEMPERATURE. AVOID TEMPERATURES ABOVE 86°F (30°C). KEEP BOTTLE TIGHTLY CLOSED.
KEEP THIS AND ALL DIETARY SUPPLEMENTS OUT OF THE REACH OF CHILDREN.

CENTRUM ST. JOHN'S WORT

This natural product is derived from the flowers and leaves of the St. John's Wort plant. It has been shown in clinical studies to:
• Help maintain healthy emotional balance and a positive outlook.*

Supplement Facts	
Serving Size: 2 Softgels	
Amount Per Serving	
St. John's Wort Extract - Standardized to 0.3% Total Hypericin Compounds (Hypericum perforatum) Aerial Part	400 mg†
† Daily Value not established.	

Other Ingredients: Soybean Oil, Gelatin, Maltodextrin, Glycerin, Sorbitol, Yellow Wax, Lecithin, Water, Silicon Dioxide, Titanium Dioxide, FD&C Red #40, FD&C Blue #1, Propylene Glycol, Hydroxypropyl Methylcellulose.

Directions: Adults—Take two softgels two times daily with a full glass of water. Take consistently each day for at least four weeks for best results.

Precautions: Use only as directed. Do not exceed recommended dosage. While using this product, avoid excessive exposure to sun. As with any supplement, if you are taking a prescription product, or if you are pregnant or are nursing a baby, contact your physician before taking this product.
STORE AT ROOM TEMPERATURE. AVOID TEMPERATURES ABOVE 86°F (30°C). KEEP BOTTLE TIGHTLY CLOSED.
KEEP THIS AND ALL DIETARY SUPPLEMENTS OUT OF THE REACH OF CHILDREN.

YOUNGEVITY
THE ANTI-AGING CO.
3227 SKYLANE DRIVE
DALLAS, TEXAS 75006

Direct Inquiries to:
Website: www.youngevity.com
eMail: asd@youngevity.com
Corporate Fax: 972-404-3067
Corporate Tel: 972-239-6864 ext. 108

OUR ANTI-AGING, LIFE-CHANGING PRODUCTS ARE MANUFACTURED TO PHARMACEUTICAL STANDARDS

The Anti-Aging System contains 3 products: VIAOC, Super Anti-Oxidant Cell Protector and HGH—Turn Back the Hands of Time

The 10-Lbs-N-10 Days System contains 3 products: FM+, Chitosan Fat Snatcher and Super Food Soy Shake

Every Capsule Contains Our Patented Anti-Aging Miracle Minerals: Proprietary Blend: Potassium, Calcium, Magnesium, Zinc, Chromium, Selenium, Iron, Copper, Molybdenum, Vanadium, Iodine, Cobalt and Manganese.

CHITOSAN FAT SNATCHER
ALL NATURAL
With Patented Anti-Aging
Miracle Minerals

EACH CAPSULE CONTAINS:
13 Anti-Aging Patented Amino Acid Chelated Minerals

Continued on next page

Chitosan Fat Snatcher—Cont.

4 Fat Snatching Supplements
Chitosan - From Shellfish Shells (Crustacean) Aloe Vera Leaf, Citric Acid, & Iso-Ascorbic Acid

Directions: 4 Capsules Before Meals

How Supplied: 120 Capsules

FAT METABOLIZER +
Energy Booster
With Patented Anti-Aging
Miracle Minerals

EACH CAPSULE CONTAINS:
13 Anti-Aging Patented Amino Acid Chelated Minerals
8 Anti-Aging Super Supplements:
Cats Claw, Ephedra Sinica Herb, White Willow Bark, Caffeine, Kelp, Pantothenic Acid, Chromium Chelavite & Manganese Chelazome

Directions: 2 Capsules—10 AM
                2 Capsules— 2 PM

How Supplied: 120 Capsules

HGH—TURN BACK THE HANDS OF TIME
HGH Precursor
Naturally Stimulates the Release of HGH
With Patented Anti-Aging Miracle Minerals

EACH CAPSULE CONTAINS:
13 Anti-Aging Patented Amino Acid Chelated Minerals
5 Anti-Aging Amino Acids:
Stacked in a Proprietary Blend
L-Lysine HCl, L-Arginine, L-Ornithine, L-Glutamine & L-Tyrosine

6 Anti-Aging Supplements:
Glycine, GABA, Vitamin B6, Manganese, Chromium & Kelp Plant

Directions: 6 Capsules—Bedtime

How Supplied: 180 Capsules

SUPER ANTI-OXIDANT CELL PROTECTOR
Grape Seed Extract
With Patented Anti-Aging Miracle Minerals

EACH CAPSULE CONTAINS:
13 Anti-Aging Patented Amino Acid Chelated Minerals
1 Super Anti-Oxidant Cell Protector:
OPC's (Oligomeric Proanthocyanidins) (from grape seed extract)
11 Anti-Oxidant Actives:
Garlic Acid, Catechin, Epicatechin, OPC's B-1, B-2, B-3, B-4, Trimres, Tetramer B-2 Gallate, Dimer, Di-Gallate, & Oligomers

Directions: Take 1 Capsule Per 50 lbs. of Body Weight Daily

How Supplied: 90 Capsules

Super Food Soy Shake
Meal Replacement
With Patented Anti-Aging Miracle Minerals

EACH SCOOP CONTAINS:
13 Anti-Aging Patented Amino Acid Chelated Minerals
3 Mega Nutrients:
Protein from Soy, Carbohydrates from Whole Grains, Molasses, "Friendly oils" from Sunflowers, 80% monounsaturates!
13 Essential Vitamins:
Vitamins A, B1, B2, B3, B5, B6, B12, C, D, E, K, Folic Acid & Biotin

3 Colon Health Conditioners:
Lactobacillus Acidophilus, Soy Lecithin & FOS
4 Patented Chelated Amino Acids:
Phosphorus, Sulfur, Chloride, Sodium
6 Anti Aging Plant Enzymes:
Paypaya, Protease, Bromelain, Amylase, Lipase & Cellulase
6 Fiber Rich Foods:
Soy, Rice, Barley, Oats, Prunes & Citrus
5 Balancing Herbs:
Alfalfa, Capsicum Fruit, Chlorella Garcinia Fruit & Licorice Root

Directions: 2 Scoops Per Meal

How Supplied: Powder

VITALITY IMMUNITY ANTI-OXIDANT COMPLEX

A Complete Multi-Vitamin Multi-Mineral Herbal Supplement with Patented Anti-Aging Miracle Minerals

EACH CAPSULE CONTAINS:
13 Anti-Aging Patented Amino Acid Chelated Minerals
28 Anti-Aging Proprietary Complex-Anti-Oxidants, Synergistic Vitamins, Synergistic Herbs & Digestive Enzymes:

Vitamin A, C, E, Alpha Lipoic Acid, Folic Acid, Vitamin B1, B2, B3, B5, B6, B12, Biotin, Vitamin D3, Chromium, Selenium, Protease (Proteins), Lipase (Fats), Amylase (Carbohydrates), Cellulase (Fiber), Grape Seed Extract (95% Proanthocyanidins), Horsetail Grass, Kelp Powder, Licorice Root, Garlic Bulb, Rose Hips, Broccoli, Alfalfa Leaf, & Ginkgo Biloba Leaf

Directions: 3 Capsules Daily—after first meal of day

How Supplied: 90 Capsules